THE PHYSIOLOGY AND MEDICINE OF DIVING

AND COMPRESSED AIR WORK

The Physiology
and Medicine of Diving

and Compressed Air Work

SECOND EDITION

EDITED BY

P. B. BENNETT AND D. H. ELLIOTT

BAILLIÈRE TINDALL · LONDON

BAILLIÈRE TINDALL
7 & 8 Henrietta Street, London WC2E 8QE

Cassell & Collier Macmillan Publishers Ltd, London
35 Red Lion Square, London WC1R 4SG
Sydney, Auckland, Toronto, Johannesburg

The Macmillan Publishing Company Inc.
New York

First published 1969

Second edition 1975

ISBN 0 7020 0538 X

Published in the United States of America by
The Williams & Wilkins Company, Baltimore

Printed by William Clowes & Sons, Limited, London, Beccles and Colchester

Contributors

ARTHUR J. BACHRACH, PhD Director, Behavioral Sciences Department, Naval Medical Research Institute, National Naval Medical Center, Bethesda, Maryland 20014, USA.

ALBERT R. BEHNKE, BA, MD, MS (Hon.) Captain, Medical Corps, United States Navy (Retired). 2241 Sacramento Street, San Francisco, California 94115, USA.

PETER B. BENNETT, BSc, PhD Professor of Anesthesia and Biomedical Engineering, Co-Director, F. G. Hall Environmental Research Laboratory, Director Diving Research, Duke University Medical Center, Durham, North Carolina 27710, USA.

ROBERT C. BORNMANN, MD Captain, Medical Corps, United States Navy, Bureau of Medicine and Surgery, Department of the Navy, Washington D.C. 20372, USA.

RALPH W. BRAUER, MSc, PhD Director, Wrightsville Marine Biomedical Laboratory, 7205 Wrightsville Avenue, Wilmington, North Carolina 28401, USA.

ALBERT A. BÜHLMANN, MD Professor of Physiology, Chief of Cardio-Pulmonary Laboratories, Department of Medicine, University Hospital, Zurich, Switzerland.

DAVID H. ELLIOTT, OBE, DPhil, MB, MFCM Surgeon Commander, Royal Navy. Environmental Stress Division, Naval Medical Research Institute, National Naval Medical Center, Bethesda, Maryland 20014, USA, on exchange service. Since returned to Institute of Naval Medicine, Alverstoke, Hants., England.

A. EVANS, BSc Senior Research Associate, Medical Research Council Decompression Sickness Team, Department of Surgery, Royal Victoria Infirmary, Newcastle upon Tyne NE1 4LP, England.

JOSEPH C. FARMER, MD Assistant Professor, Division of Otolaryngology, Department of Surgery, Duke University Medical Center, Durham, North Carolina 27710, USA.

PHILIP D. GRIFFITHS, MD Senior Research Associate in Medical Charge. Medical Research Council Central Registry, Department of Surgery, University of Newcastle upon Tyne, 21 Claremont Place, Newcastle upon Tyne NE2 4AA, England.

JOHN M. HALLENBECK, MD Lieutenant Commander, Medical Corps, United States Navy. Environmental Stress Division. Naval Medical Research Institute, National Naval Medical Center, Bethesda, Maryland 20014, USA.

ROBERT de G. HANSON, BA, MD, BCh, BAO Surgeon Commander, Royal Navy. Royal Naval Physiological Laboratory, Alverstoke, Hants., England.

ANDREW F. HAXTON, BSc, FICE Director (Retired), Charles Brand & Son Ltd, Civil Engineering Contractors, Tempsford Hall, Sandy, Bedfordshire, England.

H. V. HEMPLEMAN, MA, PhD Superintendent, Royal Naval Physiological Laboratory, Alverstoke, Hants., England.

BRIAN A. HILLS, MA, BSc, PhD Professor of Physiology; Chief, Hyperbaric Physiology Section, Marine Biochemical Institute, University of Texas Medical Branch, Galveston, Texas 77550, USA.

DEREK J. KIDD, MB, BS, MRCS, LRCP   Surgeon Captain, Canadian Armed Forces. Command Surgeon, Maritime Forces Pacific Headquarters, FMO Victoria, British Columbia, Canada.

JOHANNES A. KYLSTRA, MD   Professor of Medicine and Associate Professor of Physiology, Duke University Medical Center, Durham, North Carolina 27710, USA.

EDWARD H. LANPHIER, MD   Research Associate Professor of Physiology, Department of Physiology, Capen Hall, State University of New York at Buffalo, New York 14214, USA.

R. IAN McCALLUM, MD, DSc, FRCP   Reader, Nuffield Department of Industrial Health, University of Newcastle upon Tyne, 21 Claremont Place, Newcastle upon Tyne NE1 4LP, England.

ALISTER G. MACDONALD, BSc, PhD   Lecturer, Physiology Department, Marischal College, Aberdeen AB9 1AS, Scotland.

JOSEPH B. MACINNIS, MD   Undersea Research Limited, 21 McMaster Avenue, Toronto, Ontario, Canada.

JOHN N. MILLER, MD   Department of Anesthesiology, University of Washington, Seattle, Washington, USA.

JAMES B. MORRISON, BSc, PhD, ARCST, CEng   Associate Professor, Department of Kinesiology, Simon Fraser University, Burnaby 2, British Columbia, Canada.

KARL E. SCHAEFER, MD   Chief, Biomedical Sciences Division, Naval Submarine Medical Research Laboratory, United States Naval Submarine Base, New London, Groton, Connecticut 06340, USA.

WILLIAM THOMAS, PhD   Associate Professor, Division of Otolaryngology, Department of Surgery, University of North Carolina, Chapel Hill, North Carolina, USA.

DENNIS N. WALDER, MD, ChM, FRCS   Professor of Surgical Science, Honorary Consultant Surgeon, Royal Victoria Infirmary, Newcastle upon Tyne, England. Chairman, Medical Research Council, Decompression Sickness Panel.

PAUL WEBB, MD   Principal Associate, Webb Associates, Box 308, Yellow Springs, Ohio 45387, USA.

HAROLD E. WHYTE, BSc, FICE   Director, Charles Brand & Son Ltd, Tempsford Hall, Sandy, Bedfordshire, England.

SYRL WILLIAMS, Senior Scientific Officer, Admiralty Underwater Weapons Establishment, Portland, Dorset, England.

JAMES D. WOOD, BSc, PhD   Professor and Head of Department of Biochemistry, University of Saskatchewan, Saskatoon, Saskatchewan, Canada.

ROBERT D. WORKMAN, BSc, MS, MD   Captain, Medical Corps, United States Navy (Retired). Director of Research, Taylor Diving and Salvage, 795 Engineers Road, Belle Class, Louisiana 70037, USA.

J. MURRAY YOUNG, DPhil, MRCS, MFCM   Surgeon Commander, Royal Navy. Experimental Stress Division, Naval Medical Research Institute, National Naval Medical Center, Bethesda, Maryland 20014, USA.

Foreword

The Changing Face of Manned Undersea Activity

C. J. LAMBERTSEN

During the few years since the publication of the first edition of this book we have embarked upon a new phase in undersea research and operations. This is a phase of challenge, rapid advance in method, and consolidation of scientific information. Until now, in spite of intensive investigation, open-sea diving has been limited largely to depths of about 400 feet of seawater. Only in the past few years have operational leaders sought to extend work to beyond the depths of the continental shelves.

The expansion of interest in the advancement of diving, predicted by the Foreword of the previous volume, was, however, stimulated by a peculiar episode of history and not by steady development of understanding among industrial and scientific leaders. The critical episode was an embargo on oil shipments from the Middle East—an embargo imposed by oil-producing nations to influence political support patterns in an Israeli–Arab war. Now, with little or no experience in work at depths greater than 400 feet of seawater, oil producers have been stimulated to explore for (and produce) oil at depths to 1500 feet of seawater in 1975, with hopes of reaching 3000 feet within a few years and 6000 feet by 1980.

In a single step of awakened interest, industrial and naval leaders have accepted the physiological feasibility of diving effectively to depths of at least 1000 feet of seawater, and are asking to know the 'limits' of human performance. Clearly there are ways in which the highly advanced physiological research of the past several years can be immediately exploited to guide the desired work at intermediate depths. Moreover, man has been exposed for long periods to pressures equivalent to 2000 feet of seawater and has been found able to breathe well at rest and moderate work even when the density of respired gas was equivalent to that to be expected with helium at pressures of more than 5000 feet of seawater. The detailed studies which will allow practical diving to these depths have not been done. This is the time for investment by the industrial users of this critically important information, sought after and being obtained in step-by-step investigations of immense technical difficulty. The next phase of research and application cannot be carried out without such investment by industry, especially as the traditional unilateral supporting role of the naval organizations is being caused to change by the very expansion of industrial undersea operations. The need now is for a coalition of university, industrial and federal scientific and technical leaders to carry effective manned undersea activity to its varied limits. These advances must include gross improvement in the methods of shallow and intermediate depth diving as well as in deep extensions. They must also include the development of systems engineered to contain and protect man for work at depths so great that he could not tolerate direct exposure to the pressures involved. It is time to join forces for the exploration of important undersea reaches of our planet.

In seeking to advance the scope of diving and other pressure research, operations and development must continue to be broad for as long as man works in the sea. Therefore, a volume such as this must concern itself not only with classical air diving and deep helium–oxygen diving, but with the breath-holding diver, self-contained helium or nitrogen mixed-gas diving, pure oxygen diving, saturation and excursion diving methods, diving from submersible craft, and the use of submerged habitats to facilitate maximum extension of depth or to attain extreme extension of duration in shallow exposures. It will never be sensible to concentrate exclusively upon any one of these approaches, since each method will continue to be important indefinitely, and there will emerge the use of gas mixtures as yet untried. Continued basic and applied research as well as continued engineering development is necessary because in extending each situation, special problems are generated, not only by depth and the gases breathed, but by the exact nature of the equipment used.

At this moment, men work and dive around the world, at depths still incompletely studied, using almost in full the available basic information upon which further advance must depend. However, the oscillations of attention from practical to scientific accomplishment have been increasing in frequency—from decades to years, and now to months—and it should finally be possible to blend these into a phase of tight and fruitful collaboration between science and operations. Such collaboration is vital if the problems presented to modern diving are to be overcome. As described in introducing the previous edition, the high pressure, cold, dark, turbid, wet, dense and buoyant undersea environment imposes gross limitations upon human performance not imposed upon the astronaut. The stresses are physical and biophysical as well as chemical and toxic, and they exist in the natural working state as well as in conditions of accident or overexposure. Communication of information from diver to diver by both vision and hearing is impaired. The current, the viscosity and even the buoyancy of water restrict mobility and increase energy expenditure, as does the low water temperature. There still remains, with increasing rather than diminishing importance, a need for understanding and the means for overcoming the limitations imposed by decompression, by narcosis, by oxygen toxicity, and by the difficult pulmonary ventilation imposed by high gas density. It is even probable that limits may be imposed by hydrostatic effects, and certainly time presents the ultimate obstacle in any circumstance of physiological stress. These and other effects, as with a variety of the lesser physiological stresses imposed by space flight, are not independent. Extremely complex interactions of factors vary with depth, with exposure duration and with the method of diving employed.

One striking example of the intricate and troublesome physiological interactions at great depth is represented by the narcosis which, produced primarily by inert gas effects upon central nervous system function, can reduce the diver to mental ineffectiveness and even unconsciousness. The narcosis is added to by O_2, CO_2 and, of course, by any lowering of deep body temperature. The inefficient mobility of the diver in water and current increases CO_2 production per unit of useful work. At the same time an increased airway resistance exaggerates respiratory work, limits alveolar ventilation, interferes with metabolic carbon dioxide elimination, and furthers the auto-intoxication by carbon dioxide which grossly deepens the narcotic influence of the inert gas. These factors (exercise, narcosis, alveolar hypoventilation, and carbon dioxide retention) similarly interact to exaggerate the poisoning by oxygen. These continue to be fields for quantitative physiological exploration, since they impose obstacles to extension of practical diving. From this point on it is quantitation of physiological disturbances that is required, as in current attempts to define the degree of narcotic impairment of various human abilities when the 'dose' of an inert gas is increased. These studies show that a narcotized diver can still hear and see at depths where he cannot remember what he went down for, cannot deduce the nature of the tasks and has lost the neuromuscular coordination required for the needed manipulation. Quantitative studies are similarly necessary to define the limits of tolerance of various organs and tissues to the supranormal oxygen pressures which provide such benefit in shortening decompression.

Approaches to solving these problems have taken two important paths, each heavily dependent upon the design and construction of large and expensive equipment. One approach has been the development of new pressure laboratories which simulate the wide range of conditions encountered in undersea work to aid extension of fundamental and applied research. These laboratories have been successful only when they have been part of the extensive scientific assets of a university or federal research system. Isolated facilities are useless. It has proven more difficult to gather the necessary, broadly skilled scientific staffs for these large systems than to construct them in the first place, and a 'critical mass' of investigators is necessary for effective interdisciplinary study. Major advances have also been achieved by collaborative investigations, in which investigators gather at special centers in one or another country. The work of these laboratories is now being aided by extensive use of modern computers, which can rapidly solve problems of physiological or performance measurement of decompression theory and can extend them to include the influences of alternation of inert gases and the purposeful fluctuation of high and low oxygen levels.

Such studies on man and animals are one path of progress. The second involves attempts to utilize new information and to circumvent physiological limitations upon diving by developing new diving concepts. Extensive engineering development is providing gradually improved methods for work in the open sea. The deep diver, once required to hang on his stage for many hours of decompression after each descent, has had his range and effectiveness extended by saturation diving, with a single decompression after days or weeks of undersea work. Additionally, the diver now can descend to his work site in a pressure compartment, use it as a work station, and then can be brought back to the surface, still under pressure, to effect his long decompression after pressurized transfer to the relative comfort of a large, surface decompression chamber. These supporting systems are very recent in the evolution of manned undersea activity. While they provide marked improvement in effectiveness, in safety and in comfort of the overall diving operation, the eventual performance of specific useful work is normally still carried out by an individual diver who must leave the relative comfort and safety of the submerged compartment, enter the water and breathe his gases at the existing ambient pressure in order to bring his energy, skill and judgment to bear upon the task at hand.

For the immediate future it must be recognized that it is the systems supporting the isolated diver which are the limiting factor, as they provide his respiratory gases and warm him, improve his vision and speech, and aid his movement. Of all the many subsea oil wells that have been completed to date, only one has not in some way utilized man underwater as an aid to completion of the well system. It is unreasonable to expect the further advance, now being sought, to be obtained by engineering development alone. It will in many ways require detailed and fundamental investigation of man himself at pressure extremes. The understanding of safe and efficient undersea and high pressure operations is greatly aided by this exceptionally complete and purposeful book.

ACKNOWLEDGEMENT

The material for the Foreword is adapted from a part of the report series of the Institute for Environmental Medicine, University of Pennsylvania.

Preface

Since the publication of the first edition of this book in 1969, there have been many advances covering the whole field of underwater physiology and medicine. Thus it is now time for a further review of the biomedical problems of life at high pressure and it is the purpose of this edition to summarize, in a form convenient for reference, the present state of knowledge in this area.

Although manned submersibles or armoured suits may be necessary for man to work at great depths, so far as continental shelf depths are concerned, man himself will continue to be the cheapest and most versatile means of completing underwater tasks for the foreseeable future.

This volume is an edited collection of reviews each written by an internationally recognized authority. Nearly every chapter has been re-written and a number of new topics, such as underwater performance, problems of thermal balance and underwater accidents, has been introduced. Thus the format of this volume is similar to that of the previous edition, but contains much that is new.

Respiratory abbreviations and symbols again follow the recommendations in *Fedn Proc. Fedn Am. Socs exp. Biol.* **9**, 602–605 (1950). The units for pressure remain a problem, for while the United Kingdom has now adopted the metric system (1 bar = 100 kN m^{-2} = 100 kPa) there is still no international agreement. We have decided to retain atmospheres as the primary standard and therefore throughout the text conversions have been made so that all pressures are also given in atmospheres (ATS) or atmospheres absolute (ATA).

The pressure of 1 atmosphere is considered to be equivalent to 14·696 pounds per square inch (psi: lb/in^2) and 1·033 kilograms per square centimetre (kg/cm^2) and to the pressure exerted by 33·072 feet or 10·08 metres of seawater assuming a specific gravity of 1·025. Within the limits 1·010 and 1·030 the adoption of a specific gravity for the conversion of pressure to depths of seawater is not consistent in the published literature. The standard atmosphere equals 101·325 kN m^{-2}. A pressure conversion table is to be found in the journal, *Undersea Biomed. Res.*

July 1974

P. B. BENNETT
D. H. ELLIOTT

ACKNOWLEDGEMENTS

Grateful acknowledgements to many other sources for permission to reproduce the numerous figures and tables in this volume are made by the contributors and a considerable effort has been made to ensure that, where not original, reference has been made to the source of each illustration. Any omission of the appropriate reference in the text is unintentional and it is hoped that, should it have occurred, the author or publisher concerned will accept this apology.

Acknowledgements and thanks are also due to the French Navy for permission to publish details of the DC55 constant ratio breathing apparatus.

Contents

DISCLAIMER

The opinions or assertions, contained herein are the private ones of the various authors and are not to be construed as official or reflecting the views of the Naval Department of any nation or of any Naval Service at large.

1

A Short History of Man in the Sea

A. J. BACHRACH

For the first time in history, a dream of living and working at the bottom of the ocean approaches realization. The modern diver, equipped with specially developed gear, housed in vehicles that are products of a burgeoning technology, is a proud inheritor of the years—indeed centuries—of exploration that prepared the way. The purpose of this chapter is to review, in brief compass, some of that history and the current prospects for diving technology. It is patently not intended to be an intensive and complete review.

Excellent histories of diving have been written by Larson (1959), Dugan (1965) and Davis (1962). These works cover developments through the various stages of diving up to 1957, when saturation diving, a method to allow man to work in the sea at greater depths for longer periods, emerged from experimentation by a team of US Navy researchers at New London, Connecticut and the concepts developed by Jacques-Yves Cousteau and Edwin A. Link.

Man goes into the sea today, as through the centuries, for food, treasure, military operation, sport, and exploration. Treasure hunting is illustrated by Beebe (1934) in his book, *Half Mile Down*, in which he reports an archaeological dig in Bismaya (Mesopotamia) yielding mother-of-pearl inlays (which must have been gathered by divers and fashioned by artisans) dated *c.* 4500 B.C. Beebe also relates that pearl shells were used in quantity for carved ornaments at Thebes in 3200 B.C., and that Emperor Yu of China received an oyster pearl tribute from tribes, *c.* 2250 B.C.

These artifacts are among the earliest indica-tions of free diving or breath-hold diving and the first technique of man at work in the sea. Fig. 1.1 depicts the principal periods in diving develop-ment, beginning with free diving in unrecorded times to approximately the fourth century B.C. when Aristotle mentioned a type of diving machine (Larson 1959), and continuing to the beginning of the nineteenth century. These stages of develop-ment are:

1. Free or breath-hold diving.
2. Diving bells.
3. Surface support or helmet, the so-called hard-hat diving.
4. SCUBA (self-contained underwater breath-ing apparatus; scuba).
5. Saturation diving.

FREE DIVING

Greek mythology is filled with references to the underwater world. Hephaestus (Rome's Vulcan), because of his ugliness, was thrown from Olympus into the sea, built a smithy in a submerged cave and (according to Dugan 1965), might well be the god of submarine engineers. Aphrodite (goddess of love and beauty), who was brought forth, according to some legends, on ocean foam, was forced by Zeus to marry Hephaestus.

Herodotus tells the story of Scyllias, who was hired by Xerxes to dive for treasure on sunken Persian vessels. When Xerxes detained Scyllias upon completion of his mission, Scyllias dived into the sea at Apaetae during a storm, cut the moorings on Xerxes' galleys, causing great havoc,

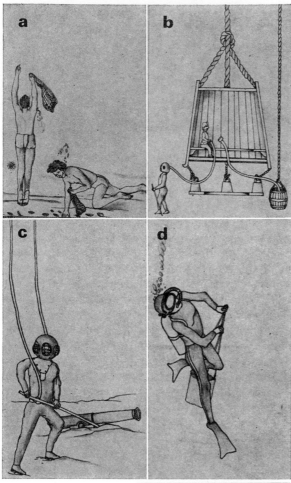

then emerged from the sea at Artemisium—9 miles distant.

Another Greek historian, Thucydides, also mentions use of divers in the Athenian attack on Syracuse to saw barriers which the Syracusans had built below the surface to obstruct and damage Greek ships. A similar use of divers to destroy submarine defences is found in the siege of Tyre, where Alexander the Great ordered divers to do underwater demolition. On another occasion, Alexander himself is supposed to have descended into the sea in a machine, a primitive diving bell called the *Colimpha* (Beebe 1934; Davis 1962).

Free diving has continued to be a major work method among divers. In 1913, a Greek sponge diver, Georghios, placed a line on the lost anchor of the Italian battleship, *Regina Margharita*, at a depth of 200 ft (7 ATA) (Dugan 1965). The Ama of Japan wear goggles or masks to breath-hold dive as deep as 145 ft (5·4 ATA), to search for pearls. In 1969, the US Navy diver, Bob Croft, made the current world's record breath-hold dive to 247 ft (8·4 ATA). The advantage of free diving is its mobility. The obvious disadvantage is the marked limitation of air available to the diver—he has only what he inhales on the surface before diving.

DIVING BELLS

Alexander's descent in the primitive diving bell *Colimpha* (around 330 B.C.) is one of the earliest reports of a device by which man could enter the ocean with protection and an air supply (*Encyclopaedia Britannica*, 1968). An account of this legendary dive appeared in a thirteenth century French manuscript, *La vrai Histoire d'Alexandre*. Aristotle, in his *Problemata*, spoke of diving appliances in use: '... they contrive a means of respiration for divers, by means of a container sent down to them; naturally the container is not filled with water, but air, which constantly assists the submerged man ...' (Aristotle 1927; Davis 1962).

Developments from Aristotle's time (384 to 322 B.C.) to the Middle Ages are few. In 1240 Roger Bacon referred to 'instruments whereby men can walk on the sea or river beds without danger to themselves' (*Encyclopaedia Britannica*, 1968) but it was not until 1535 that Guglielmo de

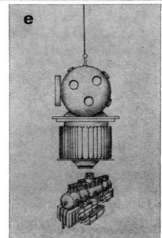

FIG. 1.1. Principal periods in diving development:

(a) ancient; (b) 4th century B.C.–c. 1800; (c) c. 1800–c. 1930; (d) c. 1930–c. 1957; (e) 1957–. Types (a), (c), (d) and (e) are still being employed today.

(Illustrations by M. Yeager.)

Lorena developed the first 'diving bell'. A diver worked for about an hour in Lake Nemi near Rome with this diving apparatus resting on his shoulders, much of the weight supported by slings (Larson 1959; Davis 1962).

In 1691 the noted astronomer, Sir Edmund Halley, built and patented a forerunner of the modern diving bell. Halley, in a report to the Royal Society of London, described his bell. It was made of wood, coated with lead, approximately 60 cu ft in volume, with a glass at the top which allowed light into the bell; it also had a valve to vent air and a barrel to provide replenished air (Larson 1959; Davis 1962). Somewhat earlier (1620) Cornelium van Drebbel, a Dutch inventor, developed the first successful submarine (propelled by oars), cruising approximately 15 ft below the surface of the Thames. Legend has it that King James I was one of his passengers.

HELMET DIVING

Although the diving bell provided air and protection to the diver, the supply of air and the mobility of the diver were severely limited. What was needed was a means of allowing a diver to move more freely with a good supply of air.

In the seventeenth and eighteenth centuries numerous contraptions, usually made of leather, were developed to provide air to divers. Most of these could not really have worked because a long tube feeding air to a diver from the surface cannot function, as it lacks a means to equalize the pressure exerted by the surrounding water.

A real step forward in the development of surface-support diving systems occurred when Freminet, a French scientist, devised a system whereby air was pumped from the surface with a bellows to provide a constant flow of air through a hose to the diver in the water. Some historians consider this system to be the first true helmet-hose diving apparatus. Using this system, Freminet is credited with diving to a depth of 50 ft (2·5 ATA) in 1774 and remaining for one hour (Larson 1959; Davis 1962).

The first major breakthrough in diving dress was the invention of an 'open' diving dress in 1819 by Augustus Siebe. Siebe's diving dress consisted of a waist-length jacket and metal helmet; air under pressure supplied from the surface to the helmet by a force-pump could escape freely at the diver's waist. In 1837 Siebe modified his 'open' dress into the 'closed' type, retaining the helmet and force-pump, and enclosing the diver in a continuous airtight dress, the air vented by a valve, the basis of modern 'hard-hat' diving gear. (William H. Jones is credited with the first design for a self-contained diving dress in 1825. His dress provided its own supply of compressed air in a metal belt around a diver's waist. Historians report the device should have been workable, but seemingly never was tested.) Siebe's diving gear was used in 1839 when the British began the salvage of the *Royal George*, a 108-gun Royal ship which, in 1782, capsized during repair operations and sank to 65 ft below the surface, creating a menace to navigation (Davis 1962).

The adaptation of 'hard-hat' gear to the use of mixed gases, particularly helium–oxygen, which allowed deeper dives, appeared in the twentieth century. A major open-sea application of helium and oxygen as a breathing mixture was in the salvage of the submarine, USS *Squalus*, in 1939. Its implications for diving technology appear in a later section of this chapter.

As advances were made in helmet diving, the diver gained more air, more protection, and more mobility, but it was not till the development of SCUBA (self-contained underwater breathing apparatus) that he was afforded the freedom of the breath-hold diver to move about, coupled with an air supply that enabled him to stay down longer than a free diver.

SCUBA

Compressed air rigs originated around 1808 when Friedrich von Drieberg devised a bellows-in-a-box system worn on the diver's back which supplied the diver with compressed air from the surface. Von Drieberg's *Triton* did not actually work, but it brought recognition to the application of compressed air as an underwater technique —an application suggested as early as 1716 by Halley in his paper on diving bells (Larson 1959). Around 1830 an American, Charles Condert, successfully dived a compressed air suit that used a portable air reservoir to depths up to 20 ft (1·6 ATA), but drowned in 1832 when his system malfunctioned. Condert's successful application of the principle of the use of compressed air was an important contribution at a critical period in diving development.

In 1865 two Frenchmen, Rouquayrol and Denayrouse, invented a suit which, while they called it 'self-contained', was in fact a helmet, surface-supported system with a reservoir of air mounted on the diver's back that gave him air, on demand, for one breathing cycle (Larson 1959; Davis 1962). The development of an automatic demand valve was a major advance for breathing apparatus. The diver now had a full breath of air when wanted, instead of the continuous and sometimes unreliable flow of air provided by a hose from the surface. Of particular interest to diving historians is the reference to this apparatus which appeared in Jules Verne's (1875) classic, *Twenty Thousand Leagues Under the Sea*. This book, written in 1869, four years after the Rouquayrol–Denayrouse gear had been developed, described the apparatus and its use in a conversation between Captain Nemo and Professor Aronnax:

"You know as well as I do, Professor, that man can live under water, providing he carries with him a sufficient supply of breathable air. In submarine works, the workman, clad in an impervious dress, with his head in a metal helmet, receives air from above by means of forcing pumps and regulators."

"That is a diving apparatus," said I.

"Just so, but under these conditions the man is not at liberty; he is attached to the pump which sends him air through an india-rubber tube, and if we were obliged to be thus held to the *Nautilus*, we could not go far."

"And the means of getting free?" I asked.

"It is to use the Rouquayrol apparatus, invented by two of your own countrymen, which I have brought to perfection for my own use, and which will allow you to risk yourself under these new physiological conditions, without any organ whatever suffering. It consists of a reservoir of thick iron plates, in which I store the air under a pressure of fifty atmospheres. This reservoir is fixed on the back by means of braces, like a soldier's knapsack. Its upper part forms a box in

which the air is kept by means of bellows, and therefore cannot escape unless at its normal tension. In the Rouquayrol apparatus such as we use, two india-rubber pipes leave this box and join a sort of tent which holds the nose and mouth; one is to introduce fresh air, the other to let out the foul, and the tongue closes one or the other according to the wants of the respirator. But I, in encountering great pressures at the bottom of the sea, was obliged to shut my head, like that of a diver, in a ball of copper; and it is to this ball of copper that the two pipes, the inspirator and the expirator, open."

"Perfectly, Captain Nemo; but the air that you carry with you must soon be used, when it only contains fifteen per cent of oxygen, it is no longer fit to breathe."

"Right! but I told you, M. Aronnax, that the pumps of the *Nautilus* allow me to store the air under considerable pressure, and on these conditions, the reservoir of the apparatus can furnish breathable air for nine or ten hours."

What is remarkable in this passage is not the often noted foresight of Verne as much as his keen awareness of contemporary science and engineering. Verne would undoubtedly have been delighted to see J. E. Williamson's motion picture of the novel which was filmed in 1915. In this motion picture 'oxylite' (discovered in 1897 by Georges Jaubert) was used in the divers' self-contained diving units to renew and purify the air supply (Larson 1959) thus fulfilling Captain Nemo's hope of divers moving freely for extended periods in the ocean around the *Nautilus*.

Some controversy surrounds credit for the first successful self-contained underwater breathing apparatus (SCUBA) which emerged early in the twentieth century. Until then SCUBA had utilized compressed air by various means allowing the diver to inhale air usually supplied from the surface, which was then exhaled into the water. This loss of air into the water necessitated a large air supply, even for a dive of short duration.

Attempts to regenerate air, thereby allowing the diver more time in the water, can be traced to around 1680, when Giovanni Borelli, an Italian physicist, devised a self-contained diving apparatus, with helmet and tubes, based on a principle of air regeneration. He theorized that exhaled air could be purified by running it through a tube cooled by sea water (the impurities supposedly would adhere to the condensation along the sides of the tube). Borelli also supplied the diver with claw-like foot fins, suggesting his diver to be a 'swimmer' rather than a vertical 'walker'. Freminet, prior to the success of his helmet-hose-bellows system in 1774, developed an apparatus based on the same principle as Borelli's, adding a small bellows in the air reservoir to assist circulation of the air. Their system of air purification was entirely invalid, yet the concept of purifying a diver's breathing supply, and hence extending his time and mobility underwater, was to become a reality (Larson 1959).

In 1879 Henry Fleuss, an English merchant seaman, developed a self-contained underwater breathing apparatus using oxygen compressed to 450 psig which was equipped with a chamber of caustic potash for purification of exhaled breath. His 'closed circuit oxygen-rebreather SCUBA' proved itself dramatically when a diver wearing his apparatus entered a flooded tunnel being built under the Severn River in England to close an iron door jammed open and to make repairs. A diver in helmet-hose gear could not have done the work in such twisted, jagged surroundings (Larson 1959; Davis 1962).

In the 1920s, Captain Yves Le Prieur, a French naval officer, sought to combine the best features of traditional helmet-hose diving and swimming underwater without apparatus. Each method had its own limitations. Helmet-hose diving limited freedom of lateral movement, but allowed reasonably long periods of time under water. Skin-diving, with no heavy equipment, afforded underwater mobility but limited the time a diver could stay under water.

Le Prieur and a fellow countryman patented in 1926 the 'Fernez–Le Prieur self-contained diving apparatus', which consisted of a steel cylinder of compressed air worn on a diver's back with an air hose leading to a mouthpiece and a pressure gauge protruding over the left shoulder. The diver wore a nose clip and small, tight goggles (Larson 1959). The goggles protected the eyes and improved visual acuity in the water, but probably limited diving to shallow water because they provided no equalization of pressure. The cylinder on the first model provided a bit less than 2000 psi

of air (3 L) and less than a quarter of an hour in the water; while the second model (containing 6·5 L of air) allowed longer dives at shallow depths (30 min at 23 ft (1·7 ATA) reducing to 10 min at 40 ft (2·2 ATA)).

Swim-fins made their appearance in 1930, the first since Borelli's claw-like fins in 1680. These fins, designed by a Frenchman, Commander de Carlieu, when coupled with the cylinder/goggles/nose clip gear of Le Prieur, further emphasized the diver as a 'swimmer'. This was a new conception of the diver who with SCUBA became mobile and free for lateral movement and was not simply lowered into the water in a bell, or in hard-hat equipment.

Le Prieur improved his equipment in 1933 to allow a half hour at depths of approximately 20 ft (1·6 ATA), dropping to around 10 min at 40 ft (2·2 ATA). He replaced the goggles of his earlier equipment with a single lens full-face mask, which allowed the diver to equalize pressure more effectively. However, Le Prieur's equipment had a major problem with its steady air flow from the tank, which wasted the limited air supply. What was needed was the application of a demand valve, controlled by the diver, such as the early one developed by Rouquayrol and Denayrouse.

In 1943 the Jacques-Yves Cousteau and Emile Gagnan 'Aqua Lung' was successfully demonstrated. It employed a demand intake valve drawing from two or three cylinders containing over 2500 psig (each cylinder having 5 L), thus increasing time in the water by eliminating the wasteful steady air flow of previous SCUBA gear. The Cousteau–Gagnan valve is the basis for modern open circuit SCUBA gear.

Now that a demand valve gave the diver control over his air flow, the next emphasis was on a breathing apparatus in which air could be truly regenerated and not wastefully vented into the water upon exhalation. By rebreathing the air (or any other breathing mix, e.g. helium/oxygen) there would be greatly reduced gas consumption, and time could be extended significantly. What was needed was a filter to scrub out the exhaled carbon dioxide, thus purifying the air to be recycled. Earlier it was mentioned that such a 'scrubber', oxylite, was invented in 1897 by a Frenchman, Georges Jaubert, but oxylite proved to be dangerous when it came into contact with water. Other chemical agents such as baralyme and lithium hydroxide are now used successfully as filters.

REBREATHERS

Today the goal of developing an effective re-breather is well within sight. Two types of breathing gear—*closed* and *semi-closed circuit* rigs—are in the process of being perfected for open-sea use. Open circuit breathing gear usually contains compressed air as the breathing mix; it has a demand regulator which provides air when the diver inhales and the air is vented into the water upon exhalation. To conserve the breathing mix and extend time at depth, closed circuit and semi-closed rebreathers have been developed. Closed circuit apparatus can employ pure oxygen (originally *only* O_2 was used, limiting depth to prevent O_2 toxicity) or a mixed gas, as in recent models, with oxygen and a diluent gas such as nitrogen or helium. The development of semi-closed recirculating diving systems followed upon the closed circuit O_2 equipment (such as the Emerson). As early as 1940 C. J. Lambertsen had developed a semi-closed steady flow O_2 rebreather system which he believed could be modified for nitrogen/oxygen use.

The risks inherent in pure oxygen, primarily oxygen toxicity, create a limitation of operating depths to about 35 ft (2 ATA) or 60 ft (2·8 ATA) resting. Modern semi-closed circuit SCUBA have been developed and used successfully in such operations as Sealab II and Sealab III as discussed later.

So far we have seen the diver advance from an extremely time-limited breath-hold diver to a self-contained operator (still time-limited) who carried his air with him to the ocean floor. The next development in increasing his effectiveness on the bottom required a means of allowing the diver to be more than a transient from the surface to the ocean floor—it needed a way by which the diver could live and work for extended periods. This goal required advances in biomedical science and diving technology never before systematically attacked. It set the occasion for the fifth and current phase—saturation diving.

SATURATION DIVING

Physiological background

Because the time required for a diver to decompress is often longer than time spent on the bottom, the ratio of diver work time to decompression time is not always a favourable one. This price that a diver must pay for staying deeper and longer led investigators in the mid-1950s to develop a concept that has become known as *saturation diving*.

This high ratio of decompression time to work time is well illustrated by the salvage work on the submarine, USS *Squalus*, mentioned earlier, which sank in May, 1939 in the North Atlantic Ocean to a depth of 243 ft. Divers from the USS *Falcon* attached a rescue chamber to the submarine's hatch, and in four trips brought 33 crew members to the surface. During the salvage operation (from May to September) divers made over 600 dives, yet because of the time required for decompression, they could work only approximately 10 min on the bottom each time they dived. Had saturation been available in 1939, it is very likely that an underwater work station or habitat could have been lowered to the salvage site and a job that required many months could have been accomplished in weeks by divers living and working on the bottom (Bachrach 1968).

Development of the techniques

In 1957, US Navy officers Bond, Mazzone and Workman experimented with the concept of saturation diving, coinciding with work by Cousteau and Link (see Chapters 21 and 22 in the first edition of this book). These investigators reasoned that after a certain period of time under pressure (for practical purposes, 24 hours), the diver has absorbed into his tissues all the inert gases that he is capable of absorbing. These gases have been compressed into solution in his body and he is effectively saturated. This diver also must decompress, but the navy investigators assumed that once he was saturated, he could stay down and be decompressed only once instead of the many times required by other techniques of diving, thus adding the advantage of mini-mizing the physical risks of decompression.

Basic animal research in hyperbaric chambers provided these navy researchers with a basis for developing the concept of saturation diving. From the mid-1950s until 1962, the principles and techniques were carefully developed and tested, first on animals, then on human volunteers, who spent long periods of time in hyperbaric chambers performing specific tasks for physiological measurement, as well as participating in simulated open-sea dives.

As with many technologies, diving research balances field and laboratory programmes, with open-sea operations illuminating problems that may be better approached in a laboratory situation. Hyperbaric chambers can provide the opportunity for simulated dives where manipulation of relevant variables, such as depth and gas mix, can be accurately controlled and measurements (including physiological parameters) can be carefully made. Many hyperbaric chambers have dry and wet chambers ('pots') where diving variables such as water and cold temperatures may be studied. Diving research can systematically proceed from dry lab to wet lab under simulated chamber conditions and finally to the open sea.

In the last several years, as discussed in later chapters of this book, a number of important hyperbaric chamber dives have produced data of crucial value to deep diving. Among the more significant have been the Royal Naval Physiological Laboratory 1500 ft (46·4 ATA) dive in 1970 at Alverstoke, England, the 1700 ft (52·4 ATA) COMEX dive later in 1970 at Marseille, France and the 1971 University of Pennsylvania 1200 ft (37·2 ATA) dive in the United States. The deepest chamber dive to date, to 2000 ft (61 ATA) was accomplished by the French at COMEX, Marseille, in 1972.

This orchestration of methodologies contributes to the knowledge needed to place man to work in the sea for longer periods, at deeper depths, with increasing safety, comfort, and efficiency. Table 1.1 presents the major open-sea saturation dives beginning with the first in 1962 by Link followed shortly by Cousteau after experimentation started in hyperbaric chambers by Bond and his co-workers. Such techniques are discussed in further detail in Chapter 2.

ONE ATMOSPHERE (ARMOURED) DIVING SUITS

As early as 1715 an English inventor, John Letheridge, designed a one atmosphere diving suit, described by Davis (1962) as 'little more than a watertight barrel, with two holes for the arms and a glass window'. Letheridge successfully dived the suit to around 60 ft (2·8 ATA) and even to 72 ft (3·2 ATA) but pressure proved a problem for the arms. Davis (1962) describes a series of armoured diving suits in the years following Letheridge but it was not until the period between the First and Second World Wars that the concept of the one atmosphere diving dress became a reality.

Several systems were developed and tested. The most successful were ones designed by Neufeldt and Kuhnke in Germany in 1913 and 1920, the Peress Tritonia diving suit tested by the Admiralty in 1933 and systems designed by the Italian, Roberto Galeazzi. The Neufeldt and Kuhnke suit, modified, was effectively used in 1930 in the salvage of the SS *Egypt* sunk in 400 ft (13 ATA) of water off the coast of France. The Peress suit was used in the discovery of the QSTS *Lusitania* sunk off the coast of Ireland in 300 ft (10 ATA) of water. Nonetheless, a decline in interest in the 1 ATS suit occurred around the Second World War for a variety of reasons, probably not the least of which was the development of the aqualung by Le Prieur, improved by Gagnan and Cousteau, as discussed earlier in this chapter and which made certain kinds of underwater work feasible as a supplement to the hard-hat systems already in use. The less expensive systems such as the hard-hat and the SCUBA rigs were also more flexible.

The most significant problem encountered in systems such as the Neufeldt and Kuhnke was the articulation of the joints. These consisted of a partial ball and socket with one part sliding into the other, both separated by ball bearings and kept watertight by a thin strip of rubber. This did not allow for ideal flexibility of limb movement and, as Gisborne and Morrison (1973) observe, it is believed that below 500 ft (16 ATA) the joints could not be moved at all, reducing movement in the water as well as productive work.

TABLE 1.1

Major open-sea saturation dives

Year	Project	Site	Depth	Duration	Habitat	No. of divers
1962	Man-in-Sea I (Link)	Mediterranean	200 ft (7 ATA)	24 hours	Cylinder 3 × 10 ft	1
1962	Conshelf I (Cousteau)	Mediterranean	33 ft (2 ATA)	7 days	'Diogene' cylinder 8 × 17 ft	2
1963	Conshelf II (Cousteau)	Red Sea	36 ft (2·1 ATA)	30 days	'Star Fish House' 34 ft at widest	5
			90 ft (3·7 ATA)	7 days	'Deep Cabin' vertical cylinder 7·5 × 16 ft	2
1964	Man-in-Sea II (Link)	Bahamas	432 ft (14 ATA)	49 hours	'SPID' (submersible, portable, inflatable dwelling)	2
1964	Sealab I	Bermuda	193 ft (6·9 ATA)	11 days	Sealab I 9 × 40 ft cylinder	4
1965	Conshelf III (Cousteau)	Mediterranean	330 ft (11 ATA)	22 days	Sphere 18 ft diameter on 48 × 28 ft chassis	6
1965	Sealab II	La Jolla California	205 ft (7·2 ATA)	45 days (15 days per team)	Sealab II cylinder 12 × 57 ft	3 teams, 10 men each 28 divers (2 did 2 team-dives)
1969	Tektite I Multi-Agency (Dept of Interior Proj. Mgmt)	Virgin Islands	50 ft (2·5 ATA)	60 days	Habitat of 2 vertical cylinders, 18 × 12·5 ft; joined by 4·5 ft diameter tunnel	4
1970	Makai Range	Hawaii	520 ft (16·7 ATA)	5 days	'Aegir' 15 × 50 ft	6
1970	Tektite II Multi-Agency (Dept of Interior Proj. Mgmt)	Virgin Islands	50 ft (2·5 ATA)	12–30 days each team	Same as Tektite I	11 teams, 5 divers each
1971–1972	Makai Range/ Navy	Hawaii	80 ft (3·4 ATA) 200 ft (7 ATA)	Bounce 10 days	'Aegir'	6

Because work is being done at depths deeper than is feasible with SCUBA or standard hard-hat, the saturation mode and the Personnel Transfer Capsule have proved successful in deep diving. But the alternative approach of a 1 ATS diving suit has again been proposed after a quiescent period of some 30 years. The advantages of an armoured diving dress are apparent; paramount is the fact that the diver breathes air at normal pressure of 1 ATS throughout the dive, no matter what the operational depth. This means that there is no physiological limitation to the dive and no decompression upon surfacing. The physiological costs of diving are thus enormously reduced.

In 1969 a British company, DHB Construction, Ltd was formed to re-examine the problems encountered in previous armoured diving suits following some earlier developmental work in 1967. The design produced a suit named 'Jim' with an operational capability of 1000 ft (Fig. 1.2) now undergoing systematic assessment by the Royal Navy at such laboratories as Alverstoke's Royal Naval Physiological Laboratory, as well as open sea testing, in 1972 trials from HMS *Reclaim* to a depth of 440 ft (14·3 ATA).

The suit provides a cast body, hinged dome and articulated limbs which have marked flexibility of movement. There is a life support system

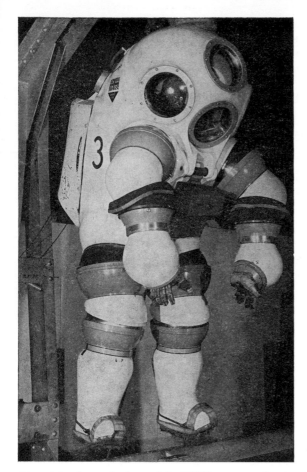

Fig. 1.2. General view of the DHB armoured suit

'Jim' has been tested in the water to simulated pressure chamber depths of 1000 ft (31 ATA) and, in recent trials, 5 individual divers performed successful water tank operations at that depth. In addition to walking on straight bottom surfaces, successful trials of walking ladders at angles of 45° have been achieved, as well as tests of manoeuvrability where the diver rolled about the floor of the tank to demonstrate flexible movement and could bend over at an angle of 60°. The manipulators attached to the suit are potentially interchangeable to provide for different tool use. Gisborne and Morrison (1973) report preliminary experiments on assembly of nuts and bolts, dismantling shackles and similar tasks, with divers requiring up to 15 periods of near an hour to acquire proficiency. With further tests, the one atmosphere diving system appears to be a promising addition to the diver's armamentarium.

PROSPECTS FOR THE FUTURE

Today the modern diver is free from the limitations of a restricted air supply, is housed in vehicles that can transport him to the ocean bottom and provide a base of operations for his work, and uses breathing apparatus that is a product of centuries of research and invention. Where do we proceed from here?

> A man in armour is his armour's slave.
> Robert Browning: *Herakles*

There have been investigations and speculations about physiologically adapting the man to the underwater environment without the use of cumbersome equipment for protection which always involves a certain loss of mobility. Two major suggestions have been:

1. The use of artificial gills (Paganelli, Bateman & Rahn 1967) for gas exchange in water, hopefully enabling divers to obtain oxygen by diffusion from the water.
2. Liquid breathing in which flooding the lungs of the diver can oxygenate them as gills (see Chapter 9).

While these physiological possibilities are exciting, it is much more likely that the advances

contained in the design which will provide for working missions up to 4 hours with an emergency reserve of from 8 to 16 hours, depending upon the level of activity of the diver. The body and dome are magnesium alloy RZ5 castings, this being the metal of choice to provide optimal strength-to-weight ratio within a compact design. Gisborne and Morrison (1973) note that the operational working depth limit of 1000 ft (31 ATA) is matched by a proof test pressure of 890 psi, equivalent to a depth of 2000 ft (61 ATA), providing a safety factor of 2. The suit is 6 ft 6 in in height and, on the surface, weighs 1100 lb with the diver inside. The articulated joints are made of aluminium alloy with a range of movement of approximately 20° about the axis. Rotary joints are used at the wrist.

will be in the area of bioengineering with improved man/machine interactions; more effective underwater heating, lighting, and communication; and the improved use of lock-in/lock-out submersibles to transport divers to depth with increasing mobility. The engineering of cryogenic gear is also a possibility to be considered. Finally, the interaction between underwater man and marine mammal working as a team is a promising area now under intensive exploration.

Man at work in the sea has a proud past and a brilliant future.

REFERENCES

ARISTOTLE (1927) Problems. In *Aristotle: Works. The Oxford Translation.* Ed. J. A. Smith & W. D. Ross. London: Oxford University Press.

BACHRACH, A. J. (1968) Man in the sea. *Interplay, The Magazine of International Affairs.* December, p. 41.

BEEBE, W. (1934) *Half Mile Down.* New York: Duell, Sloan & Pearce, Inc.

DAVIS, R. W. (1962) *Deep Diving and Submarine Operations,* 7th edition. Parts 1 and 2. Chessington, Surrey: Siebe Gorman & Co., Ltd.

DUGAN, J. (1965) *Man Under the Sea.* New York: Collier Macmillan.

Encyclopaedia Britannica (1968) S.V. Diving Apparatus. In Vol. 7.

GISBORNE, A. B. & MORRISON, J. B. (1973) *Preliminary Report of DHB Armoured Suit.* Royal Naval Physiological Laboratory Report 8–73.

LARSON, H. E. (1959) *A History of Self-Contained Diving and Underwater Swimming.* Washington, D.C.: NAS/NRC Publication 469.

PAGANELLI, C. V., BATEMAN, N. & RAHN, H. (1967) Artificial gills for gas exchange in water. In *Proc. 3rd. Symp. on Underwater Physiology.* Ed. C. J. Lambertsen. Baltimore: Williams & Wilkins.

VERNE, J. (1875) *Twenty Thousand Leagues Under the Sea.* Boston: George M. Smith & Co.

2

The Compressed Air Environment

A. F. HAXTON & H. E. WHYTE

There is little doubt that the diving bell was the first practical means whereby men engaged on engineering construction were enabled to perform their tasks under water in a compressed air environment. The first recorded use of a pressurized diving bell is by Smeaton while repairing the foundations of a bridge over the River Tyne at Hexham in 1778. In 1819 Augustus Siebe invented the supply of pressurized air to a diving dress.

The technique of using compressed air in tunnels and caissons to balance the pressure of water in the subsoil and thus to exclude it from the workings was first conceived and patented by Sir Thomas Cochrane in 1830. The basic principle of Cochrane's patent constitutes, in effect, the modern air lock to be described later. The method was used intermittently from 1839 onwards for shaft-sinking and caisson work but it was not until 1879, when compressed air tunnels were being driven simultaneously in Antwerp under the Scheldt and in New York under the Hudson River, that it began to be used extensively for tunnelling. The first medical lock was used by the late Sir Ernest Moir in the same Hudson River Tunnel in 1889.

Since then the basic principles have remained unaltered and improvements in use have been confined to details of application. Some modern research, for instance, has been devoted to the practicability of keeping workers in a raised environmental pressure for periods extending to days, weeks and even months, with a view to holding men available for work at all times and gaining an overall saving in decompression time. Whilst prolonged immersion of this nature has been proved possible it is unlikely that civilian workmen will ever readily accept conditions whereby during their 24-hour day they are deprived of social and family contacts in a normal atmospheric environment.

This chapter is therefore compiled against a background of normal shiftwork with a regular daily return to atmospheric conditions.

GENERAL APPLICATION

The general practice at present is to fill the whole of the workings with air at a pressure sufficiently greater than atmospheric to exclude the ground water, and for the workmen to carry out their duties in this raised environmental pressure. Experimental work, however, has recently been initiated in which it is attempted to confine the compressed air to the tunnel face. Excavation is performed entirely by mechanical means and the completed tunnel and the tunnel operatives therefore remain in normal atmospheric conditions. These experiments have not yet advanced sufficiently to permit further discussion.

Whereas in underwater work it is possible to provide divers with compressed gases produced under factory-controlled conditions, in tunnels and caissons the large volumes involved render it necessary to produce compressed air on the site of the works (Fig. 2.1). Since this air is to be breathed by the workmen during the whole of

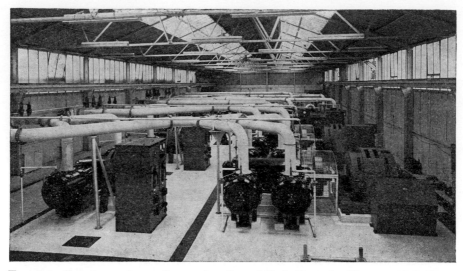

FIG. 2.1. Compressor house for construction of Clyde Tunnels, Glasgow, 1958. Low-pressure air capacity is 29 000 cu ft of free air per minute

their working period, special care must be taken to ensure that it is clean, dry and cool.

PLANT FOR THE PRODUCTION OF COMPRESSED AIR

The pressurized atmosphere is produced by mechanical compressors which may be of a variety of types. Air is drawn down into the compressors through filters placed outside the building, and through underfloor ducting. The compressed air is delivered by overhead piping through after-coolers and oil-separators at a temperature of about 70°F to the mains leading to the workings. The compressed air required for pneumatic tools within the workings and generated at a higher pressure is cleaned, cooled and purified in the same way.

In the vast majority of cases installations such as this are relatively temporary and refinements will naturally be scaled down in accordance with their utility. For instance, where the fresh air is pure there will obviously be no need for elaborate filtration.

One essential provision which must however remain, except possibly when tunnelling in rock, is the constant maintenance of pressure within the working chambers. In order to guard against breakdown of compressor plant or failure in electricity supply, adequate stand-by arrangements must be provided to be brought into operation in an emergency either manually or automatically. It is generally accepted that the minimum capacity of such stand-by should be 50% of the designed requirement. In the case of electrically driven plant an alternative prime mover must be provided to the full extent specified. This can be accomplished in three ways: by auxiliary engines to replace electric motors in case of failure; by emergency generating sets to supply current to installed electrical mains equipment; or by a reliable alternative mains electricity supply. The advantage of a fully electrical stand-by as in the second and third ways allows other vital plant such as cranes, hoists and pumps to remain in operation during the period of the mains failure.

For the prevention of panic it is highly desirable that some means are provided to allow essential lighting to be restored immediately. This is easily done by the installation of a small stand-by automatic generating set.

Compressors should be capable of operation at pressures up to 4 to 4·5 ATA and the pressure should be capable of being controlled over the whole range to the fine limit of $\pm\frac{1}{4}$ lb psi (0·5 ft seawater; 0·016 ATS). The design should be such that the delivered air is virtually oil-free.

The volumetric capacity of the compressor plant to be installed is a matter of judgement arising largely from experience and careful study of the available geological records of the strata to be encountered. The minimum requirement for ventilation given in the British compressed air regulations (Work in Compressed Air, Special Regulations, 1958) is a volume, at the pressure in the chamber, of 10 cu ft of fresh air per minute per person. It will be found in practice that unless the ground is practically impervious this volume is considerably exceeded by air losses through the working face and elsewhere and by the normal operation of the air locks leading to the working chambers.

For tunnels there is an empirical formula often used as an approximate guide to the compressed air requirements of one face:

$$C = nD^2$$

where C is the capacity in cubic feet of free air per minute, D is the diameter of the face of the tunnel in feet, and n is a factor related to the ground conditions; the value of n has been found by experience to vary between 12 for average open ground and 24 for open sand and gravel.

The pressure required is normally determined by the depth of the workings below standing water level. In practice the pressure is varied between fine limits so as to balance the appearance of water in the working face.

In the case of tunnels where the diameter of the tunnel is large compared with its depth below the ground-water level, it may not be possible to exert pressure to balance the full hydrostatic head at the lowest part of the tunnel, the tunnel invert, because of the danger of creating a 'blow' of compressed air to the surface due to the considerable excess of pressure in the highest part, the soffit of the tunnel. In this event the balance of pressure must be adjusted to some safe level in the face and water entering the tunnel below this level dealt with by other means.

CONVEYANCE OF COMPRESSED AIR TO WORKING CHAMBERS

The compressed air is normally conveyed to the working chambers by pipeline. Whenever possible these pipelines should be duplicated to guard against accidental damage to one, and they should be fitted with a non-return flap-valve at the point of discharge within the working chamber in order to conserve as much as possible of the working pressure in case of breakage.

Where the pipeline is extensive it should preferably be designed for a maximum air velocity of 30 ft/sec to avoid an excessive drop in pressure between the compressors and the working chamber.

Despite some loss in mechanical efficiency it is advantageous to generate at a slightly higher pressure than required in the working chamber and to introduce a pressure-reducing valve into the pipeline to regulate the working pressure precisely. The advantages of this procedure are that it avoids variations in pressure as the compressors cut in and out and it silences the compressor pulsations in the working chamber. Further, it ensures that the maximum pressure to which the workmen have been exposed is known with certainty.

It is essential that all pressure gauges used in the works should be accurate at all times both for technical and medical reasons. These should be checked regularly and, when necessary, recalibrated. For proper control it is important to have pressure gauges in the compressor house or control room connected directly to each working chamber. Continuous records should be kept of pressure in the working chambers, the air locks and the medical locks. This can be done conveniently by the use of pressure recorders with circular dials and a capacity of 24 hours' duration. The dials may be graduated with zero pressure either at the centre or the margin of the dial. For air locks and medical locks, where the zero end of the scale is important in registering decompressions, 'outside zero' gauges should be used. 'Inside zero' gauges may be used for working chambers when the pressures are virtually static over long periods.

AIR LOCKS, COMPRESSION AND DECOMPRESSION

Working chambers have to be sealed off from ordinary atmosphere and this is achieved by means of a concrete or steel bulkhead of sufficient strength to withstand the considerable loading applied by the higher pressure contained in the working chamber. Men and materials have to be passed in and out through this bulkhead and for this purpose one or more air locks are incorporated. In Fig. 2.2 are illustrated vertical locks such as are used for caissons and shafts, whereas an arrangement of three horizontal locks—two for materials and one for men—is commonly used to gain access to a tunnel under construction.

steel sections embedded in the bulkhead so that it protrudes on the free air side. This ensures that, when under stress, the metal is in tension and, if damaged, repairs can more easily be effected. The end doors are both hinged to open into pressure. For man-locks the design of the hinges is important since it is vital for decompression purposes for the door at the free air end to remain sealed until the moment the pressures are equalized.

When it is required to put the lock under

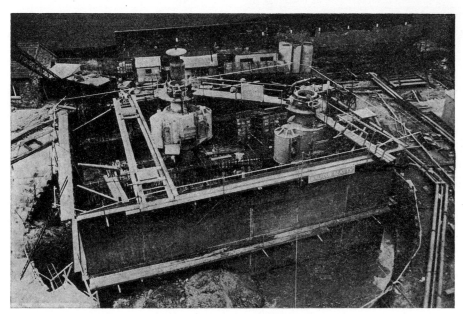

FIG. 2.2. Vertical locks for the sinking of the caisson for the North Access Shaft of the Blackwall Tunnel Duplication, London, 1962

The vertical shaft lock consists of a cylindrical materials lock with a swinging door at the bottom end and a quick-release cover at the top end which is lifted off with the hoisting rope. Two man-locks each capable of receiving four men are provided as 'blisters' on the outside of the casing of the materials lock. Vertical man-locks are of necessity small so they are not generally used for extended decompressions. The men are decompressed as rapidly as is practicable and transferred to a detached horizontal lock where they are re-compressed to the full working pressure and then decompressed by stages.

A horizontal lock is generally built of cylindrical

pressure, air is supplied from the working chamber. This operation must however be under the control of the lock keeper on the free air side and piping must be installed for this purpose, as shown in Fig. 2.3, to allow for the handling of materials and for the compression and decompression of personnel. The diameters of the pipes are usually 4 in for materials and 1 in for men.

The operation of the valves is as follows:

a is normally kept open and is provided purely as a safeguard.

b and c are normally kept shut and used only when men inside the lock are compressing themselves without the help of the lock keeper in order to enter the pressurized working chamber. Valve b is first opened by the lock keeper and eventually closed by him when the men have passed through the lock.

d is a safeguard and is generally left open.

e is operated by the lock keeper and can be used by him to control decompression. Ideally, this valve is opened to initiate the first rapid stage of decompression. At point f automatic gear

air space per man should be allocated. Timber is the most widely used material for the floor decking and seats but because of the added fire risk in compressed air, all timber within the lock must be fire-proofed and non-inflammable materials substituted wherever possible.

Good lighting is essential and this is most conveniently provided by bulkhead fittings with low voltage lamps, the wiring being run in conduit. Means of communication between the inside of

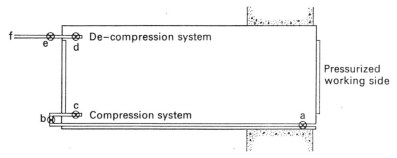

Fig. 2.3. Pipe connections through an air lock for men

is installed to control the second slow stage in accordance with whatever requirements are given in the regulations. British regulations require that an additional small bore exhaust pipe shall be installed 'which shall be operated only in emergency and which shall normally be sealed or protected'. Obviously this pipe would have a valve within the lock only to be operated if something happened to the lock keeper resulting in interruption of the normal process of decompression. Equally there should be a provision requiring another small bore pipe with a valve on only the free air side to prevent anyone inside the lock, either from inadvertence or design, shutting themselves inside the lock by closing valves c and d. The position of the open end of this pipe within the lock should be made as inaccessible as possible (e.g. underneath the floor decking).

During decompressions from the higher pressures, men will have to spend long periods, up to 2 hours or more, in the lock and careful consideration must be given to their comfort. A level floor and adequate seating should be provided. Not less than 18 in width of seating should be given to each man and a minimum of 25 cu ft of

the lock and the lock attendant are essential. In addition, the lock doors should be fitted with glass portholes so that the lock keeper can see what is happening in the lock and the men in the lock can observe the lock keeper's clock and pressure gauge. This is a requirement of the British regulations. The pressure recorders mentioned earlier will provide a permanent record of all decompressions.

Decompression under the present British regulations is initiated by a rapid drop in pressure to half absolute pressure. This results in a quick temperature drop in the lock and the formation of dense fog due to condensation of water vapour held in the air. In order to combat both of these effects thermostatically controlled high-powered fan-heaters should be placed in the lock, preferably in an inaccessible position. The thermostatic control should be set to an upper limit equal to the temperature in the working chamber, with a lower limit only a few degrees below. The electrical capacity should be about 1 kilowatt for each 200 cu ft of lock space.

For all decompressions involving a large number of men and for all decompressions of extended duration, fresh air for ventilation must be supplied to the lock during decompression. This can be provided conveniently by tapping the main pipeline supplying the working chamber and running a perforated pipe controlled by a stop-valve under one or both bench seats in the air lock. Consideration must also be given in these circumstances to the provision of toilet facilities within the man-lock.

Man-lock keepers have to be trained for their position and they must above all be reliable. As well as being required to control all decompressions, they must keep a complete record of the entry and exit of each man. When any man presents himself at the man-lock for decompression, the lock keeper must be able to ascertain quickly from the records how long the man has been exposed to pressure, in order to determine the time of decompression.

It is possible that there may be two working chambers at different pressures and connected by an intermediate lock. Although it is probable that the pressure difference between the two chambers will not be such as to require a controlled decompression, nevertheless the main man-lock keepers must be kept informed of the passage of individuals through the intermediate lock, so that, if necessary, the individual will be decompressed from the higher of the two pressures even if he presents himself for final decompression at the main man-lock connected to the lower pressure working chamber. This requirement necessitates having a lock keeper in attendance on the intermediate lock. Certain personnel, such as engineers, foremen and maintenance men, may, in the course of their duties, have to enter the working chamber more than once in any one day. Care must be taken by the man-lock keeper to ensure that all decompressions therefore take account of the history of previous exposure to pressure during the period specified according to whatever regulations may be in force. This is relatively simple where there is only one man-lock, but where there is more than one, the man-lock keepers must check with each other about previous exposures of all such personnel.

The process, mentioned earlier, of rapid decompression in a vertical lock, transfer to a horizontal lock, followed by recompression and a controlled decompression, is known as 'decanting'.

It is permissible when the vertical lock is too small, as it usually is, to permit controlled decompression. It is also permissible when, because of the dimensions of the access available, it is only possible to provide one horizontal lock, which then has to be used for the passage of both men and materials. A lengthy decompression in such a lock would mean a hindrance to the progress of the work, as it would not be possible to pass materials through the lock while it was occupied by men.

The process of rapid decompression in the main lock, transfer to the decanting lock and recompression to previous working pressure should not occupy more than 5 min. Decanting has never been regarded as a completely satisfactory method of decompression, and it should be avoided wherever it is possible to make a lock available solely for personnel, particularly at pressures of 2·5 ATA and above.

Regulations vary between countries but should require that personnel applying for employment in compressed air must be given, in writing, advice as to precautions to be taken in connection with such work. Where the pressure to which the man is to be exposed is never going to exceed 2 ATA, this advice need consist only of instruction in compression procedure, of a warning not to attempt compression if suffering from a severe cold or earache, and of a warning that all requirements of the examining doctor and of the man-lock keeper must be obeyed. Where the pressure is to exceed 2 ATA, the man must also be given, again in writing, a warning that he may develop compressed air sickness and that he must be recompressed in order to cure this. Instructions must be given as to how he is to arrange to return to the site for recompression should he be off the site when the sickness develops. He should also be warned that he is exposing himself to the risk of later bone damage and that, despite all the precautions which will be taken to safeguard his health, an absolute guarantee that he will not suffer cannot be given.

With a working pressure above 2 ATA, every man should be required to carry a label indicating that he is employed in compressed air and that, if he is found in a state of collapse, he should be returned to the site for recompression. The police, ambulance service and hospitals in the vicinity should be notified of the fact that work under compressed air at a pressure exceeding 2 ATA is being undertaken and that men may be found in a state of collapse suffering from compressed air sickness necessitating their return to the site for recompression without delay.

MEDICAL LOCKS

Recompression is carried out in a medical lock, which must be kept solely for the treatment of men suffering from compressed air sickness. All air valves must be capable of being operated from outside *and inside* the medical lock so that, in case the attendant has to enter the lock to attend to the patient, he may still control the rate of pressure variation. For the same reason, gauges placed outside the lock and showing the pressures in both main compartments must be visible also from inside either compartment. Ventilation or fresh air supply is best supplied by small valves (pet-cocks) again capable of operation from either outside or inside the lock. Heating and lighting arrangements should be similar to those in a man-lock.

In all probability, a medical lock will be situated on the surface. In hot weather, therefore, either shade should be provided or the outer surface can be water cooled.

Care must be taken to provide an adequate air supply to a medical lock. The pressure of the air for the working chamber may not be sufficiently high for medical lock purposes, since it is sometimes necessary to recompress a patient to a pressure higher than that at which he has been working. Further, during conditions of reducing pressure in the working chamber, such as during tide work, the generated pressure when a man returns for treatment may be considerably less than the highest pressure to which he has been exposed during his shift. It is therefore essential to be able to augment the generated pressure at the medical lock. Furthermore, it must be possible to supply air continuously to the medical lock even in cases of compressor breakdown or pipeline fracture. In order to cover these eventualities, a receiver filled with high-pressure air (at 7 to 9 ATA) should be positioned near the medical lock. Its capacity should be such that the inner chamber of the

medical lock can be filled at least twice with air at the working pressure or slightly above. The receiver should be fitted with a non-return valve on the supply side and a pressure-reducing valve, set to deliver air at a pressure slightly above the working pressure, on the delivery side. The low-pressure line (i.e. at working chamber pressure) should also be fitted with a non-return valve in this vicinity and both it and the line from the high-pressure receiver should be led through an additional filter before entering the medical lock.

The food lock shown in Fig. 2.4 is for the purpose of passing food and hot drinks to the patient. The dimensions should be as small as possible to avoid variations in the rate of pressure drop resulting from its use during decompression. The attendant must learn whenever possible to confine the use of the food lock to periods outside the controlled section of the decompression.

A pressure recorder should be connected to each of the two compartments of the medical lock, so that a complete record of each and every treatment is available. The first aid attendants should also write into a log book a detailed record of all circumstances relating to each treatment, with details of the previous period at work in compressed air, details of the patient's symptoms and the time at which they began, the time of entry into the medical lock, details of how he responded to treatment, when it was completed and how he felt afterwards. Such records are invaluable not only for medical purposes but also in some cases for legal evidence.

The medical lock must be situated adjacent to the first aid room, with all the normal equipment for dealing with accidents.

WAITING PERIOD AFTER DECOMPRESSION

For serious cases of decompression sickness immediate recompression is vital. Fortunately, symptoms usually develop during decompression or within a short time afterwards. In order to be reasonably certain that such cases will occur on the site, where immediate treatment is available, British regulations require all men, where the working pressure is above 2·2 ATA, to remain on the site for at least 1 hour after decompression

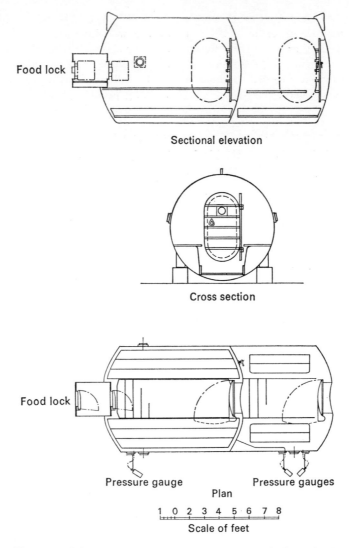

Sectional elevation

Cross section

Food lock

Pressure gauge   Pressure gauges

Plan

1 0 2 3 4 5 6 7 8
Scale of feet

FIG. 2.4. Diagrammatic arrangement of a typical medical lock

has been completed, and this period is increased to a minimum of $1\frac{1}{2}$ hours for pressures above about 3·5 ATA.

Because of this enforced waiting period, British regulations require that a suitable shelter be provided for the men, and accommodation for changing and washing. Such facilities should be of relatively high standard and should include one hot shower and one wash basin for every four or five men of the maximum number who are likely to be involved in one decompression. It is desir-

able to provide drying racks for working clothes to ensure that the men always go to work in dry clothing.

COMPRESSED AIR RECORDS

In addition to the register kept by the man-lock keepers, the individual medical record cards and the medical lock treatment-book, the current percentage relationship of total recompressions to decompressions should also be available. This is

TABLE 2.1

An example of the table produced for Type I cases only. It is a direct measure of the efficiency of the decompression process

For week ending 28 May 1967

	For week	*To date*
Shift workers		
Decompressions	479	22 163
Recompressions	2	169
Percentage	0·42	0·76
Others		
Decompressions	295	9 654
Recompressions	1	49
Percentage	0·34	0·51

generally calculated for two groups, shift workers and others. Shift workers should include all men who are regularly exposed to compressed air for more than 4 hours per day, whether or not they are actually working on a shift basis. 'Others' should be those men who are not normally exposed to compressed air for more than 4 hours per day except on isolated occasions. Such a report may take the form shown in Table 2.1.

In conclusion it must be strongly emphasized that the conduct of civil engineering works under compressed air requires an expertise which can be acquired only by practical experience. It is essential therefore that those in authority supervising the day-to-day operations should have this experience, should be fully aware of the dangers involved and should appreciate to the very highest degree the precautions which must be exercised to allow the work to proceed in safety for the structure and, more important, for the men.

Even with a lifetime of experience there is still much to be learnt to ensure the same safety for man in compressed air as he enjoys in his natural environment.

Acknowledgements

Acknowledgements are due for permission to publish the photograph of Fig. 2.1 to the Corporation of the City of Glasgow and to their consulting engineers, Sir William Halcrow and Partners, and of Fig. 2.2 to the Greater London Council, to their consulting engineers, Messrs Mott, Hay and Anderson, and to the main contractors, Messrs Balfour, Beattie and Co. Ltd.

3

Open-sea Diving Techniques

J. B. MACINNIS

Man may descend into the ocean as the occupant of a submarine, or as a mobile diver. In the former he is protected by a shield of unyielding armour, and in the latter he is directly exposed to ambient pressure and its effects. In both modes he is severely constrained by the harsh laws of his temporary environment.

Open-sea diving techniques are the special arrangement of skills that allow an individual to descend safely and work effectively as a free-diver beneath the sea. The return journey is also critical, and frequently the most important and demanding operational techniques are necessary to allow safe transport back to the surface.

It is evident that any diving technique involves critical interactions between the diver and his diving equipment. Whatever its nature, this equipment (or system) is used to minimize exposure to the stresses of the sea such as cold, wetness and pressure; and to maximize the control of life-supporting factors, such as oxygen, temperature, carbon dioxide and pressure. Therefore, the successful diver must have extensive knowledge of the physical and chemical laws of the sea related to diving; the medical consequences of disregarding these laws; and the principles and skills necessary to operate his surface and underwater equipment. These three avenues of knowledge are the foundation of effective open-sea diving techniques.

PRIMARY CONSIDERATIONS

Fundamental laws

Awareness of the laws covering diving, and the result of disobedience, has fostered the development of a combination of systems and techniques that today allow men to safely submerge to increasingly greater depths. The laws are:

Ideal Gas Law	(behaviour of gases at low pressures)
Boyle's Law	(volume inversely proportional to pressure)
Charles's Law	(volume directly proportional to temperature)
Real Gas Law	(behaviour of gases at high pressures)
Dalton's Law	(law of additive partial pressures)
Graham's Law	(diffusion rate proportional to molecular rate)
Amagat's Law	(law of additive partial volumes)
Thermal Laws:	specific heat; conductive and convective; heat transfer
Acoustical Laws:	conduction, diffraction and speed of sound
Density Laws:	Archimedes' Principle
Optical Laws:	curvature of light, absorption of colour

It is important to recognize that a direct line can be drawn from any existing technique to at least one of these fundamental laws. Another important fact is that all of these laws and their physiological relationships and implications are under constant scrutiny by a large group of laboratory investigators. Thus, any success in an open-sea system or technique has its genesis in the hours spent in laboratories and on the design board.

Dive profile

There are countless diving techniques currently used in the open sea. Their relevance and application are better understood if a typical dive is examined (Table 3.1). In this table, a deep commercial dive is used to illustrate the essential elements. Short duration dives are the most common deep underwater activity today. At least 10 000 such dives are made each year by divers working for oil exploration companies.

For example, two men descend in a diving bell to about 100 m (11 ATA) to work briefly at an oil well-head. Normally the average time at maximum pressure is less than 30 min, and the task involves light or moderate effort. Only one diver exits to the work site, while the other monitors his activity and stands by to assist.

Since compression rates are normally in the range of 30 m/min (3 ATS/min), this phase of the dive is of extremely brief duration. Life-support requirements and their attendant techniques reach a peak at maximum pressure and during decompression.

It can be seen that each phase of the dive has its major human stresses, vital life-support requirements, and critical mechanical sequences. Each of these is interdependent and must flow along a carefully planned and coordinated time frame.

Underwater tasks

Some of the major underwater work tasks conducted by commercial and scientific divers will now be outlined. It has been estimated that about four-fifths of manned underwater work in excess of 30 m (4 ATA) is carried out by commercial divers. The remainder is accomplished by military and scientific divers. Although considerable exertion sometimes accompanies their activities, sport divers are not included in this work estimate. Each different work task requires its own assortment of tools or other work support system and each device has its own technique of utilization. It is important to recognize that as demands enlarge, and confidence increases, all three groups of divers will be required to expand their work into deeper and colder waters. Supporting tool systems and techniques will have to develop accordingly.

Commercial tasks

1. Fixed structures. Work on fixed structures such as oil drilling and production platforms, towers, bridges, intakes, outfalls, reservoirs, tunnels, pulp mills, saw mills, and dams (including inspection and photography of damage by impact or corrosion; construction, repair, cleaning, removal, replacement of damaged elements). Work on mobile structures such as ships, barges and small vessels (including inspection and photography of damage; repair, cleaning, removal, replacement of damaged elements).

2. Cables and pipelines. Work on cables and pipelines including inspection and photography for damage and fouling. Location and repair of cable loops and suspensions. Burying by jetting, blasting, air-lifting, mechanical digging, hydraulic dredging. Construction and repair by underwater welding and joining. Installation and monitoring of cathodic protective devices.

3. Search and recovery. Work on search and recovery involving ships, aircraft, missiles, submersibles, transducers.

4. General tasks. These include repair and maintenance of valves and transducers, patching of leaks, placing, bolting, welding of parts, attaching of life devices, locating buried objects, placing explosive charges, site selection surveys, cutting, inducing buoyancy, rigging, excavation, erosion control, berth dredging, coating, grouting, core-drilling, scour control, data acquisition, damage surveys, logging, mining, and fish farming.

Scientific tasks

1. Biology. Observation and photography of animals and plants of the sea floor and water column. Measurements of living resource inventories, productivity, bio-scattering population density, influence of foreign objects, biological fouling, response to physical and chemical stress, bio-luminescence, bio-acoustics.

2. Physics and chemistry. Measurement of dissolved gases and solutes, gravimetric and magnetic data, acoustic data, pollution time and location distributions, pollution impact on available gases and solutes. Study of formation, configuration, aging, movement, and break up of ice.

3. Geology. Observation and photography of

TABLE 3.1

Phases of a deep, short-duration dive

Phases	Pre-dive	Observation	Compression	On-the-bottom	Decompression	Post-dive
Pressure status	Sea-level	Sea-level	Rapidly increasing	Maximum	Decreasing	Sea-level
Mechanical sequences	Prepare the diving system and subsystems	Lower bell to work site and maintain bell at work site	Maintain bell at work site	Diver(s) open hatch and exit to work site Monitor diver performance Diver(s) enter and secure hatch	Maintain seal Lift bell from work site and mate to surface decompression chamber Diver(s) transfer to decompression chamber	Inspect diving system
Psycho-physiological stresses	(Non-specific stress and tension)	(Non-specific stress, e.g. confinement)	(Non-specific stress) Noise hazard Heat Ambient pressure rise	(Non-specific stress) Cold Breathing gas density Exertion of work Urgency of the task	(Non-specific stress) Gas wash-out Rewarming Cold	Any task failure imposing a greater urgency to the next dive
Life support	General physical and mental condition Fluid balance	O_2 CO_2 elimination Temperature Humidity Communications	O_2 CO_2 elimination Inert gas Cooling Communications	O_2 CO_2 elimination Inert gas Heat Monitor for toxic contaminants Communications Helium voice processing	O_2 CO_2 elimination Decompression schedule Communications Fire prevention Monitor for toxic contaminants Heat	Rest Diet Fluid balance

sediments and outcrops of the sea-floor and slopes. Recovery by grab and core samples of sediments and outcrop material. Measurement of slope angles, surface dynamics, bearing strength, stability, sheer strength, density, thickness layering, change with depth, chemistry, scouring effects, sound velocity and mass physical properties.

4. Archaeology. Observation, measurement and recovery of artifacts from shipwrecks and former land sites.

Bio-engineering and human performance

1. Study of the performance of new non-diving equipment such as mass-spectrometers, cameras, hand coring devices and fish traps.

2. Study of the performance of new diving equipment such as closed circuit breathing systems, heated suits, mobile laboratories, navigation systems, and diver tools.

3. Study of new underwater salvage and construction techniques such as airlifts, water jets, buoyant spheres, and hydraulic systems.

4. Confirmation of hyperbaric laboratory studies.

5. Measurement of human performance under various stress conditions.

OPERATIONAL DIVING SYSTEMS

Since other chapters in this book describe specific systems, such as breathing and life support, no mechanical or physiological detail is given here. This section illustrates only the vital and complex interaction between open-sea diving systems and their technique of operation.

Breathing apparatus

Breathing systems offer a variety of operational options, which in turn reflect the complexity of manned diving. Each type of breathing system used has its own technique. Some, like open circuit SCUBA, are simple to use and maintain while at sea. Others, like semi-closed and closed circuit, are complex, and operationally difficult. For example, some closed circuit systems require a full-time technician to support their use in open-sea operations.

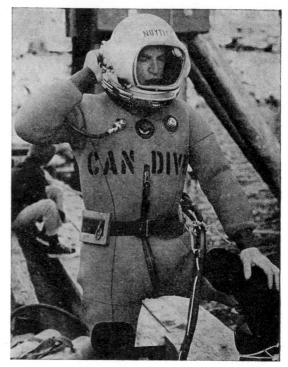

FIG. 3.1. A commercial diver checking out his helmet and suit prior to the dive

Thermal protection

Cold is probably both the most common and insidious of all the factors contributing to diving accidents. Attempts at thermal protection of the skin are as old as diving itself; but even the available diving dress of today has a definite time span of effective protection (Fig. 3.1). Beyond a certain period, cold begins to exert its rapidly debilitating and often unrecognized effects. The only readily available diving suit which offers an exception to this time limit is the open circuit hot water suit. This device provides an endless source of heat energy in the form of hot water which continuously bathes the skin of the diver. All the diving suits described require maintenance, but fortunately the techniques of their open-sea use are usually quite simple.

Recent investigations confirm the need to provide supplementary heat to the respiratory system of the diver when oxygen–helium is breathed at depths in excess of 200 m (22 ATA). Since these findings hold true for temperate waters, similar protection will also be necessary for shorter and shallower dives in polar waters. Several devices are under development to solve this problem and prototypes of both active and passive breathing gas heaters have been successfully used operationally in both deep and arctic seas.

Support platforms

There are many varieties of surface and underwater platforms used to support open-sea diving (Table 3.2). Surface platforms are critically important because their operation directly influences the use of whatever manned diving system is on board. For example, the techniques of mechanically operating a diving bell are quite different on an ad hoc rescue vessel, than on a semi-submersible drilling rig. However, the procedures used to support physiological requirements are usually the same. Underwater platforms range from a simple two-man diving stage to complex manned stations or lock-out submersibles. Each underwater platform has its own technique of employment. However, many of the life-support and mechanical subsystems are similar.

TABLE 3.2

Open-sea diving platforms—operational alternatives

	Description	Operational examples	Primary users	Approximate number in use	Maximum depth (m)
Surface					
Monohull	Conventional surface ship	Offshore supply boat	All groups	Many hundreds	
Catamaran	Twin hull vessel	USN–ASR's 21 and 22	Military	3	
'SPAR'	Long submerged columns with centre of gravity below centre of buoyancy	FLIP	Scientific	3	
'SWATH'	Small water plane area twin hull platforms which are semi-submerged on station	Semi-submersible oil drilling rig	Oil explorations companies	225	
Underwater					
Stage	Open two-man platform which is lowered to work site	USN deep dive stage	Military		100
Diving bell	Closed two-man pressure chamber which is lowered to work site	ADS–IV MK–4 Seachore	Commercial	200	330
Lock-out submersible	Twin-chambered small submarine. Forward chamber carries pilot and observer. Aft chamber similar to a diving bell	Deep diver Shelf diver SDL–I Johnson (Sea-Link) (VOL–I)	Scientific	6	300
Manned station	Large semi-permanent sea-floor dwelling maintained at ambient pressure. Usually life-support tethered to surface	SEATOPIA Helgoland	Scientific	10	200
Manned workshop	Small semi-portable sea-floor structure maintained at ambient pressure. Surface tethered	SUBIGLOO	Scientific	4	10
Welding chamber	Portable structure placed over pipelines for welding	Submerged pipeline repair system (SPRS)	Commercial	10	150

Diving bells

Tethered diving chambers, or diving bells, originated in the 1930s with the invention of the Davis submersible decompression chamber in Great Britain. Although this chamber and its several international counterparts had a transfer-under-pressure capability, they were normally used to pick up divers who had reached the work

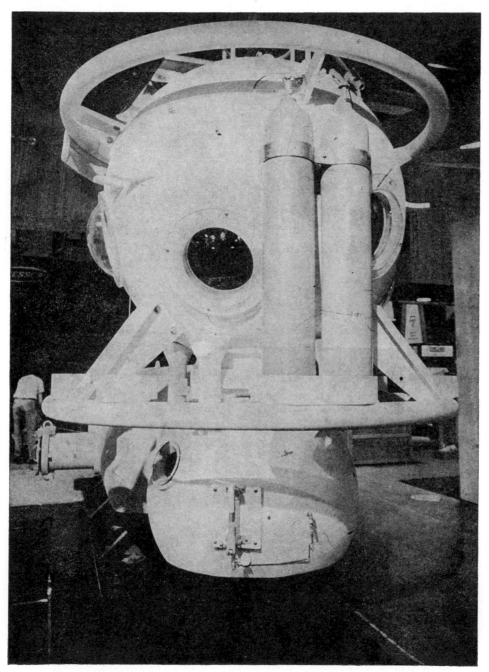

FIG. 3.2. 950 ft diving bell for 950 ft system, resting on deck chamber

site by conventional means. Current bell systems with internal and external pressure integrity began their most recent phase of evolution with Edwin Link's 1960 invention. His submersible decompression chamber was constructed of aluminum and was used for the first open-sea saturation dive in 1962. Since then, diving bell design has considerably advanced, and several hundred of these systems are currently operational. Most diving bells are used by commercial companies, and almost all are mated with deck-mounted decompression chambers for the decompression phase of the dive (Fig. 3.2). In 1972 the US Navy conducted the deepest open-sea dive to date, 1010 ft (31·5 ATA) using their DDS (Deep Diving System) MK II system.

Submersibles

Lock-out submersibles are three-dimensional extensions of diving bell capability. Instead of being tethered, the submersible and its lock-out chamber carries its divers directly to any location.

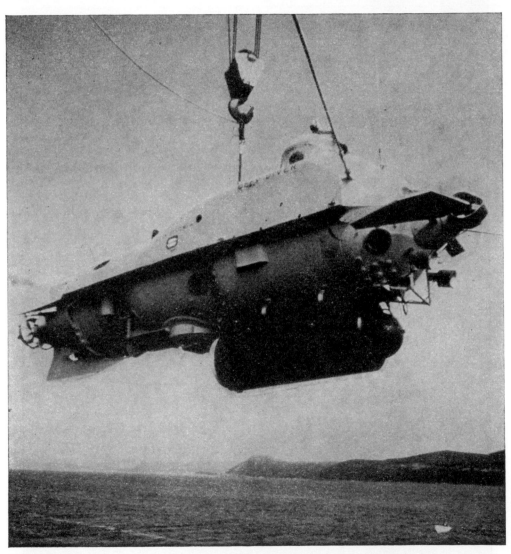

FIG. 3.3. Deep diver, a lock-out submersible. The exit hatch may be seen halfway along the underside

At the work site, the submersible is negatively ballasted, and the divers pressurize and control their chamber by techniques similar to those required to operate a diving bell (Fig. 3.3).

Two basic disadvantages of a diving bell are that its surface supporting platform requires a semi-permanent anchorage, and the bell itself is strictly limited to vertical dives. Attempts to provide tethered bell systems with propulsive motors have resulted in only a limited degree of horizontal movement and a high entanglement potential. Lock-out submersibles avoid the surface vessel anchoring requirement, and permit horizontal as well as vertical excursions. For these and other reasons, it appears that these types of submersibles, even with their current limitations on payload and gas storage capability, will be increasingly used in future deep diving operations.

Underwater stations

Since Cousteau's Conshelf I habitat, almost 50 manned underwater stations and workshops have been built and utilized. Due to high operating costs these systems are normally operated on a periodic basis and a number are presently stored and inactive. Table 3.3 shows the small number of manned stations that were operated in 1972–73. The most frequently used was Hydrolab which saw almost continuous occupation beneath Bahamian waters during 1972 (Fig. 3.4). The first nitrogen–oxygen saturation excursion dives were carried out to 180 ft (6·5 ATA) from La Chalupa during its 1973 operations off the coast of Puerto Rico.

Underwater workshops

Manned underwater workshops are smaller seafloor structures that are not designed for overnight accommodation. Their normal function is to provide a base for the storage, refuge, and communication elements of shallow dives. They are most frequently used by small teams of scientist divers studying and working at a specific site. Manned workshops are particularly useful in shallow polar seas where ice cover is a serious operational hazard. They extend the effective bottom-time and increase the safety of such open-sea dives.

Support equipment

The greatest variety of operational possibilities is found in the work-support equipment and

TABLE 3.3
Operational underwater stations: 1972–1973

Name	Country	Owner	Operational depth (m)	Atmosphere	Crew
Hydrolab	US Bahamas	Bahamas Undersea Research Foundation	13	Air	3
Chernomor	USSR	USSR	15	O_2He	4
Edalhab	USA	University of New Hampshire	15	Air	3
Sadko	USSR	USSR	25	O_2He	6
Kraken	UK	UK	30	O_2N_2	2
Seatopia	Japan	Marine Science Centre	100	O_2He	10
SDM Two	UK	UK	6	Air	2
La Chalupa	USA	Puerto Rico Marine Science	30	O_2N_2	4
Helgoland	W. Germany	Dräger	23	Air	5
Operational underwater workshops					
Sublimnos	Canada	MacInnis Foundation	10	Air	2–4
Lora I	Canada	Memorial University	10	Air	3
Subigloo	Canada	MacInnis Foundation	10	Air	2–4
Lakelab	USA	University of Michigan	10	Air	2–3
Uriuh	USA	University of Rhode Island	10	Air	2

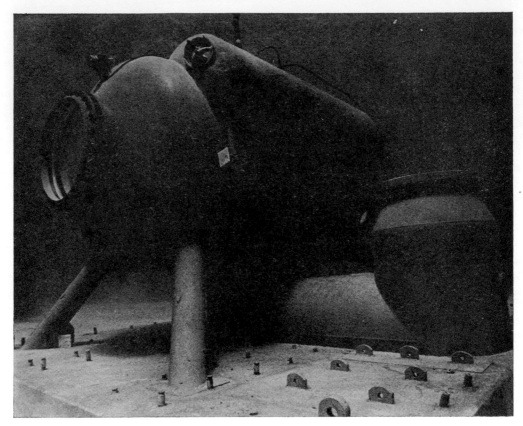

FIG. 3.4. The Hydrolab manned station in the waters off Freeport, Grand Bahama

systems outlined in Table 3.4. These range from simple hand tools to complicated propulsion vehicles. These technical devices are essentially non-life supporting, but strongly influence diver performance and safety. Consequently the technique of their use is an important component in dive management.

CHARACTERISTIC MODES OF OPEN-SEA DIVING

There are four generic types of mobile divers: military, industrial, scientific, and sport. The basic objective of the first three is work, while the primary aim of the sport diver is pleasure. There is constant overlap and interchange between all four types. One of the most impressive aspects of free-diving activity today is its growth in complexity and participation. Both these elements appear to be on a steady increase. On a world basis there are several thousand commercial, scientific, and military divers, and at least two million sport divers. Members of the former group make daily excursions to increasingly greater depths, use intricate systems, and breathe manifold and complicated gas mixtures. One vital key to their survival, success and performance effectiveness is the equipment they use. Even more important is the wide variety of open-sea diving techniques that they employ.

It is evident from the previous discussion that a great number of system and technique options are available to conduct free-diving activities. This, plus the continuously changing nature of the ocean, ensures that no two open-sea dives are identical. However, study of the four generic dive types reveals frequently repeated pressure–time profiles and recurring use of certain systems

TABLE 3.4

Work-support systems operational alternatives

Type of support	Sub-type	Basic use
Communication	Hand	SCUBA hand signals
	Wired intercom	Surface-to-diver
	Wireless	Diver-to-diver-to-surface
Navigation	Magnetic	Direction
	Acoustic	Target finding
Propulsion	One-man	Diver delivery systems for extending operational range
	Two-man	
Work-tools	Hydraulic	Rotary power
	Compressed air	Impact tools
	Electric	Welding
	Manual	Multiple uses
Documentation	Visual	Inspection and action recording
	Audio	Voice recording

and techniques. Table 3.5 displays some of these essentially average features of typical open-sea dives.

Sport divers

The population of sport divers is over a million in North America alone and they carry out tens of thousands of dives each year. By far the most common breathing system is open circuit SCUBA delivering compressed air. A short jacket of neoprene is often used to ward off the chill of long or repeated dives even in tropic waters. Most sport diving descents are usually shallow, and last for less than half an hour since almost all sport divers attempt to avoid decompression stoppages. Work on the bottom is usually a light activity such as photography or spear fishing.

Scientific divers

Scientific divers are the most active group in the use of lock-out submersibles, and manned stations and workshops (see Fig. 3.4). However, all of the systems currently operational are only utilized on a periodic basis. For most of the year these devices are under repair, being modified, or being prepared for the next expedition.

Naval divers

Although naval divers constitute the largest single group of military divers, deep oxygen–helium diving is rare and is restricted to critical search, salvage and rescue tasks. For example, in spite of the fact that the US Navy has three diving bell systems, normal manned operations are confined to depths less than 100 m (11 ATA). Heavy equipment and the traditional diving stage are used for depths down to this level for some tasks; self-contained free-swimming is necessary for other tasks.

Commercial divers

Most commercial divers work in water depths less than 30 m (4 ATA). The vast majority carry out construction and repair work during exposures of about 40 min. Most breathe surface supplied air, although SCUBA is commonly used for some tasks. A typical deep dive for commercial work is outlined in Table 3.5. Such an exposure normally involves the use of a diving bell and surface decompression chamber, and is usually conducted from an offshore supply vessel or oil drilling rig.

TABLE 3.5

Some basic features of typical open-sea dives

Generic type	Breathing gas	Breathing system	Thermal protection	Typical depth/time (m/min)	Approximate decompression time (minutes)	Usual support platforms	Comments
Commercial	Air	Tethered Open circuit demand	Neoprene wet suit	20/30	60	Vessel Surface chamber	Usually construction, repair, or well-head maintenance
	Oxygen–helium	Tethered Open circuit demand or semi-closed circuit	Variable volume dry suit	70/30	150	Vessel Diving bell Surface chamber	Diving bells, normally used for well-head operations
Military	Air	Tethered Open circuit demand	Neoprene wet suit	15/30	40	Vessel Surface chamber	Ship repair or search and salvage
	Oxygen	Closed circuit: constant flow or demand	Neoprene wet suit or dry suit	6/90	None	Vessel	Mine clearance
	Oxygen–helium	Tethered Open circuit demand or semi-closed circuit	Variable volume dry suit	60/30	120	Vessel Stage Surface chamber	Diving bell is used only occasionally
Scientific	Air	SCUBA Open circuit demand	Neoprene wet suit	15/30	30	Small boat	Observations, photography or sample collection
Sport	Air	SCUBA Open circuit demand	Neoprene wet suit	15/20	Usually none	Small boat	Observations, photography or spear fishing

TECHNIQUE SELECTION

The most important first step in any open-sea dive is careful definition and planning of the mission. The basic elements of this decision process are: water depth, nature of the work, and the time estimated to complete the work.

Water depth is the critical factor which determines the type of breathing gas and its delivery system. If oxygen–helium is used, further consideration is then given to the use of a support system such as a diving bell. The water temperature at depth forces the choice of thermal protection, while the nature of the work to be performed dictates the use of a specific work-support system. The estimated time required to complete the task is often the most important of the three basic decision elements. It influences the kind of decompression, the support system required and the total technique approach. It is important to recognize that an operational dive can vary from a simple breath-hold swim from a sea-floor station to a diving bell, or can be a deep multi-week pipeline repair task.

Field supervisors have long recognized that the ideal technical solution to an undersea task almost never exists. Even if all decision elements point to a specific set of systems and techniques, the work is usually completed using the personnel and equipment on hand. Ocean remoteness and weather factors always impose severe constraints on time, money, and system availability. In the past this has led to the unwritten principle of open-sea compromise: 'the job gets done with what's available'. Obviously this approach to dive management can reduce safety and is not to be recommended. Fortunately it is an axiom rapidly receding from the foreground of free-diving operations today.

Once there is a systems and subsystems decision, a new planning stream begins and careful consideration is given to system alternatives, and operational time requirements. The latter is divided into periods of mobilization, dive operations, demobilization, and possible contingencies.

Every successful ocean dive depends upon the skills and experience of the operating personnel. Early attention must therefore be given to the number of men required, their qualifications and responsibilities, and their physical and mental condition. Diving accident studies show that the latter factor is the one most often ignored, and that fatigue is its commonest element.

SAFETY TECHNIQUES

Theoretically all the techniques used in open-sea diving support safety. However, some are more obvious and specific than others, and will be described in this section.

One essential safety step, taken well in advance of any dive, is the engineering certification of the system to be used. In the case of diving chambers this can be as formal as adherence to American Bureau of Shipping or other Standards. With less critical equipment such as diving suits it can be as informal as knowing that a reliable manufacturer's product has been used successfully many times under identical circumstances.

There must be similar confidence in the quality of the dive methods and procedures. For example, no working dive should be carried out unless there has been extensive laboratory verification of the decompression schedules. However, at present there is a growing problem of standards for open-sea diving procedures. Although men can agree on engineering criteria for diving systems, they cannot agree on the appropriate methods of use. Much of the problem stems from industrial competition and resultant proprietary information. However, it is a situation which cannot be tolerated for long.

In complex dives the personnel are divided into a surface support team and a dive team. However, for most sport and scientific dives no such division takes place, and frequently all functions are carried out by the same men. This is another situation which contains the seeds of its own destruction.

Each diving system or subsystem has its specific mode of operation. The complete collection, known as standard operating procedures, is functionally shared by the surface and dive teams. For example, the surface team operates the life-support systems of a deck decompression chamber, but the divers operate the same systems in the diving bell. The same division of labour should occur when emergency procedures are initiated.

However, there is often the problem that the resolution of serious accidents requires co-ordinated actions that are poorly understood and rarely practised. Commitment to the pre-dive check list is an essential safety element as is a critical status evaluation of ocean and weather factors, system and procedure readiness, and personnel fitness and condition.

One of the most neglected aspects of open-sea diving is accident management and prevention. A recent survey of active participants in all four generic groups confirms that insufficient time is spent in anticipation, study and rehearsal of possible accidents. Repeated success can lead to carelessness and over-confidence; two character-istics of many diving accidents. It is an obvious truism that diving accidents are too frequent. Most deaths occur in the sport group and are related to the large number of participants and their inexperience with the exacting laws of the sea. However, each of the other groups has had its own share of fatal accidents which unfortunate-ly tend to attract local and even international headlines. Many deep diving accidents could prob-ably be avoided if there is adequate preparation for system or personnel failure and adequate real-time information about physiological and environ-mental conditions available to the surface team.

The most frequent, and often only channel of information, from the diver to the surface, is voice communication. Divers are usually quiet when working in the water and their respiratory rate and depth can be heard distinctly. The alert surface crew recognizes each diver's normal breathing profile, and voice pattern, and urges caution when they change significantly. Diver monitoring systems are able to provide much post-dive physiological information. It is un-fortunate that these instruments are rarely used in open-sea dives and most are in various stages of development or are used only for special scientific missions. However, the NASA life-support rationale is equally applicable to man-in-sea. Thus each participant in a deep or prolonged dive should have vital sign information relayed to a competent interpreter on the surface support team; although before this goal is attained more reliable and economic monitors will have to be developed.

There has now been sufficient experience with various deep diving systems to allow the evolution of certain operational stratagems. These are learned supporting actions which the operators have discovered to make the system or technique run more smoothly or safely. Some are known to be essential, such as diver physical fitness and helium conversion. Others are thought to be helpful, such as audio-visual distractions, e.g. television, during long decompressions.

Each diver inevitably assembles a portfolio of skills to bring into play within the dive profile. These skills are his personal adaptation to the specific work and pressure environment. Included among these skills are techniques of ear clearing, descent through water, and wordless anticipation of buddy needs. This type of activity must rest on firm practical ground or serious problems can occur. In the early days of helium–oxygen use, many commercial dives modified the USN de-compression schedules on an ad hoc basis. Many were successful; others were not.

Open-sea diving technology has expanded rapidly in the past two decades. Previously there was a significant time lag between an invention and widespread user adaptation. For example, it took 10 years, and the development of the wet suit, before the aqualung became popular in the mid-1950s. Today, an advance such as the open circuit hot water suit is in production within months of its invention. Manned underwater activities are expanding rapidly. There is a con-tinuous search for new technological solutions.

There still remain many unexplored relation-ships between man and the under-ocean environ-ment. One of the most important of these is the combination of drugs and diving. Use of 'conscious-ness-expanding' drugs now involves more than a small number of divers. While general incompati-bility is certain, little is known about the acute or chronic effects as they relate to diving. How-ever, there is the certainty that neither cigarette smoking, nor the taking of cannabis and harder drugs, improves diver performance and safety.

Trends indicate an increasing number of open-sea diving systems and techniques being employed in the future. World factors will assure that more scientific and military divers take to the water. Recreational diving is certain to increase as more leisure time is available. The result will be deeper and colder dives as the search for energy expands into polar seas. More diving systems will be needed to support the 600 mobile drilling rigs expected by 1980. Lock-out submersibles and manned stations will also increase as basic and applied marine science activities expand.

The next two decades will see a growing need for improved techniques and consolidation of the information which is extended from the laboratory through simulation and open-sea trials. This is the only way to ensure safe and effective open-sea work.

Acknowledgements

Acknowledgements are due for permission to publish the photograph of Fig. 3.1 to Oceaneering International, and of Fig. 3.2 to Perry Submarine Builders.

4

Engineering Principles of Underwater Breathing Apparatus

The simplest equipment that could be used for breathing underwater is an inverted bucket. With this placed over the head one could take brief but hazardous excursions underwater gaining first-hand experience of some of the problems involved in the design of breathing apparatus. The intrepid diver would soon discover that the volume of his air bubble was diminishing due to the increasing pressure with depth. This would be followed by noticeable effects on his respiration due to accumulation of carbon dioxide. If this were insufficient to terminate the experiment, then hypoxia would result as the limited amount of oxygen was depleted. The diver would be disappointed with his field of vision and would need to ballast the bucket correctly so as to be able to descend at all. Ballasting, however, can only be correct for one particular volume of the air bubble and should this be compressed any more by further descent, the diver will become relatively heavy and accelerate towards the bottom with the added possibility of experiencing nitrogen narcosis.

FREE FLOW APPARATUS

Many of these potential hazards awaiting the naive diver could be avoided by the fitting of an air pipe to the bucket and supplying it with air from the surface. Apart from the lack of a field of vision, this would be a workable apparatus in which exists the essentials of the diving bell and the diving helmet. The diving bell is merely a

very large inverted bucket and both it and the diving helmet have a long history and are still in use today. From the point of view of breathing apparatus, the only problem to be considered is the rate at which air must be pumped into them. The prime consideration is usually the provision of an adequate ventilation rate to ensure the removal of carbon dioxide. Sufficient oxygen will be supplied if the air flow is enough to prevent the carbon dioxide concentration from rising above a certain level. The flow required depends on the rate of carbon dioxide production by the diver and on the tolerable upper limit of this gas in the respired air. It would be desirable to have zero carbon dioxide, but as this requires a flow rate approaching the infinite, it is clearly impracticable. A commonly allowed upper level is 3% of 1 ATS partial pressure (0·03 ATS) and if the rate of production of carbon dioxide at STP is 3 cu ft/hr (medium work rate) then a pumping rate of 100 cu ft/hr of air is required. This simple sum assumes perfect mixing of the incoming and outgoing air and applies equally to the small volume of a helmet or the large volume of a diving bell. It is just that, in the latter case, it takes longer to reach the steady state level. It is not difficult to achieve this ventilation rate in shallow diving, but for deep diving it presents a problem. The volume must be maintained at the pressure at which the diver is working, so that at 200 ft (7 ATA) seven times the surface flow is required in order to have the same ventilation. This has set a practical limit for this type of apparatus. For example, it is recorded that during the British record-breaking dives to over 200 ft (7 ATA) in 1905, the six men required to man the pumps had to be changed every 5 min because the work was so hard.

Nowadays the use of powered pumps would eliminate the fatigue but not the wasteful pumping of gas and means have been sought to reduce the volume required. This is achieved by fitting a canister of carbon dioxide absorbent to the helmet with a venturi device to re-circulate a subsidiary flow from the helmet through the canister and back to the helmet. The venturi is powered by the fresh gas supply, the quantity of which can now be reduced by a factor of 10 or even 20 because it no longer has to ventilate the helmet directly. The gas supply problem then becomes one of providing sufficient oxygen. This problem is general to a class of apparatus known as semi-closed circuit breathing apparatus, and will be considered later under that heading.

OPEN CIRCUIT APPARATUS

By far the most commonly used underwater breathing apparatus is the aqualung or SCUBA (self-contained underwater breathing apparatus) (Fig. 4.1). The aqualung consists of one or more cylinders of compressed air connected by a manifold and this air is supplied by means of a sensitive 'demand' valve, actuated by the breathing of the diver. In a relatively short time it has reached a state of development where it is reasonably priced and may be used by almost anyone with only a minimum of training. Technically, the major interest is the construction of the demand valve (Fig. 4.2). This can be thought of as a flat circular tin with a diaphragm of rubber in place of the lid. If a suction is applied within such a tin, the rubber diaphragm will be drawn inward and this motion in the demand valve is made to operate a lever, or series of levers, which opens a valve allowing a flow of air from the high-pressure cylinders. This flow will continue so long as the suction is applied and the pressure of the issuing air will be that to which the diaphragm is exposed (i.e. to the corresponding pressure of the depth of the diver).

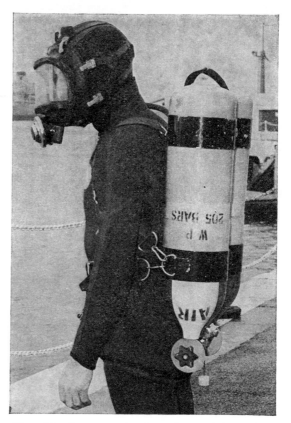

FIG. 4.1. An open circuit underwater breathing apparatus. The demand valve is mounted on the face mask

In considering the performance of demand valves, the questions to be asked are:

How much suction has to be applied to obtain a given flow?
How does this flow vary with the depth?
How does the flow vary with the pressure in the cylinders?

It is, as may be expected, easier to state the ideal than to cover the wide variations found in practice. Ideally the demand valve should dispense a flow equal to the maximum peak demand for a minimum of suction. There are no agreed standards of performance and a glance at Fig. 4.3 for three different types will show the wide variation found. These graphs show the amount of suction, expressed in centimetres of water, that must be applied to obtain the indicated flow.

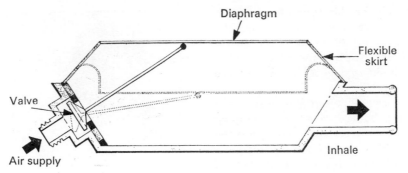

FIG. 4.2. Schematic diagram of one type of demand valve. The diaphragm is drawn inwards on inhalation, rocking the valve off its seat and allowing air to flow. On exhalation the valve is closed by the pressure of the air supply assisted sometimes by a spring (not shown). The exhaled air is released at a point close to the diaphragm

However, it must be pointed out that they were obtained on the bench in the laboratory and do not necessarily indicate the actual resistance that would be felt underwater. This is complicated by the position of the demand valve relative to the 'centre of breathing pressure' ('eupnoeic pressure') of the immersed human body.

The two most common positions for mounting the demand valve are somewhere near the back of the neck or held in the mouth. Advantages are commonly claimed for both positions. It will be obvious that the back-mounted valve will have an added resistance on inhalation when the swimmer is face downwards, but that the exhalation will be reduced by a like amount.

Apart from back-mounted and mouthpiece types, demand valves can be divided into two general classes, having somewhat different characteristics. In one class is the demand system which has an intermediate pressure reduction valve to reduce the cylinder pressure to around 100 psi (6·8 ATS) at which the demand valve operates. In the second class the demand valve operates directly from the cylinder pressure. Various aspects of performance can be predicted when the type is known. For example, in the two-stage system one would not expect the flow to be very much influenced by the cylinder pressure and this expectation is confirmed by the graph. In the single-stage system the flow does depend on the supply pressure and this is again shown in the graph. This drop in flow is not of consequence because at full-cylinder pressure the demand valve

will pass a flow greatly in excess of ordinary needs. It is only at relatively low cylinder pressures that gas starvation will occur.

The advantage of the one-stage system is simplicity and the saving of the cost of the reducer. A further prediction that can often be made is the fall in flow with increasing depth of the use of the apparatus. Approximate maximum flow at depth can be found by dividing the maximum surface flow by the number of ATS pressure at the operating depth. This implies that the demand valve is delivering a roughly constant mass flow of gas which is a feature of orifices under certain operating conditions. This feature will be seen to be of considerable importance in another type of apparatus to be described later. Two-stage systems tend to have a rising mass flow with increasing depth because the reducer is deliberately exposed to the ambient pressure and its output therefore rises in absolute terms. However, it is possible to design the reducer in such a way that the pressure rises more than the increase in the ambient pressure and this helps to maintain a good volume flow at depth.

Inhalation resistance is reduced in many demand valves by the addition of a venturi which causes a pressure drop at the demand valve and aids the suction produced by the diver. Both the single-stage and mouthpiece demand valves shown in the graphs (Fig. 4.3) have such devices, as illustrated by the falling resistance characteristics. Venturis cannot, however, reduce the initial opening resistance of the valve.

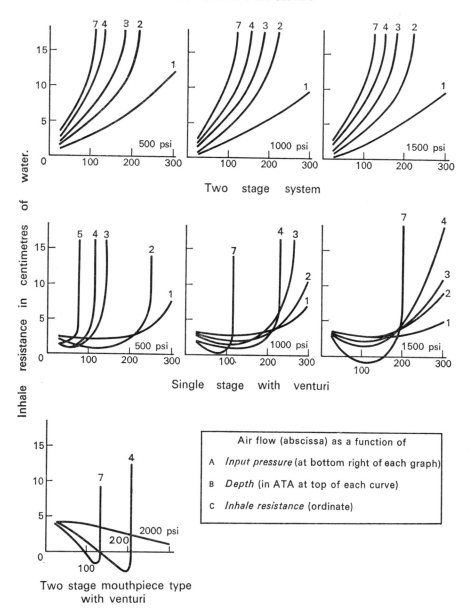

FIG. 4.3. Air flow in L/min (abscissa) from various types of demand valve

The aqualung can also be supplied with air from the surface by means of a pipe thereby ensuring virtually unlimited endurance. Such systems are variously called 'Hookah', 'Airline' or 'Surface Demand'. In many cases this method is, largely because of its convenience, replacing the free flow or standard diving system. It can also be more economical in air consumption.

SEMI-CLOSED CIRCUIT BREATHING APPARATUS

Constant mass

This is a class of breathing apparatus of growing importance in the diving industry but which was originally developed for purely military purposes. The apparatus (Figs 4.4 and 4.5) consists

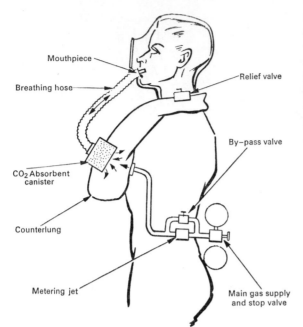

essentially of a breathing bag or counterlung and a supply of compressed gas with means for metering this into the breathing bag. In addition, a canister of absorbent is provided to remove carbon dioxide from the breathing circuit. Various valves are required to prevent over-pressurization of the breathing bag, to allow for by-passing the metered supply in case of need and to provide on-off arrangements for the apparatus. The user breathes to and from the counterlung into which a steady stream of gas is passed and the surplus escapes from the set via a relief valve.

In principle this type of set is a development of the pure oxygen apparatus (see later) for use at depths greater than about 30 ft (1·9 ATA), its chief advantage, in civil diving, being a much greater economy in the use of breathing gas com-

FIG. 4.4. Schematic diagram of a single hose semi-closed circuit breathing apparatus

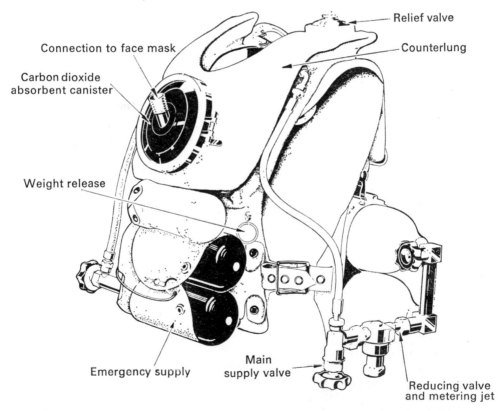

FIG. 4.5. A single hose semi-closed circuit breathing apparatus. Alternatively this type of apparatus may be designed with separate inhale and exhale hoses, each with one-way flow

pared with an open circuit apparatus. The increased depth makes it necessary to dilute the oxygen with nitrogen (or other inert gas such as helium) so that the P_{O_2} is kept below 2 ATS which leads to the problem of deciding the actual composition of the mixture to be used and the flow rate for supplying it to the set. In solving this problem, account has to be taken of the depth of the dive and the oxygen consumption rate of the diver. The depth will usually be known but not, in general, the oxygen consumption rate as it depends on the diver's work rate. However, the likely maximum and minimum rates are known and these are taken as 3 L/min and 0·25 L/min at STPD respectively. If the gas supply takes care of these two extremes, all other oxygen consumption rates will automatically be satisfied. The requirement of the body for oxygen is perhaps best stated in weight per unit time because it is then invariable under ambient pressure change. This is the reason for metering breathing gas as a constant mass per unit time flow. However, when calculating mixtures and flows it is usual to work in terms of volume at surface pressure.

For the purposes of calculation the system can be represented as in Fig. 4.6. This shows a breathing bag into which a source of gas is supplying L L/min of a mixture whose composition is $x\%$ oxygen and $(100-x)\%$ inert gas. This gas is lost from the system via two outlets. The first is the diver himself who consumes y L/min of the oxygen. The second is the relief valve through which passes the balance of the oxygen and all of the inert gas. (The solution of any inert gas in the body of the diver can be neglected.) The problem is to calculate the composition of the mixture in the counterlung and to ensure that it is always within safe limits. The constraints are:

1. The mixture in the counterlung must never contain less than 0·2 ATS partial pressure of oxygen.
2. The oxygen level in the counterlung must never rise above 2·0 ATS partial pressure (sometimes a lower figure is adopted, especially when the diver will be subject to a high level of physical activity as in continuous swimming).

The basis of the calculation is that the composition of the gas passing into the sea via the relief valve is the same as that in the counterlung.

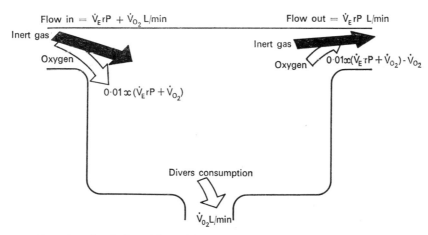

FIG. 4.6. Semi-closed breathing apparatus supplied by a constant mass flow rate of gas

A. The apparatus is supplied with L L/min of an oxygen–inert gas mixture containing $x\%$ oxygen.
B. The diver consumes y L/min of the oxygen and therefore $(L-y)$ L/min of mixture escapes via the valve.
C. This $(L-y)$ volume contains $0·01\,xL-y$ litres of oxygen so that the partial pressure of the oxygen in ATS at any depth, d (feet), is

$$\frac{0·01xL-y}{L-y}\left(\frac{d+33}{33}\right) \tag{1}$$

Further, the calculation is made for the two extremes of maximum and minimum oxygen to ensure that these two requirements are achieved. This will result in two equations each containing the same pair of unknowns. This can then be solved. An example may help to make this clear:

Example. What is the optimum oxygen percentage in an oxy–nitrogen mixture and what is the appropriate flow rate for a dive to 99 ft (4 ATA)?

Substituting in equation (1) (Fig. 4.6) 0·2 ATS partial pressure of oxygen for the worst condition leading to a low oxygen level (i.e. $d=0$, $y=3$) then

$$0{\cdot}01xL - 3 = 0{\cdot}2(L-3)$$

or

$$xL - 20L = 240 \qquad (2)$$

Substituting in equation (1), 2 ATS partial pressure of oxygen for the worst condition leading to a high oxygen level (i.e. $d=99$, $y=0{\cdot}25$) then

$$0{\cdot}02xL - 0{\cdot}5 = L - 0{\cdot}25$$

or

$$xL - 50L = 12{\cdot}5 \qquad (3)$$

Solving equations (2) and (3) simultaneously, we have that

$$30L = 227{\cdot}5$$

or

$$L = 7{\cdot}6 \text{ L/min (approx.)}$$

whence from equation (2)

$$7{\cdot}6x = 392$$

that is

$$x = 52\% \text{ approx. oxygen}$$

This practical result can now be compared with the consumption of the 'open circuit' diver at the same depth, whose average requirement at the surface is of the order of 20 L/min and therefore 80 L/min at 99 ft (4 ATA). Further, this open circuit consumption could be considerably increased by hard work.

It is not very practical to have different gas mixtures for all possible diving depths in military diving. In the Royal Navy, three mixtures have been standardized which contain 60, 40 and $32\frac{1}{2}\%$ of oxygen. The leanest oxygen mixture is used for diving to 180 ft (6·5 ATA).

The method for metering the constant mass flow of gas, in spite of the varying ambient pressure found during diving, depends on the fact that when an orifice or jet is supplied at sufficient pressure so that the issuing gas has the velocity of sound, the mass of gas issuing in unit time is constant and unaffected by variations of the ambient pressure (Payne 1952). This is true for ambient pressures up to about half that of the supply pressure. Above that pressure there is a fall in flow.

Since the supply pressure has to be kept constant, in absolute terms, in order to achieve constant mass flow, it follows that the reducer must be of the sealed variety upon which the ambient pressure does not act. In the Royal Navy it is the practice to have only one orifice size, diameter about 0·010 in, for oxy–nitrogen mixtures and to obtain the required flow, depending on which of the three standard mixtures is to be used, by setting an appropriate supply pressure.

Constant ratio

In semi-closed circuit breathing apparatus a flow of oxygen-rich gas is maintained into the apparatus and a large part of the oxygen is extracted while the remainder is passed into the water. In the Royal Navy and United States Navy equipment the flow is maintained on a constant mass basis, arrived at by consideration of maximum and minimum oxygen requirements.

A very different and ingenious system is employed in the equivalent French Navy apparatus. Here the counterlung is a large bellows having a smaller bellows arranged concentrically within the larger (Fig. 4.7). On expiration both bellows are inflated with the exhaled gas, but on the next inspiration part of the contents of the smaller bellows, depending on the length of the stroke, is expelled into the water by an arrangement of valves. Thus, a constant fraction of each breath independent of its volume, is ejected from the apparatus. This intermittent loss of gas is replaced, also intermittently, when the top of the bellows contacts a supply valve mounted in the base during the inhalation stroke.

On analysis, it will be seen that the success of this apparatus depends on the fact that the ventilation coefficient K (which is the ratio of the

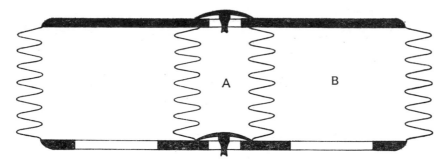

FIG. 4.7. Constant ratio bellows system
Cross-sectional diagram on the diameter. Spaces A and B are filled on exhalation
into the bellows. On inhalation the volume in A is expelled from the set.

respiratory minute volume, $\dot{V}_E$ to the oxygen consumed in 1 min, $\dot{V}_{O_2}$) has a limited range of values in spite of the great variability in breathing patterns from individual to individual and in the same individual from resting to working conditions.

To analyse the working of the set, let $\dot{V}_E$ be the minute volume at standard temperature and pressure (STP) and let r be the ratio of the volume of the small bellows to that of the large bellows. Then the action of the small bellows is such that a volume, $\dot{V}_E$ times r, is ejected into the water in 1 min at 1 ATA. At an absolute pressure P, the STP volume ejected is therefore

$$\dot{V}_E \times r \times P \qquad (4)$$

This is not the only loss from the set since $\dot{V}_{O_2}$ L/min is consumed and replaced by carbon dioxide which is removed by absorbent. Hence the loss of gas from the set and therefore the amount of fresh gas replacing it is

$$(\dot{V}_{Er}P) + \dot{V}_{O_2} \qquad (5)$$

measured at 1 ATA.

In order to find the oxygen partial pressure in the gas rebreathed, similar arguments can be used as for the constant mass flow apparatus. In this case, it may not be strictly true to consider that the composition of the gas rebreathed is identical to that ejected into the water at any instant. In this situation (Fig. 4.8) it will be seen that the oxygen partial pressure is given by

$$P_{O_2} = \frac{x(\dot{V}_{Er}P + \dot{V}_{O_2}) - 100\dot{V}_{O_2}}{\dot{V}_{Er}P} \times \frac{P}{100} \qquad (6)$$

where x is the oxygen percentage in the gas supply.

In order to calculate the limits between which the oxygen level will vary it is necessary to know the relationship between $\dot{V}_{O_2}$ and $\dot{V}_E$. This relationship can be written as $\dot{V}_E = K\dot{V}_{O_2}$ where K may be called the ventilation coefficient. K is here assumed to lie between 15 and 30 (see Chapter 5).

Rewriting equation (6) to replace $\dot{V}_E$ by $K\dot{V}_{O_2}$, $\dot{V}_{O_2}$ is eliminated and the equation becomes

$$P_{O_2} = \frac{x(KrP + 1) - 100}{KrP} \times \frac{P}{100} \qquad (7)$$

In determining the oxygen percentage to be used in the supply and the appropriate bellows ratio to be adopted for a dive to any given depth, the same considerations as for the constant mass apparatus will apply, that is, the oxygen partial pressure to be at least 0·2 at the surface in the worst case, and not more than 2 ATS partial pressure of oxygen at the maximum depth also in the worst case. A little consideration will show that the worst cases are $K = 15$ at the surface and $K = 30$ at depth. This may be compared with the constant mass case where maximum and minimum oxygen uptake had to be considered.

By way of illustration, an example will be worked for a dive to 99 ft (4 ATA). Putting $K = 15$, and the fact that the oxygen partial pressure is to be at least 0·2, equation (7) gives for $P = 1$ ATA

$$15xr - 300r + x - 100 = 0 \qquad (8)$$

Putting $K = 30$ and the requirement that the oxygen partial pressure is to be not more than 2 ATS, equation (7) gives for $P = 4$ ATA (99 ft)

$$120xr - 6000r + x - 100 = 0 \qquad (9)$$

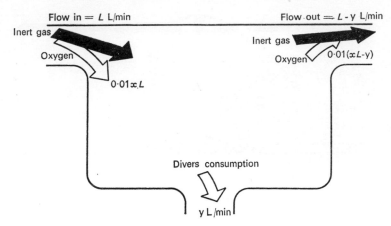

FIG. 4.8. Semi-closed breathing apparatus supplied by a constant ratio of gas

A. The apparatus is supplied with $\dot{V}_{Er}P + \dot{V}_{O_2}$ L/min of an oxygen–inert gas mixture containing $x\%$ oxygen.
B. The diver consumes $\dot{V}_{O_2}$ L/min of oxygen and therefore $\dot{V}_{Er}P$ L/min of mixture is ejected from the set.
C. This contains the following percentage of oxygen

$$\frac{x(\dot{V}_{Er}P + \dot{V}_{O_2}) - 100\dot{V}_{O_2}}{\dot{V}_{Er}P}$$

D. The partial pressure of the oxygen at absolute pressure, P, is

$$\frac{x(\dot{V}_{Er}P + \dot{V}_{O_2}) - 100\dot{V}_{O_2}}{\dot{V}_{Er}P} \times \frac{P}{100}$$

Subtracting (8) from (9) gives

$$r(7x - 380) = 0$$

Whence

$$x = 54\% \text{ approx.}$$

and therefore

$$r = 1/11$$

CONSTANT PARTIAL PRESSURE OXYGEN SUPPLY

Semi-closed breathing apparatus using a pre-mixed gas supply metered on a constant mass basis have a depth limit of about 180 ft (6·5 ATA). Beyond this depth the gas mixture required would be so lean in oxygen (in order to keep the partial pressure below 2 ATS) that the flow rates (to supply the necessary mass of oxygen) would become uneconomically large. Development work is currently being carried out to achieve means for supplying a semi-closed apparatus with a variable gas mixture—one in which the oxygen partial pressure is constant. (Note that the supply has a constant P_{O_2}; the gas rebreathed will not

necessarily have a constant partial pressure in this type of apparatus.)

The partial pressure of the oxygen in the mixture supplied at any absolute pressure P is given by:

$$P_{O_2} = \frac{V_{O_2} \times P}{V_{O_2} + V_{inert}}$$

where $V_{O_2} =$ volume of oxygen supplied at pressure P
and $V_{inert} =$ volume of inert gas supplied at pressure P.

If the oxygen is supplied on a fixed mass basis then

$$P \times V_{O_2} = \text{Constant (Boyle's law)}$$

so therefore

$$V_{O_2} + V_{inert} = \text{Constant}$$

that is, the gas mixture to be supplied consists of a fixed mass of oxygen plus a variable mass of inert gas such that the total volume of the gases is kept constant independent of the ambient pressure.

A relatively simple way of approximating to this type of flow is by the use of two reducing valves and two jets. The first valve and jet is a conventional constant mass arrangement to supply the oxygen. The second reducer to supply the inert gas would be a special kind known as over-compensated. In a reducing valve, the output pressure acts on a diaphragm and the resulting force is balanced against some fixed force, usually a spring. When the diaphragm is exposed to the ambient pressure then this pressure must be added to the output pressure (as indicated by a gauge) to arrive at the absolute output pressure.

Such a valve, if taken underwater, would give a rising absolute output pressure—the pressure rising by the amount of the increase in the ambient pressure. If this reducer were supplying a fixed orifice a rising mass flow would be obtained but the volume measured at ambient pressure would be found to be falling. In order to obtain a slightly rising volume of inert gas which, with the falling oxygen volume, will give a constant sum, it is necessary to multiply the ambient pressure increase by some factor between two and three. This can be done by loading the reducer diaphragm with a second diaphragm or piston which has an area two or three times that of the reducer diaphragm and exposing this to the ambient pressure. This will give the increase in output pressure necessary for constant volume flow.

An apparatus having a constant Po_2 supply is being developed at the RNPL (Morrison & Mayo 1973) in which a constant mass flow of oxygen is metered with a make-up flow of inert gas to give a constant volume flow of the mixture, independent of depth, by means of a laminar flow device. This consists of a series of small bore tubes arranged in parallel. For laminar flow through a small bore tube, physics textbooks give an equation of the form

$$\Delta P = A\mu V$$

where ΔP = pressure drop across the tube, μ = viscosity of the gas, A = a constant dependent on geometry of tube and V = volume flow. From this it is seen that, apart from geometry considerations, the resistance to flow is purely due to the viscosity of the gas and since this is independent of the ambient pressure so too is the flow. The

inert gas is passed with the constant mass of oxygen through the laminar flow device and the pressure drop developed is fed back to the regulator controlling the flow of the inert gas which acts in such a way as to keep this pressure drop constant. This therefore keeps the volume measured at the ambient pressure constant. An experimental model has been tested to a depth of 200 ft (7 ATA) and found to work well in practice. The laminar flow device has been much reduced in size since the reference was published and is now no larger than a pencil.

The apparatus just described makes use of the energy of the stored gas to control the mixture and no external power supplies are needed. Another apparatus using similarly the energy of the compressed gas to control the mixture is being developed at the Defence and Civil Institute of Environmental Medicine (Stubbs 1972). In this apparatus a pneumatic flowpath consisting of a 'viscous pneumatic resistor' and a 'linear pneumatic resistor' in series is used to monitor and control the mixture. The viscous resistor could be a small bore tube and the linear resistor a porous membrane. When a gas is passed through this combination the pressure drop across the pair of resistors will be apportioned across the linear and viscous resistors in a manner which is characteristic of the particular gas. This arises because the pressure drop across the viscous resistor is proportional to the molecular weight of the gas whilst that across the linear resistor is proportional to the square root of the molecular weight. So for two different gases with the same driving pressure the pressure at the junction of the two elements will be different. To quote from the specification, 'Thus if the inlet pressure is 115 psi absolute (7·8 ATA) and the outlet pressure is 15 psi absolute (1 ATA), then the pressure at the junction will vary from 61·6 psi absolute (4·2 ATA) for pure oxygen to 36·6 psi absolute (2·5 ATA) for pure helium'. For a mixture of these two gases at the same driving pressure the junction pressure will lie between these two values depending on the proportion of the two gases in the mixture. This difference in pressure is used to operate regulators which, by means of closed feed-back loops, control the composition of the gas mixture. For details of how this is done and, in particular, how a constant Po_2 is achieved the original specification should be consulted.

At less than 180 ft (6·5 ATA) the case for adopting a constant Po_2 supply in semi-closed circuit apparatus as opposed to the simpler single mixture constant mass supply is debatable. However, should it be found desirable to reduce the upper allowable oxygen partial pressure in the breathing bag from the present 2 ATS (in the Royal Navy) to say 1 ATS then it would be found that the constant mass supply system would be restricted to very shallow depths on economic grounds. If equations (2) and (3) are reworked using an upper limit of 1 ATS Po_2 it will be found that the optimum oxygen percentage would be 26 and the flow rate about 40 L/min which would certainly be regarded as uneconomic. An apparatus with a constant Po_2 supply under the same conditions would have a flow rate of 3·5 L/min oxygen and 10 L/min of inert gas making a total flow of 13·5 L/min.

CLOSED CIRCUIT BREATHING APPARATUS

Pure oxygen

A closed circuit apparatus, as its name implies, forms with the user a closed system into which oxygen is admitted as it is consumed and from which no gas is vented except in the case of excess pressure. Carbon dioxide is absorbed chemically in most such apparatus of which the simplest is the pure oxygen type. This has been used for submarine escape, mine rescue, and for many types of work on the surface such as fire-fighting. Construction has often been little more than basic, consisting of a counterlung, carbon dioxide absorbent and a source of oxygen, usually as gas stored in a cylinder at high pressure. The oxygen flow may be entirely controlled by the user in opening a valve from time to time as the volume of oxygen in the counterlung falls or there may be a continuous flow of about 0·7 L/min and the user replenishes the counterlung as necessary by means of a by-pass valve. In another type a specially shaped counterlung operates a demand valve to admit more oxygen when the bag contains less than one breath of gas. The use of a pure oxygen apparatus underwater is severely restricted by the risk of oxygen poisoning to depths of less than about 30 ft (1·9 ATA).

Oxygen sensor

The ideal self-contained breathing apparatus from several points of view would appear to be a closed circuit mixed gas type in which the partial pressure of the oxygen was controlled at some predetermined level. Such an apparatus would be the most economical in the use of the stored gas, the flow being merely the amount of oxygen actually consumed. One apparatus of this type has been developed by the General Electric Company in the USA. In many respects this apparatus does not differ from conventional semi-closed sets. It has a similar sort of breathing circuit consisting of mouthpiece, hoses, carbon dioxide absorbent canister and breathing bags as well as the usual cylinders of compressed gas. The difference lies in the addition of equipment to measure and control the oxygen level.

The control of the oxygen partial pressure is achieved by the use of a specially developed sensor which is, in effect, a small electric cell. A tiny part of the oxygen in the breathing circuit continuously diffuses across a thin membrane into the cell and reacts at the sensing electrode with the electrolyte to give hydroxyl ions which drift across to the counter electrode reacting with it to form a metal oxide. The electrode is thus consumed which limits the life of the cell to about 6 months. The reactions taking place in the cell give rise to an electric current which is proportional to the oxygen concentration, i.e. the partial pressure and this current develops a proportional voltage across a load resistor. The voltage is used to actuate a solenoid valve which admits oxygen as the Po_2 falls. An interesting feature is the provision of a switch for selecting either a high or low level of Po_2, the former being useful to speed decompression. Inert gas is admitted to the breathing circuit as required by a demand type valve which comes into operation when the breathing bags are deflated. This happens when there is an increase in the ambient pressure, for example, when the diver descends. A certain amount of redundancy is provided by the use of three oxygen sensors and safety is further ensured by having an independent read-out of Po_2, indicators of power supply voltage and gross departure from sensor operating level, and means for manually controlling Po_2 in the event of failure of the automatic system.

Cryogenic closed circuit

In principle a simple way to achieve constant Po_2 is to make use of the relationship between the temperature and vapour pressure of a liquid, the liquid in this case being oxygen. For example, at a temperature of $-195°C$ the vapour pressure of liquid oxygen is 0·2 ATS. If helium is passed through a vessel containing oxygen at this temperature, the discharge will contain oxygen at a partial pressure of 0·2 ATS and this will be almost independent of the ambient pressure. By varying the temperature, a range of partial pressures can be obtained. At least one apparatus on this principle has already been developed (Fischel 1970).

In this apparatus the exhaled gas is passed via the exhale bag through a counterflow heat exchanger into the liquid oxygen vessel, then back through the heat exchanger and inhale bag to the diver with the oxygen level fully restored and the carbon dioxide removed. The counterflow heat exchanger cools the breathing gas from ambient down to near liquid oxygen temperature on exhalation, whereas as the gas retraces its path through the heat exchanger on inhalation it picks up heat and is rewarmed. Carbon dioxide is deposited as a solid by condensation in the heat exchanger in which there is room for several hours' use. Basically this apparatus is strikingly simple but a considerable amount of effort and ingenuity was required to make it work in practice. The chief problem was to keep the temperature of the liquid oxygen constant which was accomplished by having a separate cooling system. Other problems include heat exchanger design and coping with the use of the set in any diver attitude.

SOME OTHER POSSIBLE SYSTEMS

The development of underwater breathing apparatus is a steady field of endeavour for inventors, but sometimes one finds ideas put forward which ignore simple physical or practical considerations. Take, for example, an apparatus based on the electrolysis of water into its constituent gases, hydrogen and oxygen, with a view to utilizing the oxygen in some manner in a closed circuit system. If 2 g moles of hydrogen and 1 g mole of oxygen are combined to produce water, then approximately 136 kcal of heat are liberated. To reverse the process, 136 kcal is the least amount of energy that must be supplied. This will give 1 g mole of oxygen or 22·4 L at STP, and if a rate of consumption of 3 L/min is assumed, the energy requirement will be approximately 18 kcal/min, or 1260 watts. This is not so large as to be completely impractical but is effectively so for an autonomous breathing apparatus.

Another possibility considered is the use of semi-permeable membranes which will permit the extraction of the dissolved gases from sea water. A little consideration will show that the tension of the dissolved gases cannot be greater than 1 ATS since this is the pressure at which solution takes place at the surface. Hence, in order to extract any gas at depth it will be necessary to make use of a vacuum pump to maintain a partial pressure of less than 1 ATS of oxygen and nitrogen behind the membrane. Having extracted the gas it will then be necessary to compress this to the ambient pressure so that it can be supplied to a diver. Such complication does not seem to point the way to producing an effective breathing apparatus, although the semi-permeable membrane may be of use in eliminating carbon dioxide without the use of absorbents.

What, at first sight, seems an attractive proposition is the use of the peroxides of sodium and potassium to provide both the oxygen required by the diver and, at the same time, to remove the carbon dioxide exhaled. Unfortunately, these chemicals also react with moisture to produce oxygen and any leakage in the apparatus could produce a violent reaction, which would make an apparatus based on this principle hazardous for use under water.

In conclusion, it should be stated that the first requirement in underwater breathing apparatus is extreme reliability and the second is robustness. Divers often work under conditions of great discomfort and may be cold, not to mention suffering from seasickness and fatigue. It cannot therefore be expected that they will treat their equipment with the delicacy necessary for laboratory apparatus. Hence, the sophistication of equipment aimed at economy of gas, increase of endurance, reduction of weight, etc., must always take its place after these first two essentials are achieved.

REFERENCES

FISCHEL, H. (1970) Closed circuit cryogenic Scuba. In *Equipment for the Working Diver*, p. 229. Washington D.C.: Marine Technology Society.

MORRISON, J. B. & MAYO, I. C. (1973) Gas-mixture supply at constant Po_2 for semi-closed circuit breathing apparatus. *Underwater J.*, **5**, 23–27.

PAYNE, P. F. (1952) A supersonic regulator for divers' breathing apparatus. *Jl R. nav. scient. Serv.*, **7**, 12.

STUBBS, R. A. (1972) Pneumatic devices for the measurement of composition of binary gases. British Patent 1360172.

5

Physiological Principles of Underwater Breathing Apparatus

J. B. MORRISON

It will be obvious from the description of the mechanics of breathing apparatus presented in the previous chapter, that in order to design an equipment to satisfy the divers' requirements, knowledge of respiratory physiology is essential. In particular, it is necessary first to understand the effects of both increased pressure and underwater breathing apparatus on the physiological state of the diver, and, secondly, to specify in a quantitative manner suitable physiological design parameters.

The physiological requirements which must be realized may be summarized as follows. Firstly, the equipment must supply the diver with adequate ventilation at all levels of physical exertion. Secondly, the partial pressures of oxygen and carbon dioxide present in the breathing gas mixture must be maintained within tolerable limits. Finally, any increase in the work of breathing due to either gas density or equipment design must not become excessive.

At first glance it would appear a relatively simple task to satisfy the above conditions. A more detailed study of the problem, however, reveals a situation in which much of the physiological information required is either unestablished or controversial in nature. For example, there is a paucity of experimental information available regarding the work of breathing which is tolerable to the diver. Consequently, the actual ventilatory power requirement of equipment in service is usually unspecified and its effects on divers'

respiration under operational conditions quite unknown.

In the following paragraphs aspects of pressure physiology relevant to the design of breathing apparatus are described. On this basis the limitations imposed on the diver by some current equipment designs are outlined and the necessary design specifications for various types of underwater breathing apparatus are discussed.

EXERTION UNDERWATER

Oxygen uptake

At normal barometric conditions, the maximum exertion of healthy subjects is usually limited by circulatory factors and is reached only during extremely vigorous exercise (Cotes 1968). It is unlikely that such levels of exertion are attained underwater. At increased pressure, however, maximum oxygen uptake may become restricted by ventilatory limitations due to the combined effects of increased gas density and breathing apparatus. In the design of underwater breathing apparatus, it is relevant to consider the exercise intensity commonly achieved by divers.

The most comprehensive study of oxygen uptake underwater is that of Donald and Davidson (1954) who investigated both fin swimming and booted divers. The highest values of oxygen uptake were recorded when fin swimming at high speeds (31 to 42 m/min) over a period of 10 min. In this activity the mean oxygen uptake was 3·1 L/min STPD and a maximum value of 4·2 L/min was recorded. When wearing boots and operating in 1 to 2 ft of mud, the oxygen uptake associated with maximum movement varied between 1·2 and 2·5 L/min STPD. The oxygen uptake of fin swimmers measured by Lanphier (1954) was approximately $2·5 \pm 0·5$ L/min STPD when swimming at a speed of 1·2 knots (36 m/min). Above this speed the swimmers tired rapidly. Goff, Frassetto and Specht (1956) measured oxygen consumption in the range of 1·3 to 2·5 L/min STPD in divers fin swimming at various speeds below maximum effort over distances of 450 to 1850 m. The above studies were confined to shallow water, less than 10 m (2 ATA), using closed circuit oxygen equipment. Oxygen consumptions were calculated using the pressure drop method of measurement (Donald & Davidson 1954). In a later study at depths of 2 to 54 m (1·1 to 6·4 ATA) Morrison (1973) measured the oxygen uptake of divers breathing oxygen–nitrogen mixtures from semi-closed circuit equipment. Oxygen uptake was calculated from the gas equilibrium equation of the counterlung. The mean oxygen uptake when fin swimming against a trapeze with maximum effort was calculated to be 2·6 L/min STPD and individual values of up to 3·4 L/min were recorded.

These studies, which are in good agreement, indicate that it is possible for the average fin swimming diver to maintain oxygen uptakes of 2·5 to 3·0 L/min STPD, and it is conceivable that individual values of up to 4 L/min may be achieved. In contrast, it would appear that the booted diver is unlikely to attain an oxygen uptake greater than 2·5 L/min. Whilst it is undesirable that divers should work to exhaustion during normal operations, it is necessary that in an emergency the diver should be limited by his physical effort rather than by equipment design. Hence it is considered that the above limits of exertion form a suitable basis for the design of breathing apparatus.

In most types of semi-closed circuit underwater breathing apparatus, the supply of oxygen to the apparatus is independent of the diver's ventilation and thus the range of oxygen uptake ($\dot{V}_{O_2}$) is an essential parameter of the design. It is likely that oxygen uptakes in excess of 3·0 L/min would only be maintained for a few minutes and could nor-

mally be met by the reserve volume of oxygen contained in the counterlung of the apparatus. Hence in this type of apparatus it would seem reasonable to assume as a standard that the equipment should provide the diver with not less than 3·0 L/min STPD oxygen uptake during exertion. In the case of booted divers, this figure might be reduced to 2·5 L/min STPD. Minimum oxygen uptake must also be specified. Although it is unlikely that a diver will achieve a true resting state, a resting value of 0·25 L/min STPD oxygen uptake is normally assumed. It should be noted that these standards are referred to STPD conditions and in practice where flow rates are measured at ambient conditions, the appropriate correction must be applied.

Some equipments currently in use are designed to considerably lower standards than quoted above (e.g. $\dot{V}_{O_2} \leqslant 2·0$ L/min). It is evident that in such equipment there is a great risk of the diver breathing a hypoxic gas mixture, especially when swimming or working close to the minimum depth limit of the equipment (Morrison 1973).

Ventilation

In open circuit underwater breathing apparatus the supply of oxygen is available on demand and depends only on the diver maintaining adequate ventilation. The ventilation of the diver, therefore, becomes the relevant parameter in these designs. In the studies of underwater exertion already described, ventilation was not measured. However, having established the exertion possible, ventilation requirements can be deduced with reasonable accuracy from investigations conducted in pressure chambers under dry conditions.

In various studies of exercise at increased ambient pressure, a reduction of the ventilation equivalent for oxygen, $\dot{V}_E/\dot{V}_{O_2}$, compared with that at surface has been observed. In conjunction with this reduction of ventilation, equivalent various degrees of carbon dioxide retention have been measured (Lanphier 1963; Hesser, Fagraeus & Linnarsson 1968; Broussolle et al. 1970; Salzano, Rausch & Saltzman 1970). This subject is discussed in detail in a later chapter by Lanphier. The ventilatory insufficiency observed at pressure has been demonstrated by Lanphier (1963) and Hesser, Fagraeus and Linnarsson (1968) to be due partly to increased oxygen partial pressure and partly to increased gas density. Additional ventilatory effort due to breathing equipment may further reduce ventilation equivalent (Silverman et al. 1951; Salzano, Rausch & Saltzman 1970; Morrison et al. 1975).

In the Cooperative Underwater Swimming Project (CUSP 1953), divers performed static swimming against a 9 lb force whilst breathing air from open circuit breathing apparatus. At 4 ATA the mean ventilation measured was 19·4 L/min compared with a 'subsurface' value of 30·5 L/min (BTP, dry gas), a decrease of 37%. A similar US Navy study was also reported by CUSP (1953) involving weight lifting underwater, in which the mean ventilation measured at 4 ATA was some 20% less than the corresponding value at 1 ATA.

Fig. 5.1 shows the separate effects of hyperbaric oxygen–nitrogen gas mixture and underwater breathing apparatus on ventilation (Morrison et al. 1975). A reduction in exercise ventilation of approximately 20% resulted when breathing from underwater breathing apparatus at 4 ATA. In addition, in contrast to exercise at 1 ATA, end-tidal P_{CO_2} showed a significant increase in relation to exercise intensity, reaching a mean value of 50 mm Hg at an oxygen uptake of 2·5 L/min. Presumably this undesirable increase in end-tidal P_{CO_2} with exercise will be largely dependent on values of oxygen partial pressure, gas density and resistance of breathing equipment, all of which are factors of breathing apparatus design. When breathing oxygen–helium mixtures, effects of increased gas density and breathing apparatus comparable to those of Fig. 5.1 would be expected at approximately 30 ATA (300 m).

The 4 divers represented in Fig. 5.1 demonstrated an essentially normal ventilatory response to exercise at 1 ATA. As discussed later by Lanphier, there is evidence that certain trained divers classed as 'carbon dioxide retainers' have a reduced ventilatory response to exercise even under normal conditions. It is probable that this group of divers would have considerably lower ventilatory equivalents for oxygen than indicated. Fig. 5.1 suggests that when operating under pressure, the maximum ventilation of divers will probably not exceed 65 L/min BTPS at an oxygen uptake of 3·0 L/min STPD whereas at surface and in the absence of breathing apparatus, the equivalent ventilation would be of the order of 80 L/min.

Ventilation equivalent

In semi-closed circuit underwater breathing apparatus operating on the constant ratio principle, the ventilation equivalent for oxygen $(\dot{V}_E/\dot{V}_{O_2})$ is an essential design parameter. From the data of Kao (1963), Schaefer (1967) and Davies, Tuxworth and Young (1970) limits for the value of ventilation equivalent, K, of $15 \leqslant K \leqslant 30$ have been suggested by Young (1969). In the experiments described in Fig. 5.1 the individual ventilatory equivalents for oxygen measured ranged from a maximum of 35 when resting to a minimum of 18 during exercise at 4 ATA. However, one diver, classed as a carbon dioxide retainer and considered to be an extreme example of the group, who was also investigated as part of the above study, exhibited a ventilatory equivalent of 10 to 15 during exercise at 4 ATA (Morrison et al. 1975). Ventilation equivalents in excess of 30 were measured under ideal resting conditions such as are unlikely to occur during operational diving.

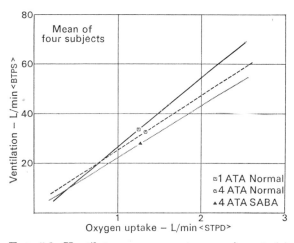

FIG. 5.1. Ventilatory response to exercise at (a) 1 ATA breathing air; (b) 4 ATA breathing oxygen–nitrogen mixture $(P_{O_2} = 0.42$ ATS); (c) 4 ATA breathing oxygen–nitrogen mixture from open circuit underwater breathing apparatus (Swimmers Air Breathing Apparatus, *RN Diving Manual* 1964). Each regression line represents the mean results of four subjects measured at rest and four levels of exercise

Ventilation equivalents of less than 15 were measured at depth in the presence of a high Po_2. It can be seen from the relevant design equations that $K < 15$ would only produce critical (i.e. hypoxic) conditions close to the surface. Hence the limits of ventilation equivalent proposed by Young (1969) would appear practical for this type of equipment.

Volume flow of gas mixture on demand

In open circuit breathing apparatus, the volume flow of gas available to the diver on demand is a function of the demand valve design. As discussed in the previous chapter the volume flow will be reduced as ambient pressure increases. In addition, the volume flow may also be adversely affected by a reduction of cylinder pressure.

For safety, it would seem reasonable to design open circuit equipment such that the average diver will demand no more than 80% of the maximum volume flow available. For example, if it is assumed that the average diver will require a maximum ventilation of 65 L/min when breathing dense gases, then a suitable standard would be that the breathing apparatus should be capable of supplying a ventilation of 80 L/min under these conditions. The corresponding limit of ventilatory power requirement is discussed in a subsequent section.

As respiration involves pulsatile flow approximately sinusoidal in nature (Cooper 1960a; Riegel & Harter 1969) the equipment must be capable of supplying instantaneous gas flow rates of much greater magnitude than the specified mean volume flow per minute. In experiments at 1 ATA, Silverman et al. (1951) found that the maximum inspiratory and expiratory flow rates were 2·5 to 3·0 times greater than corresponding minute volumes during heavy exercise. In general, maximum expiratory flows were slightly greater than maximum inspiratory flows. The addition of inspiratory and expiratory resistance caused both maximum flow rates and minute volume to be reduced, but did not appreciably affect the ratio of these two quantities.

Assuming a ventilation of 80 L/min, the data of Silverman et al. (1951) and Cooper (1960a) suggests that breathing apparatus should be tested with a gas flow approximately sinusoidal

in form having a maximum flow rate (i.e. amplitude) of 240 L/min and a frequency of 20 to 30 cycles/min. As the volume flow available from a demand valve decreases as ambient pressure is increased, it is essential that the apparatus is tested at maximum operating depth for a given gas mixture.

TABLE 5.1

Maximum voluntary ventilation at pressures of 1 to 8 ATA when breathing air from atmosphere with minimum resistance (Normal) and from RN Swimmers Air Breathing Apparatus (SABA)

Depth ATA	Maximum ventilation L/min (BTPS)		Percentage of normal ventilation
	Normal	SABA	
1	175·2	151·2	86
2	133·6	126·1	94
4	104·5	95·6	92
8	83·7	73·1	87

It can be seen from Table 5.1 that the RN Swimmers Air Breathing Apparatus (*Royal Navy Diving Manual* 1964) must be capable of meeting such a specification at gas densities of at least 6 times that of air. There is reason to doubt, however, whether some open circuit equipment available could meet this standard at all gas densities and cylinder pressures at which they are normally operated. In the previous chapter it is suggested that single stage demand valves would be particularly suspect at low cylinder pressures and high gas densities.

Counterlung volume

As closed and semi-closed circuit equipment operate on a rebreathing principle, the volume flow of gas is dependent primarily on respiratory effort. As the diver is rebreathing from a counterlung, however, the design may affect the tidal volume available to the diver.

It has been shown by Hey et al. (1966) that tidal volume is linearly related to ventilation up to a maximum tidal volume of approximately 50% of vital capacity. Tidal volume then remains constant and further increase of ventilation is achieved by increase in respiratory frequency.

This relationship is essentially unaltered by variations in $P_{A_{CO2}}$, $P_{A_{O2}}$ or exercise. In the presence of increased gas density, tidal volume tends to be increased in relation to ventilation and there is a corresponding reduction in respiratory rate. In experiments at 4·5 ATA, Hesser et al. (1968) measured a reduced respiratory frequency in 7 subjects breathing air both when resting and at various intensities of exercise. During a simulated oxygen–helium dive to a maximum pressure of 46·5 ATA, Morrison and Florio (1971) measured the relationship of ventilation to tidal volume at rest and moderate exercise. Tidal volume increased with pressure, and the resultant reduction in the slope of the relationship suggested a possible correlation with increasing gas density. Although the relationship is affected by an increase of gas density (or pressure), it is not clear whether the fraction of vital capacity at which ventilation becomes independent of tidal volume (i.e. the mean maximum tidal volume during exercise) is also altered. During heavy exercise, tidal volumes may vary from breath to breath, and values of up to 75% of vital capacity are not uncommon.

It is preferable that the mean maximum tidal volume of the diver is somewhat lower than the volume of the counterlung system in order to prevent increased resistance to breathing as the bag becomes flat. In order to ensure comfortable ventilation, therefore, it would be appropriate that the counterlung should contain a volume of breathing gas equivalent to the full vital capacity of the diver. As the vital capacity of young adult males (European) tends to be in the range of 5 ± 1 L (Cotes 1968) this would infer that prior to inspiration the counterlung should have a minimum collapsible volume of 6 L.

The collapsible volume of the counterlung is the effective volume as regards ventilation. This may be considerably less than the total counterlung volume. For example, a counterlung having both inspiratory and expiratory bags should contain a device to prevent total collapse of the inspiratory bag which would isolate the diver from the supply of breathing gas in the expiratory bag. In certain positions of the diver, the setting of the relief valve may prevent the breathing bags from becoming fully inflated. In addition, in some apparatus the relief valve setting may be altered depending on the position of the diver in order to achieve the most comfortable breathing characteristics. It is essential that such features are considered and the total volume of the counterlung increased proportionally. Hence, in order to ensure an effective volume of 6 L, a counterlung may require a total capacity of 8 to 10 L.

DEPTH LIMITATIONS OF BREATHING GASES

Ventilation limitation

A useful index of breathing capacity is maximum voluntary ventilation (MVV). The relationship of MVV to gas density is described by Lanphier in Chapter 8. In relating this index to maximum sustained breathing capacity, $\dot{V}_E$ max, of the working diver, two further factors must be considered. Maximum ventilation which can be comfortably maintained during a prolonged period of exercise may be somewhat lower than that attained during a short MVV manoeuvre. A reduction of both MVV and $\dot{V}_E$ max would be expected as a result of external resistance to ventilation imposed by underwater breathing apparatus, the extent being dependent on the particular apparatus used.

In a recent study shown in Table 5.1 it was found that breathing from open circuit underwater breathing apparatus (RN Swimmers Air Breathing Apparatus) effected a reduction of 5 to 15% in mean maximum voluntary ventilation when breathing air (Morrison & Butt 1972). The maximum voluntary ventilations achieved were on the whole higher than expected and considerably greater than predicted values based on data of breathing apparatus resistance (Lanphier 1969). The results presented in Table 5.1 are considered to be fairly representative of well-designed open circuit breathing apparatus. The breathing characteristics of semi-closed and closed circuit equipment differ considerably from those of open circuit equipment, breathing effort being very much influenced by the location of the counterlung and the orientation of the diver. In the ideal position, breathing characteristics of semi-closed circuit breathing apparatus may be as good as or superior to those of open circuit equipment, but in other orientations, considerable decrement in performance is likely to occur.

Assuming that a diver may require up to 65 L/min from his breathing set, the relationship of MVV to absolute pressure would not appear to limit SABA down to a depth of 8 ATA where average results give a value of 73 L/min (see Table 5.1). If, however, $\dot{V}$E max is somewhat lower than MVV, safe diving would be limited to shallower depths. None of the subjects considered that they could do useful work and sustain the ventilations achieved in these experiments. Broussolle et al. (1970) and Miller, Wangensteen and Lanphier (1970) have found that some subjects could maintain an exercise ventilation equivalent to their MVV when breathing air at 6 to 8 ATA. However, at 8 ATA the maximum voluntary ventilations of these subjects were 25 to 30% lower than the comparable values given in Table 5.1. In a more recent study, Fagraeus and Linnarsson (1973) found that at 6 ATA the mean $\dot{V}$E max of 8 divers was 82% of MVV.

Although it may be possible for divers to work at their MVV, in order to allow a margin of safety it would seem prudent that ventilation should not exceed 80% of this value. Assuming, therefore, that $\dot{V}$E max will not exceed 65 L/min when breathing dense gas mixtures, one might postulate that a particular breathing apparatus should be limited to the depth at which mean MVV is reduced to 80 L/min. For example, applying this criterion to SABA, Table 5.1 would indicate that when breathing air a safe limit for the working diver would be in the region of 6 ATA (50 m), and beyond this depth a less dense gas should be introduced. As most of the decrement in MVV shown in Table 5.1 is due to gas density rather than the resistance of the breathing apparatus, it is unlikely that gases of density greater than 6 times that of air could be used in other breathing apparatus if the above specification was to be utilized. In the absence of more comprehensive information this limit might be applied to other underwater breathing apparatus, although a lower limit of gas density would be more appropriate in equipment having less favourable breathing characteristics.

Divers who exhibit a relatively low ventilatory response to exercise (Lanphier 1969) would not experience problems of ventilation limitation as defined above. However, the adverse effects of the associated carbon dioxide retention, which is accentuated by increased gas density and a high Po_2 must be considered. Lanphier (1969) suggests that 'carbon dioxide retainers' are more susceptible to severe inert gas narcosis, oxygen poisoning and carbon dioxide intoxication. Incidents involving oxygen poisoning (Lanphier 1969) and loss of consciousness underwater (Morrison, Florio & Butt 1974) have been associated with markedly reduced ventilatory responses to carbon dioxide. The available information indicates that it would be unwise for divers who have a low ventilatory response to exercise to exceed the limit of gas density suggested. In addition it may be necessary to restrict the more extreme 'carbon dioxide retainer' to even lower limits of gas density and oxygen partial pressure than others. Although not strictly a parameter of breathing apparatus design, this subject merits further investigation.

Oxygen partial pressure

There is a great deal of information available on oxygen toxicity and this subject is discussed by Wood in Chapter 10. Information is derived mainly from studies carried out under chamber conditions and the combined effects of cold water, exertion and carbon dioxide retention by the diver, all of which may promote oxygen toxicity (Wood 1969; Lanphier 1969), are difficult to assess. However, an oxygen tolerance curve of a conservative nature has been recommended for the diving situation (Lanphier 1955). This curve (see Fig. 10.3), specifies the maximum safe time for which a given oxygen partial pressure (Po_2) may be breathed by the diver. A similar but more comprehensive curve is to be found in the *US Navy Diving Manual* (1970). On the basis of this curve, an upper limit of Po_2 of 1·8 ATA or less is normally assumed (Wood 1969). The lower limit of Po_2 is normally taken as in air at 1 ATA.

In the absence of conclusive evidence of inert gases affecting oxygen toxicity (Wood 1969), these limits are normally applied to both pure oxygen and oxygen in the presence of inert gases. However, due to the possible involvement of carbon dioxide retention when breathing dense gas mixtures (Lanphier 1955, 1969) it may be prudent to adopt a lower limit of $Po_2 \leqslant 1\cdot5$ ATA (Riegal & Harter 1969; *US Navy Diving Manual* 1970) under these conditions. It can be seen from the oxygen tolerance curve that it is necessary to specify not only the limit of oxygen partial pressure but also the duration in minutes for which it may be safely breathed. When breathing air on demand, oxygen tolerance limits do not affect dives of up to 4 hours' duration to 50 m or less. However, if oxygen–nitrogen or oxygen–helium gas mixtures are used, the oxygen tolerance curve will most probably dictate both the maximum depth and safe time limit of the equipment. This factor is often overlooked in current breathing apparatus specifications. For example, if the limits of $0\cdot21 \leqslant Po_2 \leqslant 1\cdot8$ ATA are followed, the duration of the apparatus at maximum depth (i.e. $Po_2 = 1\cdot8$ ATA) would be restricted to 60 minutes (Lanphier 1955). For semi-closed circuit breathing apparatus operating on the constant mass principle, calculations are complicated in that the Po_2 breathed by the diver varies with oxygen uptake. In this case, the upper limit of Po_2 (i.e. resting condition) or alternatively the supply gas Po_2 (Penzias & Goodman 1973) should be assumed in calculating maximum depth and duration.

The depth and time limits for the use of oxygen given in the oxygen tolerance curve are specifically designed for working dives. More liberal limits are often introduced in the calculation of decompression schedules, particularly under dry chamber conditions.

Inspired carbon dioxide

The effects of inspired carbon dioxide on respiration are discussed by Lanphier and Schaefer in Chapters 8 and 11. The presence of inspired carbon dioxide will normally result in an increase of ventilation and alveolar carbon dioxide partial pressure (Pa_{CO2}) both of which are detrimental to the diver's efficiency, particularly during exercise. However, if Pa_{CO2} were to remain unchanged at 40 mm Hg, an inspired carbon dioxide partial pressure Pi_{CO2} of 10 mm Hg ($1\cdot3\%$ of 1 ATS) would produce an increase of 33% in alveolar ventilation (Lanphier 1969). Although tolerable at rest, this would represent an unacceptable respiratory burden during heavy exercise. A more acceptable limit would be $Pi_{CO2} \leqslant 0\cdot5\%$ of 1 ATS

($3\cdot8$ mm Hg), which would effect a 10% increase in alveolar ventilation under the above conditions.

Added respiratory deadspace of breathing apparatus will contribute to the effective Pi_{CO2} of the breathing gas. For example, if $Pa_{CO2} = 40$ mm Hg, then an apparatus deadspace of 100 ml would be approximately equivalent to a Pi_{CO2} of 1% of 1 ATS at a tidal volume of $0\cdot5$ L (i.e. resting conditions) and a Pi_{CO2} of $0\cdot2\%$ of 1 ATS at a tidal volume of $2\cdot5$ L (i.e. during heavy exercise).

When using open circuit breathing apparatus, the Pco_2 of the gas supply would be approximately $0\cdot2\%$ of 1 ATS when breathing air at 6 ATA, and negligible when breathing oxygen–helium gas mixtures. Thus if apparatus deadspace did not exceed 100 ml, the total effective Pi_{CO2} due to both deadspace and supply gas composition would remain less than $0\cdot5\%$ of 1 ATS during heavy exercise, even in the presence of elevated Pa_{CO2}.

In re-breathing apparatus, the amount of carbon dioxide inspired will be dependent on both apparatus deadspace and the efficiency of the carbon dioxide absorbent system. An efficient scrubbing unit using baralyme or sodasorb absorbent will maintain the Pco_2 of the breathing mixture at less than $0\cdot2\%$ of 1 ATS for a considerable duration (Lower 1970; Penzias & Goodman 1973) Hence it should be possible for re-breathing equipment to maintain an effective $Pi_{CO2} \leqslant 0\cdot5\%$ of 1 ATS. However, the efficiency of the carbon dioxide absorbent is very much dependent on the environmental conditions and may be seriously affected by variations in temperature and possibly pressure (Lower 1970). It is essential that tests of carbon dioxide absorbent efficiency are carried out under operational conditions and insulation or auxiliary heating of the absorbent canister may be necessary. The pendulum breathing principle in which the diver breathes to and from the counter lung via a single breathing hose necessitates a large apparatus deadspace and is not recommended.

In free flow apparatus, helmet $Pco_2 \leqslant 3\%$ of 1 ATS is commonly allowed. This standard must impose a severe respiratory burden on the diver, particularly during exertion and in the presence of increased gas density. The use of carbon dioxide absorbent with a device to circulate the helmet atmosphere offers considerable improvement in this type of equipment.

WORK OF BREATHING

The work of breathing underwater will be dependent on the design of the breathing apparatus and the properties of the breathing gas mixture. The effects of breathing gas mixture have been discussed and it is considered that densities up to 6 times that of air at 1 ATA may be acceptable.

A common measure of breathing effort is ventilatory power requirement, which represents the work done on the equipment per unit time and is normally measured in kg-m/min. There are two major components which contribute to the external work of breathing. Firstly, the hydrostatic pressure (normally measured in cm H_2O) represented by the differential water pressure existing between the lungs and the gas supply. Secondly, the aerodynamic resistance represented by the pressure differential across the airway required to induce gas flow. Resistance is normally expressed in terms of centimetres of water pressure per unit of gas flow (i.e. cm $H_2O.L^{-1}.sec$). The elastic component of work output is generally less significant in external work of breathing, but becomes more significant if the total work of breathing (i.e. intrinsic and extrinsic) is considered.

Air flow resistance

One of the earlier studies of the effects of external resistance on respiration was carried out by Silverman et al. (1945, 1951). This investigation was primarily concerned with protective respiratory equipment and therefore does not comment on effects of gas density or hydrostatic pressures. Silverman et al. (1945) defined their resistances in terms of the pressure differential occurring at a constant flow rate of 85 L/min. On this basis they recommended a maximum tolerable pressure differential at the above flow rate to be 6·4 cm H_2O during inspiration and 4·1 cm H_2O during expiration. These limits assumed the equipment would be used during heavy exercise. This represents an apparatus having a resistance of 4·5 cm.L^{-1}.sec (inspiratory) and 2·9 cm.L^{-1}.sec (expiratory) measured at a flow rate of 1·42 L/sec.

Silverman and his co-workers also calculated the work of breathing against fixed external resistances and recommended that the 'rate of external respiratory work' should not exceed 0·6% of the total body work rate.

On the basis of Silverman's experiments, Mead (1955) estimated that total respiratory resistance should not exceed a value of 12 cm $H_2O.L^{-1}.sec$. Experimental data suggested that when breathing air, intrinsic resistance would remain below this value to a depth of 9 ATA. Mead measured the resistance of two open circuit systems at the surface and predicted from his results that when used at increased air pressures they would have resistance characteristics far in excess of his recommended value. Miles (1969) extended the predictions of Mead to include re-breathing apparatus and again concluded that the resistance at increased pressures would be unacceptable. The theory on which Miles bases his calculations, however, is not quite clear.

Table 5.2 shows the resistance measured when breathing air at 4 ATA from a currently used

TABLE 5.2

The inspiratory resistance of open circuit underwater breathing apparatus (RN Swimmers Air Breathing Apparatus) measured at peak flow rate, when breathing oxygen–nitrogen mixture during rest and heavy exercise at 4 ATA

SABA: O_2–N_2 mixture at 4 ATA	Resting	Working
Ventilation L/min (BTPS)	9·5	45·9
Peak inspiratory flow rate L/min (BTPS)	40·8	116·6
Inspiratory pressure at peak flow rate, cm H_2O	−3·9	−8·3
Expiratory pressure at peak flow rate, cm H_2O	+1·3	+8·0
Inspiratory resistance at peak flow rate, cm H_2O . L^{-1} . sec	5·8	4·3

open circuit demand valve (*Royal Navy Diving Manual* 1964). Measurements were made at peak recorded respiratory flow rates when resting and during heavy exercise requiring an oxygen uptake of approximately 2 L/min. It is notable that unlike turbulent flow characteristics, due to the action of the demand valve, inspiratory resistance does not increase in relation to gas flow rate. The resistances of Table 5.2 appear to be much lower than the values quoted by Mead (1955) and Miles (1969), and during heavy exercise at 4 ATA, resistance is not incompatible with the recommendations of Silverman et al. (1945). However, it should be noted that the pressures given in Table 5.2 do not take account of hydrostatic effects normally associated with underwater breathing apparatus.

Hydrostatic pressures

The effects of immersion on respiratory mechanics was investigated by Paton and Sand (1947). The hydrostatic pressure at which respiration was considered to be most comfortably maintained, termed the eupnoeic pressure, was determined subjectively. In the erect position, Paton and Sand fixed the eupnoeic pressure plane at 5 to 10 cm and 10 to 15 cm below the external auditory meatus when resting and exercising respectively. In all other positions the eupnoeic pressure was at the level of the suprasternal notch. Deviations of -15 to $+20$ cm H_2O pressure from the eupnoeic pressure did not effect minute volume, tidal volume or the shape of the respiratory cycle. When immersed vertically in water, vital capacity was depressed and tidal volumes were substantially closer to the limit of expiration. Paton and Sand (1947) noted the difference between eupnoeic pressure and the centre of pressure or 'centroid' of the chest. They suggested, first, that the difference might represent a compromise between the sensations of inflation and deflation throughout the respiratory tract from the mouth to the base of the lungs imposed by the hydrostatic pressure gradient; and second, that it was possible that compression of the thoracic cage might partially compensate increased external pressures, and hence affect the value of eupnoeic pressure.

Jarrett (1965) measured pulmonary pressure–volume relaxation curves of subjects when breath-holding in air and when immersed in water. Immersion in water resulted in a marked increase in intrapulmonary pressure, the relationship being shifted along the pressure axis. From these experiments Jarrett estimated the centre of pressure of the immersed chest to be 19 cm below

and 7 cm behind the suprasternal notch. Jarrett used an oronasal mask in these experiments, but also noted that it was not possible to achieve relaxation of the chest and retain a mouthpiece. He suggested therefore that the difference between his measurements of centre of pressure and the eupnoeic pressure of Paton and Sand (1947) must represent a compensation in muscular effort between the chest and the cheeks required to retain a mouthpiece comfortably. Jarrett concluded that the ideal position for a demand regulator is theoretically at the position of the lung centroid. As this is not possible, it is necessary to compromise and the practical location will then depend on the position most commonly adopted by the diver.

Penzias and Goodman (1973) and O'Neill (1970), discussing hydrostatic influences on respiration, adopt Jarrett's standards for the centre of pressure. They further extend his conclusions that, ideally, breathing gas should be supplied to the diver at lung centroid pressure to include apparatus in which the diver rebreathes from a counterlung.

O'Neill (1970) studied the hydrostatics of various counterlung systems currently in use. The end exhalation pressure differential between lung centroid pressure and breathing gas supply (i.e. counterlung pressure) was calculated for equipment having the counterlung positioned either on the chest or back. Pressure differentials ranged from extremes of -20 to $+50$ cm H_2O depending on the position of the diver and valve setting. In the most common positions, i.e. erect and prone, the hydrostatic pressure differential varied from $+15$ to -20 cm H_2O. O'Neill showed that breathing characteristics can be much improved by incorporation of a mass-spring system in the relief valve of the breathing bag. This valve, known as a cardioid valve, would automatically alter the relief pressure in relationship to the position of the diver and hence reduce the extremes of end expiratory pressure differential experienced to 0 to $+25$ cm H_2O. O'Neill also suggested that significant improvement could be obtained if 2 valves, situated on the chest and back at the level of the lung centroid, were used together with toroidal-type breathing bags. With this design, the hydrostatic pressure of the gas supply could be restricted to within ± 7 cm H_2O of lung centroid pressure.

Power requirements of ventilation

Cooper (1960a, b) measured the external work of breathing using various respiratory equipments. The work of breathing was calculated using pressure–volume diagrams obtained from exercising subjects and also from a sine wave pump employed to simulate ventilation. The results of the two methods were in good agreement, and Cooper concluded that his pump was suitable for testing respiratory equipment.

Cooper noted that Silverman's estimate of external expiratory work rate was based on mean respiratory pressures and flow rates. Assuming a sinusoidal respiratory wave form and laminar flow conditions for Silverman's fixed resistors, Cooper (1960b) recalculated the recommended external respiratory work rate to be 0·74% of total body work rate. On the basis of his own work and that of Silverman et al. (1945), Cooper constructed

standards defining external respiratory work rate. These standards shown in Fig. 5.2 indicate the maximum tolerable power requirement above which serious discomfort and physiological embarrassment may occur (solid line) and the recommended limit of external ventilatory power to ensure comfortable breathing. Although limits are represented by a straight line relationship, in practice the relationship would be non-linear in nature as shown in Fig. 5.3 and the critical value is most likely to occur at maximum ventilation.

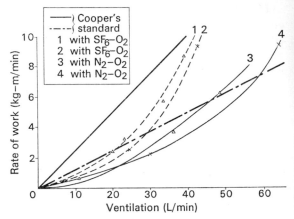

FIG. 5.3. The ventilatory power requirements of two semi-closed circuit underwater breathing apparatus (Bradley et al. 1970) when breathing N_2-O_2 and SF_6-O_2 gas mixture. The safe and ideal standards of Cooper (1960b) are also shown

Cooper's published data on pressures and flow rates (1960a) suggest that an apparatus having a ventilatory power requirement of 10 kg-m/min at a ventilation of approximately 70 L/min would have inspiratory and expiratory resistances of 2·9 and 3·9 cm.L^{-1}.sec respectively at peak flow rates of 3·5 L/sec. These are similar to the resistance values of Silverman et al. (1945) with the exception that expiratory resistance exceeds inspiratory resistance and resistances are measured at peak flow rate.

The ventilatory power requirements of two US Navy semi-closed circuit underwater breathing apparatus were studied by Bradley et al. (1970), who measured both the intrinsic and extrinsic work of breathing air and O_2–SF_6 gas mixture when exercising on a bicycle ergometer at various work loads. In addition, the contributions to

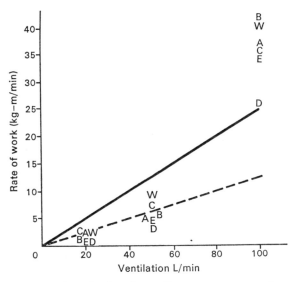

FIG. 5.2. Standards of ventilatory power requirement of breathing apparatus (Cooper 1960b). Cooper recommends that apparatus should meet these standards up to 100 L/min ventilation. The full line represents the limit above which serious discomfort and physiological embarrassment may be expected, the dotted line represents the 'ideal' limit for comfortable breathing. The letters indicate the power requirement measured at 1 ATA of mine rescue apparatus (A to E) and underwater apparatus (W)

total work load of the individual components of the breathing apparatus were also measured. In their calculations, Bradley et al. (1970), in common with Silverman et al. (1945), used the mean pressure times mean gas flow rate to approximate power output. Cooper (1960b) has noted that if laminar flow exists and respiration is taken to be sinusoidal, the theoretical work of breathing would be 23% greater than estimated by mean values. Similarly it can be shown that, for turbulent flow conditions, the theoretical work of breathing would be approximately 33% greater than estimated. Hence, the calculations of Bradley et al. may considerably underestimate the ventilatory power requirements of the equipment. Further, as the experiments were carried out under dry conditions, the hydrostatic pressure effects normally associated with semi-closed circuit underwater breathing apparatus would be absent. In practice, hydrostatic effects would substantially increase the breathing effort (Sterk 1973).

Despite the limitations discussed above, the work of Bradley et al. (1970) is of great value in assessing the power requirements of underwater breathing apparatus, as it is the only detailed investigation to date which has been carried out for this specific purpose. On the basis of their experiments, the authors concluded that the work of breathing from both underwater breathing equipments was unacceptably high. The extrinsic ventilatory power requirements when breathing air and oxygen–sulphur hexafluoride gas mixture from these equipments are shown in Fig. 5.3, and the results are compared with the standards of Cooper (1960b).

As a result of their investigations and a search of the available literature, Bradley et al. recommended as standards for underwater breathing apparatus that the equipment should meet the resistance limitations of Silverman et al. (1945) and the maximum power requirements as defined by Cooper (1960b). It was estimated that during heavy work, this would involve an external respiratory work rate of 6 kg-m/min. In addition it was suggested that hydrostatic pressure should not exceed ± 15 cm H_2O and should preferably be half of this value.

The work of breathing from semi-closed circuit

underwater breathing apparatus was measured by Sterk (1973) in the underwater situation, measurements being made in both the prone and upright position. Unfortunately the study was limited to relatively low levels of ventilation (< 24 L/min) but even during quiet breathing the ventilatory power requirements were unacceptable when compared with the standards of Cooper (1960b). Significantly, the major component of the work of breathing was attributed to hydrostatic pressure, and Sterk concluded with justification that, in order to obtain realistic results, tests of underwater breathing apparatus must therefore be carried out underwater. Sterk measured the external work of breathing with reference to pressure at the mouth rather than the centre of pressure as recommended by Jarrett (1965) and considered this to be justified to an extent by the subjective feeling of the divers. If respiratory pressures were referred to the centre of pressure the ratio of inspiratory to expiratory work would be very different and the total power requirement might also be considerably altered. Sterk estimated values of airway resistance and compliance using a linear lung model (i.e. fixed compliance and resistance) but conceded that such a model would become inaccurate in the presence of turbulent flow.

As the gas flow in underwater breathing apparatus is mainly turbulent, the airway resistance will be essentially non-linear in nature (i.e. resistance is a function of gas flow rate). Hence it is difficult to define resistance as a constant for design purposes. The power output required to ventilate the equipment offers a more comprehensive standard. However, it is inadequate to define power requirement alone. As the pressure generated by the respiratory muscles varies with both lung volume and gas flow rate (Agostoni & Fenn 1960) limits of extrinsic pressure should also be defined.

On the basis of the available information, the following standards are suggested for the work of breathing. At a ventilation of 65 L/min underwater breathing apparatus should preferably conform to Cooper's recommended limit of comfort of 8 kg-m/min when used in the normal working positions and should not exceed his safe limit of 16 kg-m/min power requirement under any operational conditions (Cooper 1960b). Hydrostatic pressure effects should not exceed ± 15 cm H_2O (Bradley et al. 1970). This represents the degree of positive or negative pressure breathing to be tolerated by the diver and is normally the pressure differential occurring at the end of inspiration and expiration (i.e. zero flow conditions). The total extrinsic pressure differential due to airway resistance, hydrostatic pressure and other effects should not exceed 25 cm H_2O at maximum flow rate. These pressures should be measured relative to the hydrostatic pressure at the lung centroid. Assuming approximately sinusoidal flow rates, at a ventilation of 65 L/min these standards would limit resistance of equipment to a maximum of $7 \cdot 5$ cm $H_2O . L^{-1}$. sec in the absence of hydrostatic pressures, or approximately $3 \cdot 0$ cm $H_2O . L^{-1}$. sec in the presence of the maximum additive hydrostatic effect, resistances being referred to maximum flow rate.

These standards are derived to a certain extent from independent investigations and it is of interest to consider whether the values given are in fact compatible. Theoretical analysis, based on turbulent flow conditions and a sinusoidal ventilatory wave form, suggests that in the presence of a hydrostatic pressure differential of -15 cm H_2O and a total pressure of -25 cm H_2O the extrinsic inspiratory power requirement alone would be approximately 14 kg-m/min at a ventilation of 65 L/min. If underwater breathing equipment were to operate at the recommended limits of breathing pressures throughout the complete respiratory cycle, therefore, it is unlikely that it would comply with the standards of external ventilatory power. However, in most underwater breathing apparatus the maximum pressures above would be experienced only for a part of the respiratory cycle. For example, when breathing from a demand valve situated on the back, the diver is constantly breathing from a negative pressure in both the upright and swimming positions. Hence the limiting value of external pressure might be reached during inspiration, but during expiration resistive pressure would be partially or totally overcome by the counter action of hydrostatic pressure. Similarly, in rebreathing equipment, maximum hydrostatic pressure differentials tend to occur only at end inspiration or end expiration. Thus it is probable that equipment conforming to the limits of pressure given above would also be capable of meeting the standards of safe power requirement.

It is considered unlikely that current underwater breathing apparatus can comply with Cooper's limit of comfort and it is probable that many equipments do not satisfy his safe limit of ventilatory power requirement (Bradley et al. 1970; Sterk 1973). The limits of extrinsic pressures and ventilatory power recommended above are clearly derived from inadequate data and can be considered at best an approximate guide to breathing apparatus requirements. In order to provide satisfactory standards the whole subject requires much further investigation.

REFERENCES

AGOSTONI, E. & FENN, W. O. (1960) Velocity of muscle shortening as a limiting factor in respiratory air flow. *J. appl. Physiol.* 15, 349–353.

BRADLEY, M. E., VOROSMARTI, J., MERZ, J., HECKERT, P. J. & KLECKNER, J. C. (1970) *Breathing Impedence of the Mk VIII and Mk XI semi-closed Underwater Breathing Apparatus.* U.S. Navy Submarine Development Group One Research Report, 1–70.

BROUSSOLLE, B., BENSIMON, E., MICHAUD, A. & VEGEZZI, P. (1970) *Comparison of Ventilatory Responses and of Partial Alveolar Pressures of CO$_2$ in Trained Divers and in Non-diving Subjects during Muscular Activity in Hyperbaric Atmosphere.* Les Troisièmes Journées Internationales de Physiologie Hyperbare. Ed. X. Fructus, pp. 80–87. Paris: Doin.

COOPER, E. A. (1960a) A comparison of the respiratory work done against an external resistance by man and by a sine-wave pump. *Q. Jl exp. Physiol.* 45, 179–191.

COOPER, E. A. (1960b) Suggested methods of testing and standards of resistance for respiratory protective devices. *J. appl. Physiol.* 15, 1053–1061.

COTES, J. E. (1968) *Lung Function Assessment and Application in Medicine.* Oxford: Blackwell Scientific.

CUSP (1953) *Report of the Co-operative Underwater Swimming Project.* Washington: Natl Res. Council Committee on Amphibious Operations, NRC: CAO: 0033.

DAVIES, C. T. M., TUXWORTH, W. & YOUNG, J. M. (1970) Physiological effects of repeated exercise. *Clin. Sci.* 39, 247–258.

DONALD, K. W. & DAVIDSON, W. M. (1954) Oxygen uptake of 'booted' and 'fin swimming' divers. *J. appl. Physiol.* **7**, 31–37.

FAGRAEUS, L. & LINNARSSON, D. (1973) Maximum voluntary and exercise ventilation at high ambient air pressures. *Förvarsmedicin* **9**, 275–278.

GOFF, L. G., FRASSETTO, R. & SPECHT, H. (1956) Oxygen requirements in underwater swimming. *J. appl. Physiol.* **9**, 219–221.

HESSER, C. M., FAGRAEUS, L. & LINNARSSON, D. (1968) *Cardio-respiratory Responses to Exercise in Hyperbaric Environment*. Report. Laboratory of Aviation and Naval Medicine, Karolinska Institutet, Stockholm.

HEY, E. N., LLOYD, B. B., CUNNINGHAM, D. J. C., JUKES, M. G. M. & BOLTON, D. P. G. (1966) Effects of various respiratory stimuli on the depth and frequency of breathing in man. *Resp. Physiol.* **1**, 193–205.

JARRETT, A. S. (1965) Effect of immersion on intrapulmonary pressure. *J. appl. Physiol.* **20**, 1261–1266.

KAO, F. F. (1963) An experimental study of the pathways involved in exercise hypernoea employing cross circulation techniques. In *The Regulation of Human Respiration*. Ed. D. J. C. Cunningham & B. B. Lloyd, pp. 461–502. Oxford: Blackwell.

LANPHIER, E. H. (1954) *Oxygen Consumption in Underwater Swimming*. US Navy Experimental Diving Unit, Washington D.C. Report 14–54.

LANPHIER, E. H. (1955) Use of nitrogen–oxygen mixtures in diving. In *Proc. Symp. Underwater Physiology*. Ed. L. G. Goff, pp. 74–78. Washington D.C.: Natl Acad. Sci.-Natl Res. Council (Publ. 377).

LANPHIER, E. H. (1963) Influence of increased ambient pressure upon alveolar ventilation. In *Proc. 2nd Symp. Underwater Physiology*. Ed. C. J. Lambertsen & L. J. Greenbaum, Jr., pp. 124–133. Washington D.C.: Natl Acad. Sci.-Natl Res. Council (Publ. 1181).

LANPHIER, E. H. (1969) Pulmonary function. In: *The Physiology & Medicine of Diving and Compressed Air Work*. Ed. P. B. Bennett & D. H. Elliott, pp. 58–112. London: Baillière Tindall & Cassell.

LOWER, B. R. (1970) Removal of CO_2 from closed circuit breathing apparatus. In *Equipment for the Working Diver*, pp. 261–282. Washington D.C.: Marine Technology Society.

MEAD, J. (1955) Resistance to breathing at increased ambient pressures. In *Proc. Symp. Underwater Physiology*. Ed. L. G. Goff, pp. 112–120. Washington D.C.: Natl Acad. Sci.-Natl Res. Council. (Publ. 377).

MILES, S. (1969) *Underwater Medicine*, 3rd Edition. London: Staples.

MILLER, J. N., WANGENSTEEN, O. D. & LANPHIER, E. H. (1970) *Respiratory Limitations to Work at Depth*. Les Troisièmes Internationales d'Hyperbarie et de Physiologie Subaquatique. Ed. X. Fructus, pp. 118–123. Paris: Doin.

MORRISON, J. B. (1973) Oxygen uptake studies of divers when fin swimming with maximum effort at depths of 6–176 feet. *Aerospace Med.* **44**, 1120–1129.

MORRISON, J. B. & BUTT, W. S. (1972) Effect of underwater breathing apparatus and absolute air pressure on divers' ventilatory capacity. *Aerospace Med.* **43**, 881–886.

MORRISON, J. B. & FLORIO, J. T. (1971) Respiratory function during a simulated saturation dive to 1500 ft. *J. appl. Physiol.* **30**, 724–732.

MORRISON, J. B., FLORIO, J. T. & BUTT, W. S. (1974) *Loss of Consciousness Under Water: 1 and 2*. Royal Naval Physiological Laboratory Reports 1–74 & 2–74.

MORRISON, J. B., FLORIO, J. T., BUTT, W. S. & MAYO, I. C. (1975) *The Effects of Underwater Breathing Apparatus and Absolute Pressure on the Respiratory Response to Exercise*. Royal Naval Physiological Laboratory Report. (In press.)

O'NEILL, W. J. (1970) A study of the breathing hydrostatics of various bag-type diving apparatuses and description of the two-valve Toroidal and Abalone back-mounted design. In *Equipment for the Working Diver*, pp. 183–211. Washington D.C.: Marine Technological Society.

PATON, W. D M. & SAND, A. (1947) The optimum intrapulmonary pressures in underwater respiration. *J. Physiol., Lond.* **106**, 119–138.

PENZIAS, W. & GOODMAN, M. W. (1973) Underwater breathing apparatus. In *Man Beneath the Sea*, pp. 512–585, Canada: John Wiley.

RIEGEL, P. S. & HARTER, J. V. (1969) Design of breathing apparatus for diving to great depths. *Proc. Design Engng Div. Conf.*, New York N.Y.: Am. Soc. Mech. Engrs.

Royal Navy Diving Manual (1964) *Swimmers Air Breathing Apparatus*. Part 3, Chap. 23. BR 155.

SALZANO, J., RAUSCH, D. C. & SALTZMAN, H. A. (1970) Cardiorespiratory responses to exercise at a simulated seawater depth of 1000 ft. *J. appl. Physiol.* **28**, 34–41.

SCHAEFER, K. E. (1967). *Adaptation to CO_2 with Particular Reference to CO_2 Retention in Diving*. Report 489. US Naval Submarine Med. Res. Center.

SILVERMAN, L., LEE, G., PLOTKIN, T., SAWYERS, L. A. & YANCEY, A. R. (1951) Air flow measurements on human subjects with and without respiratory resistance at several work rates. *Archs ind. Hyg.* **3**, 461–478.

SILVERMAN, L., LEE, G., YANCEY, A. R., AMORY, L., BARNEY, L. J. & LEE, R. C. (1945) Report No. 5339. Washington D.C.: Office of Scientific Research and Development.

STERK, W. (1973) *Respiratory Mechanics of Diver and Diving Apparatus*. R. Neth. Navy Diving Med. Centre, Den Helder.

US Navy Diving Manual (1970) NAV Ships. 0994–001–9010. Washington D.C.: Navy Dept.

WOOD, J. D. (1969) Oxygen toxicity. In *The Physiology and Medicine of Diving and Compressed Air Work*. Ed. P. B. Bennett & D. H. Elliott, pp. 113–143, London: Baillière Tindall & Cassell.

YOUNG, J. M. (1969). Contribution to Williams, S. Underwater breathing apparatus. In *The Physiology and Medicine of Diving and Compressed Air Work*. Ed. P. B. Bennett & D. H. Elliott, pp. 28–31, London: Baillière Tindall & Cassell.

6

Life Support Systems

J. N. MILLER

The term 'life support system' has been adopted from the new jargon of space technology. In fact, the concept goes back a century and more to the realization that man is a homeostatic animal. He can live only within narrow limits of oxygen partial pressure, is poorly tolerant to raised levels of carbon dioxide, has a narrow range of thermal stability, is required to maintain a very stable osmotic equilibrium, is prone to atmosphere-borne infection and is readily intoxicated by many chemical compounds and elements, some of which are formed by his own metabolic processes. In principle, therefore, the whole raison d'être of a life support system is to maintain the standard of life both quantitatively and qualitatively that was present before the life support system was required. This broad concept has applications ranging from environmental pollution in the widest sense through to diving as a more narrow application. It is with diving applications that this chapter is concerned.

Compressed air work of relatively short duration in diving and tunnel construction represents by far the greatest proportion of exposure to increased pressure that man currently encounters; and in such work the main life support requirement is merely to ensure a sufficient flow of fresh air to maintain adequate blood oxygenation and low levels of carbon dioxide. By such simple means men have been able to work under pressure for considerable periods.

With the engineering advances that made manned space flight possible, a new technology of life support engineering and physiology de-

veloped and spilled over into the diving and submarine fields. New chemical processes are available which simultaneously reduce carbon dioxide and produce oxygen; cryogenic and even thermonuclear processes have been employed in atmosphere control. Over the same period, gas analysis equipment to monitor closed compartment atmospheres has changed from simple volumetric apparatus to highly sophisticated mass spectrometry and gas chromatography. With more extensive and more efficient methods of maintaining a stable atmosphere, and with more effective equipment to monitor the atmosphere, man has stayed in space for a few weeks, submarines now patrol submerged for several months, and divers can live at depth for many weeks.

Life support requirements for diving depend very much upon the duration of the exposure to increased pressure. Deep dives require prolonged decompression and the logistics of maintaining a stable respirable atmosphere by simple ventilation alone are frequently not feasible in terms of gas storage or cost, especially if special gas mixtures or expensive gases, such as helium or neon are employed. Carbon dioxide is usually removed chemically and oxygen added as required by the metabolic demands of the diver. In saturation diving, where the exposure to increased pressure may last from several days to many weeks, not only must carbon dioxide be removed and oxygen added but thermal equilibrium must be maintained, humidity carefully controlled, and other noxious gases produced by metabolism eliminated. With such requirements has grown the need for more specialized and more sophisticated gas analytical techniques. Such diving procedures are indeed a far cry from the open circuit ventilation methods employed most commonly, but despite the complexity and the expense they are now dominating the field of commercial diving.

CARBON DIOXIDE REMOVAL

Carbon dioxide in solution is weakly acidic, and as such is readily neutralized by strong alkalis to form a carbonate salt and water. When potassium or sodium hydroxide are used by themselves to absorb CO_2, the reaction is strongly exothermic, and the heat generated may become a hazard in itself. Both materials are also highly deliquescent and are prone to deterioration during storage. They are so highly caustic and unstable that it is usual for them to be mixed with other less caustic alkalis such as hydrated barium hydroxide and calcium hydroxide.

Traditionally, a mixture of barium hydroxide, calcium hydroxide and potassium hydroxide, known as 'baralyme', has been favoured by the US Navy; while 'soda lime', a mixture of sodium hydroxide, potassium hydroxide and calcium hydroxide, has been favoured by the Royal Navy. In addition, particularly in space vehicles where weight considerations play a major role, lithium hydroxide (LiOH) is used. It has approximately half the weight for the same volume as the others at 8 to 10 times the cost. All three absorbent materials are packaged in granular form and provide little difficulty in handling in operational circumstances. The primary disadvantage with these materials is that they can be used once only. They are heavy to transport and bulky to store. Soda lime and baralyme particularly, are in general use throughout the diving industry, being the primary means of CO_2 absorption in high pressure chambers, saturation diving systems, underwater habitats and many types of underwater breathing apparatus. Their efficiency increases as the partial pressure of CO_2 rises, being quite inefficient at partial pressures below about 10 mm Hg. In addition, their efficiency diminishes at decreased relative humidities.

Passive absorption systems

Provided sufficient gas convection can be maintained within a closed compartment there is no strict necessity to maintain forced ventilation through chemical CO_2 absorbent beds. Open boxes of baralyme or soda lime placed on the deck plates of a high pressure chamber have been used quite successfully in relatively short duration oxyhelium dives. Specially fabricated panels containing CO_2 absorbent material placed in position to catch convective air currents have themselves provided the sole means of carbon dioxide removal for 2 months during the voyage of the *Ben Franklin* (Haigh 1971). A similar panel can readily be constructed from two blankets sown together to form a number of small pockets containing soda lime or baralyme.

Active absorbing systems

In general, forced ventilation scrubbing systems used with high pressure chambers are either internal or external. Each type has its advantages and disadvantages. At the present time all systems in use employ chemical absorbent material—soda lime, baralyme or lithium hydroxide—through which chamber air is either drawn or forced by a fan. Numerous means have been used over the years to drive the fan: electricity, hydraulics, pneumatics and magnetically coupled drive units.

Power systems used depend very much upon prevailing conditions. At sea, for example, in a diving bell, electricity may be the most suitable power source, despite the inherent danger of fire from sparking in atmospheres containing high partial pressures of oxygen, or the risk of electrocution in the water. Non-sparking, brushless motors encased in metal and purged with nitrogen venting to the outside of the bell are the type of choice.

Within static chambers, particularly where there is no shortage of low pressure compressed air, a pneumatically powered system is extremely effective. Such an internal CO_2 scrubbing system is in use in the high pressure chambers at the Royal Naval Physiological Laboratory (Eaton 1970) and is shown in Fig. 6.1. It employs standard submarine soda lime canisters through which chamber gas is drawn by a 'squirrel cage' fan powered via a magnetic coupling by a compressed air motor venting outside the chamber. Noise is minimized and the efficiency of the motor is regulated by the compressed air pressure outside the chamber. Gas flow through the scrubber decreases with increasing gas density, but this can be offset to

a scrubber fan has been developed (Canty et al. 1972; see Fig. 6.2). This employs a magnetic coupling passing directly through the chamber wall in such a way that the non-ferrous cup between the inner and outer magnets forms in effect a part of the chamber wall. The outer magnet is rotated by a belt drive from an electric motor

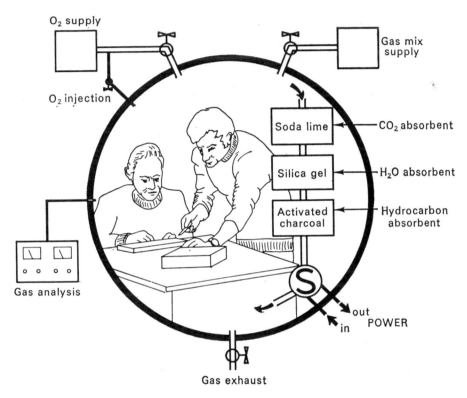

FIG. 6.1. Diagram of an internal scrubbing system of the type used at RNPL. In practice, power transmission to the blower is mediated via a magnetic coupling driven by a sealed compressed air motor, vented externally. Chamber air is drawn through the appropriate absorption beds

some degree by increasing the fan speed. In practice, this system has proved extremely reliable and the changing of soda lime canisters has been reduced to a single rapid operation. Replenishment of canisters during a very long exposure can be made via the medical lock as it is large enough to take the standard submarine canister. Each submarine canister has been found to provide efficient CO_2 removal for two men for a minimum period of 12 hours.

Another method for providing power to drive

outside the chamber, and the drive is transmitted magnetically through the cup to the inner magnet inside the chamber. Either a direct drive shaft or a flexible shaft from the inner magnet is used to rotate the scrubber fan.

Other attempts to provide abundant non-electrical power inside high pressure chambers have included hydraulic systems. Vane-type pumps have been used effectively at low pressures, but are relatively inefficient, being prone to leaks at the shaft seal while under pressure and to

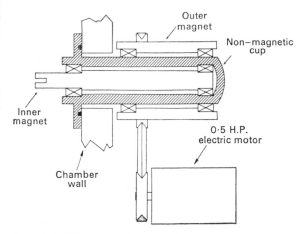

FIG. 6.2. Diagram of magnetically coupled power unit designed to transfer high-torque power drive directly through the wall of a pressure vessel. The outer magnet is driven via a 'V' belt from a suitable electric motor, and transfers its energy across a non-magnetic cup, the interior of which is at chamber pressure, to the inner magnet which, itself, acts as a rotary drive shaft to power tools and equipment such as scrubber motors

corrosion in cast-iron pump housings. Positive displacement hydraulic pumps are effective alternatives to other hydraulic systems, but require a driven impellor to impart rotary movement to a fan.

A low resistance liquid potassium hydroxide CO_2 scrubbing system was developed by Margaria, Galente and Cerretelli (1959), for physiological experiments. The system (Fig. 6.3) is basically a miniature adaptation of a large scale industrial scrubbing unit. In this system liquid KOH is sprayed from a reservoir over ceramic rashig rings in a glass fibre tower. Air is pumped through the tower near the bottom, passes up through the wet rashig rings and loses its carbon dioxide. The method could certainly be adapted for use in a high pressure chamber, especially where the application required a very low resistance to gas flow.

The main disadvantage with internal CO_2 scrubbing systems is the requirement for the men at pressure to replenish the absorbent. If a chamber environment became contaminated at extreme depth, access to the scrubbing system could be denied to fresh personnel from the outside. Thus, there is the ever present risk of irretrievable loss

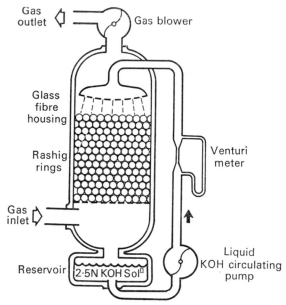

FIG. 6.3. Liquid potassium hydroxide scrubbing system (after Margaria, Galente & Cerretelli 1959). Liquid 2·5 N KOH is continuously pumped over a vertical bed of ceramic rashig rings of appropriate size at a flow rate sufficient to keep the bed wet. At the same time, CO_2-containing air is drawn up through the moistened bed, losing its CO_2 in passage

of control of the chamber atmosphere. With an external scrubbing system, control of chamber atmosphere is assured at all times.

External scrubbing systems operate on a closed loop with piping attached to the chamber (Fig. 6.4). Gas is drawn from one or more dependent places in the chamber, and is passed through the absorbent bed and pumped back to the chamber near the overhead. Replenishment of the absorbent is relatively simple as the loop can be closed off and decompressed. The canisters are then exchanged at surface pressure and the whole system repressurized.

With an external system provision can readily be made for scrubbing other noxious gases, for example carbon monoxide, methane and hydrogen sulphide, which build up during long exposures in closed atmospheres. Appropriate absorbent beds, for example silica gel for water vapour, activated charcoal for the removal of hydrogen sulphide and ammonia, can replace soda lime canisters. In addition, appropriate catalytic

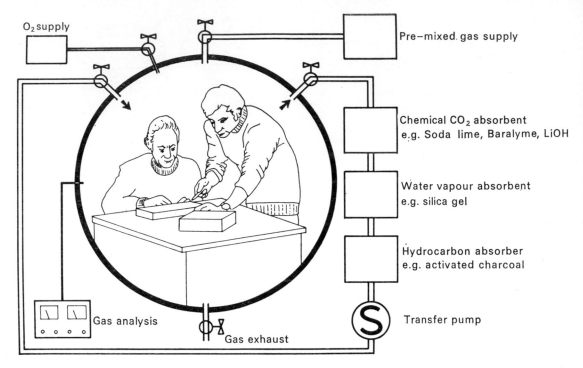

O₂ supply

Pre-mixed gas supply

Chemical CO₂ absorbent
e.g. Soda lime, Baralyme, LiOH

Water vapour absorbent
e.g. silica gel

Hydrocarbon absorber
e.g. activated charcoal

Transfer pump

Gas analysis

Gas exhaust

FIG. 6.4. Diagram of an external scrubbing system employing conventional absorption methods, of the type in use at the US Naval Experimental Diving Unit. Each absorption unit is separately housed in an external pressure vessel coupled to the chamber and to each other by high pressure piping and valves. In addition, to facilitate rapid replacement of absorption beds, two systems in parallel are commonly used: one shut down for replacement of chemicals and cleaning, while the other is in use. Not only is the system bulky and expensive, considerable problems have occurred in maintaining effective shaft seals on the transfer pumps against the persistently high head of pressure

burners can also be placed in series within the loop. Certainly it is true that the internal system in use at the Royal Naval Physiological Laboratory (RNPL) can also employ absorbent beds other than soda lime packed in appropriate canisters, but there is no effective internal way of removing hydrocarbons, carbon monoxide or other trace contaminants.

The disadvantages with external scrubbing systems are that they tend to be bulky, as the components are exposed to full chamber pressure. Difficulties in practice have been noted with drive-shaft seals failing to hold pressure in the system. With the recent development of suitable magnetic couplings this latter disadvantage may well disappear. A third disadvantage is one of cost. External systems are very much more expensive to build and install than their internal counterparts. Separate pressure vessels are re-

quired to house the absorbent canisters and wide bore high pressure piping is required to close the loop. Expensive chamber modifications may have to be undertaken if provision for such a system has not been included in the design stage.

OXYGEN ADDITION

Just as carbon dioxide is produced by the men under pressure, oxygen is consumed. The tolerable limits of oxygen partial pressure to which divers may be exposed depends very much upon the duration of the exposures. Obviously, the lower limit is that partial pressure which is sufficient to support life, about 0·1 ATS (70 mm Hg Po_2). but a more reasonable lower limit for general use should lie between 0·18 and 0·2 ATA. The upper limit for Po_2 is exposure-dependent, and for prolonged exposure, that is days to weeks, should probably not exceed 0·5 ATS. A recent report from the Institute for Environmental Medicine at the University of Pennsylvania (Clark & Lambertsen 1971) presents basic information on the tolerance of the lungs to increased partial pressures of oxygen in normal men. Fig. 6.5 depicts one of the pulmonary oxygen tolerance curves presented in the report, and represents the upper limit of oxygen exposure as a function of duration sufficient to cause some detectable effect of pulmonary with chamber gas. Intermittent injections are made when the oxygen partial pressure falls below a predetermined minimum level established during the planning of the dive. Provided calibration procedures are available, and a triple electrode system is used, a temperature-compensated polarographic method may be employed, the current-flow suitably amplified, and used both to give a meter read-out and to power a solenoid valve system governing the injection. During the

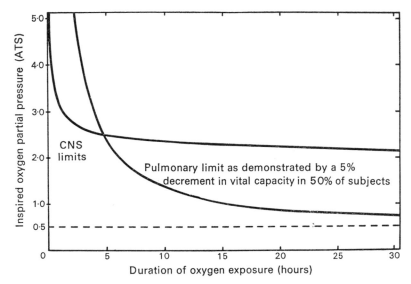

Fig. 6.5. A practical tolerance limit in normal man to pulmonary oxygen toxicity (after Clark & Lambertsen 1971)

oxygen toxicity in 50% of normal subjects. It must always be remembered that the effect of increased oxygen partial pressures upon lung tissue is cumulative, and if a high Po_2 has been used during the dive itself the pulmonary tolerance limits may easily be exceeded during decompression, particularly if the oxygen partial pressure is increased still more, for example, with the use of pure oxygen inhaled intermittently between 15 m (2·5 ATA) and the surface.

Oxygen supply to make up for metabolic consumption during saturation diving must only be made under conditions of strict control. Perhaps the best system in use at the present time employs the injection of small quantities of oxygen into the chamber at high pressure through a venturi, thus ensuring adequate mixing of the oxygen 1500 ft (46 ATA) simulated dive at RNPL in 1970, chamber Po_2 was thus maintained within 0·43 and 0·45 ATA (Eaton 1971).

The addition of large volumes of oxygen while at pressure and without effective means of instantaneous gas mixing should never be employed. If no suitable injection system is available, then the chamber gas should be replaced with fresh premixed gas.

OXYGEN REMOVAL (OXYGEN DUMPING)

Pure oxygen breathing is frequently used during decompression to facilitate the elimination of inert gas. Oxygen also is frequently used as a breathing medium during therapeutic recompression in the treatment of decompression sickness. Exhaled oxygen contaminates the chamber atmosphere unless arrangements have been made for its removal. Most commonly, frequent flushing of the chamber atmosphere with fresh air is used to reduce the oxygen levels, but by such means it is not practicable to reduce the level of oxygen

weight tubing connected to the chamber wall via a needle valve. The needle valve is used to control the degree of inflation of a four litre anaesthetic bag connected to the fitting immediately downstream from the dump line. The bottom end of the bag is open to chamber atmosphere via a non-return valve so that if the needle valve is open

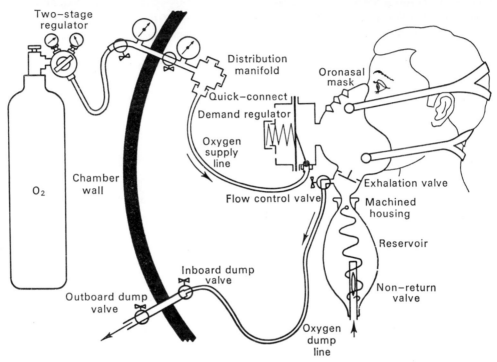

FIG. 6.6. Richard A. Morin's oxygen dump system. Oxygen is delivered via a demand regulator and exhaled gas is collected for dumping in a reservoir bag attached to the exhaust port of an oronasal mask. Exhaust flow in the oxygen dump line is controlled manually in such a way that the reservoir bag is kept partially filled. With moment to moment changes in pulmonary ventilation, constant adjustment of the exhaust flow control valve is required

much below 0·25 ATS. A fully effective, automatic, inexpensive and reliable method for dumping exhaled gas has yet to be devised, but several workable compromises are available.

The system currently in use at RNPL is similar to that designed by Richard A. Morin of the State University of New York at Buffalo (Fig. 6.6). Oxygen is delivered via a single-hose regulator from the built-in breathing system through a comfortable, well-fitting oronasal mask. Exhaled gas passes out through a non-return valve and thence is 'dumped' through a length of light-

too wide, the bag deflates and chamber gas is drawn up through the non-return valve in the bag, thereby preventing the lungs from being exposed accidentally to any large pressure gradient. A coiled spring held inside the bag prevents its collapse when fully deflated. The main disadvantage with the system is the need for frequent adjustment of the needle valve to cater for changes in ventilation rate, which soon becomes irritating. The system in use at the Deep Trials Unit of the Admiralty Experimental Diving Unit is similar, except that a much larger bag is employed, obviating the necessity of having the safety relief valve at the bottom of the bag.

A third system available (Fig. 6.7) is in use at the Virginia Mason Research Center, and depends upon the use of a large high gas-flow pressure regulator mounted inside the chamber and operating at differential pressures of 5 to 7 psi. Small-bore pressure hose is used to couple the exhalation valve of the breathing system to the

cost of a large precision-built regulator capable of simultaneously handling the exhaled gas from several divers.

CONTROL OF TEMPERATURE

As discussed in a later chapter (16), inadequate control of thermal balance is one of the prime contributory factors in many diving accidents. In

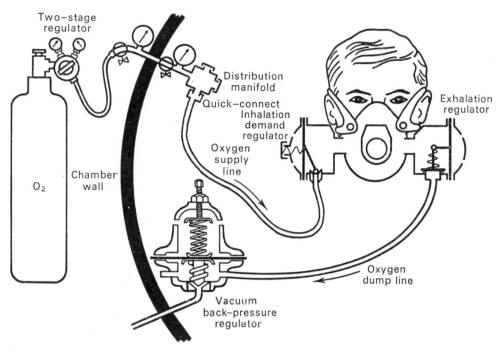

Two-stage regulator

Distribution manifold

Quick-connect Inhalation demand regulator

Oxygen supply line

Chamber wall

O₂

Exhalation regulator

Oxygen dump line

Vacuum back-pressure regulator

FIG. 6.7. Automatic oxygen dumping system of the type in use at the Virginia Mason Research Center, Seattle. Oxygen is delivered via a demand regulator and exhaled gas passes to the oxygen dump line via a special exhalation regulator and thence to the outside via a large vacuum back-pressure regulator set to maintain a constant pressure-drop of 5 to 7 psi across its diaphragm. Variations in pulmonary ventilation have little effect on the system

in-flow side of the regulator, and the gas is vented externally through the chamber wall. Such a system has the advantage of being automatic once the regulator has been set. Moreover, variable ventilation rates are automatically catered for by the regulator itself, and several divers can be accommodated simultaneously. Its disadvantages are that the exhalation tubing tends to be bulky and may cause difficulty in maintaining an adequate face-seal of the oronasal mask. Furthermore, it is expensive, primarily because of the

saturation oxy-helium diving, particularly in the open sea, the problem is a prime limiting factor to the performance of the divers. In general, cold is the more important factor in operational diving, but excessive overheating can also become a problem.

The range of temperatures covering a zone of comfort at 1 ATS in an air environment is quite wide, particularly if the subjects are allowed a free selection of clothing. In oxy-helium atmospheres under pressure, however, the zone of comfort becomes progressively narrower as the pressure increases. From $20°C \pm 10°C$ at 1 ATS in air, the comfort zone narrows to about $29°C \pm 1°C$ at about 500 m (50 ATA) in an oxy-helium atmosphere, regardless of the choice of clothing. The problem, then, is to maintain an internal temperature inside a steel shell weighing several tons within such a narrow range, with the shell perhaps suspended in an aqueous environment representing an infinite heat sink at a temperature as much as 26°C lower than the internal temperature.

Deck-mounted chambers on board ship or in the laboratory can readily be insulated against heat loss by means of a suitable insulating jacket. Moreover, heating of the steel shell can be facilitated by means of electrically powered heat tapes encircling the chamber as for the system employed at RNPL (Eaton 1971). This system utilizes 24 1000 watt heat tapes arranged in 12 individual circuits distributed around the outside of the chamber wall, each heat tape being held to the chamber wall by adhesive tape. A close-fitting insulation jacket of glass-fibre wool encased in woven glass cloth, manufactured in sections, lies exterior to the heat tapes. The arrangement is such that sections of the jacket are readily removable, thus allowing cooling. With the jacket firmly in place and all tapes switched on, it is possible to raise the internal temperature of the chamber containing an oxy-helium atmosphere, 1°C per minute. With this system, the whole chamber (approximately 16 tons of mild steel) reaches the required temperature and heats the gas simultaneously by conduction, radiation, and convection. The divers, therefore, live in an atmosphere of even temperature distribution.

Evaporative heat loss from the divers depends upon the level of water vapour in the atmosphere. It has been found, however, that at about 500 m (51 ATA) the range of comfort was so narrow that one diver performing light work became uncomfortably hot while the attendant was feeling chilled (Broussolle et al. 1975). Although Webb (1975) has made an attempt to solve this problem with an automatically regulated suit controlled by sensors attached to the subject, the solution is cumbersome. However, without some individually tailored personal micro-environment, such as Webb suggests, working dives to extreme depths may not be practicable.

With ship-board systems, operating in the sea, an account of the heating and insulation system employed in the US Navy Mk I Deep Diving System Personnel Transfer Capsule has been published by Majendie (1970) and by Riegel and Glasgow (1970). Basically, the system employs a number of heating elements distributed around the external shell of the capsule and cemented closely to its surface in a manner rather similar to that employed at RNPL. Insulation is provided externally by a 1 inch thick layer of thin syntactic foam cemented in sections to the surface of the capsule. By such means, constant internal temperatures of 35°C in an oxy-helium atmosphere have been maintained at about 260 m (27 ATA) depth with a water temperature of 13°C (55°F). However, despite the insulation, the heat loss at the shell may be such that a high degree of internal gas mixing would be required to keep the gas temperature uniform. Heat requirements even with heavy insulation are large, particularly at depths in excess of 200 m (21 ATA) in water temperatures below 10°C where oxy-helium mixtures are used. With external heating elements used on a chamber in the water, it is necessary to ensure that the elements are adequately electrically insulated in the event of a short circuit. No data is yet available about the electrical hazard to a diver underwater in the event of such a short circuit, but it is wise at the present time to assume that the risk of electrocution is high for any diver in close proximity to the chamber.

Hot water and even steam circulating systems either internally or externally placed have been used effectively over the years, but seem to have been superseded recently by the development of better forms of electrically heated elements. Internal heating systems have several disadvantages; they tend to be bulky, are localized sources of heat by radiation and conduction, and distribute heat poorly by passive convection. Apart from the power requirements of internal electrical, hot water, or steam heating systems an efficient forced convection system must also be provided, requiring in its turn a further source of power. In oxy-helium conditions, the heating elements of such an internal system are too hot to touch and, therefore, present the possible hazard of burns. Non-insulated, electrically resistive heating elements should be avoided at all times, on account of their attendant fire hazard, potential source of electric shock and risk of causing burns. They have been used, however, during quite deep dives where the oxygen content of the atmosphere was below fire risk threshold.

CONTROL OF WATER VAPOUR

Only in dives of long duration, i.e. in excess of 48 hours, does the control of humidity become important. Especially during decompression, the main problems seem to arise from the condensation of water vapour within the chamber so that the chamber walls, items of equipment, utensils, clothing and blankets become damp. Apart from the discomfort of living in a damp and sometimes dripping environment, the skin of the divers themselves becomes more than usually prone to infection. Fungal infections of the skin, and infections of the external ear are common, particularly in chambers containing a water-filled compartment.

Because of the large quantity of water contained in the chamber atmosphere its removal poses a significant problem with certain types of scrubbing systems. Just as large quantities of CO_2 can choke the system by freezing out at relatively high temperatures in cryogenic scrubbing systems, so too may the system be choked by frozen water vapour. In scrubbing systems relying upon molecular sieve material, moisture drastically reduces the efficiency of the material. It is therefore usual to interpose between the moist gas of the chamber and the scrubbing system a replenishable canister of silica gel to remove a large proportion of the water before the gas passes into the scrubbing system. It is possible by frequent replacement of the silica gel to maintain humidity levels within the chamber of between 50 and 70% of the saturated water vapour pressure at the particular chamber temperature.

Accurate analysis of water vapour content has proved in practice to be extremely difficult, but in most circumstances is fortunately not really necessary. In general, within shore-based facilities it has not been found too difficult to maintain a satisfactory relative humidity and, of course, temperature, within the narrow band of comfort required by the divers. Excessive evaporative cooling at constant chamber temperature, particularly in oxy-helium atmospheres, is soon brought to the attention of the chamber operating staff and is readily controlled by an increase in chamber temperature accompanied by the removal of silica gel from the scrubbing system.

OTHER GASES

In the course of digestion, particularly in the large intestine, small quantities of toxic gases may be produced by bacterial fermentation. Of these, the two most common are methane (CH_4) and hydrogen sulphide (H_2S), the actual quantities produced being a function of the diet. Many carbohydrates, particularly those with high bulk content, such as cereals, are responsible for the production of CH_4, whereas highly spiced proteins and egg materials may lead to production of H_2S. Over a considerable period of time, which may be regarded as weeks rather than days in an entirely closed environment, concentrations of these gases may approach maximal permissible levels.

Methane itself is non-toxic but highly inflammable in the presence of oxygen. In addition, small quantities of hydrogen are produced, which further contribute to a fire potential, although concentrations in excess of 4% by volume would be required.

Hydrogen sulphide is a highly toxic gas, even in low concentrations, acting as a central nervous system poison at concentrations of 700 p.p.m. at 1 ATS or greater, and as a pulmonary irritant in concentrations as low as 70 p.p.m. with prolonged exposure. The maximal permissible concentration for prolonged exposure is the surface equivalent of 10 p.p.m. or less.

Bacterial action on nitrogenous material in the bowel and particularly in urine may produce *ammonia*, a highly toxic gas which is irritant to the lungs and mucous membranes in low concentrations. The maximal concentration of ammonia should not exceed the surface equivalent of 50 p.p.m. *Acetone* and some volatile compounds are eluted from urine, but only very small amounts actually contaminate the chamber atmosphere.

Red blood cells have a mean life of approximately 120 days with a constant input of new cells balancing the destruction of the old. As a by-product of the degradation of haemoglobin from these destroyed cells, small quantities of *carbon monoxide* are produced each day and over a lengthy period may exceed the maximal permissible concentration of 50 p.p.m.

The production of CH_4 and, to a greater extent, H_2S can largely be controlled by appropriate choice of diet for the divers. The production of NH_3 can be reduced to a minimum by adequate daily cleanliness, which includes not only personal hygiene, but daily changing of underclothing, and meticulous attention to the handling and removal from the chamber of collected urine and faecal material. Toilet buckets, their seats, canisters and also the area around the toilets should be scrubbed daily to prevent the build-up of NH_3. It should also be remembered that if such material is spilt some may seep beneath the deck plates where an ideal environment always exists for a high level of bacterial activity.

In general, the majority of noxious gases produced by metabolic breakdown in the gut and urine can largely be removed by activated charcoal, frozen out of the gas by a cryogenic system, or readily removed by molecular sieve material. Provision should therefore be made in each type of scrubbing system for their removal. In this respect a catalytic furnace has proved extremely effective. Carbon monoxide, on the other hand, is poorly absorbed by activated charcoal, but is readily removed cryogenically by molecular sieve material or by catalytic furnace.

Traditionally, hopcalite has been used as the reagent in such catalytic furnaces, and is a mixture of 50% manganese dioxide, 30% copper oxide, 15% cobalt oxide and 5% silver oxide. It is most frequently used as a catalyst to oxidize the carbon monoxide in air. However, finely divided platinum is now superseding hopcalite as the catalyst in such furnaces, as it is more efficient and can deal with a wider range of contaminants.

Further breakdown products of faecal materials include indole compounds and other complex combinations of hydrocarbons and nitrogen, some of which may be halogenated with chlorine. In addition, chemicals used in many sanitary pans as oxidants or cleansing agents may also contain chlorine. For example, buffered solutions of hypo-chlorite evolve small quantities of chlorine gas. The maximal permissible concentration of chlorine at 1 ATS is 1 p.p.m.

Many of the materials used in the construction of diving chambers (paints, lagging, electrical insulation materials, lubricants on door hinges, and even materials such as synthetic clothing and some toilet articles) are subject to out-gassing of noxious materials. Most out-gassing products tend to consist of carbon dioxide and volatile hydrocarbons, many of which, being aromatic in nature, are quite toxic to liver, bone marrow and central nervous tissue. The most hazardous hydrocarbons belong to the halogenated groups, particularly those containing fluorine, and when oxidized in the presence of sulphur-containing compounds may form highly toxic by-products indeed. Such a compound is sulphur tetrafluoride, lethal at 10 p.p.m.

In normal circumstances, provided time has been allowed, for example, for new paint work to cure thoroughly, little problem from such materials may be expected in diving conditions. They do, however, represent a potential problem in nuclear submarines where crews may be required to live in a totally closed environment for periods in excess of 3 months, or perhaps, in long-term underwater habitat experiments. Some such materials may be absorbed onto active charcoal, but all may be removed cryogenically or by molecular sieve material. In the event of a dive continuing longer than several weeks, it would perhaps be advisable to exchange the chamber gas completely at least once during the dive.

The greatest potential hazard from out-gassed solvent materials is by their accidental introduction to the chamber environment. Noxious solvent chemicals such as trichlorethylene and petroleum by-products such as kerosene (paraffin) have been introduced at different times by accident into high pressure chamber environments. High pressure valves with Teflon or nylon seats pose a potential hazard. Such a valve may be opened inadvertently so that supersonic gas-flow is permitted across a critical orifice with an attendant rise in temperature at the edge of the valve seat in excess of the vapourizing temperature of the material forming the seat (approximately 450°C in the case of nylon, 600°C in the case of Teflon). The vapour given off is highly toxic even in low concentrations. The presence of any such materials in high concentration would, of course, constitute a major chamber accident. Indeed, the removal of the products in very low concentration presents difficulties if some oxidative process such as a high temperature catalytic furnace is used. Cryogenic and molecular sieve systems handle such materials adequately.

GAS ANALYSIS

Clearly, the requirement for gas analysis varies with the type of work being undertaken at pressure. During long-term experimental saturation dives within the high pressure laboratory, fully detailed knowledge of all components of the chamber atmosphere is required. Whereas, for short-term oxy-helium dives to 200 m (21 ATA) or less, using a submersible decompression chamber locking onto a deck decompression chamber, the main gas analysis requirements are merely for oxygen and carbon dioxide. Moreover, relatively simple but robust equipment will suffice in such cases. In the laboratory, however, highly sophisticated analytical equipment is necessary.

As it is not always possible to be certain of the components within the chamber atmosphere during a prolonged laboratory experiment, mass spectrometry, covering a wide mass range is advisable, in order to obtain an indication of the range of compounds present, either from their mass numbers directly or by their cracking patterns. In addition, such analysis should give an order of magnitude of the concentration of the compounds present. For more detailed analysis of the components of the chamber gas, the most accurate method available is by gas chromatography. Such instruments are expensive but must ultimately be the arbiters of the concentrations of all gases present. With the advent of the quadrupole non-magnetic mass spectrometer, greater flexibility of use for a lower capital cost can be achieved than with previous types. Some models can be used both as a chamber gas analyser of high resolution and accuracy, covering mass ranges from 2 to 200 overall, and by switching modes can rapidly be employed as fast-responding respiratory gas analysers.

Under routine operating conditions, the primary monitoring requirements are for oxygen and carbon dioxide. For continuous oxygen analysis two methods are principally in use, paramagnetic analysis and polarography.

The paramagnetic method exploits the fact that the oxygen molecule, consisting as it does of two atoms each with an unpaired electron in its outer shell, has strong magnetic susceptibility. Instruments operating on this principle are accurate, linear, though until recently were relatively slow responding.

The polarographic method depends on the reduction of oxygen at the cathode of an electrochemical cell, the output of which is proportional to the oxygen partial pressure of the gas surrounding the cell.

While paramagnetic systems are inherently more accurate, the operating mechanism is fragile and therefore subject to damage in transit. Polarographic systems on the other hand, are extremely robust and highly portable, but require frequent calibration to ensure accuracy. They are, perhaps, better employed as sensors of relative changes in oxygen concentration, rather than as arbiters of absolute concentration and, as such, lend themselves to the sensor side of an oxygen injection system, as described above.

The most common means employed to analyse carbon dioxide content is by infra-red absorption analysis, which is adequate for most operational circumstances. The accuracy of such analysers is inversely proportional to the rate of response: fast response instruments, i.e. 95% response in less than 1 second, are somewhat less accurate than slower responding instruments.

In addition, spot checks on carbon dioxide and oxygen content can be made by a chemical absorption method, used in such instruments as the Lloyd–Haldane or micro-Scholander apparatus. These techniques, however, require considerable skill on the part of the operator.

The more exotic gases encountered are for the most part better left to mass spectrometry and gas chromatographic analysis, with the possible exception of carbon monoxide which is difficult to detect by mass spectrometry. However, many such gases can be detected, although not necessarily positively quantified, by the use of appropriate chemical detector tubes. For instance, a large range of specific Draeger tubes is available to detect specific volatile compounds ranging from carbon monoxide to various types of mineral oil.

HELIUM RECLAMATION

The bulk of the helium used in the western world is produced in the United States of America and Canada, and the cost to the user in different parts of the world varies but is relatively expensive. Therefore, depending upon the quantity used, it is often advantageous to avoid wasting the helium vented during decompression. After the removal of carbon dioxide, water vapour, carbon monoxide, micro-organisms and other trace contaminants, the remaining components of the gas mixture are helium, oxygen and some nitrogen, usually 1% or less. The partial pressure of oxygen

present tends to depend upon the depth of the dive.

The simplest means of re-using the gas collected is to accept a small degree of nitrogen contamination and either to add more oxygen to the mixture to make up a given higher Po_2 oxygen–helium mix, or to add fresh helium to the mixture to make up a given lower Po_2 oxygen–helium mix. With each transfer of gas in such a cascade method some will be lost, but the method is quite cost effective if extremely large volumes of gas are not required over the year.

If the cost-effectiveness of the cascade method is outweighed either by the cost of helium lost or the time taken to reconstitute mixtures within the cascade, the impure helium mixture may be scrubbed of both oxygen and nitrogen. Industrially, two methods are employed: cryogenic freezing-out of O_2 and N_2 by passing the gas

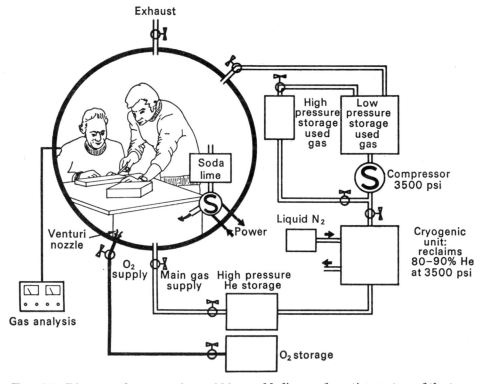

FIG. 6.8. Diagram of a cryogenic scrubbing and helium reclamation system of the type at present in use at the Deep Trials Unit, Admiralty Experimental Diving Unit. To avoid choking the cryogenic unit with solid CO_2, the CO_2 is scrubbed separately by an internal system. The bulk of water vapour condenses out during transfer stages. Helium and oxygen mixtures are produced within the chamber, mixing being by venturi nozzle

mixture through heat exchanger coils cooled with liquid nitrogen, or multiple molecular sieve columns. In both methods, some helium is again lost.

Fig. 6.8 represents schematically the cryogenic helium reclamation system in use at the Deep Trials Unit of the Admiralty Experimental Diving

and require a constant drain on expenditure due to the usage of liquid nitrogen. In addition, the need to rely upon a ready supply of liquid nitrogen reduces the general usefulness of such equipment to shore-based facilities within reasonable transporting distance of a supplier of the bulk gas in liquid form.

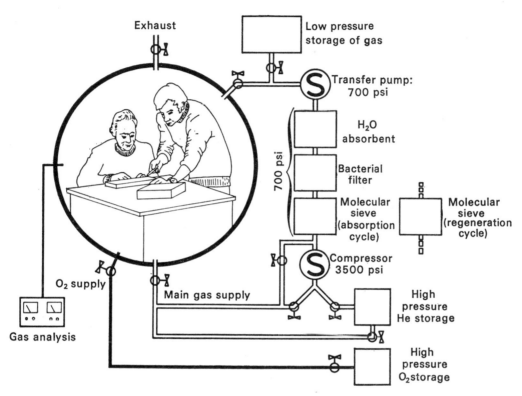

FIG. 6.9. Diagram of a molecular sieve scrubbing and reclamation system. No internal CO_2 scrubber is required, although provision must be made for water vapour removal before gas enters the molecular sieve bed to prevent caking of the bed. At the end of a given scrubbing cycle, the bed material is regenerated simply by back-flushing with scrubbed gas, and the impure flushed gas from the regenerated sieve material can either be dumped or passed back through the bed at its next scrubbing cycle

Unit. Carbon dioxide, water vapour and some other noxious materials are scrubbed out of the chamber atmosphere first and then the gas is bled down to large, helium-tight bags, from which it is pumped through the cryogenic unit into the high pressure helium storage bank. Although 90 to 95% recovery by the unit is claimed, some additional helium is lost in the storage bags and pipework, making the overall recovery somewhat lower. The capital costs of such units are high

Molecular sieve reclamation appears, at least superficially, to be more attractive in terms of lower overall capital cost and of reducing running costs. The columns of sieve material may be regenerated, and require replacement at infrequent intervals. Fig. 6.9 shows schematically the type of system that could be applied to a diving context. A positive benefit is the ability of the system to scrub out of the chamber atmosphere all contaminants except water, which should be removed independently to prevent choking of the bed with wet, caked, molecular sieve material. It is true that some helium is lost when the beds are reverse-flushed with pure helium to regenerate the molecular sieve material, and, in addition, some is lost in pipework and storage vessels. In normal industrial practice, however, better than 80 to 85% recovery of helium may be expected.

RECENT ADVANCES

In conventional diving systems oxygen is delivered from high pressure gas storage cylinders and CO_2 is removed chemically by an absorption system. As a result of the heavy fuel penalties imposed by the weight of high pressure gas cylinders and CO_2 absorbent in manned space vehicles, much effort has been expended in developing more economical ways of delivering oxygen to, and removing CO_2 from, closed environments. Two main developments are worthy of note.

Peroxide/superoxide systems

In these systems oxygen is carried as a superoxide or peroxide, for example, potassium superoxide (KO_2), sodium superoxide (NaO_2) or sodium peroxide (Na_2O_2). These compounds react with water and carbon dioxide either simultaneously or successively in a variety of ways. The simple overall reactions can be written as:

$$8KO_2 + 4CO_2 \longrightarrow 4K_2CO_3 + 6O_2 \qquad (1)$$

$$8NaO_2 + 4CO_2 \longrightarrow 4Na_2CO_3 + 6O_2 \qquad (2)$$

$$2Na_2O_2 + 2CO_2 \longrightarrow 2Na_2CO_3 + O_2 \qquad (3)$$

Broken down into its component parts, the superoxide reacts in the presence of moisture, e.g. water vapour from the breath or in the chamber:

$$4KO_2 + 2H_2O \longrightarrow 4KOH + 3O_2$$

The potassium hydroxide thus formed, absorbs the carbon dioxide by the reaction:

$$CO_2 + 2KOH \longrightarrow K_2CO_3 + H_2O$$

Thus there is absorption of the carbon dioxide and generation of oxygen. In theory at least, the quantity of oxygen produced by the reaction should be a direct function of the concentration of CO_2.

Such a system has been produced commercially by L'Air-Liquide in France who claim that under normal conditions of relative humidity between 50 and 70% at 20°C, the potassium superoxide system keeps the composition of the atmosphere constant at the initial composition of oxygen and CO_2 and, furthermore, adjusts the rate of the reactions to correspond with the level of activity of the divers. Quantitatively, the reaction should deliver 190 litres of oxygen at atmospheric pressure, per kilogram of potassium superoxide present. In addition, the chemical reactions are exothermic, the quantity of heat liberated being about 1 kcal/L oxygen. Using this system, two divers were entirely supported at 30 m simulated depth in a high pressure chamber for $1\frac{1}{2}$ hours. This dive was followed by a simulated saturation dive in which three divers were supported in an oxy-helium environment at 100 m simulated depth for 3 days. The system as marketed by L'Air-Liquide is used as an internal life support system with an external power requirement sufficient to drive the blower fan drawing air through the superoxide reactor.

A further advantage of potassium superoxide lies in its high reactivity as an oxidizing agent. Many of the noxious products formed metabolically in low concentration during prolonged dives, such as carbon monoxide, ammonia, indoles and mercaptans, are readily oxidized, and held in solution within the superoxide bed. The very reactivity of potassium superoxide is, however, a disadvantage in that it is extremely caustic to human tissue, which creates a potential hazard, particularly in handling and storage of the material. Moreover, within such an internal life support system, efficient filtration must be provided for gas on the outflow side, to prevent such caustic materials from entering the chamber atmosphere and being deposited on skin, clothing, bedding or equipment, or being inhaled by the divers. The end product formed, potassium carbonate (K_2CO_3), tends to be deliquescent, which may cause the granular bed of KO_2 to cake and solidify at its most reactive parts, thereby reducing the overall activity of the bed and decreasing the efficiency of the gas circulation blower.

For larger volume oxygen production and CO_2

absorption, sodium peroxide (Na_2O_2) and sodium superoxide (NaO_2) react with moisture to form caustic soda (NaOH) and hydrogen peroxide (H_2O_2), which itself decomposes to oxygen and water. The caustic soda solution thus produced is transferred to a second reactor where it absorbs the carbon dioxide from the atmosphere, with the formation of sodium carbonate. Although a more complex system than the potassium super-oxide one described above, the reactions are more readily controlled to match oxygen consumption requirements within the environment, and can handle large volumes of gas. This system is, perhaps, more applicable as a life support system in a submarine, submersible or underwater habitat than in conventional diving operations.

The prime disadvantage with such systems is that a non-regenerable carbonate salt is formed, and, like soda lime, the superoxides and peroxides have a once-only capability. L'Air-Liquide claim durations for their system of 24 hours per man per 3·75 kg of potassium superoxide; 16 hours per man per 3·2 kg, and 8 hours per man per 2 kg, thus relying upon average oxygen consumptions between 0·5 L/min for the 24-hour duration, and 0·8 L/min for the 8-hour duration.

High temperature solid electrolyte systems

In these systems (Weissbart, Smart & Wydeven 1969) a doped zirconia ceramic membrane is employed at a temperature of 1000°C. If a potential is applied to the two faces of the membrane by the use of suitable electrodes, oxygen ions pass across the membrane from anode to cathode. The reactions are: at the anode, $CO_2 \rightarrow CO + O_{(S)}$, at the cathode, $2O_{(S)} \rightarrow O_2$. At a lower temperature, and using a suitable catalyst, carbon monoxide disproportionates into carbon dioxide with the deposition of graphitic carbon: $2CO \rightarrow CO_2 + C$. On recirculation of the gas, the carbon dioxide is reduced by the zirconia electrolytic cell into oxygen and carbon. The Faradaic efficiency of the system is claimed to be high, particularly if small amounts of water are present with the carbon dioxide, enough to decrease the reduction of the electrolyte itself. Such a system is largely self regenerating, but has the grave disadvantage in the diving situation of operating at very high temperatures.

Photosynthetic systems

In the presence of appropriate ultra-violet light intensity and a suitably nutrient environment, green algae convert carbon dioxide into oxygen. Within the marine environment such purely biological systems may find a place in the future. In addition, by slight alteration in the nutrient medium and level of ultra-violet light, specialized forms of algal growth can be encouraged which are in themselves highly nutritious, if perhaps monotonous, sources of food.

APPLICATIONS OF LIFE SUPPORT AT SEA

The limitations of ship-board isolation impose restrictions upon the type and size of the life support system used, and perhaps upon the level of sophistication attainable in the analysis of chamber gas. There is clearly a limit to the bulk and weight of the life support system employed.

With the advent of effective designs for an efficient, compact, molecular sieve life support system, the problems of conventional external systems may be overcome. The bulky pipework and massive canister housings right next to the chamber can be replaced by a self-contained unit including, if necessary, its own power supply and compressor, housed remotely from the chamber area and coupled to it by narrow bore pipes and small valves. In addition, the molecular sieve material is regenerated and has an overall life in excess of 6 months. Moreover, the molecular sieve system enables a better than 80% recovery when used for helium reclamation. The combined capabilities of life support and helium reclamation built into a readily transportable modular unit make the design extremely attractive for both ship-board and shore-based use. It is envisaged that the external molecular sieve life support system would be supported by a small scrubbing system inside the chamber capable of removing CO_2, water vapour and perhaps some of the hydrocarbons. This system would be used in an emergency where the molecular sieve system was not functioning for some hours.

In the meantime, the choice of life support system for ship-board use centres around the advantages and disadvantages of internal versus external systems. Both are based upon the chemical removal of CO_2 by a granular alkaline bed, the removal of water vapour by silica gel and by the scrubbing of other noxious compounds by activated charcoal. The advantages of the internal system are primarily ones of cost and of saving in space in the region immediately around the chamber, coupled with some enhancement to gas circulation within the chamber. As such, it is a very useful system, particularly on dives of relatively short duration to depths shallower than 200 m, where access to the interior of the chamber by external control staff is a practical proposition in an emergency.

In general, for greater safety and flexibility in operation an external system is to be preferred. With an external loop it is possible to include a catalytic furnace to remove carbon monoxide and other noxious products, thus allowing significantly prolonged durations of bottom time and decompression. The main disadvantages are the bulk and the cost. The bulk encroaches upon useful deck space within the ship, and, as in the case of some diving ships where the chambers are mounted relatively high in the superstructure, the increased mass may significantly raise the centre of gravity of the ship. In addition, a bulky external life support system, mounted next to the chamber and coupled to it by wide bore high pressure steel piping, increases the problems should the chamber need to be moved as it is virtually an integral part of the chamber structure.

Shore-based facilities generally do not have a major problem with space and unless geographically isolated, provide no great logistical problem for the supply of fresh soda lime, silica gel, activated charcoal, liquid nitrogen, or, for that matter, replenishment of molecular sieve material. In addition, the electrical requirements for a shore-based facility can be virtually limitless, whereas, at sea, the use of electrical power may be restricted. Moreover, the power supplies to shore-based facilities are in general mains voltage, whereas at sea electrical voltages on-line may differ greatly.

FIRE HAZARDS

Three factors combine to cause any fire: the partial pressure of oxygen must be sufficiently high to support both ignition and combustion, some form of inflammable material must be present, and there must be an active source of ignition. For obvious reasons, matches and cigarette lighters must not be allowed in high pressure chambers.

As a general rule, it is wise to prevent equipment or lighting operated from mains voltages from being exposed to high pressure chamber atmospheres. Although methods for encasing electrical equipment in an explosion-proof housing purged with an inert gas such as nitrogen are in common use, a potential hazard nonetheless exists. It is worthwhile, as far as possible, to exclude combustible materials such as paper, loose clothing, and excess bedding, but not to the detriment of the diver's welfare. It is now well known that despite somewhat increased partial pressures of oxygen, a sufficiently high partial pressure of inert gas provides a significant blanketing effect to ignition and propagation of a fire (Dorr & Schreiner 1969). In deep oxy-helium dives where the oxygen partial pressure is maintained at 0·5 ATS or lower, the fire hazard is insignificant. Only during the shallow phases of a decompression where oxygen partial pressures are raised does the risk increase. Therefore, it is advisable to employ some form of exhaled gas dumping outside the chamber, particularly when the divers are breathing pure oxygen either during a normal decompression or during recompression therapy.

Although much discussion has centred upon the best ways of combating fires in high pressure chambers, one of the simplest and most effective ways of handling the situation is simply to repressurize the chamber with an appropriate inert gas thus reducing the oxygen concentration. It is fortunate that the intensity of a fire will diminish to manageable levels, or even be extinguished, with oxygen partial pressures remaining sufficient to maintain life. The resultant increase in total pressure will, of course, add somewhat to the decompression time, but the problems so caused are relatively minor.

Once the fire has been extinguished, the major hazard is from smoke and fumes generated by combustion. A damp cloth held over the nose and mouth can act as a very efficient filter screening the lungs and mucous membranes from heavy contamination. As soon as possible the divers should breathe a respirable gas mixture delivered via the built-in breathing system, thus allowing adequate ventilation of the chamber and subsequent restitution of an internal respirable mixture. In competent hands all this could be done very quickly, allowing early assessment of the damage and, hopefully, an early return to a stable state. In chambers lacking a considerable margin for pressurization above the pressure at which the fire breaks out the same method could be employed, with judicious simultaneous venting of chamber atmosphere through the exhaust valve, the controlling factor being the Po_2 inside the chamber as judged by the activity of the fire. Again, a built-in breathing system with a respirable gas mixture on-line must be readily available to the divers.

On the other hand, emergency decompression of the chamber may prove catastrophic for the divers, without necessarily diminishing the problems of extinguishing the blaze.

Water sprinkler systems have, in the main, proved ineffective. However, a weak (100:1) solution of high grade household detergent in water forced under pressure across a fine mesh screen placed in front of a high volume air blower has proved very effective in putting out test fires in chambers (Dorr & Schreiner 1969). Smoke and other solid particles adhere to the surface of the bubbles formed leaving a respirable, if soapy, gas mixture in the chamber.

The majority of fires in high pressure chambers have involved some fault in electrical equipment operated either from mains supply, or drawing a relatively large current—the energy for ignition being volts × amperes. If such equipment must be used inside a high pressure chamber then, apart from internal protection of the equipment by a housing purged with inert gas, the active power line should be fitted outside the chamber with a circuit-breaking device having a current loading very little above the operating level of the equipment, so that even a small surge of current lasting longer than a few seconds would be sufficient to break the circuit. At no time should electrical fuses or circuit-breakers be employed inside the chamber, as the potential energy sufficient to cause ignition would still lie in contact with the chamber environment.

In addition, isolation of the chamber from earth via an isolation transformer, has advantages, particularly when employed with a warning system coupled between the input side of the transformer and earth, such that an alarm is sounded should an electrical potential greater than a given pre-set level be recorded. With such a system in use, all equipment capable of conducting electricity must similarly be isolated from earth, and any electrical equipment operated ancillary to the chamber be earthed to the chamber. It is seldom practicable that all such criteria can be met.

REFERENCES

BROUSSOLLE, B., CHOUTEAU, J., HYACINTHE, R., de la PECHON, J. C., BURNET, H., BATTESTI, A., CRESSON, D. & UMBERT, G. (1975) Cardio-respiratory function during 1640 ft (51 ATA), helium–oxygen simulated dives. In *Underwater Physiology. Vth Symp. Underwater Physiology*. Ed. C. J. Lambertsen. Bethesda: Fedn Am. Socs exp. Biol.
CANTY, J. M., LANPHIER, E. H., MORIN, R. A. & MILLER, J. N. (1972) A new facility for studies at very high pressure. *Third International Conference on Hyperbaric and Underwater Physiology*, pp. 56–62. Ed. X. Fructus. Paris: Doin.
CLARK, J. M. & LAMBERTSEN, C. J. (1971) Pulmonary oxygen toxicity: A review. *Pharmac. Rev.* **23**, 37–133.
DORR, V. A. & SCHREINER, H. R. (1969) *Combustion Safety in Diving Atmospheres: Region of Noncombustion, Flammability Limits of Hydrogen–Oxygen Mixtures, Full-scale Combustion and Extinguishing Tests, and Screening of Flame-resistant Materials*. Ocean Systems, Inc. Report. ONR Contract N00014–66–CO149, pp. 26–28.
EATON, W. J. (1970) The pressure vessel and its life support systems. In *Interim Report on Some Physiological Studies during 1500 ft Simulated Dive*, pp. 26–28. Royal Naval Physiological Laboratory Report 1–70.
HAIGH, K. R. (1971) Results from the Gulf Stream drift mission—Part 1. *Underwat. J.* **2**, 13–21.
MAJENDIE, J. (1970) Diver heating. In *Equipment for the Working Diver*, pp. 95–118. Washington, D.C.: Marine Technology Society.
MARGARIA, R., GALENTE, E. & CERRETELLI, P. (1959) An efficient CO_2 absorber for experiments on metabolism. *J. appl. Physiol.* **14**, 1066–1068.
RIEGEL, P. S. & GLASGOW, J. G. (1970) Experimental determination of heat requirements for the Mark I P.T.C. In *Equipment for the Working Diver*, pp. 119–128. Washington, D.C.: Marine Technology Society.
WEBB, P. (1975) Thermal stress in undersea activity. In *Underwater Physiology. Vth Symp. Underwater Physiology*. Ed. C. J. Lambertsen. Bethesda: Fedn Am. Socs exp. Biol.
WEISSBART, J., SMART, W. & WYDEVEN, T. (1969) Oxygen reclamation from carbon dioxide using a solid electrolyte. *Aerospace Med.* **40**, 136–140.

7

Hydrostatic Pressure Physiology

A. G. MACDONALD

This chapter is concerned with hydrostatic pressure, which exerts important physiological effects in deep dives. The effects of high partial pressures of gases and the problems of pulmonary ventilation at high pressure are dealt with in other chapters.

In the first edition of this book the late Professor Wallace Fenn made an important contribution to diving physiology by discussing the effects of hydrostatic pressure at both the physical–chemical and physiological levels. He drew two shrewd conclusions. One rounded off a summary of some observations of the effects of hydrostatic pressure on the nervous system of test animals thus: 'All these results confirm the opinion recently expressed by the author that pressure effects are likely to be of special importance as a limiting factor in deep dives (Fenn 1969).' The second conclusion followed closely, and out of context it may appear paradoxical: 'Although the high pressures encountered in deep dives may cause symptoms, it is by no means certain that they will be severe enough to be prohibitive.'

The continental shelf lies at a depth of 200 m and is already within reach of oxy-helium divers. It occupies approximately 5% of the area of the sea floor (Defant 1961). The continental slope covers 10% of the sea floor and extends from 200 m down to the floor of the ocean which is normally at least 3000 m deep and accounts for 85% of the sea floor. The greatest depth in the ocean is 10 790 m in the Challenger Deep. It will be apparent from this chapter that man's ultimate depth range might conceivably approach

2000 m (200 ATS), a guess which leaves man confined to about 10% of the total sea floor unless otherwise protected.

The extension of the depths to which operational divers can safely penetrate is proceeding at a rapid pace. In 1966 actual and simulated dives to pressures of 20 ATA were undertaken and 6 years later a simulated dive to a pressure of 60 ATA was successfully completed by the French. Hydrostatic pressure of this magnitude is sufficient to exert direct physiological effects but it is probably far short of the maximum pressure which humans may safely endure for a period of days. In the next few years it is anticipated that divers will experience pressures which exert more serious effects on their physiology and eventually a practical depth and duration limit to diving will be reached.

Descent to greater depths requires that men are confined to deep sea submarines, of which many have been built to operate at depths of several thousands of metres (Sweeney 1970).

There exists the special case of the submariner who needs to escape from a foundered submarine. He may need to expose himself briefly to a much higher hydrostatic pressure than would be reasonable for a normal dive. It is going to be extremely difficult to predict the survival of men making submarine escapes from great depths.

The first part of this chapter is concerned with examples of the effects of hydrostatic pressure on a wide variety of physiological systems. It will be confined to pressures of several hundred atmospheres although special attention will be given to the 1 to 100 ATA range, which is of prime interest in diving physiology.

In the second part, the molecular basis of the physiological effects of pressure will be discussed. It will be shown that these effects are becoming increasingly amenable to rigorous, physical–chemical interpretation. Indeed, the effects of pressure are such that pressure itself is an important analytical tool which is capable of assisting understanding of many fundamental biological processes. A limited number of physiologists have demonstrated this over the years but the development of deep diving is proving a particularly valuable stimulus in high pressure research from which many branches of the biological sciences and medicine will eventually benefit.

EFFECTS OF PRESSURE AT THE PHYSIOLOGICAL LEVEL

The whole animal

Invertebrates and vertebrates. Aquatic animals show marked locomotor changes when hydraulically compressed. This was first shown by Regnard (1885) who observed small Crustacea, *Copepoda*, *Amphipoda* and *Cladocera*, in a pressure vessel fitted with quartz windows. He noted how pressures immobilized them. When decompressed such animals recovered normal activity promptly. Regnard's pioneering studies were described in a monograph on underwater life (Regnard 1891) but failed to stimulate further work. In 1935 Ebbecke described similar effects in several marine animals and at the present time a number of workers are independently repeating and extending these observations.

In order to make comparisons with deep sea crustacea living at several hundred atmospheres pressure, Macdonald (1972) has quantitatively described both the hyperexcitable and inhibitory effects of pressure in the seashore crustacean *Marinogammarus marinus*. Fig. 7.1 shows the relatively simple apparatus required for the purpose and also Regnard's remarkable early vessel. The development of plastic high pressure windows is making observational pressure equipment generally available. Fig. 7.2 shows the increase in the locomotor activity of *Marinogammarus* which takes place when it is subjected to various

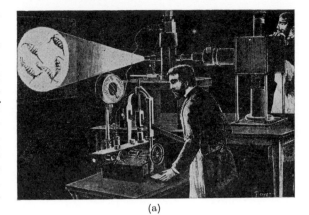

(a)

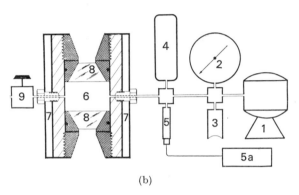

(b)

FIG. 7.1. Observational high pressure apparatus

(a) shows Regnard's (1885) apparatus.
(b) (Macdonald, unpublished) shows the modern equivalent. 1, air-powered hydraulic pump, with water reservoir (not illustrated); 2, pressure gauge; 3, bursting disc (fuse); 4, gas-filled accumulator to smooth pressure pulses from the pump; 5, pressure transducer, connecting to 5a a potentiometric controller; 6, pressure vessel enclosed in a water jacket, 7; 8, plastic high pressure window; and 9, bleed valve. The proportions of the vessel and window are suitable for pressures up to 700 ATS at room temperatures. The bleed valve, 9, allows water to flow through the apparatus. The initial loss of water from the pressurized vessel causes a slight pressure drop which is detected by the transducer, which connects to the potentiometric controller. This in turn actuates the hydraulic pump which raises the pressure to the selected level. A continuous flow of water at high pressure $\pm 2\%$ is achieved.

compression rates. As pressure increases, movement becomes jerky and at pressures around 50 ATS at 3°C the whole body undergoes spasms or convulsions. The increase in locomotor activity fades at constant high pressure and fails to appear when the rate of compression is sufficiently slow, although body spasms have been observed at 85 ATS in the slow compression experiments

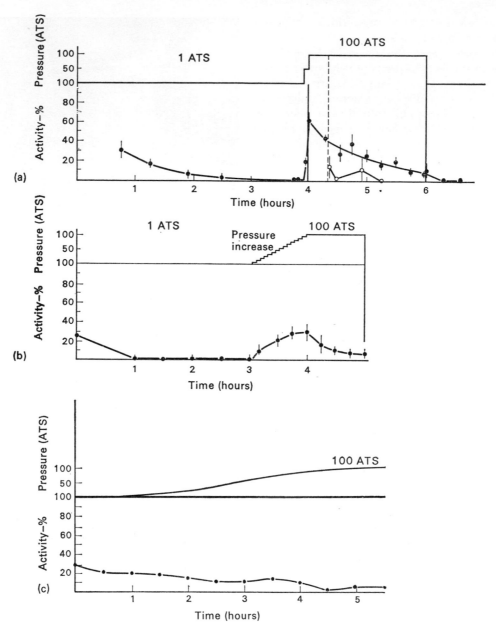

FIG. 7.2. Hyperexcitable effect of moderate pressure on the crustacean *Marinogammarus marinus*

Each graph shows time in hours on the horizontal axis and activity and pressure separately on the vertical axis. Activity is defined as the percentage of a 3-minute period of observation during which an individual was seen to move in the pressure vessel. Each point represents the mean ±S.E. of at least 6 results using different animals, at 3°C.

Pressure is applied stepwise by a handpump in (a) and (b), but smoothly in (c) by means of heat applied to a second pressure vessel.

(a) shows the hyperexcitable effect of 100 ATS which is rapidly reversed on decompression (open circles and vertical dashed line).

(b) shows less activity than (a), and (c) shows how the animals fail to respond to very slow compression (Macdonald 1975b).

(Fig. 7.2c). At 100 ATS pressure and 3°C *Marino-gammarus* respires oxygen at a normal rate, and remains apparently healthy for many days.

Compression to 200 ATS causes a rapid inhibition of locomotor activity. *Marinogammarus* may be immobilized for several days at 200 ATS and yet recover within minutes of decompression. It appears that in crustacea the temporary paralysis caused by 200 ATS is accompanied by little progressive injury, but tolerance to anoxia seems to be a prerequisite for recovery. Compression of *Marinogammarus* to higher pressures results in prolonged recovery times.

We may therefore distinguish several types of reversible effects in locomotor activity at high pressure: Type I, hyperexcitable; Type II, inhibition by 200 ATS, rapidly reversed after decompression, recovery independent of the duration of pressure treatment; and a Type III response, inhibition, slowly reversed after only a few minutes' high pressure treatment at around 500 ATS (Macdonald 1972). Other invertebrates, and vertebrates which live at or near atmospheric pressure, exhibit broadly similar responses to pressure.

The lethal dose of pressure for a wide variety of marine animals has been determined by Naroska (1968) and Menzies and George (1972).

Of acute interest to high pressure physiologists are those deep sea animals which are tolerant to high pressure. The locomotor responses of two such animals have been observed at pressures up to 500 ATS. One is an Ostracod, *Gigantocypris mülleri*, whose pressure tolerance is reported by Macdonald (1972), the other is an amphipod, *Lanceola sayana*, which like *Gigantocypris* continues normal locomotion at 300 ATS (Macdonald & Teal, in press).

Shallow water vertebrates, amphibia and fish, have also been hydraulically compressed. Larvae of *Rana sylvatica* and *Amblystoma*, for example, show increased swimming movements at pressures up to 150 ATS. At higher pressures, spasms and a rigid paralysis occur (Johnson & Flagler 1951). Fish have been included in extensive studies by Brauer (1972) and the pressure–convulsion thresholds for several shallow water species are compared with thresholds determined in air-breathing vertebrates in Brauer's own chapter (see Fig. 13.1).

The hyperexcitable effects of hydrostatic pressure in mammals, including the human diver, are discussed by Brauer and Bennett in Chapters 13 and 14. Here we may bridge the gap between aquatic and air-breathing animals by considering hydraulically compressed, liquid-breathing mammals. In a decisive experiment Kylstra and his colleagues (1967) used mice breathing a fluorocarbon liquid in which oxygen is highly soluble, at a body temperature of between 17 to 25°C. Rapid compression elicited tremors and spasms in the limbs over the pressure range 50 to 80 ATS and tonic convulsions were seen at higher pressures. The muscular spasms faded at constant pressure. Similarly, hypothermic mice, which were compressed with the appropriate heliox gas mixture, showed tonic convulsions at pressures in the range 69 to 86 ATS. The spasms appeared to be caused by some central disturbance as spinal transects blocked spasms in the posterior half of the body.

Pressure was shown to kill the liquid-breathing mice by paralyzing the respiratory muscles, providing Ornhagen and Lundgren (1975) in a later study, with a convenient end-point with which to measure the tolerance of mice to hydrostatic pressure. These workers made the surprising observation that the rate of compression had little effect on pressure tolerance, but a low body temperature (17°C) yielded a pressure limit of breathing of 150 ATS, compared to 125 ATS at 32°C. Convulsions were seen in the range of 80 to 100 ATS; lowering the body temperature intensified the convulsions. Respiratory frequency and heart rate both declined with increase in pressure. Thus liquid-breathing, hypothermic mice and marine crustacea show marked similarities at high hydrostatic pressure.

The threshold values for the pressure convulsions in a wide range of mammals are summarized in Fig. 13.1 from Brauer (1972). These were obtained with animals breathing gas in otherwise relatively normal conditions. There is no reason to suppose that the convulsions are caused by factors other than pressure, but temperature, the partial pressure of respired gases and other factors can influence the action of pressure. The same is true for hydraulically compressed animals.

The sensation of hydrostatic pressure. Some animals appear equipped to sense small changes in hydrostatic pressure. Fish, for example, may obtain sensory information about their ambient pressure from the distension of their gas-filled swim bladders (Qutob 1962). Other animals, including fish which lack a swim bladder, and crustacea which also lack a bulk gas phase, respond to small changes in hydrostatic pressure, and pose an intriguing problem in sensory-transduction physiology. *Synchelidium* (Crustacea), for example, appears to respond to an increase in hydrostatic pressure of 0·01 ATS (Enright 1962).

Another interesting case is the water flea *Daphnia* which may be induced to swim up and down a water column in response to a diurnal light regime. The movement of a group of animals in a 45 cm high pressure vessel was monitored by Lincoln (1970) who showed that the animals sensed an abrupt pressure change of 4 ATS. Several physiological mechanisms held to be capable of detecting small changes in hydrostatic pressure have been postulated by different authors, including piezo-electric phenomena, the differential compressibility of tissues and a pressure-sensitive film of electrolytically generated gas on a tissue surface (Digby 1972).

Protozoa. The effects of pressure on Protozoa were first seen by Ebbecke (1935b) who achieved a magnification of thirty-fold to view the freshwater ciliate *Paramecium* through a high pressure window. A pressure of 50 ATS reduced Paramecium's swimming speed and 600 ATS soon stopped the majority of cells. The recovery of normal movement was seen to occur soon after decompression. Kitching has confirmed this observation in *Paramecium aurelia* but notes that other ciliates (*Colpoda cucullus, Holophyra* sp.) swim more rapidly on compression (Kitching 1970).

The effect of pressure on cell structures may be readily seen in certain Protozoa. Irregularly shaped amoeboid forms round up at high pressure and so to a lesser extent do the highly structured ciliates. The rounding up is due to a liquefaction of the cytoplasm, which will be discussed shortly.

Pressure may change the swimming speed of ciliates by acting specifically on the cilia rather

than the cell as a whole; other microtubular systems in Protozoa exhibit marked sensitivity to pressure and these are also considered in the next section.

Cytoplasmic rigidity, contractility and muscular contraction

Cytoplasm. Bulk cytoplasm in relatively undifferentiated cells may be regarded as a gel which, in all cases examined, liquefies under a pressure of several hundred atmospheres (Marsland 1970). In amoeboid cells, a rounding up occurs, whilst in certain invertebrate eggs the centrifugal displacement of pigment granules is greatly enhanced at high pressure. Lowering the temperature of such cells also liquefies their cytoplasm. Thus high pressure and low temperature both appear to weaken the cohesiveness of sub-units of the cytoplasm. Fig. 7.3 shows how the cohesiveness (gel strength) is related to the capacity of a cleaving cell to constrict into two.

Cleavage is but one of the several forms of cytoplasmic activity which pressures of several hundred atmospheres inhibit. Cytoplasmic streaming in plant and amoeboid cells (Marsland 1938; Landau, Zimmerman & Marsland 1954) and the

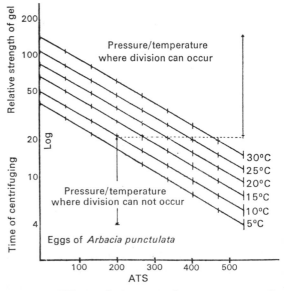

FIG. 7.3. Effects of pressure and temperature on the gel strength of the cortical cytoplasm in the egg of *Arbacia punctulata*. Centrifuge times are a measure of gel strength (after Marsland 1950)

movement of chromosomes (Pease 1946) are also pressure labile. Provided the pressure treatment is limited, recovery from the effects of high pressure is usually both rapid and complete.

Pressure undoubtedly affects the biochemistry of those cells whose mechanical activities are suspended through liquefaction of the cytoplasm. In the case of cultured amnion cells the initial application of pressure causes a transient contraction in the cell cortex (Landau 1961). Pressure therefore appears to stimulate mechanical activity prior to inhibiting it. Alternatively it may be argued that by initially weakening the gel, pressure reveals the underlying tendency of cytoplasm to contract.

A transient contraction in amoeboid cells (*Amoeba proteus*, cultured embryonic chick heart fibroblasts, and cultured human amnion cells) which have been held at a liquefying pressure and then decompressed, is also seen (Landau, Zimmerman & Marsland 1954; Landau 1960, 1961). The observation suggests an accumulation of reactants which are involved in a contractile process. Attempts to follow levels of ATP have revealed rather complicated results and in any case the role of ATP in either cytoplasmic rigidity or its contraction is by no means clear (Landau & Peabody 1963).

Cells may be prevented from progressing through their cell cycle by the application of pressure during interphase or during cleavage (Zimmerman & Silberman 1965). *Arbacia* (sea urchin) eggs normally cleave on a predictable schedule after fertilization. If prevented from so doing by a fairly long exposure to high pressure and then decompressed, the eggs undergo two simultaneous cleavages to achieve the 4-cell stage on schedule (Marsland 1938). The ciliated protozoan *Tetrahymena pyriformis* shows a strong tendency to continue growth in cell volume when prevented from cleaving by a pressure of 175 ATS (Fig. 7.4). Zimmerman and co-workers have also used *Tetrahymena* in a series of pressure studies and, most recently, have induced synchronous division by means of pulses of high pressure (Zimmerman 1971).

A number of ultrastructural components of cells are pressure labile. Examples include certain kinds of microtubule arrays, notably the mitotic

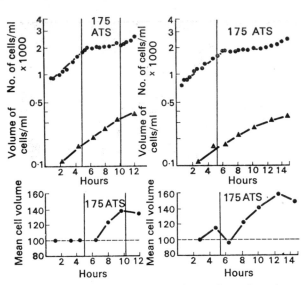

FIG. 7.4. Inhibition of cell division and continuation of cell growth in *Tetrahymena pyriformis* at 175 ATS. Results of a typical experiment are shown. They were obtained with a Coulter counter apparatus, the probe of which was mounted within a pressure vessel

Upper graph shows numbers and total volume of cells per millilitre against time in hours. Lower graph shows mean cell volume as percentage of the pre-compression volume (Macdonald 1967a).

apparatus in the cleaving *Arbacia* egg (Zimmerman & Marsland 1964; see also Pease 1946); the long axonemes which support the axopodia of the protozoan *Actinosphaerium* (Kitching 1957; Tilney, Hiramoto & Marsland 1966); and microtubules both in the cell cortex and in the basal part of the cilia in *Tetrahymena* (Kennedy & Zimmerman 1970). In all these cases pressure reversibly disaggregates microtubules. The microvilli in the small intestine of the salamander and the pinocytosis channels in amoeba are also reversibly disrupted by pressures in the range of 200 to 500 ATS (Tilney & Cardell 1969; Zimmerman & Rustad 1965). Polysomes are also susceptible to high pressure treatment and these are discussed in the section dealing with macromolecular synthesis.

In view of the action of pressure on both chromosome movement within cells and the amoeboid movement of whole cells, it is not surprising that pressure distorts morphogenesis in tadpoles (Fig. 7.5) and fish embryos (Rugh & Marsland 1943; Draper & Edwards 1932).

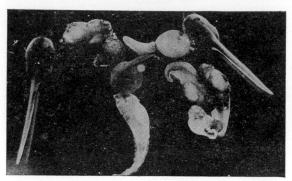

Fig. 7.5. Abnormal development of *Rana pipiens* tadpoles. The animals are 2 weeks old and experienced 400 ATS for 20 min, 1 hour after fertilization. Of individuals treated in this way 44% hatched. The tadpole on the left developed normally at atmospheric pressure (Rugh & Marsland 1943)

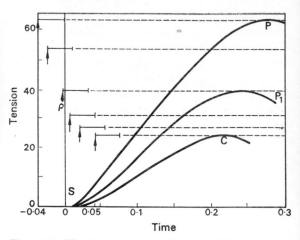

Fig. 7.6. The increase in tension caused by pressure applied at different stages in the contraction cycle of striated muscle. C, myogram at atmospheric pressure P, the myogram obtained when 272 ATS is applied 15 sec before stimulation at S. P_1, the myogram obtained when 272 ATS is applied with electrical stimulation at S. Horizontal dashed lines indicate the tension developed following compressions at the times (sec) indicated by the arrows (Brown 1936)

Ultrastructure elements which are stable at high pressure include some of the components of cilia, mitochondria, and most membranes. The latter, as will be seen, are by no means unaffected in their function at high pressure.

Muscle. Whereas liquefaction is a major feature of many cells at high pressure, the structure of muscle cells seems to remain stable, with contraction able to take place at several hundred atmospheres pressure. Indeed an important effect of pressure on muscle is to enhance its contraction. This section is concerned with the performance of isolated but otherwise intact muscles.

The frog gastrocnemius muscle and the retractor penis muscle of the turtle, both striated, are caused to contract slowly by the application of hydrostatic pressure. Curare fails to inhibit the effect and no action potential accompanies the contraction, which may be induced repeatedly and is accordingly known as a reversible contracture (Ebbecke 1914, 1935c; Brown & Edwards 1932). In an early review by Cattell (1936), pressure contracture was also reported in smooth muscle. Pressure thus bypasses the excitation stage in muscular contraction and acts at or close to the fundamental contractile process.

In the case of the retractor penis muscle which functions conveniently slowly at 4°C, 130 ATS elicits an increase in tension, which becomes maximal at 530 ATS. Tension fades at constant pressure

and much higher pressures act deleteriously and irreversibly.

Pressure and electrical stimuli act jointly to cause a twitch tension greater than normal at room temperature. Maximum tension is, however, developed more slowly at pressure. By combining electrical stimulation and rapid pressure changes Brown (1934, 1936) was able to show that pressure need act only at an early stage in the contraction cycle, apparently to mobilize compounds, which augment the final tension (Fig. 7.6). Twitch tension is also reduced if continuous pressure is applied to a muscle at low temperature. Tetanic tension is little affected by pressures which enhance the twitch tension.

Brown and Goodall (1956) have measured the relationship between pressure and the tension developed at 22°C in both the retractor penis muscle of the turtle and the glycerinated rabbit psoas muscle, under precisely controlled reaction conditions. The results were strikingly similar, and Brown (1957) suggests that pressure acts in both to activate acto-myosin in readiness for contraction. This complex phenomenon awaits further study.

The isolated frog heart increases its amplitude

and rate of contraction at 60 ATS at room temperature (Edwards & Cattell 1928; Yasuda 1959). The isometric contraction of the isolated ventricle from the terrapin at room temperature alters its rate of contraction at 107 ATS only slightly but it generates 47% more tension and relaxes more slowly than at atmospheric pressure. As in skeletal muscle the effect of pressure at low temperature is to reduce twitch tension (Edwards & Cattell 1930).

Cultured heart cells which exhibit rhythmic contraction are also inhibited by pressure at low temperature but are accelerated by pressure at higher temperatures. Following the application of pressure at room temperature there is a transient steep rise in the rate of beating of such cells which is followed by equilibration to a rate characteristic of the prevailing temperature and pressure (Landau & Marsland 1952; Fig. 7.7). A

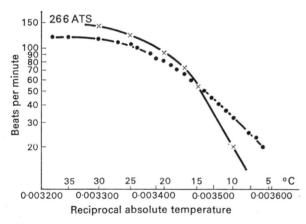

FIG. 7.7. The effect of 266 ATS pressure on the rate of beating of cultured heart cells measured over the temperature range 6 to 38°C. Each point is based on the values derived from 6 different heart preparations. For details see text and Landau and Marsland (1952)

kinetic interpretation of this observation is considered separately later as it has been invoked to account for the pressure–temperature relations of several physiological systems.

In diving physiology it is important to know how muscles respond to prolonged exposures to a moderate pressure, but only rather severe conditions have been studied in animal experiments. When frog striated muscle is held at pressures in the range of 250 to 450 ATS it shows an increased

consumption of oxygen. In the case of the skeletal muscle of the eel a tendency to acidify its medium and to increase its wet weight, presumably by osmosis, has been noted (Fenn & Boschen 1969; Fontaine 1928). These muscles resemble tetanized muscles.

Frog gastrocnemius muscles held at pressures between 67 to 130 ATS and electrically stimulated, show a parallel rise in isometric twitch tension and heat production. At higher pressures relatively more heat is evolved, until at pressures greater than 300 ATS both the tension and the amount of heat which is liberated, decline (Cattell 1935).

The electrical properties of muscle at high pressure were first investigated by Ebbecke and Schaefer in 1935. In the frog sartorius muscle they found the amplitude of the action potential was reduced slightly by 200 ATS and halved by 400 ATS. Only a slight decrease in the threshold to subliminal stimuli was detectable. Terrapin auricle, undergoing natural stimulation from the sinus, shows increased action potentials at pressures up to 300 ATS, in parallel with the increase in tension (Cattell 1936). Some evidence also shows that the excitability of the isolated frog heart may be increased by pressure.

An experiment by Ebbecke and Schaefer (1935) comes close to answering the obvious question; which is more sensitive to pressure, the muscle or its peripheral innervation? A frog gastrocnemius muscle was stimulated by its motor nerve at 100 ATS. In those experiments which showed enhanced excitability, it seemed that the nerve was responsible. At pressures in the region of 300 ATS the performance of the frog muscle declined but could be offset by the increased stimulation of the motor nerve. Although a great deal of work remains to be done it appears that a moderate pressure elicits changes in muscular activity by way of the nerve supply and perhaps also by intensifying contractions elicited by normal innervation (Type I response). Higher pressures may induce abnormal nervous stimulation or cause a contracture (Type II response).

Pressure may affect contraction by acting at the muscle membrane, perhaps by affecting its selectivity for ions. Substitution of Cl^- for NO_3^- in the bathing Ringer mimics the pressure-enhanced isometric twitch of the frog sartorius muscle (Podolsky 1956). NO_3^-, like hydrostatic pressure, had no effect on tetanic tension.

Membranes

Excitable membranes. The results of early studies of nerves have to be treated with some caution because the experimenters ignored the heat emitted during compression and in the case of liquid paraffin, in which the preparations were often immersed, the heat may be considerable. Perhaps the same reservation should apply to the results of the early experiments on muscle at high pressure.

The following effects were seen in nerves during exposures to high pressure.

Amphibian motor nerve bundles showed an increased response to submaximal stimuli at 100 ATS, reaching a four-fold response as judged by the height of the compound action potential at 400 ATS (Ebbecke & Schaefer 1935). This effect was seen in nerves which were maintained at 200 ATS for 5 hours (Grundfest 1936) and is therefore independent of the heat of compression. The same preparation shows a diminished response to supramaximal stimuli at high pressure although even at 1000 ATS a response was elicited. Pressures in the region of 300 ATS had the effect of spreading the action potential and, in particular, of prolonging the descending part of the spike. Complex after-potentials were frequently observed. A single stimulus sometimes caused a repetitive firing of action potentials, an effect which Grundfest (1936) compared to that seen in nerves treated with veratrine. This phenomenon may be important in the high pressure nervous syndrome in human divers.

In contrast, amphibian gastrocnemius muscles showed no increased excitation to submaximal stimuli and no after-effects following the propagation of an action potential at high pressure. The muscles' response to supramaximal stimuli was diminished by pressure to a greater extent than the motor nerve.

Motor fibres from *Bufo marinus* have been studied at high pressure and room temperature by Spyropoulos (1957a), who avoided serious heating effects during compression. The falling phase of the action current proved the most pressure-sensitive feature of the nerve (Fig. 7.8).

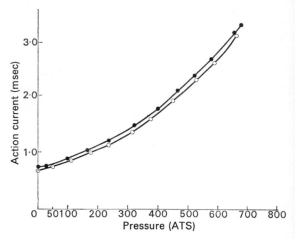

FIG. 7.8. Effects of hydrostatic pressure on the duration of the action current of the node of Ranvier at 23 to 25°C. Data from two different nerve fibres are plotted (after Spyropoulos 1957)

Rheobase voltage, conduction velocity and the amplitude of the action current were only affected slightly by a brief exposure to pressures up to 400 ATS and none more than by 10 to 15%. Prolonged exposures markedly raised the rheobase.

The squid giant axon has also been studied at high pressure by Spyropoulos (1957b). Its resting potential was affected very little but the action potentials were prolonged at approximately 300 ATS (10 to 15°C). Threshold current and potential were reduced by a pressure of 7 ATS or more, and at 200 ATS the nerve fired spontaneously. As in the myelinated vertebrate nerve the conduction velocity and the amplitude of the action potentials were little affected by pressure.

The efflux of K^+ and the influx of Na^+ in unstimulated toad sciatic nerves are both increased by a 3-hour exposure to 160 ATS at 25°C (Gershfield & Shanes 1959). This condition has also been compared to the veratrine-treated nerve. Pressure enhances the action of cocaine, a local anaesthetic, on amphibian motor nerves, whereas the action of general anaesthetics such as nitrous oxide and ethanol are reversed either in part or totally by a moderate pressure (Spyropoulos 1957b; Roth, Smith & Paton 1975). Although some of the effects of veratrine may resemble those of pressure, the two agents do not appear to act synergistically (Gershfield & Shanes 1959).

Synaptic transmission is likely to be an important site of action of pressure but no experiments with nerves seem to be reported. The action of acetylcholine ($4 \cdot 8 \times 10^{-6}$ M) on the rabbit duodenum is impaired by 30 ATA at 37°C, which delays the appearance of the maximum response of the muscle to the transmitter (Akers & Carlson 1975). The authors speculate that a change in the receptor molecule is responsible.

There is a great deal to learn about excitable tissue at pressure. The only general conclusion which can be made at present is that membranes show a variety of effects and probably do not behave as a simple compressible phase. Molecular changes of the type, to be discussed later, are presumably at work.

Inexcitable membranes. Pressure doubtless affects the normal functioning of membranes by numerous indirect routes, simply because it affects so many biochemical processes. However, three rather direct and specific effects of pressure on membrane physiology have been discussed in the literature.

Erythrocytes of the cat exhibit a reduced efflux of sodium at 80 ATS which Podolsky (1956) tentatively attributed to a change in the hydration of Cl^- ions. Interestingly, this effect, like the pressure-enhanced isometric twitch in the frog muscle, is mimicked by substituting NO_3^- for Cl^- in the Ringer. In some way NO_3^- ions at 1 ATS resemble Cl^- ions at 80 ATS.

The very much more complicated isolated frog skin preparation undergoes first a transient depolarization, then a prolonged hyper-polarization when it is subjected to 100 ATS (Brouha et al. 1970). The authors' interpretation of this and other experiments, is that 100 ATS pressure increases the permeability of the skin to sodium. For a full discussion of more recent experiments with the isolated frog skin see Macdonald and Miller (1975). These examples remind us that both the blood and the kidney may be directly influenced by hydrostatic pressure in deep simulated dives with human subjects.

The active uptake of the amino acids, glutamic acid, glycine, phenylalanine and proline into a marine bacterium was found to be reversibly inhibited by 100 ATS or more at an appropriately low temperature (Paul & Morita 1971). The subsequent metabolism of the incorporated amino acids was little affected, so it was reasoned that pressure acts on the transport mechanism situated in the cell membrane.

Metabolism

The synthesis of RNA and DNA in both prokaryote and eukaryote cells is less sensitive to high pressure than protein synthesis. The scheme shown in Fig. 7.9 illustrates a number of stages in protein synthesis. Amino acids become converted to the amino-acyl adenylate which binds with an appropriate molecule of transfer RNA. Peptide bond formation between amino acids takes place when t-RNA complexes with messenger RNA which thus determines the amino acid sequence in aggregated ribosomes. These aggregates or polysomes are the functional unit of protein synthesis in both prokaryote and eukaryote cells, and seem to be affected by high pressure. A recent study of the effect of pressure on the synthesis of polyphenylalanine mediated in vitro by the synthetic messenger polyuridylic acid has consolidated some earlier reports on several synthesizing systems (Pollard & Weller 1966; Landau, 1967, 1970; Albright & Morita 1968; Yayanos & Pollard 1969; Arnold & Albright 1971; Hilderbrand & Pollard 1972). Pressure inhibits the aminoacylation of transfer RNA, the effect being first apparent at 200 ATS; 600 ATS reduces the rate of the process to 20% of the control level. The rate at which the phe-t-RNA-polyuridylic acid-ribosome-complex is formed is, however, greatly reduced by 200 ATS. The formation of this complex is highly sensitive to the concentration of Mg^{++} ions and, it was argued, pressure may act on the magnesium equilibrium. The fidelity with which polyphenylalanine was assembled was improved by pressures of up to 200 ATS but deteriorated at higher pressures. The net synthesis of polyphenylalanine in the presence of excess magnesium ions was reduced by high pressure (640 ATS) but increased by 100 ATS (Fig. 7.10). At lower concentrations of Mg^{++} ions it was reduced at all pressures. The authors argued that the ribosome is probably the major site at which pressure acts in this in vitro system, which they also regard as similar to the protein synthesizing machinery which has been studied at pressure in

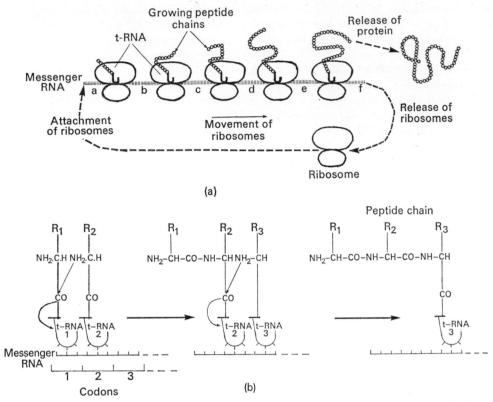

FIG. 7.9. Simplified scheme of protein synthesis, by (a) polysomes and (b) by peptide bond formation from amino-acyl t-RNA (after Arnstein 1965)

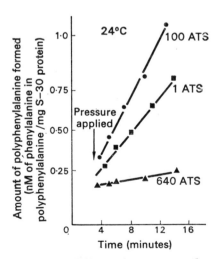

FIG. 7.10. Effects of pressure on the in vitro synthesis of polyphenyl-alanine. The reaction mixture is described in Hildebrand and Pollard (1972)

living organisms, specifically *E. coli*, *Vibrio marinus* (both bacteria) and *Hela* cells. In the ciliate *Tetrahymena pyriformis* pressure inhibits the incorporation of labelled phenylalanine into protein (Zimmerman 1969).

Polysomes have been shown to be pressure labile at certain late stages of the cell cycle in synchronized *Tetrahymena pyriformis* (Hermolin & Zimmerman 1969). Ribosomes which were isolated from *Tetrahymena* and pulsed with 1000 ATS pressure for 5 minutes proved unaltered in their ability to participate in the synthesis of polyphenylalanine at atmospheric pressure. Either the pressure effect was rapidly reversed or, as Letts and Zimmerman (1970) suggest, pressure affects protein synthesis by way of m-RNA or the m-RNA-ribosome interaction. Ribosomes from sea urchin eggs are dissociated to sub-units by the hydrostatic pressure which is generated during centrifugation (Infante & Krauss 1971).

Bacteria lend themselves to a wide range of biochemical studies at high pressure. In general, if sufficient pressure is applied for long enough then a reduction of enzyme activity is found. Many enzymes functioning in intact cells show a change in activity at about 200 ATS in the temperature range 20 to 35°C. They include succinic, formic and malic dehydrogenases and aspartase in *E. coli*, and phosphatase and urease in marine bacteria and *Micrococcus* sp. respectively. ZoBell's recent review should be consulted for further examples (ZoBell & Kim 1972).

A characteristic response of bacteria growing at a moderate pressure is the formation of filaments, due to the suppression of new septa. Thus pressures of several hundred atmospheres inhibit the division of both prokaryote and eukaryote cells but probably by different mechanisms. Interestingly, some deep sea bacteria exhibit the ability to grow preferentially at high pressures which correspond to their natural habitat (Zobell & Kim 1972).

The respiration of whole organisms, tissues and cells has been measured at high pressure, principally by determining the rate of oxygen consumption. In a crustacean whose movements were greatly stimulated by pressure, Macdonald (1975b) found a significant rise in respiration which was not seen in animals which were compressed slowly to avoid stimulation. Fenn and Boschen (1969), as we have already noted, found that isolated frog muscles consumed more oxygen at pressures which induced contracture. In the ciliate *Tetrahymena* respiration is much more resistant to high pressure than, for example, the division mechanism in the cell (Macdonald 1965).

In the anaerobic bacterium *Streptococcus faecalis*, glycolysis and growth in mass have been observed in enclosed cultures, which permit the overall molar volume change (ΔV) of growth and metabolic processes to be measured (Marquis & Fenn 1969; Marquis, Brown & Fenn 1971). Pressures of up to 400 ATS failed to stop the culture growing in volume by some 15/mole lactate produced. It will be shown later in this chapter that pressure affects the rate, but not the equilibrium point, of chemical changes, not in relation to overall volume changes, ΔV, but in accordance with the volume changes in critical rate determining steps within the overall process.

Dissolved gases

Henry's Law states that the mass of gas dissolved in a liquid is determined by the partial pressure of the gas and its solubility coefficient. Hydrostatic pressure decreases the solubility of atmospheric gases, causing their equilibrium or partial pressures to increase with increase in hydrostatic pressure. The effect has been experimentally demonstrated by Enns, Scholander and Bradstreet (1964) who employed a pressure-resistant plastic tube which passed through the wall of a pressure vessel. Inside the pressure vessel the exterior of the plastic tube was subjected to hydrostatic pressure applied by water. The water contained dissolved gas which was previously equilibrated with gas at atmospheric pressure. On compression to a maximum of 100 ATS hydrostatic pressure, the partial pressure of the dissolved gas was increased, with the result that it diffused through the wall of the plastic tube to the atmosphere where it would be detected. Dissolved O_2, N_2, Ar, He and CO_2 all showed an increase in partial pressure of approximately 14% at 100 ATS. It was argued that this increase would be expected to reach 400% at 1000 ATS hydrostatic pressure. Fenn (1972) posthumously published a stimulating essay on this phenomenon but little is known of its physiological implications in diving.

Pressure has been shown to influence the interaction between oxygen and haemoglobin (Wells 1975). Haemoglobin from human erythrocytes was studied at pH 6·8 and at 25°C. At 100 ATS hydrostatic pressure and at oxygen concentrations of less than 20% normal saturation, haemoglobin showed an increased affinity for oxygen. At higher oxygen concentrations the converse was found. Pressures higher than 100 ATS and up to 1000 ATS reduced the affinity for oxygen at all concentrations.

Independently, Kiesow, Bless and Shelton (1973) have studied the effect of high pressures of helium on intact red blood cells at pH 7·1. They concluded a helium pressure of 100 ATS slightly increased the affinity of haemoglobin for oxygen. This effect is probably due to pressure rather than helium. There are no data to show the extent of this phenomenon in divers.

Chemically inert gases such as nitrogen and the

clinical anaesthetics show a change in their potency with increase in hydrostatic pressure. The potency of these substances is normally related to their physical properties, notably the ease with which they dissolve in oils and, in particular, their solubility in solvents whose solubility parameter is approximately $9(\text{cal cm}^{-3})^{1/2}$ (Smith 1969). Hydrostatic pressure alters the potency of inert narcotics in two ways.

The first type of potency change is seen in the following preparations: bioluminescent bacteria (Johnson, Brown & Marsland 1942); intact animals (Johnson & Flagler 1951; Lever, Miller Paton & Smith 1971; Miller 1972); nerve preparations (Spyropoulos 1957b; Roth, Smith & Paton 1975); and liposomes (Johnson & Miller 1970). In these, pressure reverses in whole or in part the action of the narcotic at all doses. The change in potency is attributed to the compressive effect of hydrostatic pressure which counteracts the molar volume expansion caused by the dissolution of narcotic molecules in a hydrophobic phase.

A second way in which pressure affects narcotic potency is seen in dividing *Tetrahymena* cells. Here an ineffective dose of narcotic (halothane, n-propane, nitrogen) is rended effective by 100 ATS hydrostatic pressure which alone has no effect on the dividing cells. High doses of narcotic are counteracted by 100 ATS pressure (Kirkness & Macdonald 1972, 1973). In this unusual biphasic action of pressure on narcotic potency is seen a curious and unexplained similarity with the way in which pressure affects the oxyhaemoglobin equilibrium. Pressure enhances the action of an anaesthetic-like substance applied to frog sciatic nerves (Hsia & Boggs 1973).

CAUSES—PHYSICAL EFFECTS OF HIGH PRESSURE

'The only way tissue can possibly "know" that it is being compressed is through a volume change' (Cattell, in Grundfest 1936).

Introduction

Any effect of pressure can only come about by way of a change in molecular volume. In physiological systems it is the solvent water molecules

surrounding solute particles which are the prime source of changes in molecular volume and therefore in this section we have to concern ourselves mainly with solute–water interactions.

First, compare the effect of high pressure on a gas with its effect on pure water. Argon, at room temperature for example, shows an increase in density in line with a rise in pressure over a range of 3000 ATS. Its viscosity, however, only increases six-fold over the same pressure range (Lazarre & Bodar 1956). In contrast, water shows an increase in density of only 4% with an increase in pressure of 1000 ATS. Its viscosity varies with pressure and temperature in a complicated way, as seen in Fig. 7.11. Under certain conditions viscosity may

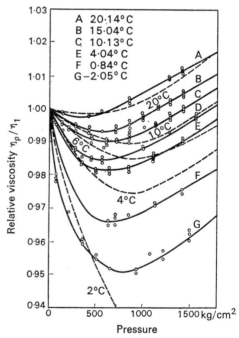

Fig. 7.11. Effects of pressure on the relative viscosity of seawater of 19·375‰ chlorinity (Horne & Johnson 1966)

actually decline while density increases. Water molecules are closely packed ('precompressed'), compared to the molecules comprising a gas, and they must exist in various kinds of clusters to give rise to the anomalous viscosity shown in Fig. 7.11 and indeed to the many other properties of bulk water (Drost-Hansen 1972; Horne 1969). Most of the changes in molecular volume with which we are concerned are ultimately derived from the peculiar properties of water.

The compression of the free volume of solutes such as lipids, macromolecules or solvents is a second source of change in volume in the range of pressures relevant here, but before we consider the changes which hydrostatic pressure induces at the molecular level some formal thermodynamic framework is necessary.

At constant temperature, pressure affects an equilibrium in accordance with the difference in volume between the two sides of the equilibrium:

$$\frac{\delta \ln K}{\delta P} = \frac{\Delta V}{RT} \qquad (1)$$

where P is pressure, K is the equilibrium constant, T is temperature, ΔV is the volume change in the process and R is the gas constant.

The extent to which pressure will favour one side of an equilibrium is dependent on the magnitude of ΔV, the difference between the partial molal volumes of the two constituents of the equilibrium. We therefore need to know values of ΔV for the various solute–solvent interactions of physiological importance.

The rate of a chemical reaction proceeding at high pressure is influenced by the volume change which takes place in the rate determining activation step.

Thus the rate constant k is related to pressure in the following simplified way:

$$\frac{\delta \ln k}{\delta P} = \frac{\Delta V\dagger}{RT} \qquad (2)$$

A reaction which proceeds with a volume increase in the activation stage $(+\Delta V\dagger)$ is inhibited by high pressure. A convenient way of treating experimental data is to plot the logarithm of the reaction velocity against pressure and from the slope calculate the activation volume by

$$\Delta V\dagger = 2\cdot3RT \left[\frac{\log k_1 - \log k_2}{P_2 - P_1}\right] \qquad (3)$$

k_1 and k_2 are the rate constants at pressure P_1 and P_2. R, the gas constant, is $82\cdot07$ cm^3/mole^{-1}, yielding $\Delta V\dagger$ in cm^3/mole^{-1}. If the data yield a straight line plot then the activation volume is unaffected by high pressure.

The concept of activation volume is not an easy one. The analogy with the action of temperature on the rate at which a chemical reaction proceeds may be helpful here. As temperature increases a greater number of molecules acquire the necessary energy to react, the temperature coefficient of the reaction being given by the familiar Arrhenius equation:

$$\mu = 2\cdot3R \left[\frac{\log k_1 - \log k_0}{1/T_0 - 1/T_1}\right] \qquad (4)$$

where μ is the activation energy, and k_1 and k_0 the rate constants at temperatures T_1 and T_0. The analogy with temperature has, however, a serious failing. Whereas an increase in temperature accelerates most reactions within well-understood limits, no such generalization applies to the effects of pressure. The volume of the activated complex may be larger or smaller than the reactants, that is, the change in volume upon activation may be positive or negative. Pressure may therefore retard or accelerate chemical reactions. Johnson, Eyring and Polissar (1954) provide an authoritative exposition of this subject in their outstanding monograph.

Equilibria and chemical change

Water molecules are attracted and compressed by the electrical field around ions. Thus ionization is generally favoured by an increase in pressure. Those salts which are completely dissociated under normal conditions will clearly not alter the extent of their dissociation at high pressure but the zone of electrostricted water around the individual ions may show changes in properties, as for instance in the case of Cl$^-$ ions and the red cell membrane at high pressure. Fig. 7.12 shows how pressure enhances the electrical conductance of hydrogen chloride over a wide temperature range, but depresses that of potassium chloride at 75°C. At lower temperatures pressure exerts both effects on potassium chloride. Such complicated effects seem to arise from the different behaviour of the clusters of water molecules around potassium and hydrogen.

Substances which are only weakly ionized under normal conditions show the expected shift in their dissociation constant with increase in pressure. Table 7.1 compiled by Disteche (1972) lists some

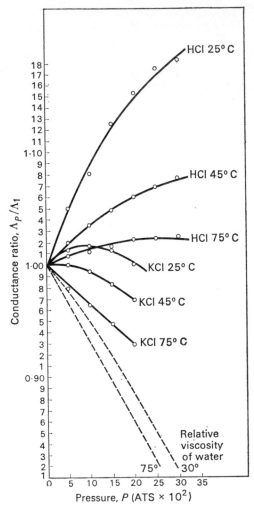

FIG. 7.12. Relative conductance of 0·01M HCl and 0·01M KCl at different pressures and temperatures (Hills, Overden & Whitehouse 1965)

come together to form an apolar or hydrophobic 'bond' (strictly an interaction), the water which is released from around each group is more voluminous than the previously bound water. Pressure therefore also favours the separation of unchanged groups (Table 7.2). In contrast to both ionic and hydrophobic 'bonds', hydrogen bonds form with a volume decrease in a number of cases which Suzuki and Taniguchi (1972) discuss.

Macromolecules are sensitive to moderate pressures because hydrophobic (apolar), ionic and hydrogen bonds play an important part in their higher order structure. The covalent peptide bond has interesting volumetric properties (Linderstrom-Lang & Jacobsen 1941) but it is not broken by pressures which are of interest in the present context.

The volume of water which a protein displaces when in aqueous solution is determined by the volume of its constituent amino acids, the additional volume due to voids within its structure, and the volume change arising from solute–solvent interactions at the surface of the molecule (McMeekin, Groves & Hipp 1954; Zamyatnin 1972). The effect of pressure on an equilibrium may be predicted when we have volumetric data (equation (1)) but the complexity of proteins and the effect of pressure itself on molal volumes greatly limits useful predictions. Yayanos (1972) has shown that the apparent molal volume of the amino acid glycine increases as the pressure is raised to 1000 ATS. The electrostriction of the solvent water at high pressure is less than at atmospheric pressure, as the bulk water structure is changed by the pressure. In this respect glycine behaves qualitatively like sodium and chloride ions whose partial molal volumes also increase with increase in pressure.

The reversible reaction

$$2 \text{ glycine} \rightleftharpoons \text{glycylglycine} + H_2O \qquad (5)$$

at 25°C and atmospheric pressure involves a volume change of +8 cm³/mole⁻¹ going to the right. At 500 ATS the volume change is +7·5 cm³/mole⁻¹. Pressure thus favours the separation of glycine molecules (but to a lesser extent with increase in pressure). Changes in the conformation and in the degree of aggregation of macromolecules are particularly important in the physio-

examples of the change in volume caused by the ionization of weak acids, including water. It will be recalled that the dissociation of magnesium salts by pressures in the 200 ATS range has been invoked to account for the inhibition of protein synthesis in vitro.

The formation of ionic bonds, the converse of dissociation, involves a volume increase and in general is opposed by high pressure.

Apolar or unchanged groups interact with water molecules in a way which leads to a localized decrease in volume. Thus when two apolar groups

TABLE 7.1

Volume changes for the ionization of some weak acids and buffers at 1 atmosphere and 22°C
(from Disteche 1972)

Acids and buffers	Glass electrode $-\Delta V_1\infty$ $(cm^3\ mole^{-1})$	Density $-\Delta V_1\infty$ $(cm^3\ mole^{-1})$	Conductivity $-\Delta V_1\infty$ $(cm^3\ mole^{-1})$
Acetic acid	11·6	12·5	12·2
Acetate buffer	10·7		
Formic acid	9·2	8·0	8·8
Formate buffer	7·4		
Carbonic acid ($K_{(1)}$)	26·6	29·0	26·5
Bicarbonate buffer ($K_{(1)}$)	25·4	27·8	
Carbonate buffer ($K_{(2)}$)	25·6		
Phosphoric acid ($K_{(1)}$)	17·7		15·5
Phosphate buffer ($K_{(1)}$)	15·7		
Phosphate buffer ($K_{(2)}$)	24·0	28·1	
Adenosine triphosphate (pH 7·0)	24·0	24·1	
Phosphorylcreatine (pH 7·0)	21·2		
Borate buffer (H_3BO_3 + borax; pH 8·0)	32·1		
Water (25°C) (K_w)	20·4	20·55	
Tris amine buffer ($K_{bh} = K_w/K_b$)	−2·5		
Tris amine buffer (K_b)	17·9		

TABLE 7.2

ΔV of bonds involved in the structure of macromolecules (data compiled from various authors, Suzuki & Taniguchi 1972)

Bond (interaction)	Volume change $(cm^3/mole^{-1})$
Ionic bond as in the association of H^+ with	
(a) acetic acid	+11·8
(b) glutamic acid	+12·7
Hydrophobic 'bond', as in the transfer of CH_4 from aqueous phase to hydrophobic solvent	+22·7
Hydrogen bond, as in formic acid in H_2O	−4·1

logical effects of moderate pressures. Colloids which are stabilized by hydrogen bonds set more firmly with an increase in pressure and a decrease in temperature, and are termed exothermic gels. Examples include polyvinyl alcohol and gelatin. Endothermic gels such as methyl cellulose are liquefied by high pressure and low temperature because such gels are stabilized by hydrophobic 'bonds' (Heyman 1936; Freundlich 1937; Marsland 1970; Suzuki & Taniguchi 1972). As we have seen, living cytoplasm and some ultrastructure liquefy at high pressure, an effect which may be regarded as an equilibrium shift, the ΔV probably being derived in part from the dissociation of hydrophobic groups.

$$\text{Monomeric sol} \underset{-\Delta V}{\overset{+\Delta V}{\rightleftharpoons}} \text{Polymerized gel} \qquad (6)$$

DNA is a particularly stable macromolecule at high pressure because of its hydrogen-bonded, double helical structure. Proteins undergo denaturation at very high pressures which are without effect on DNA. Examples of proteins which undergo reversible depolymerization or disaggregation under the influence of a moderate hydrostatic pressure include poly-valyl-ribonuclease (PVRN-ase) (Kettman et al. 1966), β-casein, (Payens & Hermens 1969), fibrin and sickle cell haemoglobin (Murayama & Hasegawa 1970), myosin and a number of enzymes (Penniston 1971). This list includes a fairly well-understood system, PVRN-ase, and others in which depolymerization merely seems the most reasonable explanation for the observed effect of pressure. PVRN-ase aggregates by forming hydrophobic interactions. Fig. 7.13 shows how 150 ATS re-

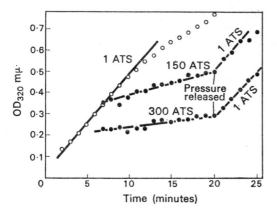

FIG. 7.13. Effect of hydrostatic pressure on the thermal aggregation of PVRN-ase (Kettman et al. 1965)

duces the rate at which the thermally driven reaction proceeds. Equation (3) yields a $\Delta V\dagger$ of 203 cm^3/mole^{-1} in 0·6M NaCl medium. As the reaction is akin to a phase change there is a close match between $\Delta V\dagger$ and ΔV, the latter being the overall volume change in the reaction. Another protein whose degree of aggregation is highly sensitive to pressure is rabbit myosin. In the

conditions of the experiments carried out by Josephs and Harrington (1968), pressures of 100 ATS or less shifted the monomer ⇌ polymer equilibrium to the left. ΔV was calculated at −380 cm^3/mole^{-1} monomer formed, the volume change being attributed mainly to ionization.

Proteins which undergo depolymerization with a significant volume change at atmospheric pressure, and which are potentially pressure labile, include TMV protein (Lauffer 1964), actin (Ikkai & Ooi 1966), flagellin (Gerber & Noguchi 1967), and collagen (Cassel & Christensen 1967). Data for the change in volume and opacity accompanying the aggregation of collagen are shown in Fig. 7.14. The authors regarded the process as a phase transition with no change taking place in the conformation of the individual sub-units. As in the case of PVRN-ase the volume change on aggregation is mainly attributed to the exclusion of solvent water from the sub-units.

Biochemical processes

It is convenient to start the interpretation of the effects of high pressure on biochemical reactions with the Michaelis–Menten treatment of an enzymic reaction. This assumes that the reaction proceeds at a fairly low temperature with the enzyme in the native state. The reaction is envisaged in two stages; first the formation of the enzyme–substrate complex takes place and then

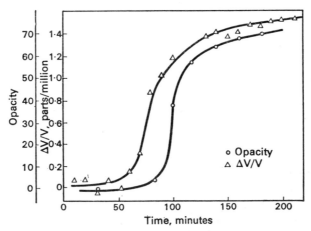

FIG. 7.14. Volume change and change in opacity during aggregation of tropocollagen in solution at 16°C (Cassell & Christensen 1967)

it subsequently becomes activated and decays to form products.

$$E + S \underset{k_{-1}}{\overset{k_1}{\rightleftharpoons}} ES \qquad (7)$$

$$ES \overset{k_2}{\longrightarrow} products \qquad (8)$$

Note that the rate constant k_2 applies to the irreversible and final step in the reaction.

It may be shown that when the substrate concentration is high, irrespective of the velocities of k_1 and k_{-1}, the rate constant determining the overall reaction is k_2 (Laidler 1951). This is limited at high pressure by its activation volume $V_2\dagger$, corresponding to the activation step $ES \rightarrow ES\dagger \rightarrow$ products.

At low concentrations of substrate the situation is more complicated. When k_{-1} is faster than k_2 the important rate determining volume change is $\Delta V\dagger \, (= \Delta V_2\dagger + \Delta V)$, i.e. the $ES \rightarrow ES\dagger$ activation volume plus the overall volume change of the reaction, $E + S + ES$. When k_2 is faster than k_{-1} the rate determining volume change is $\Delta V_1\dagger$, corresponding to the activation step in forming the enzyme–substrate complex ($E + S \rightarrow ES\dagger \rightarrow ES$).

For the purpose of investigating pressure effects in detail, high substrate concentrations are convenient to use, as in the experiments of Laidler and Beardell (1955) who studied the ATP-ase activity of myosin at high pressure. They found $\Delta V_2\dagger$, the activation volume for the $ES \rightarrow ES\dagger$ step, to be negative and in the range of -25 to -32 cm^3/mole^{-1}, depending on the potassium chloride concentration. Activation steps in several enzyme-catalysed reactions involve a volume decrease, suggesting that activation commonly involves the appearance of charges and hence the electrostriction of solvent.

Table 7.3 lists values of $\Delta V_2\dagger$ quoted by Laidler and Beardell (1955) and by subsequent workers. Penniston (1971) found negative values for some enzymes but those listed in Table 7.4 are enzymes in which the $ES \rightarrow ES\dagger$ step is inhibited by high pressure. $\Delta V_2\dagger$ seems to involve a volume increase in these cases. Penniston points out that with the exception of 5′ nucleotidase, the other two enzymes studied by him and listed in Table 7.3 are known to be monomeric (the state of 5′ nucleotidase is not known) whereas those in Table 7.4 are multimeric. It is argued that the enzyme monomer–polymer equilibrium shifts to the left at high pressure in those enzymes listed in Table 7.4, irrespective of the substrate concentration. We have therefore to consider the structure of an enzyme before adopting a Michaelis–Menten treatment of high pressure kinetic data.

Pancreatic ribonuclease acting on cytidine-2′, 3′-phosphate undergoes activation of the ES complex at an accelerated rate at high pressure

TABLE 7.3

The sign and magnitude of the $\Delta V_2\dagger$ of some enzymic reactions. (For details see text and original accounts)

Enzyme	$\Delta V_2\dagger$ $(cm^3/mole^{-1})$	
Myosin ATP-ase	-32 to -25	Laidler & Beardell 1955
Trypsin	$-13 \cdot 7$	Talwar, Macheboeuff & Bassett 1954
Chymotrypsin	$-13 \cdot 5$	Werbin & McLaren 1951
Sucrase	-8	Laidler 1951
Amylase (salivary)	-22	Laidler 1951
Anylase (pancreas)	-28	Laidler 1951
Pancreatic ribonuclease	$-20 \cdot 0$	Williams & Shen 1972
Fructose diphosphatase	-40	Hochachka, Schneider & Moon 1971
5′ Nucleotidase	Negative	Penniston 1971
Peroxidase	Negative	Penniston 1971
Myokinase	Negative	Penniston 1971
Lysozyme	Negative	Neville & Eyring 1972

TABLE 7.4

Multimeric enzymes exhibiting an apparent $+\Delta V_2$†
(from Penniston 1971)

Creatine kinase
DPN-ase
Alkaline phosphatase
Argininosuccinase
Pyruvic carboxylase

ATP-ases
  Beef heart mitochondria
  ETP_H
  Purified mitochondrial ATP-ase
  Rat liver mitochondria
  Erythrocyte ghosts
  Sarcotubular vesicles

ATP–^{32}Pi exchanges
  Beef heart mitochondria
  ETP_H
  Rat liver mitochondria

(Table 7.3). In this case there is evidence from other sources for the appearance of charges in both the substrate and the enzyme prior to their decay to products. Lysozyme from hen eggs acting on the dried cells of *Micrococcus luteus* yields a negative value of ΔV_2† which is influenced by the concentration of sodium chloride in the reaction mixture (Table 7.3). With increase in the concentration of sodium chloride it was found that the activation volume diminished, because, it was argued, salts become incorporated into the activated complex and presumably diminish the extra electrostriction it may exert on the solvent water during activation.

Although ΔV_2† is important to know from the standpoint of chemistry, it will be shown that it may be of secondary importance in physiological conditions.

Values of ΔV† for myosin ATP-ase obtained by Laidler and Beardell (1955) range from $+22\cdot7$ to $7\cdot7$ cm^3/mole^{-1}. It is not possible to pinpoint the precise reaction step to which ΔV† applies, the relative magnitudes of the separate rate constants not being known. But the volume increase is consistent with charge neutralization occurring in the association of enzyme and substrate, with the release of bound water.

The Michaelis–Menten treatment, it will be recalled, assumes the enzyme to be at low temperature and in the native state. When the tempera-

ture of a number of physiological systems is raised, a change in the action of pressure occurs, as is seen in the rhythmic beating of heart cells and in the action of pressure on the isometric tension of muscle. In these cases and in a third, biolumines-cence, high pressure enhances the process at high temperature but retards it at low temperature. Bioluminescence may be conveniently measured in bacterial cell suspensions and under standard conditions the intensity of the light emitted is a measure of the rate of the photogenic reaction. Fig. 7.15 shows that in the bacterium *Photo-*

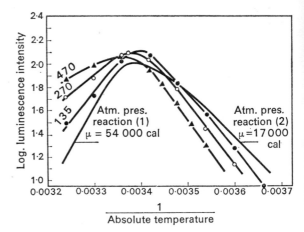

FIG. 7.15. Pressure-temperature relations in the intensity of the bioluminescence from *Photobacterium phosphoreum* at 470, 270 and 135 ATS (Brown, Johnson & Marsland 1942)

bacterium phosphoreum pressure diminishes the light emission at 10°C or less, but increases at higher temperatures. Raising the temperature is thought to cause a shift to the right in a reversible, thermal denaturation of some critical enzyme, $EN \underset{-\Delta V}{\overset{+\Delta V}{\rightleftharpoons}} ED$. If the volumetric changes are as indicated in this hypothetical equilibrium, then pressure will favour the enzyme in the native state. Thus pressure may accelerate a reaction by increasing the concentration of the effective enzyme at high temperature. When that concentration is not rate determining, as at low temperature, pressure may exert the opposite net effect on the reaction by inhibiting the new rate determining step (Johnson, Eyring & Polissar 1954).

Factors other than temperature normally modulate the activity of enzymes in physiological conditions. Attempts have been made to study the interaction between selected enzymes and their regulator molecules at high pressure. Here we may consider the case of the enzyme fructose diphosphatase (FDP-ase) which was extracted from the liver of the trout (Hochachka, Schneider & Moon 1971). The hydrolysis of fructose diphosphate (FDP) to fructose-6-phosphate and inorganic phosphate is catalysed by this enzyme which is inhibited by high concentrations of AMP, and activated by FDP and Mg^{++} ions.

The experiments were carried out at 3°C because comparisons with the enzymes from deep sea fish were being attempted in the study. Kinetic constants for the two activating agents were determined at high pressure. The K_m for FDP was doubled by 400 ATS, suggesting that such a pressure reduced the affinity of the enzyme for its substrate. The K_a for Mg^{++} was doubled by 800 ATS, and the K_i for AMP was halved by the

same pressure. Fig. 7.16 shows how varying substrate concentration leads to an acceleration or an inhibition of the FDP-ase reaction at pressure. At high substrate concentration the ΔV_2† is −40 $cm^3/mole^{-1}$ (Table 7.3).

The general conclusion is that high pressure affects the rate of reaction of FDP-ase in physiological conditions (low substrate concentrations), by way of the ΔV of the enzyme–regulator interaction. However, the fact should not be overlooked that if a trout was subjected to pressure treatment sufficient to affect its liver metabolism then drastic changes would simultaneously occur in its nervous and cardiovascular systems!

CONCLUSIONS

In many cases high pressures act to exert a physiological effect, not by compression, but by dissociation. Pressure affects all aspects of physiology and biochemistry to some extent. Table 7.5 summarizes some of the physiological effects of moderate pressures, indicating the kind of research necessary to extend man's safe depth range. The effects listed are manifestations of subtle molecular changes which are of considerable academic interest.

The response of excitable tissue to high pressure seems a particularly important area for future work. The physiology of marine animals, whose adaptations to high pressure are beginning to be studied, has obvious comparative interest in diving physiology. Those animals which do not live particularly deep but which undergo long-range vertical migrations also have special properties of interest. The Weddell seal, not yet a laboratory mammal, would appear to have a nervous system well suited to diving. It can descend to 500 m (51 ATA) in a few minutes and hunt, presumably without experiencing tremor or convulsions.

Our understanding of the multivarious ways in which hydrostatic pressure affects human divers should make substantial progress if we apply high pressure techniques to otherwise well-studied physiological preparations and take advantage of the comparative experiments which Nature has provided.

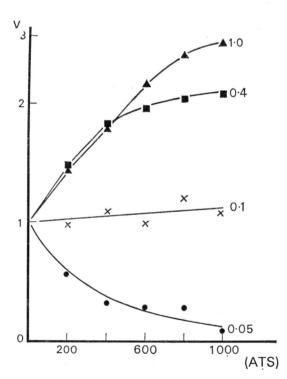

FIG. 7.16. Effect of pressure on the relative reaction velocity of trout liver FDP-ase at different concentrations of FDP, shown in millimoles on each curve (after Hochachaka, Schneider & Moon 1971)

TABLE 7.5

Some physiological effects of moderate hydrostatic pressures. Rate of pressure change and other conditions are ignored in this summary (for details and references see text)

Pressure in atmospheres above atmospheric	Effect
0·01	Threshold pressure to elicit swimming response in *Synchelidium*. Other crustacea are less sensitive.
7	Reduction in threshold current squid axon
20	Change in EEG in humans undergoing simulated dives
30	Increased latency in rabbit duodenum response to acetylcholine
50	Marked hyperexcitability in animals
	Disaggregates sickle cell haemoglobin
	Significant shift in monomer–polymer equilibria in proteins, e.g. myosin
	Greatest depth (pressure) to which the Weddell seal normally dives
60	Experienced by humans with no ill effects
	Increase in tension produced by striated and cardiac muscle
	Approximately halves potency of narcotic gases and other agents in newts, with lesser effects in mice
80	Na^+ efflux from erythrocytes reduced
	Exceeds convulsion threshold for primates
100	Frog skin hyperpolarized
	Amphibian motor nerves increase their response to submaximal stimuli
	Affects oxyhaemoglobin equilibrium slightly
	Tolerated for hours by mammals and for days by invertebrates
	10% change in K for equilibrium involving ΔV of 23 cm^3/mole^{-1} at 30°C

Acknowledgements

This chapter was completed during a sabbatical term at the Institute of Marine Biomedical Research, University of North Carolina at Wilmington. The author is grateful to the Director, Dr. R. Brauer, for commenting constructively on the manuscript.

REFERENCES

AKERS, T. K. & CARLSON, L. D. (1975) The changes in smooth muscle receptor coupling of acetylcholine and norepinephrine at high pressure. In *Underwater Physiology. Vth Symp. Underwater Physiology*. Ed. C. J. Lambertsen. Bethesda: Fedn Am. Socs exp. Biol.

ALBRIGHT, L. J. & MORITA, R. Y. (1968) Effect of hydrostatic pressure on synthesis of protein, ribonucleic acid and deoxyribonucleic acid by the psychrophilic marine bacterium *Vibrio marinus*. *Limnol. Oceanogr.* **13**, 637–643.

ARNOLD, R. M. & ALBRIGHT, L. J. (1971) Hydrostatic pressure effects on the translation stages of protein synthesis in a cell free system from *E. coli*. *Biochim. biophys. Acta* **238**, 506–512.

ARNSTEIN, H. R. V. (1965) Mechanism of protein biosynthesis. *Br. med. Bull.* **21**, 217–222.

BRAUER, R. (1972) In *Barobiology and the Experimental Biology of the Deep Sea*, pp. 1–13. Chapel Hill: University of North Carolina Sea Grant Program.

BROUHA, A., PEQUEUX, A., SCHOFFENIELS, E. & DISTECHE, A. (1970) The effects of high hydrostatic pressure on the permeability characteristics of the isolated frog skin. *Biochim. biophys. Acta* **219**, 455–462.

BROWN, D. E. S. (1934) The effect of rapid changes in hydrostatic pressure upon the contraction of skeletal muscle. *J. cell. comp. Physiol.* **4**, 257–281.

BROWN, D. E. S. (1936) The effect of rapid compression upon events in the isometric contraction of skeletal muscle. *J. cell. comp. Physiol.* **8**, 141–157.

BROWN, D. E. S. (1957) In *Influence of Temperature on Biological Systems*. Ed. F. G. Johnson. American Physiological Society.

BROWN, D. E. S. & EDWARDS, D. J. (1932) A contracture phenomenon in cross-striated muscle. *Am. J. Physiol.* **101**, 15–16.

BROWN, D. E. S. & GOODALL, M. C. (1956) Reversal of relaxing mechanism in muscle fibre systems by hydrostatic pressure. *Nature, Lond.* **178**, 1470–1471.

BROWN, D. E. S., JOHNSON, F. G. & MARSLAND, D. A. (1942) The pressure, temperature relations of bacterial luminescence. *J. cell. comp. Physiol.* **20**, 151–168.

CASSELL, J. M. & CHRISTENSEN, R. G. (1967) Volume change on formation of native collagen aggregate. *Biopolymers* **5**, 431–437.

CATTELL, M. (1935) Changes in the efficiency of muscular contraction under pressure. *J. cell. comp. Physiol.* **6**, 277–290.

CATTELL, M. (1936) The physiological effects of pressure. *Biol. Rev.* **11**, 441–475.

DEFANT, A. (1961) *Physical Oceanography.* Vol. 1. Oxford: Pergamon Press.

DIGBY, P. S. B. (1972) Detection of small changes in hydrostatic pressure by Crustacea and its relation to electrode action in the cuticle. *Symp. Soc. exp. Biol.* **26**, 445–472.

DISTECHE, A. (1972) Effects of pressure on the dissociation of weak acids. *Symp. Soc. exp. Biol.* **26**, 27–60.

DRAPER, J. W. & EDWARDS, D. J. (1932) Some effects of high pressure on developing marine forms. *Biol. Bull.* **63**, 99.

DROST-HANSEN, W. (1972) Effects of pressure on the structure of water in various aqueous systems. *Symp. Soc. exp. Biol.* **26**, 61–101.

EBBECKE, U. (1914) Action of pressure on frog muscle. (In German.) *Pflügers Arch. ges. Physiol.* **157**, 79–116.

EBBECKE, U. (1935a) On the effects of high pressures on marine organisms. (In German.) *Pflügers Arch. ges. Physiol.* **236**, 648–657.

EBBECKE, U. (1935b) The behavior of *Paramecium* under the influence of high pressures. (In German.) *Pflügers Arch. ges. Physiol.* **236**, 658–661.

EBBECKE, U. (1935c) Muscle spasm and tetanus under the influence of compression. (In German.) *Pflügers Arch. ges. Physiol.* **236**, 669–677.

EBBECKE, U. & SCHAEFER, H. (1935) Effect of high pressure on the action potential in muscle and nerve. (In German.) *Pflügers Arch. ges. Physiol.* **236**, 679–692.

EDWARDS, D. J. & CATTELL, M. (1928) The stimulating action of hydrostatic pressure on cardiac function. *Am. J. Physiol.* **84**, 472–484.

EDWARDS, D. J. & CATTELL, M. (1930) The action of compression on the contraction of heart muscle. *Am. J. Physiol.* **93**, 80–96.

ENNS, T., SCHOLANDER, P. F. & BRADSTREET, E. D. (1964) Effect of hydrostatic pressure on gases dissolved in water. *J. phys. Chem., Ithaca* **69**, 289–391.

ENRIGHT, J. T. (1962) Responses of an Amphipod to pressure changes. *Comp. Biochem. Physiol.* **7**, 131–145.

FENN, W. O. (1969) The physiological effects of hydrostatic pressures. In *The Physiology and Medicine of Diving and Compressed Air Work.* Ed. P. B. Bennett & D. H. Elliott. London: Baillière Tindall & Cassell.

FENN, W. O. (1972) Partial pressures of gases dissolved at great depths. *Science, N.Y.* **176**, 1011–1012.

FENN, W. O. & BOSCHEN, V. (1969) Oxygen consumption of frog tissues under high hydrostatic pressure. *Resp. Physiology.* **7**, 335–340.

FONTAINE, M. (1928) Sur les analogues existant entre les effets d'une tetanisation et ceux d'une compression. *C.r. hebd. Séanc. Acad. Sci., Paris* **186**, 99–101.

FREUNDLICH, H. (1937) Some recent work on gels. *J. phys. Chem., Ithaca* **41**, 901–910.

GERBER, B. R. & NOGUCHI, H. (1967) Volume change associated with the G–F transition of flagellin. *J. molec. Biol.* **26**, 196–210.

GERSHFIELD, N. L. & SHANES, A. M. (1959) The influence of high hydrostatic pressure on cocaine and veratrine action in a vertebrate nerve. *J. gen. Physiol.* **42**, 647–653.

GRUNDFEST, H. (1936) Effects of hydrostatic pressure upon the excitability, the recovery and the potential sequence in the frog nerve. *Cold Spring Harb. Symp. quant. Biol.* **4**, 179–187.

HERMOLIN, J. & ZIMMERMAN, A. M. (1969) The effect of pressure on synchronous cultures of *Tetrahymena*: a ribosome study. *Cytobios.* B, 247–256.

HEYMAN, E. (1936) Studies on sol–gel transformations. *Trans. Faraday Soc.* **32**, 462–473.

HILDEBRAND, C. E. & POLLARD, E. C. (1972) Hydrostatic pressure effects on protein synthesis. *Biophys. J.* **12**, 1235–1250.

HILLS, G. J., OVENDEN, P. J. & WHITEHOUSE, D. R. (1965) Proton migration in aqueous solution. *Discuss. Faraday Soc.* **39**, 207–215.

HOCHACHKA, P. W., SCHNEIDER, D. E. & MOON, T. W. (1971) The adaptation of enzymes to pressure. 1. A comparison of trout liver Fructose Diphosphatase with the Homologous enzyme from an off-shore benthic fish. *Am. Zool.* **11**, 479–490.

HORNE, R. A. (1969) *Marine Chemistry.* New York: Interscience.

HORNE, R. A. & JOHNSON, D. S. (1966) The viscosity of compressed seawater. *J. geophys. Res.* **71**, 5275–5277.

HSAI, J. C. & BLOGGS, J. M. (1973) Pressure effect on the membrane action of a nerve-blocking spin label. *Proc. natn. Acad. Sci. U.S.A.* **70**, 3179–3183.

IKKAI, T. & OOI, T. (1966) Actin: volume change on transformation of G-form to F-form. *Science, N.Y.* **152**, 1756–1757.

INFANTE, A. A. & KRAUSS, M. (1971) Dissociation of ribosomes induced by centrifugation: evidence for doubting conformational changes in ribosomes. *Biochim. biophys. Acta.* **246**, 81–99.

JOHNSON, F. G., BROWN, D. E. S. & MARSLAND, D. A. (1942) Pressure reversal of the action of certain narcotics. *J. cell. comp. Physiol.* **20**, 269–276.

JOHNSON, F. G., EYRING, H. & POLISSAR, M. J. (1954) *The Kinetic Basis of Molecular Biology.* New York: John Wiley.

JOHNSON, F. H. & FLAGLER, E. A. (1951) Activity of narcotized amphibian larvae under hydrostatic pressure. *J. cell. Comp. Physiol.* **37**, 15–25.

JOHNSON, S. M. & MILLER, K. W. (1970) Antagonism of pressure and anaesthesia. *Nature, Lond.* **228**, 75–76.

JOSEPHS, R. & HARRINGTON, W. F. (1968) On the stability of myosin filaments. *Biochemistry, N.Y.* **7**, 2834–2847.

KENNEDY, J. R. & ZIMMERMAN, A. M. (1970) The effects of high hydrostatic pressure on the microtubules of *Tetrahymena pyriformis*. *J. Cell Biol.* **47**, 568–576.

KETTMAN, M. S., NISHIKAWA, A. H., MORITA, R. Y. & BECKER, R. R. (1965) Effect of hydrostatic pressure on the aggregation reaction of poly-L-valyl-ribonuclease. *Biochem. biophys. Res. Commun.* **22**, 262–267.

KIESOW, L. A., BLESS, J. W., SHELTON, J. B. (1973) Oxygen dissociation in human erythrocytes: its response to hyperbaric environments. *Science, N.Y.* **179**, 1236–1238.

KIRKNESS, C. M. & MACDONALD, A. G. (1972) Interaction between anaesthetics and hydrostatic pressure in the division of *Tetrahymena pyriformis* W. *Expl Cell Res.* **75**, 329–336.

KIRKNESS, C. M. & MACDONALD, A. G. (1973) Effect of helium pressure on the narcotic potency of nitrogen in dividing cells. *Försvarsmedicin* **9**, 310–313.

KITCHING, J. A. (1957) Effects of high hydrostatic pressures on *Actinophrys sol* (Heliozoa). *J. exp. Biol.* **34**, 511–517.

KITCHING, J. A. (1970) Some effects of high pressure on Protozoa. In *High Pressure Effects on Cellular Processes*, pp. 155–177. Ed. A. M. Zimmerman. New York: Academic Press.

KYLSTRA, J. A., NANTZ, R., CROWE, J., WAGNER, W. & SALTZMAN, H. A. (1967) Hydraulic compression of mice to 166 atmospheres. *Science, N.Y.* **158**, 793–794.

LAIDLER, K. J. (1951) Influence of pressure on the rates of biological reactions. *Archs Biochem. Biophys.* **30**, 226–236.

LAIDLER, K. J. & BEARDELL, A. J. (1955) Molecular kinetics of muscle adenosine-triphosphatase III influence of hydrostatic pressure. *Archs Biochem. Biophys.* **55**, 138–151.

LANDAU, J. V. (1960) Sol-gel transformations in fibroblasts of embryonic chick heart tissue: A pressure–temperature study. *Expl Cell Res.* **21**, 78–87.

LANDAU, J. V. (1961) The effect of high hydrostatic pressure on human cells in primary and continuous culture. *Expl Cell Res.* **23**, 538–549.

LANDAU, J. V. (1967) Induction, transcription and translation in *E. coli*—a hydrostatic pressure study. *Biochim. biophys. Acta* **149**, 506–512.

LANDAU, J. V. (1970) In *High Pressure Effects on Cellular Processes*. Ed. A. M. Zimmerman. New York: Academic Press.

LANDAU, J. V. & MARSLAND, D. A. (1952) Temperature–pressure studies on the cardiac rate in tissue culture explants from the heart of the tadpole. *J. cell. comp. Physiol.* **40**, 367–381.

LANDAU, J. V. & PEABODY, R. A. (1963) Endogenous adenosine triphosphate levels in human amnion cells during application of high hydrostatic pressure. *Expl. Cell Res.* **29**, 54–60.

LANDAU, J. V., ZIMMERMAN, A. M. & MARSLAND, D. A. (1954) Temperature–pressure experiments on amoeba proteus; plasmagel structure in relation to form and movement. *J. cell. comp. Physiol.* **44**, 211–232.

LAUFFER, M. (1964) In *Symposium on Foods: Proteins and their reactions*. Ed. H. W. Schultz & A. F. Anglemain. Westport, Connecticut: A.M.I. pub. Co.

LAZARRE, R. & BODAR, B. (1956) Measurement of the viscosity of argon compressed to 3000 kg/cm². (In French.) *C.r. hebd. Séanc. Acad. Sci., Paris* **243**, 487–489.

LETTS, P. J. & ZIMMERMAN, A. M. (1970) Polypeptide synthesis with microsomes from pressure-treated *Tetrahymena*. *J. Protozool.* **17**, 593–596.

LEVER, M. J., MILLER, K. W., PATON, W. D. M. & SMITH, E. B. (1971) Pressure reversal of anaesthesia. *Nature, Lond.* **231**, 368–371.

LINCOLN, R. J. (1970) A laboratory investigation into the effect of hydrostatic pressure on the vertical migration of planktonic crustacea. *Mar. Biol.* **6**, 5–11.

LINDERSTROM-LANG, K. & JACOBSEN, C. F. (1941) The contraction accompanying enzymatic breakdown of proteins. *C.r. Trav. Lab. Carlsberg* **24**, 1–46.

MACDONALD, A. G. (1965) The effect of high hydrostatic pressure on the oxygen consumption of *Tetrahymena pyriformis* W. *Expl Cell Res.* **40**, 78–84.

MACDONALD, A. G. (1967a) Delay in the cleavage of *Tetrahymena pyriformis* exposed to high hydrostatic pressure. *J. cell. Physiol.* **70**, 127–129.

MACDONALD, A. G. (1967b) The effect of high hydrostatic pressure on the cell division and growth of *Tetrahymena pyriformis*. *Expl Cell Res.* **47**, 569–580.

MACDONALD, A. G. (1972) The role of high hydrostatic pressure in the physiology of marine animals. *Symp. Soc. exp. Biol.* **26**, 209–231.

MACDONALD, A. G. (1973a) *Physiological Aspects of Deep Sea Biology*. Monograph of the Physiological Society. Cambridge: Cambridge University Press (In press.)

MACDONALD, A. G. (1973b) Locomotor activity and oxygen consumption in shallow and deep sea invertebrates exposed to high pressure and low temperature. In *Underwater Physiology. Vth Symp. Underwater Physiology*. Ed. C. J. Lambertsen. Bethesda: Fedn Am. Socs exp. Biol.

MACDONALD, A. G. & MILLER, K. (1975) Biological membranes at high hydrostatic pressures. In *Biophysical and Biochemical Perspectives in Marine Biology*, III. Academic Press (In press.)

MARQUIS, R. E. & FENN, W. O. (1969) Dilatometric study of streptococcal growth and metabolism. *Can. J. Microbiol.* **15**, 933–940.

MARQUIS, R. E., BROWN, W. P. & FENN, W. O. (1971) Pressure sensitivity of Streptococcal growth in relation to catabolism. *J. Bact.* **105**, 504–511.

MARSLAND, D. A. (1938) The effects of high hydrostatic pressure upon cell division in Arbacia eggs. *J. cell. comp. Physiol.* **12**, 57–70.

MARSLAND, D. A. (1950) The mechanism of cell division: temperature pressure experiments of the cleaving eggs of *Arbacia punctulata*. *J. cell. comp. Physiol.* **36**, 205–227.

MARSLAND, D. A. (1970) In *High Pressure Effects on Cellular Processes*. Ed. A. M. Zimmerman. New York: Academic Press.

MCMEEKIN, T. L., GROVES, M. L. & HIPP, N. J. (1954) Partial specific volume of the protein and water in Betalactoglobulin crystals. *J. Polym. Sci.* **12**, 309–315.

MENZIES, R. J. & GEORGE, R. Y. (1972) Hydrostatic pressure–temperature effects on deep sea colonization. *Proc. R. Soc. Edinb.* **B 73**, 195–202.

MILLER, K. W. (1972) Inert gas narcosis and animals under high pressure. *Symp. Soc. exp. Biol.* **26**, 363–378.

MURAYAMA, M. & HASEGAWA, F. (1970) Effect of hydrostatic pressure on the aggregation reaction of human fibrin. *Fedn Proc. Fedn Am. Socs exp. Biol.* **29**, 401.

NAROSKA, V. (1968) Comparative investigations into the influence of hydrostatic pressure on the viability and metabolic rates of marine invertebrates and telecosts. (In German.) *Kieler Meeresfors.* 24, 95–123.

NEVILLE, W. M. & EYRING, H. (1972) Hydrostatic pressure and ionic strength effects on the kinetics of lysozyme. *Proc. natn Acad. Sci. U.S.A.* 69, 2417–2419.

ORNHAGEN, H. C. & LUNDGREN, C. E. G. (1973) Hydrostatic pressure tolerance in liquid breathing mice. In *Underwater Physiology. Vth Symp. Underwater Physiology.* Ed. C. J. Lambertsen. Bethesda: Fedn Am. Socs. exp. Biol.

PAUL, K. L. & MORITA, R. Y. (1971) Effects of hydrostatic pressure and temperature on the uptake and respiration of amino acids by a facultatively psychrophilic marine bacterium. *J. Bact.* 108, 835–843.

PAYENS, T. A. J. & HERMANS, K. (1969) Effects of pressure on the temperature-dependent association of B-casein. *Biopolymers* 8, 335–345.

PEASE, D. C. (1946) Hydrostatic pressure effects upon the spindle figure and chromosome movement. II Experiments on the meiotic divisions of *Tradescantia* pollen mother cells. *Biol. Bull.* 91, 145–169.

PENNISTON, J. T. (1971) High hydrostatic pressure and enzymic activity: Inhibition of multimeric enzymes by dissociation. *Archs Biochem. Biophys.* 142, 322–332.

PODOLSKY, R. L. J. (1956) A mechanism for the effect of hydrostatic pressure on biological systems. *J. Physiol.* 132, 38P.

POLLARD, E. C. & WELLER, P. K. (1966) The effect of hydrostatic pressure on the synthetic processes in bacteria. *Biochim. biophys. Acta* 112, 573–580.

QUTOB, Z. (1962) The swimbladder of fishes as a pressure receptor. *Archs néerl. Zool.* 15, 1–67.

REGNARD, P. (1885) Phenomenes objectifs que l'on peut observer sur les animaux soumis aux hautes pressions. *C.r. Séanc. Soc. Biol.* 37, 510–515.

REGNARD, P. (1891) *Recherches experimentales sur les conditions physiques de la vie dans les eaux.* Paris: Mason.

ROTH, S. H., SMITH, R. A. & PATON, W. D. M. (1975) Pressure reversal of nitrous oxide conduction failure in peripheral nerve. In *Underwater Physiology. Vth Symp. Underwater Physiology.* Ed. C. J. Lambertsen. Bethesda: Fedn Am. Socs exp. Biol.

RUGH, R. & MARSLAND, D. A. (1943) The effect of hydrostatic pressure upon the early development of the frog's egg (Rana pipiens). *Proc. Am. Phil. Soc.* 86, 459–466.

SMITH, E. B. (1969) The role of exotic gases in the study of narcosis. In *The Physiology and Medicine of Diving and Compressed Air Work.* Ed. P. B. Bennett & D. H. Elliott. London: Baillière Tindall & Cassell.

SPYROPOULOS, C. S. (1957a) Response of single nerve fibres at different hydrostatic pressures. *Am. J. Physiol.* 189, 214–218.

SPYROPOULOS, C. S. (1957b) The effects of hydrostatic pressure upon the normal and narcotized nerve fibre. *J. gen. Physiol.* 40, 849–857.

SUZUKI, K. & TANIGUCHI, Y. (1972) Effect of pressure on biopolymers and model systems. *Symp. Soc. exp. Biol.* 26, 103–124.

SUZUKI, K., TANIGUCHI, Y. & ENOMOTO, T. (1972) The effect of pressure on the sol–gel transformation of macromolecules. *Bull. chem. Soc. Japan.* 45, 336–338.

SWEENEY, J. B. (1970) *A pictorial history of oceanographic submersibles.* New York: Crown publishers.

TALWAR, G. P., MACHEBOEUFF, M. A. & BASSETT, J. (1954) Some aspects of the influence of hydrostatic pressures on reactions catalysed by enzymes. *J. Colloid Sci.* 9, Suppl.

TILNEY, L. G. & CARDELL, R. R. (1969) The determination of cell polarity as exemplified by the reformation of micro villi and terminal web after pressure induced disassembly. *J. Cell Biol.* 43, 46. (Abstract.)

TILNEY, L. G., HIRAMOTO, Y. & MARSLAND, D. (1966) Studies on microtubules in Heliozoa. III A pressure analysis of the role of these structures in the formation and maintenance of the axopodia of *Actinosphaerium nucleofilum.* *J. Cell Biol.* 29, 77–95.

WELLS, J. M. (1975) Hydrostatic pressure and hemoglobin oxygenation. In *Underwater Physiology. Vth Symp. Underwater Physiology.* Ed. C. J. Lambertsen. Bethesda: Fedn Am. Socs exp. Biol.

WERBIN, H. & McLAREN, A. D. (1951) The effect of high pressure on the rates of proteolytic hydrolysis. 1. Chymotrypsin. *Archs Biochem. Biophys.* 31, 285–293.

WILLIAMS, R. K. & SHEN, C. (1972) The effect of pressure on the activity of ribonuclease. *Archs Biochem. Biophys.* 152, 606–612.

YASUDA, H. (1959) Effects of high hydrostatic pressure on the cardiac muscle. Part 1. On the isolated frog heart. *J. Okayama med. Soc.* 71, 5855.

YAYANOS, A. A. (1972) Apparent molal volume of glycine, glycolamide, alanine, lactamide and glycylglycine in aqueous solution at 25°C and high pressure. *J. phys. Chem., Ithaca* 76, 1783–1792.

YAYANOS, A. A. & POLLARD, E. C. (1969) A study of the effects of hydrostatic pressure on macromolecular synthesis in *Escherischia coli. Biophys. J.* 9, 1464–1482.

ZAMYATNIN, A. A. (1972) Protein volume in solution. *Prog. Biophys. molec. Biol.* 24, 109–123.

ZIMMERMAN, A. M. (1971) High pressure studies in Cell Biology. *Int. Rev. Cytol.* 30, 1–47.

ZIMMERMAN, A. M. & MARSLAND, D. A. (1964) Cell division: effects of pressure on the mitotic mechanisms of marine eggs (*Arbacia punctulata*). *Expl Cell Res.* 35, 293–302.

ZIMMERMAN, A. M. & RUSTAD, R. (1965) Effects of high pressures on pinocytosis in *Amoeba proteus. J. Cell Biol.* 25, 397–400.

ZIMMERMAN, A. M. & SILBERMAN, L. (1965) Cell division, the effect of hydrostatic pressure on the cleavage schedule in *Arbacia punctuluta. Expl Cell Res.* 38, 454–464.

ZIMMERMAN, A. M. (1969) In *The Cell Cycle,* pp. 203–225. Ed. G. M. Padilla, G. L. Whitson & I. L. Cameron. New York: Academic Press.

ZOBELL, C. E. & KIM, J. (1972) Effects of deep sea pressures on microbial enzyme systems. *Symp. Soc. exp. Biol.* 26, 125–146.

8

Pulmonary Function

E. H. LANPHIER

The ability of divers to do useful work underwater and the safety of such work at various depths both depend in large part upon respiratory variables. The purpose of this chapter is to examine some of these variables, to explore their interrelationships with environmental conditions and diving equipment, and to assess their implications.

Energy for life and activity is obtained almost solely from the chemical reactions of oxidative metabolism. The 'fuel' for metabolism is derived from food and is readily stored by the body, but oxygen must be supplied to the sites of metabolic reactions on a moment-to-moment basis closely matched to need. Similarly, carbon dioxide must be eliminated at essentially the same rate as it is being produced by these reactions.

When the delivery of oxygen or the removal of carbon dioxide is hampered by disease, environmental factors, or breathing apparatus, physical activity will be restricted proportionally. Severe restriction of the exchange of these gases will threaten life.

Respiratory gas exchange includes many steps. It begins with inspiration of a suitable gas that can give up oxygen to the blood in the lungs. It includes the processes of blood–gas transport and diffusion that carry oxygen to the actual places of metabolic oxidation in the active tissue cells. Respiratory exchange can be so defined as to include the energy-producing reactions within the cells. It must, in any case, include transport of carbon dioxide from the cells to the lungs and the process whereby the appropriate quantity of CO_2 is finally exhaled.

This chapter is entitled Pulmonary Function because its focus of attention is upon the process of gas exchange within the lungs. Other aspects of the respiratory process will be mentioned, but it is within the lungs that the effects of the underwater environment and of increased ambient pressure are most clearly evident.

The discussion will begin with the metabolic cost of different types and degrees of activity. A given level of energy expenditure in turn entails a corresponding rate of oxygen consumption and carbon dioxide production. These, in turn, call for a certain rate of alveolar ventilation. Factors such as respiratory dead space and presence of CO_2 in the inspired gas determine what rate of total pulmonary ventilation will yield the required volume of effective alveolar ventilation per unit time.

The most common disorder of pulmonary function in the high pressure-underwater environment is simple insufficiency of alveolar ventilation. The most important consequence is elevation of alveolar and arterial carbon dioxide pressure.

Increased gas density is the environmental factor that most commonly causes deficiency of pulmonary and alveolar ventilation. Increased work of breathing or restriction of expiratory flow, or both, may be responsible for limitation of ventilatory capacity. Whether abnormalities of intrapulmonary gas distribution or diffusion become important at higher pressures is less clear.

This chapter will attempt to summarize current knowledge concerning respiratory effects encountered underwater and under high pressure and what is known about their influence upon the work capacity and safety of divers. A background of basic physiological information is provided in the hope of making the whole subject intelligible.

Several closely related topics are covered elsewhere in this volume and will be mentioned only as necessary to clarify their relationship to pulmonary function. Among other subjects considered beyond the scope of this chapter are breath holding and breath-hold diving. These have been reviewed (Rahn & Yokoyama 1965) and are the subject of continuing study.

OXYGEN CONSUMPTION

The level of physical activity is the most important factor that determines the body's need for oxygen. In turn, oxygen consumption provides the most useful index of exertion.

Energy equivalent to about 5 kilocalories (kcal) is derived in the course of consuming one litre of oxygen. In this chapter, oxygen consumption will be abbreviated $\dot{V}_{O_2}$ [1] and expressed in litres per minute corrected to standard conditions (L/min STPD).[2]

Fig. 8.1 presents two widely utilized classifications of work. Parallel scales are provided as a means of relating several potentially confusing ways in which activity is often quantified. Indications of maximum oxygen uptake ($\dot{V}_{O_{2max}}$) in different groups are also presented.

At rest and in many activities, body size influences $\dot{V}_{O_2}$. A simple and often adequate way of taking this factor into account is to assume that $\dot{V}_{O_2}$ is proportional to body weight. Some of the values in Fig. 8.1 have been expressed in ml/kg.min, assuming the traditional 70 kg (154 pound) 'average man'. Multiples of assumed basal and resting $\dot{V}_{O_2}$ values have also been indicated.

Values of $\dot{V}_{O_2}$ for a wide variety of activities are presented in Fig. 8.2. Some of the few available values for underwater work are included. Fig. 8.3 assembles most of the available data on the O_2 cost of underwater fin swimming. Morrison

(1973) reports a study of maximum effort in stationary fin swimming against a submerged 'trapeze' at various simulated depths. His maximum values closely approximate the mean and range reported by Lanphier (1954) for swimming at 1·2 knots.

Study of an actual submerged long-distance ocean swim was reported by Hunt, Reeves and Beckman (1964). $\dot{V}_{O_2}$ was not measured directly, but values between 1·3 and 1·8 L/min can be surmised from other measurements. Speeds were estimated to be between 1·0 and 1·2 miles per hour.

Aerobic capacity

At any given moment, an individual's $\dot{V}_{O_2}$ must necessarily lie somewhere between his minimum or basal value and the highest $\dot{V}_{O_2}$ of which his body is capable. Allowing for body size and completeness of relaxation, minimum adult values of $\dot{V}_{O_2}$ can be as low as 0·2 L/min. A commonly used 'average resting' value is 0·3 L/min.

Every individual has an upper limit oxygen uptake that can be reached in very heavy work involving major muscle groups. $\dot{V}_{O_{2max}}$ (maximum $\dot{V}_{O_2}$ or 'aerobic capacity') is governed in healthy men at sea level by the ability of the circulatory system to transport oxygen from the lungs to the working muscles (see, for example, Ouellet, Poh & Becklake 1969). As will be seen, ventilatory restrictions can limit $\dot{V}_{O_{2max}}$ at depth (Cook 1970; Miller, Wangensteen & Lanphier 1971).

As indicated in Fig. 8.1, $\dot{V}_{O_{2max}}$ varies widely even among healthy young males. With allowance for body size and constitutional factors, $\dot{V}_{O_{2max}}$ depends mainly upon the individual's state of athletic training. $\dot{V}_{O_{2max}}$ is almost universally accepted as the best available index of cardiovascular and respiratory 'fitness'.

For a diver of average size and reasonable 'fitness', a $\dot{V}_{O_{2max}}$ of at least 3·0 L/min can probably be expected. Values as high as 6 L/min are reported only rarely (Wilmore & Haskell 1972; Hanson 1973). A diver who has an unusually high value of maximum oxygen uptake for his size has

---

[1] In standard respiratory symbols (Pappenheimer 1950), V represents a gas volume while $\dot{V}$ represents volume per unit time, or flow. The subscript indicates the volume at issue. For example, $\dot{V}_{O_2}$ represents the rate of oxygen consumption by the body while $\dot{V}_E$ signifies the volume of gas expired per unit time.

[2] Standard Temperature (0°C) and Pressure (760 mm Hg), Dry gas. This correction is applied to $\dot{V}_{O_2}$ and $\dot{V}_{CO_2}$, where the number of molecules involved in metabolic reactions per unit time depends upon the level of activity and is essentially independent of ambient pressure and other environmental factors.

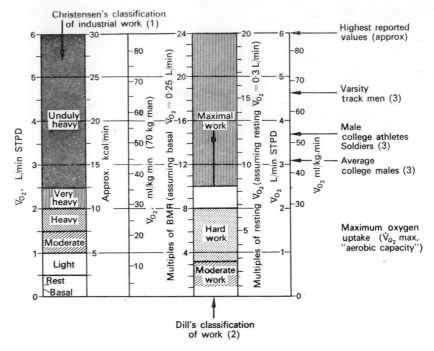

FIG. 8.1. Oxygen costs of activity

Parallel scales are provided to relate the often-confusing ways in which metabolic costs of activity are sometimes expressed. The primary unit used in this chapter is $\dot{V}_{O_2}$ in L/min. Another commonly used unit is the equivalent number of kilocalories, kcal (energy in units of heat). The relationship between kcal and litres of O_2 varies somewhat with the respiratory quotient (RQ), but the factor 5 kcal/L of O_2 is sufficiently accurate for usual purposes. The kcal/min scale given here is based on this factor. Expression of $\dot{V}_{O_2}$ in ml/kg of body weight is frequently desirable. The ml/kg scale given here applies, in its relationship to the $\dot{V}_{O_2}$ L/min scale, only to a 70-kg man. Scales representing O_2 uptake in multiples of basal and resting $\dot{V}_{O_2}$ are also provided, based on assumed values of 0·25 L/min for basal $\dot{V}_{O_2}$ and 0·3 L/min for resting $\dot{V}_{O_2}$.

In addition to the scales, two major classifications of work are presented: (1) that of Christensen (1953), in terms of $\dot{V}_{O_2}$ L/min or kcal/min, and (2) that of Dill (1936), expressed in multiples of basal $\dot{V}_{O_2}$. At the right, approximate values of maximum $\dot{V}_{O_2}$ ($\dot{V}_{O_2max}$ or 'aerobic capacity') are indicated for different groups. The values (3) were derived from data presented by Taylor et al. (1963)

special advantages in diving, especially in terms of his ventilatory requirements at high work rates. By the same token, a man whose state of fitness is poor will be under serious disadvantages in diving as will become apparent later in this chapter.

The influence of the aqueous environment on $\dot{V}_{O_2max}$ is potentially important. Holmér (1972) reported inability of surface swimmers to match, in flume swimming, the $\dot{V}_{O_2max}$ they could achieve in dry land exercise. Dixon and Faulkner (1971) reported similar findings in untrained swimmers doing tethered swimming but found the

same $\dot{V}_{O_2max}$ in trained swimmers whether in running or swimming.

Moore et al. (1970) reported no decrement in performance when non-swimming leg work was performed during total submergence. Morrison (1973) reports results suggestive of a limitation of $\dot{V}_{O_2max}$ in fin swimming against a 'trapeze', but breathing apparatus effects may have influenced the findings.

The influence of inspiratory oxygen pressure ($P_{I_{O_2}}$)[1] is also important. Lowered $P_{I_{O_2}}$ drops $\dot{V}_{O_2max}$ significantly and dramatically reduces endurance time (Gleser & Vogel 1973). Elevation

[1] Standard respiratory symbols let P indicate the partial pressure of a gas. Here, the subscripts indicate that the pressure at issue is that of oxygen in the inspired gas.

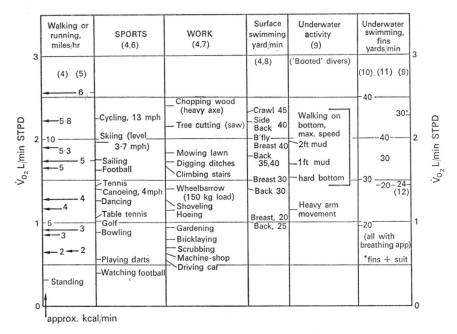

F IG. 8.2. Oxygen costs of activity

Oxygen cost of various types and levels of activity. Approximate average values are indicated (in terms of $\dot{V}o_2$ L/min and kcal/min) to help put known and probable underwater requirements into perspective. Many of the values given would be subject to considerable variation depending upon the actual level of activity, size of individual, proficiency, etc.

Sources are indicated by numbers in parenthesis: (4) from a large compilation from many sources by Passmore and Durnin (1955); (5) averages from data of Margaria et al. (1963); (6) data of Covell et al. (1965); (7) from a compilation by Mayer (1959); (8) derived from data of Karpovich and Millman (1944); (9) data of Donald and Davidson (1954); (10) from Lanphier (1954), see also Fig. 8.3; (11) approximate average values derived from open-water swimming data of Goff et al. (1956), see also Fig. 8.3.

Much higher values of $\dot{V}o_2$ are reported for some forms of work and sport than are shown here. However, most of the higher values (as, for example, in surface swimming at higher speeds) apply to relatively brief bursts of activity involving varying proportions of O_2 debt

of P_{IO_2} has relatively minor effects in increasing maximal oxygen uptake. Margaria (1972) administered oxygen at 1 ATA and found an increase of about 8%. Fagraeus et al. (1973) studied $\dot{V}o_{2max}$ with air at different pressures. They found an increase of 9% at 1·4 ATA and no further improvement at 2·0 or 3·0 ATA. Ventilation was markedly reduced at the higher pressures.

Taunton et al. (1970) reported improved work capacity with both air and oxygen at pressures to 2·0 ATA, but actual $\dot{V}o_2$ was not measured. Deroanne et al. (1973) report a 3% increase in $\dot{V}o_{2max}$ with oxygen at 1 ATA and no further

improvement at 2 ATA. Hyperoxic convulsions interfered with measurements at 3 ATA. Cook (1970) maintained a normoxic Po_2 in nitrogen–oxygen mixtures at 2 and 3 ATA. He found marked reductions in pulmonary ventilation and endurance time as well as significant reductions in $\dot{V}o_{2max}$. Moore and his associates (1970) report higher $\dot{V}o_2$ and $\dot{V}E^1$ at all workloads submerged, but it is extremely difficult to be sure that submergence does not alter the actual effort involved in a given task.

In general, it seems safe to assume that submergence and pressure produce no basic change

1. Volume expired per unit time: the usual measure of total pulmonary ventilation. Lung volumes and volumes of pulmonary ventilation are corrected to BTPS Body Temperature (37°C unless otherwise specified), existing barometric Pressure, gas Saturated with water vapour at body temperature. BTPS values are about 1·08 times average ambient (ATPS) room-temperature values. STPD values are roughly 0·8 of BTPS values if the barometric pressure is 760 mm Hg.

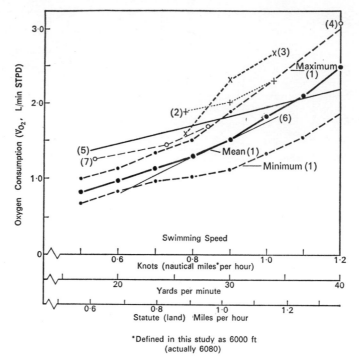

FIG. 8.3. Oxygen consumption in underwater swimming

Values of $\dot{V}_{O_2}$ at various swimming speeds are presented for underwater swimming with fins. The primary data presented (1) are from the USN Experimental Diving Unit (EDU) study reported by Lanphier (1954). The unit of speed in that study was a 'rounded knot' (upper horizontal scale), but more common units of speed are given in parallel scales.

Other sources of data: (2 to 4) points from Donald and Davidson (1954) representing (2) low, mean and high values obtained at speeds of 26 to 34 yards/min in swimmers not wearing protective suits; (3) comparable values in suited swimmers; (4) mean $\dot{V}_{O_2}$ of suited swimmers studied at 34 to 46 yards/min. (5) Approximate average values obtained in two open-water field studies by Goff et al. (1956). (6) Approximate average values from two model-basin studies (circulating water, stationary swimmer) reported by Goff et al. (1957). (7) Approximate average values from 'CUSP' Project (Committee on Amphib. Ops. 1953).

All studies were conducted at shallow depths. (There is no known reason to expect that steady state values for $\dot{V}_{O_2}$ would be different at a given speed at greater depth except perhaps because of increased work of breathing.) Except where noted, swimmers wore minimal protective clothing. In general, only experienced underwater swimmers participated. Different types of fins were employed, and this is known to have an effect on swimming efficiency and thus on $\dot{V}_{O_2}$ at a given speed. Different types of closed circuit scuba were also used, and the configuration of the types probably influenced the swimmers' total 'drag'. None of the apparatus had notably 'streamlined' configuration.

The range of speeds shown here represents the practical range of this form of underwater propulsion with the equipment used (Lanphier 1954). Below 0·7 knot, there was insufficient headway to maintain adequate depth-control. Above 1·2 knots, the swimmers tired rapidly

in the oxygen requirements associated with a given physiological workload. Attention can be focused instead upon ways in which the environment or factors such as breathing apparatus affect the individual's ability to meet his respiratory needs.

Oxygen debt

Most measurements of gas exchange associated with work are made after 4 or 5 minutes of con-tinuous exertion, when the subject is assumed to have reached a *steady state* of respiratory and circulatory adjustment. Variables such as $\dot{V}_{O_2}$, $\dot{V}_E$, and heart rate increase very rapidly at the onset of exertion, but they do not reach steady levels at once. Whipp and Wasserman (1972) report that in leg work $\dot{V}_{O_2}$ reached steady state within 3 minutes at low work rates but that steady state was progressively delayed at higher loads. During very strenuous work, exhaustion may occur before anything approaching a steady state is reached.

Energy is required for muscle contraction from the moment work begins, so the lag in $\dot{V}o_2$ signals an *oxygen deficit* in the first few minutes of even mild exertion. The energy not supplied by aerobic metabolism in this period is derived for the most part from high-energy phosphates (adenosine triphosphate, ATP; creatine phosphate, CP) stored in limited amounts in the muscles themselves. The ATP and CP are resynthesized when work ceases, and resynthesis requires oxygen. The repayment of this kind of *oxygen debt* is seen in that fact that $\dot{V}o_2$ does not drop at once to the resting level but remains elevated briefly during recovery. This form of oxygen debt is always repaid within a very few minutes at most.

Rapidly repaid oxygen debt is also called *alactic* or *alactacid* debt. This distinguishes it from the form of oxygen debt associated with elevation of blood lactic acid levels. *Lactacid* O_2 debt develops primarily when the work rate approaches or exceeds the individual's aerobic capacity, $\dot{V}o_{2max}$. Increasing blood lactate levels signify that energy is being derived from *anaerobic glycolysis*, a metabolic pathway that yields energy inefficiently but without concurrent use of oxygen and whose end-product is lactic acid.

Ability to contract an oxygen debt provides a very desirable safety factor in permitting limited periods of exertion beyond the moment-to-moment or 'pay as you go' limits for the individual or for particular muscles concerned. An alactacid debt is incurred at the onset of work of almost any degree (di Prampero et al. 1970). Some differences of opinion remain concerning the development of lactacid debt in submaximal work (Margaria 1972; Wasserman et al. 1973), but not about the fact that blood lactate increases in continued exertion beyond $\dot{V}o_{2max}$.

For practical purposes, we can accept Shephard's view (1972) that a disproportionate increase in ventilation—presumably reflecting accumulation of acid metabolites in the blood and corresponding to the *anaerobic threshold* of Wasserman et al. (1973)—can be expected at work rates equivalent to between 50 and 80% of the individual's maximal oxygen uptake. Exactly at what work rate the disproportionate increase

occurs will depend upon the type of exercise at issue, the strength of the muscle groups being used, and the state of training of the subject.

Figures provided by Margaria (1972) indicate that the energy available from anaerobic glycolysis in an average man is equivalent to that derived from consumption of less than 4 L oxygen. The ability to mobilize this energy rapidly may be very important in an emergency, but the cost in terms of subsequent performance may be high.

Intermittent work

Information concerning oxygen debt has important applications in connection with intermittent work. Åstrand et al. (1960) reported that a higher total amount of work can be accomplished over a given period with brief bursts of heavy exertion than with maximum sustained effort. Many forms of underwater work are inherently intermittent rather than steady in nature, and it is likely that optimal patterns of intermittent work could be found and exploited for underwater purposes.

Margaria et al. (1969) reported that no lactic acid is found in supramaximal exercise so long as the demand for energy can be met by the alactic phosphagen-splitting mechanism. They confirmed that repayment of this fraction is a fast process. If the debt contracted during the working period is completely paid during the rest period, very heavy intermittent exercise can be carried out indefinitely. Margaria and his co-workers (1969) based their study on treadmill running at a speed and slope that could be maintained continuously for less than 40 sec. When the same work was performed in 10 sec bursts between 30 sec rest periods, this schedule could be kept up indefinitely.

Lactic acid effects

There are several reasons for wishing to limit the production and accumulation of lactic acid. One is its local relationship to muscular fatigue and the very long period required to regain normal work capacity. Where it can be applied, the principle of intermittent work should be useful in accomplishing maximal work without lactacid debt. Otherwise, maintaining steady work at a level that can be kept up for a long time is much better than producing lactic acid in the course of ill-conceived episodes of heavy exertion.

An even more important aspect of lactacid debt underwater is its relationship to respiration. Disproportionate increases in pulmonary ventilation can be very troublesome and quite possibly hazardous for a diver whose $\dot{V}E$ is already close to its limits because of breathing apparatus or increased gas density or both.

Most studies of underwater work to date have been based upon 'steady state' measurements. Observations with more realistic work patterns, longer periods of work, intermittent effort, and more attention to lactic acid levels might yield valuable insights.

Importance of fitness

As mentioned earlier, a good state of cardiovascular and respiratory fitness is considered almost synonymous with having a high aerobic capacity or $\dot{V}O_{2max}$. Other things being equal, this in turn reflects the individual's background of athletic training. It is self-evident that a diver with high aerobic capacity will be able to work harder and will have greater endurance under given conditions underwater. He has an advantage even at a given submaximal work rate since he is less likely to accumulate lactic acid and develop a disproportionate increase in ventilation. He is also less subject to general fatigue in most kinds of work. The ability to work efficiently, systematically and decisively can no doubt overshadow brute strength and work capacity in importance, as many older divers no doubt can prove. Nevertheless, aerobic capacity deserves more attention in the selection, training, and maintenance of divers than it has yet received.

CARBON DIOXIDE PRODUCTION

Carbon dioxide is the end-product of the same metabolic process in which oxygen is consumed. Oxygen consumption and carbon dioxide production at the cellular level are thus very closely related variables. The relationship is expressed by the respiratory quotient (RQ):

$$RQ = \frac{CO_2 \text{ production}}{O_2 \text{ consumption}} \quad (1)$$

The value of RQ is determined primarily by the diet and can range from 0·7 (fat) to 1·0 (carbohydrate). Protein and an averaged mixed diet yield an RQ of about 0·8.

In view of this close relationship, carbon dioxide production can never differ greatly from oxygen consumption. However, it is important to distinguish the true RQ, reflecting the actual metabolic process, from the relative values of $\dot{V}O_2$ and $\dot{V}CO_2$ obtained from external measurements. The body's carbon dioxide stores are large and labile, and the amount of carbon dioxide expired in a given period may be much smaller or much larger than the amount actually being produced at that time.[1] To make clear the distinction between 'true' and 'apparent' RQ, the latter has been designated the *respiratory gas exchange ratio* with the symbol R.

$$R = \frac{\dot{V}CO_2}{\dot{V}O_2} \quad (2)$$

For many purposes, the $\dot{V}CO_2$ can be estimated accurately enough if the probable or actual $\dot{V}O_2$ is known and the value of R can be approximated. In a normal individual at rest or during light work under ordinary conditions, $\dot{V}CO_2$ will probably be about 0·8 of $\dot{V}O_2$. During very prolonged exertion, or in work done without normal recent food intake, R may drop toward 0·7 with increased mobilization of fat stores for energy production. R can fall below 0·7 during retention of carbon dioxide. In acute exertion, RQ and R will generally rise toward 1·0. R can rise above 1·0 if accumulation of lactic acid is causing metabolic acidosis with displacement of carbon dioxide from plasma bicarbonate and compensatory increase in ventilation. Lowering of the arterial carbon dioxide pressure (Pa_{CO2})[2] tends to restore the pH toward normal.

In many instances it is sufficiently accurate to assume that $\dot{V}CO_2 = \dot{V}O_2$ ($R = 1·0$). However, it is necessary to recognize situations in which this is likely not to be the case and where the difference may be important.

---

[1] Because $\dot{V}CO_2$ can vary at a given work rate, $\dot{V}O_2$ is a more reliable index of exertion and actual metabolic activity.
[2] P signifies the partial *P*ressure of the gas identified by the subscript (usually expressed in mm Hg or torr). The location at issue is also specified by a subscript: small capital letters indicate a gas phase (I = inspired, E = expired, A = alveolar) while lowercase letters indicate blood-gas values (a = arterial, v = venous, v̄ = mixed venous).

Measurement of $\dot{V}o_2$ and $\dot{V}co_2$

In considering the physiological demands of a specific task, it is seldom entirely sufficient to apply existing data concerning $\dot{V}o_2$ and $\dot{V}co_2$ at various levels of activity. Actual determinations must often be made. Methods applicable underwater or under high pressure are basically like those used on dry land. Information concerning such methods is compiled in a number of sources such as Consolazio, Johnson and Pecora (1963).

The environment introduces several problems. The usual apparatus for 'closed circuit' determination of $\dot{V}o_2$ cannot be used underwater, but Donald and Davidson (1954), Lanphier (1956a), and Goff, Brubach and Specht (1957) have described applicable methods utilizing the same principle. Pure oxygen is normally used, but this becomes potentially hazardous for determinations involving exertion at pressures approaching 2 ATA. Use of gases other than pure oxygen in a closed circuit involves risk of hypoxia and requires unusual precautions. The change in volume on which the usual closed circuit determination is based is reduced in proportion to the absolute pressure, and this reduces the accuracy of determinations at depth.

The 'open circuit' approach is based on the volume of gas respired per unit of time and on the differences in oxygen and carbon dioxide concentrations between inspired and expired gas. These differences are reduced in proportion to the absolute pressure, which places a burden on the precision of gas analysis if accurate results are to be obtained in studies conducted under high pressure with analysis of gas samples at normal pressure. Use of carefully calibrated electrode-type analyzers at the pressure of the experiment is potentially more precise.

ALVEOLAR VENTILATION

The most common respiratory abnormalities in diving are those involving insufficient ventilation of the lungs with resulting elevation of alveolar carbon dioxide pressure (PA_{CO2}) and consequent disturbance in arterial carbon dioxide tension (Pa_{CO2}).

PA_{CO2} depends upon the fractional concentration of carbon dioxide in the alveolar gas (FA_{CO2})[1] and the total 'dry gas' pressure in the alveoli[2]:

$$PA_{CO2} = FA_{CO2} \times (PB - 47) \qquad (3)$$

PB is a property of the environment. By definition:

$$FA_{CO2} = \frac{\text{volume of } CO_2 \text{ in alveolar gas}}{\text{total volume of alveolar gas}} \qquad (4)$$

It is useful to consider these volumes not as volumes *in* the alveolar space but as volumes *leaving* the alveolar space. It is helpful to visualize the alveolar space as a box of unspecified size (see Fig. 8.4) with carbon dioxide flowing in at a given rate at one end and fresh air flowing in at another rate at the other end. The carbon dioxide and fresh air mix together completely in the box and flow out through another opening. The crucial values are the relative volumes of carbon dioxide entering and of the mixed gas leaving per unit time.

Let us say that the inflow of carbon dioxide is at a rate of 1·0 L/min and that the outflow of the mixture of fresh air and carbon dioxide is at 20 L/min (both volumes corrected to the same conditions). All of the carbon dioxide entering must also leave. The carbon dioxide must therefore represent 1·0/20 of the outflowing gas. Its fractional concentration must be 0·05, equivalent to 5%. The Pco_2 of this gas would be 0·05 × ($PB - 47$).

This crude model is a useful representation of alveolar ventilation and carbon dioxide dilution. The inflow of carbon dioxide is the $\dot{V}co_2$. The outflow of 'mixed' gas is the alveolar ventilation, $\dot{V}A$. The fraction of carbon dioxide in the mixture, whether flowing out or still in the box, is FA_{CO2}. It does not matter, in per-minute terms, that alveolar ventilation is actually in-and-out through the same passages rather than continuous. The

---

[1] *F* signifies *Fractional* concentration. The subscripts are as described earlier. Thus, FA_{CO2} indicates the fraction of carbon dioxide in alveolar gas.

[2] The value of 'total' pressure required here is that of 'true gases' present (excluding water vapour). The total alveolar pressure, including water vapour pressure, will be essentially equal to the barometric or ambient pressure (PB). The water vapour pressure must be subtracted from this. It depends upon the alveolar temperature and is 47 mm Hg at 37°C.

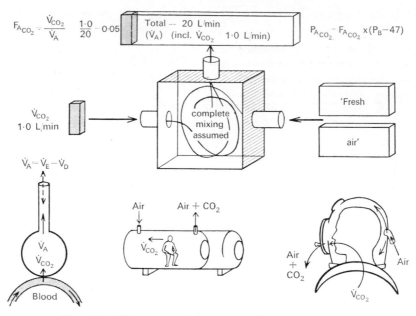

FIG. 8.4. Diagrammatic representation of CO_2 dilution

The box (center) can represent the alveolar space, the volume of a diving helmet, or the interior of a pressure chamber. In the example given, 1·0 L/min of CO_2 enters the box along with an unspecified flow of 'fresh air'. These volumes mix together and emerge as 20 L/min of 'alveolar' gas containing 1·0 L/min of CO_2. The fractional concentration of CO_2 in this gas must be 1/20 or 0·05. In the usual situation, the incoming 'fresh air' must supply the volume of oxygen being removed from the system per unit time. (See text for further details)

model could as well have been built in the form of a bellows. The crucial relationship is this:

$$F_{A_{CO2}} = \frac{\dot{V}_{CO2}}{\dot{V}_A} \qquad (5)$$

Note, however, that this expression is valid only if $\dot{V}_{CO2}$ and $\dot{V}_A$ are expressed in the same units and corrected to the same conditions.

The different corrections normally applied to $\dot{V}_{CO2}$ and $\dot{V}_A$ are particularly important when dealing with $P_{A_{CO2}}$ under increased pressure. Correction of $\dot{V}_{CO2}$ and $\dot{V}_{O2}$ to STPD is appropriate because both result from chemical reactions that proceed on a molecular basis. Corrected to STPD, $\dot{V}_{O2}$ and $\dot{V}_{CO2}$ are proportional to the number of molecules involved and remain essentially the same for a given level of activity regardless of wide variations in ambient pressure.

Pulmonary and alveolar ventilation are logically corrected to BTPS, conditions actually existing in the lungs when they were measured. At any specific level of exertion, ventilation remains much the same (when measured at the pressure concerned) over a wide range of ambient pressures. Unless other factors intervene, a diver doing the same amount of work would take about the same size of breaths about the same number of times per minute at 3 ATA as at 1 ATA.

Why pulmonary and alveolar ventilation should behave in this way is best seen by referring back to the box model of Fig. 8.4. From the physiological standpoint, the $P_{A_{CO2}}$ should remain unchanged with changes in ambient pressure. But how can the box be taken to 10 ATA, for example, without changing the $P_{A_{CO2}}$? Equation (3) indicates that if $P_{A_{CO2}}$ is to remain the same while P_B is multiplied by 10, $F_{A_{CO2}}$ must drop to about one-tenth of its original value. When the box is taken to 10 ATA, the $\dot{V}_{CO2}$ of 1·0 L/min remains the same in number of molecules (or STPD volume) per minute, but its actual volume at 10 ATA will be only about 0·1 L/min. If $\dot{V}_A$ is maintained at 20 L/min (as measured at 10 ATA), $F_{A_{CO2}}$ will be 0·1/20, or 0·005 which is one-tenth of its value at 1 ATA. $P_{A_{CO2}}$ thus remains nearly constant.

As pointed out by Rahn and Fenn (1955), expressions such as equation (5) can be employed easily if a factor is added to correct both values to the same units and conditions. In most respiratory work, $\dot{V}_A$ is expressed in L/min BTPS while $\dot{V}_{O_2}$ and $\dot{V}_{CO_2}$ are in ml/min STPD. The factor that will correct ml/min STPD to L/min BTPS is $0.863/(P_B-47)$. In this chapter, $\dot{V}_{O_2}$ and $\dot{V}_{CO_2}$ have been expressed in L/min STPD, so the corresponding factor is $863/(P_B-47)$. Entering this factor, equation (5) becomes:

$$F_{A_{CO_2}} = \frac{863}{P_B-47} \times \frac{\dot{V}_{CO_2}(\text{L/min STPD})}{\dot{V}_A(\text{L/min BTPS})} \quad (6)$$

This expression for $F_{A_{CO_2}}$ can now be substituted in equation (3). Note that P_B-47 cancels, leaving

$$P_{A_{CO_2}} = 863 \frac{\dot{V}_{CO_2} \ (\text{L/min STPD})}{\dot{V}_A \ (\text{L/min BTPS})} \quad (7)$$

This means that whatever the ambient pressure, $P_{A_{CO_2}}$ depends upon the ratio between $\dot{V}_{CO_2}$ corrected to standard conditions and $\dot{V}_A$ corrected to the actual conditions existing in the lungs. If the work rate remains the same, the value of $\dot{V}_{CO_2}$ can be assumed to remain constant at any reasonable pressure.[1] Concern can then be focused on $\dot{V}_A$. If $\dot{V}_A$ does *not* remain the same when the diver changes depth while doing the same work, then it is certain that constant $P_{A_{CO_2}}$ is not being maintained. The usual abnormality at depth is a decrease in $\dot{V}_A$ with consequent elevation of $P_{A_{CO_2}}$ and $P_{a_{CO_2}}$. This represents *hypercapnia* or what is sometimes called *carbon dioxide retention*.

The relationship indicated by equation (7) is a very simple one. For example, if $\dot{V}_{CO_2}$ remains constant but $\dot{V}_A$ drops to half its original value, $P_{A_{CO_2}}$ must double. The relationship is also rather critical. The usually stated 'average normal' value of $P_{A_{CO_2}}$ is 40 mm Hg, where the ratio is approximately 1/20 (or 0.05). The 'average normal range' is usually considered to be 35 to 45 mm Hg. A rise to 80 mm Hg ($\dot{V}_A$ half-normal for a given $\dot{V}_{CO_2}$) would be incapacitating in most

individuals. Definite signs of carbon dioxide toxicity are usually evident at $P_{A_{CO_2}}=60$ mm Hg. There is reason to believe that oxygen toxicity and nitrogen narcosis would be enhanced significantly even at 50 mm Hg. At the opposite extreme, most individuals would begin to show effects of *hypocapnia* (low $P_{A_{CO_2}}$) at values below 30 mm Hg and would approach incapacitation at 20 mm Hg ($\dot{V}_A$ twice-normal for a given $\dot{V}_{CO_2}$).

Calculation of $P_{A_{CO_2}}$ is simple when $\dot{V}_{CO_2}$ and $\dot{V}_A$ are known, and equation (7) is readily rearranged to solve for $\dot{V}_A$ or $\dot{V}_{CO_2}$. However, graphical presentation of equation (7) is useful in visualizing the relationships and in making rapid estimates. Fig. 8.5 is such a presentation. It can be used in the following example:

An average underwater swimmer is proceeding at 0.9 knot and has a $\dot{V}_{O_2}$ of 1.5 L/min STPD according to Fig. 8.2 or 8.3. His $\dot{V}_{CO_2}$ is probably very close to 1.5 L/min also. You wish to know what alveolar ventilation would be required to maintain $P_{A_{CO_2}}=40$ mm Hg at $\dot{V}_{CO_2}=1.5$ L/min. Finding 1.5 L/min on the horizontal scale and locating the diagonal line for $P_{A_{CO_2}}=40$, the corresponding value of $\dot{V}_A$ can be read off the vertical scale. It is found to be about 32 L/min BTPS. Note that the swimmer's depth does not need to be known for this determination. If the same man's actual $\dot{V}_A$ was known to be only 26 L/min, his $P_{A_{CO_2}}$ could be estimated by locating 26 L/min on the vertical scale and seeing what $P_{A_{CO_2}}$ diagonal corresponds to this value of $\dot{V}_A$ when $\dot{V}_{CO_2}$ is 1.5 L/min. Here, the $P_{A_{CO_2}}$ would be about 50 mm Hg.

Alveolar ventilation is a highly useful concept, but it does not tell the full story of respiratory needs. Achieving a given $\dot{V}_A$ requires the somewhat larger volume of total pulmonary ventilation represented by $\dot{V}_E$.[2] The difference involves respiratory dead space, which will be discussed shortly.

The statement that the diver's depth does not need to be known in considering $\dot{V}_A$ also requires clarification. It does not need to be known as long

---

[1] At a given work rate, $\dot{V}_{CO_2}$ will be constant in terms of actual metabolic carbon dioxide production assuming that there is no change in the substrate or proportion of anaerobic metabolism. If $\dot{V}_A$ were to drop markedly, there would be a period of carbon dioxide retention with some drop in $\dot{V}_{CO_2}$ until new equilibria were reached. The effect of such a change would generally be small enough to be neglected.

[2] $\dot{V}_E$ literally represents the expired volume per unit time. Total pulmonary ventilation is generally measured by collecting the expired gas over a specified interval.

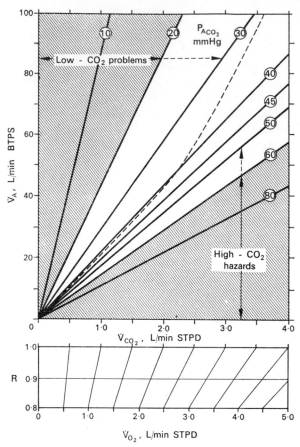

FIG. 8.5. Relationships determining $P_{A_{CO_2}}$

The figure is a graphic presentation of equation (7):

$$P_{A_{CO_2}} = 863 \frac{\dot{V}_{CO_2}}{\dot{V}_A}$$

(where $\dot{V}_{CO_2}$ is in L/min STPD and $\dot{V}_A$ is in L/min BTPS). The horizontal and vertical scales, respectively, represent these two variables. The diagonal lines represent the indicated values of $P_{A_{CO_2}}$. For example, the $P_{A_{CO_2}} = 40$ mm Hg line gives all the possible combinations of $\dot{V}_{CO_2}$ and $\dot{V}_A$ that yield $P_{A_{CO_2}} = 40$.

Shaded areas indicate values of $P_{A_{CO_2}}$ so far above or below the normal range as to present distinct problems. The dashed line shows typical relationships for increasing levels of exertion. At lower values of $\dot{V}_{CO_2}$, a certain $P_{A_{CO_2}}$ (here 40 mm Hg) is maintained quite constantly. But at some level (usually corresponding to about 70% of the individual's $\dot{V}_{O_{2max}}$) $\dot{V}_A$ begins to increase out of proportion to further increases in $\dot{V}_{CO_2}$. As a result, $P_{A_{CO_2}}$ must fall.

The scales below the $\dot{V}_{CO_2}$ scale represent corresponding values of $\dot{V}_{O_2}$ at different values of R. Find the value of $\dot{V}_{O_2}$ on the appropriate R scale, then read the $\dot{V}_{CO_2}$ directly above this point.

The graph as a whole can be used in place of calculation for several types of determinations and permits the relationships to be visualized. (See text for further details)

as $\dot{V}_A$ is expressed in L/min BTPS. But, for example, achieving a given $\dot{V}_A$ BTPS requires moving twice as many gas molecules at 2 ATA as at 1 ATA. If a diver is using closed circuit scuba, this makes little difference except in the greater respiratory work of moving the denser gas at depth. It has great practical importance if the diver's ventilation is being supplied on open circuit from self-contained cylinders or by airhose. In such case, the mass (or 'surface equivalent' volume) of air that must be supplied to maintain a given $\dot{V}_E$ or $\dot{V}_A$ is directly proportional to the pressure in ATA. Consequently, for example, the cylinders of an aqualung last only about half as long at a given level of exertion at 2 ATA as at 1 ATA. This and related questions will also be discussed more fully.

Arterial v. alveolar P_{CO_2}

The foregoing discussion has concentrated on $P_{A_{CO_2}}$, but it is the arterial carbon dioxide tension, $P_{a_{CO_2}}$, that is of primary physiological concern. $P_{A_{CO_2}}$ is important because it is the main factor that normally determines the $P_{a_{CO_2}}$. It has been assumed tacitly here that $P_{A_{CO_2}}$ and $P_{a_{CO_2}}$ are equal to each other. In some pathological states, $P_{a_{CO_2}}$ can be significantly higher than $P_{A_{CO_2}}$. To date, there is little or no evidence that important differences between $P_{A_{CO_2}}$ and $P_{a_{CO_2}}$ are likely to be found in normal individuals exposed to pressures in the usual range. However, possible differences related to very high gas density will be discussed in a later section.

Effects of inspired carbon dioxide

The discussion of alveolar ventilation has thus far been based on the assumption that the inspired gas is free of carbon dioxide. In practical underwater situations, this assumption can seldom be made. The matter is important because few external factors can have a more serious effect on the adequacy of alveolar ventilation than even relatively small amounts of carbon dioxide in the inspired gas.

'Fresh' air contains about 0·04% carbon dioxide ($F_{I_{CO_2}} = 0·0004$). Even at 10 ATA, this would yield a $P_{I_{CO_2}}$ of only about 3 mm Hg. Unfortunately, a diver is seldom certain that he is receiving 'fresh' air; and in many situations he certainly is not. The $P_{I_{CO_2}}$ is almost certain to be above a negligible level in a diving helmet, in much rebreathing equipment, and in many pressure chambers. One way of looking at excessive dead space in breathing apparatus is to consider the effective $P_{I_{CO2}}$ attributable to carbon dioxide 'given back' on inspiration.

The effect of inspired carbon dioxide on $P_{A_{CO2}}$ and required $\dot{V}_A$ is illustrated by an approximate expression based on equation (7):

$$P_{A_{CO2}} = 863 \frac{\dot{V}_{CO_2}}{\dot{V}_A} + P_{I_{CO2}} \qquad (8)$$

$\dot{V}_{CO_2}$ and $\dot{V}_A$ are corrected to STPD and BTPS as usual. $P_{A_{CO2}}$ is calculated in the usual way except that $P_{I_{CO2}}$ must be added to the resulting value. Likewise, Fig. 8.5 can be employed by adding $P_{I_{CO2}}$ to the value of $P_{A_{CO2}}$ obtained graphically.

$P_{A_{CO2}}$ cannot remain lower than $P_{I_{CO2}}$. All that alveolar ventilation can do is to decrease the *difference* between $P_{I_{CO2}}$ and $P_{A_{CO2}}$. Maintaining $P_{A_{CO2}} = 40$ in the face of $P_{I_{CO2}} = 20$ mm Hg would require the ventilation ordinarily needed to maintain $P_{A_{CO2}} = 20$: twice the usual $\dot{V}_A$ for a given $\dot{V}_{CO_2}$. With $P_{I_{CO2}} = 30$, $P_{A_{CO2}} = 40$ could be maintained only with four times the usual $\dot{V}_A$. Especially during exertion when $\dot{V}_A$ is already large, maintaining normal $P_{A_{CO2}}$ in the face of much elevation of $P_{I_{CO2}}$ would require enormous volumes of ventilation. Such increases in ventilation will not occur, and elevation of $P_{A_{CO2}}$ is an almost inevitable result of elevation of $P_{I_{CO2}}$.

$P_{I_{CO2}}$ must be kept as low as possible, but it is difficult to define an acceptable limit. A limit of 10 mm Hg is sometimes suggested, and it is interesting to see what this implies. Take as an example a diver doing moderate work with $\dot{V}_{CO_2} = 1 \cdot 5$ L/min STPD. With $P_{I_{CO2}} = 0$, he needs $\dot{V}_A = 32 \cdot 4$ L/min BTPS to maintain $P_{A_{CO2}} = 40$ mm Hg. If $P_{I_{CO2}} = 10$, maintaining $P_{A_{CO2}} = 40$ would now require $\dot{V}_A = 43 \cdot 2$ L/min. The increase is 33% of the normal $\dot{V}_A$ and could represent a considerable

respiratory burden. At a higher work rate, a 33% increase in $\dot{V}_A$ could be impossible. In actual situations, there would be a lesser increase in $\dot{V}_A$ and some increase in $P_{A_{CO2}}$. The actual levels would depend largely upon the diver's inherent response to carbon dioxide and the work of breathing and cannot readily be predicted. One can say only that the $P_{A_{CO2}}$ in such situations will be somewhere between the $P_{A_{CO2}}$ ordinarily maintained by the diver and that value plus the $P_{I_{CO2}}$. Considerable elevations are possible, and even rather small elevations can have serious implications under some circumstances. The matter will be discussed more fully in a later section.

Helmet ventilation

A prime source of excessive $P_{I_{CO2}}$ in diving is inadequate helmet ventilation. The same problems and principles also apply to ventilation of pressure chambers.[1] The situation is almost identical to that shown in the box model used in discussing alveolar ventilation (Fig. 8.4).[2] The diver adds carbon dioxide to the helmet space at a rate equal to his $\dot{V}_{CO_2}$. Air entering through the airhose mixes with the carbon dioxide and flows out with it through the exhaust port. The same approach to calculation can also be applied, using equation (7) for approximations. Here, the P_{CO_2} within the space is the diver's $P_{I_{CO2}}$ and must therefore be kept much lower than his $P_{A_{CO2}}$. $\dot{V}_A$ becomes helmet ventilation expressed in L/min BTPS. (For precise calculations, the actual temperature and water vapour content of the ventilating air would have to be taken into account.)

In the example used above, the diver's $\dot{V}_{CO_2}$ was $1 \cdot 5$ L/min, corresponding to moderate work. What must his helmet ventilation be in order to maintain $P_{I_{CO2}} = 10$ mm Hg? Without calculation, it can be seen that $P_{I_{CO2}} = 10$ will require helmet ventilation equal to four times the $\dot{V}_A$ normally required for $P_{A_{CO2}} = 40$. In this example,

---

[1] The size of the enclosure does not affect the basic relationship or the final value of P_{CO_2}. It does influence the rate at which P_{CO_2} rises to its final (equilibrium or steady state) level. The ambient pressure does not influence the rate-of-rise or final level of P_{CO_2} so long as $\dot{V}_{CO_2}$ and ventilation are constant in standard and ambient terms, respectively, as in equation (7).

[2] The assumption of complete mixing may be grossly incorrect in diving helmets according to a study reported by Muren and Wulff (1972). Incomplete mixing will ordinarily impair the efficiency of helmet ventilation. Muren and Wulff found that drawing the exhaust from the region of highest CO_2 concentration improved the effectiveness of ventilation and markedly lowered the diver's inspiratory P_{CO_2}.

helmet ventilation would have to be 130 L/min BTPS. Note that in order to determine equivalent volumes as measured at the surface, such values must be multiplied by the depth pressure in ATA. If this diver were working at 99 ft (4 ATA), helmet ventilation for moderate work would thus require pumping in the order of $130 \times 4 = 520$ L/min (about 18 cu ft/min) of 'surface' air to his helmet. Helmet ventilation is seldom abundant for working dives.

Substituting a suitable 'open circuit' demand type breathing system would reduce the air requirement to the diver's actual $\dot{V}_E$ BTPS. The need for air would be roughly one-quarter of that required for desirable helmet ventilation. A high price, either in air or in carbon dioxide levels, is paid for whatever advantage helmets and comparable arrangements may seem to have.

Alveolar oxygen pressure

Before leaving the subject of alveolar ventilation, $P_{A_{O2}}$ deserves mention. The problem of dangerously low alveolar oxygen pressure is unusual in diving and other forms of high pressure exposure. Hypoxia can, of course, occur in failure of gas supply or other serious equipment malfunction. The $P_{A_{O2}}$ is also of major interest in breath-hold diving, but these topics are outside the scope of this chapter.

Accurate calculation of $P_{A_{O2}}$ is more complex than calculation of $P_{A_{CO2}}$. Correct equations are presented by Rahn and Fenn (1955). For most purposes, a very simple statement suffices:

$$P_{A_{O2}} = P_{I_{O2}} - 863 \frac{\dot{V}_{O2}}{\dot{V}_A} \qquad (9)$$

where $\dot{V}_{O2}$ and $\dot{V}_A$ are in L/min and corrected to STPD and BTPS respectively. Note that when $R = 1 \cdot 0$, the subtracted quantity is equal to the $P_{A_{CO2}}$. For rough estimates of $P_{A_{O2}}$ where $P_{A_{CO2}}$ is known, one can say that $P_{A_{O2}}$ is about as much below $P_{I_{O2}}$ as $P_{A_{CO2}}$ is above $P_{I_{CO2}}$.

In usual circumstances underwater, as when breathing air at depth, the $P_{I_{O2}}$ is sufficiently high that inadequate $\dot{V}_A$ would increase the $P_{A_{CO2}}$ to a troublesome level while $P_{A_{O2}}$ remained quite safe. A possible exception exists when the $P_{I_{O2}}$ is deliberately kept near the normal 'air-at-surface' value of about 150 mm Hg. This is done, for example, in prolonged saturation dives where the

possible harmful effects of long-term exposure to elevated $P_{I_{O2}}$ are of concern. Even in this situation, subnormal alveolar ventilation would presumably cause high carbon dioxide problems before low oxygen became hazardous. However, there are some indications that a $P_{I_{O2}}$ which is adequate at normal pressure may not always be adequate under high pressure. This possibility will be brought up again in a later section.

TOTAL VENTILATORY REQUIREMENTS

Knowing the optimal $\dot{V}_A$ for a given level of activity is not very useful unless it permits the corresponding *total* pulmonary ventilation, $\dot{V}_E$, to be estimated. The difference between $\dot{V}_A$ and $\dot{V}_E$ is variable and represents ventilation of *respiratory dead space*.

For practical calculations, $\dot{V}_E$ is assumed to consist of two separate volumes of different kinds of gas. One, the alveolar ventilation, $\dot{V}_A$, accounts for all of the exchange of oxygen and carbon dioxide between blood and gas that has taken place during collection of the expired volume. The other, $\dot{V}_D$, is assumed to have come entirely from the dead space. It accounts for none of the gas exchange and has the same composition as inspired gas.

$$\dot{V}_E = \dot{V}_A + \dot{V}_D \qquad (10)$$

Dead space ventilation ($\dot{V}_D$) represents the effective volume of the respiratory dead space, V_D, multiplied by the number of times this has been ventilated during the minute of collection: the respiratory frequency, f, in breaths per minute.

$$\dot{V}_D = V_D \times f \qquad (11)$$

The frequency is readily ascertained, and if a reasonable value for V_D can be obtained, $\dot{V}_D$ can be estimated. This volume can then be added to $\dot{V}_A$ to obtain $\dot{V}_E$ or subtracted from $\dot{V}_E$ to obtain $\dot{V}_A$.

The subject of dead space in the human respiratory tract has been surrounded by a great deal of confusion and controversy, and some questions remain to be settled. Accounts by Bouhuys (1964) and Dejours (1966), among others, can be consulted for details.

Actual determination of V_D is possible by several methods but is seldom practical in diving situations. The usual approach is therefore to estimate V_D as well as possible. Two kinds of dead space usually have to be considered in diving: the diver's own 'personal' dead space and the dead space of his breathing apparatus.

There is now fairly general agreement about respiratory dead space volumes to be expected in normal individuals at rest. The volume is influenced by such factors as body size, and Radford (1955) has noted that in adults the volume of the dead space in millilitres usually is roughly equal to the individual's weight in pounds. Much dispute has centred about changes in dead space in exercise, and the matter is not entirely settled. Probably the best available information comes from a study of healthy young males by Asmussen and Nielsen (1956). They found average values of total or 'physiological' dead space ranging from 170 ml at rest to 350 ml during heavy exercise. The highest value recorded was 450 ml. The increase with exercise was approximately linear in its relationship to the tidal volume of breathing, which went from about 0·5 to 3·3 L/breath.

Similar determinations have not been made under diving conditions, so there is no real alternative to assuming that such values are applicable. It is convenient and reasonable to assume that a working diver's 'personal' dead space is 300 ml (0·3 L) BTPS.

The breathing apparatus can add a considerable volume of dead space. Any part of a breathing apparatus that has to-and-fro ventilation is 'dead' until proved otherwise. One way of phrasing the question is 'Will this part contain expired carbon dioxide at the end of expiration and then give it back on inspiration?' An almost unavoidable dead space is presented by the usual mouthpiece-and-check-valve assembly. The volume of such dead space usually approaches 0·1 L, and reducing it greatly would risk making the passages too small.

The volume of an obvious dead space can be determined either by water-filling or by measurement and calculation. Sometimes, it is not possible to be sure by inspection whether a certain space is 'functionally dead' or not, or partially so. In such cases, a method of measurement like those used to determine dead space in man must be used. Full-face masks present a problem from this standpoint. In most, the entire internal gas volume between the mask and the face represents dead space and can amount to 0·5 L in some examples. In a few, where there is good separation between the oronasal and eye areas, inspired and expired gases may not mix throughout the whole volume, and the dead space may be relatively small.

The main liability of very large apparatus dead space is not so much that it increases the ventilatory requirements but that the diver will not compensate fully and will thus permit his $P_{A_{CO2}}$ to increase. It was found in one study that addition of 0·5 L of dead space to an underwater breathing system raised the average $P_{A_{CO2}}$ 6 mm Hg (Lanphier 1963). This is a consequential increase, especially when $P_{A_{CO2}}$ is already high.

It is important in considering ventilatory requirements to know whether the apparatus to be used has an inordinate amount of dead space or not. It is better to make sure that it does not. In the discussion to follow, it will be assumed that breathing apparatus is used but that its dead space is only 0·1 L. Adding this to the diver's assumed V_D of 0·3 L gives a total of 0·4 L. This is probably more than the actual value for a healthy young diver doing light work with a well-designed breathing apparatus. It cannot be more than necessary to account for less favorable situations.

Fig. 8.6 is based on $V_D = 0·4$ L. It represents the vertical $\dot{V}_A$ scale of Fig. 8.5 with additions to indicate the corresponding estimated values of $\dot{V}_E$ at respiratory frequencies up to 50 breaths/min. Such values can be calculated readily, but Fig. 8.6 aids visualization of the relationships and permits rapid comparisons.

LIMITS OF VENTILATION AT DEPTH

Useful application of information like that presented in foregoing sections entails obvious difficulties. These underscore continuing need for data from divers doing real work under actual conditions. The difficulty of making completely realistic measurements remains very great, so the physiologist and engineer must continue their efforts to obtain and piece together accessible

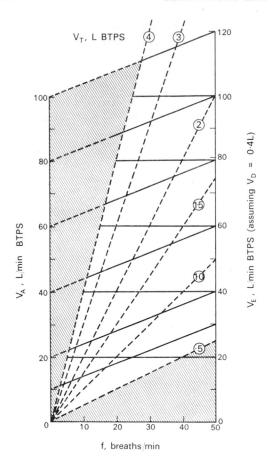

FIG. 8.6. Relationships between $\dot{V}_A$ and $\dot{V}_E$

The difference between $\dot{V}_A$ and $\dot{V}_E$ is the dead-space ventilation, $\dot{V}_D$. This, in turn, is equal to the product of the dead-space volume, V_D, and the respiratory frequency, f.

The graph relates $\dot{V}_A$ and $\dot{V}_E$ in terms of an assumed constant value of $V_D = 0.4$ L (see text) and values of f up to 50 breaths/min. The dashed diagonal lines represent different values of tidal volume, V_T, required to achieve given values of $\dot{V}_E$ at different values of f. V_T is not likely to be less than 0·5 L or more than 4·0 L, so values beyond these extremes are shaded and can be considered improbable or impossible.

Example: Find $\dot{V}_A = 40$ L/min on the left-hand scale and follow the upward-sloping line as f (bottom scale) increases. $\dot{V}_A = 40$ cannot be achieved at less than $f = 11$ unless V_T exceeds 4·0 L. At $f = 11$, V_D must equal $0.4 \times 11 = 4.4$ L/min. Consequently, $\dot{V}_E$ must be $40 + 4.4 = 44.4$ L/min, as shown on the vertical scales at the level of the point at issue. At the other extreme, $f = 50$ would involve a V_T between 1·0 and 1·5 L and requires $\dot{V}_E = 60$ to achieve $\dot{V}_A = 40$ L/min

information. One of the physiologist's most important functions is the continuing attempt to foresee the physiological implications of conditions that are not yet familiar in actual diving experience.

Understanding of basic respiratory needs assists appreciation of limitations imposed on a diver's capability by respiratory factors in the underwater environment. One of the most prominent factors is restriction of ventilatory capacity by the increased density of gas at depth. The limitations are most immediate when the breathing medium is air or any relatively dense gas mixture, but similar restrictions can be expected with lighter gases at some greater depth—assuming that other physiological factors permit such depths to be reached.

Several groups of investigators have studied the effect of depth pressure on maximum breathing capacity (MBC) or maximal voluntary ventilation (MVV) and other variables.[1] The findings in these studies are remarkably similar, especially if expressed in actual volumes of ventilation. (Most of the results were reported originally in terms of per cent change from surface control values, but in some cases very similar values at depth are made to appear dissimilar because the surface values differed.) Fig. 8.7 presents average values of MVV derived from the most important early studies of ventilatory capacity with air at pressures corresponding to various depths.

Maio and Farhi (1967) used high and low pressure (0·5 to 7·5 ATA) and gas mixtures (He–O$_2$ and SF$_6$–O$_2$) as well as air to study the effects of gas densities ranging from 0·21 that of air at 1 ATA to over 12 times the 1 ATA air value. The carbon dioxide and water vapour content of the actual rebreathed test gas was taken into account, which is particularly important at low relative densities. Whether a given relative density was achieved with a gas mixture, with altered pressure, or both, made no consistent difference in MVV or related variables.

The curve in Fig. 8.7 was drawn by eye for best fit to the majority of points. The MVV with air

[1] MBC and MVV are defined variously, but in most instances they refer to essentially the same determination and can be used interchangeably. MVV is the most widely accepted term at present. Basically, the procedure involves breathing as much as possible for a short period, usually 15 sec. Sometimes a prescribed frequency such as 100 breaths/min is maintained. The results are expressed in L/min BTPS.

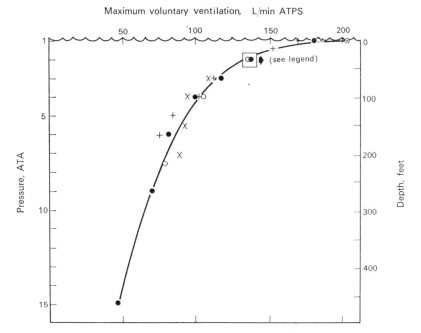

FIG. 8.7. Maximum voluntary ventilation with air at various depths

Values for MBC or MVV are plotted against depth/pressure at various levels. Values were derived from four different studies, the most extensive of which were the USN EDU study (Wood 1963) and that of Maio and Farhi (1967). Original L/min mean values were obtained from Maio and Farhi's basic data and are shown as open circles ◯. Wood's values were presented in terms of percentage change from 1·0 ATA values and in percentage predicted MBC. However, the predicted and actual 1·0 ATA values were given. Mean L/min values for the different pressures were derived from these and are shown as solid circles ●.

The results of the other two studies (Miles 1958; Seusing & Drube 1960) were given only in percentage change with no indication of actual values in L/min. It was noted that the greatest difference between Maio's and Wood's values was at 1·0 ATA, while agreement was almost perfect (both about 135 L/min) at 2·0 ATA. For purposes of comparison, it was assumed that Miles's and Seusing and Drube's 2 ATA means were also 135 L/min. The points plotted were obtained by this manipulation: × = Miles (1958); + = Seusing and Drube (1960).

The curve was drawn by eye for best fit, attaching greatest importance to the values of Wood and Maio and Farhi. In any case, only two of the plotted mean values differ from the curve by as much as 10 L/min (about 5% of the 1 ATA value).

ATPS values were used because of the lack of information needed for correction of some of the values. Judging from Maio and Farhi's original data, chamber temperatures were generally quite high. Factors for correction to BTPS would be rather small

drops very rapidly as pressure is increased and reaches about half of the 'surface control' value as pressure approaches 4 ATA. Beyond this level, the drop is much less abrupt. Possible explanations for this pattern are discussed by Maio and Farhi (1967), and the whole question of density-related flow limitation will be discussed in a later section. As observed by R. D. Workman and reported by Wood (1963), the MVV at increasing depth is roughly proportional to the reciprocal of the square root of the gas density.

Three recent studies contribute additional points for MVV with air at pressure to 6 and 8 ATA. The L/min values of Morrison and Butt (1972) and Fagraeus and Linnarsson (1973) are within the 'envelope' of plotted points in Fig. 8.7. The 'per cent change' values of Ohiwa (1969) also correspond very closely when converted by the method described in the legend of Fig. 8.7. The upper portion of the curve of Fig. 8.7 seems very well-established, but the deeper portion lacks sufficient confirmatory data.

MVV is not of much interest for its own sake in diving, but it provides one (and very possibly the best) index of the relative effects of various pressures and gas densities on the respiratory system. The effects on other variables such as maximum inspiratory and expiratory flow and timed vital capacity measures are similar but present interesting differences, as will be seen. The most practical use of MVV is in attempts to predict the average $\dot{V}_{E_{max}}$ [1] in exertion at depth.

At least at normal pressure, ventilation equal to MVV is not likely to be maintained for very long. Zocche, Fritts and Cournand (1960) found that the maximum $\dot{V}_E$ dropped to 53% of MVV during 15 min of sustained respiratory effort even when excessive loss of CO_2 was prevented. Tenney and Reese (1968) concluded that ventilation could be sustained at about 55% of MVV.

Shephard (1967) reported more optimistic conclusions. He studied young men during near-maximal exercise on a treadmill and found that the subjects were able to maintain ventilation at 70 to 80% of MVV throughout 15 min of such work and were still able to reach almost 100% of MVV just before the end of the period. Leith (see Bradley 1973) found that specific respiratory training made it possible for subjects to maintain 95% of MVV for 15 min at 1 ATA. An increase in strength of respiratory muscles can be inferred from the findings of Wright et al. (1973) in a study of men who spent 2 weeks at 4 ATA. A late increase in MVV was one of the apparent consequences. None of this evidence should be taken as proof that useful work can be done at depth while maintaining pulmonary ventilation that approaches 100% of MVV.

Miller, Wangensteen and Lanphier (1971, 1972) present theoretical grounds and limited experimental evidence for the contention that 100% of MVV can be sustained for reasonable periods of exercise at increased pressure. This view is challenged by Fagraeus and Linnarsson (1973), who measured the actual ventilation associated with very heavy work at 1, 3, and 6 ATA. The work was tolerated only for a few minutes at 3 and 6 ATA and was accompanied by severe CO_2 retention. The ventilation achieved by their subjects was almost certainly greater than what has been defined here as $\dot{V}_{E_{max}}$, but it averaged only

about 80% of MVV at each pressure. The range at 6 ATA was 60 to 97% of MVV. The investigators concluded that the highest workload that can be maintained adequately at pressures to and including 6 ATA is that which requires, at sea level, ventilation not exceeding 60% of the 15 sec MVV observed at the pressure in question.

The difference in findings between Miller et al. (1972) and Fagraeus and Linnarsson (1973) has not been explained, but it might be sought in individual differences. That these can be important is indicated by the spread of Fagraeus's values and by the fact that Miller's main subject had an unusually small MVV at 7.8 ATA. A factor emphasized by Miller et al. (1972) is that their contentions clearly would hold true only with very low-resistance breathing systems.

Effects of breathing apparatus. Many available breathing units would probably reduce $\dot{V}_{E_{max}}$ to a small fraction of MVV at a given depth. The fact that $\dot{V}_{E_{max}}$ represents *sustainable* ventilation deserves emphasis. Morrison and Butt (1972) report achieving 85 to 95% of normal 15 sec MVV while using open circuit demand scuba in 15 sec maneuvers at 8 ATA of air. These results are in line with the observations of Vorosmarti and Lanphier (1975) concerning the effects of external resistance on forced expiratory flow values. The effort required to overcome very great external resistance can be made, but it would be perilous to assume that such effort can be exerted repeatedly for more than a very short period. As will be shown, important limitations of the human airway are effort-independent and can be tested meaningfully in very short-term procedures. In contrast, limitations of breathing apparatus are inclined to be effort-related. Respiratory fatigue over a period of time is thus often the dominant factor in determining $\dot{V}_{E_{max}}$ under practical circumstances.

Determination of $\dot{V}_{E_{max}}$ during extended periods of heavy work with optimal respiratory equipment would probably provide the most useful index of a man's own practical respiratory capacity at depth. This would also provide a very

---

[1] $\dot{V}_{E_{max}}$ is used here in the sense of 'maximum sustainable pulmonary ventilation under given conditions', as opposed to MVV, which relates to a specific test performed (at rest unless otherwise specified) with low-resistance measuring equipment, etc.

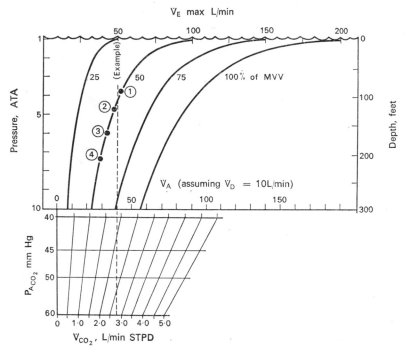

FIG. 8.8. Relationships between depth, $P_{A_{CO_2}}$, and work capacity

The diagram permits ventilatory restrictions imposed by air at increased pressure to be assessed in terms of corresponding limitations of $\dot{V}_{CO_2}$ at specified levels of $P_{A_{CO_2}}$, or of $P_{A_{CO_2}}$ levels at specified values of $\dot{V}_{CO_2}$. The upper portion is like Fig. 8.7 except that curves for 25, 50 and 75% of MVV are given to suggest possible values of $\dot{V}_{E_{max}}$ (upper horizontal scale).

The derivation and use of the diagram are illustrated by the following example (see vertical dashed line): A diver breathing air is at about 100 ft. His MVV is 100 L/min but his $\dot{V}_{E_{max}}$ is only 50% of MVV. If his $\dot{V}_D$ happens to be 10 L/min, his $\dot{V}_A$ is given directly by the $\dot{V}_A$ scale. Following the dashed line into the lower part of the diagram, it is found to cross the '$P_{A_{CO_2}}=40$' scale at a point corresponding to $\dot{V}_{CO_2}=1\cdot85$ L/min. It crosses the scales for higher values of $P_{A_{CO_2}}$ at higher values of $\dot{V}_{CO_2}$. (Once $\dot{V}_A$ is known, the same information could be obtained from Fig. 8.5.) The illustrated limitations of $\dot{V}_{CO_2}$ are not very severe in terms of practical work capacity (consult Figs 8.1 to 8.3). However, very severe limitations are seen if $\dot{V}_{E_{max}}$ is as little as 25% of MVV. For example, 25% MVV at 100 ft allows $\dot{V}_{CO_2}=1\cdot0$ L/min only if $P_{A_{CO_2}}$ is nearly 60 mm Hg.

Another example of use of the diagram involves the numbered points: If a certain task requires $\dot{V}_{CO_2}=2\cdot0$ L/min and $\dot{V}_{E_{max}}$ is 50% MVV, it is simple to estimate the depths at which this level of exertion is possible at given values of $P_{A_{CO_2}}$. Finding $2\cdot0$ L/min on the $P_{A_{CO_2}}=40$ scale of the lower graph, note that a line drawn vertically would intersect the 50% MVV curve at point (1). This corresponds to about 89 ft ($3\cdot7$ ATA). Point (2) indicates the corresponding value for $P_{A_{CO_2}}=45$, point (3) for 50, and point (4) for 60 mm Hg. The apparent gains in working depth are considerable (see text)

valuable baseline for the evaluation of breathing equipment for actual use in the field.

Fig. 8.8 relates ventilatory restrictions imposed by air at increased pressure to corresponding limits of activity in terms of $\dot{V}_{CO_2}$. As the figure and examples given in the legend make clear, the limitation of activity depends in large part upon the level of $P_{A_{CO_2}}$ that the diver can and will accept. For instance, one example indicates that $\dot{V}_{CO_2}=2\cdot0$ L/min might be maintained at less than 100 ft or at more than 200 ft depending upon

maintenance of $P_{A_{CO_2}}=40$ or $P_{A_{CO_2}}=60$ mm Hg. Other implications of such differences in CO_2 levels will be taken up in a later section.

Use of lighter gases

Fig. 8.9 indicates the relative density of various helium–oxygen mixtures compared to that of air. While pure helium is only one-seventh as dense as air, the relative density increases markedly as the fraction of oxygen in helium–oxygen mixtures is

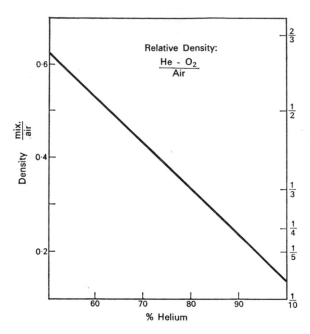

Fig. 8.9. Relative density of He–O_2 mixtures

The density of various He–O_2 mixtures is expressed in relation to the density of air. For example, relative density 0·5 or $\frac{1}{2}$ indicates a mixture one-half as dense as air. A 63% He to 37% O_2 mixture (63% He on horizontal scale) fits this description. (For further applications, see text.) (Reproduced, by permission, from *Underwater Physiology*, Ed. C. J. Lambertsen. Baltimore: Williams & Wilkins, 1967)

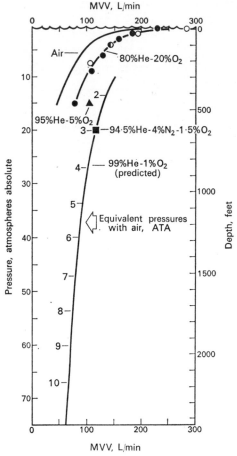

Fig. 8.10. Actual and predicted values of MVV with He–O_2 mixtures

The graph has the same form as Fig. 8.7, but the vertical scales are extended to much greater depth/pressures. The curve labelled 'air' is the same as in Fig. 8.7 and is reproduced to facilitate comparisons. Mean values with 80% He–20% O_2 are derived from the data of Wood (1963), solid circles ●, and of Maio and Farhi (1967), open circles ○. Wood's percentage change and percentage predicted MBC values were converted to L/min as explained in the legend of Fig. 8.7. The triangular point ▲ represents Wood's data for 95% He–5% O_2 at 15 ATA. The solid square ■ represents values obtained by Hamilton et al. (1966).

The curve labelled 99% He–1% O_2 is a slight revision of the predicted curve of Lanphier (1967). It is based on the air curve of Fig. 8.7, relative density of 0·15 (1/6·7), and the assumption that MVV at a given pressure with this mixture would be the same as that with air at 0·15 × this pressure.

The numbers on the predicted curve ('equivalent pressures with air') indicate the pressures where the predicted MVV values are the same as with air at the indicated lesser pressures. If the predicted curve is correct this implies, for example, that a diver's respiratory status at 67 ATA with 99% He should be about the same as with air at 10 ATA

increased. An 80% helium to 20% oxygen mixture is one-third as dense as air.

As mentioned earlier, Maio and Farhi (1967) concluded that the work of breathing, MVV, and related measures are all essentially the same at a given *relative density* whether that density is reached by means of increased pressure or by the use of gas mixtures. If so, knowing the relative density of a gas mixture should permit prediction of MVV, etc., with that mixture at various depths on the basis of known values with air at other depths. For example, the MVV at a given absolute pressure with a mixture one-third as dense as air should be the same as the MVV with air at one-third the absolute pressure.

Fig. 8.10 presents actual and predicted MVV values for helium–oxygen mixtures at various depths. Remarkable deep-diving experiments have been conducted since the first such graph was published (Lanphier 1967) and since this figure was included in the first edition of this book (Bennett & Elliott 1969). Unfortunately, it is still impossible to be sure whether the bold extrapolation of MVV values is reasonably correct or not. Most of the very deep simulated dives of recent years have neither included comparable measurements nor entailed exertion heavy enough to confirm or deny estimates of $\dot{V}_{E_{max}}$ that could be based on the predicted curve of Fig. 8.10.

A single reported value from a 1600 ft dive (50 ATA) (Spaur 1973) suggests that the curve underestimates breathing capacity at that depth. MVV at 1600 ft was reported to be 55% of the unspecified surface value. The curve of Fig. 8.10 indicates about 77 L/min or about 38% of the surface-air MVV.

One of the most ambitious diving studies of recent years included extensive respiratory measurements in two subjects at gas densities equivalent to the range from helium–oxygen at sea level to helium at 150 ATA (Wright, Peterson & Lambertsen 1972). A curve of MVV v. density is presented for one subject. It differs somewhat in shape from the basic curve of Figs 8.7 and 8.10, indicating lower values of MVV at densities below the equivalent of air at about 10 ATA and higher values beyond that point. The point equivalent to air at 15 ATA in Fig. 8.7 is particularly important for predictions extending to great depths. It stands in Fig. 8.7 at about 46 L/min. Wright's data suggest a value of about 58 L/min.

Another careful study (Anthonisen et al. 1971) indicates that subjects were able to ventilate at 40 to 50 L/min at a relative gas density equivalent to air at 15 ATA. These values do not necessarily represent MVV, but they bracket the plotted value of Fig. 8.7.

The greatest density studied in the work reported by Wright, Peterson and Lambertsen (1972) was 25·2 g/L, equivalent to almost 22 times the density of air at 1 ATA. The values of MVV reported at this density average about 50 L/min. This value is about 15 L/min above the figures that can be extrapolated from Fig. 8.7 or 8.10. The values of Wright and his colleagues lead to very optimistic predictions. For example, they suggest that moderate work should be practical, with appropriate He–O$_2$ mixtures and optimal breathing apparatus, at 150 ATA (about 5000 ft)

and probably considerably beyond. All such predictions assume, of course, that other physiological factors will not set limits at shallower depths. There is no clear indication at this time of writing whether they will or not.

If gas density and its effects upon ventilation do become true limiting factors at some depth, they may do so either by restricting exertion to levels below the minimum required for safety and essential activity or by interaction with other factors (Lanphier 1967). Possible interactions between respiratory limitation and the high pressure neurological syndrome were suspected in a study that included the highest pressure reached by man to this time of writing (Agarate & Jegou 1973).

Applicability of hydrogen. If density-related problems become consequential with helium at greater depths, or if helium becomes too costly or too difficult to obtain, one important solution may lie in the use of hydrogen (Edel et al. 1972). Lanphier (1972) reviewed work related to various aspects of this possibility. His prediction of MVV with hydrogen at great depths was based purely upon relative gas density (Fig. 8.11) although he discussed possible implications of the low viscosity of this gas.

Until 1973, no respiratory studies with hydrogen could shed light on the validity of predictions like those of Lanphier (1972). A series of dives conducted by Edel in the firm of Michel Lecler afforded the opportunity for comparative measurements with hydrogen, helium, and nitrogen at chamber pressures equivalent to 200 ft of depth (7 ATA). Results of respiratory measurements in that series were reported by Dougherty (1974). The MVV with 97% hydrogen–3% oxygen at 200 ft was 152% greater than the MVV with 97% N$_2$–3% O$_2$ and 32% greater than that with 97% He–3% O$_2$ at the same depth. The value with H$_2$–O$_2$ at 200 ft was also 16% higher than the MVV with air at normal pressure. Comparison of Dougherty's values with predictions like those of Fig. 8.10 and 8.11 indicate that Lanphier's predictions (1972) may be conservative rather than overoptimistic. The importance of the question clearly warrants further study.

French investigators have reported unfavorable effects of hydrogen in deep animal studies

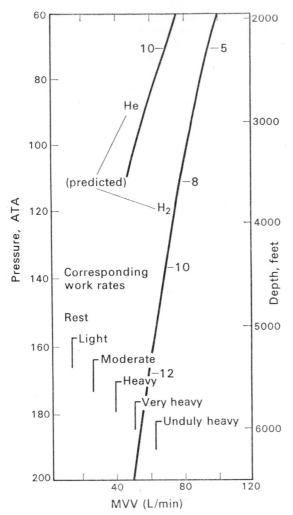

FIG. 8.11. Predicted MVV with hydrogen at great depth

The graph represents an extension of Fig. 8.10 into still-greater depths. The line for H_2 is based on the assumption that only relative gas density needs to be considered in predicting MVV and that the density of the H_2 breathing medium is $\frac{1}{14}$ that of air. The indications of work load are based on normal values of pulmonary ventilation for the indicated severity of work (Christensen's classification) and are valid here only to the extent that MVV provides a direct index of sustainable ventilation during exertion at depth (after Lanphier, 1972)

(Balouet et al. 1971; Michaud et al. 1973). Their experience has no parallel in American studies and has not been explained.

The potential of neon. Neon or 'crude neon' (about 75% neon, 25% helium) is receiving increasing attention as a possible substitute for pure helium in breathing mixtures (Schreiner,

Hamilton & Langley 1972; Strauss et al. 1972). Neon is relatively dense, but it has desirable properties. Crude neon is probably suitable for dives at least to 700 ft (22·2 ATA) (Schreiner 1972).

Measures other than MVV

The MVV has obvious shortcomings as an index of working capacity at depth. Its uncertain relation to $\dot{V}_{E_{max}}$ has been discussed. Varène et al. (1974) raise the possibility that airway conductance may not be the same during exercise as during resting measurements. MVV can also be criticized on the basis of the effort required and the possible influence of motivation and other factors on reproducibility. Such considerations have led increasing numbers of investigators to focus attention upon other measures instead of MVV or in addition to it. A suitable record of forced vital capacity (FVC) can be analyzed in terms of several recognized indices, and the maximum expiratory flow–volume curve can be plotted. Inspiratory values are also readily measured. If oesophageal pressure is recorded together with spirometry, values for resistance and the work of breathing can be computed.

All of these indices and variables show changes consistent with each other and with alterations in MVV at increasing density, but they are not by any means completely comparable. Physiological reasons for some of the differences have become apparent and will be discussed in a later section. All such measures have in common the fact that they are at least as far removed from actual working capacity as is the MVV.

In a particularly thoughtful study, Varène et al. (1974) proposed means of computing maximum work from flow measurements. The approaches appear useful, but several important assumptions must be made. Relative limitation of exertion was predicted at about 50 ATA for He–O_2. Computation of MVV from forced expiratory measurements is not notably successful (J. Vorosmarti, personal communication 1972).

Studies of pulmonary mechanics at depth with emphasis on measures other than MVV (and not already mentioned) include the work of Anthonisen et al. (1971), Hyacinthe and Broussolle (1972), and Wood and Bryan (1969). Schaefer, Carey and Dougherty (1971) reported that several flow-related variables decreased during compression but recovered significantly during saturation at depths of 600 to 800 ft (19·2 to 25·2 ATA). Several possible explanations were advanced.

Work studies at depth

A number of investigators have made a direct approach to limits of exertion at depth by having their subjects work at measured rates, usually with a bicycle ergometer. Most have been satisfied to establish the fact that mild or moderate work can be handled uneventfully at the depth in question. While such information is worth having, its applicability is very small in terms of real limits and prediction of work capacity at other depths.

An important study in which subjects were taken to their limits was reported by Strauss et al. (1975). The greatest gas density in that study was obtained with a neon–helium–oxygen mixture at a pressure equivalent to 1200 ft of sea water (38·5 ATA), density equivalent to helium at 5000 ft (153 ATA). Two young male subjects were able to pedal a bicycle ergometer during consecutive 6 min periods at increasing work loads of 300, 600 and 900 kilopond-meters/min but were unable to complete 6 min at 1200 kp-m/min. The 1200 kp-m/min workload represented about 80% of the subjects' normal maximal work capacity. The 900 kp-m/min load is equivalent to about 150 watts. At 25% net efficiency, it would entail a $\dot{V}_{O_2}$ of about 2 L/min.

Other studies with measured work can be summarized briefly: Bradley et al. (1971), 19·2 ATA, density = 3·7 × air at 1 ATA, approximate $\dot{V}_{O_2}$ = 2·0 L/min; Salzano, Rausch & Saltzman (1970), 4·4 ×, 1·6 L/min; Morrison & Florio (1971), 46 ATA, 6·7 ×, 0·9 L/min; Broussolle et al. (1972), 51 ATA, 7·5 ×, 1·5 L/min. In some of these observations, CO_2 retention occurred; but in none of them was there evidence that a respiratory limit had been reached. Large individual variability was noted especially by Bradley et al. (1971).

CONTROL OF BREATHING

As has just been seen, there is some uncertainty about the ability of divers to ventilate their lungs sufficiently at given work rates at certain depths and with different breathing media. Such uncertainty would exist even if we could assume that the breathing apparatus is optimal. The closer we approach realistic diving conditions, the less certain everything becomes. Difficulty can be encountered even when the requirements appear to lie entirely within the limits of known capability.

Carbon dioxide retention

In the usual diving situation, inadequate ventilation of the lungs (*hypoventilation*) will manifest itself in insufficient elimination of carbon dioxide, and this results in excessive levels of CO_2 in the blood and tissues (*hypercapnia*) before lack of oxygen (*hypoxia or anoxia*) becomes an important problem. The term *carbon dioxide retention* has come to be applied particularly to forms of hypoventilation and hypercapnia in which the individual is presumably capable of eliminating CO_2 in a normal manner but for some reason fails to do so.

US Naval Experimental Diving Unit (EDU) studies reported by Lanphier (1955, 1963) provide insight into problems of pulmonary function that can arise even under seemingly favorable diving conditions. Attention at EDU had been focused on respiratory problems by the unexpected toxicity of presumably safe nitrogen–oxygen mixtures when these were tested at depth. The levels of $P_{I_{O_2}}$ concerned had been tolerated for long periods when tested with 100% oxygen at lesser depths. In nitrogen–oxygen mixtures at 4 ATA, they caused symptoms of oxygen poisoning in remarkably short exposures. Elevation of $P_{A_{CO_2}}$ offered the only plausible explanation, and high values of $P_{A_{CO_2}}$ were found in subsequent experiments under very similar conditions. When divers breathed 55% N_2–45% O_2 during standardized moderate exertion at 4 ATA in a 'wet' pressure tank, their average $P_{A_{CO_2}}$ was nearly 55 mm Hg. Individual values as high as 70 mm Hg were found.

The effect of inspired carbon dioxide on oxygen toxicity is well known, and it was reasonable to suppose that retention of endogenous carbon dioxide could produce similar acceleration of oxygen poisoning. High $P_{A_{CO_2}}$ in these subjects clearly arose from insufficiency of pulmonary ventilation, so the immediate question was simply 'Why don't these divers breathe enough?'

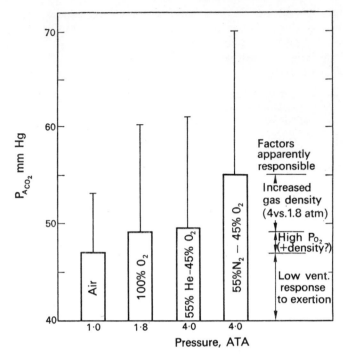

FIG. 8.12. Elevation of $P_{A_{CO2}}$ in Experimental Diving Unit studies

Pressures are indicated at the bottom of the graph. Breathing media are indicated within the graph bars. The height of each bar represents the mean value of $P_{A_{CO2}}$. The extended line above each bar represents the highest individual value obtained under each set of conditions.

The tabulation 'Factors apparently responsible' is based on differences between the various experimental conditions and the corresponding differences in mean $P_{A_{CO2}}$ (see text for interpretation)

The partial answers obtained can be summarized:

1. *High $P_{I_{O2}}$* accounted for not more than 25% of the elevation of mean $P_{A_{CO2}}$ at 4 ATA above the values found at the same work rate when breathing air just below the surface. (Fig. 8.12 presents the average and 'high man' values of $P_{A_{CO2}}$ obtained with different breathing media at different pressures.)

2. *Increased work of breathing* accounted for most of the elevation of $P_{A_{CO2}}$ above 1 ATA values, as indicated by results when helium was substituted for nitrogen at 4 ATA. Further experiments indicated that resistance in the breathing apparatus was only partially responsible. Resistance in the divers' own airways appeared to be important. (The possibility of depression of ventilation by narcotic effects of nitrogen could not entirely be ruled out, but it could not have been a major factor.)

3. *Inadequate respiratory response to exertion* was indicated by the fact that, despite resting values in the normal range, $P_{A_{CO2}}$ rose markedly with exertion even when the divers breathed air at a few feet of depth. Some of the divers, who became known as 'carbon dioxide retainers', showed particularly marked increases in $P_{A_{CO2}}$ with exertion, and these men generally had the highest values at depth also.

Several of these 'carbon dioxide retainers' were studied further with Lambertsen in his laboratory at the University of Pennsylvania (Lanphier 1956b). They were found to have marked increases in $P_{A_{CO2}}$ and $P_{a_{CO2}}$ with moderate exertion even with optimal low-resistance breathing apparatus on dry land. Their average $P_{A_{CO2}}$ went from 42 mm Hg at rest to over 48 mm Hg at work. The 'high man' value was nearly 57 mm Hg at work. Determinations of $P_{a_{CO2}}$ agreed closely with the values obtained by end-tidal gas sampling using the EDU method. Most of these divers showed a combined metabolic and respiratory acidosis during exercise instead of the mild, largely compensated metabolic acidosis that is ordinarily expected at the work rate concerned.[1]

In view of these findings, the earlier question could have been restated: 'Why do *some* divers fail to breathe adequately when they *work*?' The 'carbon dioxide retainers' had shown most of the toxic reactions in the original trials of nitrogen–oxygen mixtures. Such observations led Lambertsen and his associates (1959) to wonder whether the long-accepted acceleration of oxygen toxicity by exercise might not occur *only* when carbon dioxide retention accompanies exertion.

Individuals with characteristics like the carbon dioxide-retaining divers are found occasionally in the general population of athletic young men, but the proportion among EDU divers was extraordinarily high. From all usual medical standpoints, these men were completely healthy. They were also in a good state of 'fitness' with high exercise tolerance. Only one resting physiological measurement conducted at EDU appeared to correlate highly with carbon dioxide retention in exercise: the respiratory response to inspired carbon dioxide (Lanphier 1956b) (Fig. 8.13).

Men with remarkably low ventilation in exercise were also encountered by Goff and his associates (1957) in studies conducted at shallow depth with good breathing apparatus. Jarrett (1966) reported findings like those of the EDU study in diver subjects exercising with air at increased pressure. Schaefer (1969) has reported extensive studies in submarine escape training tank instructors. He found very similar characteristics. In substance, Schaefer believes that this status represents adaptation to carbon dioxide. This presupposes extensive exposure to high levels of carbon dioxide. In the tank instructors, high alveolar and arterial P_{CO_2} is inherent in the daily routine of deep breath-hold diving. It is only

slightly less easy to pinpoint high carbon dioxide exposure in divers. However, Froeb (1961) did not find distinctly abnormal carbon dioxide response in a group of long-term civilian scuba divers. Carbon dioxide adaptation in diving has been considered at greater length elsewhere (Lanphier 1964).

More recent studies in which individual differences related to CO_2 retention were noted include those reported by Salzano, Rausch and Saltzman (1970), Bradley et al. (1972), Broussolle et al. (1971), and Varène et al. (1974). The matter is discussed at some length by Bradley et al. (1971). Most but not all such reports confirm a close relationship between CO_2 retention and years of diving experience.

Whatever its etiology, *the individual tendency to retain carbon dioxide during exertion* appears to be the most important single factor in the problem of abnormal $P_{A_{CO_2}}$ and its potentially serious consequences. Other factors, such as increased work of breathing, high $P_{I_{O_2}}$, carbon dioxide in the inspired gas, and excessive apparatus dead space all remain important; but their effects appear to be magnified greatly in men who do not maintain normal carbon dioxide values even under optimal conditions of work. The 'carbon dioxide retainers' are difficult to separate as a distinct group. The tendency appears to be present, in varying degrees, in a large proportion of experienced divers, so it is not easy to 'draw a line'. However, it seems desirable, in large diving activities, to employ a standardized test that would detect and quantify this tendency, permit its development to be followed, and permit special surveillance at least in the most extreme cases.

A diver will seldom stop work just because he cannot keep his $P_{A_{CO_2}}$ at 40 mm Hg (Lanphier 1963). It has, in fact, been argued that the best diver is a man who can tolerate high levels of $P_{A_{CO_2}}$. This is certainly true from the standpoint

---

[1] The usual situation would include a modest degree of lactic acid production resulting in mild metabolic acidosis. The body's normal compensatory response to this state is an increase in alveolar ventilation. This is usually sufficient to return the blood pH to a near normal level by virtue of lower P_{aCO_2} and some loss of plasma bicarbonate. This describes the 'disproportionate increase in ventilation' ordinarily seen at the 'anaerobic threshold' as described by Wasserman et al. (1973) (see Fig. 8.5). In the 'CO_2 retainers', lactic acid production occurred, but the compensatory response did not. In fact, alveolar ventilation was and remained abnormally low for the work concerned. As a result, the $P_{A_{CO_2}}$ and P_{aCO_2} were above normal levels and remained so. Elevated P_{aCO_2} by definition constitutes respiratory acidosis, which in this instance was present together with mild metabolic acidosis.

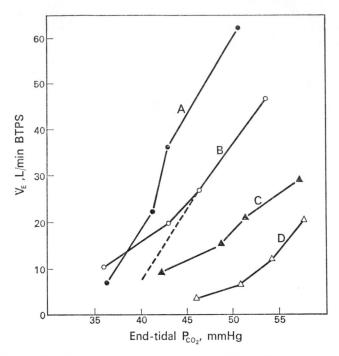

FIG. 8.13. CO$_2$-response in Experimental Diving Unit subjects

Men who had been subjects in EDU studies reported by Lanphier (1963) (see Fig. 8.12) were investigated at rest when breathing air and various CO$_2$ mixtures in the laboratory. Values of $\dot{V}$E were plotted against the $P_{A_{CO2}}$ (end-expiratory measurements) existing when $\dot{V}$E reached a steady level.

Representative examples of curves obtained are shown here. Curve A was obtained from the subject who generally had the lowest $P_{A_{CO2}}$ values in the underwater experiments. He was also the least experienced diver. D gives values obtained from the subject who had reached $P_{A_{CO2}} = 70$ mm Hg. An experienced diver who characteristically showed high values and who had experienced an oxygen convulsion during presumably safe exposure is represented by Curve C. B was obtained from a subject classed as a 'CO$_2$ retainer' but whose CO$_2$ response appears to be well within the normal range. (The dashed extension of his curve would qualify it as a 'typical normal response'.)

Curves A to C are from Lanphier (1956b). Curve D was obtained a few weeks later under similar circumstances (Lanphier, unpublished data)

of depth and work capacity, but this author's observations indicate that such a man is also the most likely to develop oxygen poisoning, severe inert gas narcosis, and frank carbon dioxide intoxication (as in the original interpretation of 'shallow water blackout'). It is possible that such individuals are the only ones who develop oxygen toxicity much more readily during exertion than at rest (Lambertsen et al. 1959). If high $P_{a_{CO2}}$ also increases the incidence of decompression sickness, the 'carbon dioxide retainer' is a bad risk from that standpoint also.

An important outgrowth of the EDU study discussed above is recognition that helium–oxygen mixtures have considerable value in reducing respiratory complications that arise even at

relatively shallow depths. Since open circuit equipment is impractical for use with helium, this has formed an additional argument for development of safe and practical closed and semi-closed circuit 'mixed gas' scuba and related systems.

Schaefer (1969) reports unexplained retention of carbon dioxide and related abnormalities in men exposed to a helium–oxygen–nitrogen mixture under presumably optimal conditions at 7 ATA. His findings suggest that previously unsuspected factors may exist and that much further work is required in this area of pulmonary function under increased pressure. Hamilton et al. (1966) and Hamilton (1967) report evidence of carbon dioxide retention with 94·5% helium at 20 ATA. MVV was approximately the same as with air at 2·0 ATA (see Fig. 8.10). Whether the increased work of breathing at this level or other recognized factors were sufficient to explain the elevation of $P_{A_{CO2}}$ is not entirely certain. The most interesting suggestion is that respiratory regulation is affected by increased ambient pressure per se. This possibility will be discussed.

Control mechanisms

A detailed discussion of respiratory regulation is beyond the scope of this chapter, but the subject cannot be ignored. Most of the problems of 'pulmonary function' discussed thus far are more closely related to pulmonary ventilation than to local pulmonary effects. Increased gas density increases the work of moving gas through the pulmonary airways and sets limits to maximum flow and ventilation. This is a 'local' effect. But why, when an adequate reserve of ventilatory capacity remains, do the respiratory muscles not always simply do the extra work required to maintain normal values of $P_{A_{CO2}}$ and Pa_{CO2}?

The regulation of respiration does not present many difficulties in divers at rest or during very mild work, but divers are generally in the water for purposes that require consequential exertion. The regulation of breathing during work remains a controversial topic in physiology, but a period of growing agreement is represented in papers by important investigators in symposium proceedings edited by Chapman (1967). More recent work will be discussed under appropriate headings.

Neurogenic v. humoral factors

Increased P_{CO2} and hydrogen ion concentration and decreased P_{O2} have been known for a long time to cause increases in ventilation. However, demonstrable changes in such 'humoral factors' are not sufficient singly or together to explain normal levels of ventilation during exercise. It has been necessary to postulate an additional 'work factor' that either stimulates ventilation in its own right or perhaps alters the effective sensitivity or set-point of the basic control system. Under normal conditions, the net result is a remarkably precise matching of $\dot{V}_A$ to $\dot{V}_{CO2}$ so that the $P_{A_{CO2}}$ remains virtually unchanged up to work rates

where blood lactic acid begins to rise above resting levels (see Fig. 8.5). At higher work rates, $P_{A_{CO2}}$ normally falls.

Asmussen and Nielsen (1946), Dejours (1964, 1967), and more recently D'Angelo and Torelli (1971), have focused attention on the fact that the increase in ventilation in exercise, and the decrease in recovery, have distinct fast and slow components. There is an almost instantaneous increase in ventilation at the onset of dynamic exercise. No central or chemoreceptor mechanism that depends upon changes in the blood could explain this. A similar fast drop in ventilation occurs when exercise ceases. The fast changes must depend on neurogenic mechanisms. The slower changes that follow are compatible with humoral mechanisms.

The fast or neurogenic component accounts for a considerable portion of the total increase in ventilation in exercise. Like the slower changes, it is essentially proportional to the intensity of exertion. Although the neurogenic mechanisms have not been fully identified, there seems to be no doubt that proprioceptors in the active regions are involved. There may also be a cortical component.

No specific attempts have yet been made to determine whether abnormalities encountered in diving can be related entirely to 'neurogenic' or 'humoral' mechanisms. However, existing information provides some basis for discussion.

Response to carbon dioxide

One of the definite 'humoral' factors in the control of ventilation is the response to carbon dioxide. This can be demonstrated and quantified by adding carbon dioxide to the inspired gas and measuring the ventilation that results. The most common presentation of such data is simply a plot of $\dot{V}_E$ against either $F_{I_{O2}}$ or measured $P_{A_{CO2}}$, as in Fig. 8.13.

The respiratory response to carbon dioxide, as illustrated by such 'dose-response curves', can be reduced in a number of ways as, for example, by narcotic drugs (Lambertsen & Wendel 1960), marked elevation of $P_{I_{O2}}$ (Lambertsen et al. 1963), or by deliberate adaptation of subjects to carbon dioxide (Kellogg 1960). As has been mentioned, Schaefer suggests that 'carbon dioxide retainers' have, in one way or another, become acclimatized to high P_{CO_2} (see also Lanphier 1964).

Hydrostatic pressure effects. Questions about the effect of hydrostatic pressure on respiratory regulation may have arisen first in connection with a 1000 ft chamber dive (Salzano, Rausch & Saltzman 1970). In a later study, Saltzman et al. (1971) found a high coefficient of correlation between Pa_{CO_2} and ambient pressure while no correlation appeared to exist between Pa_{CO_2} and gas density in resting subjects. Saltzman (1973) has reported further observations suggesting that a 'normal' Pa_{CO_2} may include considerably higher values at increased pressure than at 1 ATA. It remains to be seen what proportion of phenomena that have been attributed to increased gas density are actually due to 'hydrostatic re-setting of the CO_2-stat'. This question might be asked, for example, about the study of Gelfand and Peterson (1975) concerning CO_2 reactivity with neon at high pressure. Its possible relevance in 'Chouteau hypoxia' and suspected high pressure gas diffusion effects will be discussed.

P_{O_2} effects. The reduction of ventilation in exercise by high $P_{I_{O_2}}$ may be related in part to improved blood oxygen transport leading to decreased anaerobic metabolism with less production of lactic acid. This is one possibility suggested by the work of Asmussen and Nielsen (1946, 1958) and of Salzano et al. (1967). The decrease is perhaps more likely to be related to the alteration of response to carbon dioxide by high $P_{I_{O_2}}$ as shown by Lambertsen et al. (1963).

Respiratory work. The effect of increased work of breathing on ventilation can probably also be explained in terms of the response to carbon dioxide. Studies like those of Cherniack and Snidal (1956) and Milic-Emili and Tyler (1963) indicate that the basic response to increased PA_{CO_2} or Pa_{CO_2} is a corresponding increase in the *work output of the respiratory muscles*. In experiments with added external airway resistance, Milic-Emili and Tyler (1963) found that the carbon dioxide response in terms of $\dot{V}_E$ decreased with added resistance but that there was good correlation between the PA_{CO_2} and the *inspiratory work* performed. In such terms the actual ventilation achieved at a given PA_{CO_2} depends not only upon 'CO_2 sensitivity' but upon the relationship between ventilation and respiratory work: how much ventilation a given amount of respiratory work can produce.

In experiments conducted during exercise Cerretelli, Sikand and Farhi (1969) found similar relationships between the respiratory stimulus and the response in terms of respiratory work. They were able to express the total respiratory drive at various levels of exertion in terms of an equivalent PA_{CO_2}. If the work of breathing was increased by addition of external airway resistance, the ventilation was correspondingly reduced and the actual PA_{CO_2} rose accordingly. Cerretelli, Sikand and Farhi (1969) also found that increased work of breathing could limit the capacity for physical exertion to levels below those associated with anaerobic metabolism. Their subjects were unable to continue exercise when the algebraic sum of inspiratory and expiratory pressures reached about 100 cm H_2O. This presumably represented maximum dynamic respiratory effort (and thus maximum respiratory work at a given level of $\dot{V}_E$).

Effects of added resistance

Classical studies on the effects of added external resistance are those of Cain and Otis (1949) and Zechman, Hall and Hull (1957). Both teams recognized effects upon CO_2 elimination. Cain and Otis (1949) summarized the situation admirably in saying, 'The retention of CO_2 during resistance breathing indicates a compromise by the body. The body tolerates some rise in CO_2 tension in preference to expending the effort that would be required to keep it at the original level.'

More recent studies include those of Barnett and Rasmussen (1970), who found that the ventilatory response to CO_2 was influenced more markedly by the resistive work of breathing than was the response to equivalent hypoxia. Demedts and Anthonisen (1973) report a study conducted at 1 ATA in which subjects tolerated remarkably high resistance in 5 min bouts of exertion without impairment of work capacity or much reduction of ventilation. At the point of exercise limitation with still higher resistance, the response varied markedly among individuals and correlated with the resting ventilatory response to CO_2. Maximum exercise ventilation in this series was about 70% of the 15 sec MVV attained with the same resistance.

Changes in respiratory pattern with added external resistance tend to keep respiratory work to a minimum. They will be discussed further in the section on mechanics of breathing. A common change is a decrease in frequency with an increase in tidal volume.

It is reasonable to expect that relationships and limits like those seen with external resistance will be found when the work of breathing is increased in other ways, as by gas density or the effects of submergence. If further research establishes such relationships, understanding of $P_{A_{CO2}}$ elevation in underwater work will be greatly simplified. It is useful to recapitulate some of the factors apparently involved:

1. *Inherent response to respiratory stimuli.* How much respiratory work will the diver's respiratory muscles ordinarily perform in response to a given level of exertion or $P_{A_{CO2}}$?

2. *Modification of ventilatory response.* Will any environmental factor, like $P_{I_{O2}}$ or ambient pressure, alter the inherent response?

3. *Work of breathing and related factors.* How much ventilation will result from a given increase in respiratory work output?

Although quantitative answers cannot yet be supplied, it is not difficult to see in a general way why $P_{A_{CO2}}$ tends to rise during underwater work. In the first place, the diver is likely to have a below-average inherent ventilatory response to carbon dioxide and exertion. His response is likely to be impaired further by high $P_{I_{O2}}$ and perhaps by other factors in the environment. Finally, the work of breathing is increased by breathing apparatus and gas density and perhaps by submergence. As a result, the amount of respiratory work that his muscles perform will produce even less actual pulmonary ventilation than on dry land. With $\dot{V}_{CO2}$ at a given value and with $\dot{V}_E$ and $\dot{V}_A$ decreased, $P_{A_{CO2}}$ and $P_{a_{CO2}}$ must increase. The problem is aggravated further by carbon dioxide in the inspired gas or by excessive apparatus dead space. The diver's ability to compensate for such factors will be similarly impaired.

Effects of inspired CO_2

Effects of CO_2 in the inspired gas were mentioned in the discussion of Equation (8), and the likelihood of divers encountering elevated $P_{I_{CO2}}$ was discussed in connection with helmet ventilation. $P_{A_{CO2}}$ cannot remain lower than $P_{I_{CO2}}$. Even when $P_{I_{CO2}}$ is well below 40 mm Hg, a considerable increase in ventilation may be required to keep the $P_{A_{CO2}}$ close to its normal value. The statement of Cain and Otis (1949) about CO_2 in resistance breathing (above) also applies here. In almost no case will $P_{A_{CO2}} = 40$ mm Hg be maintained in the face of consequential values of $P_{I_{CO2}}$ even at rest. How much $P_{A_{CO2}}$ will rise with a given $P_{I_{CO2}}$ depends largely upon the individual's inherent response to CO_2.

The more complex question of elevated $P_{I_{CO2}}$ during exercise is the subject of several recent studies. Menn, Sinclair and Welch (1970) studied moderate and heavy exercise (2/3 $\dot{V}_{O2max}$) of 30 min duration with $P_{I_{CO2}}$ values to 30 mm Hg. The subjects experienced no difficulty up to 15 mm Hg and were able to complete the work at 30 mm despite dyspnea and intercostal pain. $\dot{V}_E$ increased with increasing $P_{I_{CO2}}$, mainly by virtue of larger tidal volume. At 2/3 $\dot{V}_{O2max}$, $P_{I_{CO2}} = 15$ produced values of $P_{A_{CO2}}$ between 45 and 52 mm Hg. The corresponding values with $P_{I_{CO2}} = 30$ were 49 and 61 mm Hg. Average values of $\dot{V}_E$ for this work rate were 76 L/min at zero inspired CO_2, 81 at 15, and 103 at 30 mm Hg. In a stepwise approach to maximum exertion, the $\dot{V}_E$ reached a maximum of about 140 L/min and did not vary with the $P_{I_{CO2}}$. Blood-gas measurements were not conducted in this phase, but marked hypercapnia and acidosis were considered a real possibility with $P_{I_{CO2}} = 21$ mm Hg or more.

Elliott et al. (1970) reported that maximal work capacity was reduced by inspiratory CO_2 pressures of 15 mm Hg or more. They concluded that inspired CO_2 at such levels interferes with the elimination of excess CO_2 that is necessary to compensate for the effects of fixed-acid metabolites (e.g. lactic acid). As a result, acid–base balance is seriously disturbed at the limits of ventilatory capacity. Sinclair, Clark and Welch (1971) summarized the situation by saying that when $P_{I_{CO2}}$ reaches 21 mm Hg in exercise '... alveolar ventilation does not increase sufficiently to compensate for its reduced effectiveness in CO_2 elimination.'

Clark (1973) reported work with R. D. Sinclair and J. B. Lenox concerning effects of hypercapnia on exercise tolerance. Clark (1973) also presented graphical and mathematical descriptions of acid–base, arterial gas, and ventilatory changes in work. Responses to $P_{I_{CO_2}}$ levels up to 40 mm Hg were studied in nine subjects doing treadmill exercise at average $\dot{V}_{O_2}$ values to over 3·5 L/min (80% of $\dot{V}_{O_{2max}}$ for the subjects concerned). One of the simplest of Clark's diagrams, reproduced in Fig. 8.14,

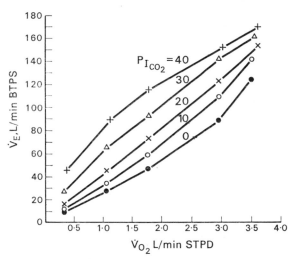

FIG. 8.14. $\dot{V}_E$ in exercise with increased $P_{I_{CO_2}}$

Mean values of $\dot{V}_E$ in a group of nine subjects during graded exercise with different levels of $P_{I_{CO_2}}$ (after Clark 1973)

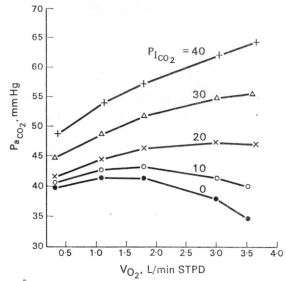

FIG. 8.15. Pa_{CO_2} in exercise with increased $P_{I_{CO_2}}$

Mean values of arterial P_{CO_2} in a group of nine subjects during graded exercise with different levels of $P_{I_{CO_2}}$ (after Clark 1973)

shows the average values of $\dot{V}_E$ encountered in this study. The combination of the highest work rate and the highest $P_{I_{CO_2}}$ forced the subjects very close to MVV. Fig. 8.15 shows that despite such respiratory responses, the Pa_{CO_2} rose substantially above control values. The normal compensatory decrease in Pa_{CO_2} above 50% of $\dot{V}_{O_{2max}}$ is clearly shown in the $P_{I_{CO_2}} = 0$ curve. A small compensatory drop is still seen when $P_{I_{CO_2}}$ is 10 mm Hg, but such a drop is essentially absent at $P_{I_{CO_2}} = 20$.

None of the information on effects of increased inspiratory CO_2 summarized above was obtained under circumstances that included such diving problems as unusual inherent responses, modification of response, exceptional work of breathing, or fixed limitation of expiratory flow. It is not difficult to surmise that combinations of high $P_{I_{CO_2}}$ with such factors could have very unfavorable effects.

Preventive measures

Whether the suggested analysis is correct in all details or not, elevation of PA_{CO_2} in diving seems almost inevitable. The use of lighter gases can, up to a point, circumvent the increase in work of breathing with breathing apparatus and at greater depths. Beyond this, only respiratory assistance (and perhaps not even that) could maintain fully normal alveolar ventilation and PA_{CO_2} in diving. For the present, there seem to be only five useful courses of action: (1) keep the work of breathing as low as possible and minimize other causes of impaired ventilation; (2) avoid carbon dioxide in the inspired gas and keep dead space to a minimum; (3) recognize that some elevation of PA_{CO_2} will probably occur and that such carbon dioxide-related hazards as oxygen toxicity and narcosis should be avoided by a wide margin; (4) avoid unnecessarily heavy exertion; and (5) pay particular attention to carbon-dioxide-retaining divers, keeping in mind that they may develop carbon dioxide intoxication or related difficulties where others may not.

Narcosis and ventilation

A question never completely answered is

whether inert gas narcosis can depress respiratory control as it does other neurological functions. This is a potentially important question. The effect of elevated Pa_{CO_2} on pre-existing narcosis is impressive (Case & Haldane 1941; Lanphier 1963; Behnke 1965; Bennett, this volume). If increased narcosis can, in turn, further depress ventilation and thus cause a greater elevation of Pa_{CO_2}, a vicious circle might sometimes develop with disastrous results.

Very severe narcosis does not abolish the respiratory drive (Lanphier 1963), but the possibility of some depression of ventilation by narcosis is extremely difficult to rule out in studies at high pressure. Density and narcotic effects are essentially inseparable. If helium is substituted for nitrogen to relieve narcosis, the density is also changed greatly, and vice versa.

Fagraeus and Hesser (1970) report a study in which changes in the CO_2 response curve were used in an effort to evaluate the relative importance of gas density (via increased work of breathing) and the narcotic action of high nitrogen pressures in causing reduction of the response to CO_2. The conclusion, based on a change in slope rather than in position of the response curve, was that increased density rather than narcosis was responsible for the change.

Two studies were based on the fact that nitrous oxide in relatively low concentration (e.g. 30%) at 1 ATA produces an effect subjectively indistinguishable from narcosis with air at depth. Bradley and Dickson (1975) found that nitrous oxide inhalation caused significant increases in $\dot{V}_E$ and respiratory frequency with decreases in tidal volume and PA_{CO_2} during both rest and work. These changes are opposite to those seen with air at depth and were thought to be the result of nitrous-oxide sensitization of the pulmonary stretch receptors.

Webber (1969) also reported an increase in frequency, but his calculations indicated no significant net change in alveolar ventilation. None of the studies to date actually permit us to rule out the possibility of ventilatory effects of inert gas narcosis at depth. Hydrostatic effects upon respiratory control mechanisms could make this question harder to answer but perhaps less important.

Carbon dioxide and narcosis

The physiological effects of CO_2 excess are the subject of another chapter in this volume (Chapter 11), and only a few such effects warrant specific mention here.

Almost all of the foregoing discussion concerns relatively brief exposure to increased PI_{CO_2} or to other conditions that can elevate Pa_{CO_2}. Neff and Petty (1972) describe patients with chronic pulmonary disease who have values of Pa_{CO_2} in the 75 to 110 mm Hg range and who tolerate this degree of hypercapnia with very few symptoms. Such levels have developed over a long period of time, and the patients are kept well oxygenated. Acute development of arterial CO_2 pressures in the 75 to 110 mm Hg range would produce, among other effects, loss of consciousness or severe impairment of mental function in most individuals.

A longstanding and recurrent debate has concerned the role of CO_2 in inert gas narcosis. Definitive answers now appear to be available. Hesser, Adolfson and Fagraeus (1971) analysed compressed air narcosis into its 'CO_2' and 'N_2' components. They concluded that (1) Pa_{CO_2} values below 40 mm Hg had a negligible effect in contributing to narcosis, and (2) that high alveolar N_2 and CO_2 pressures are simply additive in their effects on performance.

Bennett and Blenkarn (1974) studied four subjects at rest at 6·7 and 9·6 ATA, alternating between air and He–O_2. Definite decrements in mental performance were found during air breathing, but no evidence of hypoxemia or elevation of Pa_{CO_2} was seen under any of the experimental conditions. In this situation, narcosis was evidently due to raised nitrogen pressure alone. This does not alter the fact that accompanying elevation of carbon dioxide levels can markedly enhance the degree of narcosis (Case & Haldane 1941; Lanphier 1967).

MECHANICS OF BREATHING

The foregoing discussion indicated that the most prominent disorder of pulmonary function in diving is inadequate ventilation of the lungs during exertion. One of the important causes of hypoventilation is excessive work of breathing.

The mechanics and .work of breathing are covered at length in chapters by several leading investigators in the Respiration volumes of the *Handbook of Physiology* (Fenn & Rahn 1964, 1965). Less detailed but very valuable discussions are provided by Comroe (1965) and Dejours (1966). Only a summary of some of the aspects most important in diving and of some pertinent newer information can be attempted here.

The work of breathing can be analyzed in terms of the mechanical work done against forces that *oppose changes in lung volume* and those that *resist the movement of air*. The most important aspects are those related to the elasticity of the chest–lung system, and those concerned with resistance to gas flow in the airways. These are also the factors most affected by forces present in underwater work. Increased gas density increases airway resistance while submergence involves hydrostatic pressure differences that interact with the elastic properties of the system.

Lung volumes

The left-hand portion of Fig. 8.16 presents the standard subdivisions of lung volume. The values indicated are round numbers and are somewhat larger than those usually presented for 'average' healthy young males. They are probably close to the average for divers, but individual variability is great.

An important volume-landmark of the chest–lung system is the resting or relaxation volume (V_R) that it seeks when the respiratory muscles are relaxed and the airways are open. The lung volume at V_R is the functional residual capacity (FRC). The level of V_R is generally at about 30% of the vital capacity (VC).

During rest or mild work under normal conditions, only the inspiratory muscles are active. They increase the lung volume above V_R and then relax, most often gradually, to allow elastic recoil to return the system to V_R.

Tidal volume (V_T) represents the volume of any

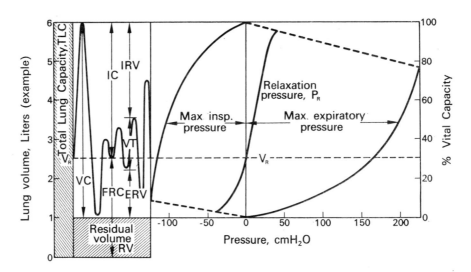

FIG. 8.16. Lung volumes and the static pressure–volume diagram

The left-hand portion of the figure presents standardized subdivisions of lung volume together with a scale in liters from which roughly approximate 'normal' values for the individual volumes can be derived. Details are discussed in the text. Abbreviations not explained in the text include IC (inspiratory capacity), IRV (inspiratory reserve volume), and ERV (expiratory reserve volume). IC is a 'fixed' value, representing the volume that can be inspired above V_R. IRV and ERV depend entirely upon the size and 'position' of the tidal volume (V_T). As indicated, V_T can vary greatly. It does so particularly at different levels of exertion.

The right-hand portion of the figure is a representative pressure–volume diagram of the chest–lung system. This type of diagram was originally used by Rohrer (1915) and has since been utilized and modified by numerous authors. The sloping dashed lines at top and bottom represent compression and expansion of lung gas as + or − pressure is applied, as in reaching maximum inspiratory or expiratory pressure. This effect is magnified at altitude but becomes negligible at depth. (See text for further details)

individual breath. The traditional average resting value is 0·5 L, but actual V_T varies greatly with the individual's pattern of breathing and with the level of activity. V_T can be as large as VC, but it scarcely ever reaches this limit and does not often exceed about 50% of VC even during exertion. As activity increases, V_T ordinarily increases first by virtue of larger end-inspiratory volumes. Increase of V_T by expiration beyond V_R requires activation of expiratory muscles and generally occurs only at higher levels of exertion.

Maximum respiratory pressures

Much can be learned about the properties of the respiratory system and its muscular and elastic forces by measuring pressures developed at the mouth under various static conditions. Typical results of such measurements are shown in the pressure–volume diagram at the right of Fig. 8.16. The vertical scale represents lung volume as shown at the left. The horizontal scale indicates positive and negative pressures (in cm H_2O) as might be indicated by a water manometer at the mouth with the glottis open and the nose closed.

The outer curves indicate the pressures that can be produced by maximum inspiratory and expiratory effort at various lung volumes. The greatest positive pressure is produced by maximum expiratory effort when the lungs are full. At the lung volume of maximum expiration, expiratory effort yields no pressure; but inspiratory effort at this volume can produce maximum negative pressure. The maximum positive and negative pressures shown here can be maintained only in static manoeuvres. With inspiratory or expiratory flow, maximum pressures are reduced.

Relaxation pressures

The curve in the centre of the pressure–volume diagram of Fig. 8.16 represents static 'relaxation pressures'. These are the pressures that develop at various lung volumes when the respiratory muscles are relaxed as completely as possible. Relaxation pressure (P_R) reflects the elastic properties of the system, derived from the characteristics of the lung and 'chest wall' acting together. Functionally, 'wall' includes not only the rib cage but also the diaphragm, abdominal contents, and abdominal wall. The 'elastic'

properties of the wall include not only the inherent elasticity of the structures concerned but also the effects of gravity and, when submerged, of buoyancy. The elasticity of the lungs is attributed in large part to surface tension at the gas–liquid interface in the alveoli.

The lungs tend to collapse to a volume considerably smaller than the residual volume (RV). The chest seeks its own 'resting volume' at about 70% of VC. At V_R the forces of the chest (tending to expand) and of the lungs (tending to collapse) are equal and opposite. Below V_R, the elastic recoil of the chest predominates, so P_R is negative. Above V_R, lung recoil predominates, so P_R is positive. Above about 70% VC, the lungs and chest are both seeking smaller volumes and thus contributing to positive P_R.

Pleural pressure

There is no actual space between the lungs and the chest wall in normal individuals, but the outer covering of the lungs and the lining of the chest can be separated if a small amount of air is admitted to the potential space between them. If this is done, 'pleural pressure' (P_{pl}) can be measured in the space that has been created. Such direct measurements of P_{pl} are seldom made in man, but a satisfactory approximation of P_{pl} can be obtained by measuring pressure in the esophagus by means of a pencil-shaped balloon on the end of a long, slender tube. Having an index of intrapleural pressure as well as of P_R permits the lung and chest components of P_R to be quantified separately. Measurement of esophageal pressure is also very useful in estimation of the work of breathing.

Respiratory work

Mechanical work is defined in physics and engineering as the product of force × displacement. The product of mean pressure-change × volume-change is equivalent. Areas on a pressure–volume diagram are therefore proportional to work, and respiratory work can be determined by simultaneous plotting of these variables in appropriate units and measuring the resulting area.

The work of breathing can be visualized most readily from the standpoint of a mechanical respirator applied to the mouth of a relaxed

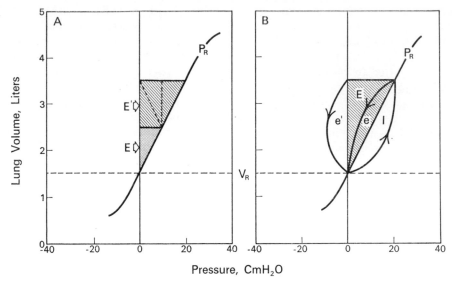

FIG. 8.17. Elastic and 'airway' work of breathing

A. The diagonal line represents the linear portion of a P_R curve (see Fig. 8.16). The lightly-shaded area E represents work done against chest–lung elasticity in inspiring 1·0 L of air above V_R. The cross-hatched area E′ represents the additional 'elastic' work of inspiring a second litre of air (see text).

B. Area E is the same as the total area shown in diagram A. It represents the elastic work of inspiring 2 L of air above V_R and also indicates the stored energy of elastic recoil. Area I represents additional work done against airway resistance on inspiration. Area (e) indicates 'airway' work in quiet expiration, completely supplied by elastic recoil. All of area E is available for expiratory work, but forceful expiration (using expiratory muscles) involves extra expiratory 'airway' work such as that indicated by area ($e′$). (See text for details.) The 'airway work' areas can become much larger in forceful respiration or in the presence of high airway resistance

subject. The work done by the respirator must be essentially equal to the less readily measured work that would be done by the respiratory muscles in producing the same flow and volume-change.

Elastic work

Fig. 8.17A is based on an enlarged P_R curve and represents the work done against the elastic properties of the system. The lightly-shaded area E represents the elastic work of inspiring 1·0 L of gas starting at V_R. To increase the lung volume 1·0 L, the respirator had to develop a final pressure of +10 cm H_2O. The mean pressure was +5·0 cm H_2O. Therefore, the shaded area E has the dimensions 1000 ml × 5·0 cm H_2O, equivalent to 5000 gram-centimetres (g-cm) or 0·05 kilogram-metres (kg-m) of work.[1]

The cross-hatched area E′ in Fig. 8.17A represents the additional work of inspiring another 1·0 L of gas to achieve $V_T = 2·0$ L above V_R. This requires a final respiratory pressure of +20 cm H_2O. Note that the total area E + E′ is equal to four times the area of E alone. In other words, doubling V_T required four times as much 'elastic' work. This suggests that the work of breathing should be considerably less with small tidal volumes than with large ones. This is basically true, but other factors can offset the advantage.

Fig. 8.17A treats the mid-portion of the P_R curve as a straight line with a slope such that 1 cm H_2O increase in pressure causes an increase of 100 ml in lung volume. The *compliance* of the system is thus 100 ml/cm H_2O, which is about average for normal individuals in the range of

[1] If a gram is defined as a force equal to the weight of 1 ml of water, a pressure of 1·0 cm water can be expressed as 1·0 g/cm². If this pressure were exerted on a piston having a cross-sectional area of 1·0 cm², the total force would be 1·0 g; and if the piston were moved 1·0 cm to displace 1·0 cm³ (1·0 ml) of volume, the work done (force × displacement) would be 1·0 g-cm. It could also be expressed in kg-m (100 000 g-cm = 1·0 kg-m). The forces concerned are more correctly expressed in dynes; but the approach indicated here is clearer to non-physicists and leads to the same ultimate conclusions.

lung volumes where breathing normally occurs. At the upper and lower ends of the P_R curve, compliance is decreased: a greater change in pressure is required to produce a given change in lung volume.

Work against airway resistance

In the examples given, the respirator must not only do work against the elastic recoil of the system when it increases the lung volume but it must also overcome airway resistance.[1] At the beginning and end of inspiration there is no gas flow, and no extra pressure is required at these points. The respirator must supply additional positive pressure to produce inspiratory flow, and this involves additional work related to the rate of flow and to the airway resistance. This work can be shown on a pressure–volume diagram as in area I of Fig. 8.17B.

The energy of work represented by area I cannot be utilized further. The elastic work (shaded area E) is stored as the potential energy of elastic recoil and can be utilized during expiration. In quiet breathing, overcoming expiratory

airway resistance requires a quantity of work like that represented by area e, and the energy of elastic recoil is more than sufficient to provide for this work. The work represented by the remainder of area E is accounted for by opposing 'negative work' done by the inspiratory muscles as they relax gradually to maintain smoothly controlled expiration (see Yamashiro & Grodins 1971).

Forceful expiration or high airway resistance may require active expiratory effort. In such case, the work could include not only all of area E but also additional pressure developed by the expiratory muscles and represented by an area such as e′.

Fig. 8.18 shows actual 'work loops' from a study of respiratory limitations at depth (Miller, Wangensteen & Lanphier 1972). The orientation of the figure is opposite to that of Figs 8.16 and 8.17 because the focus of interest is upon esophageal pressure during breathing rather than upon relaxation pressures measured at the mouth.

Wasted respiratory work

'Negative work', mentioned above, requires energy and could be classed as wasted effort; but it appears to be characteristic of many respiratory patterns. Forms of 'wasted work' that are probably much more important in exercise and diving arise in connection with work against airway resistance. Two prime examples can be cited. One is encountered with demand-type breathing apparatus if maximum flow is reached at a level below that desired by the user. Further inspiratory effort will not increase the flow but the average individual will instinctively make such an effort. If he does so, his total inspiratory work may be much greater than is necessary or productive.

A similar situation may develop on expiration, particularly with increased gas density. As will be seen, maximum expiratory flow is 'effort-independent' over a large range of lung volumes. If the individual reaches maximum flow and tries to exceed it, a considerable portion of his total expiratory effort may be wasted. The $\dot{V}_{O_2}$ and $\dot{V}_{CO_2}$ of wasted respiratory work will, in effect, subtract from the individual's capacity for other work.

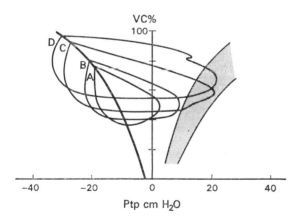

FIG. 8.18. Pressure–volume loops during work at depth

Representative 'pressure–volume loops' (transpulmonary pressure v. %VC) recorded in one subject during exercise breathing air at pressures between 1 ATA (A) and 7·8 ATA (D). The actual ventilation was 60 to 70 L/min in each case, but in C and D the required $\dot{V}_E$ was at or above MVV. The shaded area represents the 'P_{max} region' (see text) where increased expiratory pressure no longer increases expiratory flow (after Miller, Wangensteen & Lanphier 1972)

[1] Airway resistance is covered in greater detail in a later section of this chapter.

Measurement of respiratory work

Measurement of the total work of breathing under realistic conditions is not completely simple. One of the main difficulties is the fact that the muscles concerned are part of the elastic system.

For some purposes, it is sufficient to record 'work loops' of volume change v. esophageal pressure. The area of such a loop reflects work against airway resistance and lung elasticity. It neglects work done on the 'chest wall'. This has been considered to be a relatively small, or at least rather constant, part of total work. However, Goldman (1973) calls attention to the discovery that *distortional work*, associated with deformation of the chest wall from its relaxed configuration, can account for 25 to 30% of the total mechanical work of breathing at high values of $\dot{V}E$. Above 40 L/min, the method that takes distortional work into account consistently yields higher values than the traditional approach. Neglect of this factor no doubt has introduced important errors into the quantification of respiratory work.

Inadequate estimation of mechanical work is almost certainly one of the reasons why very low values have often been reported for the *efficiency* of respiratory work.

$$\text{Efficiency} = \frac{\text{mechanical work done}}{\text{energy required to do this work}} \quad (12)$$

Measurement of *energy required* is also difficult to accomplish with precision since it depends upon determining, by one strategem or another, the fraction of total $\dot{V}O_2$ that is actually attributable to respiratory work. It is not surprising that estimates of the oxygen cost of breathing vary widely.

Attempting to quantify the mechanical work of breathing makes it obvious that the physical definition of work leaves as much to be desired when dealing with the 'elastic' work of breathing as it does in other physiological forms of work[1].

EFFECTS OF SUBMERGENCE

On dry land, we assume that pressures in the alveoli will be zero (equal to the surrounding air pressure) when the respiratory muscles are relaxed and the chest returns to its resting end-expiratory position at the 'relaxation volume,' VR (see Fig. 8.16). The same kind of relationships hold true when the individual is submerged. Upon relaxation, the pressure of surrounding water and the action of buoyant forces combine to produce a certain pressure within the lungs. This pressure will be the same as the pressure at some specific depth in the surrounding water, and this depth can be indicated in terms of its distance above or below a stable anatomical landmark like the suprasternal notch. In this discussion, we will designate as the *balance point* that depth where the pressure is the same as the alveolar pressure of the relaxed chest–lung system when the individual is submerged in a specified position.

Pressure and buoyant force

It should not be surprising to learn that the exact locations of 'balance points' are not completely certain. Especially when a diver is vertical, standing or sitting underwater, the forces acting upon him are quite complex. Anatomically, the thoracic cage and diaphragm present a structure that is irregular not only in shape but also in pliability. The pressure of surrounding water is different at every level subtended by the structures concerned. Buoyant force cancels the effect of gravity upon the abdominal contents, whose weight ordinarily tends to pull the diaphragm down. The buoyancy of the air-filled chest probably tends to elevate the rib cage to some small degree, tending to lower the pressure within. Buoyant force clearly offsets the usual tendency of blood to pool in the lower portions of the body, so we can expect to find a larger-than-usual volume of blood in the great veins and pulmonary vessels.

---

[1] Quantification of work in terms of force × displacement or $1/2\,\Delta P \times$ volume-change often appears grossly inadequate from the physiological standpoint. If there is no displacement or volume change, no work is done according to this definition; yet holding a weight at some height, isometric exercise, or maintaining a given lung volume against elastic forces or external pressure clearly requires energy. The definition also fails to account for the duration of effort or for the negative work of 'braking' when a weight is lowered slowly or when a lung volume is gradually returned to VR. Tension × time is sometimes used, but this also leaves much to be desired in terms of correlation with energy cost.

Hydrostatic imbalance

Other interacting factors in submergence probably remain important, but it is natural to focus attention on the mean or 'effective' pressure represented by the balance point. This concept can assist our thinking even while the precise location of the point is unclear. Let us say, for example, that a diver is trying to breathe through a long snorkel and that his balance point is 40 cm below the surface. This is the same as saying that the effective pressure around his chest will be 40 cm H_2O greater than the pressure of the air he is trying to breathe. When his glottis is open, the air pressure is also the pressure in his lungs.

Some of the implications of such 'hydrostatic imbalance' in the respiratory system can be visualized with the aid of pressure–volume diagrams like those of Figs 8.16 and 8.17. In this example, the relaxation volume V_R will in effect be displaced down the P_R curve 40 cm in the negative (expiratory) direction. When the diver relaxes his respiratory muscles with his glottis open, his lung volume will become roughly the same as that normally associated with maximum expiration. Maintaining his normal range of lung volumes would require the diver to exert constant extra inspiratory effort equivalent to about 40 cm H_2O.

Even if the diver accepts the new level of V_R, the work of inspiration will be increased because of lower compliance at the low end of the P_R curve and because of increased airway resistance related to the smaller lung volume (Agostoni et al. 1966; Hong et al. 1969). If the effective depth were equal to his maximum inspiratory pressure (Fig. 8.16), the diver would not be able to inspire at all. At intermediate levels, his inspiratory capacity could be limited severely. If the hydrostatic imbalance were very large, lung damage (in the form of 'thoracic squeeze') and cardiovascular effects would probably outweigh ventilatory problems in importance.

Imbalance in breathing apparatus. Swimmers using snorkels effectively are seldom more than barely awash, and gross discomfort rules out prolonged snorkel-breathing when the chest is more than a foot or so underwater. Even head-out immersion is not a major feature of realistic diving. Nevertheless, hydrostatic imbalance pre-sents important problems. It is a built-in feature of many types of breathing apparatus and can have important physiological implications as will be seen. Having a demand valve or breathing bag that is too high in relation to the chest has a negative-pressure-breathing effect like that of head-out immersion or snorkeling. Locating such components too far below the balance point has the opposite effect and leads to the abnormal necessity of having to use the expiratory muscles to exhale even at rest. It seems highly desirable to determine where the balance points are located for various body positions under water and to design breathing apparatus accordingly.

Eupneic pressure. The classical work in this area is that of Paton and Sand (1947). They approached the problem by having submerged subjects select the most comfortable (eupneic) pressure of the respiratory gas in terms of depth related to body landmarks. With remarkable consistency and uniformity, their subjects chose the level of the suprasternal notch in all positions except head-up vertical posture. Here, eupneic pressure was above the notch at rest and approached the notch during hyperpnea.

Although Paton and Sand's actual findings can scarcely be faulted, it seems illogical to find the balance point so far above the theoretical 'center of pressure' of the chest. This apparent paradox has rightly led subsequent investigators to ask whether the level indicated by comfort is necessarily optimal from other standpoints. Jarrett (1965) found the balance point at the 'centroid' of the chest, and Thompson and McCally (1967) give support to his contention that the subjective choice is influenced by pressure sensations in the upper airways.

Important changes in the work of breathing do not seem likely to result from a moderate displacement of V_R up or down the P_R curve, provided that the diver accepts it. If discomfort impels him to seek some other base-line volume, a great deal of respiratory effort might be wasted. If such reactions are common, then comfort might remain the best criterion. Otherwise, the most evidence suggests that the optimal respiratory pressure corresponds to a balance point somewhat deeper than the eupneic level selected in the upright position.

Even if the balance point were accurately known, the effects of hydrostatic imbalance on the work and energy cost of breathing would be difficult to predict accurately. The most important factors are among those least adequately taken into account by the physical definition of work. The problem is complicated by the fact that divers confronted by uncomfortable imbalance are apt to adopt unusual respiratory patterns. These apparently alleviate discomfort and probably reduce the total work of breathing, but they are difficult to analyze. One response to 'negative' imbalance is to inspire rapidly and deeply, then to close the glottis so that the inspired volume can be maintained through a long pause without muscular effort. Subsequent expiration may be unrestrained or may be 'braked' by the glottis rather than by the inspiratory muscles. The role of the larynx in regulation of gas flow is too often overlooked (Rattenborg 1961) and may be particularly important underwater.

Mechanical effects

A number of recent studies have investigated the effect of head-out immersion. In most respects the findings are applicable to breathing apparatus with 'negative' imbalance. The work of Hong et al. (1969) examined immersion to the neck using immersion to the xiphoid as the control. Like several previous investigators, they found the P_R curve shifted to the right about 16 cm H_2O in 'steady state' immersion. The shift was only about half as great in brief immersions, and the possibility that involuntarily maintained inspiratory tonus made the difference was suggested. Gastric pressure increased gradually from 0 to about 40 mm Hg. VC was reduced about 8% while ERV dropped to about 30% of its control value in steady state immersion. The shift of blood into the thorax was about 220 ml after 10 sec and did not increase much thereafter. Work of breathing increased about 60% with most of the change attributable to increased elastic work. Increased airway resistance at low lung volumes was also implicated.

Balldin, Dahlbäck and Lundgren (1971) reported that in head-out immersion with oxygen breathing, the VC dropped an average of 22·4% in 13 subjects. The change was attributed largely to

atelectasis formation. With air, the VC dropped only 7·8%. Dahlbäck and Lundgren (1972) report that pulmonary air trapping occurs in immersion unless lung volume is increased to about 40% of VC.

McKenna et al. (1973) studied the oscillation mechanics of subjects immersed to the neck, found no change in resistance or resonant frequency, and concluded that immersion per se produced no significant load on the respiratory system. According to this, 'moving the water out of the way with each breath' does not require consequential extra work.

The MVV of submerged divers at various depths was investigated by Wright and Crothers (1973). At 1 ATA MVV was 11% less submerged than dry. At 1000 ft the MVV of the submerged diver was only 5% less than that of the dry subject. The investigators felt that the findings supported extrapolation of dry studies to open water conditions and pointed to breathing apparatus, rather than effects of submergence on the pulmonary system, as the chief limiting factor in underwater respiration.

Flynn, Camporesi and Nunneley (1974) used an advantageous but unusual method of applying a positive-pressure difference to the airways of immersed subjects. They kept the airways at ambient pressure while lowering the mean hydrostatic pressure of the water in which the subjects were immersed. Immersion to the 7th cervical vertebra decreased VC by 3%, RV by 7%, ERV by 53%, and TLC by 3%. The P_R curve was shifted almost 20 cm H_2O to the positive side. Presumably, applying the equivalent of about 20 cm H_2O positive pressure to the airway would restore the curve to its original position and bring the measured variables back to their normal values. In fact, pressures of 25 cm H_2O or more were required. Bringing FRC up to its normal value required 8 to 9 cm H_2O more than the P_R shift suggested. One possible explanation is that involuntary end-expiratory muscle tone developed in opposition to the effective positive airway pressure. Recalling the high abdominal (gastric) pressures reported by Hong et al. (1969), it might not be surprising that relatively high pressures are required to oppose effects of submergence on the abdomen and diaphragm.

Cardiovascular effects

Even if a diver is comfortable and has negligible respiratory effects, it remains possible that a physiologically significant imbalance of respiratory pressures exists. Important earlier studies of submergence and comparable negative-pressure breathing include those of Hong, Ting and Rahn (1960) and Ting, Hong and Rahn (1960). They did not report consequential disturbances of circulation with pressures to -30 cm H_2O.

Diuresis. Interest in imbalance of respiratory pressures was further aroused by attempts to use head-out immersion to simulate certain aspects of prolonged weightlessness. The subject has been reviewed by McCally (1965). Such immersion produces a marked salt and water *diuresis*, and this can produce notable debilitation if it is allowed to continue. Stimulation of cardiac stretch receptors appears to be a major factor. This occurs with an increase in intrathoracic blood volume attributable to attenuation of gravitational effects on the circulation system and negative transthoracic pressure difference.

Maintenance of eupneic airway pressure does not eliminate diuresis, and McCally (1965) calls attention to the likelihood that diuresis is common in most forms of diving. It was present in the long underwater swim reported by Hunt, Reeves and Beckman (1964). Korz, Fischer and Behn (1967) used immersion to simulate hypervolemia in a study of the renin–angiotensin system.

Diuresis can be prevented by maintaining respiratory pressures above the eupneic level (Howard et al. 1967; Hunt 1967). This should be taken into consideration in apparatus design especially where long periods of use are probable. Pressure too much above eupneic pressure can apparently cause the opposite problem of water retention (Sladen, Lauer & Pontoppidan 1968).

Hemodynamic changes. Arborelius et al. (1972a) report that head-out immersion produced a 32% increase in cardiac output with little change in heart rate. Right atrial and pulmonary arterial pressure gradients increased about 13 mm Hg. Central blood volume increased about 0·7 L. The increase in cardiac output is probably responsible for the acceleration of nitrogen elimination in immersion reported by Balldin and Lundgren (1972) and for the more uniform distribution of pulmonary perfusion found by Arborelius and his co-workers (1972b). That hydrostatic imbalance in the opposite direction (passive lung inflation) can impair diffusing capacity and reduce pulmonary blood flow is suggested by animal experiments reported by Fisher and Hyde (1969).

Interference with pulmonary gas exchange is indicated by increase in the alveolar–arterial O_2 pressure difference, (A–a) DO_2, in immersed subjects as reported by Cohen et al. (1971). Flynn, Saltzman and Summitt (1972) found a smaller change in immersion during exercise at 19 ATA than under control conditions. Although indicative of ventilation/perfusion abnormality or true venous admixture, such limited changes do not threaten to impair work capacity or produce significant hypoxemia or hypercapnia. Hydrostatic imbalance greater than that associated with immersion to the neck presumably could do so.

Effects in breathing apparatus

A large proportion of the problems that could be inferred from the foregoing discussion appeared in practical form in work with breathing apparatus as reported by Sterk (1970, 1973). Sterk dealt primarily with a newly developed semi-closed circuit apparatus that had encased breathing bags mounted relatively high on the back. Sterk's observations included neither exertion nor very high gas density. Nevertheless, they showed clearly how breathing apparatus can not only oppose the diver's respiratory efforts but also put his chest and airways at a disadvantage. Sterk sees no substitute for studying apparatus and man together in water, under conditions as realistic as possible, and for long enough periods to permit time-dependent problems to become evident.

In Sterk's apparatus, 'negative' imbalance brought the diver's lung volume to a level characterized by low chest–lung compliance and high airway resistance. The rubber suit and scuba harness further impaired the diver's ability to inspire. The location of the exhaust valve was beneficial in one body position and detrimental in another. Lack of information on balance point location hampers analysis of apparatus behaviour. Lack of acceptable standards for imbalance, resistance, and total respiratory work hampers the entire enterprise.

One of Sterk's most useful analytical app-roaches is shown in Fig. 8.19. The quasi-static compliance curve shows graphically both the lowered vital capacity and diminished compliance that characterized use of this apparatus. Sterk attributed loss of vital capacity in the upper part of the diagram to factors that act against the inspiratory muscles: hydrostatic forces, suit and

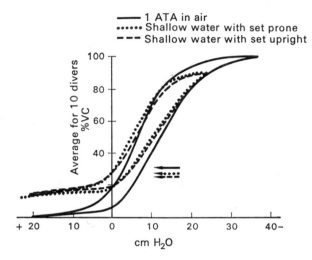

FIG. 8.19. Quasi-static compliance curves with breathing apparatus

'Quasi-static' compliance curves (mean of values from 10 divers) obtained in air at 1 ATA (solid lines) and in shallow water wearing a breathing apparatus. With this particular breathing unit, prone and upright positions (broken lines) yielded essentially the same values, including significantly diminished VC. Arrows indicate resting end-expiratory levels, V_R. Pressures are 'eso-phagus-to-mouth' (transpulmonary), volumes are percent of air-control VC (after Sterk 1973)

harness, and the weight of the apparatus. The decrease at the lower end of the scale probably resulted from closure of lung units together with an increase in intrathoracic blood volume.

Utilization of hydrostatic imbalance. There are several reasons to believe that a small positive-pressure 'bias' might be desirable in underwater breathing apparatus (D. E. Leith, personal communication 1974). This could be provided simply by judicious location of components. So also could inspiratory assistance of any desired degree. Few if any possibilities of this kind have ever been exploited deliberately.

AIRWAY FACTORS[1]

Work done against resistance in the airways is an important fraction of the total work of breathing. This work, and the related phenomenon of expiratory flow limitation, are particularly important when $\dot{V}_E$ is high, as in exercise; and their importance is greatly magnified by increased gas density, as in work at depth. The effect of gas density in limiting ventilatory capacity has been discussed. Here, we will look more closely at the reasons for such limitations. Much work remains to be done in this area of underwater physiology, but relatively recent findings have done much to illuminate the matter. A number of important factors and relationships can be pointed out.

Airway resistance

The concept of electrical resistance is familiar. 'Airway resistance' represents a similar relation-ship and can be expressed:

$$R = \frac{\Delta P}{\dot{V}} \qquad (13)$$

where ΔP is the pressure-drop between two points along the course of an airway, $\dot{V}$ is the flow in volume per unit time, and R is the resistance expressed in units of pressure-drop per unit of flow.

Electrical resistance is normally thought to have a constant value. Airway resistance seldom does. Except at very low values of flow and gas density, it increases as flow increases. In part for this reason, the term 'resistance' is often used loosely while attention is focused on the actual value of ΔP at a given flow.

In considering the human respiratory tract as a whole, ΔP represents the difference between alveolar pressure (P_{alv}) and pressure at the mouth (P_m, ordinarily zero unless breathing apparatus is being used). ΔP is most readily visualized on a pressure–volume diagram like Fig. 8.17B or in work-loops as in Fig. 8.18.

In a classical paper, Rohrer (1915) suggested that total ΔP in the human respiratory tract can be viewed as the sum of two components:

$$\Delta P = K_1 \dot{V} + K_2 \dot{V}^2 \qquad (14)$$

[1] Basic material for this section in the first edition was prepared by F. A. Furgang.

This formulation oversimplifies the problem greatly. Jaffrin and Kesic (1974) regard it as an empirical attempt to describe the transition between the low-flow regime of constant resistance and that of resistance increasing with flow, and they find no fluid mechanical significance in Rohrer's coefficients. Nevertheless, equation (14) remains more useful for such purposes as introductory discussion and rough prediction than are some of the more adequate mathematical models.

Equation (14) indicates that for practical purposes the system behaves as if it consisted of two parts in series: one in which resistance is constant and ΔP is simply proportional to $\dot{V}$ and another in which resistance increases with flow and ΔP is more or less proportional to $\dot{V}^2$. It has often been assumed that the $K_1\dot{V}$ factor represents laminar flow, following the Hagen–Poiseuille relationship, while $K_2\dot{V}^2$ accounts for turbulent flow. Turbulent flow can be expected in an airway when the *Reynolds number* exceeds about 2000:

Reynolds number

$$= \text{velocity} \times \text{diameter} \times \frac{\text{density}}{\text{viscosity}} \quad (15)$$

where velocity represents the average gas velocity in an airway in cm/sec, diameter is in cm, density is in g/cm^3, and viscosity is in poises.[1]

ΔP can be nearly proportional to $\dot{V}^2$ even when flow is not grossly turbulent. Examples include the pressure drops of convective acceleration, flow with change in cross-sectional area of airways, and flow with changes in direction.

The 'constants' K_1 and K_2 must take into account the pertinent characteristics of the airways: length, diameter, number of parallel passages, roughness of walls, etc. The pertinent characteristics of the gas are its *viscosity* (in K_1, if this represents purely laminar flow) and its *density* (in K_2, if this represents turbulence and other 'non laminar' forms of flow). Another apparent factor is the *proportion* of the system that conforms to K_1 or K_2, respectively. As flow or density increases beyond certain limits, the proportions must change; so the Rohrer 'constants' cannot very well have constant values. This probably accounts for the poor predictive value of equation (14) when large changes in the relevant variables occur.

Equation (14) remains useful as a frame of reference in considering the work of breathing at depth. For example, Maio and Farhi (1967) found that changes in gas density influenced ΔP even at low levels of flow. This indicated that flow was not strictly laminar at such levels. At the same time, computed Reynolds numbers for the various parts of the airway system were so low that gross turbulence could not be involved. Subsequent studies (e.g. Wood & Bryan 1969) emphasize the importance of convective acceleration and other forms of flow in which ΔP is proportional to $\dot{V}^2$ and density.

The viscosities of most practical respiratory gases are rather closely similar, and viscosity is not much influenced by ambient pressure. Neither the low viscosity of hydrogen nor the high viscosity of neon appear to have much practical influence on the work of breathing at depth. Strictly laminar flow, in which viscosity is important, contributes little to the total ΔP under most diving conditions. Lanphier (1972) suggested that the effect of viscosity on the Reynolds number might have some practical consequences, but there appears to be no evidence that this is the case.

Jaffrin and Kesic (1974) present a concise review of earlier studies in terms of an analysis of the fluid mechanical aspects of pulmonary gas flow. They conclude that 'flow in the lungs obeys approximately the same general law as the flow in a single rough pipe and that a universal correlation of resistance data with flow rate and the nature of the gas can be achieved from dimensional analysis'. They present laws of similitude which permit extrapolation of results from one gas to another. When certain assumptions can be

[1] In an airway of given diameter the velocity will be proportional to flow ($\dot{V}$) in that airway. The Reynolds number will thus be proportional to both $\dot{V}$ and density.

Turbulent flow is believed to be present in the trachea under usual conditions. It is much more likely to develop in the larger airways of the respiratory tract than in small ones. The Reynolds number is lower in a small airway not only because its diameter is smaller but because velocity is decreased by the greater total cross-sectional area of the respiratory tract at the level of small airways.

made, their basic equation takes a relatively simple form, of which they say 'i.e., the normalized pressure drop along the airway is a function of Reynolds number only'. On inspiration with air at 1 ATA, Jaffrin and Kesic (1974) find constant resistance (indicating laminar flow) up to about 0·5 L/sec, and resistance proportional to flow above about 2·0 L/sec. The most important range of flows, a transitional phase, exists between these values. Jaffrin and Kesic's calculations on gas density changes produce satisfactory agreement with data of Maio and Farhi (1967).

Kylstra (1973) has also reported a mathematical model that comes very close to describing the actual behaviour of the human airways under various conditions.

The geometry of the mouth, pharynx and larynx can vary from moment to moment. Their contribution to total ΔP is therefore not only large but also quite variable (Spann & Hyatt 1971). A major portion of 'upper' airway resistance is ordinarily in the larynx.

Maximum expiratory flow

It once seemed obvious that respiratory flows were limited by airway resistance and by the ability of the respiratory muscles to produce large positive or negative alveolar pressures. If reaching a certain flow rate requires a greater P_{alv} than muscular strength and endurance can muster, the flow would obviously be limited to some lower value. Maximum values of MVV and $\dot{V}_E$ were considered to be reflections of limitations of flow. All of this is probably quite true in inspiration and in the use of breathing apparatus that presents substantial external airway resistance. The findings of Cerretelli, Sikand & Farhi (1969) with external resistance, mentioned earlier, are consistent with such a view.

It is now generally recognized that airway resistance and the ability to perform respiratory work are not the only limiting factors for exercise ventilation when resistances in the respiratory tract itself are concerned, as with high gas density. Papers by Fry and Hyatt (1960), Mead et al. (1967), and Pride et al. (1967) did much to crystallize a concept that is almost certainly important in explaining respiratory limitations at depth. This has to do with maximum rates of expiratory gas flow and is often referred to as *dynamic airway compression*.

Even under ordinary conditions in normal individuals, maximum expiratory flow is *effort-independent* over a large range of lung volumes: the very important range from about 75% of VC down to about 25% of VC. Effort is required to reach maximum flow; but once this level is reached, further elevation of P_{alv} does not produce any further increase in flow. Maximum expiratory flow is seldom required or reached by normal individuals under usual circumstances, but it can be reduced sufficiently by increased gas density to become important in limitation of work capacity at depth (Lord, Bond & Schaefer 1966; Maio & Farhi 1967; Varène, Timbal & Jacquemin 1967; Wright, Peterson & Lambertsen 1972).

The maximum expiratory flow concept is not entirely simple, and the basic papers mentioned deserve direct study. As advanced by Mead et al. (1967), the explanation hinges upon existence, somewhere along the length of the respiratory tract, of an equal pressure point (EPP) where pressure within the airway is equal to pressure surrounding the airway.

During forceful expiration, the driving pressure P_{alv} is derived from the pressure of static elastic recoil of the lung itself (P_{stl}) and from contraction of expiratory muscles. Expiratory muscular effort produces positive pleural pressure, P_{pl}. Airways within the thorax are surrounded by pressure essentially the same as P_{pl}. If EPP is in an intrathoracic airway, the pressure both inside and outside the airway must by definition be essentially equal to P_{pl}.

P_{alv} is the sum of P_{pl} and the 'recoil' pressure P_{stl}. Therefore, ΔP in the 'upstream segment' (between the alveoli and EPP) must be equal to P_{stl}. P_{stl} must therefore represent the driving pressure for flow in the upstream segment. The actual value of P_{stl} depends upon the compliance of the lung and the lung volume. The higher the lung volume, the higher P_{stl} will be and the greater the flow in the upstream segment can be.

If P_{alv} is increased by voluntary expiratory effort at a given lung volume, the increase represents only an increase in P_{pl}. If flow increases, P_{stl} will be expended in a shorter distance, so EPP must move upstream. As a result, a greater portion of the intrathoracic airway will be down-stream from EPP and will have higher pressure outside than inside. At some point downstream from EPP, the airway will actually be compressed. Normal cartilage-supported airways are not actually flattened, but the ends of the cartilage semi-rings can be forced together and overlapped in such a way that the lumen is markedly reduced (Olsen et al. 1967; Olsen, Stevens & McIlroy 1967).

Once airway compression has begun, further increases in expiratory effort, reflected in increasing P_{pl}, will produce further compression of the airway rather than any further increase in flow.

In the situation described, maximum expiratory flow is determined by P_{stl} and by the resistance P_{stl} must overcome in the upstream segment between the alveoli and EPP. Because P_{stl} is governed by lung volume, maximum expiratory flow falls as lung volume decreases in the course of expiration. Under usual conditions, maximum expiratory flow is 'effort-dependent' at high and low lung volumes but 'effort-independent' in the range of volumes where breathing normally takes place.

Maximum expiratory flow determined by airway compression is clearly shown in forced vital capacity maneuvers and doubtless influences the MVV even in normal individuals. Values are low in emphysema patients because pulmonary elasticity is impaired and upstream segment resistance is usually increased. Frank closure of smaller airways can be expected at higher lung volumes when elasticity is impaired. (The effects of gas density on *closing volumes* and their possible importance in diving have not yet been demonstrated.)

Limitation of $\dot{V}_{E_{max}}$ by maximum expiratory flow is probably one of the factors involved at 1 ATA in the study reported by Craig, Blevins and Cummins (1970). Divers at depth are rendered similar to emphysema patients by increases in resistance in the upstream segment. This resistance depends upon the same factors discussed in connection with equations (14) and (15). Density is important not only in turbulent flow but also in convective acceleration, which refers to the acceleration of the air stream that must occur when the total cross-section of the airways decreases in the direction of flow (Hyatt & Wilcox 1963).

Mead et al. (1967) concluded that at high lung volumes and high flow rates, convective acceleration accounted for nearly all of the ΔP in the upstream segment. Wood and Bryan (1969) studied maximum expiratory flow at 6 different lung volumes and at pressures from 1 to 10 ATA. At lung volumes greater than 25% VC, they found that maximum flow was proportional to gas density $^{-0.45}$—for all practical purposes the same relationship as the 'reciprocal of the square root of the density' discussed earlier in connection with MVV at depth. This value was also consistent with convective acceleration (and/or other 'non-laminar' flow factors) as the main source of upstream segment resistance. The fact that calculated Reynolds numbers are low favors explanations other than turbulence.

The contributions in this area of Albano (1970) and Vail (1971a, b; 1973) are difficult to summarize adequately and are best appreciated in the original publications.

Two figures from Miller et al. (1972) will help to show the implications of expiratory flow phenomena at depth. Fig. 8.20 shows (left) a maximum expiratory flow v. lung volume (MEFV) curve obtained in a forced VC maneuver with air at 1 ATA. Peak flow of over 9 L/sec is reached at about 85% VC. Flow falls progressively as lung volume decreases. The right-hand portion of the diagram shows pressure–flow relationships at each of several lung volumes. At 80% VC, the curve suggests that greater transpulmonary pressure from greater expiratory effort might have produced somewhat greater flow, but this is clearly close to the effort-independent range. At each of the lower lung volumes, flow reached a plateau despite increasing transpulmonary pressures. P_{max} signifies the pressure that yielded maximum flow at a particular lung volume.

Fig. 8.21 shows (left) MEFV curves for 1, 2, 4, and 8 ATA. A very marked reduction not only of peak flow but of maximum flow at all lung volumes is seen. The plot (right) of maximum flow at 60% VC v. ambient pressure shows the same type of curve-shape that was noted for MVV v. depth (Fig. 8.7). The reductions with

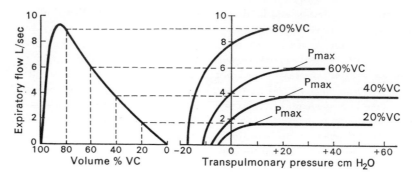

FIG. 8.20. MEFV and pressure–flow curves at 1 ATA

Left: maximum expiratory flow–volume (MEFV) curve from one subject breathing air at 1 ATA. Right: pressure–flow relationships at several lung volumes in the same subject (after Miller, Wangensteen & Lanphier 1972)

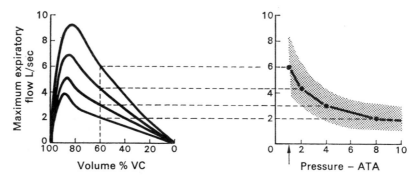

FIG. 8.21. MEFV curves at depth; maximum flow v. depth

Left: MEFV curves obtained in one subject at pressures of 1, 2, 4, and 7·8 ATA breathing air. Right: flow values obtained at 60% VC plotted against ambient pressure (after Miller, Wangensteen & Lanphier 1972)

increased density are striking. Flow–pressure plots like Fig. 8.20 have also been produced at various depths. There is no evidence that values of P_{max} are greatly modified by increased density in healthy young divers. Older men, heavy smokers, and individuals with small-airway disease may have density-dependent values of P_{max} (J. N. Miller, personal communication 1974).

External resistance

The dynamic compression concept has given rise to a number of theories about the relationships between respiratory tract limitations and the effects of external expiratory resistance.

It might be argued that added external resistance would simply add to the total resistance to be overcome and would further reduce effort-independent maximum expiratory flow. Such a view overlooks the fact that the governing resist-ance is in the 'upstream segment' and not else-where. Analysis in terms suggested by Mead et al. (1967) leads to a different conclusion: addition of external resistance would require greater effort and a higher value of P_{pl} to maintain a given flow. However, pressure in the intrathoracic airways would rise to the same extent as P_{pl}, and the net tendency of airways to collapse should not be altered. Maximum expiratory flow should remain unchanged provided that the individual can per-form the extra expiratory work imposed by added external resistance.

The work of Vorosmarti and Lanphier (1975) showed that remarkably high resistances can, in fact, be added in brief maneuvers without reduction of effort-independent maximum expira-tory flow. In no true sense can added expiratory resistance be accommodated without correspond-ing effort. The only situation in which added resistance can be accepted without *additional* effort arises when an individual is already doing 'wasted work' in attempting to increase flow above the maximum by developing expiratory pressures above P_{max} during effort-independent flow.

The fact that maximum flow rates can be maintained briefly despite added resistance could be vital in a short-term emergency situation, but it offers no excuse for poor design of breathing apparatus. No amount of *inspiratory* resistance can be added without potential penalties even though the inspiratory phase is seldom the primary limiting factor. Inspiratory flow is believed by most investigators always to be effort-dependent.

Suggestions have been made to the effect that added external expiratory resistance might *increase* the level of effort-independent expiratory flow. The thought behind such suggestions is that elevation of airway pressure would tend to prevent airway compression. It is difficult to see how this could be the case. Although the whole system would be operating at a higher pressure, the pressure differences and pressure drops responsible for airway compression would be essentially unchanged.

The alleged benefits of 'pursed-lips breathing' (PLB) in emphysema give apparent support to the expectation of higher flows with added resistance. Actually, no study of PLB has shown improved maximum flow or decreased work of breathing. Mueller, Petty and Filley (1970) suggest that the source of symptom benefit reported by some patients has to do with a more effective pattern of breathing (slower, larger tidal volume) and perhaps decreased airway compression.

Decreased airway compression in this case is almost certainly achieved by close regulation of expiratory flow, allowing it to approach maximum without quite reaching critical levels. Such fine regulation may perhaps be achieved more readily by modulation of upper airway resistance than by close regulation of expiratory effort and P_{pl}. If so, the larynx probably provides primary regulation (Rattenborg 1961; Clément, Stănescu & van de Woestijne 1973). Perhaps PLB provides 'fine control'. It would not be surprising to find such forms of regulation in divers who are obliged

to work close to effort-independent maximum expiratory flow. Wood and Bryan (1969) report that 'choking dyspnea' can be associated with airway compression at depth.

Respiratory assistance

Recurrent suggestions concern the possibility of providing mechanical respiratory assistance to overcome respiratory limitations imposed by gas density at depth. Again, consideration along lines suggested by Mead et al. (1967) leads to interesting conclusions. Application of pressure around chest or abdomen would increase P_{pl} and could substitute for voluntary expiratory effort, but it would have no more effect on effort-independent maximum expiratory flow than does added effort.

Applying negative pressure at the mouth could also supplement (or substitute for) muscular effort, but it would lower pressure in the airways and cause compression to occur at lower values of P_{pl}. It would thus be no more beneficial than an increase in P_{pl}, and it involves special disadvantages of its own akin to those of head-out immersion. In addition, it would tend to collapse extrathoracic airways (Sterk 1973).

When an individual's $\dot{V}_E$ becomes limited by maximum expiratory flow under a given set of conditions, there are only a few ways of increasing the total volume of gas that he can inspire and expire per minute or per respiratory cycle. One is to *breathe at higher lung volumes* where the maximum effort-independent flow is greater. Doing so would require greater inspiratory work against elastic forces, but this could be offset by a modest continuous 'positive-pressure bias' (D. E. Leith, personal communication 1974). A more obvious measure is to *allow more time for expiration* by increasing inspiratory flow so as to shorten the inspiratory phase of the cycle. This is a natural response to interference with the expiratory phase, and inspiration is normally not limited. Nevertheless, some well-engineered inspiratory assistance would probably be welcome and valuable.

Breathing apparatus

It seems pointless to discuss existing 'standards' for breathing apparatus when the needs of the present—not to mention the future of diving—

cry out for equipment so much better than anything presently available. A man can tolerate astonishing respiratory obstacles and yet survive (Uhl et al. 1972), but there is no reason why optimal equipment should continue to elude us. At the very least, a breathing unit should, in effect, 'take care of its own work': it should be designed so as to perform the added work that its use would otherwise entail. A more worthy objective is a breathing apparatus that not only does its own work but helps, rather than hinders, the diver's respiratory efforts (see Bradley 1973).

It is not yet certain whether the practical limits of ventilatory capacity at depth will ultimately be set by effort-independent flow or by the work of breathing, even with ideal breathing apparatus or none. With existing respiratory equipment, the work factor will almost surely set the limit at some level below that of flow limitation. The importance of prolonged bouts of respiratory work must not be underestimated.

ALVEOLAR EXCHANGE

Airway resistance, effects of submergence, obstacles presented by breathing apparatus, and all the rest must be overcome by respiratory work in order to achieve 'adequate' pulmonary ventilation. Unfortunately, ventilation that would ordinarily be adequate does not always ensure satisfactory exchange of oxygen and carbon dioxide within the lungs. Such circumstances are common in pulmonary disease, but only a few of the possible mechanisms are known to be important in healthy divers at depth or are suspected of being important enough to deserve discussion here.

Regional inhomogeneity: $\dot{V}A/\dot{Q}$ relationships

The ultimate purpose of 'pulmonary function' is to permit the blood to take up oxygen from the 'alveolar' gas and to deliver excess CO_2 into this gas. It is easy to see that this objective requires that there be reasonably good matching of alveolar *ventilation* ($\dot{V}A$) and blood flow (*perfusion*, $\dot{Q}$) in individual regions of the lungs. Ideally, the ratio of $\dot{V}A/\dot{Q}$ would be close to 1·0. To use extreme examples, it is clear that no exchange of gas would occur either in a region that

was ventilated but had no blood flow ($\dot{V}A/\dot{Q}=$ infinity) or in one that was perfused but had no ventilation ($\dot{V}A/\dot{Q}=$zero). The former region would constitute *respiratory dead space*, wasting ventilation, while the latter would represent a *right-to-left shunt*, putting unchanged venous blood into the systemic arterial stream. Ordinarily, only small portions of the lungs would be at either of these extremes; but abnormal $\dot{V}A/\dot{Q}$ relationships short of the extremes can have very serious effects (West 1965; Farhi 1966). They represent the central problem in several types of pulmonary disability.

Gravity affects lung tissue as well as blood within the lungs. In the erect position, the upper portions of the lungs can change their volume more freely and thus receive more ventilation. At the same time, a much higher proportion of blood flow goes to the lower parts of the lungs. A normal individual standing at rest might have a $\dot{V}A/\dot{Q}$ ratio of 3·0 in the upper region and only 0·5 in the lower parts. Exercise ordinarily improves the uniformity of both ventilation and perfusion.

There is no reason to expect submergence to cancel gravitational effects within the lungs because these involve gas–liquid relationships entirely within the confines of the thorax. Nevertheless, the anti-gravity effect in the periphery tends to shift blood from the limbs into the thorax, as has been noted. This helps to improve the uniformity of perfusion. On the other hand, the gradient of external pressure and the effect of buoyancy both tend to raise the diaphragm in vertical submerged subjects. To the extent that this further reduces the expansion of lower parts of the lungs, it can contribute to $\dot{V}A/\dot{Q}$ inequality.

Impairment of oxygen transfer, manifested in an increased alveolar–arterial oxygen pressure difference, (A–a) DO_2, is usually the chief consequence of $\dot{V}A/\dot{Q}$ abnormality. West (1971) has pointed out that CO_2 retention can also be an important result.

A question not yet fully answered is what effect major changes in gas density have on the distribution of ventilation. It seems reasonable, for example, to suppose that increased density would cause a greater portion of inspired gas to go to regions having somewhat lower airway resistance than others. A study reported by Miller and Winsborough (1973) points to a more optimistic view. Their conclusion was that in healthy young men altered $\dot{V}_A/\dot{Q}$ in heavy exertion at depth was attributable to inadequate total ventilation rather than to an important increase in regional inhomogeneity of ventilation.

Intrapulmonary diffusion

Stratified inhomogeneity is a term applied to incomplete mixing of 'new' inspired gas (the tidal volume, VT) with 'old' gas in the terminal airways and gas exchange units of the lungs (the functional residual capacity, FRC). It is clear that gross flushing is incomplete and that the process of renewal of gas in the alveolar region must include mixing by diffusion (Cumming et al. 1966). This factor is ordinarily not an important barrier to gas exchange, but diffusion is bound to be slower in denser gas. Consequently, there was some anxiety about possible impairment of diffusion at depth.

Diffusion dead space. Liquid breathing experiments reported by Kylstra, Paganelli and Lanphier (1966) called attention to an extreme form of apparent diffusion limitation. They found very large P_{O_2} and P_{CO_2} differences between 'alveolar' liquid and arterial blood. These differences could best be explained on the basis of a large *diffusion dead space* related to the slow diffusion of gases through the liquid-filled spaces between a central bolus of fresh inspired liquid and the alveolar-capillary membrane.

Further consideration of this concept led Kylstra, Paganelli and Rahn (1966) to speculate upon its possible significance in gas breathing. Their formulations were adapted by Lanphier (1967) to make tentative predictions about intrapulmonary O_2 and CO_2 diffusion with air and helium–oxygen mixtures at depth. One interpretation pointed to the possibility that maintaining near-normal inspiratory oxygen pressure might lead to hypoxia, at least during exertion, with helium–oxygen mixtures at practical working depths. If this occurred, it presumably could be offset by increasing the $P_{I_{O_2}}$—except that pulmonary oxygen toxicity might then become a problem.

'Chouteau hypoxia'. Meanwhile, in France,

Chouteau and his associates encountered difficulties in deep chamber dives conducted with goats in a nearly normoxic He–O_2 atmosphere (Chouteau 1972). The animals developed a syndrome that was interpreted as being of hypoxic origin. This was dramatically abolished by relatively modest elevation of $P_{I_{O_2}}$—only to recur if the ambient pressure was raised further. Again, the syndrome was abolished by raising the $P_{I_{O_2}}$. In one series, this sequence was repeated several times on the way to a final pressure of over 100 ATA, where some animals succumbed to what might have been pulmonary oxygen damage. Experience in deep animal studies in several French laboratories has been summarized by Chouteau and Imbert (1971). Chouteau, Imbert and LePechon (1972) reviewed experience with different species. Berry (1972) describes somewhat contradictory findings in a minipig taken successfully to 1100 m (109 ATA).

It is not surprising that 'Chouteau hypoxia' was tentatively attributed to gas-diffusion difficulties. Several groups of investigators attempted to reproduce the circumstances of Chouteau's experience by exposing animals to gas of equal density using heavier gases at lower pressures. At least some of these investigators lost sight of the fact that it is not *density* per se but the *binary diffusion coefficient* for oxygen in the diluent gas that is most likely to be crucial. None matched the binary coefficients of Chouteau's studies.

Almost uniformly, the attempts to reproduce Chouteau's findings produced results opposite from the expectations. The values of (A–a) D_{O_2} fell with increased density—as if higher density improved diffusion rather than impaired it. Since such is clearly not the case, the explanation had to be sought elsewhere. The situation was reviewed by Lanphier (1972).

Intrapulmonary gas mixing. Meanwhile, considerable light has been shed on the normal processes of mixing that must occur within the lungs for oxygen to be delivered and CO_2 to be removed effectively. Studies by Knelson, Howatt and DeMuth (1970) and Bondi and Van Liew (1973) called attention to the fact that an inspiratory pause increases the efficiency of breathing. In terms already discussed, the increased efficiency can be visualized in terms of decreased respiratory dead space, V_D. An important aspect of this must be improved mixing between the tidal volume (VT) of 'fresh' gas and the functional residual capacity (FRC) of 'old' gas that remains in the lungs between breaths.

Papers by Engel et al. (1973) and Johnson and Van Liew (1974) provide a good review of the subject together with relevant experimental findings. It is probably easiest to focus attention on the transport of O_2 from the ambient air to the alveolar–capillary membrane. The mixing of gas between the VT and FRC must include at least three processes. The most obvious is *convection:* inspiratory gas flow carries some of the inspired oxygen molecules directly into the FRC. There is reason to believe, however, that only 10 to 15% of the VT is mixed with the FRC in this way during each resting respiratory cycle.

The importance of the mixing effect of *cardiac action* is emphasized by the work of Engel et al. (1973). For example, they concluded that the heart beat was responsible for about one-fourth of the reduction in dead space volume (V_D) in the first 10 sec of breath holding. They speculated that the mechanism for the cardiac effect 'may involve both Taylor diffusion and convective mixing due to eddy currents and secondary motions'.

Taylor diffusion is thought to be particularly important in middle-sized airways. *Longitudinal dispersion* is another term for this process, in which one finds a combination of convection with flow along the length of the airway and radial diffusion from the center of the stream toward the walls. When flow is more or less laminar, radial diffusion would tend to take oxygen out of the faster moving flow laminae in the center of the airway. When flow becomes turbulent, the parabolic front of the laminar flow velocity profile is replaced by a blunt profile. The composition of gas in turbulent flow is more nearly uniform across the airway, so radial diffusion becomes less important.

Faster flow in the center of a laminar gas stream is probably responsible for an important part of the delivery of oxygen to or toward the terminal gas exchange units of the lung. Once there, in any event, oxygen must still make its way to the alveolar–capillary membrane by molecular gas diffusion.

Even in this simplified account, it is evident that gas diffusion operates in at least two ways. Diffusion within the gas exchange units is an essential factor in delivery of oxygen to the blood. Taylor diffusion within the airways, on the other hand, tends to decrease the penetration of oxygen toward the terminal exchange units by mixing more oxygen with 'old' gas that remains in the airways. Development of turbulence decreases the importance of Taylor diffusion but also abolishes oxygen delivery by faster central flow-layers.

The role of gas density in this situation is clearly not simple. There is no question that an increase in gas density will diminish the rate of molecular gas diffusion. This will tend to impede the diffusion of oxygen to the alveolar–capillary membrane, but it will also reduce the role of Taylor diffusion in dispersing oxygen before it can reach the gas-exchange units. The net effect could be either favorable or unfavorable. A further increase in density may cause turbulence to develop in certain generations of airways, and again the consequences may be difficult to predict.

In the light of such contradictory actions, increases in gas density may not only have effects that are unpredictable in the light of present knowledge but observed effects may perhaps be reversed by further changes. In attempting to explain Chouteau hypoxia, we have already mentioned the importance of binary diffusion coefficients as opposed to values of density alone.

It is important, finally, to recall that apparent hypoxia in near normoxic exposures at depth may find its ultimate explanation in something other than (or in addition to) gas density. The possibility that pressure per se may affect the respiratory control system was mentioned in an earlier section. It is also possible that the neuromuscular phenomena of the high pressure neurological syndrome can include interference with coordinated respiratory movements.

Such questions as these may appear extraordinarily theoretical at this point, but it seems more than likely that they will soon come to have vital importance in determining man's ability to penetrate great depths as a useful diver.

Acknowledgements

The author acknowledges support of his work over a long period by the Office of Naval Research under Contract Nonr 969 (03) and more recently under Contract No. N00014-71-C-0342.

Revision of this chapter was carried out while the author was on leave-of-absence from the State University of New York at Buffalo and in training for Anglican holy orders at Nashotah House, a theological seminary of the Episcopal Church. He owes thanks to the faculty and fellow seminarians, whose patience and encouragement made the work possible under unusual circumstances.

REFERENCES

AGARATE, C. A. & JEGOU, A. J. (1973) A simulated dive at 2001 feet. In *1973 Offshore Technical Conference, Houston, Texas*. Preprints, Vol. I, pp. 511–513. Published by the conference.

AGOSTONI, E., GURTNER, G., TORRI, G. & RAHN, H. (1966) Respiratory mechanics during submersion and negative pressure breathing. *J. appl. Physiol.* **21**, 251–258.

ALBANO, G. (1970) *Principles and Observations on the Physiology of the Scuba Diver*. Arlington: Office of Naval Research, Dept. of the Navy (ONR Report DR-150).

ANTHONISEN, N. R., BRADLEY, M. E., VOROSMARTI, J., & LINAWEAVER, P. G. (1971) Mechanics of breathing with helium–oxygen and neon–oxygen mixtures in deep saturation diving. In *Underwater Physiology. Proc. 4th Symp. Underwater Physiology*. pp. 339–345. Ed. C. J. Lambertsen. New York: Academic Press.

ARBORELIUS, M., Jr., BALLDIN, U. I., LILJA, B. & LUNDGREN, C. E. G. (1972a) Hemodynamic changes in man during immersion with the head above water. *Aerospace Med.* **43**, 592–598.

ARBORELIUS, M., Jr., BALLDIN, U. I., LILJA, B. & LUNDGREN, C. E. G. (1972b) Regional lung function in man during immersion with the head above water. *Aerospace Med.* **43**, 701–707.

ASMUSSEN, E. & NIELSEN, M. (1946) Studies on the regulation of respiration in heavy work. *Acta physiol. scand.* **12**, 171–188.

ASMUSSEN, E. & NIELSEN, M. (1956) Physiological dead space and alveolar gas pressures at rest and during muscular exercise. *Acta physiol. scand.* **38**, 1–21.

ASMUSSEN, E. & NIELSEN, M. (1958) Pulmonary ventilation and effect of oxygen breathing in heavy exercise. *Acta physiol. scand.* **43**, 365–378.

ÅSTRAND, I., ÅSTRAND, P.-O., CHRISTENSEN, E. H. & HEDMAN, R. (1960) Intermittent muscular work. *Acta physiol. scand.* **48**, 448–453.

BALLDIN, U. I. & LUNDGREN, C. E. G. (1972) Effects of immersion with the head above water on tissue nitrogen elimination in man. *Aerospace Med.* **43**, 1101–1108.

BALLDIN, U. I., DAHLBÄCK, G. O. & LUNDGREN, C. E. G. (1971) Changes in vital capacity produced by oxygen breathing during immersion with the head above water. *Aerospace Med.* **42**, 384–387.

BALOUET, G., BARTHELEMY, L., LEROY, J. P., MICHAUD, A. & PARC, J. (1971) Étude des lesions provoquées par l'utilisation de mélanges respiratoires oxygène-hydrogène dans des conditions hyperbares. *C.r. Séanc. Soc. Biol.* **165**, 1750–1753.

BARNETT, T. B. & RASMUSSEN, B. (1970) Ventilatory responses to hypoxia and hypercapnia with external airway resistance. *Acta physiol. Scand.* **80**, 538–551.

BEHNKE, A. R., Jr. (1965) Inert gas narcosis (Chap. 41, pp. 1059–1065, in Fenn & Rahn 1965).

BENNETT, P. B. & BLENKARN, G. D. (1974) Arterial blood gases in man during inert gas narcosis. *J. appl. Physiol.* **36**, 45–48.

BENNETT, P. B. & ELLIOTT, D. H. (Eds) (1969) *The Physiology and Medicine of Diving and Compressed Air Work*, p. 83. London: Baillière Tindall & Cassell.

BERRY (1972) *Animal Tests on a Small Hog at Depth: 1100 meters*. Toulon: Groupe d'Études et de Recherches Sous-marines, Rep. GERS 07–71 (NAVSHIPS transl. 1337).

BONDI, K. R. & VAN LIEW, H. D. (1973) Fluxes of CO_2 in the lung gas studied by continuously recorded arterial pH. *J. appl. Physiol.* **35**, 42–46.

BOUHUYS, A. (1964) Respiratory dead space (Chap. 28, pp. 699–714, in Fenn & Rahn, 1964).

BRADLEY, M. E. (Ed.) (1973) Respiratory limitations of underwater breathing equipment. In *Second Undersea Medical Society Workshop*. Bethesda: Undersea Medical Society.

BRADLEY, M. E. & DICKSON, J. G., Jr. (1975) The effects of nitrous oxide narcosis on the physiologic and psychologic performance of man at rest and during exercise. In *Underwater Physiology. Vth Symp. Underwater Physiology* (1972). Ed. C. J. Lambertsen. Bethesda: Fedn Am. Socs exp. Biol.

BRADLEY, M. E., VOROSMARTI, J., ANTHONISEN, N. R. & LINAWEAVER, P. G. (1971) Respiratory and cardiac responses to exercise in subjects breathing helium–oxygen mixtures from sea level to 19·2 atmospheres. In *Underwater Physiology. Proc. 4th Symp. Underwater Physiology*. Ed. C. J. Lambertsen, pp. 325–337. New York: Academic Press.

BROUSSOLLE, B., HYACINTHE, R.. BURNET, H., BATTESTI, A. & GRESSON, D. (1972) *Exchanges gazeux respiratoires et mecanique ventilatoire au cours d'une plongée fictive a 51 ATA (500 metres) en mélange helium-oxygène*. Cent. Mar. Biophys. Rep. on Cont. CNEXO 71–343 NAVSHIPS transl. 1367).

CAIN, C. C. & OTIS, A. B. (1949) Some physiological effects resulting from added resistance to respiration. *J. Aviat. Med.* **20**, 149–160.

CASE, E. M. & HALDANE, J. B. S. (1941) Human physiology under high pressure. I. Effects of nitrogen, carbon dioxide and cold. *J. Hyg. Camb.* **41**, 225–249.

CERRETELLI, P., SIKAND, R. & FARHI, L. E. (1969) Effect of increased airway resistance on ventilation and gas exchange during exercise. *J. appl. Physiol.* **27**, 597–600.

CHAPMAN, C. B. (Ed.) (1967) *Physiology of Muscular Exercise*. New York: American Heart Association (Monograph No. 15).

CHERNIACK, R. M. & SNIDAL, D. P. (1956) The effect of obstruction to breathing on the ventilatory response to CO_2. *J. clin. Invest.* **35**, 1286–1290.

CHOUTEAU, J. (1972) Experimentation animale de plongée profonde en mélanges synthetiques realisée au CEMA, au GERS, et au CERTSM. In *Third International Conference on Hyperbaric and Underwater Physiology*. Ed. X. Fructus, pp. 8–12. Paris: Doin.

CHOUTEAU, J. & IMBERT, G. (1971) La limitation hypoxique de la plongée profonde de longue durée. In Medecine de la plongée. Ed. J. Chauderon. *Maroc Méd.* **51**, 229–230.

CHOUTEAU, J., IMBERT, G. & LePECHON, J. C. (1972) Physiologie comparée de divers mammiferes aux hautes pressions en atmosphère oxygène–helium. *Maroc. Méd.* **52**, 448–449.

CHRISTENSEN, E. H. (1953) Physiological valuation of work in the Nykroppa Iron Works. *Ergonomics Soc. Symp. on Fatigue*. Ed. W. F. Floyd & A. T. Welford, pp. 93–108. London: Lewis.

CLARK, J. M. (1973) Tolerance and adaptation to acute and chronic hypercapnia in man. In *Proc. 1973 Divers' Gas Purity Symp.* pp. I–1 to I–20. U.S.N. Supervisor of Diving. Rep. 2–73.

CLARK, J. M., SINCLAIR, R. D. & LENOX, J. B. (1974) Effects of hypercapnia on exercise tolerance and symptoms in man. *J. appl. Physiol.* (In press.)

CLÉMENT, J., STĂNESCU, D. C., & VAN DE WOESTIJNE, K. P. (1973) Glottis opening and effort-dependent part of the isovolume pressure–flow curves. *J. appl. Physiol.* **34**, 18–22.

COHEN, R., BELL, W. H., SALTZMAN, H. A. & KYLSTRA, J. A. (1971) Alveolar–arterial oxygen pressure difference in man immersed up to the neck in water. *J. appl. Physiol.* **30**, 720–723.

COMMITTEE ON AMPHIBIOUS OPERATIONS (1953) *Report of the Cooperative Underwater Swimmer Project*. Washington: National Research Council Committee on Amphibious Operations, NRC: CAO: 0033.

COMROE, J. H., Jr. (1965) *Physiology of Respiration*. Chicago: Year Book Medical Publishers.

CONSOLAZIO, C. F., JOHNSON, R. E. & PECORA, L. J. (1963) *Physiological Measurements of Metabolic Functions in Man*. New York, Toronto, London: McGraw-Hill.

COOK, J. C. (1970) Work capacity in hyperbaric environments without hyperoxia. *Aerospace Med.* **41**, 1133–1135.

COVELL, B., NASR EL DIN & PASSMORE, R. (1965) Energy expenditure of young men during the weekend. *Lancet* **1**, 727–728.

CRAIG, A. B., Jr. & DVORAK, MARIA (1969) Comparison of exercise in air and in water of different temperatures. *Medicine and Science in Sports* **1**, 124–130.

CRAIG, F. N., BLEVINS, W. V. & CUMMINGS, E. G. (1970) Exhausting work limited by external resistance and inhalation of carbon dioxide. *J. appl. Physiol.* **29**, 847–851.

CUMMING, G., CRANK, J., HORSFIELD, K. & PARKER, I. (1966) Gaseous diffusion in the airways of the human lung. *Resp. Physiol.* **1**, 58–74.

DAHLBÄCK, G. O. & LUNDGREN, C. E. G. (1972) Pulmonary air-trapping induced by water immersion. *Aerospace Med.* **43**, 768–774.

D'ANGELO, E. & TORELLI, G. (1971) Neural stimuli increasing respiration during different types of exercise. *J. appl. Physiol.* **30**, 116–121.

DEJOURS, P. (1964) Control of respiration in muscular exercise (Chap. 25, pp. 631–648, in Fenn & Rahn 1964).

DEJOURS, P. (1966) *Respiration*. New York: Oxford University Press.

DEJOURS, P. (1967) Neurogenic factors in the control of ventilation during exercise (pp. 1–146 to 1–153, in Chapman 1967).

DEMEDTS, M. & ANTHONISEN, N. R. (1973) Effects of increased external airway resistance during steady-state exercise. *J. appl. Physiol.* **35**, 361–366.

DENISON, D. M., WAGNER, P. D., KINGABY, G. L. & WEST, J. B. (1972) Cardiorespiratory responses to exercise in air and underwater. *J. appl. Physiol.* **33**, 426–430.

DEROANNE, R., DUJARDIN, J., LAMY, M., MARÉCHAL, R., PETIT, J. M. & PIRNAY, F. (1973) Effect of hyperbaric oxygenation on maximum aerobic work capacity. *Försvarsmedicin* **9**, 352–356.

DILL, D. B. (1936) The economy of muscular exercise. *Physiol. Rev.* **16**, 263–291.

DILL, D. B., EDWARDS, H. T., NEWMAN, E. V. & MARGARIA, R. (1936). Analysis of recovery from anaerobic work. *Arbeitsphysiol.* **9**, 299–307.

DI PRAMPERO, P. E., DAVIES, C. T. M., CERRETELLI, P. & MARGARIA, R. (1970). An analysis of O_2 debt contracted in submaximal exercise. *J. appl. Physiol.* **29**, 547–551.

DIXON, R. W., Jr. & FAULKNER, J. A. (1971) Cardiac outputs during maximum effort running and swimming. *J. appl. Physiol.* **30**, 653–656.

DONALD, K. W. & DAVIDSON, W. M. (1954) Oxygen uptake of 'booted' and 'fin swimming' divers. *J. appl. Physiol.* **7**, 31–37.

DOUGHERTY, J. H., Jr. (1974) Pulmonary functions during hydrogen–oxygen breathing at pressure equivalent to 200 feet of sea water. Presented at the Undersea Medical Society Annual Scientific Meeting, Washington.

EDEL, P. O., HOLLAND, J. M., FISCHER, C. L. & FIFE, W. B. (1972) Preliminary studies of hydrogen–oxygen breathing mixtures for deep sea diving. In *The Working Diver*. (Proceedings of Symposium, Columbus, Ohio, February 1972.) pp. 257–270. Washington, D.C.: Marine Technology Society.

ELLIOTT, J. C., FINKELSTEIN, S., ROBERTS, A. P. & LUFT, U. C. (1970) Gas exchange and acid–base balance breathing low concentrations of CO_2 during exercise and recovery. In *Aerospace Medical Association, Preprints of Scientific Program, 1970 Annual Scientific Meeting, St. Louis, April 27–30, 1970*. Published by the Association.

ENGEL, L. A., MENKES, H., WOOD, L. D. H., UTZ, G., JOUBERT, J. & MACKLEM, P. T. (1973) Gas mixing during breath holding studied by intrapulmonary gas sampling. *J. appl. Physiol.* **35**, 9–17.

FAGRAEUS, L. & HESSER, C. M. (1970) Ventilatory response to CO_2 in hyperbaric environments. *Acta physiol. scand.* **80**, 19A–20A.

FAGRAEUS, L. & LINNARSSON, D. (1973) Maximal voluntary and exercise ventilation at high ambient air pressures. *Försvarsmedicin* **9**, 275–278.

FAGRAEUS, L., KARLSSON, J., LINNARSSON, D. & SALTIN, B. (1973) Oxygen uptake during maximal work at lowered and raised ambient air pressures. *Acta physiol. scand.* **87**, 411–421.

FARHI, L. E. (1966) Ventilation–perfusion relationship and its role in alveolar gas exchange. In *Advances in Respiratory Physiology*. Ed. C. G. Caro. pp. 148–197. London: Edward Arnold.

FENN, W. O. & RAHN, H. (Eds) (1964) *Handbook of Physiology, Section 3: Respiration*, Vol. I. Washington: American Physiological Society.

FENN, W. O. & RAHN, H. (Eds) (1965) *Handbook of Physiology, Section 3: Respiration*, Vol. II. Washington: American Physiological Society.

FISHER, A. B. & HYDE, R. W. (1969) Decrease of diffusing capacity and pulmonary blood flow during passive lung inflation. *J. appl. Physiol.* **27**, 157–163.

FLYNN, E. T., CAMPORESI, E. M. & NUNNELEY, S. A. (1974) Cardiopulmonary function during positive pressure breathing in water. (In preparation.)

FLYNN, E. T., SALTZMAN, H. A. & SUMMITT, J. K. (1972) Effects of head-out immersion at 19·18 ATA on pulmonary gas exchange in man. *J. appl. Physiol.* **33**, 113–119.

FROEB, H. F. (1961) Ventilatory response of SCUBA divers to CO_2 inhalations. *J. appl. Physiol.* **16**, 8–10.

FRY, D. L. & HYATT, R. E. (1960) Pulmonary mechanics. *Am. J. Med.* **29**, 672–689.

GELFAND, R. & PETERSON, R. (1975) The effects on CO_2 reactivity of breathing crude neon at high pressures. In *Underwater Physiology. Vth Symp. Underwater Physiology* (1972). Ed. C. J. Lambertsen. Bethesda: Fedn Am. Socs exp. Biol.

GLESER, M. A. & VOGEL, J. A. (1973) Effects of acute alterations of $\dot{V}_{O_{2max}}$ on endurance capacity of men. *J. appl. Physiol.* **34**, 443–447.

GOFF, L. G., FRASSETTO, R. & SPECHT, H. (1956) Oxygen requirements in underwater swimming. *J. appl. Physiol.* **9**, 219–221.

GOFF, L. G., BRUBACH, H. F. & SPECHT, H. (1957) Measurements of respiratory responses and work efficiency of underwater swimmers utilizing improved instrumentation. *J. appl. Physiol.* **10**, 197–202.

GOLDMAN, M. (1973) Effect of chest wall configuration on the mechanical work of breathing. (See Bradley 1973.)

HAMILTON, R. W., Jr. (1967) Physiological responses at rest and in exercise during saturation at 20 atmospheres of He–O_2. In *Proc. 3rd Symp. Underwater Physiology*. Ed. C. J. Lambertsen. pp. 361–373. Baltimore: Williams & Wilkins.

HAMILTON, R. W. & LANGLEY, T. D. (1971) Exercise in high pressures of neon, helium and nitrogen. *Physiologist, Wash.* **14**, 157.

HAMILTON, R. W., Jr., MacINNIS, J. B., NOBLE, A. D. & SCHREINER, H. R. (1966) *Saturation Diving to 650 Feet* (Technical Memorandum B-411), Ocean Systems, Inc., Tonawanda, N.Y.

HANSON, J. S. (1973) Maximal exercise performance in members of the U.S. Nordic ski team. *J. appl. Physiol.* **35**, 592–595.

HESSER, C. M. & LINNARSSON, D. (Eds) (1973) Proceedings of the first annual scientific meeting of the European Undersea Biomedical Society. *Försvarsmedicin* **9**, 227–529.

HESSER, C. M., ADOLFSON, J. & FAGRAEUS, L. (1971) Role of CO_2 in compressed-air narcosis. *Aerospace Med.* **42**, 163–168.

HOLMÉR, I. (1972) Oxygen uptake during swimming in man. *J. appl. Physiol.* **33**, 502–509.

HONG, S. K., TING, E. Y. & RAHN, H. (1960) Lung volumes at different depths of submersion. *J. appl. Physiol.* **15**, 550–553.

HONG, S. K., CERRETELLI, P., CRUZ, J. C., & RAHN, H. (1969) Mechanics of respiration during submersion in water. *J. appl. Physiol.* **27**, 535–538.

HOWARD, P., ERNSTING, J., DENISON, D. M., FRYER, D. I., GLAISTER, D. H. & BYFORD, G. H. (1967) Effects of simulated weightlessness upon the cardiovascular system. *Aerospace Med.* **38**, 551–563.

HUNT, H., REEVES, E. & BECKMAN, E. L. (1964) *An Experiment in Maintaining Homeostasis in a Long Distance Underwater Swimmer*. U.S. Navy Med. Res. Inst., Bethesda, Maryland, Research Report MR 005.13–4001.06. No. 2.

HUNT, N. C. (1967) Positive pressure breathing during water immersion. *Aerospace Med.* **38**, 731–735.

HYACINTHE, R. & BROUSSOLLE, R. (1972) Étude de la mecanique ventilatoire au cours d'une plongée fictive à 51 ATA en helium-oxygène. *Bull. Medsubhyp.* **8**, 4–6.

HYATT, R. E. & WILCOX, R. E. (1963) The pressure–flow relationship of the intrathoracic airway in man. *J. clin. Invest.* **42**, 29–39.

JAFFRIN, M. Y. & KESIC, P. (1974) Airway resistance: a fluid mechanical approach. *J. appl. Physiol.* **36**, 354–361.

JARRETT, A. S. (1965) Effect of immersion on intrapulmonary pressure. *J. appl. Physiol.* **20**, 1261–1266.

JARRETT, A. S. (1966) Alveolar carbon dioxide tension at increased ambient pressures. *J. appl. Physiol.* **21**, 158–162.

JOHNSON, L. R. & VAN LIEW, H. D. (1974) Use of arterial P_{O_2} to study convective and diffusive gas mixing in the lungs. *J. appl. Physiol.* **36**, 91–97.

KARPOVICH, P. V. & MILLMAN, N. (1944) Energy expenditure in swimming. *Am. J. Physiol.* **142**, 140–144.

KELLOGG, R. H. (1960) Acclimatization to carbon dioxide. *Anesthesiology* **21**, 634–641.

KNELSON, J. H., HOWATT, W. F. & DeMUTH, G. R. (1970) Effect of respiratory pattern on alveolar gas exchange. *J. appl. Physiol.* **29**, 328–331.

KORZ, R., FISCHER, F. & BEHN, C. (1967) Renin-angiotensin system in simulated hypervolemia induced by immersion. *Klin. Wschr.* **47**, 1263–1268.

KYLSTRA, J. (1973) Estimate of maximum expiratory flow based on the EPP concept and Weibel's lung model. (See Bradley 1973.)

KYLSTRA, J. A., PAGANELLI, C. V. & LANPHIER, E. H. (1966) Pulmonary gas exchange in dogs ventilated with hyperbarically oxygenated liquid. *J. appl. Physiol.* **21**, 177–184.

KYLSTRA, J. A., PAGANELLI, C. V. & RAHN, H. (1966) Some implications of the dynamics of gas transfer in water-breathing dogs. In *Ciba Foundation Symposium on Development of the Lung.* Ed. A. V. S. de Reuck & R. Porter. pp. 34–58. London: Churchill.

LAMBERTSEN, C. J. (Ed.) (1975) *Underwater Physiology. Vth Symp. Underwater Physiology* (1972). Bethesda: Fedn Am. Socs exp. Biol.

LAMBERTSEN, C. J. & WENDEL, H. (1960) An alveolar pCO_2 control system: its use to magnify respiratory depression by meperidine. *J. appl. Physiol.* **15**, 43–48.

LAMBERTSEN, C. J., HALL, P., WOLLMAN, H. & GOODMAN, M. W. (1963) Quantitative interactions of increased P_{O_2} and P_{CO_2} upon respiration in man. *Ann. N.Y. Acad. Sci.* **109**, 731–741.

LAMBERTSEN, C. J., OWEN, S. G., WENDEL, H., STROUD, M. W., LURIE, A. A., LOCHNER, W. & CLARK, G. F. (1959) Respiratory and cerebral circulatory control during exercise at 0·21 and 2·0 atmospheres inspired P_{O_2}. *J. appl. Physiol.* **14**, 966–982.

LAMBERTSEN, C. J., GELFAND, R., LEVER, M. J., BODAMMER, G., TAKANO, N., REED, T. A., DICKSON, J. G. & WATSON, P. T. (1973) Respiration and gas exchange during a 14-day continuous exposure to 5·2% O_2 in N_2 at pressure equivalent to 100 FSW (4 ATA). *Aerospace Med.* **44**, 844–849.

LANPHIER, E. H. (1954) *Oxygen Consumption in Underwater Swimming.* U.S. Navy Experimental Diving Unit, Washington, D.C. Formal Report 14–54.

LANPHIER, E. H. (1955) Use of nitrogen–oxygen mixtures in diving. In *Proc. 1st Symp. Underwater Physiology.* Ed. L. G. Goff. pp. 74–78. Washington: Natl Acad. Sci.-Natl Res. Council (Publ. 377).

LANPHIER, E. H. (1956a) Physiological considerations in design of breathing apparatus. In *Submarine Medicine Practice,* NAVMED P-5054, Chap. 12, pp. 185–210. Washington: U.S. Govt Printing Office.

LANPHIER, E. H. (1956b) *Nitrogen–Oxygen Mixture Physiology, Phase 3.* U.S. Navy Experimental Diving Unit, Washington, Research Report 2–56.

LANPHIER, E. H. (1963) Influence of increased ambient pressure upon alveolar ventilation. In *Proc. 2nd Symp. Underwater Physiology.* Ed. C. J. Lambertsen & L. J. Greenbaum, Jr. pp. 124–133. Washington: Natl Acad. Sci.-Natl Res. Council (Publ. 1181).

LANPHIER, E. H. (1964) Man in high pressures. In *Handbook of Physiology, Section 4: Adaptation to the Environment.* Ed. D. B. Dill, E. F. Adolph & C. G. Wilber. Chap. 58, pp. 893–909. Washington: American Physiological Society.

LANPHIER, E. H. (1965) Overinflation of the lungs (pp. 1189–1193 in Fenn & Rahn 1965).

LANPHIER, E. H. (1967) Interactions of factors limiting performance at high pressures. In *Underwater Physiology. Proc. 3rd Symp. Underwater Physiology.* Ed. C. J. Lambertsen. pp. 375–385. Baltimore: Williams & Wilkins.

LANPHIER, E. H. (1972) Human respiration under increased pressures. In *The Effects of Pressure on Organisms* (Symposia of the Society for Experimental Biology No. XXVI.) Ed. M. Sleigh & A. Macdonald. pp. 379–394. Cambridge: Cambridge University Press.

LINNARSSON, D. & FAGRAEUS, L. (1972) Maximal work performance in hyperbaric air. In *Underwater Physiology. Proc. 5th Symp. Underwater Physiology.* Ed. C. J. Lambertsen. (In press.)

LORD, G. P., BOND, G. F. & SCHAEFER, K. E. (1966) Breathing under high ambient pressure. *J. appl. Physiol.* **21**, 1833–1838.

MAIO, D. A. & FARHI, L. E. (1967) Effect of gas density on mechanics of breathing. *J. appl. Physiol.* **23**, 687–693.

MARGARIA, R. (1967) Anaerobic metabolism in muscle. *Canad. med. Assoc. J.* **96**, 770–774.

MARGARIA, R. (1972) The sources of muscular energy. *Scient. Am.* March 1972, pp. 85–91.

MARGARIA, R., CAMPORESI, E., AGHEMO, P. & SASSI, G. (1972) The effect of O_2 breathing on maximal aerobic power. *Pflügers Arch. ges. Physiol.* **336**, 225–235.

MARGARIA, R., CERRETELLI, P., AGHEMO, P. & SASSI, G. (1963) Energy cost of running. *J. appl. Physiol.* **18**, 367–370.

MARGARIA, R., OLIVA, R. D., DI PRAMPERO, P. E. & CERRETELLI, P. (1969) Energy utilization in intermittent exercise of supramaximal intensity. *J. appl. Physiol.* **26**, 752–756.

MARSHALL, R., LANPHIER, E. H. & DuBOIS, A. B. (1956) Resistance to breathing in normal subjects during simulated dives. *J. appl. Physiol.* **9**, 5–10.

MAYER, J. (1959) Exercise and weight control. *Postgrad. Med.* **25**, 325–332.

McCALLY, M. (1965) Body fluid volumes and the renal response to immersion (pp. 253–270 in Rahn & Yokoyama 1965).

McKENNA, W. J., GRIFFIN, P. M., ANTHONISEN, N. R. & MENKES, H. A. (1973) Oscillation mechanics of the submerged respiratory system. *Aerospace Med.* **44**, 324–326.

MEAD, J. (1955) Resistance to breathing at increased ambient pressures. In *Proc. 1st Symp. Underwater Physiology* Ed. L. G. Goff. pp. 112–120. Washington: Natl Acad. Sci.-Natl Res. Council (Publ. 377).

MEAD, J., TURNER, J. M., MACKLEM, P. T. & LITTLE, J. B. (1967) Significance of the relationship between lung recoil and maximum expiratory flow. *J. appl. Physiol.* **22**, 95–108.

MENN, S. J., SINCLAIR, R. D. & WELCH, B. E. (1970) Effect of inspired CO_2 up to 30 mm Hg on response of normal man to exercise. *J. appl. Physiol.* **28**, 663–671.

MICHAUD, A., LeCHUITON, J., PARC, J., BARTHELEMY, L., BALOUET, G., GIRIN, E., CORRIOL, J. & CHOUTEAU, J. *Bilan d'une experimentation animale de plongées aux mélanges hydrogène–oxygène.* Presented at the GERS Physiology Symposium of the Marine Nationale, Toulon, France, January 1973.

MILES, S. (1958) *The Effect of Increase in Barometric Pressure on Maximum Breathing Capacity.* Med. Res. Council, R.N. Personnel Res. Committee R.N.P. 58/922, U.P.S. 174, R.N.P.L. 1/58.

MILIC-EMILI, J. & TYLER, J. M. (1963) Relation between work output of respiratory muscles and end-tidal CO_2 tension. *J. appl. Physiol.* **18**, 497–504.

MILLER, J. N., WANGENSTEEN, O. D. & LANPHIER, E. H. (1971) Ventilatory limitations on exertion at depth. In *Underwater Physiology. Proc. 4th Symp. Underwater Physiology.* Ed. C. J. Lambertsen. pp. 317–323. New York: Academic Press.

MILLER, J. N., WANGENSTEEN, O. D. & LANPHIER, E. H. (1972) Respiratory limitations to work at depth. In *Proc. Third International Conference on Hyperbaric and Underwater Physiology.* Ed. X. Fructus. pp. 118–123. Paris: Doin.

MILLER, J. N. & WINSBOROUGH, M. (1973) The effect of increased gas density upon $\dot{V}A/\dot{Q}$ and gas exchange during expiratory flow-limited exercise. *Försvarsmedicin* **9**, 321–331.

MOORE, T. O., BERNAUER, E. M., SETO, G., PARK, Y. S., HONG, S. K. & HAYASHI, E. M. (1970) Effect of immersion at different water temperatures on graded exercise performance in man. *Aerospace Med.* **41**, 1404–1408.

MORRISON, J. B. (1973) Oxygen uptake studies of divers when fin swimming with maximum effort at depths of 6–176 feet. *Aerospace Med.* **44**, 1120–1129.

MORRISON, J. B. & BUTT, W. S. (1972) Effect of underwater breathing apparatus and absolute air pressure on divers ventilatory capacity. *Aerospace Med.* **43**, 881–888.

MORRISON, J. B. & FLORIO, J. T. (1971) Respiratory function during a simulated saturation dive to 1,500 feet. *J. appl. Physiol.* **30**, 724–732.

MUELLER, R. E., PETTY, T. L. & FILLEY, G. F. (1970) Ventilation and arterial blood gas changes induced by pursed lips breathing. *J. appl. Physiol.* **28**, 784–789.

MUREN, A. & WULFF, K. (1972) Carbon dioxide distribution in the diver's helmet. In *Proc. Third International Conference on Hyperbaric and Underwater Physiology.* Ed. X. Fructus. pp. 99–100. Paris: Doin.

NEFF, T. A. & PETTY, T. L. (1972) Tolerance and survival in severe chronic hypercapnia. *Archs intern. Med.* **129**, 591–596.

OHIWA, H. (1969) On the ventilatory dynamics under high atmospheric pressures. *Jap. J. ind. Hlth* **11**, 469–476.

OLSEN, C. R., STEVENS, A. E. & McILROY, M. B. (1967) Rigidity of tracheae and bronchi during muscular constriction. *J. appl. Physiol.* **23**, 27–34.

OLSEN, C. R., STEVENS, A. E., PRIDE, N. B. & STAUB, N. C. (1967) Structural basis for decreased compressibility of constricted tracheae and bronchi. *J. appl. Physiol.* **23**, 35–39.

OUELLET, Y., POH, S. C. & BECKLAKE, M. R. (1969) Circulatory factors limiting maximal aerobic exercise capacity. *J. appl. Physiol.* **27**, 874–880.

PAPPENHEIMER, J. (1950) Standardization of definitions and symbols in respiratory physiology. *Fedn Proc. Fedn Am. Socs exp. Biol.* **9**, 602–605.

PASSMORE, R. & DURNIN, J. V. G. A. (1955) Human energy expenditure. *Physiol. Rev.* **35**, 801–840.

PATON, W. D. M. & SAND, A. (1947) The optimum intrapulmonary pressure in underwater respiration. *J. Physiol.* **106**, 119–138.

PRIDE, N. B., PERMUTT, S., RILEY, R. L. & BROMBERGER-BARNEA, B. (1967) Determinants of maximal expiratory flow from the lungs. *J. appl. Physiol.* **23**, 646–662.

RADFORD, E. P., Jr. (1955) Ventilation standards for use in artificial respiration. *J. appl. Physiol.* **7**, 451–460.

RAHN, H. & FARHI, L. E. (1964) Ventilation, perfusion and gas exchange—the $\dot{V}A/\dot{Q}$ concept (Chap. 30, pp. 735–766, in Fenn & Rahn 1964).

RAHN, H. & FENN, W. O. (1955) *A Graphical Analysis of the Respiratory Gas Exchange; the O_2–CO_2 Diagram.* Washington: The American Physiological Society.

RAHN, H. & YOKOYAMA, T. (Eds) (1965) *Physiology of Breath-Hold Diving and the Ama of Japan.* Washington: Natl Acad. Sci.-Natl Res. Council (Publ. 1341).

RATTENBORG, C. (1961) Laryngeal regulation of respiration. *Acta anaesth. scand.* **5**, 129–140.

ROHRER, F. (1915) Der Strömungswiderstand in den menschlichen Atemwegen und der Einfluss der unregelmässigen Verzweigung des Bronchialsystems auf den Atmungsverlauf verschiedenen Lungenbezirken. *Pflügers Arch. ges. Physiol.* **162**, 225–299.

SALTZMAN, H. A. (1973) Effects of altered environment at simulated depths on gas exchange. (See Bradley 1973.)

SALTZMAN, H. A., SALZANO, J. V., BLENKARN, G. D. & KYLSTRA, J. A. (1971) Effects of pressure on ventilation and gas exchange in man. *J. appl. Physiol.* **30**, 443–449.

SALZANO, J. V., BELL, W. H., WEGLICKI, W. B. & SALTZMAN, H. A. (1967) Metabolic, respiratory and hemodynamic responses to exercise at increased oxygen pressure. In *Underwater Physiology. Proc. 3rd Symp. Underwater Physiology.* Ed. C. J. Lambertsen. pp. 351–360. Baltimore: Williams & Wilkins.

SALZANO, J., RAUSCH, D. C. & SALTZMAN, H. A. (1970) Cardiorespiratory responses to exercise at a simulated seawater depth of 1,000 feet. *J. appl. Physiol.* **28**, 34–41.

SCHAEFER, K. E. (1969) Chap. 6 in first edition of this volume.

SCHAEFER, K. E., CAREY, C. R. & DOUGHERTY, J. H., Jr. (1971) Pulmonary function and respiratory gas exchange during saturation-excursion diving to pressures equivalent to 1000 feet of sea water. In *Underwater Physiology. Proc. 4th Symp. Underwater Physiology.* Ed. C. J. Lambertsen. pp. 357–370. New York: Academic Press.

SCHREINER, H., HAMILTON, R. W., Jr. & LANGLEY, T. D. (1972) Neon: an attractive new commercial diving gas. In: *1972 Offshore Technical Conference, Houston, Texas.* Preprints, Paper no. OTC 1561. Published by the conference.

SEUSING, J. & DRUBE, H. C. (1960) Die Bedeutung der Hyperkapnie für das Auftreten des Tiefenrausches. *Klin. Wschr.* **38**, 1088–1090.

SHEPHARD, R. J. (1966) The oxygen cost of breathing during vigorous exercise. *Q. Jl exp. Physiol.* **51**, 336–350.

SHEPHARD, R. J. (1967) The maximum sustained voluntary ventilation in exercise. *Clin. Sci.* **32**, 167–176.

SHEPHARD, R. J. (1972) *Alive Man! The Physiology of Physical Activity.* Springfield, Ill.: Thomas.

SINCLAIR, R. D., CLARK, J. M. & WELCH, B. E. (1971) Comparison of physiological responses of normal man to exercise in air and in acute and chronic hypercapnia. In *Underwater Physiology. Proc. 4th Symp. Underwater Physiology.* Ed. C. J. Lambertsen. pp. 409–417. New York: Academic Press.

SLADEN, A., LAVER, M. B. & PONTOPPIDAN, H. (1968) Pulmonary complications and water retention in prolonged mechanical ventilation. *N. Engl J. Med.* **279**, 448–453.

SPANN, R. W. & HYATT, R. E. (1971) Factors affecting upper airway resistance in conscious man. *J. appl. Physiol.* **31**, 708–712.

SPAUR, W. H. (1973) U.S.N. Supervisor of Diving Dive 1600 ft. 20 April–21 May 1973. U.S. Navy Experimental Diving Unit, Washington. (Preliminary Summary.)

STERK, W. (1970) Diver and underwater breathing apparatus: a lungmechanical study. *Neds milit.-geneesk. Tijdschr.* **23**, 322–356.

STERK, W. (1973) *Respiratory Mechanics of Diver and Diving Apparatus.* Doctoral dissertation. Utrecht.

STRAUSS, R. H., WRIGHT, W. B., PETERSON, R. E., LEVER, M. J. & LAMBERTSEN, C. J. (1975) Respiratory function in exercising subjects breathing nitrogen, helium, or neon mixtures at pressures from 1 to 37 atmospheres absolute. In *Underwater Physiology. Vth Symp. Underwater Physiology.* (1972). Ed. C. J. Lambertsen. Bethesda: Fedn Am. Socs exp. Biol.

TAUNTON, J. E., BANISTER, E. W., PATRICK, T. R., OFORSAGD, P. & DUNCAN, W. R. (1970) Physical work capacity in hyperbaric environments and conditions of hyperoxia. *J. appl. Physiol.* **28**, 421–427.

TAYLOR, H. L. (1960) Exercise and metabolism. *Science and Medicine of Exercise and Sports.* Ed. Johnson, W. R., Chap. 8, pp. 123–161. New York: Harper.

TAYLOR, H. L., WANG, Y., ROWELL, L. & BLOMQUIST, G. (1963) The standardization and interpretation of submaximal and maximal tests of working capacity. *Pediatrics* **32**, 703–722.

TENNEY, S. M. & REESE, R. E. (1968) The ability to sustain great breathing efforts. *Resp. Physiol.* **5**, 187–201.

THOMPSON, L. J. & McCALLY, M. (1967) Role of transpharyngeal pressure gradients in determining intrapulmonary pressure during immersion. *Aerospace Med.* **38**, 931–935.

TING, E. Y., HONG, S. K. & RAHN, H. (1960) Cardiovascular responses of man during negative-pressure breathing. *J. appl. Physiol.* **15**, 557–560.

UHL, R. R., VAN DYKE, C., COOK, R. B., HORST, R. A. & MERZ, J. R. (1972) Effects of externally imposed mechanical resistance on breathing dense gas at exercise: mechanics of breathing. *Aerospace Med.* **43**, 836–841.

VAIL, E. G. (1971a) Hyperbaric respiratory mechanics. *Aerospace Med.* **42**, 536–546.

VAIL, E. G. (1971b) Respiratory mechanics—airway collapse. *Aerospace Med.* **42**, 975–979.

VAIL, E. G. (1973) Pulmonary insufficiency with airway flutter, closure, and collapse. *Aerospace Med.* **44**, 649–662.

VARÈNE, P., TIMBAL, J. & JACQUEMIN, C. (1967) Effect of different ambient pressures on airway resistance. *J. appl. Physiol.* **22**, 699–706.

VARÈNE, P., VIEILLEFOND, H., LEMAIRE, C. & SAUMON, G. (1974) Expiratory flow volume curves and ventilatory limitation of muscular exercise at depth. *Aerospace Med.* **45**, 161–166.

VOROSMARTI, J. & LANPHIER, E. H. (1975) Effects of external resistance on maximum expiratory flow at increasing gas density. In *Underwater Physiology. Vth Symp. Underwater Physiology* (1972). Ed. C. J. Lambertsen. Bethesda: Fedn Am. Socs exp. Biol.

WASSERMAN, K., WHIPP, B. J., KOYAL, S. N. & BEAVER, W. L. (1973) Anaerobic threshold and respiratory gas exchange during exercise. *J. appl. Physiol.* **35**, 236–243.

WEBBER, J. T. (1969) Respiratory Effects of Nitrous Oxide Narcosis. M.A. Thesis. State University of New York at Buffalo.

WEST, J. B. (1965) *Ventilation/Blood Flow and Gas Exchange.* Philadelphia: F. A. Davis; London: Blackwell.

WEST, J. B. (1971) Causes of carbon dioxide retention in lung disease. *N. Engl J. Med.* **284**, 1232–1236.

WHIPP, B. J. & WASSERMAN, K. (1972) Oxygen uptake kinetics for various intensities of constant-load work. *J. appl. Physiol.* **33**, 351–356.

WILMORE, J. H. & HASKELL, W. L. (1972) Body composition and endurance capacity of professional football players. *J. appl. Physiol.* **33**, 564–567.

WOOD, L. D. H. & BRYAN, A. C. (1969) Effect of increased ambient pressure on flow-volume curve of the lung. *J. appl. Physiol.* **27**, 4–8.

WOOD, W. B. (1963) Ventilatory dynamics under hyperbaric states. *Proc. 2nd Symp. Underwater Physiology.* Ed. C. J. Lambertsen & L. J. Greenbaum, Jr. pp. 108–123. Washington: Natl Acad. Sci.-Natl Res. Council (Publ. 1181).

WRIGHT, W. B. & CROTHERS, J. R. (1973) Effects of immersion and high pressures on pulmonary mechanical functions in man. In: *Aerospace Medical Association, 1973 Annual Scientific Meeting.* Preprints, p. 39. Published by the Association.

WRIGHT, W. B., PETERSON, R. & LAMBERTSEN, C. J. (1972) *Pulmonary Mechanical Functions in Man Breathing Dense Gas Mixtures at Great Depths.* U.S. Navy Experimental Diving Unit, Washington, Research Report 14–72.

WRIGHT, W. B., FISHER, A. B., HENDRICKS, P. L., BRODY, J. S. & LAMBERTSEN, C. J. (1973) Pulmonary function studies during a 14-day continuous exposure to $5 \cdot 2\%$ O_2 in N_2 at pressure equivalent to 100 FSW (4 ATA). *Aerospace Med.* **44**, 837–843.

YAMASHIRO, S. M. & GRODINS, F. S. (1971) Optimal regulation of respiratory airflow. *J. appl. Physiol.* **30**, 597–602.

ZECHMAN, F., HALL, F. G. & HULL, W. E. (1957) Effects of graded resistance to tracheal air flow in man. *J. appl. Physiol.* **10**, 356–362.

ZOCCHE, G. P., FRITTS, H. W., Jr. & COURNAND, A. (1960) Fraction of maximum breathing capacity available for prolonged hyperventilation. *J. appl. Physiol.* **15**, 1073–1074.

9

Liquid Breathing and Artificial Gills

J. A. KYLSTRA

Many of the problems encountered in diving are caused by the compressibility of gases. A simple solution would be to use breathing mixtures that are not compressible: liquids. The obvious danger would be drowning. However, newborn mammals can survive in water for surprisingly long periods of time. Signs of life have been observed in puppies submerged in water for as long as 54 min (Edwards 1824). Newborn rats submerged in water at 37°C continue to make respiratory movements, can survive underwater for at least 40 min, recover when taken out of the water and develop normally into adult rats (Fazekas, Alexander & Himwich 1941).

This ability of newborn mammals to survive in an aquatic environment can partly be explained by their tolerance to anoxia (Glass, Snyder & Webster 1944). Injection of iodoacetate and fluoride shortens the survival of newborn rats in nitrogen, presumably by blocking anaerobic glycolysis (Himwich et al. 1942). This tolerance to anoxia of the newborn mammal is lost shortly after birth. Teleologically, this is understandable. Once the crucial transition from fetal life in amniotic fluid to air breathing has been made, tolerance to anoxia normally is no longer required. Conceivably, administration of the necessary enzymes to adult mammals could restore their initial tolerance to hypoxia, but this is no more than science fiction at present.

Drowning mammals often inhale water which, as a rule, has a composition different from that of blood. Net transfer of water and solutes across the alveolar walls, as a result of diffusion and osmosis, can cause tissue damage and alterations in the volume and composition of body fluids which are incompatible with life (Brouardel & Loye 1889; Swann et al. 1947). If a lung is filled with a solution containing salts in concentrations similar to those normally found in blood plasma, or with a liquid that does not mix with water, no significant net transfer of either water or solutes should occur across the blood–air barrier.

According to Henry's law, the amount of gas dissolved in a liquid is directly proportional to the partial gas pressure at equilibrium on the gas–liquid interface. Thus, it should be possible to prevent hypoxic death by having the diver breathe a pressure-oxygenated liquid.

Medical technology has produced 'artificial kidneys' and 'artificial lungs' in which the blood of a patient, flowing outside his body along a semi-permeable membrane, can exchange solutes and gases with the external environment. Thus, it would seem reasonable, at first sight, to expect that suitable extracorporeal gas exchangers could be constructed, modelled after the gills of fish. Such an 'artificial gill', enabling a diver with liquid-filled lungs to obtain oxygen by diffusion from the sea, would have obvious logistic advantages. Even more important is the fact that a diver equipped with an artificial gill, extracting oxygen like a fish from the water in which he swims, would never be exposed to toxic oxygen partial pressures. Contrary to what is still believed by some, the oxygen concentration of seawater does not appreciably increase with depth; the oxygen partial pressure in the ocean at great depths may actually be substantially less than at the surface. In conventional diving, accurately calibrated gas mixtures with a very low concentration of oxygen are essential at great depths to avoid oxygen toxicity.

It is clear that the development of liquid breathing and the construction of artificial gills, if at all feasible, could be of great importance. The possibilities of man exchanging respiratory gases directly with an aquatic environment had not been explored seriously until 1961 and it is, as yet, difficult to predict the outcome of such research.

LIQUID BREATHING

Experiments with animals

Gas exchange and ventilation. Mice and rats have been kept alive up to 18 hours while totally submerged in salt solutions equilibrated with oxygen at high pressures. The animals appeared to inhale and exhale the salt solution, responded to external stimuli when not previously anesthetized, and were obviously capable of extracting adequate amounts of dissolved oxygen from their aqueous environment. Mice submerged in a hyperbarically oxygenated balanced salt solution to which a carbon dioxide buffer, THAM (tris-hydroxymethyl aminomethane), had been added, lived markedly longer than in an identical but unbuffered salt solution (Kylstra, Tissing & van der Mäen 1962). In a tracheostomized rat submerged in plain hyperbarically oxygenated saline, the arterial carbon dioxide partial pressure was 174 mm Hg and the arterial pH was 6·61 after 30 min, but in another rat who, under otherwise identical conditions, breathed saline to which 0·4% THAM had been added, a carbon dioxide partial pressure of 50 mm Hg and a pH of 7·00 were measured in the arterial blood 30 min after the beginning of the experiment (Pegg, Horner & Wahrenbrock 1963). In anesthetized, intubated or tracheostomized, spontaneously breathing hypothermic dogs, who were submerged in hyperbarically oxygenated unbuffered saline, arterial blood gas analyses revealed adequate oxygenation, but retention of carbon dioxide (Kylstra & Tissing 1964). Intrathoracic pressure fluctuations in these saline-breathing animals reflected the

effort required to move liquid instead of air through the trachea and bronchi. The pressure in the right atrium ranged from 40 mm Hg below to 15 mm Hg above atmospheric pressure, and expiration lasted twice as long as inspiration. The pulmonary gas exchange during liquid breathing was measured in anesthetized normothermic dogs who were ventilated mechanically with a hyperbarically oxygenated modified Ringer solution (Kylstra, Paganelli & Lanphier 1966). The minute volume of liquid ventilation ranged from 1 to 4 L at respiratory frequencies ranging from 6 to 21 breaths/min. The arterial oxygen tension varied between 18 and 1790 mm Hg, and the oxygen consumption between 31 and 93 ml/min at inspired oxygen tensions ranging from 1380 to 3640 mm Hg. The respiratory exchange ratio (R) ranged from 0·3 to 0·7 at arterial carbon dioxide tensions from 43 to 80 mm Hg, indicating deficient carbon dioxide elimination. The carbon dioxide partial pressure in 'end-tidal' liquid, i.e. following exhalation of 82 to 93% of the tidal volume, ranged from 28 to 74% of the simultaneously measured partial pressure of carbon dioxide in the arterial blood, suggesting the presence of stratified inhomogeneity of dissolved alveolar gas. There was a clear, although statistically not significant, trend for the end-tidal carbon dioxide partial pressure to approach the partial pressure of carbon dioxide in the arterial blood as the respiratory frequency decreased and more time was available for the diffusive mixing of dissolved alveolar carbon dioxide.

Clark and Gollan (1966) first used a fluorinated hydrocarbon (FX–80) as a breathing fluid. The solubility, at 37°C, of oxygen in this liquid is approximately 20 times as great as in unbuffered isotonic salt solutions. That of carbon dioxide is three times as great. However, retention of carbon dioxide also occurred in fluorocarbon-breathing cats and dogs. Modell, Newby and Ruiz (1970) also reported respiratory acidosis (with arterial carbon dioxide partial pressures up to 80 mm Hg) in anesthetized dogs who were ventilated with bubble-oxygenated FX–80 fluorocarbon liquid. However, Sass et al. (1972) were able to maintain the arterial carbon dioxide partial pressure of anesthetized dogs who were ventilated mechanically with oxygenated FX–80 fluorocarbon liquid between 16 and 40 mm Hg, but the pH of the arterial blood progressively decreased to values near 7·0 at the end of 4 hours of liquid breathing.

Lundgren and Örnhagen (1972) measured the oxygen consumption of anesthetized mice who breathed oxygenated fluorocarbon liquid without mechanical assistance. The body temperature of the animals was varied between 16 and 37°C, and the oxygen pressure in the liquid ranged from 1·0 to 7·8 ATS. It was found that the oxygen uptake was not influenced by the inspired oxygen pressure, up to a body temperature of 22°C. At higher body temperatures, the inspired oxygen pressure had to be increased to 3·5 ATS in order to maintain a normal oxygen uptake. Intra-peritoneal THAM injections did not appreciably influence survival time. Oxygen uptake increased with body temperature, reaching (by extra-polation) 2·8 ml/g body weight per hour at 37°C as compared to 1·6 ml/g body weight per hour at 37°C in oxygen-breathing anesthetized mice. The difference was attributed to the greater than normal work required to breathe a liquid instead of gas.

Survival and recovery. Out of 6 dogs who had breathed a pressure oxygenated salt solution for 20 min without mechanical assistance 1 survived the experiment and was in good health for many years afterwards (Kylstra & Tissing 1964). Out of 16 dogs who had been ventilated mechanically with a hyperbarically oxygenated salt solution for up to 58 min 6 survived without grossly apparent ill after effects. Half of these surviving dogs were sacrificed 22, 90 and 116 days respectively after the experiment. Only minor patho-logical changes were found in the lungs of 2 of these animals, but masses of eosinophilic material surrounded by small round cells embedded in scarred areas, and dense eosinophilic membranes in association with chronic inflammatory cells and fibroblasts were seen in alveolar and bronchiolar lumina of the lungs of the third dog (Kylstra, Paganelli & Lanphier 1966).

All of 10 dogs who had been ventilated with hyperbarically oxygenated saline for 15 min survived (Blenkarn & Hayes 1970). After 48 hours, the arterial oxygen and carbon dioxide partial pressures were normal while the animals breathed room air. Morphologic changes observed up to

24 hours after the liquid ventilation consisted of patchy atelectasis and intrabronchial froth. Mild interstitial edema and distention of the rough endoplasmic reticulum was observed at 2 and 6 days after the experiments.

Modell et al. (1971) reported that all of a series of 36 dogs who had been ventilated for 1 hour with oxygenated fluorocarbon liquid survived. For several days afterwards, the arterial oxygen tension of these animals was lower than normal when they breathed air. This was attributed to residual fluorocarbon in the lungs and/or partial airway closure. Pathologic examination of the lungs 3 hours after the liquid ventilation had been terminated disclosed an acute exudative inflam-matory reaction which was confined to the bron-chioles. By 72 hours, the acute reaction had sub-sided and the dominant change consisted of vacuolated intra-alveolar macrophages, presum-ably containing fluorocarbon. At 10 days, the macrophages were still present, but generally in much smaller numbers. After 18 months, the lungs appeared normal. Saga et al. (1973) ventilated the lungs of 11 dogs with a highly purified fluoro-carbon liquid, Caroxin-F, for 1 hour. All animals survived the experiment. During the period of liquid breathing, there was an increase in the arterial carbon dioxide partial pressure and a decrease in the pH of the arterial blood, but these values returned to normal immediately after the animals resumed gas breathing. After a further 24 hours the mean arterial oxygen tension was 84 mm Hg and the mean partial pressure of carbon dioxide in the arterial blood was 34 mm Hg while the dogs breathed air. An increase in the airway resistance and a decrease in the lung compliance was found 24 hours after the termination of liquid breathing, but these parameters returned to normal within 72 hours. The temporary impair-ment in pulmonary function following the breath-ing of Caroxin-F was attributed to residual fluoro-carbon liquid in the lung.

Experiments with isolated lungs

Gas exchange. West et al. (1965) studied the distribution of ventilation and blood flow in excised lungs of greyhound dogs, filled with saline, suspended in a saline bath, and perfused with blood. The distribution of blood flow was measured by injecting aggregated ^{131}I-labelled albumin into the pulmonary artery and scanning the lung from bottom to top when the particles had been trapped by the small vessels. After equilibrating the alveolar saline with more inhaled iodinated albumin and scanning again, blood flow per unit alveolar volume could be calculated. At vascular pressures which had been shown to cause great topographical inequality of blood flow in the gas-filled lung, blood flow was evenly distributed, on the average, in the saline-filled preparation, presumably because the hydrostatic pressure differences in the blood vessels were balanced by corresponding pressures in the airways. The topographical distribution of a single breath of iodinated albumin in saline was found to be uniform but there was a striking stratified inhomogeneity along the airways. This was believed to be due to the slow diffusion rate of albumin in saline and similar effects were seen with inhaled radioactive oxygen and carbon dioxide dissolved in saline. Stratified inhomogeneity of dissolved radioactive xenon, persisting for more than 30 sec but less than 3 min, was demonstrated in a subsequent series of experiments. In addition to stratification of alveolar dissolved gas, there was evidence of stratification of alveolar capillary blood flow which would seem to impair the efficiency of gas transfer in saline-ventilated lungs (West, Maloney & Castle 1973).

Ventilation. Leith and Mead (1966) recorded pressure–volume and maximum expiratory flow–volume curves from air-filled and gas-free saline-filled dog and rat lungs suspended in volume or pressure plethysmographs. In the saline-filled lungs, the static recoil pressures were less than half of the ones in air-filled lungs and maximum expiratory flows were about 100 times smaller than in air-filled lungs. On the basis of these results, a maximum saline ventilation in man of about 3·5 L/min was predicted. Hamosh and Luchsinger (1968) also measured the maximum expiratory flow of saline from excised dogs' lungs and essentially confirmed the findings of Leith and Mead. Volume–flow characteristics of saline and FC–80 fluorocarbon-filled excised dogs' lungs were compared by Schoenfisch and Kylstra (1973), using volume-displacement plethysmography. In these experiments, expiratory flow started from

a lung volume at which the static recoil pressure of the same lung filled with air had been 20 cm H_2O. The maximum flows of saline and fluorocarbon were compared over the first 50% of the total volume expired. The mean flows were 121 ml/sec for the saline-filled lungs and 104 ml/sec for the fluorocarbon-filled lungs. At comparable lung volumes, the static recoil pressure of FC–80-filled lungs was found to be greater than in saline-filled lungs, indicating that alveolar surface tension is not abolished in a fluorocarbon-filled lung (Kylstra & Schoenfisch 1972).

Tolerance of liquid-breathing mammals to pressure, decompression, and change in velocity

To separate the effects of pressure from the pharmacological effects of gases, Kylstra et al. (1967) hydraulically compressed fluorocarbon-breathing mice. With partial pressures of oxygen in the fluorocarbon liquid of 700 mm Hg or less and the temperature of the liquid ranging from 17° to 25°C 40 mice were subjected to pressures up to 166 ATS. The first effect observed in most animals was trembling of the limbs, and voluntary movements became jerky and uncoordinated. When the pressure was increased further, generalized tonic convulsions were observed. These tremors, uncoordinated limb movements, and tonic convulsions occurred at pressures ranging from 50 to 100 ATS. Three mice were compressed with helium to 100 ATS. Tremors and uncoordinated movements, but not tonic convulsions, were observed. Five mice were pre-cooled in a water bath until their rectal temperature had dropped to approximately 20°C. When the animals were then compressed with helium, tonic convulsions, similar to the ones observed in hydraulically compressed mice, occurred in 3 animals at pressures ranging from 69 to 86 ATS. Örnhagen and Lundgren (1975) studied the influence of compression rate and body temperature on the pressure tolerance of fluorocarbon-breathing mice. The pressure of oxygen in the liquid was 4 ATS. The limit of pressure tolerance was defined as respiratory standstill. At a rectal temperature of 17°C, the mean limiting pressure was 150 ATS; at 21°C, 220 ATS; at 27°C, 220 ATS; at 31°C, 125 ATS. The rate of compression had no marked effect on the pressure tolerance although 6 ATS/min appeared less favorable than a slower rate. Pressure-induced convulsions began to appear at between 80 to 100 ATS. With the highest compression rate, tonic convulsions were particularly marked and long lasting (>1 min). At a body temperature of 17°C, the convulsions were long lasting (>1 min) compared to the short bursts (<10 sec) of convulsive activity seen at 27°C and 31°C. The respiratory frequency and heart rate decreased in a roughly linear fashion with increasing pressure. This was particularly evident in animals studied at a body temperature of 21°C and 27°C. For instance, at 21°C and 50 ATS, the mean heart rate was 104 beats/min and the mean respiratory frequency 17 breaths/min. At 150 ATS the mean heart rate had fallen to 77 beats/min and the respiratory frequency to 5 breaths/min. Except for a prolongation of the P–Q interval in some animals and a general tendency for the amplitude to be less at increasing pressures, the electrocardiograms were normal. Although no special emphasis was placed on saving the animals, some of them recovered and appeared normal several months after exposure to pressures of up to 250 ATS (8250 ft).

Gollan and Clark (1967) submersed mice in fluorocarbon liquid which had been bubble-oxygenated for 10 min at atmospheric pressure. The beaker containing the mouse was then encased in a gas-impermeable Mylar membrane, put into a small steel chamber, and exposed to an air pressure of 33 ATS (1124 ft) for 10 min. After decompression of the chamber, which required about 5 sec, the mouse was removed from the liquid, held head down to drain the liquid from its lungs, and placed in an atmosphere of gaseous oxygen. Of such liquid-breathing animals 14 survived, while the same number of control animals died upon removal from the chamber. Kylstra et al. (1967) reported that a fluorocarbon-breathing mouse survived uniform compression to 100 ATS for 30 sec; it was decompressed in 3 sec, resumed air breathing, and was alive and in apparent good health 1 month after the experiment. Such a rate of decompression is equivalent to surfacing from 3300 ft (1000 m) underwater at a vertical speed of 700 miles/hour (1200 km/hour) without signs of decompression sickness.

Margaria, Gualtierotti and Spinelli (1958) placed pregnant rats in an open steel cylinder containing water, and dropped the cylinder from various heights. Deceleration was computed from the depth of the indentation made by the cylinder in a strip of lead on impact. The adult rats with air-filled lungs died instantly and examination of their lungs revealed extensive damage. The fetuses, however, who were delivered surgically after calculated decelerations of up to 10 000 g, survived and developed normally. Sass et al. (1972) found that pulmonary atelectasis, arterio-venous shunting, and downward displacement of the heart did not occur in dogs who were ventilated mechanically with oxygenated fluorocarbon liquid and subjected to inertial forces on a centrifuge.

Observations in man

Gas exchange. It is now possible to 'ventilate' one lung of man with saline while the other lung is ventilated with oxygen. Such a procedure is occasionally used to treat patients with various diseases of the lung (Ramirez 1966; Kylstra et al. 1971; Rogers, Braunstein & Shuman 1972). During lavages of the lung of a patient with alveolar proteinosis and of a healthy volunteer, the partial pressures of oxygen and carbon dioxide in end-tidal liquid were found to remain virtually unchanged, as the time between the beginning of infusion to the end of drainage of a tidal volume increased from less than 30 to more than 200 sec, while the arterial and mixed venous oxygen and carbon dioxide partial pressures remained essentially the same. This suggests that diffusive gas tension equilibrium between alveolar capillary blood and alveolar contents was established within 30 sec in these saline-filled human lungs (Kylstra et al. 1973). The computed difference between the mean end-capillary and alveolar carbon dioxide partial pressures was, on the average, less than 1 mm Hg in the 28-year-old patient with alveolar proteinosis but 9 mm Hg in the 40-year-old volunteer.

Ventilation. In an anesthetized volunteer, the maximum expiratory flow of saline from the left lung was measured by applying and gradually increasing suction at the outflow tube until the rate of flow of saline ceased to increase. The minimum time required to remove 500 ml saline, starting from a lung volume of 2000 ml, was

9·4 sec. The computed total lung capacity (TLC) of the left lung ($0.45 \times$ TLC of both lungs measured the day before the experiment) was 2900 ml. Assuming that the time required for inspiration would be equal to the time required for expiration, and assuming an equal maximal expiratory flow rate for both lungs, the maximum minute ventilation of this man, if he were breathing saline, would be 3·2 L, at a tidal volume of 1 L and with expirations starting at 70% of TLC. In the patient with alveolar proteinosis, 500 ml saline was drained from the left lung in 7 sec, starting at TLC. Making the same assumptions as before, the maximum minute volume of ventilation in this patient, if he were to breathe saline, would be 4·2 L, at a tidal volume of 1 L and with expiration starting from TLC.

Recovery. In general, patients tolerate the complete filling and subsequent 'ventilation' of one lung at a time, with a physiological salt solution at normal body temperature, remarkably well. Following a lavage, the patients generally receive supplemental oxygen by mask for several hours but by the next day they are usually up and around again. Chest X-rays taken shortly after a lung lavage show a diffuse opacification of the washed lung, but the lung is clear again after 24 hours. Serial pulmonary function tests following lavage of a lung of a healthy volunteer revealed a decrease in the vital capacity, timed vital capacity, and total lung capacity, but these parameters returned to pre-lavage control levels in 72 hours and remained at these levels during the following 2 years. Static pressure–volume relationships of the left lung and chest of the anesthetized and curarized volunteer revealed a considerable decrease in compliance immediately following lavage, as compared to the measurements made just before the lavage. This was attributed primarily to a diminished volume of air in the lung, caused by the presence of residual saline, and to the surface tension at the interface between residual liquid and air (Kylstra et al. 1971).

Loss of surfactant. Kylstra and his colleagues (1971) studied the surface tension of the lavage effluent from the lungs of a normal volunteer and 4 patients with asthma. They found minimal surface tensions well in excess of 12 dynes/cm.

Rogers and Sonne (1970) examined the effluent from the lungs of 10 patients. They collected the effluent serially in 1500 ml bottles and centrifuged a 500 ml sample of each bottle. The centrifugate was resuspended in 40 ml of saline and placed in a modified Wilhelmi balance. A minimum surface tension below 13 dynes/cm was found in at least 1 bottle of the lavage effluent of each patient, and in 2 of 5 bottles in 7 patients. When all of the effluent liquid was mixed in a large container and a 500 ml centrifuged sample was examined, the minimum surface tension was similar to the one reported by Kylstra et al. (1971). Rogers, Braunstein and Shuman (1972) also noted a shift in the pressure–volume curve of the lung downwards and to the right, immediately following a lavage. However, the pressure–volume curve returned to normal by 24 to 72 hours.

Subjective acceptability of liquid-filled lungs. Ramirez (1966) initially performed lung lavage in awake patients; only the larynx and trachea were anasthetized topically. Nevertheless, the patients tolerated the procedure. Kylstra (1968) reported that a healthy volunteer whose larynx and trachea had been anesthetized to facilitate intubation, but who otherwise received no medication, did not experience unacceptably unpleasant sensations arising from the flow of saline into and out of his lungs or from the presence of residual liquid in his lung after the lavage.

The problem of carbon dioxide elimination and oxygen toxicity

In all but one of the thus far reported series of experiments with saline- or fluorocarbon-breathing animals, the elimination of carbon dioxide through the liquid-filled lungs was found to be inadequate, in spite of the fact that the animals were anesthetized. Clearly, this would seem to preclude a practical application of liquid breathing since a diver, in order to perform useful work, should be able to increase his carbon dioxide production well above resting levels without experiencing a sense of suffocation, or worse, losing consciousness, as a result of an increase in the carbon dioxide partial pressure in his blood.

The elimination of carbon dioxide through liquid-filled lungs ($\dot{V}_{CO_2}$) depends upon the solubility of carbon dioxide in the alveolar liquid

(αCO_2), the partial pressure of carbon dioxide in the arterial blood (Pa_{CO_2}) and the effective alveolar ventilation ($\dot{V}A^e$), which may be defined as the virtual volume of exhaled liquid in which the partial pressure of carbon dioxide is the same as in the arterial blood, or more conventionally, as the difference between the minute volume of ventilation ($\dot{V}E$) and the dead space ventilation ($\dot{V}D$). Thus, under steady state conditions, i.e. when the production of carbon dioxide in the tissues equals the elimination of this gas through the lungs, and assuming that the inspired liquid contains no carbon dioxide:

$$Pa_{CO2} = \frac{\dot{V}CO_2}{\dot{V}A^e . \alpha CO_2}$$

where the units of $\dot{V}CO_2$, Pa_{CO_2}, αCO_2 and $\dot{V}A^e$ are milliliters (STPD) per minute, millimeters of mercury, milliliters (STPD) per milliliter and millimeter of mercury, and milliliters per minute, respectively. If CO_2 elimination in liquid-filled lungs is inadequate, as evidenced by a greater than normal Pa_{CO_2}, either $\dot{V}A^e$ or αCO_2 or both must be deficient and should be increased.

The maximum expiratory flow of either gas or liquid is dependent upon the recoil of the lung and limited by dynamic compression of the airways (Mead et al. 1967). Therefore, the maximum expiratory flow cannot be increased by mechanical assistance, i.e. by artificially applying a greater than normal difference in pressure between the alveoli and the mouth. However, the inspiratory flow is not limited by dynamic airway compression, so that, theoretically, the inspiratory flow should continue to increase as the difference between the pressure in the alveoli and at the mouth increases. Interestingly, the inspiratory flow in spontaneously saline-breathing dogs was about twice as great as the expiratory flow (Kylstra & Tissing 1964). As a result, the minute volume of ventilation was 33% greater than would have been the case if inspiration and expiration had lasted equally long. As discussed earlier, measurements of the flow of saline from the left lung of a 40-year-old healthy volunteer would indicate a maximum minute volume of 3·2 L saline, at a tidal volume of 1 L starting at 70% of TLC, if the duration of inspiration and expiration were equal. By doubling the inspiratory flow

rate, as did the saline-breathing dog, the volunteer's maximum minute volume of saline ventilation could be increased to 4·3 L. Likewise, the maximum minute volume of ventilation in the 28-year-old patient with alveolar proteinosis, if he were breathing saline, could be 5·6 L instead of 4·2 L at a tidal volume of 1 L with expirations starting from TLC.

The addition of THAM to the inspired salt solution effectively increases αCO_2. It markedly prolonged survival of liquid-breathing mice (Kylstra, Tissing & van der Mäen 1962) and minimized respiratory acidosis in liquid-breathing rats (Pegg, Horner & Wahrenbrock 1963). In order to quantitatively evaluate the increase in αCO_2 caused by the addition of THAM to a saline breathing fluid, an isotonic 0·3 molar THAM solution, titrated to pH 7·4, was equilibrated, at 37°C, with various gas mixtures containing carbon dioxide at partial pressures ranging from 7 to 70 mm Hg. The carbon dioxide content of the gas-equilibrated THAM solution, determined by the method of Van Slyke, was approximately 390 ml (STPD) per liter. In contrast, 1 L of saline under these conditions contains only 29 ml (STPD) of CO_2; 1 L of FC–80 fluorocarbon liquid 84 ml (STPD) of CO_2 (Schoenfisch & Kylstra 1973).

The maximum effective alveolar ventilation in a liquid-breathing man will always be less than his maximum volume of ventilation. How much less depends upon the size of the anatomical dead space, the respiratory frequency, the distribution of the flow of inhaled liquid and blood in the lung, and the presence or absence of partial gas pressure gradients within the liquid-filled gas exchange units of the lung. As mentioned earlier, diffusive mixing of the liquid-filled gas exchange units of the human lung appears to be complete within 30 sec so that partial gas pressure gradients in the gas exchange units of the lung should not be a problem as long as the respiratory frequency does not exceed two breaths per minute. In addition, there was no evidence of a gross imbalance between the flows of inspired liquid and blood in saline-filled human lungs (Kylstra et al. 1973). This is in good agreement with observations in the excised lungs of dogs (West et al. 1965). It seems, therefore, reasonable to conclude that, at a respiratory frequency of two or three breaths per minute, the physiological dead space in liquid-breathing men would not be much greater than the anatomical dead space. Thus, the maximum effective alveolar ventilation of a saline-breathing diver, conservatively, may be estimated at approximately 3 L/min.

If a man were to breathe an isotonic 0·3 molar THAM solution titrated to pH 7·4, at an effective alveolar ventilation of 3 L/min, then he would be able to eliminate $3 \times 390 = 1170$ ml (STPD) of carbon dioxide per minute at an arterial carbon dioxide partial pressure of 40 mm Hg, and he would thus be able to perform work which requires an oxygen uptake of 1462 ml (STPD) per minute, assuming that $R = 0·8$. However, the solubility of oxygen in a 0·3 molar THAM solution is no greater than in saline (0·0299 ml/L/mm Hg at 37°C), so that a partial pressure of 16 300 mm Hg or 21·45 ATS of oxygen, at least, would be required in the inspired THAM solution to supply the 1462 ml of oxygen per minute. Such partial pressures of oxygen are prohibitively toxic. If the man were to breathe FX–80 fluorocarbon (assuming that his effective alveolar ventilation would be the same), his oxygen consumption, at a normal arterial carbon dioxide partial pressure, would be 315 ml (STPD) per minute. An inspired oxygen partial pressure of less than one atmosphere would suffice, but the oxygen uptake would only be enough to satisfy basal metabolic needs and leave no room for productive physical activity. In general, the carbon dioxide carrying capacity of THAM solutions would be adequate, but the solubility of oxygen in aqueous solutions is so low that prohibitively high partial pressures of inspired oxygen would be necessary. The solubility of oxygen in FX–80 fluorocarbon liquid (0·638 ml/L/mm Hg at 37°C) is high enough, but the solubility of carbon dioxide in FX–80 fluorocarbon liquid (2·105 ml/L/mm Hg at 37°C) is not, so that, even at complete rest in the water, a fluorocarbon-breathing diver would barely be able to maintain a normal arterial carbon dioxide partial pressure while breathing at his maximum ventilatory capacity.

A combination of the advantages of a fluorocarbon liquid and THAM might be a practical solution. Fluorocarbon liquids do not mix with water. However, it is now possible to make stable emulsions of fluorocarbon liquid droplets in aqueous solutions with the aid of suitable emulsifiers (Pluronics). Such emulsions have already been prepared in a number of laboratories to be used as a blood substitute in which the fluorocarbon liquid droplets would function as red blood cells, carrying oxygen from the lungs to the tissues. On calculation of the maximum possible uptake of oxygen through the lungs of a diver who would be breathing an emulsion of 30% (by volume) of FX–80 fluorocarbon liquid in an isotonic 0·3 molar THAM solution at pH 7·4, assuming again an effective alveolar ventilation of 3 L/min, it turns out that, at an arterial carbon dioxide partial pressure of 40 mm Hg, he would be able to eliminate $3 \times [(0·7 \times 390) + (0·3 \times 40 \times 2·105)] = 895$ ml (STPD) of carbon dioxide per minute. At a normal respiratory gas exchange ratio of 0·8, this diver's oxygen uptake, at a normal arterial carbon dioxide partial pressure, would thus be 1118 ml (STPD)/min. To supply this amount of oxygen each minute, the partial pressure of oxygen in the inhaled emulsion should be at least $1118/3 \times [(0·7 \times 0·0299) + (0·3 \times 0·638)] = 1755$ mm Hg, i.e. less than 3 ATS. Such an inspired oxygen partial pressure is acceptable since the mean arterial oxygen partial pressure would be appreciably lower.

ARTIFICIAL GILLS

An artificial gill is a device for the exchange of gases, by means of simple diffusion across a semipermeable membrane, between a free-swimming diver and the surrounding water.

Ideally, the membrane to be used in an artificial gill should be permeable to oxygen and carbon dioxide but impermeable to all other substances. Unfortunately, such a membrane does not exist. One can choose from three classes of semipermeable membrane. One type, such as Cellophane, has micropores. The size and surface charge of the pores determine which solutes will pass and which ones are held back. Other membranes are homogenous films and their selective permeability depends on differences between solubility and diffusion coefficients of various solutes in the film. Selectivity is based on the fact that net transfer of one molecular species along a concentration gradient within the membrane occurs at a different rate from the diffusion of another molecular species. If no concentration gradient across the membrane exists, or if the substance is insoluble in the membrane, no net transfer occurs. Several such synthetic membranes are commercially available and have been used in the construction of membrane oxygenators for medical purposes. A third category of membranes, known as 'millipore' membranes, can be used to separate a liquid from a gas phase. These membranes contain relatively large holes and are usually made of hydrophobic material. Surface tension can resist considerable hydrostatic pressure if the pores are small enough, so that no water enters a submerged air-filled container with hydrophobic millipore membrane walls. In essence, the membrane is a skeleton supporting a myriad of minute air–water interfaces. One example of a hydrophilic millipore membrane is wet woven cloth. A bubble of air trapped under the cloth is prevented by surface tension from escaping through the pores so that it can provide buoyancy for a swimmer in case of emergency.

Robb (1965) first demonstrated that mammals can exchange sufficient amounts of gas with an aqueous environment by diffusion through artificial homogeneous films. He managed to keep hamsters alive in a closed container with a silicone rubber membrane wall and completely submerged in bubble-oxygenated water. Oxygen consumed by the hamster lowered the oxygen partial pressure in the chamber and, because the oxygen tension in the water surrounding the container was much higher, oxygen diffused into the container at a rate determined by the metabolism of the hamster. Carbon dioxide produced by the animal raised the partial pressure of carbon dioxide in the closed chamber and, since the carbon dioxide partial pressure of the surrounding water was negligible, carbon dioxide diffused out through the membrane into the water.

Paganelli, Bateman and Rahn (1967) have analysed the transfer of gases into and out of a similar system using a millipore instead of silicone rubber membrane. Based on carefully measured gas fluxes at various rates of water flow along the membrane, they predict that it should be possible to keep a resting man submerged in a river for an indefinite period of time in a closed chamber with a millipore wall of 8 m², provided that the water flows along the membrane at a rate of 6 m.p.h. The oxygen partial pressure in the chamber would remain at 100 mm Hg. The total gas pressure in the chamber would be less than at the surface. Carbon dioxide elimination from the closed chamber atmosphere into the surrounding water is no problem since carbon dioxide is many times more soluble in water than oxygen.

The situation is much more complicated in an artificial gill in which, regardless of depth, the pressure must be the same as in the ambient water. One can conceive of two categories of artificial gills: one, a gas-filled gill, in which air exhaled by the diver exchanges oxygen and carbon dioxide with seawater before being re-inhaled and the other a blood-filled gill, which closely resembles the gill of fish and in which gas exchange occurs directly between the seawater and the diver's blood.

The gas-filled artificial gill

An artificial gill based on the principle of re-conditioning the exhaled air by diffusion exchange with seawater has been designed by Ayres (1966). Basically, this device is a self-contained underwater breathing apparatus incorporating a membrane gas exchanger and a source of compressed air for addition of gas to the system upon descent so as to prevent collapse of both the gill and the chest of the diver. Ayres describes a radiator-like device made of pairs of 18 inch square membranes, 1/1000 inch thick, defining 1/16 inch wide intercommunicating gas compartments alternating with 3/16 inch wide intercommunicating water compartments. A total of 48 units, stacked to a height of 12 inches, provides approximately 216 ft² of gas-permeable membrane exposed to water. Air exhaled by the diver traverses the gas compartments and flow of water through the 'gill slits' is caused by forward motion of the diver. In a photograph illustrating a newspaper report (Jones 1966), the inventor is sitting on the beach breathing into his device which is barely submerged in shallow water. Such a test is not very convincing and is not likely to reveal the inherent defect of this system, namely the in-evitable loss of inert gas into the surrounding water by outward diffusion through the membrane.

Membranes through which oxygen and carbon dioxide diffuse rapidly are also permeable to nitrogen (Simril & Hershberger 1950; Robb 1965). The partial pressure of inert gas in seawater is no greater than in the atmosphere at the surface. The partial inert gas pressure in a gas-filled artificial gill is always higher when the gas is compressed by the weight of a column of water above. If the membrane is not completely impermeable to inert gas, outward diffusion will occur along the gradient created by the hydrostatic pressure. Inert gas tension gradients across the gill membrane increase linearly with depth, and so will the loss of inert gas into the surrounding sea-water. Even at moderate depths, the loss of gas from the gill will require continuous addition of inert gas at a rate which is likely to be many times greater than the rate at which the diver consumes oxygen. Thus, paradoxically, in order to economize on oxygen, a diver would have to carry a far greater supply of inert gas. Even if a membrane which is completely impermeable to inert gas were available, the diver would continue to lose gas through his skin and the gill would eventually collapse if not refilled.

The blood-filled artificial gill

No blood-filled artificial gill has yet been designed and tested experimentally, but the successful use in medicine and surgery of artificial kidneys and heart–lung machines clearly suggests such a possibility. Silicone rubber, which can be made in sheets of only 1/1000 inch thick (Robb 1965), would seem to be by far the most suitable membrane available to date for the construction of such an artificial gill. It is beyond the scope of this book to discuss the medical problems involved in the use of extracorporeal blood oxy-genators and the technical problems encountered in the construction of a membrane oxygenator with a large membrane area. It is appropriate, however, to point out that most of the cardiac output should pass through the gill. Hemoglobin is almost completely saturated with oxygen at a partial oxygen pressure of approximately 100 mm Hg, which means that an additional pressure of, at best, 50 mm Hg, can add only negligible quantities of oxygen to the blood. If only part of the blood ejected by the heart of the diver passes through the artificial gill and a substantial fraction of his cardiac output by-passes the gas exchange area, oxygenated blood return-ing from the artificial gill will mix with oxygen-depleted venous blood by-passing the gill. This would result in a substantial drop in the oxygen partial pressure in the mixed arterial blood. In order to avoid venous admixture, it would be preferable to connect the gill with the main pulmonary artery. Even if it were possible for a surgeon to establish such a connection which would remain patent and would not restrict a diver in his activities underwater, the operation might condemn him to live the rest of his life underwater. Furthermore, carbon dioxide is approximately 25 times more soluble in water than oxygen and permeates more than 5 times as readily through silicone rubber than oxygen (Robb 1965). It can be shown that a diver who wants to maintain an arterial oxygen tension of 100 mm Hg by gas exchange with the ocean through a blood-filled silicone rubber gill must be prepared to take an arterial carbon dioxide ten-sion of less than 10 mm Hg for granted. Un-fortunately, such low arterial carbon dioxide tensions are not compatible with the require-ments of acid–base balance in man. A detailed discussion of this topic is beyond the scope of this chapter, but the reader is urged to consult the important theoretical analysis of aquatic gas exchange by Rahn (1966).

REFERENCES

AYRES, W. A. (1966) *Gill-type Underwater Breathing Equipment and Methods for Reoxygenating Exhaled Breath.* U.S. Patent No. 3,288,394, Jan. 11.

BLENKARN, G. D. & HAYES, J. (1970) Bilateral lung lavage with hyperbarically oxygenated saline in dogs. *J. appl. Physiol.* **29**, 786–793.

BROUARDEL, P. & LOYE, P. (1889) Recherches sur la circulation pendant l'asphyxie par submersion et sur le sang des noyés. *Archs Physiol. norm. path.* **5**, 449–459.

CLARK, L. C. & GOLLAN, F. (1966) Survival of mammals breathing organic liquids equilibrated with oxygen at atmospheric pressure. *Science, N.Y.* **152**, 1755–1756.

EDWARDS, W. F. (1824) *De l'Influence des Agents Physiques sur la Vie.* Paris: Crochard.

FAZEKAS, J. F., ALEXANDER, F. A. D. & HIMWICH, H. E. (1941) Tolerance of newborn to anoxia. *Am. J. Physiol.* **134**, 281–287.

GLASS, H. G., SNYDER, F. F. & WEBSTER, E. (1944) Rate of decline in resistance to anoxia of rabbits, dogs and guinea pigs from onset of viability to adult life. *Am. J. Physiol.* **140**, 609–615.

GOLLAN, F. & CLARK, L. C. (1967) Prevention of bends by breathing an organic liquid. *Trans. Ass. Am. Physns* **29**, 102–109.

HAMOSH, P. & LUCHSINGER, P. C. (1968) Maximum expiratory flow in isolated liquid filled lungs. *J. appl. Physiol.* **25**, 485–488.

HIMWICH, H. E., BERSTEIN, A. O., HERRLICH, H., CHESLER, A. O. & FAZEKAS, J. F. (1942) Mechanisms for maintenance of life in newborn during anoxia. *Am. J. Physiol.* **135**, 387–391.

JONES, S. V. (1966) Fish-like gills are designed for swimmers. *The New York Times*, Jan. 15.

KYLSTRA, J. A. (1968) Experiments in water breathing. *Scient. Am.* **219**, 66–74.

KYLSTRA, J. A. & SCHOENFISCH, W. H. (1972) Alveolar surface tension in fluorocarbon filled lungs. *J. appl. Physiol.* **33**, 32–35.

KYLSTRA, J. A. & TISSING, M. O. (1964) Fluid breathing. In *Clinical Application of Hyperbaric Oxygen.* Ed. I. Boerema, W. H. Brummelkamp & N. G. Meyne. pp. 371–379. Amsterdam: Elsevier Publishing Co.

KYLSTRA, J. A., PAGANELLI, C. V. & LANPHIER, E. H. (1966) Pulmonary gas exchange in dogs ventilated with hyperbarically oxygenated liquid. *J. appl. Physiol.* **21**, 177–184.

KYLSTRA, J. A., TISSING, M. O. & van der MÄEN, A. (1962) Of mice as fish. *Trans. Am. Soc. artif. internal Organs* **8**, 378–383.

KYLSTRA, J. A., RAUSCH, D. C., HALL, K. D. & SPOCK, A. (1971) Volume-controlled lung lavage in the treatment of asthma, bronchiectasis and mucoviscidosis. *Am. Rev. resp. Dis.* **103**, 651–665.

KYLSTRA, J. A., SCHOENFISCH, W. H., HERRON, J. M. & BLENKARN, G. D. (1973) Gas exchange in saline filled lungs of man. *J. appl. Physiol.* **35**, 136–142.

KYLSTRA, J. A., NANTZ, R., CROWE, J., WAGNER, W. & SALTZMAN, H. A. (1967) Hydraulic compression of mice to 166 atmospheres. *Science, N.Y.* **158**, 793–794.

LEITH, D. E. & MEAD, J. (1966) Maximum expiratory flow in liquid-filled lungs. *Fedn Proc. Fedn Am. Socs exp. Biol.* **25**, 506.

LUNDGREN, C. E. G. & ÖRNHAGEN, H. C. (1972) Oxygen consumption in liquid breathing mice. *Aerospace Med.* **43**, 831–835.

MARGARIA, R., GUALTIEROTTI, T. & SPINELLI, D. (1958) Protection against acceleration forces in animals by immersion in water. *J. Aviat. Med.* **29**, 433–437.

MEAD, J., TURNER, J. M., MACKLEM, P. T. & LITTLE, J. B. (1967) Significance of the relationship between lung recoil and maximum expiratory flow. *J. appl. Physiol.* **22**, 95–108.

MODELL, J. H., NEWBY, E. J. & RUIZ, B. C. (1970) Long term survival of dogs after breathing oxygenated fluorocarbon liquid. *Fedn Proc. Fedn Am. Socs exp. Biol.* **29**, 1731–1736.

MODELL, J. H., HOOD, C. I., KUCK, E. J. & RUIZ, B. C. (1971) Oxygenation by ventilation with fluorocarbon liquid (FX–80). *Anesthesiology* **34**, 312–320.

ÖRNHAGEN, H. C. & LUNDGREN, C. E. G. (1975) Hydrostatic pressure tolerance in liquid breathing mice. In *Underwater Physiology. Vth Symp. Underwater Physiology* (1972). Ed. C. J. Lambertsen. Bethesda: Fedn Am. Socs exp. Biol.

PAGANELLI, C. V., BATEMAN, N. & RAHN, H. (1967) Artificial gills for gas exchange in water. In *Underwater Physiology. Proc. 3rd Symp. Underwater Physiology.* Ed. C. J. Lambertsen. pp. 452–468. Baltimore: Williams & Wilkins.

PEGG, J. H., HORNER, T. L. & WAHRENBROCK, E. A. (1963) Breathing of pressure-oxygenated liquids. In *Proc. 2nd Symp. Underwater Physiology*, pp. 166–170. Washington, D.C.: Natl Acad. Sci.-Natl Res. Council. (Publ. 1181.)

RAHN, H. (1966) Aquatic gas exchange: theory. *Resp. Physiol.* **1**, 1–12.

RAMIREZ, R. J. (1967) Pulmonary alveolar proteinosis. Treatment by massive bronchopulmonary lavage. *Archs intern. Med.* **119**, 147–156.

ROBB, W. L. (1965) *Thin Silicone Membranes. Their Permeation Properties and some Applications.* General Electric Co. Tech. Information Series. Report No. 65–C–031, October.

ROGERS, R. M. & SONNE, J. E. (1970) Demonstration of surface active material in human lung lavage effluent. *Clin. Res.* **18**, 490.

ROGERS, R. M., BRAUNSTEIN, M. S. & SHUMAN, J. F. (1972) Role of bronchopulmonary lavage in the treatment of respiratory failure. *Chest* **62**, 95S–104S.

SAGA, S., MODELL, J. H., CALDERWOOD, H. W., LUCAS, A. J., THAM, M. K. & SWENSON, E. W. (1973) Pulmonary function after ventilation with fluorocarbon liquid P–12F (Caroxin-F). *J. appl. Physiol.* **34**, 160–164.

SASS, D. J., RITMAN, E. L., CASKEY, P. E., BANCHERO, N. & WOOD, E. H. (1972) Liquid breathing: prevention of pulmonary arterial-venous shunting during acceleration. *J. appl. Physiol.* **32**, 451–455.

SCHOENFISCH, W. H. & KYLSTRA, J. A. (1973) Maximum expiratory flow and estimated CO_2 elimination in liquid ventilated dogs' lungs. *J. appl. Physiol.* **35**, 117–121.

SIMRIL, V. L. & HERSHBERGER, A. (1950) Permeability of polymeric films to gases. *Mod. Plast.* **27**, 95–102.

SWANN, H. G., BRUCER, M., MOORE, C. & VEZIEN, B. L. (1947) Fresh water and sea water drowning: study of terminal cardiac and biochemical events. *Tex. Rep. Biol. Med.* **5**, 423–437.

WEST, J. B., MALONEY, J. E. & CASTLE, B. L. (1972) Effect of stratified inequality of blood flow on gas exchange in liquid-filled lungs. *J. appl. Physiol.* **32**, 357–361.

WEST, J. B., DOLLERY, C. T., MATTHEWS, C. M. E. & ZARDINI, P. (1965) Distribution of blood flow and ventilation in saline-filled lung. *J. appl. Physiol.* **20**, 1107–1117.

10

Oxygen Toxicity

J. D. WOOD

The toxic effects of oxygen at high pressure (OHP) were first reported by Bert (1878). In his classic work *La Pression Barometrique* he describes in detail the incidence of convulsions in various animal species exposed to OHP. Another pioneer in the field of oxygen toxicity was J. L. Smith (1899) who carried out the first extensive investigation on OHP-induced pulmonary pathology. Later workers confirmed and amplified the findings of the early investigators and the reader is referred to the review articles by Stadie, Riggs and Haugaard (1944) and Bean (1945) for detailed accounts of the studies up to the early 1940s. Reviews encompassing more recent studies are available in the excellent and comprehensive articles by Clark and Lambertsen (1971b) on pulmonary toxicity and by Haugaard (1968) on the cellular mechanisms of oxygen toxicity. The present chapter will cover the more significant findings of the early period but the emphasis will be placed on recent advances.

EFFECT OF OHP ON THE LUNGS

Most of the investigations on pulmonary pathology have been carried out within the range 0·7 to 3·0 ATA oxygen since at pressures less than 0·7 ATA oxygen the damage occurs very slowly if at all, and at greater than 3 ATA oxygen (66 ft) there is the overshadowing onset of convulsions. The overt sign of lung damage in animals exposed to OHP is the occurrence of marked dyspnoea (Hill 1912; Gesell 1923; Binger, Faulkner & Moore 1927; Paine, Keys & Lynn 1941). Examina-

tion of the lungs shows pulmonary damage consisting of extensive areas of haemorrhage and oedema (Hill 1912; Karsner 1916; Karsner & Ash 1916–17; Shilling & Adams 1933), hyaline membrane formation (Bruns & Shields 1954; Van Breeman, Neustein & Bruns 1957; Cedergren, Gyllensten & Wersall 1959), epithelial degeneration (Karsner 1916; Kaplan et al. 1969), proliferative changes in alveolar epithelial cells (Kapanci et al. 1969), thickening and hyalinization of the walls of the pulmonary arteries (Smith et al. 1932; Kydd 1967) and atelectasis (Behnke et al. 1934; Penrod 1956; Cedergren, Gyllensten & Wersall 1959; Van Den Brenk & Jamieson 1962). Pathological changes at the subcellular level have also been reported. Exposure of rats to 3·0 or 4·0 ATA oxygen for up to 6 hours produces loss of matrical density and vacuolization, swelling and rupture of mitochondria in alveolar and endothelial cells (Nasseri, Bucherl & Wolff 1967; Rosenbaum, Wittner & Lenger 1969). An increase in free ribosomes and dilation of the cisternae of the endoplasmic reticulum also occurs.

OHP-induced lung damage can be divided into two overlapping phases of progressive degeneration (Kaplan 1969; Clark & Lambertsen 1971b), an acute exudative phase involving alveolar oedema, intra-alveolar haemorrhage, fibrinous exudate, hyaline membrane formation and destruction of endothelial and type I alveolar epithelial cells, and a subacute proliferative phase involving interstitial fibrosis, fibroblastic proliferation and hyperplasia of type II alveolar epithelial cells. The acute exudative changes are completely reversible whereas the proliferative changes are more slowly reversible and may result in permanent scarring of the lung (Kapanci et al. 1969; Kaplan et al. 1969).

Human studies

The detailed examination of the lungs is precluded in human studies for obvious reasons but post-mortem examination of patients dying after prolonged oxygen therapy suggests that overlapping exudative and proliferative phases of pathology also occur in man (Nash, Blennerhassett & Pontoppidan 1967). Various investigations involving the exposure of man to OHP have also indicated that lung damage occurs (Welch, Morgan & Clamann 1963). The dominant symptom is usually described as substernal distress and the time to onset of the symptom varies inversely with the partial pressure of oxygen (Fig. 10.1).

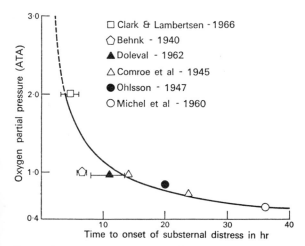

FIG. 10.1. Time to onset of pulmonary symptoms of oxygen toxicity in man

At 1 ATA oxygen the latent period is approximately 12 hours although a large individual variation is present and there has been a report (Behnke 1940) of substernal distress occurring after only 6 to 7 hours at 1 ATA oxygen.

Clark and Lambertsen (1966, 1971a) found that pulmonary irritation became detectable after 3 to 6 hours at 2 ATA (33 ft) oxygen. They describe the course of events as follows: 'Symptoms began as a mild carinal irritation with occasional cough, intensified slowly to about 8 hours, then rapidly

until the bronchial tree was painfully outlined and each inspiration was distressful, with dyspnea and uncontrollable coughing at rest.' A rapid improvement with respect to bronchitis and cough was observed within 4 hours after exposure. Although discernible irritation took some hours to develop the vital capacity began to decrease almost immediately, reaching a significant 9% decrease below normal by 8 hours. In most cases the vital capacity continued to fall for 2 to 4 hours after exposure and return to normal levels required up to 12 days. Similar exposure conditions also produce decreases in lung compliance (Fisher et al. 1968), and although the latter changes probably contribute to the reduction of vital capacity they are too small to be considered the sole cause.

The demonstrated sensitivity of vital capacity to 2 ATA (33 ft) oxygen, together with the report by Comroe et al. (1945) that the vital capacity in man is decreased by breathing 0·5 to 1·0 ATA oxygen for 24 hours, suggests that this measurement may be used as a sensitive indicator of the state of the lungs in man during exposure to OHP.

POSSIBLE MECHANISMS INVOLVED IN THE PRODUCTION OF LUNG DAMAGE

Despite the detailed documentation of OHP-induced pulmonary pathology, progress towards the delineation of the mechanisms involved has been slow. It appears that the syndrome of pulmonary oxygen poisoning consists of multiple interacting factors which include both a direct action of oxygen on lung tissue and an indirect action involving neural and hormonal factors. The various factors which may be involved in the pathogenesis will now be discussed.

Direct action of oxygen

The direct action of oxygen on lung tissue has been demonstrated in experiments where only one lung of an intact animal is exposed to increased oxygen pressure, the remaining lung being ventilated with nitrogen, helium or air. Only the lung exposed to OHP shows extensive gross and microscopic damage (Penrod 1958) and a smaller reduction in surfactant activity is observed in air-exposed lungs when the opposite lung is ventilated with oxygen (Motlagh et al. 1969). The quantitative importance of this direct action of oxygen, as opposed to that involving neural and hormonal mechanisms remains to be ascertained.

Neural and hormonal factors

Neural and hormonal factors are involved in the aetiology of both the 'slow developing' lung pathology observed at pressures less than 2 to 3 ATA oxygen and the 'fast developing' pathology associated with the onset of seizures at pressures greater than 2 to 3 ATA oxygen. In both cases a hypophyseal–adrenocortical involvement is indicated by the protective effect of hypophysectomy (Bean 1952; Bean & Johnson 1952; Bean & Smith 1953) and adrenalectomy (Gerschman et al. 1954; Bean & Johnson 1955; Smith & Bean 1955a; Taylor 1958) and by the enhancement of the pulmonary pathology following the administration of cortisone and related substances (Warshaw, Malomut & Spain 1952; Gerschman et al. 1954; Smith & Bean 1955a; Taylor 1958; Buckingham & Sommers 1960. Likewise a sympatho-adrenomedullary involvement in both types of lung damage is indicated by the enhancement of OHP-induced pulmonary damage following the administration of epinephrine (Bean, Johnson & Smith 1954; Bean & Johnson 1955; Smith & Bean 1955a). A protective effect of adrenal demedullation (Gerschman et al. 1955) and adrenergic blocking drugs (Johnson & Bean 1957) was also observed with respect to the fast developing lung pathology.

The question remains to be answered as to whether there is a relationship between fast developing pulmonary damage and CNS damage. It is perhaps significant that this type of lung damage occurs only in animals that have convulsed (Johnson & Bean 1957; Wood, Stacey & Watson 1965) and that similar lung damage occurs in animals after seizures induced by thiosemicarbazide (Tennekoon 1954) and pentamethylenetetrazol (Riechert 1941). Moreover, in keeping with the results obtained with OHP, anaesthetic agents protect against both seizures and lung damage induced by the chemical agents whereas sympatholytic agents protect against only

pulmonary pathology (Bean, Zee & Thom 1966). These observations lead Bean and his colleagues to suggest that pulmonary damage by OHP is not only secondary to the occurrence of seizures but also that this pulmonary involvement may be attributed in large part to the attendant autonomic reaction, i.e. the neuro-endocrinogenic component of the seizure.

There is insufficient evidence available at the present time to establish whether the fast developing lung damage is caused by an acceleration of the processes involved in the slow developing lung damage at lower pressures, or whether it is brought about by an entirely different mechanism. The involvement of hypophyseal–adrenocortical and sympatho-adrenomedullary factors in both pathologies does, however, suggest a similar mechanism. It is also significant in this regard that microscopic examination of the two types of lung damage reveals little qualitative difference between the two (Karsner 1916; Van Den Brenk & Jamieson 1962).

Lung surfactant

The role of surface active material in the aetiology of OHP-induced lung damage has received increasing attention in recent years. Alveoli have a natural tendency to collapse because of their physical properties but this collapse is prevented by a lining of lipoprotein material, about 50 Å thick, which lowers the surface tension of the lungs thereby stabilizing the alveoli and ensuring normal functioning of respiration (Pattle 1955, 1965). The low surface tension also prevents transudation from the capillaries which would otherwise occur (Pattle & Thomas 1961). The surface active portion of the lipoprotein material is believed to be the phospholipid, dipalmityl lecithin (Brown 1964). It follows from the above that if for any reason the amount of lung surfactant is decreased, the resulting rise in alveolar surface tension might be expected to bring about collapse of the alveoli and transudation. Since atelectasis and oedema are major signs of oxygen poisoning several workers have investigated the effect of OHP on the lung surfactant in order to evaluate the possible role of the substance in the development of OHP-induced lung pathology. A selection from the

TABLE 10.1
Effect of OHP on lung surfactant

Species	Exposure to OHP	Effect on surface tension of lung extracts*	Reference
Mouse	0·9 ATA, 5–7 days	increase	Adamson, Bowden & Wyatt (1970)
	1 ATA, 4½ days	none	Pattle & Burgess (1961)
Rat	1 ATA, 5 days	none	Giammona, Kerner & Bondurant (1965)
	2 ATA, 17–18 hours	increase	Kennedy (1966)
	4 ATA, 6 hours	increase	Webb et al. (1966)
	8 ATA, 20–45 min	none	Bondurant & Smith (1962)
Guinea pig	1 ATA, 4 days	none	Fujiwara, Adams & Seto (1964)
	4 ATA, 1–4 hours	none	Ishizuka (1966)
	4 ATA, 6 hours	increase	Webb et al. (1966)
Rabbit	1 ATA, 3 days	increase	Giammona, Kerner & Bondurant (1965)
	1 ATA, 3–4 days	increase	Collier (1963)
	3 ATA, 1–5 hours	none	McSherry & Gilder (1970)
Cat	1 ATA, 3½ days	increase	Giammona, Kerner & Bondurant (1965)
Dog	0·7 ATA, 44–52 hours†	increase	Morgan et al. (1965)
	0·7 ATA, 44–52 hours‡	none	Morgan et al. (1965)
	1 ATA, 69 hours	increase	Caldwell et al. (1963)
	2 ATA, 23 hours	increase	Ishizuka et al. (1970)
	4 ATA, 1–5 hours	none	Ishizuka (1966)

* An increase in surface tension is taken as an indication of a decrease in lung surfactant.
† Lung oedema observed.
‡ No lung oedema observed.

results published on this topic is presented in Table 10.1.

It is readily apparent that many of the results are contradictory and that the overall situation is confusing, yet a sufficient number of investigators have reported decreased amounts of surfactant to make this phenomenon 'reasonably well established'. The wide spectrum of exposures used in the experiments and the variety of experimental techniques used to extract the surfactant probably contribute to the observed inconsistencies. The difficulties encountered in equating results obtained using different surfactant extraction procedures is well illustrated in the reports of Bondurant and Miller (1962) and Morgan, Finley and Fialkow (1965).

In view of the equivocal nature of the surface tension findings it would be presumptuous to say much about the cause of the decrease in surfactant. Rather speculative hypotheses have been put forward attributing the decrease to OHP-induced changes in structures believed responsible for the synthesis of the surfactant, such as alve-

olar cell mitochondria (Giammona, Kerner & Bondurant 1965) and the lamellar bodies of alveolar epithelial cells (Morgan et al. 1965). On the other hand oedema and atelectasis per se can cause decreases in the surface activity of lung extracts (Said et al. 1965; Levine & Johnson 1965). Thus, although current results suggest an association between OHP-induced changes in surfactant activity and lung damage, at least in animals exposed to hyperoxia until death from pulmonary intoxication, the precise causal relationship remains to be established.

Carbon dioxide

The possible implication of carbon dioxide in the aetiology of OHP-induced lung damage has been suggested by Ohlsson (1947) who observed that rabbits breathing 0·8 to 0·9 ATA oxygen survive only half as long as normal, 3 days as opposed to 6 days, if 3% carbon dioxide is added to the breathing mixture. Other workers were, however, unable to confirm this finding (Smith & Bean 1955b; De Clement & Smith 1962). On the other hand protection against OHP-induced lung pathology can be obtained by the prior administration of the intracellular buffer tris (hydroxymethyl) aminomethane (THAM), an action which has been attributed to the buffering action of THAM which results in a decreased $P\text{co}_2$ and an increased pH in the tissues and blood (Nahas 1965; Haugaard 1968). The role of carbon dioxide in the development of lung damage therefore remains uncertain.

Inert gases

The influence of inert gases on lung damage has not been studied extensively but it would appear that the absence of inert gas is not a major contributory factor in the development of OHP-induced lung pathology. McGavin et al. (1966) compared the toxic effect on rats of breathing 3 ATA oxygen, 3 ATA oxygen + 3 ATA nitrogen, and 3 ATA oxygen + 3 ATA helium respectively, and found that all lungs showed the usual congestion, oedema and atelectasis although the presence of an inert gas appeared to decrease the severity of the atelectasis.

EFFECT OF OHP ON BLOOD AND CIRCULATION

Although OHP-induced changes in circulatory regulation are less well defined and less dramatic than the effects on the lungs or the central nervous system, they nevertheless must be considered in any discussion on oxygen toxicity because of the secondary effects resulting from changes in the transport of blood gases. In general it is difficult to establish a circulatory effect in quantitative terms because the changes tend to be buffered by other influencing factors (Lambertsen 1965); but certain conclusions have been reached, based on the results of various studies.

The evidence for OHP-induced changes in blood pressure and pulse rate is equivocal. The majority of studies have indicated a slight decrease in either or both of these entities, in animals (Bert 1878; Bean 1929, 1931; Shaw, Behnke & Messer 1934; McBride, Vance & Ledingham 1970) and in man breathing oxygen at 1 ATA (Parkinson 1912; Dautrebrand & Haldane 1921; Behnke 1940) and at 3 to 4 ATA (Schwab, Fine & Mixter

1936; Lambertsen et al. 1953b). On the other hand, Behnke, Forbes and Motley (1935–36) report an increase in both pulse rate and blood pressure in man exposed to 3 to 4 ATA oxygen while Kety and Schmidt (1948) found a slight decrease in pulse rate but a significant increase in blood pressure in man exposed to 1 ATA oxygen.

The observed effects of OHP on blood flow are more consistent. Significant decreases occur in the blood flow of the coronary sinus (Meijne & Straub 1966; Podlesch & Herpfer 1970), coronary artery (Winter et al. 1970) and myocardium (McBride, Vance & Ledingham 1970) in dogs breathing 2 to 4 ATA oxygen. OHP-induced decreases in the regional blood flow of dogs occur at both 1 ATA oxygen (Bergovsky & Bertun 1966) and 4 ATA oxygen (Hahnloser et al. 1966). This effect was most marked in the brain, less so in the bowel and least obvious in the limb (Bergovsky & Bertun 1966). Convincing evidence has been obtained for a decreased cerebral blood flow in man exposed to OHP. Kety and Schmidt (1948) observed a 13% decrease in cerebral blood flow in men breathing 1 ATA oxygen which compares well with the results of Lambertsen et al. (1953a) indicating 13% and 25% decreases in cerebral blood flow in men breathing 1 ATA and 3·5 ATA oxygen respectively. The latter decreases were accompanied by 25% and 55% increases in cerebral vascular resistance which Lambertsen and his co-workers consider the cause of the below normal rates of blood flow. In keeping with these findings Saltzman et al. (1964) observed a 46% decrease in the size of retinal blood vessels in men within 5 min of exposure to 3 ATA oxygen. Since cerebral vasoconstriction does not occur during OHP breathing when the alveolar $P\text{co}_2$ is held constant (Turner et al. 1957), Lambertsen (1963) suggests that the cerebral vasoconstriction is not due to a direct effect of oxygen on the vessels but rather to the arterial hypocapnia that accompanies the respiratory stimulation produced by oxygen.

The transport of carbon dioxide from the tissues to the lungs is impaired under conditions of OHP (Gesell 1923). Normally all of the oxygen utilized by the tissues is derived from oxygen taken up by and released from haemoglobin. When animals or man breathe oxygen at greater than 3 ATA, however, the oxygen requirements of the tissues can be met by the oxygen dissolved in the blood and the haemoglobin remains in the oxidized state. Since fully oxygenated haemoglobin is a less effective buffer for the hydrogen ions of carbonic acid than is reduced haemoglobin, the transport of carbon dioxide, although still occurring, does so at higher than normal levels of P_{CO_2} and $[H^+]$ (Lambertsen 1965). Compounding the problem is the decreased amount of carbon dioxide transported in combination with reduced haemoglobin as the carbamino compound.

Under certain conditions OHP can produce damage to red blood cells in vivo but the quantitative importance of this phenomenon in healthy men exposed to OHP for only short periods of time remains dubious. Haemolysis occurs in vitamin E deficient mice, but not in vitamin E supplemented mice exposed to 3 ATA oxygen (Mengel et al. 1964). Although haemolysis was not observed in the blood of dogs exposed to 5 ATA oxygen for up to 3 hours, the erythrocytes from the exposed animals showed an increased osmotic fragility (Mengel et al. 1965; Zirkle et al. 1965a). There is one reported case of a human developing haemolytic anaemia following exposure for 26 min to 2 ATA oxygen (Mengel 1965) but in contrast no haemolysis was observed in divers exposed to 2·8 ATA oxygen for 90 min (Bradley & Vorosmarti 1968). Lipid peroxide formation has been suggested as a cause of OHP-induced haemolysis (Kahn et al. 1967) while other workers hypothesize that an accumulation of aminochrome derivatives plays a major role in the destruction of the red blood cells (Houlihan et al. 1970).

EFFECT OF OHP ON THE CENTRAL NERVOUS SYSTEM

Convulsions

The most dramatic manifestation of oxygen toxicity at pressures in excess of 2 to 3 ATA (33 to 66 ft) is the onset of convulsions (Bert 1878; Bean 1945). In animals the seizures take the form of generalized convulsions which are frequently, but not always, preceded by minor twitching of the head and forelimbs. Susceptibility to OHP-induced convulsions varies greatly from one species to another (Thompson 1889; Smith 1899; Shilling & Adams 1933), and cold-blooded animals in particular are more resistant than are warm-blooded animals.

Unfortunately man is not exempt from the convulsant action of OHP. Bornstein and Stroink (1912) observed muscle spasms in the legs after an exposure of 50 min, with exercise, to 3 ATA (66 ft) oxygen, and Thomson (1935) reports twitching of the lips and face in two men exposed to 4 ATA (100 ft) oxygen for 13 to 16 min. One of these subjects subsequently convulsed while still at 4 ATA but breathing air. Convulsions in man at 4 ATA (100 ft) oxygen have also been observed by Behnke and co-workers (Behnke et al. 1934–35; Behnke 1940) who liken the seizures to those seen in epilepsy. The findings of these early investigators have been amply confirmed and our current knowledge of the progressive symptoms of oxygen poisoning is most aptly expressed by Lambertsen (1965) who describes the course of events as follows: 'The convulsions are usually but not always preceded by the occurrence of localized muscular twitching, especially about the eyes, mouth and forehead. Small muscles of the hands may be involved and incoordination of diaphragm activity in respiration may occur. These phenomena increase in severity over a period which may vary from a few minutes to nearly an hour with essentially clear consciousness being retained. Eventually an abrupt spread of excitation occurs and the rigid tonic phase of the convulsion begins. The tonic phase lasts for about 30 sec and is accompanied by an abrupt loss of consciousness. Vigorous clonic contractions of the muscular groups of head and neck, trunk and limbs then occur becoming progressively less violent over about one minute.'

The electrical activity of the animal brain during OHP-induced seizures is well documented (Cohn & Gersh 1945; Sonnenschein & Stein 1953; Batini et al. 1954a, b; Stein 1955; Rucci, Giretti & LaRocca 1967, 1968), the pattern in the fully developed seizure being similar to that observed in grand mal epilepsy. A typical effect of OHP on cortical and subcortical electrical activities is shown in Fig. 10.2. Rucci, Giretti & LaRocca (1967) using unrestrained, unanaesthetized rats showed that seizures are usually preceded by

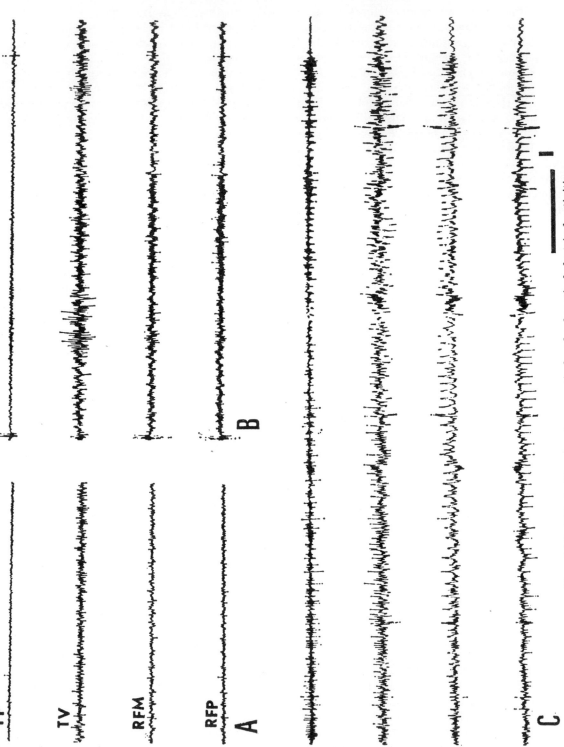

FIG. 10.2. Effect of hyperoxia on cortical and subcortical electrical activities

TF, transverse frontal lead; TV, unipolar record from right ventral nucleus of thalamus; RFM, unipolar record from left mesencephalic reticular formation; RFP, unipolar record from pontine reticular formation. A: Before hyperoxia; B: 20 min after beginning of hyperoxia (4 ATA); C: 23 min after beginning of hyperoxia, particularly evident in TV before the onset of frank seizure. Note spindle-like waves in the subcortical leads, particularly evident in TV before the onset of frank seizure. Calibrations: 6 sec and 150 μV. (Reproduced from Rucci, Giretti and LaRocca (1967) with permission of the publisher)

electrical activity, which is most evident in the subcortical centres, and which consists of increases in voltage and discharge rate and in spindle-like waves. The onset of the seizure is simultaneous in all cortical records, and the subcortical leads fire at the same time as those in the cortex. The cerebral cortex is not necessary for initiating and developing seizures since convulsions are observed in the decorticate rat. The cerebellum does not show pre-seizure activity and fires later than the extracerebellar formations (Rucci, Giretti & LaRocca 1968); it may play an inhibitory role in the development of the OHP-induced convulsion.

Tolerance limits

Much of our present information on the tolerance of man to oxygen pressures exceeding 2 ATA (33 ft) is derived from the extensive study of Donald (1947) where the time to onset of symptoms was used as a quantitative measure of susceptibility. In most cases the symptom was lip twitching but in a few instances it was nausea, vertigo or convulsions. An extremely large variation in susceptibility was observed, not only between individuals, but also in any one person from day to day. Moreover, the onset of symptoms occurred consistently sooner when experiments were done with men in water than with men in a dry chamber, and the tolerance to OHP was greatly reduced when work was carried out during the exposure.

Obviously, in the light of such observations, the same safety limits on oxygen breathing cannot be applied to diving and dry chamber work. Based on the findings of Donald it is now current practice to limit oxygen diving when work or swimming is being done to a depth of 25 ft (1·8 ATA; Miles 1962). Based on studies carried out at the US Navy Experimental Diving Unit, Lanphier (1955) constructed the oxygen limit curve (Fig. 10.3) showing the underwater working limits. A somewhat similar but more comprehensive oxygen limit curve is to be found in the US Navy Diving Manual (1970). Because of the dry conditions, absence of exercise and availability of medical personnel much more lenient limits can be imposed, in most cases, during hyperbaric oxygen therapy. Foster (1965) reported

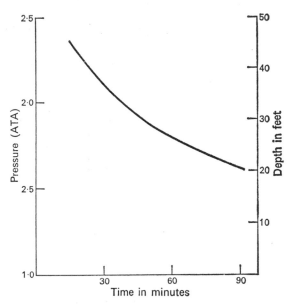

FIG. 10.3. Oxygen limit curve for man. (Reproduced from Lanphier (1955) with permission of the publisher.)

only 3 cases of convulsions in 475 exposures to 3 ATA (66 ft) oxygen for periods of 20 to 69 min during hyperbaric oxygen therapy. The results of his studies are shown in Table 10.2 together with those obtained at the US Navy Experimental Diving Unit and reported by Lambertsen (1955). It would appear that men do not run any great risk of convulsions when exposed in a dry chamber and at rest to 2·8 or 3·0 ATA oxygen for periods of 2 hours or 1 hour respectively, but that increasing the pressure above this level greatly increases the chance of oxygen toxicity. An exposure of 2 hours at 3 ATA oxygen may be the practical safe limit under these conditions although additional studies at this exposure are necessary to clarify the situation.

Carbon dioxide and OHP-induced convulsions

The possible involvement of carbon dioxide in the aetiology of oxygen toxicity has been the subject of vigorous discussion for many years. As mentioned previously, oxygen at pressures greater than about 3 ATA (66 ft) impairs the function of haemoglobin with respect to the role in the transport of carbon dioxide in the blood. Although Gesell (1923), Bean (1945) and Taylor (1949)

TABLE 10.2

Oxygen poisoning in man exposed to OHP in a dry chamber and at rest

Exposure to OHP		Cases of oxygen poisoning	Reference
Pressure (ATA)	Duration (min)	Total number of exposures	
3·0	20–29	1/118	
3·0	30–39	1/277	
3·0	40–49	1/57	Foster (1965)
3·0	50–59	0/18	
3·0	60–69	0/5	
2·8	120	0/20	
3·4	120	37/48	Lambertsen (1955)
4·0	60	26/29	

consider high tissue carbon dioxide tension a likely consequence of this impairment, Lambertsen (1965) points out that loss of the dual role of haemoglobin does not decrease the transport of carbon dioxide but only causes the transport to be carried out at lower pH and higher carbon dioxide tension due to the loss of buffering power of the haemoglobin. Carbon dioxide tension and acidity of brain tissue would not therefore be expected to show extensive change under OHP conditions.

Unfortunately, data obtained by direct measurement of brain carbon dioxide tension at greater than 3 ATA oxygen are sparse but estimates of brain carbon dioxide tensions have been made from blood gas analysis. For example, the blood carbon dioxide tension data obtained by Behnke et al. (1934) using dogs and by Lambertsen et al. (1953b) using men suggest that the elevation in brain carbon dioxide tension under 3 to 4 ATA oxygen may be small, in the range 2·5 to 6·0 mm Hg. These values are in good agreement with the maximal 4 mm Hg rise in brain carbon dioxide tension predicted by Lambertsen (1963) from theoretical considerations.

The question now arises as to whether changes of the above magnitude are sufficient to cause the convulsions observed during OHP exposures. This seems unlikely since the elevations in carbon dioxide and acidity are equivalent to those produced by the breathing of 6% carbon dioxide at normal inspired oxygen tension (Lambertsen 1966), a treatment which does not per se produce convulsions. The increased susceptibility of animals to OHP when carbon dioxide is added to the breathing mixture (Shaw, Behnke & Messer 1934; Taylor 1949; Marshall & Lambertsen 1961) is sometimes quoted as evidence for the involvement of elevated brain carbon dioxide tension in OHP-induced siezures, but it would appear more probable that the inhaled carbon dioxide produces its effect by increasing arterial carbon dioxide tension with consequent vasodilation and increase in the oxygen supply to the cerebral tissues (Lambertsen et al. 1955–56).

Thus, from the results at present available, it seems reasonable to conclude that OHP causes small but definite increases in brain carbon dioxide tension and acidity, which possibly contribute towards oxygen poisoning but which do not by themselves constitute the entire mechanism.

Inert gases and OHP-induced convulsions

This subject has not been studied extensively and the two investigations that have been reported are contradictory. Whereas Bennett (1966) reported a significant increase in susceptibility of rats to seizures when argon or nitrogen, but not helium, was present in the breathing mixture, McGavin et al. (1966) found no effect of nitrogen or helium on the survival time or convulsion times of rats breathing OHP. The pressures used by the latter workers were, however, considerably lower than those employed by Bennett and may have been insufficient for an observable effect.

POSSIBLE MECHANISMS INVOLVED IN THE PRODUCTION OF SEIZURES

In view of the well-established ionic basis of nerve transmission it seems reasonable to predict that changes in the permeability of membranes to ions such as sodium and potassium are the immediate cause of the seizures. Supporting evidence for permeability changes comes from the studies of Kaplan and Stein (1957) which showed that slices of guinea pig brain lost considerable quantities of potassium when incubated under 4 ATA oxygen (100 ft). However, changes in ion permeability probably constitute a secondary effect of OHP and current research is directed towards the elucidation of the primary effects which cause the permeability changes. The three major possibilities which have been considered in this regard are: the membrane is itself damaged, the oxidative processes which produce the energy required for the sodium and potassium ion pumps are impaired, or the metabolism and/or function of the neurotransmitter substances are deranged.

Membrane damage and related phenomena

Both of the major structural components of cellular membranes are susceptible to attack by oxygen, the lipids by oxidation of the unsaturated fatty acids and the proteins by the oxidation of the sulphydryl groups. Such changes could alter the structural integrity of the membrane (Wolman 1963) or could inhibit a variety of 'membrane associated' enzyme actions.

There is no doubt that lipid peroxides are formed in the brain of animals during exposure to OHP (Becker & Galvin 1962; Wolman 1963; Zirkle et al. 1965b). However, it is unlikely that oxidation of structural lipids with consequent damage to membranes is responsible for OHP-induced convulsions because oxygen poisoning is rapidly reversible (Lambertsen 1955)—yet repair of damaged lipids in the membranes might be expected to take a considerably longer period of time. Moreover, Becker and Galvin (1962) were

unable to find any correlation between lipid peroxidation and susceptibility to OHP-induced seizures. Membrane damage may account, however, for the signs of permanent central nervous system damage such as hind leg paralysis (Van Den Brenk & Jamieson 1964).

Zirkle et al. (1965b), while acknowledging the possible importance of cell membrane damage, suggest that oxygen poisoning may result from the inhibition of enzymes and coenzymes by the lipid peroxides per se. Evidence for such a phenomenon was obtained by Roubal and Tappel (1966a, 1966b) who demonstrated, using in vitro techniques, that proteins, enzymes and amino acids were damaged as a result of concomitant lipid peroxidation. The above concept could, of course, be invoked with equal justification to explain damage to structural proteins in the membranes. The oxidation of membrane protein sulphydryl groups, either by oxygen or lipid peroxides, may possibly be involved in the aetiology of OHP-induced seizures since the reversible nature of this oxidation is in harmony with the known reversibility of oxygen poisoning.

OHP-induced damage to membranes, if sufficiently severe, may lead to visible changes in cell ultrastructure, but there is a paucity of data in this area. Recently, Balentine (1973) showed that a single, non-convulsant, exposure of rats to OHP selectively affected neuronal dendrites. The mitochondria were enlarged and the change was associated with an increased density of the dendritic process which appeared to be due to a condensation of cytoplasmic constituents or to mitochondrial degeneration. The role, if any, which these structural changes play in the onset of the seizures remains to be elucidated.

Altered oxidative metabolism

Since the cellular ionic pumps are dependent on an adequate supply of energy, any impairment in the energy-supplying metabolism of the cell will have dire consequences with respect to the functioning of the nervous system. Although there are numerous reports on the inhibition of respiration in brain slices and homogenates exposed to oxygen pressures ranging from 1 to 8 ATA (0 to 230 ft) (Van Goor & Jongbloed 1942, 1949; Stadie, Riggs & Haugaard 1945b; Mann &

Quastel 1946; Dickens 1946), no impairment in respiration of brain preparations from animals exposed in vivo to OHP was observed by Stadie, Riggs and Haugaard (1945a). The absence of an effect may, however, be due to the rapidly reversible nature of any OHP-induced metabolic defects.

Rats exposed to 5 ATA (130 ft) oxygen for 1·5 hours had seizures and their brain ATP levels were less than half the normal concentration, but both these effects of OHP were prevented by the administration of succinate prior to the oxygen exposure (Sanders, Hall & Woodhall 1965; Sanders et al. 1966). Sanders and his co-workers therefore suggest that succinate produces its anticonvulsant action by acting as a substrate which, on oxidation, provides ATP production via flavoprotein reduction and subsequent electron transport chain function and thus helps sustain energy levels essential for cell function (Sanders, Lester & Woodhall 1968). In addition, Chance, Jamieson and Williamson (1966) found that both the reverse and forward electron transfer pathways were inhibited by OHP, the reverse pathway being the more sensitive. On the basis of their finding that glutathione, GABA and glutamate all protect animals against OHP-induced seizures, Sanders, Currie and Woodhall (1969) postulate that the pathway glutathione → glutamate → GABA → succinate may serve as a secondary support system in the maintenance of brain ATP levels (all the individual reactions of this pathway are known to exist). There are, however, certain findings which are difficult to reconcile with the above hypothesis. For example, Sanders, Cavanaugh and Woodhall (1966) found that rats exposed to 1 ATA oxygen for 2 hours did not convulse, yet their brain ATP levels were lower than those in convulsed animals. In addition, glycine, L-alanine and D-alanine were almost as effective as GABA in preventing the seizures (Wood & Watson 1964). The anticonvulsant action of these and related compounds appeared indeed to depend on their inhibitory action on neurons rather than on any role in oxidative metabolism.

In summary, it would seem that the exposure of animals to OHP does produce changes in oxidative metabolism but whether these changes play a role in the mechanism of the convulsions remains to be clearly established.

Altered neurotransmitter metabolism and function

The levels and the rate of metabolism of various neurotransmitter substances have been examined with respect to their possible role in OHP-induced seizures. The data must be interpreted cautiously, however, since the metabolism of these compounds is highly compartmentalized within and without the cells and important changes in the concentration of the neurotransmitters at a critical subcellular site, e.g. the synaptic cleft, may not be paralleled by the overall change in the level of the compound in the brain tissue. Bearing in mind this restriction, the available data will now be evaluated with respect to a possible role in the mechanism of OHP-induced seizures for the neurotransmitter substances, norepinephrine, dopamine, 5-hydroxytryptamine (serotonin) and γ-aminobutyric acid (GABA) and acetylcholine.

The enzymes responsible for the synthesis of the neurotransmitters are more sensitive to OHP-induced inhibition than are the enzymes which degrade the compounds (Table 10.3) (Tunnicliff, Urton & Wood 1973). Glutamic acid decarboxylase, the enzyme involved in the synthesis of GABA, is by far the most sensitive of all the enzymes tested. Thus it is necessary to examine the metabolism of all the neurotransmitters with respect to a role in the aetiology of OHP seizures and particular attention should be focused on GABA.

Exposure of rats and mice to OHP resulted in significantly lower brain levels of norepinephrine, dopamine and serotonin (Häggendal 1967; Faiman Heble & Mehl 1969) although this effect was not always observed (Blenkarn, Schanberg & Saltzman 1969). There was, however, no correlation between the concentration of any of the three compounds of brain and the onset of OHP-induced seizures. Moreover, drug-induced changes in the concentration of the three amines in mouse brain were without effect on the susceptibility of the animals to the seizures. However, it may be the turnover rate of the amines rather than their concentration per se which is the critical factor with respect to seizures, particularly since it has been reported by Diaz, Ngai and Costa (1968) and Neff and Costa (1967) that the turnover rates of norepinephrine and serotonin are increased in

TABLE 10.3

Effect of OHP on neurotransmitter enzymes

Enzyme	Inhibition (%)
Synthesizing	
glutamic acid decarboxylase	52
Dopa decarboxylase	11
5-hydroxytryptamine decarboxylase	11
tyrosine hydroxylase	3
tryptophan hydroxylase	2
choline acetylase	8
Degrading	
GABA-α-oxoglutarate aminotransferase	−2
acetylcholinesterase	−2
monoamine oxidase	2
catechol-O-methyl transferase	0

Activity of the enzymes was measured in chick brain homogenates which had been exposed to 3 ATA oxygen for 20 min at 25°C.
Data from Tunnicliff, Urton and Wood (1973).

animals breathing 100% oxygen at ambient pressure.

The most extensive evidence for the involvement of a neurotransmitter in the aetiology of OHP-induced seizures has been obtained with GABA. The great sensitivity of the synthesis of GABA to OHP-induced inhibition has already been pointed out (Table 10.3). Other evidence pointing to a role for GABA in the seizure process has been reviewed recently (Wood 1971) and may be summarized as follows:

1. OHP causes a decrease in the concentration of GABA in the brain.

2. The decrease in GABA level occurs prior to convulsions and is thus in keeping with a cause and effect relationship.

3. The decrease in GABA is reversible, as is oxygen toxicity.

4. The decrease in concentration is specific for GABA among the brain amino acids.

5. The critical pressure of oxygen (3 ATA) required to lower GABA levels in mice is also that required to induce seizures in the animals.

6. The administration of GABA to animals prior to their exposure to oxygen protects them against seizures.

7. Susceptibility of animals to seizures correlates well with the rate of decrease in GABA

levels for different animal species, for different pressures, for different CO_2 levels in the oxygen breathing mixture, and for different ages of the animals (Fig. 10.4).

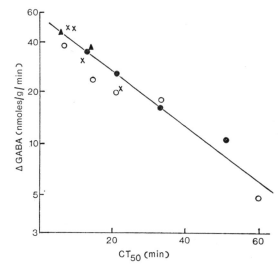

FIG. 10.4. Correlation between susceptibility to OHP seizures and the rate of decrease in brain GABA levels

○ different species; ● mice, different oxygen pressures; ▲ mice, different CO_2 levels in the oxygen mixture; X chicks, different ages. The CT_{50} value is the length of exposure to OHP which is required to induce convulsions in 50% of the animals. For further details regarding the experimental details see Wood (1970, 1971)

In summary, there is a high probability that GABA is involved in the mechanisms of OHP-induced convulsions, but the possibility that other neurotransmitters are also involved cannot be eliminated. The answer to many of the unsolved problems would seem to lie in studies at the subcellular level and it is to this area that research efforts should now be directed.

Other mechanisms

Although the aforementioned areas have attracted the greatest research effort, other possible mechanisms involved in OHP-induced convulsions have been considered. The involvement of the pentose–phosphate pathway has been examined (Brue 1967) and Russian workers have been particularly interested in the effect of OHP on ammonia and glutamine metabolism and on proteins (Gershenovich, Krichevskaya & Bronovitskaya 1964). OHP decreased glutamine levels and increased ammonia levels in the brain but no correlation was obtained between these changes and the onset of seizures.

The possible involvement of adrenochrome in the mechanism of OHP-induced seizures has also been considered. The concentration of this compound in brain increases during the clonic phase of the convulsions (Gershenovich, Krichevskaya & Alekseenko 1955) and it has been suggested by Houlihan et al. (1970) that an increased production of adrenochrome and adrenolutin may be responsible for the toxic action of oxygen, particularly since the effects of those compounds per se resemble some of the toxic effects of oxygen.

Gerschman (1964) attributes the toxic effects of oxygen to an increase in the cellular concentration of free radicals, the damaging effects on enzymes and cell function being caused by the attack of these free radicals on vital tissue constituents. The superoxide radical $(O_2{}^-)$ is inactivated in tissues by the enzyme superoxide dismutase which catalyses the following reaction: $O_2{}^- + O_2{}^- + 2H^+ \rightarrow H_2O_2 + O_2$ (McCord & Fridovich 1969). On the basis of these findings Gregory and Fridovich (1973) suggest that one facet of oxygen toxicity may be due to the production of $O_2{}^-$ in amounts greater than normal so that the capacity of the defence system, i.e. superoxide dismutase, is exceeded.

ENDOCRINES AND OHP

Exposure of animals to OHP brings about hypertrophy of the adrenals (Bean 1951; Bean & Johnson 1954). Adrenalectomy and thyroidectomy both protect against oxygen toxicity whereas the administration of adrenaline or thyroxine enhance the OHP effects (Campbell 1937; Bean & Johnson 1955). Bean (1964, 1965) points out that the usual defence mechanisms against stress, the hormone defence system (hypophysis, adrenal cortex, cortical hormones) and the nervous defence system (sympathetic nervous system, adrenal medulla, adrenaline), no longer act in this manner under OHP conditions but that, on the contrary, their increased activity augments the severity of the oxygen toxicity. There can be little doubt, therefore, that the endocrine system is involved during the course of oxygen poisoning but the exact nature of this involvement remains to be elucidated.

MICRO-ORGANISMS AND OHP

The toxic action of OHP on micro-organisms has been reported by several workers. There is not sufficient space here to give a detailed account of this aspect of oxygen poisoning but readers are referred to the Proceedings of the International Conferences on Hyperbaric Medicine (Boerema, Brummelkamp & Meijne 1964; Ledingham 1965; Brown & Cox 1966) and to the review by Gottlieb (1971).

PROTECTIVE AGENTS

A wide variety of substances have been tested for prophylactic properties against oxygen poisoning in animals but although several compounds have afforded partial protection the development of a compound giving complete protection is still awaited. A selection of some of the substances affording partial protection is listed in Table 10.4. If, as seems likely, oxygen toxicity is brought about by several mechanisms rather than by a single one the development of a truly effective protective agent will remain a most difficult task.

Although anaesthetics such as sodium pentobarbital are among the better protective agents against OHP seizures they must be used with

TABLE 10.4

Protective agents against oxygen toxicity in animals

Substance	Protection against	Reference
arginine	convulsions	Gershenovich & Krichevskaya (1960)
GABA	convulsions, lung damage	Wood, Watson & Clydesdale (1963)
		Wood, Stacey & Watson (1965)
succinate	convulsions, mortality	Sanders, Hall & Woodhall (1965)
		Sanders, Lester & Woodhall (1968)
glutathione	convulsions, mortality	Gerschman, Gilbert & Caccamise (1958)
		Sanders, Currie & Woodhall (1969)
5-hydroxytryptamine	spasticity and paralysis	Van Den Brenk & Jamieson (1964)
vitamin E	convulsions	Taylor (1965)
vitamin K	mortality	Horne (1966)
tris buffer	convulsions, lung damage	Bean (1961)
lithium	convulsions	Radomski & Watson (1973)
antioxidants	convulsions, paralysis, lung damage	Jamieson & Van Den Brenk (1964)
anaesthetic agents	convulsions, lung damage	Bean & Zee (1965)
2-mercaptoethylamine	mortality	Gerschman et al. (1954)
dimercaprol	convulsions, mortality	Van Tassel (1965)
2:4 dinitrophenol	spasticity and paralysis	Van Den Brenk & Jamieson (1964)
pargyline	convulsions	Schatz & Lal (1971)

great caution because although the overt signs of convulsions are removed the possibility exists that 'hidden' damage to the central nervous system or other tissues may still occur.

FUTURE RESEARCH

In spite of many years of extensive research the mechanisms involved in OHP-induced lung damage and seizures remain to be elucidated. What then of the future? New approaches to the problems should be devised and promising leads already obtained should be thoroughly investigated. In the latter category may be placed (1) the role of lung surfactant in the pulmonary pathology; (2) the role of neurotransmitters in the aetiology of seizures, particularly at the subcellular level; (3) the role of the endocrine system in both pulmonary and central nervous system damage; and (4) the effect of OHP on membrane structure and function.

In addition the effect of OHP on organs other than the lungs and central nervous system should be investigated. The latter organs have received most of the attention in the past because the signs of the toxic effect of OHP are so dramatic, but it seems unlikely that the other organs go unscathed.

Finally, it should be stressed that the varied nature of the physiological and biochemical events which are sensitive to OHP render it improbable that oxygen poisoning is due to one simple mechanism. More likely oxygen toxicity involves various mechanisms, some possibly interconnected, others not, and some perhaps more important than others. The slow rate of progress in delineating the causes of oxygen poisoning is probably due to this 'multiple effect' of OHP.

REFERENCES

ADAMSON, I. Y. R., BOWDEN, D. H. & WYATT, J. P. (1970) Oxygen poisoning in mice. Ultrastructural and surfactant studies during exposure and recovery. *Archs Pathol.* **90**, 463–472.

BALENTINE, J. D. (1973) Selective vulnerability of the central nervous system to hyperbaric oxygen. In *Oxygen Transport to Tissues. Adv. exp. Med. Biol.* **37A** Ed. H. Bicker & D. F. Bruley pp. 293–298. New York: Plenum Press.

BATINI, C., PARMA, M., RICCI, G. F. & ZANCHETTI, A. (1954a) Aspetti electroencefolografici della syndrome convulsive iperossica, *Archo Fisiol.* **53**, 346–353.

BATINI, C., PARMA, M., RICCI, G. F. & ZANCHETTI, A. (1954b) Meccanismi piramidali ed extrapiramidali delle con-
vulsioni iperossiche. *Archo Fisiol.* **53**, 362–369.

BEAN, J. W. (1929) Effect of high oxygen pressures on blood acidity, oxygen consumption, volume flow of blood
acidity, oxygen consumption, volume flow of blood and respiration. *Proc. Soc. exp. Biol Med.* **26**, 832.

BEAN, J. W. (1931) Effects of high oxygen pressure on carbon dioxide transport, on blood and tissue acidity, and on
oxygen consumption and pulmonary ventilation. *J. Physiol.* **72**, 27–48.

BEAN, J. W. (1945) Effects of oxygen at increased pressure. *Physiol. Rev.* **25**, 1–147.

BEAN, J. W. (1951) Adrenal alteration induced by oxygen at high pressure. *Fedn Proc. Fedn Am. Socs exp. Biol.* **10**,
11.

BEAN, J. W. (1952) The hypophysis as a determinant in the reaction of the mammal to oxygen at high pressure.
Am. J. Physiol. **170**, 508–517.

BEAN, J. W. (1961) Tris buffer, CO_2 and the sympatho-adrenal system in reactions to O_2 at high pressure. *Am. J.
Physiol.* **201**, 737–739.

BEAN, J. W. (1964) General effects of oxygen at high tension. In *Oxygen and the Animal Organism*, Ed. F. Dickens &
E. Neil. pp. 455–672. New York: Macmillan Co.

BEAN, J. W. (1965) Factors influencing clinical oxygen toxicity. *Ann. N. Y. Acad. Sci.* **117**, 745–755.

BEAN, J. W. & JOHNSON, P. C. (1952) Influence of hypophysis on pulmonary injury induced by exposure to oxygen
at high pressure and by pneumococcus. *Am. J. Physiol.* **171**, 451–458.

BEAN, J. W. & JOHNSON, P. C. (1954) Adrenocortical response to single and repeated exposure to oxygen at high
pressure. *Am. J. Physiol.* **179**, 410–414.

BEAN, J. W. & JOHNSON, P. C. (1955) Epinephrine and neurogenic factors in the pulmonary edema and CNS reactions
induced by O_2 at high pressure. *Am. J. Physiol.* **180**, 438–444.

BEAN, J. W. & SMITH, C. W. (1953) Hypophyseal and adrenocortical factors in pulmonary damage induced by oxygen
at atmospheric pressure. *Am. J. Physiol.* **172**, 169–174.

BEAN, J. W. & ZEE, D. (1965) Metabolism and the protection by anaesthesia against toxicity of O_2 at high pressure.
J. appl. Physiol. **20**, 525–530.

BEAN, J. W., JOHNSON, P. C. & SMITH, C. W. (1954) Adrenocortical and medullary factors in O_2 at high pressure.
Fedn Proc. Fedn Am. Socs exp. Biol. **13**, 9.

BEAN, J. W., ZEE, D. & THOM, B. (1966) Pulmonary changes with convulsions induced by drugs and oxygen at high
pressure. *J. appl. Physiol.* **21**, 865–872.

BECKER, N. H. & GALVIN, J. F. (1962) Effect of oxygen-rich atmospheres on cerebral lipid peroxides. *Aerospace Med.*
33, 985–987.

BEHNKE, A. R. (1940) High atmospheric pressures; physiological effects of increased and decreased pressure; application of these findings to clinical medicine. *Ann. intern. Med.* **13**, 2217–2228.

BEHNKE, A. R., FORBES, H. S. & MOTLEY, E. P. (1935–36) Circulatory and visual effects of oxygen at 3 atmospheres
pressure. *Am. J. Physiol.* **114**, 436–442.

BEHNKE, A. R., JOHNSON, F. S., POPPEN, J. R. & MOTLEY, E. P. (1934–35). The effect of oxygen on man at pressures
from 1 to 4 atmospheres. *Am. J. Physiol.* **110**, 565–572.

BEHNKE, A. R., SHAW, L. A., SHILLING, C. W., THOMSON, R. M. & MESSER, A. C. (1934) Studies on the effects of high
oxygen pressure. 1. Effect of high oxygen pressure upon the carbon dioxide and oxygen content, the acidity, and
the carbon dioxide combining power of the blood. *Am. J. Physiol.* **107**, 13–28.

BENNETT, P. B. (1966) Hyperbaric oxygen and the significance of increased cerebral oxygen and carbon dioxide
tensions. In *A Symposium on Oxygen Measurements in Blood and Tissues and their Significance.* Ed. J. P. Payne &
D. W. Hill. pp. 41–55. London: J. & A. Churchill.

BERGOFSKY, E. H. & BERTUN, P. (1966) Response of regional circulations to hyperoxia. *J. appl. Physiol.* **21**, 567–
672.

BERT, P. (1878) *La Pression Barometrique.* English Translation by M. A. Hitchcock & F. A. Hitchcock, 1943. Columbus,
Ohio: College Book Company.

BINGER, C. A. L., FAULKNER, J. M. & MOORE, R. L. (1927) Oxygen poisoning in mammals. *J. exp. Med.* **45**, 849–864.

BLENKARN, D. G., SCHANBERG, S. M. & SALTZMAN, H. A. (1969) Cerebral amines and acute hyperbaric oxygen toxicity.
J. Pharmac. exp. Ther. **166**, 346–353.

BOEREMA, I., BRUMMELKAMP, W. H. & MEIJNE, N. G. (1964) *Clinical application of hyperbaric oxygen. Proceedings
of the First International Congress on the Clinical Application of Hyperbaric Oxygen, 1963.* pp. 1–427. Amsterdam:
Elsevier Publishing Co.

BONDURANT, S. & MILLER, D. A. (1962) A method for producing surface active extracts of mammalian lung. *J. appl.
Physiol.* **17**, 167–168.

BONDURANT, S. & SMITH, C. (1962) Effect of oxygen intoxication on the surface characteristics of lung extracts.
Physiologist, Wash. **5**, 111.

BORNSTEIN, A. & STROINK, M. (1912) Ueber Sauerstoffvergiftung. *Dt. med. Wschr.* **38**, 1495–1497.

BRADLEY, M. E. & VOROSMARTI, J. (1968) Hematological changes resulting from hyperbaric oxygenation in divers
and non-divers. *Aerospace Med.* **39**, 493–497.

BROWN, E. S. (1964) Isolation and assay of dipalmityl lecithin in lung extracts. *Am. J. Physiol.* **207**, 402–406.

BROWN, I. W. & COX, B. S. (Eds) (1966) *Proceedings of the Third International Conference on Hyperbaric Medicine,
1965.* pp. 1–796. Washington D.C.: Natl Acad. Sci.-Natl Res. Council.

BRUE, F. (1967) La toxicité de l'oxygène hyperbare. Physiopathologie, cytotoxicité, protection; activation du cycle
des pentoses et autodéfense cellulaire. *Annls Anesth. fr.* **8**, 339–376.

BRUNS, P. D. & SHIELDS, L. V. (1954) High oxygen and hyaline-like membranes. *Am. J. Obstet. Gynec.* **67**, 1224–1236.

BUCKINGHAM, S. & SOMMERS, S. C. (1960) Pulmonary hyaline membranes. *Am. J. Dis. Child.* **99**, 216–227.

CALDWELL, P. R. B., GIAMMONA, S. T., LEE, W. L. & BONDURANT, S. (1963) Effect of oxygen breathing at one atmosphere on pulmonary surfactant in dogs. *Clin. Res.* **11**, 301.

CAMPBELL, J. A. (1937) Oxygen poisoning and the thyroid gland. *J. Physiol.* **90**, 91P–92P.

CEDERGREN, B., GYLLENSTEN, L. & WERSALL, J. (1959) Pulmonary damage caused by oxygen poisoning: An electron microscopic study in mice. *Acta paediat., Stockh.* **48**, 477–494.

CHANCE, B., JAMIESON, D. & WILLIAMSON, J. R. (1966) Control of the oxidation-reduction state of reduced pyridine nucleotides *in vivo* and *in vitro* by hyperbaric oxygen. In *Proceedings of the Third International Conference on Hyperbaric Medicine, 1965*. Ed. I. W. Brown & B. G. Cox. pp. 15–41. Washington D.C.: Natl Acad. Sci.-Natl Res. Council.

CLARK, J. M. & LAMBERTSEN, C. J. (1966) Rate of development of pulmonary O_2 toxicity in normal men at 2 ATA ambient. *Fedn Proc. Fedn Am. Socs exp. Biol.* **25**, 566.

CLARK, J. M. & LAMBERTSEN (1971a) Rate of development of pulmonary oxygen toxicity in man during O_2 breathing at 2·0 ATA. *J. appl. Physiol.* **30**, 739–752.

CLARK, J. M. & LAMBERTSEN, C. J. (1971b) Pulmonary oxygen toxicity: a review. *Pharma. Rev.* **23**, 37–133.

COHN, R. & GERSH, I. (1945) Changes in brain potentials during convulsions induced by oxygen under pressure. *J. Neurophysiol.* **8**, 155–160.

COLLIER, C. R. (1963). Pulmonary surface activity in O_2 poisoning. *Fedn Proc. Fedn Am. Socs exp. Biol.* **22**, 339.

COMROE, J. H., DRIPPS, R. D., DUMKE, P. R. & DEMING, M. (1945) Oxygen toxicity. The effect of inhalation of high concentrations of oxygen for twenty four hours on normal men at sea level and at a simulated altitude of 18,000 feet. *J. Am. med. Ass.* **128**, 710–717.

DAUTREBAND, L. & HALDANE, J. S. (1921) The effects of respiration of oxygen on breathing and circulation. *J. Physiol.* **55**, 296–299.

DE CLEMENT, F. A. & SMITH, C. W. (1962) Alteration of the toxicity of oxygen at atmospheric pressure by addition of CO_2 and of N_2. *Fedn Proc. Fedn Am. Socs exp. Biol.* **21**, 444.

DIAZ, P. M., NGAI, S. H. & COSTA, E. (1968) Effect of oxygen on brain serotonin metabolism in rats. *Am. J. Physiol.* **214**, 591–594.

DICKENS, F. (1946) The toxic effects of oxygen on brain metabolism and on tissue enzymes. 1. Brain metabolism. *Biochem. J.* **40**, 145–171.

DOLEVAL, V. (1962) Some humoral changes in man produced by continuous oxygen inhalation at normal barometric pressure. *Riv. Med. aeronaut spaz.* **25**, 219–233.

DONALD, K. W. (1947) Oxygen poisoning in man. *Br. med. J.* **1**, 667–672.

FAIMAN, M. D., HEBLE, A. & MEHL, R. G. (1969) Hyperbaric oxygenation and brain norepinephrine and 5-hydroxy-tryptamine; oxygen–pressure interactions. *Life Sci.* **8**, 1163–1178.

FISHER, A. B., HYDE, R. W., PUY, R. J. M., CLARK, J. M. & LAMBERTSEN, C. J. (1968) Effect of oxygen at 2 atmospheres on the pulmonary mechanics of normal man. *J. appl. Physiol.* **24**, 529–536.

FOSTER, C. A. (1965) Hyperbaric oxygen and radiotherapy. In *Hyperbaric Oxygenation*. Ed. I. M. Ledingham. pp. 380–388. Edinburgh: E. & S. Livingstone.

FRIDOVICH, I. (1972) Superoxide radical and superoxide dismutase. *Acc. chem. Res.* **5**, 321–326.

FUJIWARA, T., ADAMS, F. H. & SETO, K. (1964) Lipids and surface tension of extracts of normal and oxygen-treated guinea pig lungs. *J. Pediat.* **65**, 45–52.

GERSCHMAN, R. (1964) Biological effects of oxygen. In *Oxygen in the Animal Organism*. Ed. F. Dickens & E. Neil. pp. 475–492. New York: Macmillan Co.

GERSCHMAN, R., GILBERT, D. L. & CACCAMISE, D. (1958) Effect of various substances on survival times of mice exposed to different high oxygen tensions. *Am. J. Physiol.* **192**, 563–571.

GERSCHMAN, R., GILBERT, D. L., NYE, S. W., NADIG, P. & FENN, W. O. (1954) Role of adrenalectomy and adrenal cortical hormones in oxygen poisoning. *Am. J. Physiol.* **178**, 346–350.

GERSCHMAN, R., GILBERT, D. L., NYE, S. W., PRICE, W. E., Jr. & FENN, W. O. (1955) Effects of autonomic drugs and of adrenal glands on oxygen poisoning. *Proc. Sec. exp. Biol. Med.* **88**, 617–621.

GERSCHMAN, R., NYE, S. W., GILBERT, D. L., DWYER, P. & FENN, W. O. (1954) Oxygen poisoning. Protective effect of β-mercaptoethylamine. *Proc. Soc. exp. Biol. Med.* **85**, 75–77.

GERSHENOVICH, Z. S. & KRICHEVSKAYA, A. A. (1960) The protective role of arginine in oxygen poisoning. *Biokhimiya* **25**, 790–795.

GERSHENOVICH, Z. S., KRICHEVSKAYA, A. A. & ALEKSEENKO, L. P. (1955). Adrenergic substances of the brain and adrenals under increased oxygen pressure. *Ukr. biokhem. Zh.* **27**, 3–11.

GERSHENOVICH, Z. S., KRICHEVSKAYA, A. A. & BRONOVITSKAYA, Z. G. (1964) The ammonia–glutamine–glutamic acid system and oxidative phosphorylation in the brain during oxygen intoxication. In *Problems of the Biochemistry of the Nervous System*. Ed. A. V. Pallodin, translated by H. Hillman & R. Woodman. pp. 267–277. New York: Macmillan Co.

GESELL, R. (1923) On the chemical regulation of respiration: Regulation of respiration with special reference to the metabolism of the respiratory center and the coordination of the dual function of hemoglobin. *Am. J. Physiol.* **66**, 5–49.

GIAMMONA, S. T., KERNER, D. & BONDURANT, S. (1965) Effect of oxygen breathing at atmospheric pressure on pulmonary surfactant. *J. appl. Physiol.* **20**, 855–858.

GOTTLIEB, S. F. (1971) Effect of hyperbaric oxygen on microorganisms. *A. Rev. Microbiol.* **25**, 111–152.

HÄGGENDAL, J. (1967) The effect of high pressure air or oxygen with and without carbon dioxide added on catecholamine levels of rat brain. *Acta physiol. scand.* **69**, 147–152.

HAHNLOSER, P. B., DOMANIG, E., LANPHIER, E., & SCHENK, W. G. (1966) Hyperbaric oxygenation: Alterations in cardiac output and regional blood flow. *J. thor. cardiovasc. Surg.* **52**, 223–231.

HAUGAARD, N. (1968) Cellular mechanisms of oxygen toxicity. *Physiol. Rev.* **48**, 311–373.

HILL, L. (1912) *Caisson Sickness and the Physiology of Work in Compressed Air*. London: Edward Arnold.

HORNE, T. (1966) Protective action of some vitamin K analogues against the toxic action of hyperbaric oxygen. *Biochem. J.* **100**, 11P.

HOULIHAN, R. T., ALTSCHULE, M. D., HEGEDUS, L. & CROSS, M. H. (1970) Rheomelanin accumulation in the blood and lungs, and hemolysis in rats poisoned by hyperbaric oxygen. In *Proceedings of the Fourth International Congress on Hyperbaric Medicine*. Ed. J. Wada & T. Iwa. pp. 61–65. Tokyo: Igaku Shoin.

ISHIZUKA, R. (1966) A surface tension study of the animal lungs: influence of oxygen toxicity due to hyperbaric oxygenation. *Jap. J. thorac. Surg.* **19**, 578–584.

ISHIZUKA, R., MIYAKAWA, K., MAEKAWA, T., IMAMURA, B., AKASHI, T., TANAKA, N., KASAI, Y., JOCKIN, H. C. & BERNHARD, W. F. (1970) Pulmonary surface characteristics in oxygen toxicity. In *Proceedings of the Fourth International Congress on Hyperbaric Medicine*. Ed. J. Wada & T. Iwa. pp. 16–21. Tokyo: Igaku Shoin.

JAMIESON, D. & VAN DEN BRENK, H. A. S. (1964) The effects of antioxidants on high pressure oxygen toxicity. *Biochem. Pharmac.* **13**, 159–164.

JOHNSON, P. C. & BEAN, J. W. (1957) Effect of sympathetic blocking agents on the toxic action of oxygen at high pressure. *Am. J. Physiol.* **188**, 593–598.

KANN, H. E., MENGEL, C. E., CLANCY, W. T. & TIMMS, R. (1967) Effects of *in vivo* hyperoxia on erythrocytes. VI. Hemolysis occurring after exposure to oxygen under high pressure. *J. Lab. clin. Med.* **70**, 150–157.

KAPANCI, Y., WEIBEL, E. R., KAPLAN, H. P. & ROBINSON, F. R. (1969) Pathogenesis and reversibility of the pulmonary lesions of oxygen toxicity in monkeys. II. Ultrastructural and morphometric studies. *Lab. Invest.* **20**, 101–118.

KAPLAN, S. A. & STEIN, S. N. (1957) Effects of oxygen at high pressure on the transport of potassium, sodium and glutamate in guinea pig brain cortex. *Am. J. Physiol.* **190**, 157–162.

KAPLAN, H. P., ROBINSON, F. R., KAPANCI, Y. & WEIBEL, E. R. (1969) Pathogenesis and reversibility of the pulmonary lesions of oxygen toxicity in monkeys. I. Clinical and light microscopic studies. *Lab. Invest.* **20**, 94–100.

KARSNER, H. T. (1916) The pathological effects of atmospheres rich in oxygen. *J. exp. Med.* **23**, 149–170.

KARSNER, H. T. & ASH, J. E. (1916–17) A further study of the pathological effects of atmospheres rich in oxygen. *J. Lab. clin. Med.* **2**, 254–255.

KENNEDY, J. H. (1966) Hyperbaric oxygenation and pulmonary damage. The effect of exposure at two atmospheres upon surface activity of lung extracts in the rat. *Med. Thorac.* **23**, 27–35.

KETY, S. S. & SCHMIDT, C. F. (1948) The effects of altered arterial tensions of carbon dioxide and oxygen on cerebral blood flow and cerebral oxygen consumption of normal young men. *J. clin. Invest.* **27**, 484–492.

KYDD, G. H. (1967) Lung changes resulting from prolonged exposure to 100 percent oxygen at 550 mm Hg. *Aerospace Med.* **38**, 918–923.

LAMBERTSEN, C. J. (1955) Respiratory and circulatory actions of high oxygen pressure. In *Proc. 1st Symp. Underwater Physiology*. Ed. L. G. Goff. pp. 25–38. Washington D.C.: Natl Acad. Sci.-Natl Res. Council.

LAMBERTSEN, C. J. (1963) Physiological effects of oxygen. In *Proc. 2nd Symp. Underwater Physiology*. Ed. C. J. Lambertsen & L. J. Greenbaum. pp. 171–187. Washington D.C.: Natl Acad. Sci.-Natl Res. Council.

LAMBERTSEN, C. J. (1965) Effects of oxygen at high partial pressure. In *Handbook of Physiology*, Section 3, Vol. II. Ed. W. O. Fenn & H. Rahn. pp. 1027–1046. Washington D.C.: American Physiological Society.

LAMBERTSEN, C. J. (1966) Physiological effects of oxygen inhalation at high partial pressures. In *Fundamentals of Hyperbaric Medicine*, pp. 12–20. Prepared by Committee on Hyperbaric Oxygenation. Washington D.C.: Natl Acad. Sci.-Natl Res. Council.

LAMBERTSEN, C. J., EWING, J. H., KOUGH, R. H., GOULD, R. & STROUD, M. W. (1955–56) Oxygen toxicity. Arterial and internal jugular blood gas composition in man during inhalation of air, 100% O_2 and 2% CO_2 in O_2 at 3·5 atmospheres ambient pressure. *J. appl. Physiol.* **8**, 255–263.

LAMBERTSEN, C. J., KOUGH, R. H., COOPER, D. Y., EMMEL, G. L., LOESCHCKE, H. H. & SCHMIDT, C. F. (1953a) Oxygen toxicity. Effects in man of oxygen inhalation at 1 and 3·5 atmospheres upon blood gas transport, cerebral circulation and cerebral metabolism. *J. appl. Physiol.* **5**, 471–486.

LAMBERTSEN, C. J., KOUGH, R. H., COOPER, D. Y., EMMEL, G. L., LOESCHCKE, H. H. & SCHMIDT, C. F. (1953b) Comparison of relationship of respiratory minute volume to Pco_2 and pH of arterial and internal jugular blood in normal man during hyperventilation produced by low concentrations of CO_2 at 1 atmosphere and by O_2 at 3·0 atmospheres. *J. appl. Physiol.* **5**, 803–813.

LANPHIER, E. H. (1955) Use of nitrogen–oxygen mixtures in diving. In *Proc. 1st Symp. Underwater Physiology*. Ed. L. G. Goff. pp. 74–78. Washington D.C.: Natl Acad. Sci.-Natl Res. Council.

LEDINGHAM, I. M. (1965) *Proceedings of the Second International Congress on Hyperbaric Oxygenation, 1964*. pp. 1–472. Edinburgh: E. S. Livingstone.

LEVINE, B. E. & JOHNSON, R. P. (1965) Effects of atelectasis on pulmonary surfactant and quasi-static lung mechanics. *J. appl. Physiol.* **20**, 859–864.

McBRIDE, T. I., VANCE, J. P. & LEDINGHAM, I. M. (1970) Changes in myocardial blood flow and oxygen consumption during acute and prolonged exposure to hyperbaric oxygen. In *Proceedings of the Fourth International Congress on Hyperbaric Medicine*. Ed. J. Wada & T. Iwa. pp. 236–238. Tokyo: Igaku Shoin.

McCORD, J. M. & FRIDOVICH, I. (1969) Superoxide dismutase. An enzymic function for erythrocuprein (Hemocuprein). *J. biol. Chem.* **244**, 6049–6055.

McGAVIN, D., GUPTA, R. K., WINTER, P. M. & LANPHIER, E. H. (1966) Effect of inert gas on high-pressure oxygen toxicity in rats. *Physiologist, Wash.* **9**, 242.

McSHERRY, C. K. & GILDER, H. (1970) Pulmonary oxygen toxicity and surfactant. In *Proceedings of the Fourth International Congress on Hyperbaric Medicine*. Ed. J. Wada & T. Iwa. pp. 10–15, Tokyo: Igaku Shoin.

MANN, P. J. C. & QUASTEL, J. H. (1946) Toxic effects of oxygen and hydrogen peroxide on brain metabolism. *Biochem. J.* **40**, 139–144.

MARSHALL, J. R. & LAMBERTSEN, C. J. (1961) Interaction of increased Po_2 and Pco_2 effects in producing convulsions and death in mice. *J. appl. Physiol.* **16**, 1–7.

MEIJNE, N. G. & STRAUB, J. P. (1966) Coronary sinus blood flow during oxygen ventilation at 1 ATA and 3 ATA. *Dis. Chest* **50**, 161–172.

MENGEL, C. E., KANN, H. E., HEYMAN, A. & METZ, E. (1965) Effects of in vitro hyperoxia on erythrocytes. II. Hemolysis in a human after exposure to oxygen under high pressure. Blood 25, 822–829.

MENGEL, C. E., KANN, H. E., SMITH, W. W. & HORTON, B. D. (1964) Effect of in vivo hyperoxia on erythrocytes. I. Hemolysis in mice exposed to hyperbaric oxygenation. Proc. Soc. exp. Biol. Med. 116, 259–261.

MENGEL, C. E., ZIRKLE, L. G., O'MALLEY, B. W. & HORTON, B. D. (1965) Studies of the mechanism of in vivo RBC damage by oxygen. Aerospace Med. 36, 1036–1041.

MICHEL, E. L., LANGEVIN, R. W. & GELL, C. F. (1960) Effects of continuous human exposure to oxygen tension of 418 mm Hg for 168 hours. Aerospace Med. 31, 138–144.

MILES, S. (1962) Oxygen. In Underwater Medicine, pp. 116–139. London: Staples Press.

MORGAN, T. E., FINLEY, T. N. & FIALKOW, H. (1965) Comparison of the composition and surface activity of 'alveolar' and whole lung lipids in the dog. Biochim. biophys. Acta 106, 403–413.

MORGAN, T. E., FINLEY, T. N., HUBERAND, G. B. & FIALKOW, H. (1965) Alterations in pulmonary surface active lipids during exposure to increased oxygen tension. J. clin. Invest. 44, 1737–1744.

MOTLAGH, F. A., KAUFMAN, S. Z., GIUSTI, R., CRAMER, M., GARZON, A. A. & KARLSON, K. E. (1969) Electron microscopic appearance and surface tensions properties of the lungs ventilated with dry or humid air or oxygen. Surg. Forum 20, 219–220.

NAHAS, G. G. (1965) Control of acidosis in hyperbaric oxygenation. Ann. N. Y. Acad. Sci. 117, 774–786.

NASH, G., BLENNERHASSETT, J. B. & PONTOPPIDAN, H. (1967) Pulmonary lesions associated with oxygen therapy and artificial ventilation. N. Engl J. Med. 276, 368–374.

NASSERI, M., BUCHERL, E. S. & WOLFF, J. (1967) Lich-und electronenmikroskopische Untersuchungen uber die Strukturveränderung der Lunge nach Einwirkung hohen Sauerstoffdruckes. Virchows Arch. path. Anat. Physiol. 342, 190–198.

NEFF, N. H. & COSTA, E. (1967) The effect of oxygen on the turnover rate of biogenic amines in vivo. Fedn Proc. Fedn Am. Socs exp. Biol. 26, 463.

OHLSSON, W. T. L. (1947) A study on oxygen toxicity at atmospheric pressure with special references to the pathogenesis of pulmonary damage and clinical oxygen therapy. Acta med. scand. 190, Suppl., 1–93.

PAINE, J. R., KEYS, A. & LYNN, D. (1941) Manifestation of oxygen poisoning in dogs confined in atmospheres of 80 to 100% oxygen. Am. J. Physiol. 133, 406–407.

PARKINSON, J. (1912) The effect of inhalation of oxygen on the rate of the pulse in health. J. Physiol., Lond. 44, 54–58.

PATTLE, R. E. (1955) Properties, function and origin of the alveolar lining layer. Nature, Lond. 175, 1125–1126.

PATTLE, R. E. (1965) Surface lining of lung alveoli. Physiol. Rev. 45, 48–79.

PATTLE, R. E. & BURGESS, F. (1961) The lung lining film in some pathological conditions. J. Path. Bact. 82, 315–331.

PATTLE, R. E. & THOMAS, L. C. (1961) Lipoprotein composition of the film lining of the lung. Nature, Lond. 189, 844.

PENROD, K. E. (1956) Nature of pulmonary damage produced by high oxygen pressures. J. appl. Physiol. 9, 1–4.

PENROD, K. E. (1958) Lung damage by oxygen using differential catheterization. Fedn Proc. Fedn Am. Socs exp. Biol. 17, 123.

PODLESCH, I. & HERPFER, G. E. (1970) Coronary blood flow under high oxygen pressure. In Proceedings of the Fourth International Congress on Hyperbaric Medicine. Ed. J. Wada & T. Iwa. pp. 231–235. Tokyo: Igaku Shoin.

RADOMSKI, M. W. & WATSON, W. J. (1973) Effect of lithium on acute oxygen toxicity and associated changes in brain gamma-aminobutyric acid. Aerospace Med. 44, 387–392.

RIECHERT, W. (1941) Beitrag zum cardiazol-lungenodem. Arch. exp. Path. Pharmak. 197, 620–624.

ROSENBAUM, R. M., WITTNER, M. & LENGER, M. (1969) Mitochondrial and other ultrastructural changes in great alveolar cells of oxygen-adapted and poisoned rats. Lab. Invest. 20, 516–528.

ROUBAL, W. T. & TAPPEL, A. L. (1966a) Damage to proteins, enzymes and amino acids by peroxidizing lipids. Archs Biochem. Biophys. 113, 5–8.

ROUBAL, W. T. & TAPPEL, A. L. (1966b) Polymerization of proteins induced by free-radical lipid peroxidation. Archs Biochem. Biophys. 113, 150–155.

RUCCI, F. S., GIRETTI, M. L. & LaROCCA, M. (1967) Changes in electrical activity of the cerebral cortex and of some subcortical centers in hyperbaric oxygen. Electroenceph. clin. Neurophysiol. 22, 231–238.

RUCCI, F. S., GIRETTI, M. L. & LaROCCA, M. (1968) Cerebellum and hyperbaric oxygen. Electroenceph. clin. Neurophysiol. 25, 359–371.

SAID, S. I., AVERY, M. E., DAVIS, R. K., BANERJEE, C. M. & EL-GOHARY, M. (1965) Pulmonary surface activity in induced pulmonary edema. J. Clin. Invest. 44:458–464.

SALTZMAN, H. A., HART, L., ANDERSON, B., DUFFY, E. & SIEKER, H. O. (1964) The response of the retinal circulation to hyperbaric oxygenation. J. Clin. Invest. 43, 1283.

SANDERS, A. P., CURRIE, W. D. & WOODHALL, B. (1969) Protection of brain metabolism with glutathione, glutamate, γ-aminobutyrate and succinate. Proc. Soc. exp. Biol. Med. 130, 1021–1027.

SANDERS, A. P., HALL, I. H. & WOODHALL, B. (1965) Succinate: protective agent against hyperbaric oxygen toxicity. Science, N.Y. 150, 1830–1831.

SANDERS, A. P., LESTER, R. G. & WOODHALL, B. (1968) Hyperbaric oxygen toxicity prevention with succinate. J. Am. med. Ass. 204, 241–246.

SANDERS, A. P., HALL, I. H., CAVANAUGH, P. J. & WOODHALL, B. (1966) Effects of hyperbaric oxygenation on metabolism 1. ATP concentration in rat brain liver and kidney. Proc. Soc. exp. Biol. Med. 121, 34–36.

SCHATZ, R. A. & LAL, H. (1971) Elevation of brain GABA by pargyline; a possible mechanism for protection against oxygen toxicity. J. Neurochem. 18, 2553–2555.

SCHWAB, R. S., FINE, J. & MIXTER, W. J. (1936) The reduction of post encephalographic symptoms by the inhalation of 95% oxygen. J. nerv. ment. Dis. 84, 316–321.

SHAW, L. A., BEHNKE, A. R. & MESSER, A. C. (1934) The role of carbon dioxide in producing the symptoms of oxygen poisoning. Am. J. Physiol. 108, 652–661.

SHILLING, C. W. & ADAMS, B. H. (1933) A study of the convulsive seizures caused by breathing oxygen at high pressures. *Nav. med. Bull.* **31**, 112–121.

SMITH, C. W. & BEAN, J. W. (1955a) Adrenal factors in toxic action of O_2 at atmospheric pressure. *Fedn Proc. Fedn Am. Socs exp. Biol.* **14**, 140.

SMITH, C. W. & BEAN, J. W. (1955b) Influence of CO_2 on toxicity of O_2 at atmospheric pressure. *Am. J. Physiol.* **183**, 662.

SMITH, F. J. C., BENNETT, G. A., HEIM, J. W., THOMSON, R. M. & DRINKER, C. K. (1932) Morphological changes in the lungs of rats living under compressed air conditions. *J. exp. Med.* **56**, 79–89.

SMITH, J. L. (1899) The pathological effects due to increase of oxygen tension in the air breathed. *J. Physiol.* **24**, 19–35.

SONNENSCHEIN, R. R. & STEIN, S. N. (1953) Electrical activity of the brain in acute oxygen poisoning. *Electroenceph. clin. Neurophysiol.* **5**, 521–524.

STADIE, W. C., RIGGS, B. C. & HAUGAARD, N. (1944) Oxygen poisoning. *Am. J. med. Sci.* **207**, 84–114.

STADIE, W. C., RIGGS, B. C. & HAUGAARD, N. (1945a) Oxygen poisoning. III. The effect of high oxygen pressure upon the metabolism of brain. *J. biol. Chem.* **160**, 191–208.

STADIE, W. C., RIGGS, B. C. & HAUGAARD, N. (1945b) Oxygen poisoning. IV. The effect of high oxygen pressure upon the metabolism of liver, kidney, lung and muscle tissue. *J. biol. Chem.* **160**, 209–216.

STEIN, S. N. (1955) Neurophysiological effects of oxygen at high partial pressure. In *Proc. 1st Symp. Underwater Physiology*. Ed. L. G. Goff. pp. 20–24. Washington D.C.: Natl Acad. Sci.-Natl Res. Council.

TAYLOR, D. W. (1956) The effects of vitamin E and methylene blue on the manifestations of oxygen poisoning in the rat. *J. Physiol.* **131**, 200–206.

TAYLOR, D. W. (1958) Effects of adrenalectomy on oxygen poisoning in the rat. *J. Physiol., Lond.* **140**, 23–36.

TAYLOR, H. J. (1949) The role of carbon dioxide in oxygen poisoning. *J. Physiol., Lond.* **109**, 272–280.

TENNEKOON, G. E. (1954) Pulmonary edema due to thiosemicarbazide. *J. Path. Bact.* **67**, 341–347.

THOMPSON, W. G. (1889) The therapeutic value of oxygen inhalation with exhibition of animals under high pressure of oxygen. *Med. Rec., N.Y.* **36**, 1–7.

THOMSON, W. A. R. (1935) The physiology of deep-sea diving. *Br. med. J.* **2**, 208–210.

TUNNICLIFF, G., URTON, M. & WOOD, J. D. (1973) Susceptibility of chick brain L-glutamic acid decarboxylase and other neurotransmitter enzymes to hyperbaric oxygen *in vitro*. *Biochem. Pharmac.* **22**, 501–505.

TURNER, J., LAMBERTSEN, C. J., OWEN, S. G., WENDEL, H. & CHIODI, H. (1957) Effects of 0·08 and 0·8 atmosphere of inspired P_{O_2} upon cerebral hemodynamics at a constant alveolar P_{CO_2} of 43 mm Hg. *Fedn Proc. Fedn Am. Socs. exp. Biol.* **16**, 130.

US Navy Diving Manual (1970) Section 1.5.7, pp. 165–167.

VAN BREEMEN, V. L., NEUSTEIN, H. B. & BRUNS, P. D. (1957) Pulmonary hyaline membranes studied with the electron microscope. *Am. J. Path.* **33**, 769–789.

VAN DEN BRENK, H. A. S. & JAMIESON, D. (1962) Pulmonary damage due to high pressure oxygen breathing in rats. (1) lung weight histological and radiological studies. *Aust. J. exp. Biol. med. Sci.* **40**, 37–50.

VAN DEN BRENK, H. A. S. & JAMIESON, D. (1964) Brain damage and paralysis in animals exposed to high pressure oxygen; pharmacological and biochemical observations. *Biochem. Pharmac.* **13**, 165–182.

VAN GOOR, H. & JONGBLOED, J. (1942) The effect of oxygen tension on tissue and cellular metabolism *in vitro*. *Arch. néerl. Physiol.* **26**, 407–422.

VAN GOOR, H. & JONGBLOED, J. (1949) Oxygen poisoning. *Enzymologia* **13**, 313–324.

VAN TASSEL, P. V. (1965) Effect of dimercaprol on oxygen toxicity in rats. *J. appl. Physiol.* **20**, 531–533.

WARSHAW, L. J., MOLOMUT, N. & SPAIN, D. M. (1952) Cortisone effect on pneumonitis produced in mice by exposure to a high oxygen atmosphere. *Proc. Soc. exp. Biol. Med.* **80**, 341–344.

WEBB, W. R., LANIUS, J. W., ASLAMI, A. & REYNOLDS, R. C. (1966) The effects of hyperbaric-oxygen tensions on pulmonary surfactant in guinea pigs and rats. *J. Am. med. Ass.* **195**, 279–280.

WELCH, B. E., MORGAN, T. E. & CLAMANN, H. G. (1963) Time-concentration effects in relation to oxygen toxicity in man. *Fedn Proc. Fedn Am. Socs exp. Biol.* **22**, 1053–1056.

WINTER, P. M., WILLIAMS, B. T., RODING, B. & SCHENK, W. G. (1970) Coronary artery blood flow and oxygen transport under hyperbaric oxygen. In *Proceedings of the Fourth International Congress on Hyperbaric Medicine*. Ed. J. Wada & T. Iwa. pp. 228–230. Tokyo: Igaku Shoin.

WOLMAN, M. (1963) In *The Selective Vulnerability of the Brain in Hypoxemia*. Ed. J. P. Schade & W. H. McMenemey. p. 349. Oxford: Blackwell.

WOOD, J. D. (1970) Seizures induced by hyperbaric oxygen and cerebral γ-aminobutyric acid in chicks during development. *J. Neurochem.* **17**, 573–579.

WOOD, J. D. (1971) Oxygen toxicity in neuronal elements. In *Underwater Physiology. Proc. 4th Symp. Underwater Physiology*. Ed. C. J. Lambertsen. pp. 9–17. New York: Academic Press.

WOOD, J. D. & WATSON, W. J. (1964) Molecular structure-activity relationships of compounds protecting rats against oxygen poisoning. *Can. J. Physiol. Pharmac.* **42**, 641–646.

WOOD, J. D., STACEY, N. E. & WATSON, W. J. (1965) Pulmonary and central nervous system damage in rats exposed to hyperbaric oxygen and protection therefrom by gamma-aminobutyric acid. *Can. J. Physiol. Pharmac.* **43**, 405–410.

WOOD, J. D., WATSON, W. J. & CLYDESDALE, F. M. (1963) Gamma-aminobutyric acid and oxygen poisoning. *J. Neurochem.* **10**, 625–633.

WOOD, J. D., WATSON, W. J. & DUCKER, A. J. (1967) Oxygen poisoning in various mammalian species and the possible role of gamma-aminobutyric acid metabolism. *J. Neurochem.* **14**, 1067–1074.

WOOD, J. D., WATSON, W. H. & MURRAY, G. W. (1969) Correlation between decreases in brain γ-aminobutyric acid levels and susceptibility to convulsions induced by hyperbaric oxygen. *J. Neurochem.* **16**, 281–287.

ZIRKLE, L. G., MENGEL, C. E., BUTLER, S. A. & FUSON, R. (1965a) Effects of *in vivo* hyperoxia on erythrocytes. IV. Studies in dogs exposed to hyperbaric oxygenation. *Proc. Soc. exp. Biol. Med.* **119**, 833–837.

ZIRKLE, L. G., MENGEL, C. E., HORTON, B. D. & DUFFY, E. J. (1965b) Studies of oxygen toxicity in the central nervous system. *Aerospace Med.* **36**, 1027–1032.

11

Carbon Dioxide Effects Under Conditions of Raised Environmental Pressure

K. E. SCHAEFER

Exposure to the increased barometric pressure encountered underwater affects the mechanics of respiration and in particular the respiratory gases. Carbon dioxide plays a major role in the physiology of the high-pressure environment since the increased breathing resistance easily leads to carbon dioxide retention. The latter has been observed frequently in scuba and helmet diving.

Pulmonary gas exchange in breath-hold diving is influenced by the compression and decompression events resulting in a reversed carbon dioxide gradient during descent. The alveolar carbon dioxide level can be controlled during the ascent from depth by the speed of ascent which is of significance to both breath-hold diving and the buoyant ascents of submarine escape.

Investigations of pulmonary gas exchange in rest and exercise during exposure to high pressure while breathing helium–oxygen gas mixtures have demonstrated the existence of respiratory limitations and associated CO_2 retention for heavy exhaustive work only.

In shallow habitat air diving using combinations of air and normoxic nitrogen–oxygen breathing mixtures evidence for the development of a slight respiratory acidosis and CO_2 retention has been obtained.

BREATH-HOLD DIVING

Pulmonary gas exchange

Pulmonary gas exchange during breath-hold diving has been extensively studied in tank instructors at the 100 ft Submarine Escape Training Tank, US Naval Submarine Base, New London, Connecticut, in dives to 90 ft (3·7 ATA) (Schaefer 1955; Schaefer & Carey 1962). During descent, the ambient pressures increase rapidly resulting in a compression of chest and lungs. It was found that the carbon dioxide tension in the lungs rose quickly above the venous carbon dioxide tension and a reversed carbon dioxide gradient developed. At 90 ft (3·7 ATA) approximately 50% of the predive carbon dioxide content of the lungs had disappeared and was taken up by the blood and tissues. The influx of carbon dioxide into the lungs during ascent appeared to be rather slow and it was found possible to control the alveolar carbon dioxide level by the speed of ascent. If the ascent was fast, the alveolar carbon dioxide tension attained on reaching the surface was low, being between 30 and 35 mm Hg, but if the ascent was slow the alveolar carbon dioxide tension rose to 40 to 45 mm Hg. The alveolar oxygen tension rose from control levels of 100 mm Hg to 300 mm Hg at 90 ft (3·7 ATA) and fell on ascent rapidly during the last 10 ft (1·3 ATA) to values as low as 25 to 30 mm Hg.

The disappearance of carbon dioxide from the lungs during dives, together with the oxygen utilization and mechanical compression of the thorax as the subject descends, produce a progressive shrinkage of the total chest volume.

A diver at 90 ft (3·7 ATA) is protected to a

certain extent as the carbon dioxide tension does not rise to dangerous levels and the oxygen tension is rather high. Under these conditions, breath-holding time is considerably prolonged. However, during the last part of ascent or just at the moment the diver reaches the surface, available oxygen may become so depleted as to produce hypoxia. Thus the alveolar oxygen falls to a very low level at the end of ascent from dives to 90 ft (3·7 ATA). The author has seen one instructor become confused in the initial moments after reaching the surface during which he gave an alveolar sample, but he quickly recovered after the first breath. His alveolar oxygen concentration was 3·5% (PA_{O2} 28 mm Hg). With a very low oxygen content and a normal or below normal carbon dioxide concentration, the nitrogen content of the alveolar air at the end of the dive is markedly increased, 89% compared with a normal 79%.

These findings can be explained by the difference in rate of elimination of nitrogen compared with carbon dioxide. Nitrogen, carbon dioxide and oxygen gas tensions in the lungs are increased four-fold at a depth of 99 ft (4 ATA). Under these circumstances, nitrogen as well as carbon dioxide and oxygen diffuse from the lungs into the blood. Nitrogen follows the law of solubility of gases in liquids in relation to partial pressure. In carbon dioxide uptake by the blood and tissues, three factors play a role, namely, solubility in liquids, chemical combination with an alkaline buffer and carbon dioxide transfer between the plasma and the cell system. The reservoir to take up carbon dioxide appears much larger than that for nitrogen. During ascent, which represents a form of rapid decompression, nitrogen is rapidly released from a small store under high pressure, whereas it takes longer to release carbon dioxide from a large store. On the basis of theoretical calculations, DuBois (1955) had predicted such changes in pulmonary gas exchange during diving, and Bjurstedt and Hesser (1956) confirmed the existence of a reversed carbon dioxide gradient during compression in dog experiments simulating skin dives to 130 ft (4·9 ATA). Lanphier and Rahn (1963) investigated gas exchange during simulated breath-hold dives in man and obtained similar results, which were later confirmed in field studies on diving pattern and alveolar gas exchange in Korean diving women (Hong et al. 1963). The most comprehensive information on the physiology of breath-hold diving is contained in the symposium arranged by Rahn and Yokoyama (1965).

The influx of carbon dioxide into the lungs during ascent is regulated, at least in part, by the speed of ascent. Table 11.1 shows the alveolar carbon dioxide and oxygen tensions measured

TABLE 11.1

End–dive PA_{CO2} and PA_{O2} values following descent to 90 ft and ascent at different speeds

Dives to 90 ft (3·7 ATA)	Alveolar gas tensions	
Speed of ascent	PA_{CO2} mm Hg	PA_{O2} mm Hg
1·9 ft/sec (0·06 ATS/sec)	45·7 ± 4·1 (12)	34·8 ± 5·7 (12)
2·3 ft/sec (0·07 ATS/sec)	37·3 ± 1·2 (3)	34·7 ± 4·2 (3)
3·5 ft/sec (0·10 ATS/sec)	31·5 ± 1·3 (3)	27·3 ± 3·1 (3)
Breath-holding at surface	52·4 ± 2·4 (12)	64·8 ± 13·4 (12)

Number of dives indicated in parentheses.
Breath-holding at the surface was carried out by the same subjects who performed the dives to 90 ft and ascended at an average speed of 1·9 ft/sec. Breath-holding time of 1·5 min corresponded with the average time of breath-hold dives.

after surfacing from dives in which three different rates of ascent were used. With faster ascents the alveolar carbon dioxide tensions attained on reaching the surface decreased.

Measurements of blood gases, lactic acid, respiration and metabolism were made on four subjects before and after diving to 90 ft (3·7 ATA). The carbon dioxide content of blood rose very slightly while the oxygen content fell during the dive. The lactic acid content in the blood increased about five-fold during the dive. In this case a sample was taken 1 min after the dive. The lactic acid decreased to a level slightly above normal within 5 min. On more frequently collected venous samples, peak lactic acid concentrations were also measured after 3 min of recovery following the dive. The 1-min values were consistently lower than the 3-min values. This corresponds with similar findings obtained in pearl divers by Scholander et al. (1962). The delayed but large rise in lactic acid found during the recovery phase in man is quite similar to that observed in the seal and might, according to Scholander et al. (1962), also be interpreted as an indication of reduced muscle–blood flow during the dive.

Respiration was increased three-fold during the first minute after the dive and returned to normal level within 15 min. The excess oxygen up-take above the control level after the dive was limited to 4 min and averaged 1400 ml in four subjects. This indicates that the oxygen debt occurring during the dive of $1\frac{1}{2}$ min is in the order of 1400 ml. The excess carbon dioxide exhalation within the first 4 min after diving averaged 900 ml (Schaefer 1955).

To investigate pulmonary and circulatory adjustments which determine limits of depths in breath-hold diving, data on pulmonary gas exchange were collected in open-sea breath-hold dives to depths of 217·5 and 225 ft (7·5 and 7·8 ATA) on diver Croft who made a world-record dive to 240 ft (8·3 ATA) on 12 August 1968 (Schaefer et al. 1968b). Thoracic blood volume displacements were measured at depths of 25, 50, 90 and 130 ft (1·7, 2·5, 3·7 and 4·9 ATA), by use of the impedance plethysmograph. The open-sea dives were carried out with an average speed of descent of 3·95 ft/sec. (0·13 ATS/sec) and an average rate of ascent of 3·50 ft/sec (0·11 ATS/sec).

End-dive alveolar oxygen tensions did not fall below 36 mm Hg, while alveolar carbon dioxide tension did not rise above 40 mm Hg except in one case (Fig. 11.1). These findings indicate that

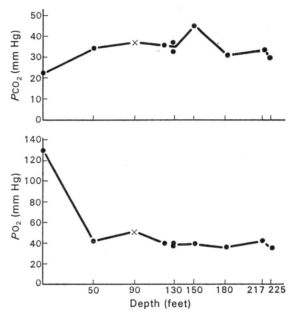

FIG. 11.1. End-dive alveolar gas tension obtained after rapid ascent at an average rate of 1·2 m/sec from various depths. Control values (on the left): alveolar gas tensions after rapid exhalation following maximal inhalation. × represents a tank dive and a solid circle an open-sea dive (after Schaefer et al. 1968b)

for diver Croft, who has an unusual lung capacity, neither hypoxia nor hypercapnea determined the depth limits under those conditions. At depths of 90 and 130 ft (3·7 and 4·9 ATA), blood was forced into the thorax, amounting to 1047 and 850 ml respectively.

Since blood-shifts into the thorax have been shown to play a significant role in allowing the breath-hold diver to go to deeper depth than could be predicted from measurements of total lung capacity and residual volume, studies were carried out in the wet and dry chamber to determine whether the blood shifts are caused by hydrostatic pressure only. Measurements of transthoracic resistance (impedance plethysmograph) made during simulated breath-hold dives to 25, 50 and 90 ft (1·7, 2·5 and 3·7 ATA) in the wet and dry chamber demonstrated that blood shifts into the thorax during breath-holding are caused by hydrostatic pressure, since no changes in thoracic resistance occurred during breath-hold dives in the dry chamber (Schaefer et al. 1972).

Paulev (1969) carried out extensive investigations of respiratory and cardiovascular effects of breath-holding. Essentially, he found that breath-holding with an intrapulmonic pressure of 20 to 40 mm Hg (Valsalva maneuver) produced a drastic reduction of limb blood flow, if the arterial blood pressure fell. On the basis of his experiments and studies on 129 persons, Paulev concluded that loss of consciousness with the risk of drowning may be caused by CO_2 narcosis in combination with the well-known hypoxia during ascent from deep breath-hold dives. Hong et al. investigated the time course of alveolar gas pressures and alveolar O_2 and CO_2 exchange together with changes in cardiac output and blood pressure during prolonged breath-hold with air. During 4 min of breath-holding the lung supplied 700 ml of O_2 into the blood while it gained only 160 ml of CO_2 from the blood, indicating a significant retention of CO_2. The CO_2 increased during the first 30 seconds and levelled off at about 50 mm Hg. $P_{A_{O_2}}$ fell continuously and reached approximately 30 mm Hg at the end of breath-holding at 4 min. Cardiac output did not change significantly. These observations on alveolar gas exchange during breath-holding confirm and extend the findings obtained previously during 1-min breath-holds by Craig and Harley (1968) and breath-holds longer than 1 min by Hong et al. (1970) and Tibes and Stegemann (1969).

Craig and Medd (1968) measured oxygen consumption and CO_2 production during single and repetitive dives to 5 and 10 m (1·5 and 2·0 ATA) and the results of these experiments were compared to those from underwater swimming and land exercise with breath-holding. CO_2 retention observed during the dive was greater after the deeper dives. It was concluded that part of the CO_2 retention was related to the effect of increased ambient pressure and lung compression. Water immersion itself must play a role, since the $P_{A_{CO_2}}$ at the end of the underwater swim was not as high as it was after the land exercise with breath-holding.

SUBMARINE ESCAPE (FREE AND BUOYANT ASCENT)

Buoyant ascent (aided by an inflated life jacket) has been successfully carried out from depths of 300 ft (10 ATA) at an ascent rate of 340 ft/min. (10·3 ATS) without respiratory distress (Bond, Workman & Mazzone 1960). Recent evaluation of alveolar gas exchange data obtained during buoyant ascent from 90 ft (3·7 ATA) have shown that the alveolar carbon dioxide tension can be kept at normal levels at the average ascent rates used (DuBois, Bond & Schaefer 1963).

A series of successful ascents made in 1965 by submariners of the Royal Navy from depths down to 500 ft (16 ATA) have been described (Elliott 1966). A theoretical depth-time curve for buoyant ascent was established, according to which it appears possible to make these ascents from 600 ft (19 ATA) without being endangered by carbon dioxide narcosis, nitrogen narcosis or anoxia (Fig. 11.2). Escape from depths of 600 ft (19 ATA) has since been accomplished by the Royal Navy in open-sea trials with a pressurization time of 20 sec, bottom time of 1·5 sec and a free ascent rate of 8·5 ft/sec (0·25 ATS/sec) to the surface (Donald 1970; Barnard 1971).

It has been proposed that the depth for submarine escape could be considerably extended by using a hyperbaric suit which enables the submariner to attain an increasing ascent rate and to maintain an overpressure for a certain period on the surface which would be equivalent to a decompression stop at 10 to 20 ft (1·3 to 1·6 ATA) (Eaton & Hempleman 1971).

It has also been suggested that to substitute carbon tetrafluoride for nitrogen as an inert gas dilutent in submarine escape procedures would double the depth capability (Gait & Miller 1973). Since carbon tetrafluoride is a more slowly saturating inert gas, oversaturation in any critical tissue can be avoided during the short exposure periods required during submarine escape procedures. These authors found in LD_{50} studies in mice exposed for 1 min to high pressure of carbon tetrafluoride or nitrogen with sufficient oxygen available in the breathing atmosphere that a greater depth for carbon tetrafluoride was demonstrated.

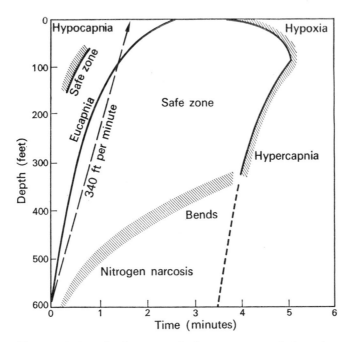

F IG . 11.2. Depth–time curve for buoyant ascent (submarine escape) from 600 ft (19 ATA) (after DuBois, Bond & Schaefer 1963)

SELF-CONTAINED DIVING

Several cases of unexplained loss of consciousness were observed with the use of oxygen closed circuit diving equipment in which canisters are employed for carbon dioxide removal (Barlow & MacIntosh 1944). Carbon dioxide intoxication was implicated as the most likely cause of a 'shallow-water blackout'. Additional investigations demonstrated that it is possible in most subjects to produce a marked carbon dioxide intoxication without severe respiratory dyspnea. In other words, the depressant effects of carbon dioxide can manifest themselves without the warning sign of a strong respiratory stimulation. Predominance of depressing carbon dioxide effects over respiratory stimulation are facilitated by physical exertion and high-oxygen tensions. However, Miles (1957) has suggested that shallow-water blackout might be caused by sudden increases in oxygen tensions leading to oxygen syncope. When an open or a closed circuit scuba is used at great depth, the direct effect of pressure produces an increased density of the breathing mixture resulting in increased resistance to breathing. Under these conditions the work of breathing is increased by the resistance developed in the breathing apparatus and in the airways of the diver (Marshall, Lanphier & DuBois 1956). Pulmonary resistance at 100 ft (4 ATA) increases two-fold compared with values at sea level (Mead 1955).

Although the underwater breathing equipment has been considerably improved over the years divers still experience difficulties during deep dives (Bradley 1974). Serious respiratory limitations have been encountered with different types of underwater breathing equipment during the Sealab III experiment, in the 1010-ft (31·5 ATA) open-sea dive and in a 640-ft (20·4 ATA) open-sea dive using neon. In the Sealab III experiment the divers were thermally unsupported and were working from a depth of 620 ft (19·8 ATA) breathing helium–oxygen with a Mark IX UBA equipment, which did not allow them to get enough gas.

It should be pointed out that carbon dioxide accumulation in the body has severe effects on thermoregulation. When higher CO_2 concentrations are reached heat production is impaired while heat loss is increased (Schaefer 1974). In the 1010-ft (31·5 ATA) open-sea dive the divers were thermally supported but encountered respiratory difficulties even during minimal exercise using a Mark II DDS, and a Kirby–Morgan Band Mask. Laboratory tests carried out with this mask showed that the mechanical work of breathing dense gas with this equipment was extremely high (Storrie 1974). In the 640-ft (20·4 ATA) open-sea dives neon–oxygen mixtures were used as breathing gases with the Kirby–Morgan Band Mask. During the working dives at this depth, the divers became hypercarbic, but did not recognize this condition. The inspired oxygen was rather high (1·6 ATA) which might have contributed to the CO_2 retention (Hamilton 1974). Physiological effects of underwater breathing equipment on ventilation and gas exchange have to be taken into consideration.

During head-out immersion in the erect position, cardiac output increases by more than 30% and perfusion of muscle tissues (anterior tibial) rises more than 100% (Lundgren 1974). The increase in circulation enhances nitrogen elimination and could in conjunction with oxygen breathing result in pulmonary atalectasis. Furthermore, recent experiments at Duke University have demonstrated that the resting arterial P_{CO_2} rises with the ambient hydrostatic pressure in the order of 0·5 mm Hg per atmosphere of ambient pressure increase (Saltzman 1974; Saltzman et al. 1971).

In dogs exposed to high pressure of helium–oxygen, a change in the electrochemical potential difference for bicarbonate between plasma and the cerebrospinal fluid (CSF) was found which is indicative of an increase in the concentration of CSF bicarbonate. Saltzman (1974) interpreted these findings as suggesting the development of central alkalosis with increasing hydrostatic pressure perhaps due to alteration of the blood–brain barrier for bicarbonate. These findings have a number of implications for diving physiology. The direct effect of the hydrostatic pressure raising the arterial P_{CO_2} independent of respiratory limitations brings up questions about a steady state arterial P_{CO_2} of a diver at 1000 or 2000 ft (31·2 or 61·4 ATA). What would be a 'normal value' under these conditions when there is no respiratory limitation? This is of particular im-

portance for the evaluation of underwater breathing equipment using physiological tests.

To verify the observations of Saltzman et al. (1971) of a positive correlation between Pa_{CO_2} and ambient pressure made in human subjects Kerem and Salzano (1974) studied the effects of 18 hours of exposure of unanesthetized dogs to a helium–oxygen mixture (3·4% or 16·6% helium) at an ambient pressure of 6·45 ATA. The gas density was only slightly raised to 1·17 relative to that of air at 1 ATA and the oxygen concentration remained at normoxic levels. Arterial and cerebrospinal fluid (CSF) P_{CO_2} increased 5 and 4 mm Hg respectively, CSF bicarbonate rose 2 mEq/L and CSF pH was not changed. Arterial pH decreased 0·04 units, the plasma standard bicarbonate did not change. These findings confirmed the observations of Saltzman et al. (1971) in humans and indicate that increased gas density and elevated inspired oxygen concentrations do not seem to play a role in the hydrostatic effect on Pa_{CO_2}.

Physiological testing methods have been proposed for underwater breathing apparatus. At the US Navy Experimental Diving Unit tests have been performed on breathing equipment at different working depths in which a limit of the arterial blood P_{CO_2} was set at 50 mm Hg. If higher levels of CO_2 were reached, the equipment was considered unsafe (Wright 1974). Another limit of 11 kg-m/min for respiratory work has been used which is based on clinical studies showing that patients with chronic pulmonary disease frequently develop 'respiratory failure' if their ventilatory work exceeds this level. Both of these limits are arbitrarily defined as a first measure to set physiological criteria for the testing of underwater breathing equipment and need further studies to confirm their validity.

Helmeted diving

In deep diving, in which the conventional suit and helmet are used, a large amount of air has to be ventilated to prevent the accumulation of carbon dioxide. Often this may not be fully accomplished. Moreover, at great depths, breathing resistance becomes very marked and may easily lead to carbon dioxide retention. Lanphier found that a considerable number of experienced helmeted divers at the US Navy Experimental Diving Unit experienced carbon dioxide retention during underwater work (Lanphier 1955a, b). The respiratory minute volume declined during work dives to moderate depth using oxygen–nitrogen mixtures. The degree of retention of carbon dioxide was related to the ventilatory response to carbon dioxide (Lanphier 1956). Those with a high tolerance to carbon dioxide retained more carbon dioxide. When breathing resistance was reduced by the use of helium–oxygen mixtures, the carbon dioxide retention was small or absent. A lowered sensitivity to carbon dioxide was frequently found in these divers (Lanphier & Morin 1961).

More recent studies carried out in the Swedish Navy by Muren and Wulff (1972) demonstrated that CO_2 retention found in the divers' helmet during heavy work is mainly caused by an unequal distribution of CO_2 and can be greatly alleviated by the insertion of an air diversion tube. Simulating the flow rates used in practical diving, 60 and 40 L/min. Pco_2 levels measured at three different locations, helmet, throat and suit were 12, 19 and 23 mm Hg with 40 L/min. ventilation during work. Considering a Pco_2 of 20 mm Hg as a critical limit, an attempt was made to improve the unequal distribution of CO_2 in the helmet. A number of symptoms occurred during heavy work, which implicated CO_2 retention as a causal factor. The divers often report a sudden lack of power occasionally associated with dizziness. It was observed that the normal reaction of an experienced diver under those conditions is to relax and take a little rest, after which the symptoms usually disappear. The young, ambitious and less experienced diver, however, insists on carrying on with heavy work with the obvious risk of losing control of himself. A very frequent symptom is the occurrence of headaches during and after the dive. These symptoms are characteristic of exposure to increased CO_2 concentrations greater than 3% CO_2 (Schaefer 1958, 1962).

When Muren and Wulff discovered by analysis of the air from the exhaust valve that the fresh air was to a great extent shunted directly from the inlet to the exhaust valve, they put an airtight metal cap around the exhaust valve and connected a 25 to 30 cm long plastic tube to the cap with the lower perforated end of the tube placed under the breast plate. Only the air from the lowest part of the compartment could enter the exhaust valve. Striking results were observed; the Pco_2 in the inspired air in the helmet was reduced 30 to 40%, the divers were relieved and experienced no headaches and less depth narcosis.

The latter finding points to additional effects of CO_2 and nitrogen narcosis, which is discussed below. The divers also chose of their own accord considerably higher working levels.

CARBON DIOXIDE RETENTION AND HYPERVENTILATION DURING PROLONGED EXPOSURE TO HIGH PRESSURE BREATHING HELIUM–OXYGEN MIXTURES

In preparation for Sealab operations, experiments were carried out in a dry chamber, in which three subjects were exposed for 12 days to 7 ATA breathing a gas mixture of 92% helium, 3·5% oxygen and 4·5% nitrogen. Maximum breathing capacity decreased 38% on the first day of compression and remained at this level for the rest of the exposure period (Lord, Bond & Schaefer 1966). Tidal volume increased significantly and alveolar carbon dioxide was markedly elevated. Pulmonary as well as urinary carbon dioxide excretion were significantly increased throughout the exposure indicating a marked carbon dioxide build-up (Schaefer 1968a). The carbon dioxide retention found under these conditions is difficult to explain. Several factors have to be considered. The increase in breathing resistance was not so large as to account for the carbon dioxide retention. There was no evidence of narcotic effects. The level of atmospheric carbon dioxide in the chamber averaged 1·17% sea level equivalent. The response to prolonged exposure to 1·5% carbon dioxide had been found to be quite different inasmuch as both pulmonary and urinary carbon dioxide excretion are reduced below control levels during 24 days of uncompensated respiratory acidosis (Schaefer et al. 1963).

Further evidence for carbon dioxide retention in the high-pressure environment has been obtained by Hamilton et al. (1965) in saturation diving at 650 ft (20 ATA). Two subjects were exposed for 48 hours in a dry chamber in which the carbon dioxide concentration was maintained at or below 1% of an atmosphere. The carbon dioxide response curves measured under these conditions were found to be shifted to the right, while the slopes were not changed. The shift to the right is part of the response observed during adaptation to increased carbon dioxide levels (Schaefer 1949). However, the decrease in slope associated with respiratory adaptation to carbon dioxide is missing in the observed changes under high pressure.

Increased alveolar CO_2 tensions during dives have also been found by Jarrett (1966) and Salzano, Rausch and Saltzman (1970) who attributed the rise in CO_2 to decreased ventilation as a result of increased gas density.

An absence of CO_2 retention in oxygen–helium dives to 1000 ft has been reported by Overfield et al. (1969). Moreover in saturation excursion dives to 800 and 1000 ft (24·2 and 31·2 ATA) Schaefer, Carey and Dougherty (1970) did not see any statistically significant changes of PA_{CO_2} during rest and exercise, although individual variations were quite large. In these experiments the ambient CO_2 level was kept below measurable levels. In the second dive to 1000 ft, the alveolar CO_2 tension tended to decrease in the two divers. This finding, together with the increased bicarbonate excretion in the urine, decrease in chloride excretion and a rise in urinary pH, was interpreted as reflecting a more alkalotic state due to hyperventilation. In line with these observations were electroencephalographic recordings, which showed in one subject throughout the saturation and decompression periods a consistent decrease in mean frequency and an increase in the percentage of slow waves, 6 to 8 Hz (theta activity) correlated with the CO_2 excretion in the urine (Proctor et al. 1972)

Figure 11.3 shows the time course in alveolar carbon dioxide tension, urinary CO_2 excretion and EEG changes during the saturation–excursion dive to 1000 ft (31·2 ATA) and the subsequent two decompression periods. The second decompression period followed a recompression from 30 to 527 ft (1·9 to 16·9 ATA) to treat persistent 'bends'.

The importance of hyperventilation in saturation–excursion dives has been emphasized by Brauer (1968) and by Bühlmann (1969), who carefully instructs his subjects not to hyperventilate during the dive.

Between 1968 and 1972, the depth of simulated dives in chambers using helium–oxygen mixtures increased from 1170 and 1189 ft to 2000 ft (36·4 and 36·9 ATA to 60·4 ATA). No evidence of CO_2

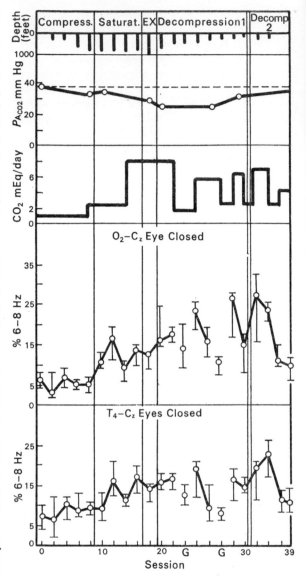

FIG. 11.3. Subject C.D. Time course in alveolar carbon dioxide tension, urinary CO_2 excretion and EEG changes (percentage 6–8 Hz frequency), two electrode positions O_2–C_z and T_4–C_z, eyes closed. (After Proctor et al. 1972)

retention was found in any of these deep dives under resting conditions. In the British dive to 1500 ft (46·3 ATA), Morrison, et al. (1975) observed that the alveolar carbon dioxide partial pressure was slightly lower at rest ($\geqslant 34$ mm Hg) and unchanged or increased during moderate exercise of 300 kg-m/min as compared with measurements made at the surface ($\geqslant 46$ mm Hg). Respiratory ventilation was increased both at rest and during exercise; tidal volume increased and respiratory rate declined with depth. Studies of cardiorespiratory functions during dives to 1640 ft (50·6 ATA) breathing helium–oxygen mixtures by Broussolle et al. (1972b) showed little changes in $P_{A_{O2}}$ and $P_{A_{CO2}}$ at 1640 ft.

There was, however, a slight increase in oxygen consumption and carbon dioxide excretion. No signs of CO_2 retention were observed during the dive to 2001 ft (60·4 ATA) (Fructus, Agarate & Sicardi 1975). In a comprehensive program of investigations of the limits of human tolerance to the gas densities of high pressures, depths of 2000, 3000, 4000 and 5000 ft of seawater (61·4, 91·6, 121·8 and 152 ATA) were simulated at a shallower depth by breathing helium, neon and nitrogen mixtures (Lambertsen 1975). During exposure to helium with oxygen at a pressure equivalent to 1200 ft (36·3 ATA) no respiratory limitations and signs of CO_2 retention were observed. When crude neon was inhaled at a depth of 1200 ft, the effects of gas density and respiratory resistance as well as respiratory work were equivalent to breathing helium at a depth of 5000 ft (152 ATA). No evidence of CO_2 retention was found under resting conditions. With heavy exercise, respiratory limitations and CO_2 retention were encountered. These effects are discussed below.

SHALLOW HABITAT AIR DIVING

Considerable efforts have been made in recent years to extend the depth of saturation diving using air or normoxic nitrogen–oxygen mixtures for working from a shallow undersea habitat. In Project Tektite, subjects were exposed for 2 months to 1·9 ATS of nitrogen (slightly less than 50 ft of seawater; 2·5 ATA) with natural oxygen tension in a habitat in the open sea. No effects were observed that would limit the ability of normal men

to work for prolonged periods at this depth (Miller and Lambertsen 1971). Subsequently a 14-day exposure to 4 ATA (corresponding to 100 ft of seawater) of a normoxic nitrogen–oxygen mixture was carried out in a chamber which allowed detailed measurements of respiration, and gas exchange (Lambertsen et al. 1973). Slight increases in Pa_{CO2} were found during exposure at rest and exercise. Although the workload during exercise was 70% of maximum capacity at 1 ATA, the subjects were able to complete the exercise at increased pressure. However, there was a marked decrease in minute ventilation during exercise and concurrent increases in Pa_{CO2} which most likely were caused by the increase in airway resistance at this pressure. Some CO_2 retention was also indicated in the slight increase in base excess and buffer base during exposure. The slopes of the CO_2 response curves measured during exposure showed a marked decrease during acute exposure, which was maintained during the chronic exposure of 14 days.

It was concluded, that the increased respiratory work due to the increased density of the N_2–O_2 mixture at 4 ATA caused the decrease in the ventilatory response to exercise and CO_2 inhalation rather than a suppression of chemosensibility. The slight respiratory acidosis found during the 14-day exposure to 5·2% O_2 in N_2 at pressure equivalent to 100 ft of seawater (4 ATA) was associated with hemoconcentration, a loss in plasma volume (-19%) and a reduction in red cell mass (-25%) (Alexander et al. 1973; Johnson et al. 1973). Hamilton et al. (1973) reported recently about two saturation–excursion dives at 90 and 120 ft (3·7 and 4·6 ATA) with descending and ascending excursions. A normoxic nitrogen–oxygen mixture was used. Pulmonary function tests and respiratory gas exchange studies did not show any significant changes. Performance tests and evoked brain responses demonstrated a definite adaptation to nitrogen narcosis in divers saturated at 90 and 120 ft. Their performance at 200 and 250 ft (7·1 and 8·6 ATA) during excursion dives showed practically no impairment from control levels. These studies demonstrated the feasibility of long duration excursions to depths of approximately 300 ft (10·1 ATA) using combinations of air and nitrogen–oxygen breathing mixtures.

Moreover, two 30-day studies using compressed air at simulated depths of 50 and 60 ft of seawater (oxygen partial pressures 0·52 ATA and 0·59 ATA respectively) were recently carried out at the US Naval Medical Research Laboratory without medical complications (Adams 1974). Pulmonary function studies did not show any significant changes. Ventilatory and pulse rate response to exercise loads of 100 and 150 watts increased during the end of the 4-week exposure. Two sets of CO_2 tolerance curves obtained for normoxic and hyperoxic conditions showed both a slight but significant reduction in slope during exposure. These findings were interpreted as indicating an effect of the increased density of gases. Acid–base balance studies carried out during the 60-ft dive (2·8 ATA) produced evidence of a mild respiratory acidosis by the second week of exposure and lasting throughout the experiment. The P_{CO_2}, actual bicarbonate and standard bicarbonate of venous blood significantly increased commensurate with a decrease in base excess. Red cell diphosphoglycerate (DPG) concentration was significantly decreased during the phase of the dive (days 9 to 20) during which shallow excursions were made and also during the second week of the post-dive period. Hematological studies revealed in both compressed air saturation dives a decline of hemoglobin, RBC count and calculation hematocrit through the compression period which became statistically significant during the first week of the post-decompression period. The fall of these hematological parameters was greater during the second dive at 60 ft (Murray 1974). Reticulocyte counts remained stable through the compression phase but increased to values statistically higher than pre-dive values during the second to fourth week following decompression.

It is of interest to compare the 14-day normoxic exposure to 100 ft (4 ATA) with the 30-day hyperoxic exposure to 60 ft (2·8 ATA) with regard to CO_2 retention. An acidosis developed under both conditions. There was an increase in base excess in the 4 ATA normoxic experiment, indicating CO_2 retention, and a decrease of base excess in the hyperoxic compressed air exposure, which would suggest the development of a metabolic acidosis. The slopes of the CO_2 response curves decreased under both conditions.

THE ROLE OF CARBON DIOXIDE IN INERT GAS NARCOSIS

If the diver is exposed to compressed air at pressures higher than 99 to 132 ft (4 to 5 ATA), he shows an impairment of performance and certain personality changes which have been referred to as narcotic effects of nitrogen (Behnke, Thomson & Motley 1935). Bean (1950) suggested carbon dioxide retention as the cause of nitrogen narcosis. His conclusion was based on findings of an acute rise in alveolar carbon dioxide associated with rapid compression of dogs. The hypothesis of Bean was supported more recently by Seusing and Drube (1960) who reported increases in alveolar carbon dioxide tension in air and helium dives in the dry chamber. Bühlmann (1961) also favoured the carbon dioxide theory of nitrogen narcosis based on measurements and calculations of breathing resistance during dives to greater depths. However, he avoided further comments on the carbon dioxide theory in a more recent paper (Bühlmann 1963). Evidence against the theory implicating carbon dioxide as the likely cause of nitrogen narcosis has been accumulating in recent years. Rashbass (1955) observed impairment of performance in divers under pressure without an associated rise in alveolar carbon dioxide tension. Moreover, Lanphier and Busby (1962) were able to demonstrate that strong subjective effects of nitrogen narcosis were present when both alveolar and arterial carbon dioxide tensions were low. Schaefer (1965a) pointed out that the symptoms of nitrogen narcosis and those of carbon dioxide effects on consciousness are distinctly different. Bennett (1963) produced the most convincing proof that the carbon dioxide theory of nitrogen narcosis is not correct. He exposed anesthetized cats to nitrogen, helium and argon under increased pressures and found a depression of evoked response in the presence of nitrogen indicating a narcotic effect, while the brain carbon dioxide tension did not change.

In more recent experiments in man Bennett and Blenkarn (1973) measured arterial blood gases and performance efficiency in 6 subjects during the decompression stages at 286 ft (9·6 ATA) and 190 ft (6·7 ATA) following a saturation oxygen–helium dive to 870 ft with excursion to 1000 ft. The arithmetic tests scores fell by 34·5% when the subjects were breathing air at 286 ft but were not different from the control values during breathing of a 20/80 helium–oxygen mixture.

The Pa_{CO_2} values obtained during breathing air or oxygen–helium at both decompression stages did not show any significant differences. They ranged between 31 and 35 mm Hg, indicating a hypocapnia. A positive base excess of 4·1 mEq/L was observed which the authors interpreted as a chronic metabolic adaptation to a mild hypercapnia of 44 to 50 mm Hg under steady state conditions. Such a mild degree of hypercapnia had been determined under steady state conditions by Saltzman et al. (1971) in three men at 200 ft and 250 ft (7·1 and 8·5 ATA) breathing alternately normoxic oxygen–nitrogen and normoxic oxygen–helium. The Pa_{CO_2} was in both cases 45 mm Hg as compared to 41 mm Hg on the surface breathing air.

When subjects breathed nitrogen–oxygen mixture, an increase in reaction time and an increase in failures to respond to the reaction time test were observed. During helium–oxygen breathing no changes were found, although the arterial CO_2 level was elevated to the same extent. From both experiments the conclusion could be drawn that the raised arterial carbon dioxide is not the direct cause of the inert gas narcosis.

Hesser, Adolfsen and Fagraeus (1971) attempted a delineation of the nitrogen and CO_2 component in compressed air narcosis by comparing the effects of inhalation of gas mixtures containing the sea level pressure equivalent of 0, 2, 4 and 6% CO_2 in air at 6·0 ATA and in O_2 at 1·3 ATA. The inspired O_2 pressures were approximately 1·2 ATA in both conditions, while the inspired N_2 tension differed by 4·7 ATA. The performance changes measured under both conditions plotted against the alveolar CO_2 tensions demonstrated clearly the nitrogen and CO_2 component. The CO_2 tension had no significant effect on the nitrogen component; however, the narcotic action of CO_2 was enhanced with increasing N_2 pressure. High alveolar N_2 and CO_2 pressures are additive in their effects on performance; below 40 mm Hg, the CO_2 component is negligible.

This investigation enlarged on the earlier observations of Case and Haldane (1941) who concluded that CO_2 might not be the cause, but might well enhance the development of nitrogen narcosis. Severinghaus (1974) recently discussed the problem of CO_2 narcosis on the basis of data obtained in experiments in which the anesthetic potency of CO_2 was determined by titrating CO_2 against N_2O in volunteers (McAleavy et al. 1961). The endpoint of performing a coordinated task, which coincided with falling asleep, was first determined by raising slowly the N_2O concentration. Then the P_{CO_2} was varied in the subjects. After reaching a steady state at P_{CO_2} of 25, 40 and 55 mm Hg, N_2O was added. The concentration of N_2O was slowly raised until the subjects fell asleep. As can be seen from Fig. 11.4 the effective concentration of N_2O was markedly lower at higher P_{CO_2}. An increase in P_{CO_2} of 10 mm Hg decreased the anesthesia endpoint by 50 mm Hg of N_2O pressure.

The results of these studies demonstrate clearly that the effects of the two anesthetic agents CO_2 and N_2O are additive. According to Severinghaus this type of analysis is applicable to nitrogen narcosis and has been carried out for nitrogen, helium and other inert gases. All of them have

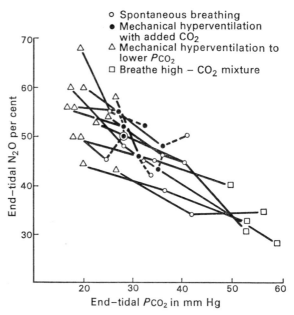

Fig. 11.4. The anesthetic potency of N_2O is altered by CO_2, such that less N_2O is required to obtain consciousness at higher P_{CO_2}, suggesting that CO_2 (or H^+) has anesthetic potency five times as great as N_2O (after Severinghaus 1974)

Control of ventilation at 4 ATA

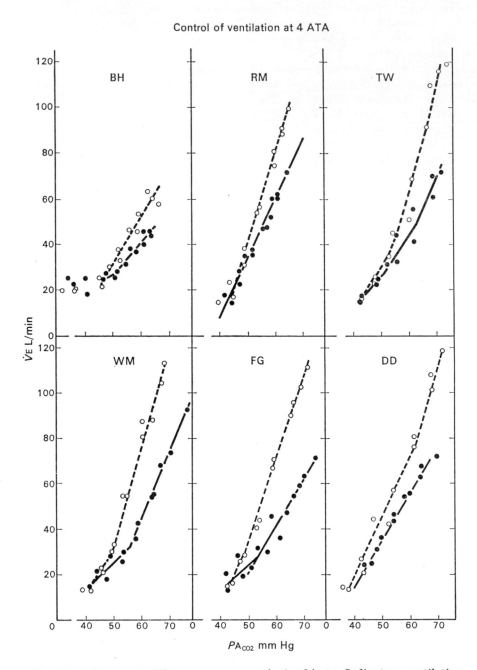

FIG. 11.5. Hyperoxic CO_2 response curves in 6 subjects. Ordinates: ventilation in L/min; abscissae: PA_{CO2} in mm Hg. Shown for each subject are data from two rebreathing runs at 1 ATA (open circles, dashed line) and two rebreathing runs at 4 ATA (solid circles, solid lines). The curves were fitted by eye (after Doell, Zutter & Anthonisen 1973)

been found to possess additive anesthetic potencies with the exception of helium. The latter has an anesthetic effect at enormous pressures of 200 ATM, but at this level pressure per se has a stimulating effect.

The CO_2 narcosis effects have been related to the extracellular pH (Eisele, Eger & Myallem 1967). The lipid-like anesthetic activity of CO_2 has not been tested because it seems to produce acidotic anesthesia at much lower levels.

RESPIRATORY RESPONSE TO CO_2 AND THE CONTROL OF VENTILATION AT HIGH PRESSURE

The marked CO_2 retention found in divers under increased pressure breathing nitrogen–oxygen mixtures (Lanphier 1963) and in divers during exposure to a helium–oxygen–nitrogen mixture at 7 ATA with an ambient CO_2 level of 1·1% (Schaefer et al. 1968a) have raised the question of whether exposure to pressure alters the sensitivity of the respiratory centre to carbon dioxide resulting in a decreased ventilation or whether an increased work of respiration at depth is responsible for the rise in Pa_{CO2} and fall in ventilation.

Wood and Bryan (1970; 1971) provided quantitative data which indicate that the sensitivity of the respiratory center to CO_2 is not changed under increased pressure. However the efficiency of the respiratory work is reduced. A CO_2 breath-hold time curve and the rebreathing CO_2 ventilatory response curve (Read test) were obtained at 1·0, 4·0, and 7·0 ATA. Moreover esophageal pressure–volume curves were measured during the Read test to derive inspiratory work. The slope in the breath-holding CO_2 response curve did not change, but the ventilatory response to CO_2 decreased at depth. For a given P_{CO2} inspirator work and tidal volume did not change with increased pressure, which has been interpreted as an indication of the unaltered sensitivity to CO_2. Because of the decrease in air flow rates and respiratory frequency at depth the same inspiratory work produces less ventilation at depth. The ventilatory response to CO_2 is therefore diminished. Similar data were obtained by Doell, Zutter and Anthonison (1973). Using a rebreathing method they examined the ventilatory responses to CO_2 and hypoxia at 1 and

4 ATA. Ventilatory responses to CO_2 were less at 4 ATA than at 1 ATA which is shown in Fig. 11.5.

Since the ventilatory responses to hypoxia were the same at 1 ATA and 4 ATA, at normal Pa_{CO2}, the conclusion was drawn that the output of the central chemoreceptors, as shown by the hyperoxic CO_2 response was expressed in inspiratory work, while the output of the peripheral chemoreceptors, as shown in the normocapnic hypoxic response, was reflected in ventilation. The authors noted that three of the subjects used slower frequencies and larger tidal volumes at depth in response to the hypercapnic stimuli resulting in a work-conserving breathing pattern. However, no change in the tidal volume–frequency combination was observed in response to the hypoxic stimuli at depth.

Fagraeus and Hesser (1970) also studied the ventilatory response to CO_2 in hyperbaric environments. When breathing low concentrations of CO_2 in oxygen at 1·7 ATA and in air at 8·0 ATA, the inspired O_2 and CO_2 pressures were approximately the same in the two conditions, whereas the inspired N_2 pressures differed by 6·3 ATA. The rise in N_2 pressure from 0 to 6·3 ATA caused a nearly 50% reduction in slope with no shift in position of the CO_2 response curve. In view of the fact that the CO_2 response curves obtained from subjects with added breathing resistance also show only a reduction in slope the authors concluded that the reduction of ventilation found under increased pressure was due to the increase in gas density and breathing resistance.

CO_2 RETENTION DURING EXERTION AT HIGH AMBIENT PRESSURES

The ventilatory limitations on heavy physical work at increased ambient pressures is one of the primary factors determining the depth limit in diving operations. Because of the increased density of the inspired gas, the work of breathing is increased, resulting in a decrease of alveolar ventilation and CO_2 retention. It is well known that the latter effect may be hazardous or fatal for a diver. A number of studies have been carried out in recent years to determine the depth at which respiratory limitations for moderate and heavy work develop. Fig. 11.6 (from Fagraeus & Linnarson 1973) is

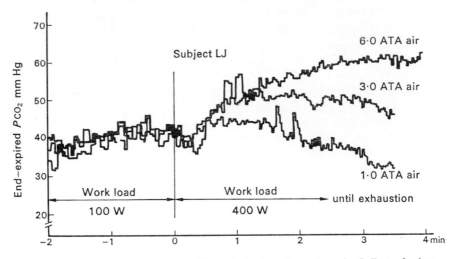

FIG. 11.6. Typical time course of breath-by-breath end-expired P_{CO_2} during submaximal and maximal exercise at 1·0, 3·0 and 6·0 ATA air (after Fagraeus & Linnarson 1973)

representative of the findings on CO_2 retention in exercise at high ambient air pressures.

It shows typical time courses of breath-by-breath end-tidal P_{CO_2} during submaximal (100 watts) and maximal exercise (400 watts) at 1·0, 3·0 and 6·0 ATA air. No changes in $P_{A_{CO_2}}$ are seen during submaximal exercise, but during maximal exercise CO_2 retention is clearly pronounced at 3·0 ATA air and $P_{A_{CO_2}}$ increases to levels of 56 mm Hg at 6·0 ATA air. These observations are characteristic and are in line with previous findings on end-tidal CO_2 during submaximal work breathing helium–oxygen mixtures at 600 ft (Bradley et al. 1971), at 800 and 1000 ft (25·2 and 31·2 ATA) (Schaefer et al. 1970) and at 1640 ft (60·6 ATA) Broussolle et al. 1975.

When higher workloads were used (1200 kilopond-meters per min, which corresponded to 80% of the subjects' maximal work capacity), subjects were unable to complete this exercise test at 1200 ft of seawater breathing a neon–helium–oxygen mixture which has a density equivalent to that of helium–oxygen at 5000 ft (152 ATA) (Strauss et al. 1975). Under these conditions there was a clearly pronounced CO_2 retention. Occasionally, an increase in alveolar $P_{A_{CO_2}}$ has been found during light work. Broussolle et al. (1969) observed in subjects exercising at 55 watts at 7 ATA in air an increase of $P_{A_{CO_2}}$ to 52·7 mm Hg from a con-

trol level of 35·8 mm Hg at 1 ATA. The subjects might have been some of the trained divers, who would rather retain CO_2 instead of increasing their ventilation sufficiently to meet the demands of the exercise. This form of adaptation to CO_2 is discussed below in more detail.

Studies of acid–base balance in arterialized blood during heavy work 1100 kg-m/min at 1 ATA and 5 ATA air showed an increase of $P_{A_{CO_2}}$ to 70 mm Hg and a decrease of pH to 7·29 during exercise at 5 ATA (Kurenkow 1973). Eklund, Kaijser and Melcher (1973) made an attempt to differentiate between metabolic factors (acidosis) and ventilatory factors (decreased working capacity of the breathing muscles) as possible causes of the respiratory limitations observed during heavy work-loads at increased pressures. They compared the effect of CO_2 inhalation (20 mm Hg) on maximal exercise of leg work at an ambient pressure of 2 ATA of a 100% O_2 atmosphere with the effect of increased CO_2 at 2 ATA during maximal forearm work. The latter condition involved a much smaller muscle mass that would not lead to great demands on oxygen uptake and ventilation, while in the former condition the oxygen and ventilation requirements might be limiting. During maximal leg work and CO_2 inhalation, the arterial P_{CO_2} rose to 55 mm Hg and the venous P_{CO_2} of the femoral vein to nearly 100 mm Hg. In both cases these values were about 10 mm Hg higher than in the condition without CO_2 inhalation, ventilation was about 10 L higher during exercise with CO_2 and the performance time significantly reduced (3·4 min as compared with 4·7 min). During forearm work CO_2 breathing produced similar changes in venous P_{CO_2} (99 mm Hg) as compared to 90 mm Hg during controls; however the venous pH fell to only 7·13 as compared with 6·99 in the leg exercise. The performance time for forearm work was not shortened. The authors concluded that under the conditions studied the increased effort of breathing was more important as a limiting factor for performance than the induced change in tissue pH. The venous pH data obtained under both conditions are not really comparable. During leg work the venous pH dropped to 6·99 where enzyme inhibitions occur (Schaefer 1974), while during forearm work the pH was above this level. However, the conclusions of the authors are supported by the results of maximal and submaximal exercise studies during acute and chronic hypercapnia. Because of the interaction of hypercapnia and exercise, they also apply to exercise at increased pressures and the concomitant increase in Pa_{CO_2}. The studies of Luft, Finkelstein and Elliott (1974) on maximal exercise at an ambient CO_2 level of 15 mm Hg (which is the highest acceptable limit for emergencies in space craft) clearly demonstrated that the respiratory discharge of CO_2 is impeded. A substantial rise in arterial P_{CO_2} during maximal exercise breathing air with CO_2 admixture was observed while the Pa_{CO_2} was reduced during maximal exercise under control conditions. Fig. 11.7 shows the acid–base changes during and after maximal exercise with and without 15 mm Hg $P_{I_{CO_2}}$. At the end of the exhaustive work Pa_{CO_2} fell to 30 mm Hg under control conditions, but rose to 41 mm Hg in the last minute of exercise. The time course of Pa_{CO_2} during CO_2 exposure and during recovery was also different. As a result of this rise in Pa_{CO_2} the metabolic acidosis generated by the anaerobic processes in the muscles can no longer be regulated by respiration. It was noted that the subjects who were pedalling at 50 rev/min were also breathing at this rate, when they were close to the maximum minute ventilation of 150 L/min. With the onset of symptoms of dyspnea, some attempted to raise the respiratory

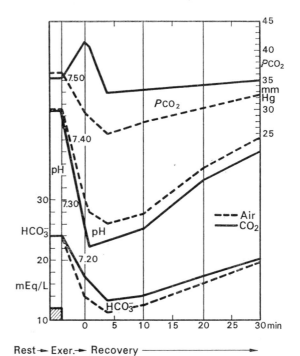

Fig. 11.7. Acid–base changes during and after exercise with and without 15 mm Hg $P_{I_{CO_2}}$ (after Luft, Finkelstein & Elliott 1974)

rate above the pedalling rate which led to a fall in tidal volume and alveolar ventilation. Clearly an example where the work of breathing becomes the limiting factor! Symptoms of intercostal muscle pain and subjective distress from the ventilatory effort were reported by subjects performing maximal exercise in 21 mm Hg P_{CO_2} (Menn, Sinclair & Welch 1970). In both studies CO_2 elimination was greatly reduced. Similar findings were obtained by Sinclair, Clark and Welch (1971).

Earlier studies of submaximal exercise during acute and chronic exposure to 3% CO_2 (21 mm Hg) had also demonstrated a reduction in CO_2 output and ventilatory efficiency (Häbisch 1949; Schaefer 1949). Lanphier (1969) and Miller, Wangensteen and Lanphier (1971) have suggested using the measurement of maximal voluntary ventilation (MVV) at pressure to predict the exercise level at which ventilation becomes insufficient and CO_2 begins to accumulate. They concluded that a ventilation at a workload at pressure which coincides with 100% of MVV is possible.

Shephard (1967), however, found that the

highest ventilation subjects were able to maintain during near-maximal exercise at sea level corresponded to 70 to 80% of their 15-sec MVV. Freedman (1970) reported that ventilation at maximal tolerable exercise corresponded to 64% of the 15-sec MVV, and Fagraeus and Linnarsson (1973) suggested on the basis of their studies of maximal exercise at 6 ATA air, the use of an exercise load of 60% of the 15-sec MVV.

ADAPTATION TO DIVING

Carbon dioxide tolerance curves were obtained by exposing subjects for 15 min to 3·3, 5·4 and 7·5% carbon dioxide. Alveolar ventilation and alveolar gas tensions were determined at the end of each exposure period. The carbon dioxide tolerance curves of experienced tank instructors showed a shift to the right and a decreased slope when compared with those of the laboratory personnel (Schaefer 1965b). As shown in carbon dioxide sensitivity tests by eight tank instructors, the high tolerance to carbon dioxide is developed during regular diving and is lost after 3 months without diving. The ventilatory response to 5% carbon dioxide is significantly larger at the end of the 3-month layoff period. The change in lung volumes, consisting of an increase in total lung capacity, vital capacity, tidal volume and a decrease in residual volume, may contribute to the reduced sensitivity to carbon dioxide because of the relationship found between large tidal volume,

low respiratory rate and low response to carbon dioxide (Schaefer 1958).

Adaptation to breath-hold and scuba diving involves an adaptation to carbon dioxide. Adaptation to breath-hold diving has been observed in instructors at the Escape Training Tank in New London, Connecticut (Schaefer 1965b).

Other parameters of adaptation to carbon dioxide have been previously established in human subjects during prolonged exposure to 1·5% carbon dioxide. They included besides changes in acid–base equilibria, an increase in red cell sodium and a decrease in red cell potassium (Schaefer, Nichols & Carey 1964). Tables 11.2 and 11.3 show the distribution of carbon dioxide in plasma and cells and the distribution of electrolytes in plasma and red cells of 11 tank instructors after periods with and without heavy underwater work. It can be seen that after a period of intensive diving, the pH is decreased, the carbon dioxide tension and bicarbonate levels are increased, and the sodium and potassium concentrations in red cells exhibit the typical changes observed in prolonged exposure to carbon dioxide. These data provide further support for an adaptation to carbon dioxide during breath-hold diving.

Evidence of an increase in carbon dioxide stores as a result of diving was obtained in instructors, following a 2-year period of diving when compared with data obtained after a 3-month period of no diving. During constant hyperventilation, lasting 1 hour, more carbon dioxide was eliminated and

TABLE 11.2

Effect of daily breath-hold dives during a 6-month period on distribution of carbon dioxide in plasma and red cells (venous blood) of 11 tank instructors

	Plasma				*Red cells*	
HCO_3 mmoles/L	H_3CO_4 mmoles/L	pH		P_{CO_2} mm Hg	HCO_3 mmoles/L	H_2CO_3 mmoles/L
After a 5-month period without water work (control)						
25·1 ± 1·5	1·34 ± 0·09	7·38 ± 0·01		44·7 ± 2·96	16·76 ± 0·87	1·12 ± 0·07
After a 6-month period with heavy water work						
28·3* ± 1·38	1·58* ± 0·18	7·35* ± 0·05		52·7* ± 6·1	18·60* ± 0·67	1·32 ± 0·15

* Differences from controls statistically significant at the 5% level.

TABLE 11.3

Effect of daily breath-hold dives for a period of 6-months on red cell and plasma electrolytes (venous blood) (11 subjects)

	Measured values									Calculated values			
	Whole blood					Plasma				Red cells			
	H$_2$O, g/L	Na, mEq/L	K, mEq/L	Cl, mEq/L	Haematocrit	H$_2$O, g/L	Na, mEq/L	K, mEq/L	Cl, mEq/L.	H$_2$O, g/L	Na, mEq/L	K, mEq/L	Cl, mEq/L
After a 5-month period without water work (control)													
	824 ±12·8	86·8 ±5·0	43·9 ±2·3	84·5 ±2·3	43·0 ±1·9	924 ±7·3	142 ±3·5	4·78 ±0·62	103·5 ±3·5	692 ±27	13·7 ±3·8	95·8 ±15·4	59·2 ±6·6
After a 6-month period with heavy water work													
	811* ±5	86·8 ±2·9	34·6* ±2·4	83·5 ±2·4	44·8 ±2·3	915† ±9·3	133* ±4·4	4·09† ±0·39	103·5 ±1·6	679 20	30·4† ±17·3	72·1* ±5·4	59·4 ±6·9

* Differences from controls statistically significant at the 1% level and better.
† Differences from controls statistically significant at the 5% level.

the end-tidal carbon dioxide tension was significantly elevated in the first condition (Dougherty & Schaefer 1962).

The adaptation to carbon dioxide in breath-hold diving is associated with an adaptation to low oxygen. Experiments with divers breathing low oxygen mixtures demonstrated that they show a lower ventilatory response and are able to utilize oxygen better than non-divers (Schaefer 1965a, b).

During skin diving, carbon dioxide intoxication does not appear to be a major problem and is certainly less likely to occur than in scuba diving. The alveolar and blood carbon dioxide levels are rather low throughout a dive and can easily be controlled by the speed of ascent. Moreover, a lowered sensitivity to carbon dioxide, as a result of adaptation, gives divers an additional protection against the acute toxic effects of carbon dioxide.

The high tolerance to CO_2 has been found to be associated with a reduced autonomic response as indicated in smaller elevations of pulse rate and blood sugar during CO_2 exposure. Blood pressure response to an injection of a cholinergic drug (mecholyl) was measured in a group of 13 divers and 19 laboratory personnel (Schaefer 1965a, b). The divers exhibited a significant smaller fall in blood pressure than the group of laboratory personnel. These findings suggest that the adaptation to breath-hold diving produces a damping effect on the cholinergic system. The stress resistance found in divers is in line with their subjective observations of increased 'relaxation' in the course of prolonged diving training. Song et al. (1963) found that the diving women of Korea had a lower ventilatory response to CO_2 than non-diving women; however, their response to hypoxia was not different.

In the majority of studies in scuba divers adaptation to CO_2 was observed, with the exception of an investigation by Froeb (1961). He compared the respiratory response to carbon dioxide in 16 professional divers using scuba equipment with those of non-divers and did not find any evidence of adaptation to carbon dioxide in the scuba divers. In studies of well-trained underwater swimmers of the US Navy and untrained swimmers (laboratory personnel) using a closed circuit oxygen breathing unit, a higher mean end-tidal carbon dioxide tension was found in the trained swimmers during swims at a speed of 1·1 to 1·8 km/hour (Goff & Bartlett 1957; Goff, Brubach & Specht 1957). During resting conditions under water, differences in end-tidal carbon dioxide tensions were negligible. Findings indicated some degree of adaptation to carbon dioxide in the trained swimmers which perhaps, in part, was related to the noted respiratory pattern with long post-inspiratory pauses. Furthermore, adaptation to increased work of the inspiratory muscles might have contributed to the elevated carbon dioxide tensions in the trained underwater swimmer because it was shown that alveolar carbon dioxide tensions increase linearly with the workload on the inspiratory muscles (Milic-Emili & Tyler 1962).

Lanphier (1963) found in a group of scuba divers end-tidal P_{CO_2} values of 50 mm Hg during moderate exercise underwater at 4 ATA breathing air.

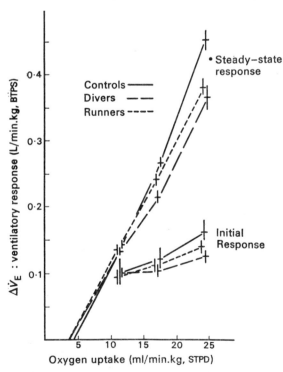

FIG. 11.8. Steady state and initial (neurogenic) ventilatory responses to exercise of the three groups of subjects as a function of $\dot{V}_{O_2}$ (after Lally, Zechman & Tracy 1973)

Some of the 'CO$_2$ retainers' of this group were subsequently studied in more detail and found to show large increases in Pa_{CO2} during moderate exercise in air at normal atmospheric pressure, although they used a low-resistance breathing apparatus.

Broussolle et al. (1968) measured the ventilatory response to increased CO$_2$ concentrations in scuba divers and found a reduction of 30% compared to non-divers. Broussolle et al. (1972) also observed in trained scuba divers a marked reduction in the ventilatory response to different workloads (55, 110 and 165 watts) associated with higher alveolar CO$_2$ values in comparison to non-divers. The CO$_2$ elimination in the trained scuba divers was less, particularly at higher workloads (110 watts). A marked reduction in the CO$_2$ response of trained divers was also found by Varène, Jacquemin and L'Huissier (1972).

Recent studies of exercise hyperpnea in divers, non-divers and runners by Lally, Zechman and Tracy (1974) showed significantly lower steady state ventilatory responses in divers as compared with controls (laboratory personnel) in exercise walking at 10% grade at 1·2 and 3 mph. Moreover, the fast (neural) component of the initial 15-sec ventilatory response was also less in divers. The values for runners were intermediate between divers and sedentary non-divers (Fig. 11.8). Both divers and athletes had higher Pa_{CO2} values and lower R values than the sedentary control group, although divers more so than athletes. End-tidal Pa_{CO2} was about 5 mm Hg higher in divers at different level of exercises as compared to those of sedentary non-divers. Divers showed a markedly slower and deeper breathing pattern than the other two groups. The authors conclude that this unusual ventilatory behaviour is not fitness related and may involve besides a reduced chemosensitivity a conditioned response phenomenon.

REFERENCES

ADAMS, G. M. (1974) Shallow Habitat Air Dive, I: Thirty days at a simulated depth of fifty feet of seawater with excursions between 5 and 235 feet. *Undersea Biochemical Research*, **1**, A30.

ALEXANDER, W. C., LEACH, C. S., FISCHER, C. L., LAMBERTSEN, C. J. & JOHNSON, P. C. (1973) Hematological, biochemical, and immunological studies during a 14 day continuous exposure to 5·2% O$_2$ in N$_2$ at pressure equivalent to 100 FSW (4 ATA). *Aerospace Med.* **44**, 850–854.

BARLOW, H. B. & MACINTOSH, F. C. (1944) *Shallow Water Blackout*. Report, Medical Research, RN Personnel Research Committee, 44/125 UPS 49(a).

BARNARD, E. E. P. (1971) Submarine escape from 600 ft (183 m). *Proc. R. Soc. Med.* **64**, 1271–1273.

BEAN, J. W. (1950) Tensional changes of alveolar gas in reactions to rapid compression and decompression and question of nitrogen narcosis. *Am. J. Physiol.* **16**, 417–425.

BEHNKE, A. R., THOMSON, R. M. & MOTLEY, E. P. (1935) The psychologic effects from breathing air at 4 atmospheres pressure. *Am. J. Physiol.* **112**, 554–558.

BENNETT, P. B. (1963) Neurophysiologic and neuropharmacologic changes in inert gas narcosis. In *Underwater Physiology. Proc. 2nd Symp. Underwater Physiology*, p. 209. Washington, D.C.: Natl Acad. Sci.–Natl Res. Council. (Publ. 1181.)

BENNETT, P. B. & BLENKARN, G. D. (1973) Arterial blood gases in man during inert gas narcosis. *Försvarsmedicin* **9**, 447–451.

BJURSTEDT, H. & HESSER, C. M. (1956) Carbon dioxide exchange during transient exposure to high atmospheric pressure under breath-holding (simulated skin diving to 40 meters). *T. milit. Hälsov* **81**, 183.

BOND, G. F., WORKMAN, R. D. & MAZZONE, W. F. (1960) *Deep Submarine Escape*. Report No. 346. New London, Connecticut: US Naval Medical Research Laboratory.

BRADLEY, M. E. (Ed.) (1974) Sealab. In *Respiratory Limitations of Underwater Breathing Equipment. Report on the Second Undersea Medical Society Workshop*. WS: 4–15–74, p. 1.

BRADLEY, M. E., ANTHONISEN, N. R. VOROSMARTI, J. & LINAWEAVER, P. G. (1971) Respiratory and cardiac responses to exercise in subjects breathing helium–oxygen mixtures at pressures from sea level to 19·2 atmospheres. In: *Underwater Physiology. Proc. 4th Symp. Underwater Physiology*. Ed. C. J. Lambertsen, pp. 325–337, New York: Academic Press.

BRAUER, R. W. (1968) Seeking man's depth level. *Ocean Industry* **3**, 28–33.

BROUSSOLLE, B., BENSIMON, E. MICHAUD, A. & LONJON, I. (1968) Sensibilité ventilatoire au gaz carbonique des plongeurs sous-marins. *J. Physiol.*, Paris, **60**, 410.

BROUSSOLLE, B., BENSIMON, E., MICHAUD, A. & VEGEZZI, C. (1972) Comparaison des reponses ventilatoires et des pressions partielles alveolaires du CO$_2$ de plongeurs sous-marins entraines et de temoins non-plongeurs au cours du travail musculaire en atmosphère hyperbare. In *Proc. Third International Conference on Hyperbaric and Underwater Physiology*. Ed. X. Fructus. pp. 80–87. Paris: Doin.

BROUSSOLLE, B., CHOUTEAU, J., HYACINTHE, R., LE PECHON, J. CL., BURNET, H., BATTESTI, A., CRESSON, D. & IMBERT, G. (1975) Cardiorespiratory function during 1640 ft (51 ATA) helium–oxygen simulated dives. In *Underwater Physiology, Vth Symp. Underwater Physiology*. Ed. C. J. Lambertsen. Bethesda: Fedn Am. Socs exp. Biol.

BUHLMANN, A. A. (1961) La physiologie respiratoire au cours de la plongée sous-marine. *Schweiz. med. Wschr.* **91**, 774.
BUHLMANN, A. A. (1963) Respiratory resistance with hyperbaric gas mixtures. *Proc. 2nd Symp. Underwater Physiology.* pp. 98–107. Washington, D.C.: Natl. Acad. Sci.–Natl Res. Council. (Publ. 1181.)
BUHLMANN, A. A. (1969) Personal communication.
CASE, E. M. & HALDANE, J. B. S. (1941) Human physiology under high pressure. I. Effects of nitrogen, carbon dioxide and cold. *J. Hyg., Camb.* **41**, 225–249.
CRAIG, A. B., JR & HARLEY, A. D. (1968) Alveolar gas exchanges during breath-hold dives. *J. appl. Physiol.* **24**, 182–189.
CRAIG, A. B., JR & MEAD, W. L. (1968) Oxygen consumption and carbon dioxide production during breath-hold diving. *J. appl. Physiol.* **24**, 190–202.
DOELL, D., ZUTTER, M. & ANTHONISON, N. R. (1973) Ventilatory responses to hypercapnia and hypoxia at 1 and 4 ATA. *Resp. Physiol.* **18**, 338–346.
DONALD, K. W. (1970). *A Review of Submarine Escape Trials from 1945 to 1970 with Particular Emphasis on Decompression Sickness.* RN Personnel Research Committee, UPS 290, 1–26.
DOUGHERTY, J. H., JR & SCHAEFER, K. E. (1962) Adjustment of carbon dioxide stores in divers during voluntary hyperventilation. *Fedn Proc. Fedn Am. Socs exp. Biol.* **21**, 441.
DUBOIS, A. B. (1955) Breath-holding. In *Proc. 1st Symp. Underwater Physiology.* Ed. L. G. Goff. P. 90. Washington, D.C.: Natl Acad. Sci.–Natl Res. Council. (Publ. 377.)
DUBOIS, A. B., BOND, G. F. & SCHAEFER, K. E. (1963) Alveolar gas exchange during submarine escape. *J. appl. Physiol.* **18**, 509–512.
EATON, W. J. & HEMPLEMAN, H. V. (1971) *Preliminary Studies to Assess the Feasibility of a Significant Extension in Depth of the Free Ascent Submarine Escape Technique.* Royal Naval Physiol. Lab. Report 3/71, 1–14.
EISELE, J. H., EIEGER, I. I. & MUALLEM, M. (1967) Narcotic properties of carbon dioxide in the dog. *Anesthesiology* **28**, 856.
EKLUND, B., KAIJSER, L. & MELCHER, A. (1973) The effect of CO_2 retention on physical performance under hyperbaric conditions. *Förvarsmedicin* **9**, 221–274.
ELLIOTT, D. H. (1966) Submarine escape: the hood inflation system. *Jl R. nav. med. Serv.* **52**, 120–130.
FAGRAEUS, L. & HESSER, C. M. (1970) Ventilatory response to CO_2 in hyperbaric environments. *Acta physiol. scand.* **80**, 19A–20A.
FAGRAEUS, L. & LINNARSON, D. (1973) Maximal voluntary and exercise ventilation at high ambient pressures. *Förvarsmedicin* **9**, 275–278.
FREEDMAN, S. (1970) Sustained maximum voluntary ventilation. *Resp. Physiol.* **8**, 20–44.
FROEB, H. F. (1961) Ventilatory response of scuba divers to CO_2 inhalations. *J. appl. Physiol.* **16**, 8–10.
FRUCTUS, X., AGARATE, C. & SICARDI, F. (1975) Postponing the High Pressure Nervous Syndrome down to 500 meters and deeper. Study of compression schedules for very deep dives. In *Underwater Physiology. Vth Symp. Underwater Physiology.* Ed. C. J. Lambertsen. Bethesda: Fedn Am. Socs exp. Biol.
GAIT, D. G. & MILLER, K. W. (1973) A novel approach to improved submarine escape performance. *Aerospace Med.* **44**, 645–648.
GOFF, L. G. & BARTLETT, R. G., JR (1957) Elevated end tidal CO_2 in trained underwater swimmers. *J. appl. Physiol.* **10**, 203–206.
GOFF, L. G., BRUBACH, H. G. & SPECHT, H. (1957) Measurement of respiratory responses and work efficiency of underwater swimmers utilizing improved instrumentation. *J. appl. Physiol.* **10**, 197–202.
HÄBISCH, H. (1949) Über den Gaswechsel bei Ruhe und Arbeit unter kurzund langfristiger Kohlensäure-Einwirkung. *Pflügers Arch. Ges. Physiol.* **251**, 594–608.
HAMILTON, R. W. (1974) Deep diving using neon. In *Respiratory Limitations of Underwater Breathing Equipment. Report on the Second Undersea Medical Society Workshop.* Ed. M. E. Bradley. WS: 4–15–74, p. 2.
HAMILTON, R. W., MACINNIS, J. B., NOBLE, A. D. & SCHREINER, H. R. (1965) *Saturation Diving at 650 feet.* Technical Memorandum B-411. Ocean Systems Inc. Tonawanda Research Laboratory, Tonawanda, New York.
HAMILTON, R. W., KENYON, D. J., SCHREINER, H. R. & EDEL, P. O. (1973) Computation and testing of no-stop decompression procedures for use from saturation in a nitrogen–oxygen habitat. Preprints of Annual Scientific Meeting of the Aerospace Med. Ass. pp. 239–240.
HESSER, C. M., ADOLFSON, J. & FAGRAEUS, L. (1971) Role of CO_2 in compressed air narcosis. *Aerospace Med.* **42**, 163–168.
HONG, S. K., RAHN, H., KANG, D. H., SONG, S. H. & KANG, D. S. (1963) Diving pattern, lung volumes, alveolar gas of the Korean diving women (ama). *J. appl. Physiol.* **18**, 457–465.
HONG, S. K., MOORE, T. O., SETO, S., PARK, H. K., HIATT, W. R. & BERNANER, E. M. (1970) Lung volumes and apneic bradycardia in divers. *J. appl. Physiol.* **29**, 689–693.
HONG, S. K., LIN, Y. C., LALLY, D. A., YIM, B. I. B., KOMINAMI, N., HONG, P. W. & MOORE, T. O. (1971) Alveolar gas exchanges and cardiovascular functions during breath-holding with air. *J. appl. Physiol.* **30**, 540–547.
JARRETT, A. S. (1966) Alveolar carbon dioxide tension at increased ambient pressure. *J. appl. Physiol.* **21**, 158–162.
JOHNSON, P. C., DRISCOLL, T. B., ALEXANDER, W. C. & LAMBERTSEN, C. J. (1973) Body fluid volume changes during a 14-day continuous exposure to 5·2% O_2 in N_2 at pressure equivalent to 100 FSW (4 ATA). *Aerospace Med.* **44**, 860–863.
KEREM, D. & SALZANO, J. (1974) Effects of hydrostatic pressure on arterial P_{CO_2}. *Undersea Biomedical Research* **1**, A–25–26.
KURENKOW, H. I. (1973) Human work performance in hyperbaric environment. *Förvarsmedicin* **9**, 332–336.
LALLY, D. A., ZECHMAN, F. W. & TRACY, R. A. (1974) Ventilatory responses to exercise in divers and non-divers. *Resp. Physiol.* **20**, 117–129.
LAMBERTSEN, C. J. (Ed.) (1975) Collaborative investigation of limits of human tolerance to pressurization with helium, neon and nitrogen. Simulation of density equivalent to helium–oxygen respiration at depths to 2000, 3000, 4000

and 5000 feet of sea water. *Underwater Physiology. Vth Symp. Underwater Physiology.* Ed. C. J. Lambertsen. Bethesda: Fedn Am. Socs exp. Biol.

LAMBERTSEN, C. J., GELFAND, R., LEVER, M. J., BODAMMER, G., TAKANO, N., REED, T. A., DICKSON, J. G. & WATSON, P. J. (1973) Respiration and gas exchange during a 14-day continuous exposure to 5·2% O_2 in N_2 at pressure equivalent to 100 FSW (4 ATA). *Aerospace Med.* **44**, 844–849.

LANPHIER, E. H. (1955a) *Nitrogen–oxygen Mixture Physiology. Phases 1 and 2.* Research Report No. 7–55, US Naval Experimental Diving Unit, Washington.

LANPHIER, E. H. (1955b) Use of nitrogen–oxygen mixtures in diving. In *Proc. 1st Symp. Underwater Physiology.* Ed. L. G. Goff., p. 74. Washington, D.C.: Natl Acad. Sci.–Natl Res. Council. (Publ. 377.)

LANPHIER, E. H. (1956) Carbon dioxide retention in working dives breathing nitrogen–oxygen mixtures at depth. *Fedn Proc. Fedn Am. Socs exp. Biol.* **15**, 116.

LANPHIER, E. H. (1963) Influence of increased ambient pressure upon alveolar ventilation. In *Proc. 2nd Symp. Underwater Physiology.* pp. 124–133. Washington, D. C.: Natl Acad. Sci.–Natl Res. Council. (Publ. 1181).

LANPHIER, E. H. (1969) Pulmonary function. In *The Physiology and Medicine of Diving and Compressed Air Work.* Ed. P. B. Bennett and D. H. Elliott, pp. 58–112. London: Ballière, Tindall and Cassell.

LANPHIER, E. H. & BUSBY, D. E. (1962) Alveolar and arterial P_{CO_2} in man under increased ambient pressures. *Proc. 22nd int. Congr. physiol. Sci.*, Vol. II, Abstract No. 301.

LANPHIER, E. H. & RAHN, H. (1963) Alveolar gas exchange during breath-hold diving. *J. appl. Physiol.* **18**, 471–477.

LANPHIER, E. H. & MORIN, R. A. (1961) Effects of gas density on carbon dioxide elimination. *Physiologist* **4**, 63.

LORD, G. P., BOND, G. F. & SCHAEFER, K. E. (1966) Breathing under high ambient pressure. *J. appl. Physiol.* **21**, 1833–1838.

LUFT, U. C., FINKELSTEIN, S. & ELLIOTT, J. C. (1974) Respiratory gas exchange, and acid–base balance and electrolytes during and after maximal work breathing 15 mm Hg $P_{I_{CO_2}}$. In *Carbon dioxide and Metabolic Regulations.* Ed. S. Nahas & K. E. Schaefer. pp. 282–293. New York: Springer.

LUNDGREN, C. (1974) Immersion and negative pressure effects on lung function and inert gas exchange. In *Respiratory Limitations of Underwater Breathing Equipment. Report on the Second Undersea Medical Society Workshop.* Ed. M. E. Bradley. WS: 4–15–74, p. 17.

MCALEAVY, J. C., WAY, W. L., ALLSTATT, A. H. GUADAGNI, N. P. & SEVERINGHAUS, J. W. (1961) The effect of P_{CO_2} on the depth of anaesthesia. *Anesthesiology*, **22**, 260.

MARSHALL, R., LANPHIER, E. H. & DUBOIS, A. B. (1956) Resistance to breathing in normal subjects during simulated dives. *J. appl. Physiol.* **9**, 4–10.

MEAD, J. (1955) Resistance to breathing at increased ambient pressures. *Proc. 1st Symp. Underwater Physiology.* Ed. L. G. Goff, p. 112. Washington, D.C.: Natl Acad. Sci.–Natl Res. Council. (Publ. 377.)

MENN, S. J., SINCLAIR, R. D. & WELCH, B. E. (1970) Effects of inspired P_{CO_2} to 30 mm Hg on responses to normal man to exercise. *J. appl Physiol.* **28**, 663–771.

MILES, S. (1957) *Oxygen Syncope.* Report, Medical Research Council. RN Personnel Research Committee, RNP 57/880, UPS 161.

MILIC-EMILI, J. & TYLER, J. M. (1962) Relationship between arterial P_{CO_2} and work of breathing in man. *Fedn Proc. Fedn Am. Socs exp. Biol.* **21**, 445.

MILLER, J. N., WANGENSTEEN, O. D. & LANPHIER, E. H. (1971) Ventilatory limitations on exertion at depth. In *Underwater Physiology. Proc. 4th Symp. Underwater Physiology.* Ed. C. J. Lambertsen. pp. 317–323. New York: Academic Press.

MILLER, J. W. & LAMBERTSEN, C. J. (1971) Project Tektite: An open sea study of prolonged exposure to a nitrogen–oxygen environment at increased ambient pressure. In *Underwater Physiology. Proc. 4th Symp. Underwater Physiology.* Ed. C. J. Lambertsen. pp. 551–558.

MORRISON, J. B., BENNETT, P. B., BARNARD, E. E. P. & EATON, W. J. (1975) Physiological studies during a deep simulated oxygen–helium dive to 1500 feet. In *Underwater Physiology. Vth Symp. Underwater Physiology.* Ed. C. J. Lambertsen. Bethesda: Fedn Am. Socs exp. Biol.

MUREN, A. & WULFF, K. (1972) CO_2 distribution in the divers' helmet. In *Proceedings of the Third International Conference on Hyperbaric and Underwater Physiology.* Ed. X. Fructus. pp. 99–100, Paris: Doin.

MURRAY, R. D. (1974) Shallow Habitat Air Dive I. Effect on selected hematological constituents. *Undersea Biomedical Research* **1**, A31.

OVERFIELD, E. M., SALTZMAN, H. A., KYLSTRA, J. A. & SALZANO, J. V. (1969) Respiratory gas exchange in normal men breathing 0·9% oxygen in helium at 31·3 ATA. *J. appl. Physiol.* **27**, 471–475.

PAULEV, P. E. (1969) Respiratory and cardiovascular effects of breath-holding. *Acta physiol. scand.* Suppl. 324. 1–116.

PROCTOR, L. D., CAREY, C. R., LEE, R. M., SCHAEFER, K. E. & ENDE, H. van den (1972) Electroencephalographic changes during saturation excursion dives to a simulated sea water depth of 1000 feet. *Aerospace Med.* **43**, 867–877.

RAHN, H. & YOKOYAMA, T. (Eds) (1965) *Physiology of Breath-hold Diving and the Ama of Japan.* Publication 1341, pp. 113–137. Washington, D.C.: Natl Acad. Sci.

RASHBASS, C. (1955) *The Unimportance of Carbon Dioxide as a cause of Nitrogen Narcosis.* Report, Medical Research Council. RN Personnel Research Committee, UPS 153.

SALTZMAN, H. A. (1974) Effects of altered environment at simulated depths on gas exchange. In *Respiratory Limitations of Underwater Breathing Equipment. Report on the Second Undersea Medical Society Workshop.* Ed. M. E. Bradley. WS: 4–15–74, p. 17.

SALTZMAN, H. A., SALZANO, J. V., BLENKARN, G. D. & KYLSTRA, J. A. (1971) Effects of pressure on ventilation and gas exchange in man. *J. appl. Physiol.* **30**, 433–49.

SALZANO, J. V., RAUSCH, J. V. & SALTZMAN, H. A. (1970) Cardiorespiratory responses to exercises at a simulated seawater depth of 1000 feet. *J. appl. Physiol.* **28**, 34–41.

SCHAEFER, K. E. (1949) Atmung und Saure Basengleichgewicht bei Langdauerndem Aufenthalt in 3% CO_2. *Pflügers Arch. ges. Physiol.* **251**, 689–715.

SCHAEFER, K. E. (1955) The role of carbon dioxide in the physiology of human diving. In *Proc. 1st Symp. Underwater Physiology*. Ed. L. G. Goff. pp. 131–139. Washington, D.C.: Natl Acad. Sci.–Natl Res. Council. (Publ. 377.)

SCHAEFER, K. E. (1958) Respiratory pattern and respiratory response to CO_2. *J. appl Physiol.* **8**, 524–531.

SCHAEFER, K. E. (1965a) *Handbook of Physiology. Section 2: Circulation.* Ed. W. F. Hamilton & P. Dow. Volume III, Chapter 51, pp. 1843–1873. Washington D.C.: American Physiological Society.

SCHAEFER, K. E. (1965b) Adaptation to breath-hold diving. In *Physiology of Breath-hold Diving and the Ama of Japan*. Publication 1314, pp. 237–251. Washington, D.C.: Natl Acad. Sci.

SCHAEFER, K. E. (1967) Diving physiology. In *McGraw-Hill Yearbook Science and Technology*. Ed. D. I. Eggenberger. p. 1. New York: McGraw-Hill.

SCHAEFER, K. E. (Ed.) (1972) CO_2 effects on consciousness. In *Environmental Effects on Consciousness*, p. 96, New York: MacMillan.

SCHAEFER, K. E. (1974) Metabolic aspects of adaptation to carbon dioxide. In *Carbon Dioxide and Metabolic Regulations*. Ed. G. Nahas & K. E. Schaefer. pp. 253–265. New York: Springer.

SCHAEFER, K. E. & CAREY, C. R. (1962) Alveolar pathways during 90 foot breath hold dives. *Science, N.Y.* **137**, 1051–1052.

SCHAEFER, K. E., CAREY, C. R. & DOUGHERTY, J. (1970) Pulmonary gas exchange and urinary electrolyte excretion during saturation excursion diving to pressures equivalent to 800 and 1000 feet of sea water. *Aerospace Med.* **41**, 856–864.

SCHAEFER, K. E., NICHOLS, G., JR & CAREY, C. R. (1964) Acid-base balance and blood and urine electrolytes of man during acclimatization to CO_2. *J. appl. Physiol.* **19**, 48–58.

SCHAEFER, K. E., HASTINGS, B. J., CAREY, C. R. & NICHOLS, G., JR (1963) Respiratory acclimatization to carbon dioxide. *J. appl. Physiol.* **18**, 1071–1078.

SCHAEFER, K. E., ALLISON, R. D., CAREY, C. R. & STRAUSS, R. (1972) *The Effects of Simulated Breath-holding Dives in the Dry and Wet Chambers on Blood Shifts into the Thorax.* Submarine Medical Research Laboratory Departmental Report 729.

SCHAEFER, K. E., BOND, G. F., MAZZONE, W. F., CAREY, C. R. & DOUGHERTY, J. H. (1968a) *Carbon Dioxide Retention During Prolonged Exposure to High Pressure Environment.* Report No. 520, US Naval Submarine Medical Center, Groton, Conn.

SCHAEFER, K. E., ALLISON, R. D., DOUGHERTY, I. H., JR, CAREY, C. R., WALKER, R., YOST, F. & PARKER, D. (1968b) Pulmonary and circulatory adjustments determining the limits of depths in breath-hold diving. *Science, N.Y.*, **162**, 1020–1023.

SCHOLANDER, P. F., HAMMEL, H. T., LE MESSURIER, H., HEMMINGSEN, E. & CAREY, W. (1962) Circulatory adjustment in pearl divers. *J. appl. Physiol.* **17**, 184–190.

SEUSING, J. & DRUBE, H. C. (1960) The significance of hypercapnia for the occurrence of depth intoxication. *Klin. Wschr.* **38**, 1088–1090.

SEVERINGHAUS, J. S. (1974) In *Carbon Dioxide and Metabolic Regulations*. Ed. G. Nahas & K. E. Schaefer. pp. 138–143. New York: Springer.

SHEPARD, R. J. (1967) The maximum sustained voluntary ventilation in exercise. *Clin. Sci.* **32**, 167–176.

SINCLAIR, R. D., CLARK, J. M. & WELCH, B. E. (1971) Comparison of physiological responses of normal man to exercise in air and in acute and chronic hypercapnia. In *Underwater Physiology. Proc. 4th Symp. Underwater Physiology*. Ed. C. J. Lambertsen. pp. 409–417. New York: Academic Press.

SONG, S. H., KANG, D. H., KANG, B. S. & HONG, S. K. (1963) Lung volumes and ventilatory response to high carbon dioxide and low oxygen in the ama. *J. appl. Physiol.* **18**, 466–470.

STORRIE, M. (1974) Mark II DDS—1010 foot open sea dive. In *Respiratory Limitations of Underwater Breathing Equipment. Report on the Second Undersea Medical Society Workshop*. Ed. M. E. Bradley. WS: 4–15–74, p. 1.

STRAUSS, R. H., WRIGHT, W. B., PETERSON, R. E., LEVER, M. J. & LAMBERTSEN, C. J. (1975) In *Underwater Physiology. Vth Symp. Underwater Physiology*. Ed. C. J. Lambertsen. Bethesda: Fedn Am. Socs exp. Biol.

TIBES, K. & STEGEMANN, I. (1969) Das Verhalten der endexpiratorischen Atemgas-Drucke, der O_2 Aufnahme und CO_2 Abgabe nach einfacher Apnoe in Wasser, auf Land und apnoeischen Tancker. *Pflügers Arch. ges Physiol.* **311**, 300–311.

VARÈNE, P., JACQUEMIN Ch. & L'HUISSIER, J. (1972) Les performances ventilatoires en plongée. In *Proc. Third International Conference on Hyperbaric and Underwater Physiology*. Ed. X. Fructus. pp. 88–94. Paris: Doin.

WRIGHT, B. (1974) Physiological testing of an air and helium hard-hat system and a closed circuit underwater breathing apparatus. In *Respiratory Limitations of Underwater Breathing Equipment. Report on the Second Undersea Medical Society Workshop*. Ed. M. E. Bradley. WS: 4–15–74, p. 8.

WOOD, L. D. H. & BRYAN, A. C. (1970) Respiratory sensitivity to CO_2 at increased ambient pressure. *Physiologist* **13**, 348.

WOOD, L. D. H. & BRYAN, A. C. (1971) Mechanical limitations of exercise ventilation at increased ambient pressure. In *Underwater Physiology. Proc. 4th Symp. Underwater Physiology*. Ed. C. J. Lambertsen. pp. 307–316.

12

Inert Gas Narcosis

P. B. BENNETT

It is now widely recognized by those associated with a hyperbaric environment that men and animals exposed to raised pressures of air exhibit signs and symptoms of narcosis and intoxication. The literature on this subject has grown enormously, especially in the last decade. For this reason a complete survey of all the relevant data is not possible in this chapter. However, additional reviews of this subject may be found elsewhere to complement the major and contemporary aspects of the narcosis problem which are considered in the chapter that follows (Rinfret & Doebbler 1961; Featherstone & Muehlbaecher 1963; Roth 1965; Welch & Robertson 1965; Bennett 1965a, 1966, 1973; Albano 1970; Lambertsen 1971).

SIGNS AND SYMPTOMS OF COMPRESSED AIR INTOXICATION

Among the first to report the occurrence of the narcosis was Junod, a Frenchman, who in 1835 noted that when breathing compressed air 'the functions of the brain are activated, imagination is lively, thoughts have a peculiar charm and, in some persons, symptoms of intoxication are present'. A little later Green (1861) described a feeling of sleepiness, accompanied by hallucinations and impaired judgement which in his estimation merited the immediate return of the diver to the safety of the surface. Another Frenchman, Paul Bert (1878), who is well known for his work in the areas of oxygen toxicity and decompression sickness, also alluded briefly to the narcotic properties of air when breathed at increased pressures.

Similar signs and symptoms were further observed by Hill and McLeod (1903) in caisson workers (or sand hogs as they are known in North America) breathing air at 5·5 ATA (150 ft). Almost 30 years later Damant (1930) noted that divers at 10 ATA (300 ft) were abnormal mentally and suffered a loss of memory. At similar depths, Hill and Phillips (1932) found that deep divers experienced difficulty in assimilating facts and making rapid decisions which they summarized as a 'slowing of the process of cerebration'. The reports of this decade were, in the main, the result of a committee appointed by the Royal Navy to study the problems of deep diving and submarine escape (Hill et al. 1933). Among their studies was a phenomenon entitled 'semi-loss of consciousness', which referred to a lapse of consciousness of the diver in 17 of 58 dives to 11 to 7·6 ATA (330 to 220 ft). Normal hand signals were acknowledged but not acted upon and amnesia of the events during the dive was common on return to the surface. Consciousness, however, returned rapidly during the decompression. A number of efforts were made to eradicate the condition, including flushing the helmet with air to remove retained carbon dioxide and the lowering of lights, plus psychological screening of the men, but they met with little or no success. At that time Hill and Phillips (1932) suggested that the cause of the mental dullness, loss of memory and difficulty in making decisions, accompanied by a dangerous overconfidence, might be due to impurities in the breathing air originating from faulty compressors.

The first inference that the nitrogen constituent

of compressed air is responsible for the narcosis was given a few years later by Behnke, Thomson and Motley (1935). They concluded that compressed air at pressures higher than 3 ATA (66 ft) exerts a narcosis characterized by 'euphoria, retardation of the higher mental processes and impaired neuromuscular coordination'. As a pressure of 4 ATA (100 ft) was reached, their divers experienced a feeling of stimulation, excitement and euphoria, occasionally accompanied by laughter and loquacity. There was a slowing of mental activity and responses to visual, auditory, olfactory and tactile stimuli were delayed, together with a limitation of the powers of association and a tendency to fixation of ideas. Memory was impaired and concentration difficult. Errors were made in recording data and arithmetical calculations and fine movements were more difficult. Intellectual functions were generally affected more severely than manual dexterity. These signs and symptoms occurred at the beginning of exposure to compressed air and did not appreciably change over periods of exposure as long as 3 hours. On decompression recovery was rapid.

At 4 ATA (100 ft) Behnke, Thomson and Motley (1935) found that increased effort could counteract the deleterious narcosis but at 10 ATA (300 ft) the signs and symptoms amounted to stupefaction with greatly impaired muscular activity.

These signs and symptoms of narcosis show similarity with those due to alcohol, hypoxia and the early stages of anaesthesia. Indeed, exposure to depths greater than 300 ft may result in loss of consciousness and at sufficient pressure there is little doubt compressed air could be used as an anaesthetic. As might therefore be expected, there is a wide individual susceptibility. Whereas one diver is not narcotic at pressures as high as 6 ATA (165 ft), another will be quite severely affected at only 4 ATA (100 ft). In this connection emotionally stable individuals are usually affected to a smaller extent than less stable subjects (Cousteau 1953).

There are also many other factors which potentiate the signs and symptoms of narcosis such as alcohol, fatigue, hard work, apprehension and any increase in exogenous or endogenous carbon di-

oxide. Frequent exposure to compressed air affords some adaptation.

EFFECTS OF COMPRESSED AIR ON PERFORMANCE

Since the first efforts of Shilling and Willgrube (1937) there have been many attempts to quantify this impairment of mental and physical capabilities (Case & Haldane 1941; Bennett & Glass 1961; Kiessling & Maag, 1962; Albano, Criscuoli & Ciulla 1962; Frankenhaeuser, Graff-Lonnevig & Hesser 1963; Adolfson 1964; Bennett 1967, 1971; Dickson, Lambertsen & Cassils 1971; Criscuoli & Albano 1971; Adolfson, Goldberg & Berghage 1972). These results indicate an increasing decrement in performance with increasing air pressure which is first apparent at 4 ATA (100 ft).

Shilling and Willgrube (1937) examined the effects of air between 3·7 and 10 ATA (90 and 300 ft) on 46 men performing addition, multiplication, subtraction and division, recording the time taken and the number of errors. Further tests used were reaction time and letter cancellation.

The results, besides providing the first quantitative evidence of the narcotic properties of compressed air, also supported earlier qualitative observations that experienced workers and individuals of high intelligence are less affected and that the severest signs and symptoms are on immediately reaching the desired pressure (Table 12.1). In addition rapid compression was found to potentiate the narcosis.

Arithmetical efficiency and manual dexterity were studied by Case and Haldane (1941) on divers breathing air at 8·6 and 10 ATA (250 ft and 300 ft). Among other factors investigated were the effects of varying nitrogen and oxygen partial pressures and the presence of carbon dioxide and cold, together with the action of other physiologically inert gases, such as argon, helium and hydrogen. At 8·6 ATA (250 ft) manual skill was virtually unaffected but errors in arithmetic increased from 6 on the surface to 22 at pressure. At 10 ATA (300 ft) the narcosis was severe and appeared during compression, reaching a maximum in 2 minutes with marked impairment of practical ability and judgement. During continued exposure at this depth, the narcosis was no worse, in

TABLE 12.1

Effect of pressure on psychometric tests (Shilling & Willgrube 1937)

Pressure (ft)	0	90	100	125	150	175	200	225	250	275	300
Mean extra time to solve problems (sec)	0·35	11·09	6·89	7·65	9·74	11·95	13·98	17·17	26·07	26·53	31·42
Mean extra errors in solving problems	0·18	0·86	0·49	0·42	0·72	0·84	1·22	0·88	2·18	2·66	3·02
Mean decrease in numbers crossed out	—	−0·59	−0·09	−2·26	−2·30	−2·49	−2·55	−4·24	−5·85	−6·43	−8·74
Average reaction time (sec)	0·214	—	—	—	0·237	—	0·242	—	0·248	—	2·257
Mean extra time to solve problems (acclimatized subjects)	1·64	2·55	3·42	3·91	4·66	8·00	11·75	15·73	16·33	17·09	24·36

fact there was some adaptation and on decompression recovery was rapid with no after effects except occasional amnesia to events while at depth.

In the next few years there were no further studies of note. Then in 1955 Rashbass tested two figures by one figure multiplication ability in men at 8·5 ATA (250 ft) in a study of the role of carbon dioxide as the cause of the narcosis. At atmospheric pressure the 26 divers achieved a mean number of problems correct of 24·12 which deteriorated at depth to only 16·81. Using the same test at 7 ATA (200 ft) Bennett and Glass (1961) measured a mean decrement from 20·34 to 15·67.

More recently Fowler and Ackles (1972) have used a paced arithmetic task in which problems are presented at a predetermined rate adjusted so that each individual produces some 25% errors at atmospheric pressure.

Kiessling and Maag (1962) have criticized the use of multiplication, letter cancellation and tests of gross motor skill. However, the arithmetic test, consisting of two figures by one figure multiplication problems excluding noughts, ones, fives and multiples of eleven has been used extensively with considerable success. The score used is the number of problems attempted and the number correct in 2 minutes.

As alternatives, Kiessling and Maag used choice reaction time, an involved test of mechanical dexterity based on the Purdue Pegboard and a test of conceptual reasoning. These studies were carried out only at the relatively low pressure of 4 ATA (100 ft). The results showed decrements of 33·46% in reasoning ability, 20·85% in reaction time and 7·9% in manual dexterity. The length of

time spent at pressure did not seem to significantly affect the narcosis (Fig. 12.1).

Similar experiments were performed by Bennett and Towse (1971) during one hour at 6·4, 7·0, 7·7 ATA (180 ft, 200 ft, and 220 ft) in subjects breathing compressed air using such tests as the Ball Bearing, Purdue Pegboard, Wechsler Bellevue Digit Symbol and Arithmetic test also without apparent indication of adaptation. This is not so surprising when one considers that during an exposure at 4 ATA (100 ft) for 14 days, the Ames Crew Evaluator, which tests the efficiency of short-term memory, indicated that adaptation started at 5 days and only by the eighth or ninth day were the results no different from pre-dive controls (Coler, Patton & Lamkin, 1971).

It is apparent, however, that there is a need for much more quantitative study into adaptation and the effects of pressures between the minimum and maximum limits of compressed air diving.

In this regard, Poulton, Catton and Carpenter (1964) suggest that mental impairment can occur at pressures considerably less than 4 ATA (100 ft) and even as low as 2 to 3 ATA (33 to 66 ATA). This is based on evidence obtained from 34 caisson workers performing a card-sorting test. Each man was required to sort packs of playing cards as quickly as possible into the four suits. Among factors measured were the mean rate of sorting and the mean percentage of very slow responses in which there was a gap of 2·3 sec or longer between sorting the cards. Novices did not seem to do as well when exposed to pressure as those who had familiarized themselves with the test beforehand. Once the task had been practised there was no

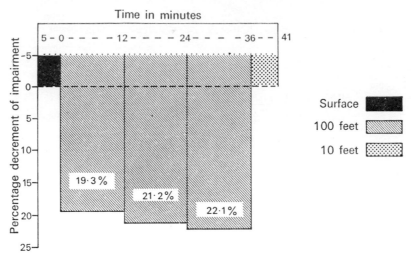

F IG. 12.1. Effect of time at 4 ATA (100 ft) on the mean loss of performance efficiency while carrying out tests of reaction time, mechanical dexterity and reasoning (Kiessling & Maag 1962)

performance decrement, even at pressures as high as 3·5 ATA (80 ft).

Since other factors could have been responsible besides the raised nitrogen partial pressure, the experiments were subsequently repeated with 80 naval subjects at 2 ATA (33 ft) and 4 ATA (100 ft) breathing either air, oxygen–helium or the same oxygen partial pressure as at depth (Bennett et al. 1967). In this double-blind experiment, the only significant deterioration in performance was in the men breathing compressed air at 100 ft, regardless of experience at the task. It was therefore concluded that the minimal partial pressure of nitrogen likely to produce an effective deterioration of performance is 3·2 ATS or that in air at 100 ft. No doubt there are very sensitive tests which, under the right conditions, will show evidence of quantitive narcosis but it would seem that such evidence is but of academic interest. Emphasis as to the difficulty of applying performance tests is shown from the work of Miles and Mackay (1959) who applied tests of arithmetic and memory to divers in the water at 6·4 ATA (180 ft), rather than in a pressure chamber.

It may be predicted, due to an increased synergistic carbon dioxide tension as a result of the breathing equipment and work of swimming, that the narcosis would be more severe in actual diving as compared with simulated pressure chamber exposures (Baddeley 1966; Davis et al. 1972). However, such was not the case in the experiments of Miles and Mackay (1959). No significant evidence of narcosis was in fact obtained, which fails to agree with the majority of findings of a quantitative decrement at 4 ATA (100 ft).

Many of these discrepancies are due to the ad hoc nature of such studies, for the dives were often primarily made to test decompression schedules or obtain other data. Further problems are the many variables of gas partial pressures, temperature, rate of compression, type, age and training of the divers and the effects of motivation and learning. With the increasing interest in this area of diving physiology and psychology it is hoped more reliable information will be obtained in the future. There is, for example, increasing interest in the deep limits of compressed air diving due to the operational requirements to reach the continental shelf with a depth of some 600 to 800 ft. However, greater standardization of the tests used by different groups is much needed, so that the results may be better correlated. At present there is a proliferation of tests, which permits little comparison of the data.

As stated earlier, it is widely believed that the limit of compressed air diving due to the hazards of narcosis is 10 ATA (300 ft). Studies of the narcosis at 4, 7, 10 and 13 ATA (100, 200, 300 and 400 ft) have emphasized the severity of the narcosis at pressures exceeding 10 ATA (300 ft) (Adolfson 1964, 1965; Adolfson & Muren 1965). Using tests of manual dexterity, attention, visual discrimination, reaction time and arithmetic, some 30 or more men were exposed to the even higher air pressure of 13 ATA (400 ft). At this depth the standard of the test of manual dexterity was reduced by 35·3% and the number of arithmetic sums correct was reduced by 61·6% with 25% more errors. Orders were appreciated but ignored. Voice reverberation and an increased intensity of vision and hearing were noted. Among the many other features were a sense of impending blackout, euphoria and dizziness, manic or depressive states, a sense of levitation, disorganization of the sense of time, and changes in facial appearance. Repeated exposure to 13 ATA (400 ft) resulted in remarkable acclimatization. These signs and symptoms were significantly greater than those found at 10 ATA (300 ft) and are more typical of those due to psychedelic drugs such as LSD, rather than alcohol, the customary analogy to narcosis.

Recently Adolfson, Goldberg and Berghage (1972) have quantified the dizziness and vertigo during exposure to increased pressures of air by means of statometry. Body sway measurements indicated in experiments to 10 ATA (300 ft) that there is a quadratic relationship between deteriorating balance and increasing depth.

It is, however, possible to be exposed to such pressures or even deeper without undue narcosis, provided the compression is rapid and the exposure brief. Normally rapid compression potentiates compressed air narcosis due to carbon dioxide retention (Shilling & Willgrube 1937; Bean 1950; Albano 1962; Adolfson 1964; Bennett 1965a), but if insufficient time is spent at depth to permit the critical concentration of nitrogen necessary for narcosis to accumulate in the brain, narcosis does not occur. Thus compression of 10 divers to 13 ATA (400 ft) and 16 ATA (500 ft) in 20 sec, followed by decompression 40 sec later, showed only a 15 to 16% decrease in two choice reaction times at 16 ATA and no significant change at 13 ATA (Bennett, Dossett & Ray 1964; Bennett 1966). One of the subjects at 16 ATA reported a hallucination of drinking a glass of beer and most of the men reported mild dizziness.

As with rapid compression, carbon dioxide retention is also believed responsible for the potentiating action of high-oxygen partial pressures (Hesser 1963; Frankenhaeuser, Graff-Lonnevig & Hesser 1963) by blocking the carbon dioxide carrying capacity of the blood (Gesell 1923).

In this connection, Frankenhaeuser, Graff-Lonnevig and Hesser (1963) used simple and four choice reaction times together with mirror drawing to study the narcotic effect of varying oxygen partial pressures at a constant nitrogen partial pressure of 3·9 ATA (100 ft). Their results showed that oxygen significantly potentiated nitrogen narcosis (Table 12.2). Work on the insect *Drosophila* even goes so far as to suggest that the synergistic action is the direct result of oxygen rather than an indirect action of carbon dioxide (Fenn 1965).

It does not, however, follow that decreasing the oxygen partial pressure will decrease the narcosis.

TABLE 12.2

Effect on 12 divers of the action of different oxygen partial pressures on the narcosis caused by a constant nitrogen partial pressure (Frankenhaeuser, Graff-Lonnevig & Hesser 1963; Hesser 1963)

| Test of narcosis | O_2 ATS | 0·2 | 0·94 | 0·22 | 1·03 | 2·60 |
	N_2 ATS	0·74	—	3·92	3·91	3·94
Simple reaction time (sec)		0·243	0·242	0·241	0·248	0·256
Choice reaction time (sec)		0·671	0·683	0·685	0·691	0·698
Mirror drawing time (sec)		9·16	9·25	9·47	9·24	8·93
Mirror drawing errors (sec)		2·89	2·85	3·39	3·11	3·34

TABLE 12.3

Comparison of the narcosis caused by breathing either air or a 96/4 nitrogen/oxygen mixture in divers at 10 ATA using an arithmetic test (Albano, Criscuoli & Ciulla 1962)

	Sums attempted			Percentage of errors				
Subject	(1) Ambient pressure	(2) 10 ATS air	(3) 10 ATS 96%, N_2, 4% O_2	(4) Ambient pressure	(5) 10 ATS air	(6) 10 ATS 96% N_2, 4% O_2	Difference (5)–(4)	(6)–(5)
A.G.	23	18	12	4·35	22·2	41·6	17·85	19·4
P.V.	24	19	15	4·25	79	86·6	74·75	7·6
R.S.	50	43	33	—	23	21·8	23·00	− 1·2
M.E.	40	20	14	10	30	42·8	20·00	12·8
S.V.	36	32	28	28	53·6	71·4	25·60	17·8
C.B.	27	24	20	7·4	50	60	42·60	10·0
C.U.	45	34	30	—	26·4	30	26·40	3·6
							$M = 32.88$	10·0
							$t = 4.30$	4·20
							$P = < 0.01$	< 0.01

For example Albano, Criscuoli and Ciulla (1962), using visual memory and arithmetic tests, found that seven subjects at 10 ATA (300 ft) breathing 96% nitrogen and 4% oxygen were quantitatively more narcotic than those breathing air (Table 12.3). Similar results were also obtained by Barnard, Hempleman and Trotter (1962) in divers performing arithmetic tasks at 10 ATA (300 ft) breathing either air or 95% nitrogen and 5% oxygen. However, reduction of the oxygen partial pressure at a constant nitrogen partial pressure does decrease the narcosis.

INERT GAS NARCOSIS

The narcosis due to breathing compressed air is not an isolated phenomenon. The noble or so-called rare gases cause the same signs and symptoms but vary in their potency (Behnke & Yarbrough 1939; Lawrence, Loomis, Tobias & Turpin 1946; Marshall & Fenn 1950; Marshall 1951; Carpenter 1953, 1954, 1955, 1956; Rinfret & Doebbler 1961; Bennett 1966, 1975; Ackles & Fowler 1971; Fowler & Ackles 1971). Many attempts have been made to correlate the narcotic potency of helium, neon, argon, krypton and xenon to properties such as lipid solubility, partition coefficients and molecular weight (Behnke & Yarbrough 1939), adsorption coefficients (Case & Haldane 1941),

thermodynamic activity (Ferguson 1939; Brink & Posternak 1948) and the formation of clathrates (Miller 1961; Pauling 1961). By far the most satisfactory correlation is, however, afforded by lipid solubility (Table 12.4).

Thus xenon is an anaesthetic at atmospheric pressure (Lawrence et al. 1964; Lazarev, Lyublina & Madorskaya 1948; Cullen & Gross 1951; Featherstone 1960; Pittinger 1962), krypton causes dizziness (Lawrence et al. 1946; Cullen & Gross 1951) and argon is narcotically some twice as potent as nitrogen (Table 12.5) (Behnke & Yarbrough 1939; Ackles & Fowler 1971; Bennett 1975).

Helium

Helium is not narcotic and for this reason is used for deep diving and saturation diving techniques (Weybrew, Greenwood & Parker 1964; Schreiner et al. 1966; Bowen, Anderson & Promisel 1966; Bennett & Towse 1971b; Fructus, Brauer & Naquet 1971). However, there are a number of disadvantages in the use of this gas such as voice distortion, the high thermal conductivity requiring the use of heated diving suits and the storage and expense of the gas. In addition recent experiments suggest there are circumstances at pressures greater than 10 to 13 ATA (300 to 400 ft) which result in the high pressure nervous

TABLE 12.4

Correlation of narcotic potency of the inert gases hydrogen, oxygen and carbon dioxide with lipid solubility and other physical characteristics

Gas	Molecular weight	Sol. in lipid	Temp. °C	Oil–water sol. ratio	Relative narcotic potency
					(least narcotic)
He	4	0·015	37°	1·7	4·26
Ne	20	0·019	37·6°	2·07	3·58
H_2	2	0·036	37°	2·1	1·83
N_2	28	0·067	37°	5·2	1
A	40	0·14	37°	5·3	0·43
Kr	83·7	0·43	37°	9·6	0·14
Xe	131·3	1·7	37°	20·0	0·039
					(most narcotic)
O_2	32	0·11	40°	5·0	
CO_2	44	1·34	40°	1·6	

TABLE 12.5

Cortical visual evoked response (VER) and performance test during first 7 minutes at 150 ft (Bennett & Towse 1972)

Test	Percentage change from surface in 20/80 oxy-argon	Percentage change from surface in air
VER	−21·9 ± 6·87	−20·1 ± 8·05
Arithmetic correct	−62·1 ± 6·54	−28·6 ± 8·80
Arithmetic attempted	−47·6 ± 8·88	−22·9 ± 6·76
Visual analogy	−33·3 ± 5·22	−0·42 ± 2·57
Ball bearing	−18·1 ± 8·91	−00·6 ± 6·89

syndrome (HPNS) which is discussed in the next chapter. The signs and symptoms of the HPNS include tremors, a marked increase in theta activity (4 to 7 c/sec) in the electrical activity of the brain, with suppression of fast frequencies, possibly accompanied by periods of somnolence in man and convulsions in animals, which seems due to the combined effect of rate of compression and the degree of hydrostatic pressure.

However, performance tests by Bennett and Towse (1971b) during a 46 ATA (1500 ft) simulated oxygen–helium dive showed that arithmetical ability was unaffected, although motor efficiency was depressed due to the hand tremors. Based on lipid solubilities, if helium were narcotic the signs and symptoms should have been similar or worse than compressed air at 10 ATA (300 ft). In fact, as discussed later in connection with the mechanism of narcosis, the failure of helium to adsorp to lipid membranes, regardless of solubility (Bennett, Papahadjopoulos & Bangham 1967) makes it unlikely that helium is a narcotic and the same applies to neon (see Fig. 12.4).

Neon

Neon is an alternative to helium of increasing contemporary interest but its high density relative to helium will cause respiratory embarrassment at much lower pressures. On the basis of animal studies, Marshall (1951) predicted that this gas would be at least three times less narcotic than nitrogen which in later years was found to agree well with the lipid solubility correlations (Ikels 1964).

The first performance tests on man were made by Hamilton et al. (1966) at 19 ATA (600 ft) using a standard pursuit rotor which demonstrated no deterioration. Similar experiments and results were obtained by Bennett (1966) at 10 ATA (300 ft) and Townsend, Thompson and Sulg (1971) at 30 ATA (1000 ft). Lambertsen (1975) studied the effects of breathing neon at 37 ATA (1200 ft) and no narcosis.

In 1970 and 1971 Schreiner, Hamilton and

Langley (1972) made the first parametric comparison of the effect of neon, nitrogen and helium on performance and neurophysiological measurements such as the auditory evoked response in dives to 7, 10 and 13 ATA (200, 300 and 400 ft) with 10% oxygen and 16 and 19 ATA (500 and 600 ft) with 7% oxygen. These studies again confirmed the lack of narcotic properties for helium and neon.

Hydrogen

Hydrogen is a further physiologically inert gas which has been considered and used for deep diving (Case & Haldane, 1941; Zetterstrom 1948; Bjurstedt & Severin, 1948; Zaltsman 1961, 1968). It is however explosive in mixtures of more than 4% oxygen and recent work (Brauer et al. 1966; Brauer, Way & Perry 1968; Brauer et al. 1971) has established that its narcotic potency is in agreement with its lipid solubility. With a relative narcotic potency of 1·83 (see Table 12.4) it is more narcotic than either helium or neon but less narcotic than nitrogen.

Brauer et al. (1971) showed that the addition of hydrogen to a helium–oxygen mixture delayed to a greater depth the onset of many of the signs and symptoms of the HPNS. Nitrogen and nitrous oxide had a similar effect. This stimulated further interest in hydrogen as a diving gas.

Thus Chouteau (1971) exposed 5 rabbits to 29 ATA (908 ft) but after 7 to 12 hours all had died. Zaltsman and his co-workers (Zaltsman 1968) compressed mice in hydrogen to 50 to 90 ATA (1654 to 3000 ft) and convulsions occurred as with helium, but deeper. A number of the animals died. Conversely Brauer et al. (1971) were successful in exposing monkeys to 58 ATA (1900 ft) for 24 hours with no difficulty and 8 further monkeys survived 6 to 20 hrs at 60 to 75 ATA (2000 to 2500 ft) and mice to 90 ATA (3000 ft). A possible reason for the discrepancy is lack of chamber heating, which may have caused the deaths.

In further studies, Rostain and Naquet (1972) compressed two monkeys to 31 ATA (1000 ft) for 24 hours resulting in convulsions and early EEG changes. The COMEX group in Marseille exposed a baboon three times in a month to oxy-hydrogen at 31, 51 and 66 ATA (1000 ft, 1650 ft and 2200 ft).

Convulsions occurred at the latter depth breathing either hydrogen or helium, and hydrogen did not, as suggested earlier, seem to alleviate the convulsions with the helium mixture.

Edel (1969, 1972) has made the only human exposures since those of Zetterstrom (1948). Two successful dives were made to 200 ft (7 ATA) for 10 and 20 min in 1967 and 12 to 200 ft for 10 to 108 min in 1970 and 1971. Dogs also were exposed to 10 ATA (300 ft) for 24 hours and 31 ATA (1000 ft) for 39 hours (Edel 1971). In all these studies there were no significant changes in biomedical data.

For the present, however, as hydrogen appears to have little practical advantage over helium to depths of 2000 ft, where the hydrostatic pressure is limiting, helium is likely to remain the gas of choice for deep diving.

CAUSES AND MECHANISMS

The cause of inert gas narcosis is complex and cannot be related to any one factor. That there are many variables has led to many suggestions for the cause of the narcosis, most of which are incorrect. Perhaps the earliest suggestion was that the narcosis is the result of pressure per se (Junod 1835; Moxon 1881). The Junod hypothesis was that increased blood flow stimulated the nerve centres because 'the increased density of the air lessened the calibre of the venous vessels, resulting in greater blood flow in the arterial system and towards principal nerve centres, especially the brain, protected by its bony case from direct pressure'. Moxon (1881), on the other hand, considered that blood was forced by the pressure from the peripheral circulation to parts of the body not accessible to respiratory exchange and the stagnant blood caused emotional disturbances.

Neither theory is correct since the narcosis is a function of the nature of the gas breathed as well as its pressure. Thus at 10 ATA (300 ft) compressed air is very narcotic whereas a 20% oxygen, 80% helium mixture is not. Further, there is no blanching of the skin as would be expected with such theories.

Early workers also considered that the cause might be due to psychological factors, such as latent suppressed claustrophobia (Hill & Green-wood 1906; Phillips 1931; Hill et al. 1933) but again the fact that different inert gases cause different degrees of narcosis at the same depth is not in support of such suggestions.

That the high oxygen tensions might be responsible was a further controversial hypothesis once in vogue (Birch 1859; Bert 1878; Binger, Faulkner & Moore 1927; Damant 1930; Smith et al. 1932). It is now well understood that oxygen is a toxic gas but it is not responsible for the narcosis which Cousteau (1953) has lyrically described as 'L'ivresse des grandes profondeurs' or rapture of the depths. Compressed air at 10 ATA (300 ft) has a partial pressure of 2 ATA (33 ft) oxygen and narcosis is severe when breathing such a mixture. However, oxygen alone at 2 ATA (33 ft) causes none of the signs and symptoms listed earlier in this chapter and can therefore be ruled out as the cause. It does, however, have synergistic properties (Hesser 1963; Frankenhaeuser, Graff-Lonnevig & Hesser 1963) which may be due to carbon dioxide retention or possibly the effect of oxygen itself (Fenn 1965).

Over recent years there have remained two major theories as to the cause of the narcosis. One is based on the early suggestions of Behnke, Thomson and Motley (1935) and Behnke and Yarbrough (1939) that the increased nitrogen partial pressure is responsible and the other, of more recent origin, argues that the cause is carbon dioxide retention (Bean 1950; Seusing & Drube 1960; Seusing 1961; Buhlmann 1963; Vail 1971).

The carbon dioxide theory

In 1947 Bean noted an acid change of 0·15 to 0·02 pH in the arterial blood of dogs during compression which was attributed to carbon dioxide retention. Subsequent measurement of alveolar carbon dioxide levels in anaesthetized dogs during short exposures to raised air pressures showed increases from the normal 5% to values as high as 10% and Bean (1950) concluded that carbon dioxide should be considered as an alternative or at least contributory cause of compressed air intoxication. Bean suggested that the retention of carbon dioxide resulted from impairment of ventilation due to the increased density of the gases breathed and the fast rate of compression

causing 'compressional inflow of gases' together with the high-oxygen pressure blocking the haemoglobin carrier mechanism. Seusing and Drube (1960) Buhlmann (1963) and Vail (1971) supported the hypothesis on similar grounds.

However, experiments by Rashbass (1955) and Cabarrou (1959, 1964), in which measurements of alveolar carbon dioxide were compared with quantitative measurements of narcosis, fail to support the carbon dioxide theory, except in regard to its synergistic properties. That respiratory embarrassment does occur at increased pressures is not disputed. Indeed, there is ample evidence in support (Miles 1957; Wood, Leve & Workman 1962; Wood 1963; Lanphier 1963). Adequate ventilation is not possible but the carbon dioxide apparently only potentiates the narcotic action of the inert gas.

More conclusive evidence against the carbon dioxide theory has been obtained by Bennett (1965c) from in vivo measurements of the brain carbon dioxide and oxygen tensions in chloralosed cats. Investigations using a variety of inert gas mixtures, with depression of auditory evoked potentials as a measure of narcosis (Bennett 1964) showed no correlation between carbon dioxide retention and the degree of the narcosis.

In addition, arterial blood measurements of oxygen and carbon dioxide (Bennett & Blenkarn 1974) in men exposed to air or 20/80 oxygen–helium at 9·6 ATA (286 ft) and 6·8 ATA (190 ft) indicated marked narcosis while breathing air but not helium. However, there was no difference in arterial carbon dioxide values between the two groups (Table 12.6). Similarly, under xenon anaesthesia, venous and arterial oxygen and carbon dioxide measurements showed no significant difference from pre-anaesthetic values (Morris, Knott and Pittinger 1955).

Hesser, Adolfson and Fagraeus (1971) also have carried out further alveolar measurements at 6 ATA (170 ft) with 1·3 ATA oxygen and correlated the results with tests of mental and motor efficiency. Both the inspired nitrogen and carbon dioxide pressures were varied simultaneously or separately. The results confirmed that high alveolar nitrogen and carbon dioxide pressures are simply additive in causing a decrement in performance but a simultaneous increase in the two

TABLE 12.6

Mean results of human mental performance and arterial carbon dioxide in air and 20/80 oxygen–helium
(Bennett & Blenkarn 1974)

	Control	20/80 O_2/He	Air
At 286 ft			
Arithmetic correct	$16 \cdot 8 \pm 1 \cdot 78$	$15 \cdot 67 \pm 2 \cdot 08$	$11 \cdot 00 \pm 1 \cdot 73$
Visual analogy test	$50 \cdot 5 \pm 5 \cdot 61$	$51 \cdot 50 \pm 5 \cdot 80$	$44 \cdot 50 \pm 1 \cdot 21$
Pa_{CO2}	—	$35 \cdot 38 \pm 4 \cdot 36$	$34 \cdot 73 \pm 3 \cdot 84$
At 190 ft			
Arithmetic correct	$16 \cdot 8 \pm 1 \cdot 78$	$18 \cdot 67 \pm 1 \cdot 53$	$15 \cdot 67 \pm 2 \cdot 08$
Visual analogy test	$50 \cdot 5 \pm 5 \cdot 61$	$50 \cdot 00 \pm 5 \cdot 42$	$51 \cdot 70 \pm 4 \cdot 19$
Pa_{CO2}	—	$35 \cdot 05 \pm 2 \cdot 56$	$32 \cdot 68 \pm 1 \cdot 60$

gas tensions results in a greater decrement than the effect of the gases alone.

The inert gas theory

The nitrogen and inert gas theory Behnke based on the Meyer–Overton hypothesis (Meyer 1899; Overton 1901) that there is a parallel between the affinity of an aliphatic anaesthetic for lipid and its narcotic potency. This also led Meyer and Hopff (1923) to state that 'all gaseous or volatile substances induce narcosis if they penetrate the cell lipids in a definite molar concentration (0·03 to 0·06 moles drug per kg of membrane) which is characteristic for each type of animal (or better, type of cell) and is approximately the same for all narcotics'. Nevertheless, arrangement of the inert gases in order of their oil–water solubilities indicates anomalies (see Table 12.4). Argon for example, is about twice as narcotic as nitrogen, although their oil–water solubility ratios are similar. This is due to argon being twice as soluble in both lipid and water. In connection with anaesthetic agents in general there are also many exceptions to this rule but so far as the noble gases are concerned there is an excellent correlation between lipid solubility and narcotic potency.

Experimental evidence from the sensitivity of mice to electro-shock further supports the Meyer–Overton hypothesis (Carpenter 1954) for at their isonarcotic partial pressures, when each gas exhibits similar pharmacological effects, the inert gas concentration in the lipid phase is remarkably similar, although the partial pressure of gas required varies from 0·045 to 163 ATS (Table 12.7).

The partial molal-free energy, derived from the fugacity of the gas, is another physical property which correlates well with narcotic potency (Ferguson 1939; Brink & Posternak 1948; Ferguson & Hawkins 1949; Marshall 1951; Carpenter 1954). Ferguson noted that activity, an expression of vapour concentration, afforded a better indication of isonarcotic potency than the Meyer–Overton moles per litre but this was qualified by Brink and Posternak who maintained that the biological system (e.g. synaptic or non-synaptic) must also be considered when expressing potency as 'activity'.

Yet another physical correlation is that of the Van der Waals physical chemical constants with narcosis and anaesthesia (Wulf & Featherstone 1957) but again there are anomalies such as the inference that argon is less narcotic than nitrogen. However, Featherstone and Muehlbaecher (1963) maintained that the majority of physical correlations with narcotic potency are in fact only extensions of the intermolecular Van der Waals attractions of these gases.

The above correlations are based on an interaction with the lipid phase of the nervous system which is generally accepted as the site of action of anaesthetics (Meyer & Hopff 1923; Butler 1950) but more recently the aqueous phase has been suggested as an alternative (Miller 1961; Pauling 1961).

The aqueous phase theories are based on the

TABLE 12.7

Comparative effect of inert and other gases on electro-shock convulsions in intact rats and transmission in isolated rat sciatic nerve related to physical characteristics of the gases (Carpenter 1954)

Gas	ED_{50} ATS	Olive oil Bunsen coeff. 37°	Olive oil Conc. mol/L	f° ATS 37°C	anar	Fibre blockade ATS	$BPED_{50}$	Δ Demarcation potential at B.P.
Cyclopropane	0·045	7·15	0·036	7·5	0·0060	1·7–1·9	36	−10%
Dichlorodifluoro-methane	0·26	5·1	0·057	7·0	0·037	3·4–4·7	18·5	−8%
Ethylene	0·47	1·28	0·026	49·0	0·0096	9·8–12·5	26	−12%
Xenon‡	0·51	1·7	0·038	52·0	0·0098		not determined	
Nitrous oxide	0·58	1·6	0·036	44·0	0·013	10–13	23	−19%
Krypton‡	1·8	0·43	0·034	215·0	0·0084		not determined	
Sulphur hexa-fluoride	1·87	0·25	0·020	20·4	0·091	≫21†	≫11	
Methane	2·9	0·28	0·043	262·0	0·011	92–110	36	−16%
Argon	12·6	0·14	0·077	725·0	0·017	310–340	27	−11%
Nitrogen	18·0	0·067	0·052	1700	0·010		not determined	
Helium	> 163·0	0·015	> 0·107				*	*

* Control at 350 ATS: no observable change in action potential or demarcation potential.
† In excess of its vapour pressure at 25°C.   ‡ Lazarev, N. (estimated ED_{50}).

formation of hydrates. Pauling (1961) suggests that clathrates are formed in which the inert gas atoms called 'guests' are held by Van der Waals forces in crystalline cages formed by the 'hosts' or molecules of a second agent. However, due to their high dissociation pressures, such hydrates would be unstable under body conditions and Pauling was obliged to infer the presence of a stabilizing factor such as the charged side chains of proteins known as 'protein binding'. Such clathrates are considered to cause narcosis by increasing the impedance of nerve tissue, trapping electrically charged ions associated with impulse conduction and decreasing metabolism.

Miller (1961) postulated an alternative but related theory which did not rely on hydrates but implied that the inert gases or anaesthetics may increase the area of highly ordered water or 'icebergs' surrounding a dissolved gas molecule. In this manner the conductance of the brain tissue would be lowered, the lipid membranes stiffened and the membranes occluded.

Dawe, Miller and Smith (1964). Miller, Paton and Smith (1965, 1967) and Eger et al. (1969) studied the anaesthetic potencies of fluorinated gases such as SF_6 and CF_4 in lipid and aqueous media in order to resolve the site of action. The evidence of these experiments provided no support for the aqueous medium as the critical phase for anaesthetic action.

Other experiments have suggested another 'bonding mechanism' in which inert gases are bound to specific sites within protein molecules (Featherstone et al. 1961; Featherstone & Meuhlbaecher 1963; Schoenborn, Watson & Kendrew 1965; Schoenborn 1965). However, the connection of the latter with mechanisms of anaesthesia remains to be elucidated.

Electrophysiological mechanisms

As regards anaesthesia by the clinical anaesthetics there are a number of reviews which have assisted in clarification of the mechanisms involved although the mechanism itself remains the subject of speculation (Butler 1950; Pittinger & Keasling 1959; Latner 1965; Paton & Speden 1965; Quastel 1965; Fink 1972). Much of this may be directly related to the mechanism of inert gas narcosis and it may be that a solution of the latter will also resolve the mechanism of anaesthesia.

So far as the inert gases are concerned, Marshall and Fenn (1950) were among the first seriously to investigate the mechanisms of inert gas narcosis. Whole frogs and mice, isolated tissues, frog reflex preparations and frog brain wave preparations were exposed to increased pressures of inert gases. After 260 min, nitrogen at 17 ATA (530 ft) and argon at 10 ATA (300 ft) reversibly blocked in vitro frog reflex preparations whereas helium had no effect even at 82 ATA (2700 ft). In vitro frog sciatic nerve was also not affected by any of the inert gases at pressures as high as 96 ATA (3135 ft). Carpenter (1954) subsequently showed that to effect a block of conduction in isolated peripheral nerve, very high pressures indeed were required such as 310 to 340 ATA with argon. However, considerably lower pressures protected mice from electro-shock convulsions (Carpenter 1953, 1954, 1955). Such experiments led to the inference that the site of action for inert gas narcosis, as with anaesthetics, is at central synapses (Larrabee & Posternak 1952; French, Verzeano & Magoun 1953; Arduini & Arduini 1954).

In vivo evidence that spinal synapses are affected by inert gases was obtained by Chun (1959) from studies of reflex inhibition in the spinal cord of 26 decerebrate cats at 7 to 9 ATA (200 to 265 ft) and by Bennett (1963a, 1966) from investigations of transmission in spinal synapses and peripheral nerve of 63 lightly anaesthetized rats. The results of the former experiments suggested that inhibitory synaptic mechanisms were affected before excitatory and the results of the latter experiments suggested that, as with anaesthesia, inert gases act on the anterior horn cell of the synapse (Austin & Pask 1952; Somjen & Gill 1963).

A correlation between changes in the mental state of divers and depression of the polysynaptic ascending reticular formation of the brain stem as shown by an abolition of the alpha blocking response (Bennett & Glass 1961) or change in the fusion frequency of flicker (Bennett & Cross 1960) also indirectly supported involvement of the synapse. The time to such changes was found to be inversely proportional to the pressure of inert gas and it was inferred that a fundamental change occurs at polysynaptic sites in the brain when a critical tension of nitrogen or inert gas is exceeded.

Subsequent experiments (Bennett 1964) on auditory induced evoked potentials at the cortex and reticular formation of chloralosed cats exposed to 12·3 ATA (373 ft) showed a significant depression of the potentials. That the initial negative evoked response was depressed before the positive was taken as further evidence that the inert gas acts at the post-synaptic rather than pre-synaptic membrane.

Further support was obtained for the concept of a critical concentration of inert gas acting at central synapses. Evidence was obtained also in support of earlier studies by French and other workers (Jullien, Roger & Chatrian 1963; Roger, Cabarrou & Gastaut 1955; Morris, Knott & Pittinger 1955) that during the onset of the narcosis at least, there is an increased excitatory state of the cortical neurones. This excitation is believed by some workers to be due to the high oxygen partial pressure (Albano, Criscuoli & Ciulla 1962; Albano & Criscuoli 1962). However, recent experiments, which suggest that narcosis is due to an intracellular increase of sodium and chloride ions in neurones, permits an alternative consideration that the hyper-excitability may be a natural function of the mechanism of inert gas anaesthesia (Bennett & Hayward 1967), or the earlier block of inhibitory synapses could result in an excitatory release (Chun 1959).

The advent of averaging computer techniques has led to the application of evoked potential measurements at the cortex of the brain in man as a method of more objective quantification of inert narcosis. Bennett, Ackles & Cripps (1969) measured the N_1P_2 spike height (as in Fig. 12.3) of 60 db auditory signals presented at 60 per minute and correlated the result with arithmetical efficiency (Table 12.8) at 50 ft increments between 100 ft (4 ATA) and 300 ft (10 ATA) in subjects breathing air and also oxygen–helium at 300 ft (10 ATA) and oxygen at surface, 2 ATA (33 ft) and 3 ATA (66 ft) (Table 12.8).

The compressed air caused decrements in both the AER and arithmetic efficiency which correlated with increasing depth (as in Fig. 12.3). Helium had no effect but oxygen caused a similar reduction of spike height (Table 12.8) although neither gas significantly depressed arithmetical performance. The effect with oxygen was taken as further evidence for narcotic properties for hyperbaric oxygen (Bennett & Ackles 1970; Bennett &

TABLE 12.8

Mean percentage changes in the auditory evoked response and arithmetic performance of divers
(Bennett, Ackles & Cripps 1969)

	Surface air (0·8 ATA N₂) (0·2 ATA O₂)	Surface oxygen (1 ATA O₂)	5 min at 33 ft oxygen (2 ATA O₂)	5 min at 66 ft oxygen (3 ATA O₂)	5 min at 300 ft air (8 ATA N₂) (2 ATA O₂)	5 min at 300 ft oxygen–helium (8 ATA He) (2 ATA O₂)	5 min at 300 ft mixture 8 ATA N₂ 1·8 ATA He 0·2 ATA O₂
Spike height N_1P_2	$-3\cdot4\pm8\cdot2$	$-11\cdot8\pm5\cdot2$	$-27\cdot8\pm8\cdot0$	$-21\cdot5\pm4\cdot9$	$-55\cdot5\pm10\cdot5$	$-29\cdot4\pm4\cdot6$	$-54\cdot1\pm4\cdot3$
Arithmetic correct	$+8\cdot5\pm5\cdot6$	$-1\cdot0\pm5\cdot2$	$+1\cdot0\pm5\cdot7$	$-6\cdot1\pm5\cdot3$	$-31\cdot2\pm10\cdot95$	$+6\cdot3\pm7\cdot1$	$-30\cdot0\pm5\cdot3$
Arithmetic attempted	$+12\cdot8\pm4\cdot2$	$-2\cdot6\pm4\cdot6$	$+1\cdot3\pm5\cdot7$	$-5\cdot9\pm4\cdot5$	$-28\cdot0\pm11\cdot8$	$+7\cdot5\pm4\cdot6$	$-23\cdot9\pm4\cdot7$

Dossett 1973) prior to enzyme changes and convulsions.

Similar studies with evoked potentials were made by Kinney and McKay (1971) using visual stimuli with remarkably similar results and Schreiner, Hamilton and Langley (1972) correlated psychomotor tests and arithmetical performance (Fig. 12.2) with auditory induced evoked potentials in men exposed to nitrogen, helium and crude neon (Fig. 12.3). These tests indicated an appreciable effect only with nitrogen. A reduction of

$63\cdot5\pm4\cdot5\%$ in the size of the N_1P_2 spike was reported also by Bevan (1971) at 10 ATA (300 ft) compressed air, who studied also the Contingent Negative Variation (CNV) or expectancy wave, which was unaffected.

Ackles and Fowler (1971) examined the effect of

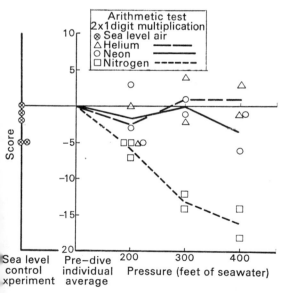

FIG. 12.2. Comparative decrement in performance at arithmetic when breathing either oxygen–helium, oxygen–neon or oxygen–nitrogen (Schreiner, Hamilton & Langley 1972)

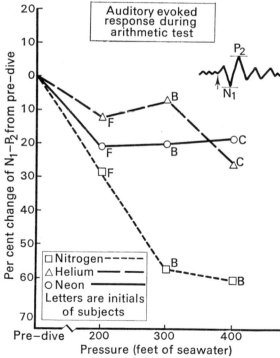

FIG. 12.3. Comparative decrement in size of N_1P_2 complex in men breathing either oxygen–helium, oxygen–neon or oxygen–nitrogen. See Fig. 12.2 (Schreiner, Hamilton & Langley 1972)

the more narcotic argon with the nitrogen in compressed air using both auditory and visual evoked potentials and performance tests. The results indicated that performance was much more seriously impaired in the men breathing argon and indicated also a non-linear reduction with increasing depth. However, the N_1P_2 response, although decreased with greater depth, showed no differential effect between argon and nitrogen (Fig. 12.4). Since a

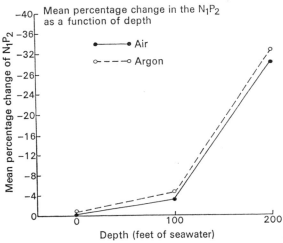

FIG. 12.4. Mean percentage change in the size of the N_1P_2 spike height of cortical evoked potentials in men breathing either compressed air or oxygen–argon. There is no differential effect between the effects of the two gases (Ackles & Fowler 1971)

reduction in potentials does not occur with helium and neon the reasons for this are not clear other than that, provided there is a narcotic effect, the decrease of evoked potential does become more severe with increasing depth.

An alternative electrophysiological approach is frequency analysis. Bennett and Dossett (1973) examined the effects of argon, nitrogen, helium and oxygen on rats at depths to 22 ATA (700 ft) and helium to 122 ATA (4000 ft) with an analyser selective for delta (2 to 4 c/sec), theta (4 to 8 c/sec) alpha (8 to 13 c/sec), beta 1 (13 to 30 c/sec) and beta 2 (20 to 30 c/sec) activities. Compressed air, argon–oxygen and oxygen alone reduced all activity bands on compression to 22 ATA (700 ft), whereas helium–oxygen and nitrogen–oxygen had little effect. At 4 ATA (100 ft) activity was augmented except for the rats in argon–oxygen or oxygen alone.

Townsend, Thompson and Sulg (1971) noted in man that there was a slight increase in alpha frequencies when reaction time was impaired by nitrogen narcosis at 8·57 ATA (250 ft), and an increase was found by Bennett and Towse (1972) in the alpha, beta 1 and beta 2 activities in men exposed to compressed air at 10 ATA (300 ft), the cause being related to activation of the reticular system as seen in Stage 1 of anaesthesia. Similar changes have been reported also by Roger, Cabarrou and Gasthaut (1955), Zaltsman (1968) and Morris, Knott and Pittinger (1955).

A comparison in rats of evoked potentials and frequency analysis (Bennett 1975) indicates that in breathing argon or nitrogen there is a significant difference between the depression of frequencies seen at 15 ATA (500 ft) and deeper but not at shallower depths, whereas with evoked potentials there is a significant difference at 4 ATA (100 ft) and 7 ATA (200 ft) but not at 10 ATA (300 ft).

Clearly much more research is required in this area and the search for a more effective means of quantifying narcosis must remain.

Cellular and membrane mechanisms

Many factors have been considered in the past to be connected with the mechanism of inert gas narcosis including a histotoxic hypoxia, depression of metabolism, cell membrane stabilization causing a block in ion permeability, inhibition of the sodium extrusion pump, increased production of inhibitors such as γ-aminobutyric acid and interference with adenosine triphosphate production (Butler 1950; Pittinger & Keasling 1959; Featherstone & Muehlbaecher 1963; Latner 1965 Bennett 1966). As with anaesthetics, the theories tend to fall into two categories, either biochemical or physical. The former implies an effect on respiratory enzyme systems and the latter solution either in, or interacting with, some part of the neurone such as the cell membrane (Featherstone & Muehlbaecher 1963; Fink 1972).

With regard to the former, no satisfactory evidence has been obtained for biochemical changes at pressures responsible for inert gas narcosis (Levy & Featherstone 1954; Carpenter 1955, 1956; Leon & Cook 1960; Thomas, Neptune & Sudduth 1963; Schatte & Bennett, 1973).

The physical theories based on the polari

ability and volume of the inert gas molecule (Featherstone & Muehlbaecher 1963) seem more likely. McIlwain (1962) has also proposed a theory linking the biochemical and physical theories which suggests that anaesthetics interact with the cell membrane, blocking ion exchange. This causes a decrease in oxygen consumption and a rise in energy stores. In addition Mullins (1954) supports the ionic block mechanism by postulating occlusion of the pores of the membrane by inert gas molecules. In a similar way Sears (1962) suggests that interaction of the inert gases within the membranes of the synaptic vesicles may prevent the release of their chemical transmitter contents.

Unsworth (1966) has proposed an alternative theory linking biochemical and physical mechanisms involving the glia. A mechanism of histotoxic hypoxia due to displacement adsorption of oxygen (Ebert, Hornsey & Howard 1958; Clements & Wilson 1962; Bennett 1966) would, it is suggested, cause a failure of the sodium pump with a delay in substrate transfer to the neurone through the glia from the capillaries.

The majority of these mechanisms involve the concept of a block of ion exchange across membrane due to adsorption of inert gas molecules. That narcotic agents, such as nitrous oxide, do have an affinity for interfacial films has been noted by Clements and Wilson (1962) who concluded that 'inert gases at partial pressures sufficient to bring about a standard effect in a biological system act on a lipoprotein–water interface to cause a standard decrease of 0·39 dyne/cm in the interfacial tension'. Experiments by the author in collaboration with Papahadjopoulos and Bangham (1967) show that inert gases at raised pressures will also penetrate a lipid monolayer (Fig. 12.5) and affect the surface tension in accordance with the rule of Clements and Wilson (1962). Further, Bangham, Standish and Miller (1965), as a result of studies with the 'n' alkyl alcohols, chloroform and ether on interfacial tension and studies of

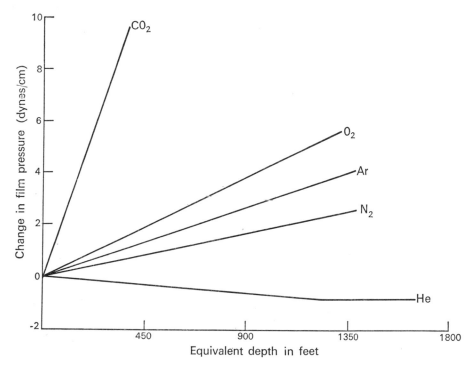

FIG. 12.5. Penetration of a lipid monolayer of egg phospholipid by inert gases, oxygen and carbon dioxide at increased pressures. An increase in film pressure indicates an equivalent fall in surface tension and increase in volume (Bennett, Papahadjoupolos & Bangham 1967)

cation permeability in model systems, suggest that such adsorption results in a transient reversible *increase* in membrane permeability to cation.

If the narcotizing or anaesthetizing concentrations in the membrane are multiplied by the free energy of adsorption a constant is obtained (Seeman 1972). This suggests that narcosis occurs when there is a drop in the free energy of the membrane.

At any event there is ample evidence of the membrane becoming more fluid and that anaesthetics increase the water permeability of membrane (Seeman et al. 1970) and increase the passive permeabilities of sodium and potassium ions (Seeman, 1972).

The inert gases are no different in this respect and comparison of in vivo potassium, sodium and chloride ions in the cerebral spinal fluid of cats over 1 hour at normal pressure with that of cats exposed to inert gas–oxygen mixtures (Bennett & Hayward 1967) showed that whereas the nitrogen and argon mixtures produced a significant fall in auditory evoked cortical response and in sodium and chloride ions, no change in either the evoked response or electrolytes was found in the animals exposed to helium or air at atmospheric pressure for a second hour (Table 12.9). Similar permeability changes have been noted in blood (Barthelemy 1963) and urine (Radomski & Bennett 1970) and in transport across frog skin (Gottlieb, Cymerman & Metz 1968).

Whereas, however, the early anaesthetic effects of narcosis indicate an increased permeability, general anaesthetics in fact display biphasic

effects. Low concentrations stimulate and higher concentrations inhibit sodium ion transport (Anderson 1972). However, the net effect on transport of sodium seems to be unrelated to the anaesthetic effect. Equipotent anaesthetic concentrations thus may either stimulate, inhibit or have no effect on sodium ion transport depending on the anaesthetic.

It is reasonable nevertheless to conclude as a broad concept that inert gas narcosis and anaesthesia are caused by the adsorption of the narcotic agent on lipid cell membranes which affects their permeability to cations. Further insight into the mechanisms have been obtained from pharmacological studies.

Pharmacological studies

The usual way of preventing inert gas narcosis for most practical purposes is to breathe oxygen–helium mixtures. Less attention has been paid in the past to the value drugs may have in either preventing the signs and symptoms of narcosis or indicating the mechanisms involved (Bennett 1972).

As both oxygen and nitrogen at raised pressures have many factors in common, such as the production of an electrolyte imbalance (Kaplan & Stein 1957) and the synergistic potentiation by carbon dioxide, Bennett (1962) examined the comparative effects of 11 drugs on nitrogen narcosis and oxygen toxicity in rats (Table 12.10). Five of the drugs chosen were effective in preventing or ameliorating nitrogen narcosis as measured by sensitivity of the rats to electro-shock, two had

TABLE 12.9

Mean change from controls of Na^+, K^+, and Cl^- (mEq) in CSF of cats exposed to 11 ATA of various inert gas/oxygen mixtures (Bennett & Hayward 1967)

	Air at atmospheric pressure		20/80 oxygen/ helium		20/80 oxygen/ nitrogen		20/80 oxygen/ argon	
	Mean	SEM	Mean	SEM	Mean	SEM	Mean	SEM
Sodium	+7·6	±4·4	+4·8	±2·1	−14·2	±3·1*	−11·2	±3·4
Potassium	−0·1	±0·22	−0·1	±0·25	−0·54	±0·18	+0·14	+0·29
Chloride	+0·6	+1·4	+0·6	±0·7	−9·6	±3·0†	−6·0	±2·7‡
No. of cats	5		5		5		5	

* $P > 0.01$;   † $P = 0.05$-0.02;   ‡ $P = 0.05$.

TABLE 12.10

Effect of 11 drugs on nitrogen narcosis and oxygen toxicity (Bennett 1962)

Drug	Mean percentage volts increase (narcotic level) at 12·2 ATA N_2 1·0 ATA O_2	Mean convulsion time at 5·4 ATA O_2	Action of drug
No drug	50%	22 min	
Carbachol	0	58	
Frenquel	2	35	
Doriden	3	33	Protective
Phenacetin	5	48	
Aspirin	28	32	
Physostigmine	49	20	No change
Adrenaline	53	22	
Scopolamine	60	30	
Methedrine	75	15	Enhances
Megimide	77	15	
Leptazol	87	9	

no effect and four enhanced the narcosis. Similar properties were found in rats exposed to high oxygen pressures and Bennett concluded that one drug should be effective in preventing both inert gas narcosis and oxygen toxicity. Further support was also obtained for the similarity of the mechanisms (Bennett 1972).

Frenquel (alpha-4-piperydyl benzhydrol hydrochloride or azacyclonal hydrochloride) was studied in greater detail in rats (Bennett 1963b) and in limited human investigations (Bennett 1961). In the rat studies, 46 animals were exposed to 13·3 ATA (400 ft) nitrogen–oxygen, argon–oxygen or helium–oxygen and after oral, intraperitoneal or intravenous administration of Frenquel an electro-shock technique was used to evaluate narcosis. Regardless of the gas used, a 40 mg dose was found effective in preventing narcosis, which suggests a biophysical action. The drug, however, was slow acting and was only at its most active some 48 hours after administration. In 12 rats the increase in voltage required to effect a response from the narcotized animals was $50\cdot2 \pm 4\%$. Forty-eight hours after oral administration of Frenquel, the value was $1\cdot21 \pm 2\cdot45\%$, indicating no difference from rats breathing air at atmospheric pressure.

In human studies a narcotic index calculated from the results of arithmetic, letter cancellation and the neuromuscular coordination ball bearing test gave a mean value in three subjects of 11·5 at 10 ATA (300 ft). As at atmospheric pressure the value was 17·5, this indicated a decrement of 34%.

A dose of 300 mg Frenquel three times a day for 7 days produced some improvement so that the decrement was only 23% with similar improvement in the subjective signs and symptoms. A dose of 1200 mg for 3 days prevented the increase in fusion frequency of flicker normally found at 10 ATA (300 ft) and markedly improved the subjective state. In both cases side effects such as hand tremor, stomach irritability and hypertension were apparent which were, however, seen less at depth than on the surface. As 1200 mg is the maximum recommended dose this is perhaps not surprising.

Since this work the proposal that narcosis is due to adsorption of inert gas molecules to preferential membrane sites with a consequent action on permeability has led to a different approach. Carbon tetrachloride poisoning causes a similar intracellular increase of sodium and chloride ions and decrease in potassium ions in liver resulting in necrosis (Bangham, Rees & Shotlander 1962). The cationic detergents stearylamine and cetyltrimethyl ammonium bromide are able to stabilize the membrane and prevent this increase of permeability and the necrosis but anionic drugs such as sodium hexadecyl and dodecyl sulphate are ineffective.

These compounds were therefore given to rats exposed to raised pressures of nitrogen and the narcosis was measured by photically induced evoked potentials (Bennett & Dossett 1970). The cationic detergents significantly prevented the depression of evoked potentials seen in the animals without the drugs. Anionic compounds had no effect (Table 12.11). It is interesting that an anti-inflammatory compound which protects erythrocytes against lysis, acetylsalicylic acid, was similarly effective. Further, as with the earlier studies, the cationic detergents markedly increased the time to convulsions in hyperbaric oxygen whereas the anionic drugs did not (Bennett & Dossett 1971).

TABLE 12.11

Effect of surface active anionic or cationic drugs on inert gas narcosis in rats at 0·9 O_2/6·41 N_2 ATA
(Bennett & Dossett 1970)

Drug	Dose	Mean percentage change in evoked response	No. of rats	Significance
1. No drug, no pressure	—	$+4 \pm 4·66$	10	—
2. No drug at pressure	—	$-29·8 \pm 3·87$	10	(1–2) $P < 0·001$
Anionic drugs				
3. Sodium hexadecyl sulphate	70 µmol/kg	$-34 \pm 3·87$	10	(2–3) Not significant
				(1–3) $P < 0·001$
4. Sodium dodecyl sulphate	80 µmol/kg	$-20 \pm 4·08$	10	(2–4) Not significant
				(1–4) $P < 0·001$
Cationic drugs				
				(1–5) Not significant
5. Stearylamine	55 µmol/kg	$-7 \pm 3·81$	10	(2–5) $P < 0·001$
6. Cetyl trimethyl ammonium bromide	14 µmol/kg	$-6·5 \pm 4·14$	10	(2–6) $P < 0·001$
				(1–7) Not significant
Anti-inflammatory drug				
7. Acetyl salicylic acid	50 mg/kg	$-1 \pm 3·68$	10	(2–7) $P < 0·001$
				(1–7) Not significant

More recently other surface active compounds have been investigated and these have been shown to be effective in preventing oxygen toxicity, too. These are lithium carbonate (Radomski & Wood 1970) and vitamin E (Taylor 1956). Thus, 500 mg/kg lithium carbonate (i.p.) in rats at 10 ATA (300 ft) compressed air reduced the normal narcotic decrement of visual evoked response from −30% of normal to only −1% but lower doses were not as effective (Bennett 1975).

Lithium ion, like the cationic detergents, is believed to produce its effects either by stabilizing nerve membranes or alternatively by active displacement of intracellular sodium (Maletzky & Blachly 1971).

Vitamin E at 400 mg/kg caused lethargy but did not affect the electrophysiological signs of narcosis. At 200 mg/kg the 30% reduction in evoked response found at 10 ATA (300 ft) compressed air was reduced to only 8·5%.

The cationic detergents are believed to be surface active and form complexes with lipid–water interfaces, especially if the former are negatively charged. Stabilization of the lipid membrane is achieved by the presence of either non-polar portions of amphipathic molecules (i.e. with a hydrophobic group and a polar group) or by the strategic positioning of positively charged groups at the water–lipid interface of the cell membrane.

Hydrostatic pressure and narcosis

The effects of hydrostatic pressure are discussed at length elsewhere in this book, but some mention needs to be made here to indicate its relevance. Antagonism between anaesthetics and high hydrostatic pressures has been known for some time (Johnson & Flagler 1950). Lever et al. (1971) extended these early studies with luminous bacteria and tadpoles to newts and mice. Halothane and Nembutal narcosis in newts could be instantaneously reversed by the application of hydrostatic pressures between 100 to 200 ATS. Similarly nitrogen narcosis, as shown by loss of righting reflex in newts at 34 ATS nitrogen was restored to normal mobility by addition of helium to 140 ATS. Mice anaesthetized by nitrogen at 45 ATS regained consciousness in a similar manner by further compression with helium.

Johnson and Miller (1970) noted that exposure of liposomes to butanol, ether and nitrogen in doses just sufficient to abolish the righting reflex of newts brought about an increased permeability of K^+ and Rb^+. A pressure of 150 ATS counterbalanced these effects. If higher doses of anaesthetic were used then higher pressures were required to counterbalance. Further, of specific interest to the cause of the High Pressure Nervous Syndrome (HPNS), application of helium pressure alone caused a fall in ion permeability. Thus it would seem that the correct combination of nitrogen/helium/oxygen should provide a diving mixture with no narcosis or HPNS. This is discussed further in Chapters 13 and 14 as regards animals and humans respectively, and recent, as yet unpublished, experiments at Duke University have confirmed that the addition of 10% nitrogen to helium/oxygen will permit rapid compressions of 33 min to 1000 ft (31 ATA) without HPNS or narcosis.

Lever et al. (1971) add that the critical anaesthetic concentration in the lipids can be estimated as 0·05 M. Such an anaesthetic dose would produce a lipid expansion of the order of 0·4% and the hydrostatic pressure required to nullify that expansion would be 100 ATS, which agrees with the experimental data. The formula used to obtain these relationships is

$$\delta = \frac{(-E^{\mathrm{vap}})^{1/2}}{V}$$

where:

δ = Solubility parameter
V = Molar volume of the solvent region
E = Energy of vapourization

Stern and Frisch (1973) have extended this work to suggest that narcotic potency of inert gases is due to their effect on the 'free volume' (or 'empty volume') possibly in the lipid of the cell membrane. Thus the anaesthetic potency of a gas depends on its lipid solubility, thermal expansivity and compressibility of the liquid phase, environmental temperature and hydrostatic pressure rather than only on the lipid solubility as in the Meyer–Overton hypothesis. Expressed in

quantitative form this 'free volume' concept is in good agreement with experimental data in the literature.

$$V_{\mathrm{f}} = V_{\mathrm{fs}} + \alpha(T - T_{\mathrm{s}}) - \beta(\pi - \pi_{\mathrm{s}}) + \gamma S p$$

where:

V_{f} = Free-volume fraction
V_{fs} = Free-volume fraction in a suitable standard
T = Temperature of the system
T_{s} = Standard temperature
π = Hydrostatic pressure of the system
π_{s} = Standard hydrostatic pressure
$\alpha = (^{\delta}v_{\mathrm{f}}/\delta T)_{\mathrm{s}}$ is the 'thermal expansion' coefficient
$\gamma = (^{\delta}v_{\mathrm{f}}/\delta v)_{\mathrm{a}}$ is the concentration coefficient
$\beta = -(^{\delta}v_{\mathrm{f}}/\delta v)_{\mathrm{s}}$ is the 'compressibility' coefficient
V = Volume fraction concentration of anaesthetic dissolved in the lipid phase
S = Solubility coefficient
p = Partial pressure of the applied anaesthetic.

Inert gas narcosis will thus occur when the concentration of dissolved inert gas causes the free volume in the lipid phase to exceed a critical free volume.

It is evident that the future solution of the mechanism of narcosis requires intensive study of the accompanying membrane physiology. However, the work discussed in this section on mechanisms of inert gas narcosis has done much in recent years to clarify how narcosis is caused. With its relationship to the mechanism of anaesthesia by general anaesthetics, which is receiving increasing attention, it may not be long before a means of prevention of narcosis is at hand and divers will be able to dive to even 10 ATA (300 ft) without the dangerous signs and symptoms of compressed air narcosis.

REFERENCES

ACKLES, K. N. & FOWLER, B. (1971) Cortical evoked response and inert gas narcosis in man. *Aerospace Med.* **41**, 1181–1184.

ADOLFSON, J. (1964) *Compressed Air Narcosis.* (Thesis.) The Institute of Psychology, University of Gothenburg, Sweden.

ADOLFSON, J. (1965) Deterioration of mental and motor functions in hyperbaric air. *Scand. J. Psychol.* **6**, 26–31.

ADOLFSON, J. & MUREN, A. (1965) Air breathing at 13 atmospheres. Psychological and physiological observations. *Särtryck ur Försvars Medicin*, **1**, 31–37.

ADOLFSON, J. A., GOLDBERG, L. & BERGHAGE, T. (1972) Effects of increased ambient air pressures on standing steadiness in man. *Aerospace Med.* **43**, 520–524.

ALBANO, G. (1962) *Influenza della velocita di discesa sulla latenza dei disturbi neuropsichici da aria compressa ne lavoro subacqueo.* Communication at 25th National Congress of Medicine, Taormina.

ALBANO, G. (1970) *Principles and Observations on the Physiology of the Scuba Diver.* (Translation from Italian.) Office of Naval Research Report DR-150, Arlington, Virginia.

ALBANO, G. & CRISCUOLI, P. M. (1962) La sindrome neuropsichica de profondita. *Boll. Soc. ital. Biol. sper.* **38**, 754–756.

ALBANO, G., CRISCUOLI, P. M. & CIULLA, C. (1962) La sindrome neuropsichica di profondita. *Lav. umano* **14**, 351–358.

ANDERSON, N. B. (1972) Dual effects of general anesthetics on active and passive sodium fluxes and on sympathetic response in toad. In *Cellular Biology and Toxicity of Anesthetics* Ed. B. R. Fink. pp. 296–303. Baltimore: Williams & Wilkins.

ARDUINI, A. & ARDUINI, M. G. (1954) Effect of drugs and metabolic alterations on brain stem arousal mechanism. *J. Pharmacol.* **110**, 76–85.

AUSTIN, G. M. & PASK, E. A. (1952) Effects of ether inhalation upon spinal cord and root action potentials. *J. Physiol., Lond.* **118**, 405–411.

BADDELEY, A. D. (1966) The influence of depth on the manual dexterity of free divers. A comparison between open-sea and pressure chamber testing. *J. appl. Psychol.* **50**, 81–85.

BANGHAM, A. D., REES, K. R. and SHOTLANDER, V. (1962) Penetration of lipid films by compounds preventing liver necrosis in rats. *Nature, Lond.* **193**, 754–756.

BANGHAM, A. D., STANDISH, M. M. & MILLER, N. (1965) Cation permeability of phospholipid model membranes: Effect of narcotics. *Nature, Lond.* **208**, 1295–1297.

BARNARD, E. E. P., HEMPLEMAN, H. V. H. & TROTTER, C. (1962) *Mixture Breathing and Nitrogen Narcosis.* Report, Medical Research Council, R.N. Personnel Research Committee, U.P.S. 208, London.

BARTHELEMY, L. (1963) Blood coagulation and chemistry during experimental dives and the treatment of diving accidents with heparin. *Proc. 2nd Symp. Underwater Physiology.* Ed. C. J. Lambertsen & L. J. Greenbaum. p. 46. Publ. 1181. Washington, D.C.: Natl Acad. Sci.-Natl Res. Council.

BEAN, J. W. (1947) Changes in arterial pH induced by compression and decompression. *Fedn Proc. Fedn Am. Socs exp. Biol.* **6**, 76.

BEAN, J. W. (1950) Tensional changes of alveolar gas in reactions to rapid compression and decompression and question of nitrogen narcosis. *Am. J. Physiol.* **161**, 417–425.

BEHNKE, A. R., THOMSON, R. M. & MOTLEY, E. P. (1935) The psychologic effects from breathing air at 4 atmospheres pressure. *Am. J. Physiol.* **112**, 554–558.

BEHNKE, A. R. & YARBROUGH, O. D. (1939) Respiratory resistance, oil–water solubility and mental effects of argon compared with helium and nitrogen. *Am. J. Physiol.* **126**, 409–415.

BENNETT, P. B. (1961) *A Preliminary Investigation into the Prevention of Nitrogen Narcosis with Frenquel.* Report, Medical Research Council, R.N. Personnel Research Committee, U.P.S. 196, London.

BENNETT, P. B. (1962) Comparison of the effects of drugs on nitrogen narcosis and oxygen toxicity in rats. *Life Sci.* No. 12, 721–727

BENNETT, P. B. (1963a) Neurophysiologic and neuropharmacologic investigations in inert gas narcosis. In *Proc. 2nd Symp. Underwater Physiology.* Ed. C. J. Lambertsen & L. J. Greenbaum. Washington, D.C.: Natl Acad. Sci.-Natl Res. Council.

BENNETT, P. B. (1963b) Prevention in rats of the narcosis produced by inert gases at high pressures. *Am. J. Physiol.* **205**, 1013–1018.

BENNETT, P. B. (1964) The effects of high pressures of inert gases on auditory evoked potentials in cat cortex and reticular formation. *Electroenceph. clin. Neurophysiol.* **17**, 388–397.

BENNETT, P. B. (1965a) The narcotic action of inert gases. In *The Physiology of Human Survival.* Ed. O. G. Edholm & A. L. Bacharach. pp. 164–182. London & New York: Academic Press.

BENNETT, P. B. (1965b) *Psychometric Impairment in Men Breathing Oxygen–Helium at Increased Pressures.* Report, Medical Research Council, R.N. Personnel Research Committee, U.P.S. 251, London.

BENNETT, P. B. (1965c) Cortical CO_2 and O_2 at high pressures of argon, nitrogen, helium and oxygen. *J. appl. Physiol.* **20**, 1249–1252.

BENNETT, P. B. (1966) *The Aetiology of Compressed Air Intoxication and Inert Gas Narcosis.* International Series of Monographs in Pure and Applied Biology; Zoology Division. Vol. 31. Oxford: Pergamon.

BENNETT, P. B. (1967) Performance impairment in deep diving due to nitrogen, helium, neon and oxygen. In *Proc. 3rd Symp. Underwater Physiology.* Ed. C. J. Lambertsen. Baltimore: Williams and Wilkins.

BENNETT, P. B. (1971) Psychological, physiological and biophysical studies of narcosis. In *Proc. 4th Symp. Underwater Physiology.* pp. 457–469. Ed. C. J. Lambertsen. New York & London: Academic Press.

BENNETT, P. B. (1972) Review of protective pharmacological agents in diving. *Aerospace Med.* **43**, 184–192.

BENNETT, P. B. (1975) Pharmacological effects of inert gases and hydrogen. In *Underwater Physiology. Vth Symp. Underwater Physiology.* Ed. C. J. Lambertsen. Bethesda: Fedn Am. Socs exp. Biol.

BENNETT, P. B. & ACKLES, K. N. (1970) The narcotic effects of hyperbaric oxygen. In *Proc. 4th International Congress on Hyperbaric Medicine.* Ed. J. Wada and T. Iwa. pp. 74–79. Tokyo: Igaku Shoin.

BENNETT, P. B. & BLENKARN, G. D. (1974) Arterial blood gases in man during inert gas narcosis. *J. appl. Physiol.* **36**, 45–48.

BENNETT, P. B. & CROSS, A. V. C. (1960) Alterations in the fusion frequency of flicker correlated with electroencephalogram changes at increased partial pressures of nitrogen. *J. Physiol.* **151**, 28–29P.

BENNETT, P. B. & DOSSETT, A. N. (1967) *Undesirable Effects of Oxygen–Helium Breathing at Great Depths.* Report, Medical Research Council, R.N. Personnel Research Committee, U.P.S. 260, London.

BENNETT, P. B. & DOSSETT, A. N. (1970) Mechanism and prevention of inert gas narcosis and anesthesia. *Nature, Lond.* **228**, 1317–1318.

BENNETT, P. B. & DOSSETT, A. N. (1971) Studies of cationic and anionic compounds on the effects of high pressures of nitrogen and oxygen. *Proc. 42nd Annual Scientific Meeting.* pp. 69–71. Washington, D.C.: Aerospace and Undersea Medical Society.

BENNETT, P. B. & DOSSETT, A. N. (1973) Alterations in EEG frequencies in animals exposed to 700 ft and 4000 ft oxygen–helium. *Aerospace Med.* **44**, 239–244.

BENNETT, P. B. & GLASS, A. (1961) Electroencephalographic and other changes induced by high partial pressures of nitrogen. *Electroenceph. clin. Neurophysiol.* **13**, 91–98.

BENNETT, P. B. & HAYWARD, A. J. (1967) Electrolyte imbalance as the mechanism for inert gas narcosis and anaesthesia. *Nature, Lond.* **213**, 938–939.

BENNETT, P. B. & TOWSE, J. E. (1971a) *Compressed Air Intoxication at 180 ft., 200 ft., and 220 ft. during Exposures of 1 Hour.* Ministry of Defence, R.N. Physiological Laboratory Report 13/71.

BENNETT, P. B. & TOWSE, J. E. (1971b) Performance efficiency of men breathing oxygen–helium at great depths between 100 ft. to 1500 ft. *Aerospace Med.* **42**, 1147–1156.

BENNETT, P. B. & TOWSE, J. E. (1972) *Electroencephalogram, Tremors, and Mental Performance during Exposure to Air or Oxygen–helium at 100 ft., 200 ft., and 300 ft.* Ministry of Defence, R.N. Physiological Laboratory Report 3/72.

BENNETT, P. B., ACKLES, K. N., and CRIPPS, V. J. (1969) Effects of hyperbaric nitrogen and oxygen on auditory evoked responses in man. *Aerospace Med.* **40**, 521–525.

BENNETT, P. B., DOSSETT, A. N. & RAY, P. (1964) *Nitrogen Narcosis in Subjects Compressed very rapidly with Air to 400 and 500 feet.* Report, Medical Research Council, R.N. Personnel Research Committee, U.P.S. 239, London.

BENNETT, P. B., PAPAHADJOPOULOS, D. & BANGHAM, A. D. (1967) The effect of raised pressures of inert gases on phospholipid model membranes. *Life Sci.* **6**, 2527–2533.

BENNETT, P. B., POULTON, E. C., CARPENTER, A. & CATTON, M. J. (1967) Efficiency at sorting cards in air and a 20 per cent oxygen–helium mixture at depths down to 100 feet and in enriched air. *Ergonomics* **10**, 53–62.

BERT, P. (1878) *La Pression Barometrique.* Paris: Masson.

BEVAN, J. (1971) The human auditory evoked response and contingent negative variation in hyperbaric air. *Electroenceph. clin. Neurophysiol.* **30**, 198–204.

BINGER, C. A. L., FAULKNER, J. M. & MOORE, R. L. (1927) Oxygen poisoning in mammals. *J. exp. Med.* **45**, 849.

BIRCH, S. B. (1859) On oxygen as a therapeutic agent. *Br. med. J.* **2**, 1033.

BJURSTEDT, T. & SEVERIN, G. (1948) The prevention of decompression sickness and nitrogen narcosis by the use of hydrogen as a substitute for nitrogen. *Milit. Surg.* **103**, 107–116.

BOWEN, H. M., ANDERSON, B. & PROMISEL, D. (1966) Studies of diver's performance during the Sealab II project. *Hum. Factors*, **8**, 183–199.

BRAUER, R. W., WAY, R. O. and PERRY, R. A. (1968) Narcotic effects of helium and hydrogen and hyperexcitability phenomena at simulated depths of 1500 to 4000 ft. of sea water. In *Toxicity of Anesthetics.* Ed. B. R. Fink. pp. 241–255. Baltimore: Williams & Wilkins.

BRAUER, R. W., JOHNSEN, D. O., PESSOTTI, R. L. & REDDING, R. W. (1966) Effects of hydrogen and helium at pressures to 67 atmospheres on mice and monkeys. *Fedn Proc. Fedn Am. Socs exp. Biol.* **25**, 202.

BRAUER, R. W., WAY, R. O., JORDAN, M. R. & PARRISH, D. E. (1971) Experimental studies on the high pressure hyperexcitability syndrome in various mammalian species. In *Proc. 4th Symp. Underwater Physiology.* Ed. C. J. Lambertsen. pp. 487–500. New York and London: Academic Press.

BRINK, F. & POSTERNAK, J. (1948) Thermodynamic analysis of relative effectiveness of narcotics. *J. cell. comp. Physiol.* **32**, 211–233.

BÜHLMANN, A. (1963) Deep diving, In *The Undersea Challenge.* Ed. B. Eaton. London: The British Sub-Aqua Club.

BUTLER, T. (1950) Theories of general anesthesia. *Pharmac. Rev.* **2**, 121–160.

CABARROU, P. (1959) *L'Ivresse des grandes profondeurs lors de la plongée à l'air.* Report, Group d'Etudes Recherches Sous-Marine. Toulon.

CABARROU, P. (1964) L'Ivresse des grandes profondeurs. *Presse méd.* **72**, 793–797.

CABARROU, P. (1966) Introduction à la physiologie de 'Homo Aquaticus'. *Presse méd.* **74**, 2771–2773.

CARPENTER, F. G. (1953) Depressant action of inert gases on the central nervous system in mice. *Am. J. Physiol.* **172**, 471–474.

CARPENTER, F. G. (1954) Anaesthetic action of inert and unreactive gases on intact animals and isolated tissues. *Am. J. Physiol.* **178**, 505–509.

CARPENTER, F. G. (1955) Inert gas narcosis. In *Proc. 1st Symp. Underwater Physiology.* Ed. L. G. Goff. Washington, D.C.: Natl Acad. Sci.-Natl Res. Council.

CARPENTER, F. G. (1956) Alteration in mammalian nerve metabolism by soluble and gaseous anaesthetics. *Am. J. Physiol.* **187**, 573–578.

CASE, E. M. & HALDANE, J. B. S. (1941) Human physiology under high pressure. *J. Hyg., Camb.* **41**, 225–249.

CHOUTEAU, J. (1971) Respiratory gas exchange in animals during exposure to extreme ambient pressures. In *Proc. 4th Symp. Underwater Physiology.* Ed. C. J. Lambertsen. pp. 385–397. New York and London: Academic Press.

CHUN, C. (1959) Effect of increased nitrogen pressure on spinal reflex activity. *Fiziol. Zh. SSSR* **45**, 605–609.

CLEMENTS, J. A. & WILSON, K. M. (1962) The affinity of narcotic agents for interfacial films. *Proc. natn. Acad. Sci. U.S.A.* **48**, 1008–1014.

COLER, C. R., PATTON, R. M. & LAMPKIN, E. C. (1971) Effects of prolonged confinement in a hyperbaric environment on short-term memory. *Proc. 41st Annual Scientific Meeting.* pp. 151–152. Aerospace Medical Association, Washington.

COUSTEAU, J. Y. (1953) *The Silent World.* London: Reprint Society.

CRISCUOLI, P. M. & ALBANO, G. (1971) Neuropsychological effects of exposure to compressed air. *Proc. 4th Symp. Underwater Physiology.* Ed. C. J. Lambertsen. pp. 471–478. New York and London: Academic Press.

CULLEN, S. C. & GROSS, E. G. (1951) The anesthetic properties of xenon in animals and human beings with additional observations on krypton. *Science, N.Y.* **113**, 580–582.

DAMANT, G. C. C. (1930) Physiological effects of work in compressed air. *Nature, Lond.* **126**, 606–608.

DAVIS, F. M., OSBORNE, J. P. BADDELEY, A. D. & GRAHAM, I. M. F. (1972) Diver performance: nitrogen narcosis and anxiety. *Aerospace Med.* **43**, 1079–1082.

DAWE, R. A., MILLER, K. W. & SMITH, E. B. (1964) Solubility relations of fluorine compounds and inert gas narcosis. *Nature, Lond.* **204**, 798.

DICKSON, J. G., LAMBERTSEN, C. J. & CASSILS, J. G. (1971) Quantitation of performance decrements in narcotised man. In *Proc. 4th Symp. Underwater Physiology*. Ed. C. J. Lambertsen. pp. 449–455. New York and London: Academic Press.

EBERT, J., HORNSEY, S. & HOWARD, A. (1958) Effect of inert gases on oxygen-dependent radiosensitivity. *Nature, Lond.* **181**, 613–616.

EDEL, P. O. (1969) Tektite I to test merits of nitrogen–oxygen breathing mix. *Ocean Industry.* **4**, 61–65.

EDEL, P. O. (1971) Dog breathes H_2–O_2 in 1000 ft. dive. *Ocean Industry.* May. 21–22.

EDEL, P. O. (1972) Preliminary studies of hydrogen–oxygen breathing mixtures for deep-sea diving. *Proc. Oceanology International.* pp. 485–489. London: Society for Underwater Technology.

EGER, E. I., LUNDGREN, C., MILLER, S. L. & STEVENS, W. C. (1969) Anesthetic potencies of sulfur hexafluoride, carbon tetrafluoride, chloroform and ethrane in dogs: Correlation with the Hydrate and Lipid Theories of anesthetic action. *Anesthesiology* **30**, 129–135.

END, E. (1938) The use of new equipment and helium gas in a world record dive. *J. ind. Hyg. Toxicol.* **20**, 511–520.

FEATHERSTONE, R. M. (1960) Anesthesia: Xenon. In *Medical Physics*. Vol. 3, p. 22. Ed. O. Glasser. Chicago: Yearbook.

FEATHERSTONE, R. M. & MUEHLBAECHER, C. A. (1963) The current role of inert gases in the search for anaesthesia mechanisms. *Pharmac. Rev.* **15**, 97–121.

FEATHERSTONE, R. M., MUEHLBAECHER, C. A., DeBON, F. L. & FORSAITH, J. A. (1961) Interactions of inert anaesthetic gases with proteins. *Anesthesiology* **22**, 977–981.

FENN, W. O. (1965) Inert gas narcosis. Hyperbaric Oxygenation. *Ann. N.Y. Acad. Sci.* **117**, 760–767.

FERGUSON, J. (1939) The use of chemical potentials as indices of toxicity, *Proc. R. Soc.* **B 197**, 387–404.

FERGUSON, J. & HAWKINS, S. W. (1949) Toxic action of some simple gases at high pressure. *Nature, Lond.* **164**, 963–964.

FINK, R. B. (Ed.) (1972) *Cellular Biology and Toxicity of Anesthetics*. Baltimore: Williams & Wilkins.

FOWLER, B. & ACKLES, K. N. (1972) Narcotic effects in man of breathing 80–20 argon–oxygen and air under hyperbaric conditions. *Aerospace Med.* **43**, 1219–1224.

FRANKENHAEUSER, M., GRAFF-LONNEVIG, V., & HESSER, C. M. (1963) Effects on psychomotor functions of different nitrogen–oxygen gas mixtures at increased ambient pressures. *Acta physiol. scand.* **59**, 400–409.

FRENCH, J. D., VERZEANO, M. & MAGOUN, H. W. (1953) A neural basis of the anaesthetic state. *Archs Neurol. Psychiat., Chicago* **69**, 519–529.

FRUCTUS, X. R., BRAUER, R. W. & NAQUET, R. (1971) Physiological effects observed in the course of simulated deep chamber dives to a maximum of 36·5 atm in a helium–oxygen atm. In *Proc. 4th Symp. Underwater Physiology*. Ed. C. J. Lambertsen. pp 545–550. New York and London: Academic Press.

GESELL, R. (1923) On the chemical regulation of respiration. *Am. J. Physiol.* **66**, 5–47.

GOTTLIEB, S. F., CYMERMAN, A. & METZ, A. V. (1968) Effect of xenon, krypton and nitrous oxide on sodium active transport through frog skin with additional observations on sciatic nerve conduction. *Aerospace Med.* **39**, 449–453.

GREEN, J. B. (1861) *Diving With and Without Armour*. Buffalo: Leavitt.

HAMILTON, R. W. (1966) Physiological responses at rest and in exercise during saturation at 20 atmospheres of He–O_2. In *Proc. 3rd Symp. Underwater Physiology*. Ed. C. J. Lambertsen. Baltimore: Williams & Wilkins.

HAMILTON, R. W., MACINNIS, J. B., NOBLE, A. D. & SCHREINER, H. R. (1966) *Saturation Diving at 650 ft*. Tech. Memo B1411. Ocean Systems Inc., Tonawanda, N.Y.

HESSER, C. M. (1963) Measurement of inert gas narcosis in man. In *Proc. 2nd Symp. Underwater Physiology*. Ed. C. J. Lambertsen & L. J. Greenbaum. Washington, D.C.: Natl Acad. Sci.-Natl Res. Council.

HESSER, C. M., ADOLFSON, J. & FAGRAEUS, L. (1971) Role of CO_2 in compressed-air narcosis. *Aerospace Med.* **42**, 163–168.

HILL, L. & GREENWOOD, M. (1906) The influence of increased barometric pressure on man. *Proc. R. Soc.* **B 77**, 442–453.

HILL, L. & McLEOD, J. J. (1903) The influence of compressed air on respiratory exchange. *J. Physiol.* **29**, 492–510.

HILL, L. & PHILLIPS, A. E. (1932) Deep sea diving. *Jl R. nav. med. Serv.* **18**, 157–173.

HILL, L., DAVIS, R. H., SELBY, R. P., PRIDHAM, A. & MALONE, A. E. (1933) *Deep Diving and Ordinary Diving*. Report of a Committee Appointed by the British Admiralty.

IKELS, K. G. (1964) *Determination of the Solubility of Neon in Water and Extracted human fat*. Task. No. 775801 SAM-TDR 64–28. USAF School of Aerospace Medicine, Brooks Air Force Base, Texas.

JOHNSON, F. H. & FLAGLER, E. A. (1950) Hydrostatic pressure reversal of narcosis in tadpoles. *Science, N.Y.* **112**, 91–92.

JOHNSON, S. M. & MILLER, K. W. (1970) Antagonism of pressure and anesthesia. *Nature, Lond.* **228**, 75–76.

JUNOD, T. (1835) Recherches sur les effets physiologiques et therapeutiques de la compression et de rarefaction de l'air, taut sur le corps que les membres isolés. *Ann. gen. Med.* **9**, 157.

JULLIEN, G., ROGER, A. & CHATRIAN, G. F. (1953) Preliminary report on variations of the EEG of the cat at various air pressures. *Riv. neurol.* **23**, 357–363.

KAPLAN, S. A. & STEIN, S. N. (1957) Sodium, potassium and glutamate content of guinea pig brain following exposure to oxygen at high pressure. *Am. J. Physiol.* **190**, 166–168.

KIESSLING, R. J. & MAAG, C. H. (1962) Performance impairment as a function of nitrogen narcosis. *J. appl. Psychol.* **46**, 91–95.

KINNEY, J. S. & McKAY, C. L. (1971) *The Visual Evoked Response as a Measure of Nitrogen Narcosis in Navy Divers*. Report No. 664. U.S. Naval Submarine Medical Center. New London.

LAMBERTSEN, C. J. (Ed.) (1971) Part XI. Influence of inert gases and pressure upon central nervous functions. In *Proc. 4th Symp. Underwater Physiology*. pp. 449–509. New York and London: Academic Press.

LAMBERTSON, C. J. (Ed.) (1975) Collaborative investigation of limits of human tolerance to pressurisation with helium, neon and nitrogen. Simulation of density equivalent to helium–oxygen respiration at depth to 2,000, 3,000, 4,000 and 5,000 ft. of sea water. In *Underwater Physiology, Vth Symp. Underwater Physiology.* Bethesda: Fed. Am. Socs exp. Biol.

LANPHIER, E. H. (1963) Influences of increased ambient pressure upon alveolar ventilation. In *Proc. 2nd Symp. Underwater Physiology.* Ed. C. J. Lambertsen & L. J. Greenbaum. Washington, D.C.: Natl Acad. Sci.-Natl Res. Council.

LARRABEE, M. G. & POSTERNAK, J. M. (1952). Selective action of anaesthetics on synapses and axons in mammalian sympathetic ganglia. *J. Neurophysiol.* **15**, 91–114.

LATNER, A. L. (1965). Possible biochemical mechanisms in anaesthesia. *Proc. R. Soc. Med.* **58**, 895–900.

LAWRENCE, J. H., LOOMIS, W. F., TOBIAS, C. A. & TURPIN, F. H. (1946) Preliminary observations on the narcotic effect of xenon with a review of values for solubilities of gases in water and oils. *J. Physiol.* **105**, 197–204.

LAZAREV, N. V., LYUBLINA, Y. I. & MADORSKAYA, R. Y. (1948) Narcotic action of xenon. *Fiziol. Zh. SSSR* **34**, 131–134.

LEON, H. A. & COOK, S. F. (1960) A mechanism by which helium increases metabolism in small mammals. *Am. J. Physiol.* **199**, 243–245.

LEVER, M. J., MILLER, K. W., PATON, W. D. M. & SMITH, E. B. (1971) Pressure reversal of anaesthesia. *Nature, Lond.* **231**, 386–371.

LEVER, M. J., MILLER, K. W., PATON, W. D. M., STREET, W. B. & SMITH, E. B. (1971) Effects of hydrostatic pressure on mammals. In *Proc. 4th Symp. Underwater Physiology.* Ed. C. J. Lambertsen. pp. 101–108. New York and London: Academic Press.

LEVY, L. & FEATHERSTONE, R. M. (1954) The effect of xenon and nitrous oxide on in vitro guinea pig brain respiration and oxidation phosphorylation. *J. Pharmac. exp. Therap.* **110**, 221–225.

McILWAIN, H. (1962) In *Enzymes and Drug Action,* Ciba Foundation Symposium jointly with Co-ordinating Committee for Symposia on Drug Action. London: Churchill.

MALETZKY, B. & BLACHLY, P. H. (1971) *The Use of Lithium in Psychiatry.* London: Butterworth.

MARSHALL, J. M. (1951) Nitrogen narcosis in frogs and mice. *Am. J. Physiol.* **166**, 699–711.

MARSHALL, J. M. & FENN, W. O. (1950) The narcotic effects of nitrogen and argon on the central nervous system of frogs. *Am. J. Physiol.* **163**, 733.

MEYER, H. H. (1899) Theoris der alkoholnarkose. *Arch. exp. Path. Pharmak.* **42**, 109.

MEYER, K. H. & HOPFF, H. (1923) Narcosis by inert gases under pressure. *Hoppe-Seyler's Z. physiol. Chem.* **126**, 288–298.

MILES, S. (1957) The effect of changes in barometric pressures on maximum breathing capacity. *J. Physiol.* **137**, 85P.

MILES, S. & MACKAY, D. E. (1959) *The Nitrogen Narcosis Hazard and the Self-contained Diver.* Report, Medical Research Council, R. N. Personnel Research Committee. U.P.S. 184, London.

MILLER, S. L. (1961) A theory of gaseous anesthetics. *Proc. natn. Acad. Sci. U.S.A.* **47**, 1515–1524.

MILLER, K. W., PATON, W. D. M. & SMITH, E. B. (1965) Site of action of general anaesthetics. *Nature, Lond.* **206**, 574–577.

MILLER, K. W. PATON, W. D. M. & SMITH, E. B. (1967) The anaesthetic pressures of certain fluorine-containing gases. *Br. J. Anaesth.* **31**, 910.

MORRIS, L. E., KNOTT, J. R. & PITTINGER, C. B. (1955) Electroencephalographic and blood gas observations in human surgical patients during xenon anesthesia. *Anesthesiology* **16**, 312–319.

MOXON, W. (1881) Croonian lectures on the influence of the circulation on the nervous system. *Br. med. J.* **1**, 491–497, 583–585.

MULLINS, L. J. (1954) Some physical mechanisms in narcosis. *Chem. Rev.* **54**, 289–323.

OVERTON, E. (1901) *Studien Über die Narkose,* Jena: Fisher.

PATON, W. D. M. & SPEDEN, R. N. (1965) Anaesthetics and the central nervous system. *Br. med. Bull.* **21**, 44–48.

PAULING, L. (1961) A molecular theory of anaesthesia, *Science, N.Y.* **134**, 15–21.

PHILLIPS, A. E. (1931) Recent research work in deep sea diving. *Proc. R. Soc. Med.* **25**, 693.

PITTINGER, C. B. (1962) Mechanisms of anaesthesia. Xenon as an anaesthetic. In *Proc. 22nd Intern. Congr. Physiol. Sci. 1.* London: Excerpta Medica Foundation.

PITTINGER, C. B. & KEASLING, H. H. (1959) Theories of narcosis. *Anesthesiology* **20**, 204–213.

POULTON, E. C., CATTON, M. J. & CARPENTER, A. (1964) Efficiency at sorting cards in compressed air. *Br. J. ind. Med.* **21**, 242–245.

QUASTEL, J. H. (1965) Effects of drugs on metabolism of brain in vitro. *Br. med. Bull.* **21**, 49–56.

RADOMSKI, M. W. & BENNETT, P. B. (1971) Metabolic changes in man during short exposure to high pressure. *Aerospace Med.* **42**, 309–313.

RADOMSKI, M. W. & WOOD, J. D. (1970) Effect of metal ions on oxygen toxicity. *Aerospace Med.* 41, 1382–1387.

RASHBASS, C. (1955) *The Unimportance of Carbon Dioxide in Nitrogen Narcosis.* Report, Medical Research Council, R.N. Personnel Research Committee. U.P.S. 153, London.

RINFRET, A. P. & DOEBBLER, G. F. (1961) Physiological and biochemical effects and applications. In *Argon, Helium and the Rare Gases.* Ed. G. A. Cook. New York: Interscience.

ROGER, A., CABARROU, P. & GASTAUT, H. H. (1955) EEG changes in humans due to changes in surrounding atmospheric pressure. *Electroenceph. clin. Neurophysiol.* **7**, 152.

ROSTAIN, J. C. & NAQUET, R. (1972) Resultats preliminaries d'une étude comparative de l'effet des mélanges oxygène–helium et oxygène–hydrogène et des hautes pressions sur le babouin Papio Papio. In *Proceedings Third International Conference on Hyperbaric and Underwater Physiology.* pp. 44–49. Paris: Doin.

ROTH, E. M. (1965) *Space Cabin Atmospheres. Part III Physiological Factors of Inert Gases.* Report 1, Part III Nat. Aeron. Space Admin., NASR-115. Albuquerque: Lovelace Foundation.

SCHATTE, C. L. & BENNETT, P. B. (1973) Acute metabolic and physiologic response of goats to narcosis. *Aerospace Med.* **44**, 613–623.

SCHOENBORN, B. P. (1965) Binding of xenon to horse haemoglobin, *Nature, Lond.* **208**, 760–762.

SCHOENBORN, B. P., WATSON, H. C. & KENDREW, J. C. (1965) Binding of xenon to sperm whale myoglobin. *Nature, Lond.* **207**, 28–30.

SCHREINER, H. R., HAMILTON, R. W. & LANGLEY, T. D. (1972) Neon: An attractive new commercial diving gas. In *Proc. Offshore Technology Conference, Houston. May 1–3.*

SCHREINER, H. R., HAMILTON, R. W., NOBLE, A. D., TROVATO, L. A. & MacINNIS, J. B. (1966) Effects of helium and neon breathing on man at 20·7 atm. pressure. *Fedn Proc. Fedn Am. Socs exp. Biol.* **25**, 230.

SEARS, D. F. (1962) Role of lipid molecules in anaesthesia. In *Proc. 22nd. Intern. Congr. Physiol. Sci. 1.* London: Excerpta Medica Foundation.

SEEMAN, P. (1972) The effects of anesthetics and tranquilizers on cell membranes. In *Cellular Biology and Toxicity of Anesthetics* Ed. B. R. Fink. pp. 149–159. Baltimore: Williams & Wilkins.

SEEMAN, P., SHAAFI, R. I., GALEY, W. R. & SOLOMON, A. K. (1970) The effect of anesthetics (chlorpromazine, ethanol) on erythrocyte permeability to water. *Biochem. Biophys. Acta* **211**, 365–373.

SEUSING, J. (1961) The problem of depth intoxication. *Wehrmed. Mitt.* **10**, 150–152.

SEUSING, J. & DRUBE, H. (1960) The importance of hypercapnia in depth intoxication. *Klin. Wschr.* **38**, 1088–1090.

SHILLING, C. W. & WILLGRUBE, W. W. (1937) Quantitative study of mental and neuromuscular reactions as influenced by increased air pressure. *U.S. nav. med. Bull.* **35**, 373–380.

SMITH, F. J. C., HEIM, J. W., THOMSON, R. M. & DRINKER, C. K. (1932) Bodily changes and development of pulmonary resistance in rats living under compressed air conditions. *J. exp. Med.* **56**, 63.

SOMJEN, G. G. (1963) Effects of ether and thiopental on spinal presynaptic terminals. *J. Pharmac. exp. Ther.* **140**, 396–402.

SOMJEN, G. G. & GILL, M. (1963) The mechanisms of the blockade of synaptic transmission in the mammalian spinal cord by diethyl ether and thiopental. *J. Pharmac. exp. Ther.* **140**, 19–30.

STERN, S. A. & FRISCH, H. L. (1973) Dependence of inert gas narcosis on lipid 'Free Volume'. *J. appl. Physiol.* **34**, 366–373.

TAYLOR, D. W. (1956) The effects of vitamin E and methylene blue on the manifestations of oxygen poisoning in the rat. *J. Physiol.* **131**, 200–206.

THOMAS, J. J., NEPTUNE, E. M. & SUDDUTH, H. C. (1963) Toxic effects of oxygen at high pressure on the metabolism of D-glucose by dispersions of rat brain. *Biochem. J.* **88**, 31–45.

TOWNSEND, R. E., THOMPSON, L. W. & SULG, I. (1971) Effect of increased pressures of normoxic helium, nitrogen and neon on EEG and reaction time in man. *Aerospace Med.* **42**, 843–847.

UNSWORTH, I. P. (1966) Inert gas narcosis—an introduction. *Postgrad. Med. J.* **42**, 378–385.

VAIL, E. G. (1971) Hyperbaric respiratory mechanics. *Aerospace Med.* **42**, 536–546.

WELCH, B. E. & ROBERTSON, W. G. (1965) Effects of inert gases in cabin atmospheres. In *Proc. 3rd. Intern. Symp. Bioastronautics and the Exploration of Space.* Ed. T. C. Bedwell & H. Strughold. Brooks Air Force Base, Texas: USAF Systems Command.

WEYBREW, B. B., GREENWOOD, M. & PARKER, J. W. (1964). *Psychological and Psycho-physiological Effects of Confinement in a High Pressure Helium–oxygen–nitrogen Atmosphere for 284 Hours.* U.S.N. Medical Research Laboratory, Report 441, New London.

WOOD, W. B. (1963) Ventilatory dynamics under hyperbaric states. In *Proc. 2nd. Symp. Underwater Physiology.* Ed. C. J. Lambertsen & L. J. Greenbaum. Washington, D.C.: Natl Acad. Sci.-Natl Res. Council. (Publ. 1181.)

WOOD, W. B., LEVE, L. H. & WORKMAN, R. D. (1962) *Ventilatory Dynamics under Hyperbaric States.* Report 1–62. Washington, D.C.: U.S.N. Experimental Diving Unit.

WULF, R. J. & FEATHERSTONE, R. M. (1957) A correlation of Van der Waals constants with anaesthetic potency. *Anesthesiology* **18**, 97–105.

ZALTSMAN, G. L. (1961) Physiological principles of a sojourn of a human in conditions of raised pressure of the gaseous medium. *Gasodarstvennoye Izdatel'stvo Meditsinskoy Literatury.* Medgiz Leningradskoye Otdeleniye.

ZALTSMAN, G. L. (Ed.) (1968) Hyperbaric Epilepsy and Narcosis (Neurophysiological Studies). pp. 1–265. Leningrad: Sechenov Institute of Evolutionary Physiology and Biochemistry, USSR Academy of Sciences.

ZETTERSTROM, A. (1948) Deep sea diving with synthetic gas mixtures. *Milit. Surg.* **103**, 104–106.

13

The High Pressure Nervous Syndrome: Animals

R. W. BRAUER

By the late 1950s diving physiologists had made great strides toward understanding and managing some of the principal hazards which beset the diver in his progress toward the depths, such as oxygen toxicity, the narcotic effects of inert gases used as oxygen diluents in high pressure environments and the mechanical effects of dense atmospheres upon respiratory work and the effectiveness of ventilation. These diverse studies held the attention of investigators to such an extent that, when the first indications of the effects of high pressures upon the central nervous system of higher vertebrates were encountered in the course of animal experiments at the Sechenov Institute in Leningrad and in human experimental dives at the Royal Naval Physiological Laboratory in England, these effects were attributed to 'helium narcosis', and were referred to as 'potentiation of the convulsant effects of oxygen by helium' (Zaltsman 1968) or as 'helium tremors' (Bennett 1967). The first recognition that high pressure itself could pose a problem in diving arose, as a by-product of studies of inert gas narcosis, independently in two laboratories. One case was during studies of the reversal of narcosis by high hydrostatic pressures (Miller et al. 1967) and the second case was when the observation of high pressure convulsions came as an unexpected complication in the course of experiments concerning the relative narcotic potencies of helium and hydrogen (Brauer et al. 1966).

In fact these several observations merely continued a chain of studies begun in the late 1880s by Regnard (1891), who first studied the effects of high hydrostatic pressures upon a variety of organisms and clearly described the now familiar sequence of hyperactivity, spasms (subsequently often miscalled tetany) and paralysis, at progressively increasing pressures. The early descriptive work by Regnard (1891) was still heavily conditioned by the technical difficulties encountered which identified changes that persisted after decompression. This was followed by the studies of Fontaine (1930) and of Ebbecke and his associates (Ebbecke 1914; Ebbecke & Hasenring 1935; Ebbecke & Schaefer 1935) who focused their attention upon the physiology of muscles under pressure. This period presently gave way to the studies of D. Brown, Johnson, Eyring and their associates (Johnson 1954) concerning the effect of pressure on simple and complex enzyme reaction chains. More recently, this work gave way as a centre of attention to the work on cell biology, and especially on cell division processes, initiated in the United States of America by Marsland (Marsland 1970) and continued especially by Zimmerman (Zimmerman 1970) and Landau and in the United Kingdom by Kitching (Kitching 1957) and his students.

Curiously, throughout this long period of more than half a century, little attention has been paid to the central nervous system. Fontaine (1930) felt that the excitement phase of the pressure syndrome depended largely on the presence of a central nervous system. A few investigators examined nerve fibers or nerve muscle preparations. Among these, Ebbecke and Schaefer (1935) noted that while the direct excitability of frog gastrocnemius is always reduced by compression, occasional nerve muscle preparations stimulated by way of the nerve showed a lowering of the threshold voltage at pressures around 100 to 200 ATS invariably resulting in lowered excitability (Grundfest 1936). Grundfest and Cattell (1935), working with single nerve fibers in paraffin oil, recorded repetitive after-discharges, increased spike potential, and spike duration at 300 to 500 ATS pressure, and noted the marked enhancement of the negative after-potential at pressures as low as 35 ATS. At pressures above 500 ATS, the threshold for stimulation rose rapidly until the preparations became unexcitable. These findings were confirmed in general by Spyropoulos (1957) under conditions which excluded the possibility of thermal artifacts. Effects upon duration of the action current were recognizable at pressures as low as 150 ATS. In squid giant axon, threshold stimulation currents were appreciably reduced at 100 ATS, and the duration of membrane impedance change was increased 50 to 100% at 200 ATS. At 200 to 500 ATS, these fibers fired spontaneously (Spyropoulos 1957). The narcotizing effect of ethanol upon this preparation could be reversed at 500 ATS. Finally, Gershfeld and Shanes (1959) demonstrated that at pressures of 150 ATS or greater, toad sciatic nerve showed an increased sodium ion content and a loss of potassium ion resembling, in this respect, the action of veratrine. Unlike the veratrine effect, however, this partial depolarization was not reversed by cocaine. In contrast to these promising results on the effect of hydrostatic pressure on axon conduction, no reports have yet dealt with synaptic transmission.

By the mid-1960s, knowledge of high pressure effects on other biological systems had made considerable progress, both on the theoretical and on the descriptive levels. Thus a reviewer could confidently say in 1970 that 'it is not so much the presence of high pressure effects in vertebrates subjected to 50 or more atmospheres that needs explaining, as the observation that effects are so relatively modest and specific' (Zimmerman 1970). Since the history of the study of hydrostatic pressure effects in general is reviewed elsewhere in this volume by Macdonald, these few historical notes will suffice here, and attention will now be turned directly to the etiology of the High Pressure Nervous Syndrome sometimes called the High Pressure Neurological syndrome (HPNS) in the higher vertebrates, and to the description of such animal experiments as are relevant.

THE HIGH PRESSURE NEURO- LOGICAL SYNDROME IN VERTEBRATES

The development of the HPNS has been followed in some detail in numerous species: Rostain and Naquet (1970) have described it for the baboon; Lever et al. (1971) have described it in mice and newts; Albano and his co-workers (Albano et al. 1972) describe the events in rats; Brauer and his co-workers have studied it in mice (Brauer, Way & Jordan 1971), in squirrel monkeys (Brauer, Jordan & Way 1972), and in 20 other vertebrate species (Brauer et al. 1974b). Zaltsman (1968) and Zaltsman, Selivra and Ponomaryer (1973) encountered events now clearly recognizable as stages of the HPNS in dogs and in mice. On the basis of this extensive material it is now possible to construct a generalized description of the stages of development of the HPNS in the higher vertebrates.

The syndrome begins with motor disturbances, which tend to be expressed in the form of enhanced, somewhat irregular motor activity in the lower vertebrates, but which in mammals and birds are seen as tremors or as somewhat jerky, ratchety movements of the head or extremities. This stage, in the mammals, is succeeded by the appearance of isolated non-volitional myoclonic jerks, again more often most noticeable in the face and upper extremities which increases in severity until it gives way to the third stage, marked by generalized clonic or tonic–clonic convulsions. If the pressure is maintained constant at this stage, and while the tremors persist, several additional seizures are seen at increasing intervals. Further increase in pressure eventually produces prolonged tonic seizures in the majority of animals. If the convulsive phase of the syndrome is suppressed pharmacologically there will eventually develop a

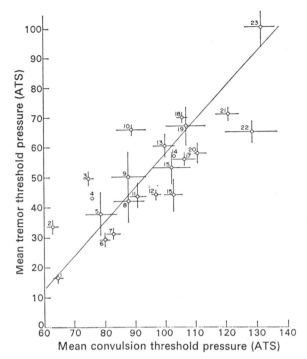

FIG. 13.1. Relation between mean HPNS tremor and convulsion thresholds for 22 species of vertebrates. The least square regression line is drawn. The correlation coefficient is 0·83 (data from Table 13.1). Horizontal and vertical bars represent standard deviation of the mean for P_C and P_T for each species

compression conditions ($T = 31–33°C$, $\dot{P} = 24$ ATS/hr, $P_{O_2} = 0·4–0·5$ ATS). The data can best be described by a simple equation:

$$\bar{P}_C = 49·6 + 0·89\ \bar{P}_T$$

where $\bar{P}_T$ and $\bar{P}_C$ are the mean tremor and the mean convulsion threshold pressures respectively (Brauer et al. 1974b). Since tremor thresholds for man under these compression conditions are known (P_T is about 26 ATS; Brauer et al. 1969), this equation allows some reasonably informed prediction of where the convulsion threshold should fall for human subjects compressed under the particular conditions of this study (helium–oxygen atmosphere, $P_{O_2} = 0·4$ ATS; compression rate, $\dot{P} = 24$ ATS/hr; chamber temperature, $31–33°C$). The most likely mean convulsion threshold for man under these conditions, as read from Fig. 13.1, is 65 ± 8 ATS, a value that is in good agreement with the baboons studied by Rostain and colleagues which developed tremors at a mean of 36 ATS and convulsions between 65 and 70 ATS (Rostain & Naquet 1970; Rostain 1973).

Within any given species, development of the HPNS is subject to a considerable degree of individual variation. Statistical analysis shows the variance is of the order of ± 5 to ± 10 ATS for either P_C or P_T, in groups as diverse as a lizard species, a mouse strain, or squirrel monkeys from the Peruvian Amazonia (Brauer et al. 1974b).

In addition, it has been shown that in monkeys individual convulsion thresholds tend to be repeated in successive exposures separated by 4 or more months of 'rest and recreation' (Fig. 13.2) (Brauer et al. 1974c). The average difference between first and second convulsion thresholds in this series was only $1·25$ ATS $\pm 1·50$. Thus, there is strong evidence to suggest that HPNS convulsion thresholds are a stable individual characteristic and that selection for high HPNS sensitivity in individuals would be of value in very deep diving operations.

The motor events described are the most readily noticed, but constitute by no means the only manifestations of the HPNS. There are, in addition, electrophysiological, and probably autonomic and perhaps cognitive changes which accompany the several stages of development of the HPNS described so far.

fourth stage, the physiological nature of which has not been fully studied. There is some reason to suspect that this stage may represent the effect of hydrostatic pressure on contractile tissues and that the inactivity and eventual death that characterize it may reflect cardiorespiratory failure (Miller et al. 1967).

The important factor in these events is comprised in the first three stages of HPNS development. Comparative studies in numerous vertebrate species suggest a definite common pattern for the relation between pressure attained and the stage of HPNS reached. This is illustrated in Fig. 13.1 which, together with Table 13.1, shows the relation between the mean pressures at which tremors (stage I) begin, to the mean convulsion threshold pressures (stage III) observed in 22 vertebrate species subjected to compression in helium–oxygen atmospheres under one particular set of

TABLE 13.1

Comparison of susceptibility to the high pressure neurological syndrome in 22 species of vertebrates shown in Fig. 13.1

Class	Order	Species	No. in Fig. 13.1
Pisces		*Achirus fasciatus*	23
		Paralichtys dentatum	19
		Anguilla rostrata	16
		Symphurus palguisa	9
Reptilia		*Thamnophis sertalis*	22
		Anolis carolinensis	18
Aves		*Serinus canarius*	21
		Streptopelia risona	20
		Gallus domesticus	15
Mammalia	Marsupialia	*Didelphys virgininiana*	5
		Choloepus hoffmanni	4
	Edentata	*Dasypus novemcinctus*	13
	Rodentia	*Epimys rattus*	10
		Mus musculus	12
		*Mus musculus**	3
		Cavia porcellus	6
	Lagomorpha	*Oryncolagus cuniculus*	16
	Ungulates	*Capra hircos*	11
	Carnivora	*Procyon lotor*	8
	Primates	*Tupaia tupaia*	1
		Saimiri sciureus	2
		Macaca mulatta	7
		Nycticebus coucang	14

* The mice were of two different strains.

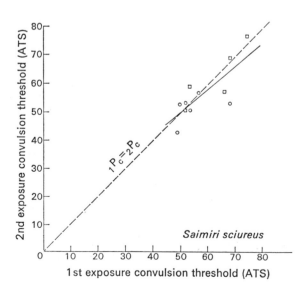

FIG. 13.2. Relation between convulsion thresholds of male squirrel monkeys in two successive exposures to high pressure heliox atmospheres, separated by 4 months' recovery. The solid line represents the computed least square regression equation $_2Pc = 8.8 + 0.83\ _1Pc$. The dashed line represents the hypothesis $_1Pc = _2Pc$. Circles represent bounce dives; squares represent saturation dives

The electroencephalographic changes accompanying compression in heliox atmospheres have been described for the baboon (Rostain & Naquet 1972), for the rat (Albano et al. 1972; Bennett & Dossett 1973), for the dog (Zaltsman, Ponomaryer & Selivra 1968; Zaltsman et al. 1973) and for the squirrel monkey (Brauer, Jordan & Way 1972; Hurd, Brauer & Wilder 1974).

During stage I in the squirrel monkey (30–40 ATS at $P = 24$ ATS/hr) bilateral slowing to the theta range was noted, associated, when present, with visible tremors (Hurd, Brauer & Wilder 1974). In the baboon Rostain (1973) reported no EEG changes below 60 ATS while tremor onset was noted between 300 and 450 ATS. In the rat Albano and his co-workers (Albano et al. 1972) observed the appearance of slow wave activity at about the time of appearance of tremors and associated with voluntary movements. They noted that these changes disappeared rapidly if the compression was stopped and the animals maintained for some time at a constant pressure. Bennett and Dossett (1973) also in the rat, confirmed this trend by the use of a Nihon Kohden frequency analyser which reveals the increased relative importance of theta and especially of delta waves in what appear to be stage I animals. The slow wave activity effect disappeared in Bennett's experiments when compression rates were slowed from 200 to 20 ATS/hr giving way to a general reduction in amplitude somewhat less marked in the delta than in the alpha range. These results differ slightly from those of other observers due to the high Po_2 of 2 ATA which was utilized throughout, and Bennett and Dossett speculated about the possible contribution of the narcotic effects of oxygen to their picture.

In dogs, Zaltsman (1968) reported increased theta wave activity at pressures which appear to represent stage I HPNS in that species.

Stage II of the HPNS in the baboon (Rostain 1973) and the squirrel monkey (Brauer, Jordan & Way 1972; Hurd, Brauer & Wilder 1974) is associated with the appearance of multifocal spiking and sharp waves, especially over the frontal rolandic areas in the baboon, and not infrequently also over the occipital regions in both primates. As pressures are raised further, these changes become more prominent and tend to spread, along with the greatly increased non-volitional, often myoclonic, motor activity. Similar changes are reported by Albano and his co-workers (Albano et al. 1972) for the rat but are curiously absent from Bennett and Dossett's animals exposed at high Po_2 (Bennett and Dossett 1973). Here, at compression rates comparable to those used in the primates or the series of Fig. 13.1, there is merely progressive depression of EEG amplitudes.

Stage III in all species is associated with paroxysmal EEG crises of the polyspike or spike and wave type. Crises of this type may either be seen to develop by generalization from isolated areas of focal activity or they may appear abruptly upon a near normal EEG background, and they may involve the entire cortex or remain partly confined to a region such as the right or left occipital cortex (Rostain 1973; Hurd, Brauer & Wilder 1974).

Post-ictal periods of coma and EEG flattening from 15 to 30 sec follow such seizures, and are succeeded by return to more normal EEG activity and clinical behaviour. If compression is continued, after the first seizure, additional seizures may occur and the EEG will tend to become increasingly disorganized. Eventually, any periods of normal activity virtually disappear and the EEG may consist of a nearly continuous series of seizures.

The overall picture which is presented by the EEG data concerning the HPNS differs in a number of important ways from that seen in epilepsy associated with definite cortical lesions and suggests strongly that the observed seizures at the cortical level are the result of abnormal electrical activity originating in subcortical structures. Using bipolar concentric electrodes implanted into various subcortical regions Hurd and his co-workers (Hurd, Brauer & Wilder 1974) detected slowing, then spiking in the mid-brain reticular formation and thalamus during stage II. Build-up of subcortical spike discharge tends to precede by several minutes the development of synchronous cortical spike discharges and the clinically recognizable motor seizure. In contrast, caudate nucleus implants failed to show significant changes in electrical activity prior to the convulsive phase, except for a progressive lowering of amplitude. The prominence of motion-associated tremors during stages I and II suggested the possibility of cerebellar involvement. Monjan, Goldberg and Brauer in unpublished work observed the development of the HPNS in rats with partial surgical or near total viral ablation of the cerebellum. The only effect noted was a significant lowering of the convulsion threshold, roughly proportional to the amount of cerebellar tissue destroyed. It is interesting to contrast these findings with Rucci's results in relation to hyperoxic convulsions (Rucci, Giretti & LaRocca, 1968).

The concept that stages I through III of the HPNS are largely dependent upon changes producing aberrant subcortical electrical activities is supported by the observation that the full syndrome of the HPNS can be observed in lower vertebrate species (Fig. 13.1) or in immature mammals. Newborn mice and rats are exceptionally susceptible to HPNS seizures (Brauer, Way & Jordan 1971; Mansfield, Brauer & Gillen 1974). Yet, in these animals cortical electrical activity cannot be recorded until the sixth and fifth day respectively after birth (Kobayashi et al. 1963), and histological development of cortical structures is likewise extremely incomplete during the first few days of independent life.

While it is thus clear that not inconsiderable changes in central nervous function are associated with pre-seizure stage II of the HPNS, the extent to which these are reflected in parallel changes in peripheral functions remains to be explored.

Development of the HPNS is not accompanied by a generalized autonomic discharge. Thus, heart rates of squirrel monkeys (Brauer, Jordan & Way 1972) and of baboons (Rostain 1973) remain virtually unchanged until the very moment of a generalized convulsion, increasing only after some moments of actual convulsive motor activity. Similarly, respiratory rates in many cases remain constant until the motor seizure is well developed. In rats a perceptible hyperpnea has been recorded, beginning about the time of onset of the tremor stage (Albano et al. 1972) and supposedly secondary to the enhanced motor tone. Whether more subtle changes in blood pressure, or regional blood flow occur remains unknown and constitutes another area where further experimental work is required.

In the primates, rectal temperatures drop dur-

ing the early stages of compression, when air is replaced by helium–oxygen at 30 to 33°C, but remain approximately constant thereafter at the new level throughout the remainder of the compression until the advent of the generalized convulsions of stage III. In mice, the severe thermal conditions of the high pressure heliox environment result in a marked decrease of rectal temperature and a similarly marked increase in metabolic rate (Fig. 13.3) which persist through the

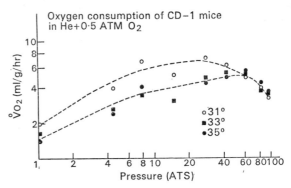

FIG. 13.3. Effect of temperature and pressure on oxygen consumption in resting CD-1 female mice in helium + 0·5 ATM O_2. Values are shown at three temperatures: 31°C (○), 33°C (■), and 35°C (●), and at nine pressures: 2·0 ATA, 4·4 ATA, 7·8 ATA, 14·6 ATA, 28·2 ATA, 41·8 ATA, 62·3 ATA, 82·6 ATA and 96·2 ATA. Mean O_2 consumption values are expressed as ml O_2/g body weight/hour

onset of the severe tremors of stage II (Sheehan & Brauer 1974). Beyond this point the metabolic rate ceases to increase with further compression, and evidence for the existence of a lower critical temperature disappears. This raises the possibility that the metabolic response to thermal challenge may have become impaired, and that this could be attributable to pressure-induced changes in hypothalamic function or in the availability of central neurotransmitters involved in thermoregulation (Feldberg 1968).

In the lizard *Anolis carolinensis* development of the HPNS is often accompanied by progressive melanophore expansion, leading to changes in skin colour from green toward brown—a kind of colorimetric index of the stages of HPNS development (Brauer & Venters, unpublished data). This colour change reflects the degree of expansion or contraction of chromatophores located in the skin of this lizard. These effects in turn are largely under humoral control in this species (Kleinholz 1938); epinephrine (and excitement causing epinephrine release) result in splotchy melanophore contraction and consequently general lightening of skin (Rahn 1956) while a pituitary melanophore-expanding hormone produces darkening of the skin. Direct neural control of skin colour response to high pressures is minimal, and isolated skin sections fail to show any colour response to high pressure. Thus, the association of skin colour changes with development of the HPNS in the Anole suggests the possibility that changes in pituitary function may be associated with the other CNS effects.

Observations of human subjects in high pressure environments have for some time suggested the possibility that vigilance performance may be impaired relatively early during development of the HPNS (Rostain, & Naquet 1974), a finding not incompatible with the observations that electrical changes occur early in centres of the reticular formation in the squirrel monkey. In the sloth there appears to be a reversal of the sleep-wakefulness cycle which is appropriately balanced in favor of sleep in this species (Goffart 1968) and this suggests the possibility that discharge from the raphe nuclei (Jouvet 1972) may be affected as animals are compressed into the tremor zone. The tremors themselves suggest changes in function of structures of the extrapyramidal motor system, a matter that has been reviewed by Bachrach and Bennett (1973). These examples must suffice for the time being to indicate that the exploration of the neurological changes which characterize the pre-seizure phase of the HPNS is a promising but as yet most incompletely developed field.

EXPERIMENTAL MODIFICATION OF THE DEVELOPMENT OF THE HPNS

It has already been mentioned that development of the HPNS is not invariable for a given species or individual, but can be modified by pharmacologic means or by varying the conditions of compression. Since these variations are of considerable interest both from a practical point of view and from their bearing on the etiology of the HPNS, they will be briefly reviewed in the following paragraphs.

Among the conditions of the compression environment, chamber temperature and noise levels appear to have only secondary effects on the HPNS. In mice, chamber temperatures between 29 and 35°C fail to affect convulsion thresholds although at the highest temperatures tremor thresholds may be decreased slightly (about 3 to 5 ATS; Sheehan & Brauer 1974). In nearly poikilothermic baby mice and in poikilothermic lizards, temperature variations between 25° and 35°C and 20° and 35°C, respectively, fail to modify the characteristic development of the HPNS. In liquid-breathing mice Lundgren and Ørnhagen (1975) report mean convulsion thresholds of 75 ± 9, 80 ± 12 and 90 ± 8 ATS for rectal temperatures of 27, 21 and 17°C. Temperatures above 35° and below 29°C are poorly tolerated by mice in high pressure heliox atmospheres and frequently kill the animals.

With regard to the effect of noise, the only data available at present refer to the relationship between audiogenic seizures and proneness to HPNS susceptibility. Audiogenic seizure-prone strains of mice are no more susceptible than resistant strains, and indeed no correlation could be detected between these two qualities (Brauer et al. 1974b). When mice of a normally audiogenic seizure-resistant strain are sensitized to such convulsions, by exposure to high decibel noise at a critical age (Henry 1967), their HPNS thresholds are no different from those of non-sensitized litter mate controls. However, during the late phases of stage II, squirrel monkeys appear to become susceptible to seizures evoked by photostimulation at the proper frequency (Brauer, Jordan & Way 1972) and the possibility that potentials evoked via other sensory modalities can produce similar effects during the pre-convulsive phase cannot yet be excluded.

All observers agree that variations in compression rate do modify the development of the HPNS in mammals (Brauer, Jordan, & Way 1972; Dossett & Hempleman 1972; Miller 1972; Rostain 1973). In mice, squirrel monkeys, and rhesus monkeys (Fig. 13.4) the general relationship between convulsion threshold and compression rate is $Pc = P_C^0 - a \log \dot{P}$ where Pc is the observed

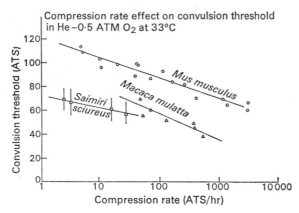

FIG. 13.4. The relation between compression rate and convulsion threshold pressure in mouse, squirrel monkey and rhesus monkey ($Po_2 = 0.4$ to 0.5 ATS $T = 31$–$33°C$)

convulsion threshold, P_C^0 and a are constants, and $\dot{P}$ is the compression rate (Brauer, Beaver & Mansfield 1974). In mice this equation is based on a range of compression rates from 1 to 1000 ATS/hr, and the constants are: $a = 16.8$ ATS, and $P_C^0 = 119$ ATS if $\log {}^{10}P$ is used and $\dot{P}$ is expressed as ATS/hr.

Unlike the convulsion thresholds, the tremor thresholds appear to vary but slightly with compression rate. Data for the squirrel monkey suggest that the onset of stage II varies with compression rate in a manner intermediate between the fine tremor and the convulsion stages.

Clinically, there is some suggestion that the syndrome that develops at high compression rates may be more severe than that seen at low compression rates. This is especially noticeable for the convulsion. At high compression rates the first generalized seizure frequently leads to full tonic seizure rather than the clonic seizure ordinarily seen first at lower compression rates. Similarly, the tremor stage appears not only reduced in time but the transition from stage I to stage II appears to come so early that not infrequently stage I is poorly marked during rapid compressions. On the other hand, the underlying syndrome does not appear to change in kind. This is suggested, not only by the continuous nature of the changes observed as compression rates are increased gradually, but also by the observation that the effect of inert gas narcosis on convulsion thresholds in mice

is quantitatively the same at a moderate compression rate of 40 ATS/hr and a fast compression rate of 600 ATS/hr (Brauer et al. 1974a; see Fig. 13.5).

Finally, it is of interest to the etiology of the HPNS that compression rate effects appear to be limited to the development of the HPNS in mature mammals. By contrast, such effects are not demonstrable in birds, reptiles, amphibians, or in young baby mice (Brauer, Beaver & Mansfield 1974) and they seem likewise to be absent in invertebrates.

With respect to the chamber atmosphere, four types of modification are possible; namely a change in relative humidity, or a change in carbon dioxide partial pressure, or a change in oxygen concentration or partial pressure, or a change in composition of the metabolically inert gas constituents. Relative humidity, while undoubtedly a factor in defining the zone of thermal comfort in high pressure atmospheres, has not been the subject of systematic study in relation to the HPNS. Perhaps the fact that liquid-breathing mice have HPNS convulsions at about the same point as heliox-breath-

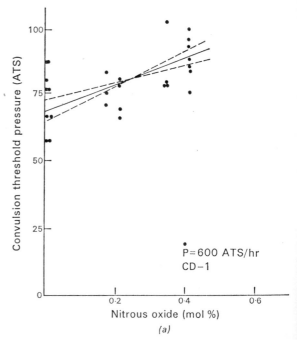

FIG. 13.5(a). Elevation of HPNS convulsion thresholds of CD-1 mice by partial substitution of helium by nitrous oxide in the compression atmosphere. Compression rate, 600 ATS/hr

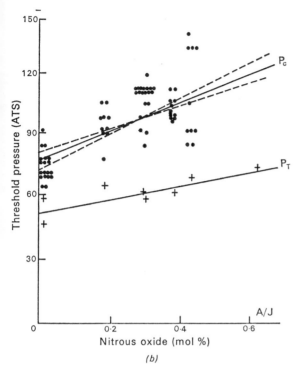

FIG.13.5 (b). Elevation of HPNS convulsion (P_C) and tremor (P_T) thresholds of A/J mice by partial substitution of helium by nitrous oxide in compression atmosphere. Compression rate, 40 ATS/hr. Dashed lines indicate variance of regression coefficient for P_C

ing dry animals (Kylstra et al. 1967) has led investigators to attach scant weight to relative humidity in this context. Carbon dioxide tensions likewise have been ignored, or rather kept at the minimum practicable level (for instance, below 0·005 ATS) by all investigators. Chance observations made on occasion of a recirculator failure now and then suggest that high CO_2 levels tend to antagonize development of the HPNS in mice and in birds. This subject clearly seems worthy of further study (Halsey, Kent & Eger 1975).

Oxygen partial pressures have been of interest since the early work on the HPNS. Zaltsman (1968) observed potentiation of the convulsant effects of oxygen in dogs by high pressures of helium. In mice, variations in the concentration of oxygen between 0·3 and 2·0% at pressures above 50 ATS failed to affect mean convulsion pressures (Brauer, Way & Jordan 1971). When concentrations reached 2·5%, however, the mean convulsion

thresholds were lowered from 92 to 77 ATS. This appears to be a clear case of synergism, since at this partial pressure of oxygen, hyperoxic convulsions in this mouse strain do not occur in less than 5 hours, while in these experiments seizures occurred after a very much shorter interval. Bennett and Dossett (1973) studied rats compressed in heliox mixtures under oxygen partial pressures maintained at 3·0 ATS. Their failure to record evidence of stages II and III contrasts with the positive findings of Albano et al. (1972); Brauer et al. (1974b); Dossett & Hempleman (1972) at lower Po_2 but under otherwise comparable conditions. This suggests the possibility that the oxygen partial pressures may have been high enough to exert a measure of anesthetic action (Bennett & Dossett 1973). From studies of lipid solubilities of oxygen and other inert gas anesthetics Paton (1967) has suggested that O_2 is about 2·8 times more effective a narcotic than nitrogen. As will be shown presently, other evidence indicates also that a nitrogen partial pressure of 10 ATS (isonarcotic with Po_2 of 3·6 ATS) does indeed raise HPNS thresholds of mice perceptibly. Chouteau and his associates working with sheep and goats (Chouteau et al. 1968; Chouteau & Lambert 1971) claim another type of effect. They report depression rather than hyperexcitability if compressions are carried out at a Po_2 of 0·2 ATS, and reversal of this effect when oxygen partial pressures were raised to 0·5 ATS or greater. While such changes have not been recorded for any other species of animal nor from any other laboratory, it is true that most experimentation to date has utilized oxygen partial pressures of 0·4 ATS or greater so that the volume of pertinent observations is limited. The possibility that change in respiratory centre function accompanies the development of high pressure effects in man has been raised also by the development of relative hypoxemias during sleep in the course of a recent deep dive (Rostain & Regesta 1973).

An interesting and potentially important effect upon the HPNS is produced by substituting other metabolically inert gases for helium in the chamber atmosphere. Very early in the development of the subject it was noted that in the rhesus monkey, substitution of hydrogen for helium seemed to increase the threshold for HPNS seizures (Brauer et al. 1966; Brauer, Way & Jordan 1971). Subsequently, more extensive work in mice showed that this effect is closely related to the calculated narcotic effectiveness of the resultant atmospheres (Brauer et al. 1974a). Increasing the proportion of narcotically active gas in the mixture gave rise to progressively higher convulsion thresholds, and substitution of narcotically more potent gases for hydrogen produced comparable effects at lower partial pressures of the added gas. Indeed, it could be shown than the increase in mean convulsion threshold was uniquely related to the narcotic effectiveness of the chamber atmosphere and independent of gas density (Fig. 13.6). Expressing the

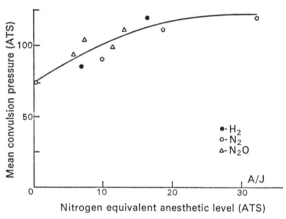

FIG. 13.6. Relation between calculated nitrogen equivalent anesthetic effectiveness of chamber gas at the time of convulsion to mean HPNS convulsion thresholds for helium–hydrogen, helium–nitrogen and helium–nitrous oxide mixtures. (Data from Figs 4–7 in Brauer et al. 1974a; Brauer & Way 1970.)

results in terms of equinarcotic nitrogen partial pressures it was found for instance that 10 ATS N_2 would raise the convulsion thresholds by about 25 ATS. This description probably underestimates the effectiveness of inert gas narcosis against the HPNS. From the opposite view, Lever et al. (1971) and Miller et al. (1967) have shown that high pressures are capable of reversing the narcotic effects of barbiturates and of inert gases, the order of effectiveness corresponding closely to that described for antagonism to HPNS convulsions (Miller et al. 1973). Thus subjects under 10 ATS of N_2 at pressures in the HPNS range are likely to show considerably less behavioral impairment or

inert gas narcosis than they would if nitrogen and oxygen were the only gases present in the chamber atmosphere.

In contrast to the convulsions, the tremor thresholds appear to be only about half as susceptible to the protective action of inert gas anesthetics (Fig. 13.7). While it is not known yet to what extent other manifestations of the pre-seizure phases of the HPNS are modified, clinically one

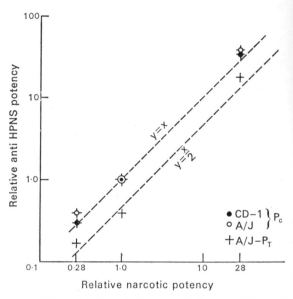

FIG. 13.7. Relation between relative anti-HPNS convulsant and tremor potencies and relative narcotic potencies of hydrogen, nitrogen, and nitrous oxide in CD-1 and A/J mice. (Data from Figs 1–3 and 4–7 of Brauer et al. 1974; Brauer & Way 1970.) Log–log plot, with lines for $y = x$ and $y = x/2$ indicated

gains the impression that squirrel monkeys at pressures in the HPNS range are far less distressed when breathing hydrogen–oxygen atmospheres than heliox. An isolated finding reported by Michaud et al. (1969) has been that pressures of 26 ATS of H_2/O_2 are lethal to rabbits within 5 to 10 hours. The suggestion of these workers that this reflects biochemical activation of hydrogen and modification of key metabolic reactions seems to be refuted by the fact that mice and monkeys safely survive far higher partial pressures of H_2 for periods as long as, or longer, than those allegedly lethal to Michaud's rabbits (Brauer, Jordan & Way 1972; Rostain 1973).

In line with what might be expected on the basis of experiments on reversal of narcosis (Lever et al. 1971), barbiturates, especially sodium phenobarbital, protect partially against HPNS convulsions (Brauer, Jordan and Way 1972). Animals thus protected can be carried to much higher pressures without lapsing into the severe convulsive syndrome.

Work with squirrel monkeys suggests that the effect of barbiturates, like that of the inert gases, is considerably more pronounced upon the convulsions than upon the tremors of stage I (Brauer et al. 1975).

In addition to the barbiturates, powerful anti-HPNS action has been found, especially in certain of the so-called central muscle relaxants with pronounced action upon transmission through polysynaptic reflex arcs, such as zoxazolamine, 2-amino-5 chlorobenzoxazole. Diazepam (Valium), an agent of somewhat related pharmacological action, is less effective but is still capable of raising HPNS convulsion thresholds by 25 to 30%. More specific antiepileptic agents, including diphenylhydantoin sodium and trimethadione, have so far given discouraging results.

Two agents which potentiate HPNS development are flurothyl and reserpine. Flurothyl, hexafluorodiethyl ether (Indoklon) is a convulsant fluoroanalogue of the general anesthetic, diethyl ether. Added to the atmosphere in amounts below those capable of producing convulsions at 1 ATS pressure, this agent is capable of lowering HPNS convulsion pressures in mice by as much as 60%.

The alkaloid reserpine is an agent of highly complex pharmacological action. Its most lasting effects, however, are linked to the depletion of monoamine transmitters, especially serotonin, from central nervous system synaptosomes. Mice, rats and squirrel monkeys pretreated with effective doses of reserpine show a profound lowering of HPNS convulsion thresholds (Fig. 13.8) (Brauer et al. 1975). In mice the relation of this effect to time elapsed between reserpine administration and compression has been studied. The depression of convulsion thresholds begins soon after reserpine administration, increases during the first 12 hours, and then remains at a steady maximum level for about a further 24 hours before gradually falling to disappear about 72 hours after the original dose. This time course parallels the concentra-

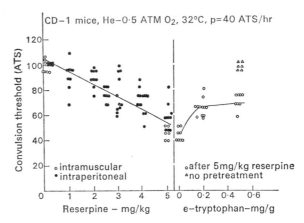

FIG. 13.8. The effect of premedication with reserpine (24 hr before dive) on HPNS convulsion thresholds in CD-1 mice and the partial reversal of this effect by the administration of L-tryptophan, dose-response relations

tion of available neurotransmitters in the brain and suggests that lowering of HPNS convulsion thresholds is causally linked to the disappearance of one or several among serotonin, norepinephrine, and dihydroxphenylalanine. Tryptophan can reverse about 20% of this effect of reserpine. Since tryptophan, administered after reserpine, speeds the restoration of normal brain serotonin levels, this finding further supports an active role for this neurotransmitter in the inhibition of HPNS convulsions.

CONSIDERATIONS CONCERNING THE ETIOLOGY OF THE HPNS

There is ample evidence, briefly touched upon in the introductory remarks, to establish the fact that at pressures of 50 to 150 ATS, the range in which the HPNS develops in vertebrates, there is a wide variety of changes in cell structure (Zimmerman & Zimmerman 1970), membrane permeability (Brouha et al. 1970), ciliary activity (Flugel 1972; Kitching 1957) axon conduction (Grundfest 1936), cell replication (Macdonald 1967; Marsland 1970), and other basic phenomena; and that even in relatively simple chemical systems changes in dissociation constants (Disteche 1972), in ion hydration (Horne & Courant 1972) and in macromolecular configuration (Becker 1972) can be detected at these or at only slightly higher pressures.

Three alternative theories of the etiology of the HPNS require comment. First is the concept that the HPNS really is merely a special case of inert gas narcosis, a phase in the overall complex of functional disintegration of brain functions during the development of high pressure epilepsy and narcosis (Zaltsman 1968). Second is the suggestion that the HPNS is merely a manifestation of central hypoxia secondary to respiratory impairment due either to excessive respiratory work or to impaired alveolar oxygen diffusion in the dense high pressure atmospheres (Chouteau, Imbert & Alinat 1969). Third is the suggestion that uneven distribution of dissolved gases between blood and tissues during rapid pressure changes results in temporary osmotic imbalance and fluid shifts which are responsible for the hyper-irritability and the compression rate dependent characteristics of the HPNS convulsions (Rostain 1973; Kylstra, Longmuir & Grace 1968).

As far as the basic events of the HPNS are concerned, all three of these hypotheses are disproved by the fact that HPNS hyperexcitability and convulsions have been produced by hydraulic compression in the absence of any gaseous atmospheres, in fluocarbon-breathing mice (Kylstra et al. 1967; Lundgren & Ørnhagen 1972), in water-breathing newts (Miller et al. 1967), and fish (Barthelemy & Belaud 1972). With respect to the third hypothesis, a further pertinent observation is that compression rate effects are absent in heliox-breathing birds weighing several times more than the mice, and about as much as the rats, in both of which compression rate effects are readily documented (Brauer, Beaver & Mansfield 1974).

Yet the HPNS is a complex entity, and the possibility that each of the above hypotheses may contain a grain of truth and contribute to the pattern of development of the syndrome under particular conditions cannot be rejected out of hand but needs to be examined in greater detail.

Actual narcotic effects of helium have not been demonstrated in mammals to date. Probably, the state of knowledge here is adequately summarized by the conclusion of Brauer and Way (1970) that 'the anesthetic effects of helium are either nil, or at least no greater than would be equivalent to 3% of the narcotic potency of nitrogen'. In a different system, a culture of *Tetrahymena pyriformis* in the logarithmic growth phase, Macdonald (1967) has recently demonstrated differences in cell division rate between preparations compressed hydraulically and preparations compressed under helium–oxygen. These results appear to be the first conclusive demonstration of narcotic effects of helium, and confirm the impression that these effects are quite small, even smaller in fact than the effects of hydrogen, which in turn is at most one fourth as potent an anesthetic as nitrogen (Brauer & Way 1970). Thus, Macdonald's data seem quite compatible with the statement quoted above. If then a value of 3:100 is accepted as the potency ratio of helium to nitrogen, then the pharmacological effects of 100 ATS of helium can hardly exceed those of 3 to 5 ATS of N_2. As shown in Fig. 13.6, such partial pressures of N_2 produce a barely perceptible increase in HPNS thresholds, and, in the absence of He and of high pressures, produce no recognizable effects on behavior of rats or mice.

The possibility of respiratory impairment in high pressure environments rests on one of two assumptions. Either the hypothesis that respiratory work increases to such an extent at high pressures that adequate respiratory exchange cannot be maintained; or the allegation that the presence of helium at high pressure interferes with oxygen diffusion to such an extent that oxygenation of blood passing through the alveolar capillaries becomes inadequate. In support of this hypothesis, its proponents refer to the reversal of the somnolence shown in sheep by the experiments increasing the chamber Po_2 (Chouteau, Imbert & Alinat 1969; Chouteau & Lambert 1971). In other studies, already discussed in conjunction with the EEG concomitants of the HPNS, oxygen partial pressures below 2 ATS were found to have a negligible effect upon the convulsion thresholds of mice, while pressures of 2 ATS or above lowered HPNS thresholds in mice (Brauer, Way & Jordan 1971), and may have raised them in rats (Bennett & Dossett 1973, compared to Albano et al. 1972 and Dossett & Hempleman 1972). In squirrel monkeys, the HPNS developed equally

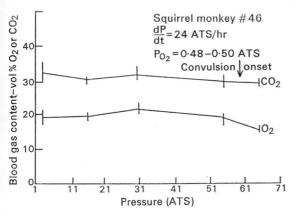

Squirrel monkey #46
$\frac{dP}{dt} = 24$ ATS/hr
$P_{O_2} = 0.48 - 0.50$ ATS
Convulsion onset

FIG. 13.9. Total blood oxygen and CO_2 content in a squirrel monkey during a simulated dive to the point of HPNS convulsions. (He-0·5 ATM O_2, 32°C)

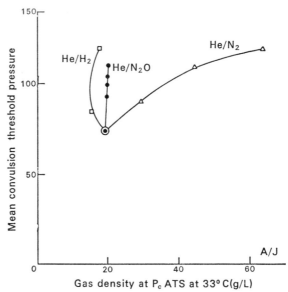

FIG. 13.10. Relation between density of chamber atmosphere at the time of convulsion to mean HPNS convulsion thresholds for A/J mice in helium–hydrogen, helium–nitrogen or helium–nitrous oxide at atmospheres. (Data from Figs 4–7 in Brauer et al. 1974a; Brauer & Way 1970)

at a P_{O_2} of 0·5 and of 1·5 ATS (Brauer, Jordan & Way 1972). The implications of these negative findings are borne out in squirrel and in rhesus monkeys (Fig. 13.9) by studies of blood gas composition which fail to reveal any consistent changes in either oxygen or CO_2 content, even in late stage II preparations on the point of convulsions. The absence of consistent changes in respiratory rate in rats (Albano et al. 1972) and squirrel monkeys (Brauer, Jordan & Way 1972) likewise fails to indicate any degree of respiratory impairment up to the convulsions of stage III. Finally, comparison of equinarcotic He/H_2, He/N_2O and He/N_2 mixtures shows that the same mean convulsion threshold pressures occur in mice in equinarcotic gas mixtures of widely different density (Fig. 13.10).

These results of animal experiments are well in keeping with the results of human experiments which have revealed that respiratory exchange is adequate for moderate exertion even at atmospheric densities corresponding to 180 ATS (Varène et al. 1971; Wright & Peterson 1975).

The possibility that blood oxygenation could become inadequate during sleep in high pressure environments as a result of an effect upon the respiratory centers has already been mentioned in conjunction with the results of the deep dives at the COMEX (Rostain & Regesta 1973).

With regard to the osmotic imbalance hypothesis, it should be noted that the original observers (Kylstra et al. 1968) recognized that the

time constants for such an effect are very short, of the order of seconds. Thus, this cause can hardly affect the results of compressions in which pressure changes occupy several, or many, hours. By contrast, the possibility cannot be excluded that such effects could come into play when compression rates are of the order of hundreds or even thousands of atmospheres per hour. This could prove to be one of the factors which underly the apparent enhancement of the severity of the several stages of HPNS at very high compression rates. Conclusive evidence on this point may have to await critical studies in liquid-breathing mammals subjected to hydraulic compression at widely different rates.

It is concluded therefore that the only interpretations which are compatible with the available data are those which focus upon the high pressures necessary to produce the HPNS as the chief etiologic factor underlying this condition. For some time the fact that compression rate does indeed modify the development of the HPNS in mammals raised the possibility that the change in pressure rather than the absolute hydrostatic pressure might be a major factor in the development of this entity. The recent discovery that the HPNS in birds, in reptiles, in newts and in young baby mice is not recognizably modified by large changes in compression rate would seem to eliminate this concept, and instead suggest that the development of the HPNS should be viewed as a dual event in the mammals, a basic change in excitability, especially pronounced along polysynaptic pathways, and a secondary development of inhibitory impulses which gain effectiveness with time and account for the higher convulsion thresholds at slow compression rates. At the present time, this can only be accepted as a working hypothesis which stands urgently in need of development of further data to render it more concrete, and which will surely have to accommodate certain facts not readily explained in the framework of this concept at present. The most significant among these would seem to be the common observation that if compression is arrested soon after the first seizure, this phase of the syndrome tends to subside, with only a few further seizures, which are spaced at progressively longer intervals.

Detailed analysis of this and other time–pressure profiles will have to reveal whether these phenomena correspond to the concept of a 'equivalent compression rate' (total pressure divided by total time elapsed from the beginning of the compression) or whether more complex relations call for modification of the working hypothesis. The basic hypothesis would suggest further that in species where compression rate effects are absent or less marked than in mammals, the time sequence of seizures, and perhaps their character, should differ from the pattern seen in mammals, tending to a more prolonged course, and perhaps a greater prominence of tonic events. While preliminary observations tend to support such a view, much remains to be done in this field, too, before more definite conclusions can be formulated.

With respect to the relatively rate-independent aspects of the HPNS, the tremors of stage I and to some extent of stage II in mammals, the most complete hypothetical formulation is that developed by Paton and Miller and their associates under the designation of the 'critical volume hypothesis of the action of inert gases and hydrostatic pressure upon the excitable cells'. Since this hypothesis is elaborated upon elsewhere in this volume (see Chapter 12), it must suffice here to indicate that the basic hypothesis and its recent confirmation are indeed most impressive and would seem to offer an attractive starting point for the explanation of many of the effects of hydrostatic pressures upon simple excitable systems. However, it may well be that no single biophysical mechanism can wholly account for the phenomena seen in a vertebrate subjected to a simulated dive to great depths, and a broad frontal attack rather than a pinpoint charge may ultimately prove to be the most effective strategy.

Finally, mention should be made of the fact that studies of the HPNS in vertebrates provide an appropriate link between the physiological study of the penetration of the oceans by man and the study of the biology of the deep sea. This raises problems of adaptation and acclimation, and of the possible relation of limitations on vertical distribution of marine organisms to HPNS-like effects. Further discussion of this subject is beyond the realm of the present chapter but has formed in part the substance of two recent conferences (Sleigh & Macdonald, 1972; Brauer 1972).

Acknowledgements

The author wishes to thank his friend, Dr. H. William Gillen, for his review of the manuscript and his helpful suggestions.

This work was supported in full by the Office of Naval Research under ONR Contract No. N00014–72–A–0320–0001.

REFERENCES

ALBANO, G. P., CRISCUOLI, M., SCAGLIONE, G. C., MAZZONE, M., LAMONACO, G. & BURMANO, G. (1972) La sindrome da estreme pressioni ambientali. Relievi EEG ed ECG su Ratti Liberi con Elettrodi da Dimora. *Ann. di Med. nav. trop.* **77**, 11–28.

BACHRACH, A. J. & BENNETT, P. B. (1973) Tremor in diving. *Aerospace Med.* **44**, 613–623.

BARTHELEMY, L. & BELAUD, A. (1972) *Constatations physiologiques et physiopathologiques faîtes sur un poisson* (Anguilla anguilla *L.*) *en conditions hyperbares.* Bulletin Medsubhyp, Service d'Hyperbare, Hôpital Salvator, Marseille. Report No. 8, November.

BECKER, R. W. (1972) Pressure effects on the properties of high molecular weight substances in solution. In *Barobiology and the Experimental Biology of the Deep Sea*. Ed. R. Brauer. pp. 269–281. North Carolina: Special Publication, North Carolina Sea Grant Program.

BENNETT, P. B. (1967) Performance impairment in deep diving due to nitrogen, helium, neon and oxygen. In *Proc. 3rd Symp. Underwater Physiology*. Ed. C. J. Lambertsen. pp. 327–340. Baltimore: Williams and Wilkins.

BENNETT, P. B. & DOSSETT, A. N. (1973) EEG activity of rats compressed by inert gases to 700 feet and oxygen–helium to 4000 feet. *Aerospace Med.* 44, 239–244.

BRAUER, R. W. (Ed.) (1972) *Barobiology and the Experimental Biology of the Deep Sea*. North Carolina: Special Publication, North Carolina Sea Grant Program.

BRAUER, R. W. & WAY, R. O. (1970) Relative narcotic potencies of hydrogen, helium, nitrogen and their mixtures. *J. appl. Physiol.* 29, 23–31.

BRAUER, R. W., BEAVER, R. W. & MANSFIELD, W. M. (1974) Compression rate effects upon HPNS and the question of etiology. (Abstrt). *Undersea Biomed. Res.* 1.

BRAUER, R. W., JORDAN, M. R. & WAY, R. O. (1972) The high pressure neurological syndrome in the squirrel monkey, *Saimiri sciureus*. In *Proc. Third International Conference on Hyperbaric and Underwater Physiology*. Ed. X. Fructus. pp. 22–30. Paris: Doin.

BRAUER, R. W., WAY, R. O. & JORDAN, M. R. (1971) Experimental studies on the high pressure neurological syndrome in various mammalian species. In *Proc. 4th Symp. Underwater Physiology*. Ed. C. J. Lambertsen. pp. 487–500. New York and London: Academic Press.

BRAUER, R. W., GOLDMAN, S. M., BEAVER, R. W. & SHEEHAN, M. E. (1974a) Antagonism of the high pressure neurological syndrome by addition of nitrogen, hydrogen or nitrous oxide to heliox atmospheres. *Undersea biomed. Res.* 1. (In Press.)

BRAUER, R. W., JOHNSON, D. O., PESSOTTI, R. L. & REDDING, R. (1966) Effects of hydrogen and helium at pressures to 67 atmospheres. *Fedn Proc. Fedn Am. Socs exp. Biol.* 25, 202.

BRAUER, R. W., JORDAN, M. R., BEAVER, R. W. & GOLDMAN, S. M. (1975) Interaction of the high pressure neurological syndrome with various pharmacological agents. In *Underwater Physiology. Vth Symp. Underwater Physiology*. Ed. C. J. Lambertsen. Bethesda: Fedn Am. Socs exp. Biol.

BRAUER, R. W., DIMOV, S., FRUCTUS, X., GOSSET, A. & NAQUET, R. (1969) Syndrome neurologique et electrographique des hautes pressions. *Revue Neurol.* 121, 264–265.

BRAUER, R. W., BEAVER, R. W., HOGUE III, C. D., FORD, B., GOLDMAN, S. M. & VENTERS, R. T. (1974b) Intra- and interspecies variability in susceptibility to the high pressure neurological syndrome in vertebrates. *J. appl. Physiol.* (In press.)

BRAUER, R. W., WAY, R. O., JORDAN, M. R., PARRISH, D. E., BEAVER, R. W. & GOLDMAN, S. M. (1974c) Repeated exposure to high pressure heliox atmospheres. *Undersea Biomed. Res.* 1. 239–250

BROUHA, A., PEGNEUX, A., SCHOFFENIELS, E. & DISTECHE, A. (1970) The effects of high hydrostatic pressures on the permeability characteristics of the isolated frog skin. *Biochim. biophys. Acta* 219, 455–462.

CHOUTEAU, J. A, & LAMBERT, G. (1971) La limitation hypoxique de la plongée profounde de longue durée. *Maroc Med.* 51, 229–236.

CHOUTEAU, J. A, IMBERT, G. & ALINAT, J. (1969) Sur une meilleure définition des phénomènes hypoxiques accompagnant la respiration du mélange oxygène–helium au cours des plongées profondes à saturation. *C.r. hebd. Séanc. Acad. Sci., Paris.* 268: 2918–2921.

CHOUTEAU, J. A., COUSTEAU, Y., ALINAT, J. & AQUADRO, C. F. (1968) Sur les limites physiologiques de la plongée à saturation à l'air et aux mélanges synthetiques. *Rev. subaq. Physiol.* 1, 38–44.

DISTECHE, A. (1972) Electrochemical devices for *in situ* or simulated deep sea measurements. In *Barobiology and the Experimental Biology of the Deep Sea*. Ed. R. Brauer, pp. 234–265. North Carolina: Special Publication, North Carolina Sea Grant Program.

DOSSETT, A. N. & HEMPLEMAN, V. (1972) The importance for mammals of rate of compression (Symp. on Effects of Pressure on Organisms). *Proc. Soc. exp. Biol.* 26, 355–361.

EBBECKE, U. (1914) Wirkung allseitigen Kompression auf den Froschmuskel. *Pflügers Arch. ges. Physiol.* 157, 75–116.

EBBECKE, U. & HASENRING (1035) Über die Kompressionsberkurzung des Muskels bei Einwirkung hoher Drucke. *Pflügers Arch. ges. Physiol.* 236, 405–415.

EBBECKE, U. & SCHAEFER, H. (1935) Über den Einfluss hoher Drucke auf den Aktionsstrom von Muskeln und Nerven. *Pflügers Arch. ges. Physiol.* 236, 678–692.

FELDBERG, N. (1968) The monoamines of the hypothalamus as mediators of temperature responses. In *Recent Advancee in Pharmacology*. Ed. J. M. Robson & R. S. Stacey. pp. 92–100. London: Churchill.

FLUGEL, H. (1972) Adaptation and acclimatization to high pressure environments. In *Barobiology and the Experimental Biology of the Deep Sea*. Ed. R. Brauer. pp. 69–89. North Carolina: Special Publication, North Carolina Sea Grant Program.

FONTAINE, M. (1930) Recherches experimentales sur les reactions des êtres vivants aux fortes pressions. *Annls Inst. océanogr., Monaco* 8, 5–97.

GERSHFELD, N. T. & SHANES, A. M. (1959) The influence of high hydrostatic pressure on cocaine and veratrine action in a vertebrate nerve. *J. gen. Physiol.* 42, 647–653.

GOFFART, M. (1968) The problem of slothfulness in the didactyl sloth (*Choloepus hoffmanni* Pet.) *Electromyography* 8, 245–251.

GRUNDFEST, H. (1936) Effects of hydrostatic pressures upon the excitability, the recovery and the potential sequence of frog nerve. *Cold Spring Harb. Symp. quant. Biol.* 4, 179–187.

GRUNDFEST, H. & CATTELL, MACKEEN (1935) Some effects of hydrostatic pressure on nerve action potentials. *Am. J. Physiol.* 113, 56–57.

HALSEY, M. J., KENT, D. W., & EGER II, E. J. (1975) Pressure studies with mice up to 270 atm. In *Underwater Physiology. Vth Symp. Underwater Physiology*. Ed. C. J. Lambertsen. Bethesda: Fedn Am. Socs exp. Biol.

HENRY, K. R. (1967) Acoustic priming of audiogenic seizures in a previously non-susceptible strain of mice. *Science, N.Y.* **158**, 938–939.

HORNE, R. W. & COURANT, B. A. (1972) Pressure-induced changes in aqueous solutions and their possible significance. In *Barobiology and the Experimental Biology of the Deep Sea*. Ed. R. Brauer. pp. 223–233. North Carolina: Special Publication, North Carolina Sea Grant Program.

HURD, R., BRAUER, R. W. & WILDER, B. J. (1974) Convulsions and tremorigenic phenomena associated with high pressure neurologic syndrome. *Trans. Am. neurol. Ass.* (In press.)

JOHNSON, F. H., EYRING, H. & POLISSAR, M. F. (1954) *The Kinetic Basis of Molecular Biology*. pp. 286–368. New York: John Wiley.

JOUVET, M. (1972) Veille, Sommeil et Rêve. *Revue Méd.* 1003–1063.

KERKUT, G. A. (1969) The use of snail neurones in neurophysiological studies. *Endeavour* **38**, 22–26.

KITCHING, J. A. (1957) Effects of high hydrostatic pressures on the activity of flagellates and ciliates. *J. exp. Biol.* **34**, 494–510.

KLEINHOLZ, L. H. (1938) Studies in reptilian colour changes II. The pituitary and adrenal glands in the regulation of the melanophores of *Anolis carolinensis*. *J. exp. Biol.* **15**, 474–491.

KOBAYASHI, T., INMAN, O., BUNO, W. & HIMWICH, H. E. (1963) A multidisciplinary study of changes in mouse brain with age. *Recent Adv. biol. Psychiatry* **5**, 293–308.

KYLSTRA, J. A., LONGMUIR, I. & GRACE, M. (1968) Dysbarism: osmosis caused by dissolved gas? *Science, N.Y.* **161**, 289.

KYLSTRA, J. A., NANTZ, R., CROWE, J., WAGNER, W. & SALTZMAN, H. A. (1967) Hydraulic compression of mice to 166 atmospheres. *Science, N.Y.* **158** (3), 793–794.

LEVER, M. J., MILLER, K. W., PATON, W. D. M. & SMITH, E. B. (1971) Pressure reversal of anesthesia. *Nature, Lond.* **231**, 368–371.

LUNDGREN, C. & ØRNHAGEN, H. (1975) Hydrostatic pressure tolerance in liquid breathing mice. In *Underwater Physiology. Vth Symp. Underwater Physiology*. Ed. C. J. Lambertsen. Bethesda: Fedn Am. Socs exp. Biol.

MACDONALD, A. G. (1967) The effect of high hydrostatic pressure on the cell division and growth of *Tetrahymena pyriformis*. *Expl Cell Res.* **47**, 569–580.

MANSFIELD, W. M., BRAUER, R. W. & GILLEN, H. W. (1974) Age dependence of seizure patterns in mice exposed to high pressure helioz atmospheres (Abstr.) *Fedn Proc. Fedn Am. Socs exp. Biol.*, April.

MARSLAND, D. (1970) Pressure temperature studies on the mechanism of cell division. In *High Pressure Effects on Cellular Processes*. Ed. A. M. Zimmerman. pp. 260–306. New York: Academic Press.

MICHAUD, A., PARC, J., BARTHELEMY, L., LECHUITON, J., CORROIL, J., CHOUTEAU, J. & LEBOUCHER, F. (1969) Premieres données sur une limitation de l'utilization de mélange oxygène–hydrogène pour la plongée profounde à saturation. *Cr. hebd. Séanc. Acad. Sci., Paris* **269**, 497–499.

MILLER, K. W. (1972) Inert gas narcosis and animals under high pressure. In *The Effects of High Pressures on Organisms*. Ed. M. A. Sleigh & A. G. Macdonald. pp. 363–378. New York: Academic Press.

MILLER, K. W., PATON, W. D. M., SMITH, R. A. & SMITH, E. B. (1973) The pressure reversal of general anesthesia and the critical volume hypothesis. *Molec. Pharmac.* **9**, 131–143.

MILLER, K. W., PATON, W. D. M., STREET, W. B. & SMITH, E. G. (1967) Animals at very high pressures of helium and neon. *Science, N.Y.* **157**, 97–98.

PATON, W. D. M. (1967) Experiments on the convulsant effects of oxygen. *Br. J. Pharmac. Chemother.* **29**, 350–366.

RAHN, H. (1956) The relationship between hypoxia, temperature, adrenalin release and melanophore expansion in the lizard *Anolis Carolinensis*. *Copeia*, 214–217.

REGNARD, P. (1891) Influence de la pression sur la vie aquatique. In *La Vie dans les Eaux*. Ed. P. Regnard. pp. 158–187. Paris: Masson.

ROSTAIN, J. C. (1973) L'effet des hautes pressions avec divers mélanges gazeux chez le singe Papio papio. MD Thesis. University of Provence.

ROSTAIN, J. C. & NAQUET R. (1972) Resultats preliminaires d'une étude comparative de l'effet des mélanges oxygène–helium et oxygène–hydrogène et des hautes pressions sur le babouin Papio-papio. In *Proc. Third International Conference on Hyperbaric and Underwater Physiology*. Ed. X. Fructus. pp. 44–49. Paris: Doin.

ROSTAIN, J. C. & NAQUET, R. (1974) Le syndrome nerveux des hautes pressions—characteristique et evolution en fonction de divers modes de compression. *Revue Neurol.* **7**. (In press.)

ROSTAIN, J. C. & REGESTA, A. (1973) Evolution du sommeil de plongeurs au cours d'un séjour prolongé sous une pressure de 31 atm de mélange helium–oxygène. *Revue EEG Neurophysiol.* **3**. (In press.)

RUCCI, F. S., GIRETTI, M. L. & LAROCCA, M. (1968) Cerebellum and hyperbaric oxygen. *Electroenceph. clin. Neurophysiol.* **25**, 359–371.

SHAPIRO, S. (1971) Hormonal and environmental influences on rat brain development and behavior. In *Brain Development and Behavior*. Ed. M. B. Sterman, D. J. McGinty, & A. M. Admolfi. pp. 307–334. New York: Academic Press.

SHEEHAN, M. E. & BAUER, R. W. (1974) Temperature regulation and energy balance in mice under high pressures. In *2nd Symp. Pharmacology of Thermoregulation II*, April, Paris.

SLEIGH, M. A. & MACDONALD, A. G. (1972) *The Effects of Pressure on Organisms—A symposium of the Society for Experimental Biology*. New York: Academic Press.

SPYROUPOULOS, C. S. (1957) The effects of hydrostatic pressure upon the normal and narcotized nerve fiber. *J. gen. Physiol.* **40**, 849–857.

SPYROUPOULOS, C. S. (1957) Response of single nerve fibers at different hydrostatic pressures. *Am. J. Physiol.* **189**, 214–218.

VARÈNE, P., SAUMON, G. G., VIELLEFOND, A. & L'HUILLIER, J. (1971) Mécanique ventilatoire en plongée profounde—resultats de l'experience PHYSALIE V. *Bull. Méd. sub. hyp.* **6**, 9–16.

WRIGHT, W. B. & PETERSON, R. (1975) Pulmonary mechanical functions in man breathing dense gas mixtures. In *Underwater Physiology. Vth Symp. Underwater Physiology*. Ed. C. J. Lambertsen. Bethesda: Fedn Am. Socs exp. Biol.

ZALTSMAN, G. L. (Ed.) (1968) *Giperbaricheskiye epilepsiya i narkoz.* Leningrad: USSR Academy Science.

ZALTSMAN, G. L., PONOMARYER, V. P. & SELIVRA, A. I. (1968) Bioelectrical activity of various centers of the brain during the process of establishment of hyperbaric narcose in the dog. In *Giperbaricheskiye epilepsiya i narkoz.* Ed. G. L. Zaltsman. pp. 206–220. Leningrad: USSR Academy Science.

ZALTSMAN, G. L., SELIVRA, A. I. & PONOMARYER, V. P. (1973) Sinchronizatsiya biopotentsialov mozga pri generalizatsii patologicheskovo vozbushdyenniya i tormozhenniya. In *Symposium: Problemi prostranstvennoi sinchronizatsii biotentsialov golovnovo mozga.* Ed. M. N. Livanov. Pushkino: Akademiya Nauk USSR.

ZIMMERMAN, A. (1970) *High Pressure Effects on Cellular Processes.* New York: Academic Press.

ZIMMERMAN, S. B. & ZIMMERMAN, A. M. (1970) Biostructural, cytokinetic and biochemical aspects of hydrostatic pressure effects on protozoa. In *High Pressure Effects on Organisms.* pp. 179–208. New York: Academic Press.

14

The High Pressure Nervous Syndrome: Man

P. B. BENNETT

Since 1965 a comparative study of the effects in animals of hydrostatic pressure, helium, hydrogen, nitrogen and other narcotic inert gases has contributed significantly to our understanding of the cause, mechanism and prevention of the High Pressure Nervous Syndrome (HPNS), as discussed in Chapter 13. Similarly the amazing progress in extension of the depth limits of human diving since the early 1960s has led first to descriptions of the signs and symptoms of HPNS in man, followed by careful measurement of these and finally, in recent years, a clearer understanding of various causes and means of prevention to perhaps permit extension well beyond the 2000 ft (61·5 ATA) limits presently defined or at least to permit descent to such depths with minimal or no HPNS (Hunter & Bennett 1974).

MEASUREMENT OF EFFECTS DURING OXYGEN–HELIUM DIVES

During the early 1960s, based on lipid solubility, helium narcosis was expected to occur in man at about 1400 ft (43 ATA) or even maybe 1000 ft (31 ATA) when considering additional factors such as carbon dioxide retention. Thus in 1965 it came as a surprise that men compressed with oxygen–helium at about 100 ft/min to 600 ft (19 ATA) for 4 hours and 800 ft (25 ATA) for 1 hour showed decrements in motor and intellectual performance. Decreases of 18% in the mental test of arithmetic ability and 25% in the

ball bearing test of fine manual dexterity were reported at 600 ft and the decrease was twice as bad at 800 ft (Bennett 1965; Bennett & Dossett 1967). These decrements were accompanied by dizziness, nausea, vomiting and a marked tremor of the hands, arms and torso which was named 'helium tremors' and is now called just tremors.

It is interesting that at this time the animal work described in Chapter 13 had yet to be done, but Zaltsman had published in 1961 a volume in Russian reporting a considerable amount of research into underwater physiology including many experiments with animals and man at high helium pressures, which only became available in the West after 1967. He reported six subjects showed rhythmic tremors with a frequency of 5 to 8 c/s (hertz) propagating to the upper extremities, torso and sometimes the lower jaw, during oxygen–helium dives to 430 to 500 ft (14 to 16 ATA), which he also called 'helium tremors'. Zaltsman noted that with continuing stay at unchanged pressure, the tremors decreased or disappeared. Similarly, the measurements of Bennett (1965) indicated recovery to normal in some 1½ hours (Fig. 14.1) and Hamilton et al. (1966) noted dizziness, hand and finger tremor were no longer present after a few minutes at constant depth during exposure of two men to a depth of 650 ft (20·6 ATA). Further experiments at depths between 300 ft to 500 ft (10 to 16 ATA) for periods of one hour confirmed the existence of the tremors but the cause remained speculative (Bennett & Dossett 1967).

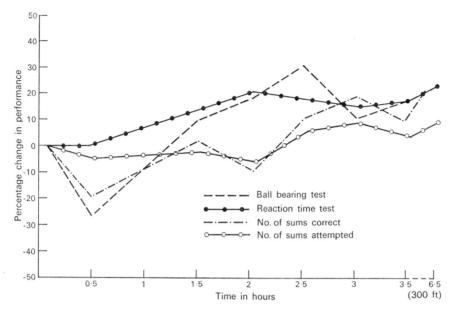

FIG. 14.1. Tests of performance efficiency on six men at 19·2 ATA (600 ft) breathing 5/95% oxygen/helium (Bennett 1965, 1967)

During this period a large number of other human deep saturation and excursion oxygen–helium dives were made (Cabarrou et al. 1966; Waldvogel & Bühlmann 1968; Weybrew & Parker 1968; Schaefer, Carey & Dougherty 1970; Proctor et al. 1971; Kelly et al. 1968; Bühlmann et al. 1970; Biersner & Cameron 1970) until the first saturation dive to 1000 ft (31 ATA) for 77 hours and 30 minutes carried out by the US Navy and Duke University in 1968 (Overfeld et al. 1969; Salzano, Rausch & Saltzman 1970; Summit et al. 1971). This latter dive showed that very slow and therefore largely impractical compressions of the order of some 40 ft/h permitted this great depth to be attained without the marked signs of tremors and mental deterioration noted in many of the early studies with compression rates of up to 100 ft/min. However, although slow rates of compression certainly help ameliorate the tremors, their undoubted relationship to the rate of increasing hydrostatic pressure rather than the pharmacological action of helium had yet to be clearly defined. Indeed, as is apparent from a recent review, even today little is known of the mechanism of tremor (Bachrach & Bennett 1973).

MEASUREMENT OF EFFECTS AT DEPTHS EXCEEDING 1000 FT (31 ATA)

It was from 1968 onward that the HPNS began to be studied in earnest. By this time some of the early animal studies were available (Brauer et al. 1971) and it was considered by the COMEX company in Marseille that with suitable 'slow' compressions, such as 10 ft/min, it should be possible to achieve depths greater than 1000 ft (31 ATA) without incapacitation due to tremors or the convulsions reported in animal studies.

In all, seven simulated dives in the 'Physalie' series were made with two subjects in each dive. Four of these dives exceeded 1100 ft (34 ATA) and on June 27 1968, a depth of 1190 ft (37 ATA) was reached but the dive aborted after only 4 minutes (Brauer 1968; Fructus, Brauer & Naquet 1971; Fructus 1972). Tremors were observed during compression, the onset occurring at between 725 and 925 ft (23 and 29 ATA), and although the compression rate was decreasing they became progressively worse with depth.

Changes in the electroencephalogram (EEG) appeared at depths close to 1000 ft (31 ATA) and were reported for the first time in man. These were characterized by the appearance of slow waves in the theta band (4 to 6 c/s) accompanied by depression of alpha activity (8 to 13 c/s). These changes became worse as the depth became greater than 1060 ft (33 ATA) and were accompanied by behavioral changes, which included intermittent bouts of somnolence, with sleep stages 1 and 2 in the EEG. If aroused the subjects woke up, but on resting lapsed again into sleep. The EEG changes persisted for 10 to 12 hours during the decompression.

These classic signs and symptoms of the HPNS were very different from those that could be expected from any narcotic effect of helium. For example, with nitrogen narcosis there are no tremors, marked psychomotor impairment, nausea and vomiting or similar EEG changes. Indeed, in the latter, the alpha and fast activities are augmented and theta unaffected at 300 ft (10 ATA) compressed air (Bennett & Towse 1972). Further, narcosis does not improve over $1\frac{1}{2}$ hours as does the HPNS.

As discussed earlier, the greater the development of the brain, the greater the sensitivity to HPNS. Squirrel monkeys show helium tremors starting at 660 to 825 ft (21 to 26 ATA) and EEG changes, such as spikes, at 1500 to 1650 ft (46 to 51 ATA) which proceed into electrical and motor convulsions at some 2050 ft (63 ATA). Since in

man the EEG changes started at some 1000 ft (31 ATA), accompanied by somnolence and tremors, there was reason to believe that convulsions might have occurred if the duration of stay at 1190 ft (37 ATA) had been prolonged, and it was considered that this was the depth limit to practical diving.

Yet a few months later three Swiss subjects were exposed to 1000 ft (31 ATA) for 3 days in a joint Swiss/British experiment by compression with helium–oxygen at 16·7 ft/min and made three excursions, two of 2 hours, duration, to a depth of 1150 ft (35·8 ATA) (Bühlmann et al. 1970). During the excursion the divers swam underwater using semi-closed apparatus and performed physical work by lifting a 20 kg weight 20 times from the floor to full arm extension over the head and appeared to have no difficulties.

Performance efficiency during both early more brief dives to 1000 ft (31 ATA) and the saturation dive did show evidence of tremors (Table 14.1) in the first $1\frac{1}{2}$ hours as revealed by the ball bearing test, which involves picking up ball bearings with tweezers and placing them in a tube of the same diameter. Other less sensitive tests, however, showed little change and there was no mental deterioration. Some nausea and vertigo were also reported with the tremor. During the excursions, performance showed no deterioration at all. It was considered, therefore, that the HPNS was prob-

TABLE 14.1

Performance impairment in deep saturation oxygen–helium and excursion dives (Bühlmann et al. 1970)

Tests	Surface	3 days at 31 ATA (1000 ft)							2 hr excursions to 36 ATA (1150 ft)
		After compression	1 hr	2 hr	3 hr	24 hr	48 hr	72 hr	
Ball bearing	12 ± 4	6 ± 5	10 ± 6	11 ± 4	12 ± 5	16 ± 6	18 ± 3	17 ± 4	19 ± 4
Dotting	69 ± 12	66 ± 9	63 ± 9	63 ± 7	62 ± 13	61 ± 6	67 ± 6	69 ± 8	63 ± 9
Dotting in squares	38 ± 4	32 ± 4	32 ± 4	34 ± 3	35 ± 5	39 ± 2	36 ± 3	41 ± 2	38 ± 3
Errors %	2	6	3	0	3	6	5	10	9
Letter code	39 ± 6	33 ± 5	30 ± 6	32 ± 4	33 ± 6	38 ± 8	35 ± 4	41 ± 5	37 ± 3
Errors %	0	7	7	2	0	0	0	2	0
Arithmetic correct	9 ± 1	—	$11·5 \pm 3$	—	11 ± 3	14 ± 2		14 ± 2	12 ± 2
Arithmetic attempted	$9·5 \pm 1$	—	$13·5 \pm 2$	—	13 ± 3	15 ± 3		17 ± 2	14 ± 2

ably a compression syndrome and a combination of the heat of compression, psychological stress and an unknown effect due to an overfast rate of change in pressure together with hyperventilation in helium.

Urine electrolyte measurements were made under these conditions together with other measurements of blood morphology and biochemistry. The urine measurements showed a reduction in sodium, calcium, magnesium and chloride ion and a diuresis of phosphorus and potassium.

Similar measurements were made also in a dive to 800 ft (25 ATA) at 3·5 ft/min with excursions at 27 and 28 ft/min to 1050 (32·7 ATA) and 1100 ft (34·2 ATA) by International Underwater Contractors Inc. and a US Navy team of scientists from the New London Submarine Medical Center (Schaefer, Carey & Dougherty 1970; Proctor et al. 1971). Tremors were observed during the excursions and as with many such early dives to 1000 ft (31 ATA) with relatively rapid compressions, arthralgia and aching muscles and joints occurred. Psychological performance was unimpaired.

Urinary pH, CO_2 and bicarbonate increased significantly; conversely to the Swiss/British dive to 1000 ft (31 ATA) sodium, potassium and phosphorus excretion increased, and calcium was unchanged while chloride decreased. The cause was believed due to hyperventilation resulting in a respiratory alkalosis and certainly this is a common finding in deep oxygen–helium diving. That Bühlmann trained his divers not to hyperventilate at depth may be important and account for the different results with the urine electrolytes of his experiments.

MEASUREMENT OF EFFECTS DURING COMPRESSION IN STAGES

Due to the excellent physical condition of the men in these dives to 1000 ft (31 ATA) and beyond it became increasingly difficult to believe that a 'barrier' existed to deep diving at 1200 ft (37 ATA). Thus in 1970 an extensive series of dives were made at the Royal Naval Physiological

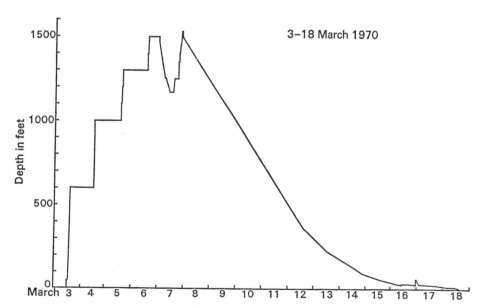

FIG. 14.2. Profile for 1500 ft (46 ATA) simulated oxygen–helium dive at RNPL. The stages on compression are shown together with recompression to 1535 ft (47·1 ATA) during the decompression in order to try to treat vestibular decompression sickness in one of the subjects. At some 30 ft, the other subject required recompression for a mild knee bend (after Bennett et al. 1971)

Laboratory (RNPL) culminating in the exposure of two men to a simulated depth of 1500 ft (46 ATA) for 10 hours. As in decompression, the exposure was made in stages instead of the usual continuous compression (Fig. 14.2). The first compression was to 600 ft (19 ATA). After 24 hours the two men were compressed at the same rate of 16·7 ft/min to 1000 ft (31 ATA) and after a further 24 hours spent one hour at 1100 ft, 1200 ft and 1400 ft (34, 37 and 43 ATA) and a further 24 hours at 1300 ft (40 ATA). During each stage a vast amount of physiological and medical data was obtained (Bennett et al. 1971; Bennett & Towse 1971a, b; Bennett & Gray 1971; Morrison & Florio,

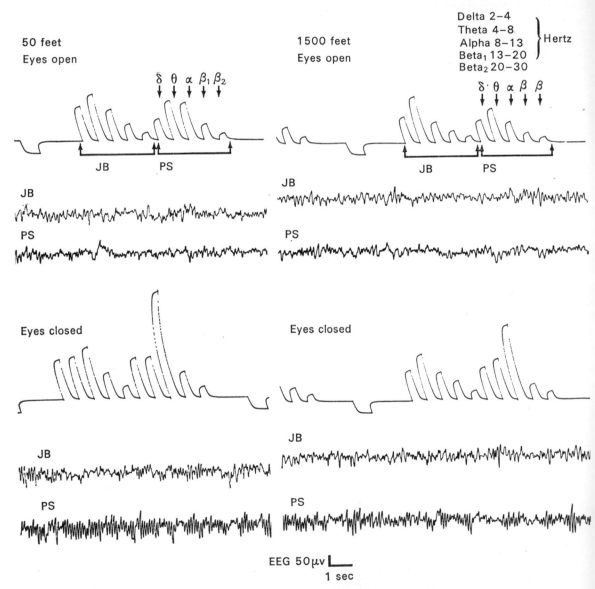

FIG. 14.3. Portions of the EEG with on-line frequency analysis of the two subjects during the 1500 ft (46 ATA) oxygen–helium dive at RNPL with eyes open and closed. Controls at 50 ft (2·5 ATA) compared with the EEG and analysis at 1500 ft indicate a reduction in EEG activity (after Bennett & Towse 1971a)

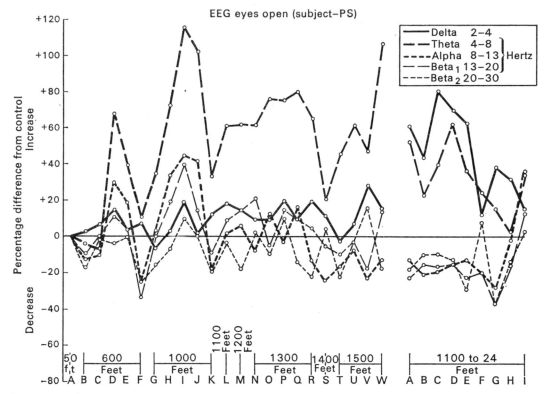

FIG. 14.4. Analysis of one of the two subjects, EEG during the 1500 ft (46 ATA) oxygen–helium dive at the RNPL at various stable stages of the dive as compared to controls at 50 ft (2·5 ATA). A marked rise in theta activity is indicated, initiated by each stage of compression. This continues to increase for 6 hours and then returns to lower levels over 12 hours (after Bennett & Towse 1971a)

1971). During this dive, for the first time the EEG was quantified by means of frequency analysis and sensory evoked potentials and postural tremors were measured by a transducer attached to the finger as well as by sensitive psychomotor tests such as the ball bearing test.

As with previous dives, the subjects reported tremors and involuntary muscle jerks and feeling dizzy with slight nausea, especially immediately on reaching the 600 ft (19 ATA) and 1000 ft (31 ATA) stages. The EEG showed a typical increase in theta activity (4 to 6 c/s) accompanied by a reduction of other activities (Figs 14.3, 14.4 & 14.5) which was delayed in one of the two subjects to 1300 ft (40 ATA) (Bennett & Towse 1971a). The EEG changes were seen most prominently when their eyes were open (Fig. 14.4). Each compression phase stimulated an increase in theta activity and this activity continued to increase for

6 hours after compression had ceased and then over some 12 hours returned to nearer normal levels. The cortical auditory evoked potentials (Fig. 14.5) showed a progressive depression with increasing depth which was at its most significant from 1300 to 1500 ft (40 to 46 ATA), when values 30% and 50% less than controls were seen in the size of the N_1P_2 complex. These results showed that there are two aspects of EEG change in the brain during HPNS in man: a rise in theta activity associated with compression and depression of overall electrical activity which is a function of increasing depth. The compression phenomena have a cycle of growth and decay of about 20 hours but the depression of overall activity shows no improvement with time and becomes progressively worse with increasing depth (Bennett & Dossett 1973).

It is pertinent that Zaltsman (1968) also

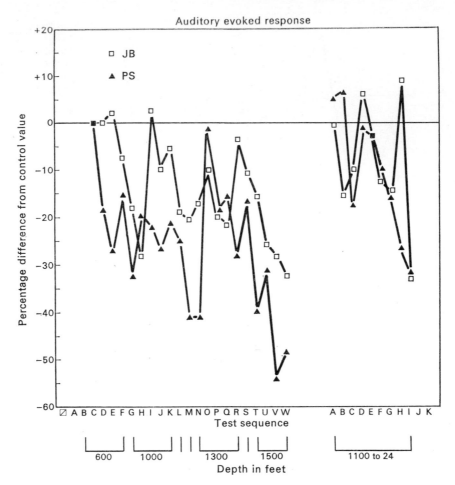

FIG. 14.5. Percentage change in the size of the N_1P_2 spike of the auditory induced averaged evoked potential at the cortex during the 1500 ft oxygen–helium
dive at RNPL in 1970. A progressive marked reduction of potentials is indicated
with increasing depth (after Bennett & Towse 1971a)

reported EEG changes with oxygen–helium compressions of 30 to 60 ft/min and compared the results with exposure to nitrogen at 70 to 350 ft (3
to 12 ATA) and argon at 30 to 200 ft (2 to 7 ATA).
Lessening of amplitude and an increase in frequency of alpha was reported. With nitrogen and
argon this was followed by intensification of fast
activity on a background of suppressed alpha until
eventually theta activity took its place. No slow
activity was seen at 630 ft (20 ATA) with helium
in spite of other signs of quite marked HPNS such
as impairment of mental efficiency, memory,
motor reflexes and dimensions of writing. There is

little doubt, however, that changes would have
been observed with the use of frequency analyses.
    The tests of performance decrement during the
1500 ft (48 ATA) exposure correlated with the
amount of tremors present (Fig. 14.6) but there
was no mental deterioration. This supported
earlier hypotheses that helium would not have
narcotic properties (Carpenter 1953; Bennett,
Papahadjopoulos & Bangham 1967). The degree
of postural tremor measured by a transducer on
the middle finger permitted the demonstration of
the interindividual variations of tremor and its
association with too fast a rate of compression and

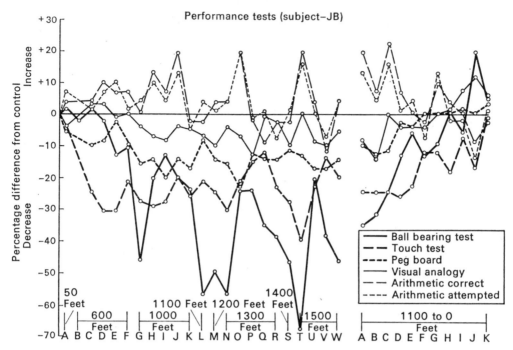

FIG. 14.6. Changes in performance tests compared with surface controls during 1500 ft (46 ATA) oxygen–helium exposure. Intellectual performance is unaffected but psychomotor tests indicate an increasing greater decrement with the sensitivity of the test. The decrement correlates with the onset of tremors elicited by each compression phase (after Bennett & Towse 1971b)

showed, in addition, that there is a more permanent tremor which appears to become worse with increasing pressure (Fig. 14.7).

In November 1970, the COMEX company carried out a further dive called Physalie V, using a similar dive profile with stages and with an increasingly slower rate of compression and three fast phases of 1 m/min between 0 to 355 ft, 1150 to 1310 ft and 1510 to 1610 (0 to 11·7, 35·7 to 40·6, 46·7 to 49·7 ATA) to attain 1706 ft (52·5 ATA) for a short time. Even so the HPNS was present but was of an ameliorated nature and considerably less than the earlier 1968 experiment. Frequency analysis of the EEG showed, however, the usual compression-related increase in theta activity and reduction of fast alpha and beta frequencies (Figs 14.8 and 14.9). Tremor appeared at 1000 to 1150 ft (31 to 40·6 ATA), became marked after 1600 ft (49·5 ATA), and was in two forms, 'static', presumably postural, and kinetic and dysmetry, presumably intentional (Fig. 14.10).

There was, too, a drop in awareness in moments of relaxation and performance tests showed reduced efficiency (Fructus 1972; Fructus, Agarate & Sicardi 1975).

The improvement compared with the earlier French dives was alluded to the application of the theory of osmotic dysbarism (Kylstra, Longmuir & Grace 1968; Hills 1971) which suggests that osmotic fluid shifts due to too fast a compression cause the HPNS. Fructus and colleagues calculated the compression rate so that a given gradient was maintained between the dissolved inert gas tension in the slowest and fastest tissues of the body, the gradient being a function of depth. That is:

$$\frac{dP}{dt} = \frac{\log 2 \times G}{T(1 - G')}$$

where G is equivalent to dG/dP, P is depth, T is tissue half time and $G(P)$ is the proposed gradient function.

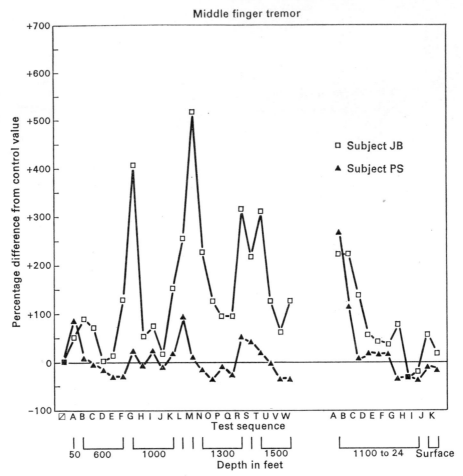

Fɪɢ. 14.7. Postural tremor measured from an accelerometer on the middle finger during a 1500 ft oxygen–helium simulated dive. Each compression phase elicits an increase in tremor which is more marked in one subject than the other. In the latter there is also a progressive increase in base-line tremor with increasing depth (after Bennett & Towse 1971b)

Similarly Chouteau, Ocana de Sentuary and Pironti (1971) formulated a relationship based on the osmotic theory and with the assumption that during compression the dissolved inert gas tension within a tissue of given half-time is not in equilibrium with the inspired inert gas partial pressure and should not exceed a certain Δp which was about 10 bar. However, there are several anomalies to this theory as well as agreements (Bennett & Towse 1972).

It would seem that compression theory is now, like decompression theory, enduring the fitting of mathematical models to calculate profiles with an

inadequate knowledge of the cause or mechanism. The one clear fact, regardless of the mathematics involved, is that, as with decompression, compression to such depths should be essentially exponential and preferably with stages to permit adaptation.

SUPPRESSION OF HPNS

Decreasing compression rate

The role of adaptation of HPNS was studied also by the COMEX organization and CNEXO (Centre National pour l'Exploitation des Oceans)

Diver A–CP

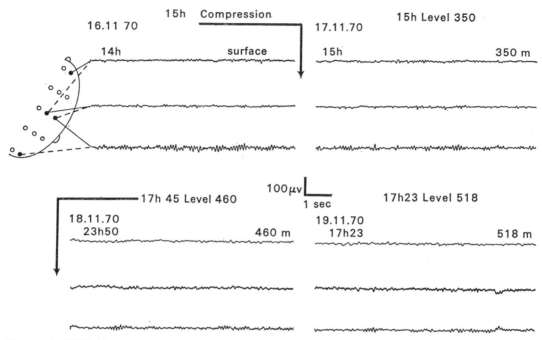

FIG. 14.8. EEG of one of the divers during various stages of the COMEX Physalie V dive to 1706 ft (52·5 ATA) illustrating the reduction in activity (after Fructus 1972)

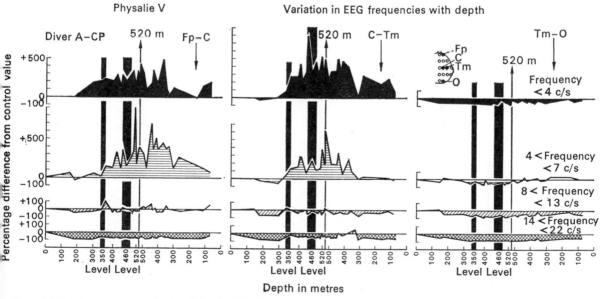

FIG. 14.9. Frequency analysis of the EEG of the same subject as in Fig. 14.8 showing the rise in theta (4 to 7 c/s) and delta (< 4 c/s) and depression of alpha (8 to 13 c/s) and beta (14 to 22 c/s) frequencies together with variations due to different electrode placement in the COMEX dive to 1706 ft (52·5 ATA) (after Fructus 1972)

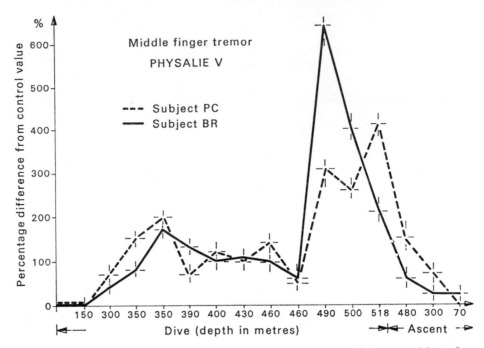

FIG. 14.10. The percentage change in the middle finger tremor of the two subjects during the COMEX dive to 1706 ft (52·5 ATA) (after Fructus 1972)

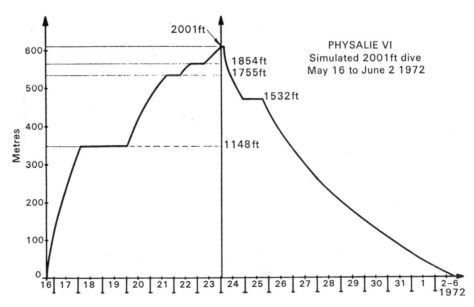

FIG. 14.11. Dive profile for the simulated deep dive to 2001 ft (60·5 ATA) in June 1972 by COMEX (after Fructus and Charpy 1972)

during a dive to 1640 ft (51 ATA) for 100 hours (Fructus, Agarate & Sicardi 1975) known as 'Sagitaire II' with a decreasing compression rate ending at 14 ft/hr on arrival. First signs of the HPNS appeared in the 1000 to 1200 ft (31 to 37 ATA) range and gradually increased with compression. After 40 hours at 1640 ft (51 ATA) the signs and symptoms stabilized and showed no adaptation over a further 60 hours. These included static (postural) tremor, muscular jerks, lack of coordination of certain movements and marked EEG changes, some of which denoted a lessening of awareness. Psychomotor performance was only slightly affected and intellectual faculties were good. No significant improvement was observed until 40 hours after decompression had started at about the 1000 ft (31 ATA) depth.

In June 1972, the deepest dive to date was made by the same French group which culminated in the exposure of two men, Patrice Chemin and Robert Gauret, to 2001 ft (60·5 ATA) for 80 min during Physalie VI.

The equivalent density of this breathing mixture to air would be found at 266 ft (8 ATA) and the compression rate involved again a slower and slower compression with stages (Fig. 14.11). The HPNS appeared at 1150 ft (35·7 ATA) and was more marked while sleeping during the stage at 1750 to 1850 ft (54 to 57 ATA) than during compression. Performance efficiency varied with the individual, one showing a decrement of 18 to 48% depending on the test, with a 20% decrement in manual dexterity, the other showing only a 16% decrement in manual dexterity. Both subjects showed an increase in reaction time (Fructus & Charpy 1972). The effects were considered to be less than those seen in the 1500 ft (46 ATA) British dive and they bode well for the success of operational diving to 1500 to 1600 ft (46 to 49 ATA). Clearly from the progression of these dives, slower compression is a significant advantage in permitting the attainment of deeper depths. A further example is given by the 1200 ft (37 ATA) simulated dive at Philadelphia (Lambertsen 1975) where the compression rate slowed from 5 ft/min between 400 ft and 900 ft to 2·5 ft/min between 900 ft and 1200 ft with stages of 4 to 2 days at 400, 700 and 900 ft (13·33 and 28 ATA). Under these conditions HPNS was not seen.

Nitrogen–helium mixtures

A further way to suppress the HPNS, as with the animal studies, is to add small amounts of a narcotic such as nitrogen or hydrogen.

Some pilot studies have been made in man by the COMEX company in France. Vigreux (1970) examined nitrogen–helium–oxygen mixtures with almost equal parts of nitrogen and helium (O_2 18%, N_2 42%, He 40%). This produced a reduction in the cost of the dive, increased thermal comfort together with an improvement in the distortion of speech due to helium.

At moderate depths of 80 m (262 ft) the results were encouraging but at 120 m (394 ft) a mixture of O_2 13%, N_2 43% and He 44% caused breathlessness and narcosis when the diver carried out moderate work. By relating the respiratory difficulties to the density of the breathing mixture, density equivalents (ED) in relation to air were obtained. Thus the 80 m (262 ft) mixed gas dive corresponds to an air dive of 53 m (174 ft) and the 120 m (394 ft) dive to that at 75 m (246 ft). On this basis 50% oxygen and 50% nitrogen mixtures, have an acceptable ED for dives not exceeding 1 hour and appropriate mixtures were proposed (Table 14.2).

TABLE 14.2

Gas mixtures for specific depths.
(Data after Vigreux 1970)

Depth	O_2		N_2		He	ED
60 m	23	:	23	:	52	31 m
80 m	18	:	18	:	64	35 m
100 m	14	:	14	:	72	38 m
120 m	12	:	12	:	76	42 m

These mixtures were satisfactory, with effective pulmonary ventilation under moderate work and no narcosis. However, there is no indication by Vigreux of scientific data in support of this contention and a quantitative titration of various percentages of gases against quantitative physiological measurements of nitrogen narcosis, oxygen toxicity and decompression sickness are required.

Zaltsman (1961) also has reported an 'antagonism' of the narcotic action of nitrogen in the presence of helium. For simplicity of operational diving, air–helium mixtures were suggested, with at depths from 60 m to 100 m (1977 ft to 328 ft) 50% by volume of helium and at depths from 101 m to 160 m (331 ft to 527 ft) 67% helium. This gave a maximum nitrogen partial pressure of 4·5 ATA and the oxygen did not exceed 2 ATA.

Under such conditions at 527 ft, heavy work between 221 and 580 kg–m/min was possible with little or no tremors or signs of the HPNS and no thermal balance or voice distortion problems. Again there is no quantitative data to support the statements of Zaltsman and much further work is required to elicit the correct ratio of helium, nitrogen and oxygen for a given depth which will effectively control the problems of nitrogen narcosis and the HPNS and at the same time not cause oxygen toxicity.

A further relevant factor, in addition to the interaction of the gases in the mixture, is the pressure itself. Smith (1969) has pointed out that anesthetic concentrations in lipid produce a uniform volume expansion of 0·4% which could be responsible for changes in permeability and that a hydrostatic pressure of 100 ATS (3300 ft) would nullify this expansion and prevent the anesthetic effect. That such a pressure reversal of anesthesia does occur in animals has been demonstrated by Lever et al. (1971). At pressures of 30 ATS or more, pre-anesthetic effects of nitrogen might also be nullified in man by the effects of the pressure, in addition to possible positive assistance from helium 'antagonism'. Further, the cause of the HPNS could well be due to the effects of hydrostatic pressure on nerve cell membranes causing a constriction of volume and, as a result, interfer-

ence with ionic perturbation in a manner opposite to that caused by nitrogen narcosis. Addition of small amounts of nitrogen or other narcotic would help to expand the membrane and counter this constriction. The measurements of penetration or adsorption of inert gases, oxygen and carbon dioxide to a lipid monolayer (Bennett, Papahadjopoulos & Bangham 1967) and the opposite effect of helium as discussed in Chapter 13 and illustrated in Fig. 13.5 suggests that a $N_2/He/O_2$ mixture should minimize both nitrogen narcosis and the HPNS.

Some quantitative indication that this is so was also obtained by Proctor et al. (1971) without their realizing it, during the 1000 ft dive described earlier. During the decompression the divers breathed a gas mixture of 3·5 ATS N_2, 1·0 to 1·5 ATS O_2 and the balance helium for 10 mins at 600 ft, 400 ft, 240 ft, and 200 ft (19, 13, 11 and 7 ATA). At 600 ft (19 ATA) there were no narcotic effects or performance deterioration but at the *shallower* depths the high nitrogen mixture caused narcosis. Presumably at 600 ft (19 ATA) the narcotic effect of the nitrogen, due to the expansion of cell membranes, was effectively balanced by the hydrostatic pressure, helium having no specific action. However, at the shallower depths, the hydrostatic pressure was insufficient to nullify the membrane expansion due to the nitrogen and narcosis occurred.

Such a mixed gas system should, if available, be much safer for short-duration deep diving, permit fast compression times and be less expensive than pure helium dives. In addition, it should overcome the problems of voice distortion and the necessity

TABLE 14.3

Characteristics of air–helium mixtures composed for humans in conditions of high pressures.
(Data after Zaltsman 1961)

Total pressure (m H₂O)	Mixture ratio %		Partial pressure of gases (ATA)			Decrease in thermal conductivity in medium as compared to helium–oxygen (number of times)	Increase in density of medium as compared to helium–oxygen (number of times)
	Air	*Oxygen*	*Oxygen*	*Nitrogen*	*Helium*		
From 60 to 100	50	10·4	0·7–1·1	2·8–4·4	3·5–11·3	2·0	2·1
From to 100	33	6·9	0·76–1·13	2·94–4·53	7·4–11·3	1·65–1·9	1·75–2

of supplying heat due to the intrinsic thermal conductivity problems of helium alone. Decompressions should be only some 4 days instead of the 14 for saturation diving.

That this may indeed be correct is supported by recent studies during 1973 at the Duke University Medical Center, North Carolina, in collaboration with the Harbor Branch Foundation and Oceaneering International Inc., in which four men were compressed in 17 min, plus 3 min of stages, to 720 ft (22·8 ATA) for 1 hour, breathing 25% nitrogen and 75% helium with 0·5 ATA oxygen throughout. The results were compared with dives to 200 ft of air and 720 ft (22·8 ATA) oxygen–helium. Intensive neurophysiological and psychological studies were made and decompression took 3 days. The same men were compressed also to 1000 ft (31 ATA) in 27 min, plus 6 min of stages,

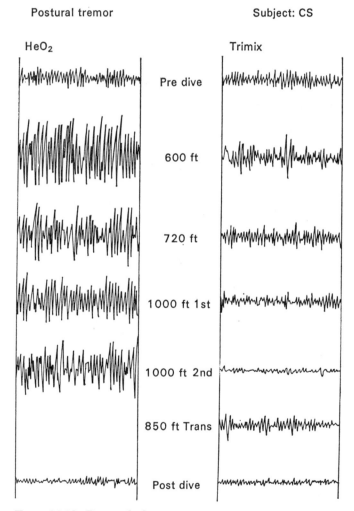

Fig. 14.12. Postural finger tremor measurements during compression to 1000 ft (31 ATA) in 27 min, plus 6 min of stages, breathing either He/O_2 or $He/N_2/O_2$ (trimix) in which the N_2 percentage is 18%. Compression with He/O_2 results in a marked increase in finger tremor. At 600 ft (19 ATA) nitrogen starts to be added in the trimix dive and the tremor is suppressed. At 850 ft (26·7 ATA) the subject returned to He/O_2 and the tremor returned (after Bennett et al. 1974)

breathing in one case trimix with 18% nitrogen and the other oxygen–helium. Decompression took 4 days.

As may be seen from Fig. 14.12 the presence of nitrogen was very effective in suppressing the tremors of HPNS. Very interestingly, removal of the nitrogen during the decompression at 850 ft (26·7 ATA) resulted in a return of the tremors. Psychomotor tests revealed a similar improvement and the nausea and dizziness, found in the dives where nitrogen was not present, ceased. Compression arthralgia was reduced.

Some decrement in performance, especially in intellectual functions, was present with the trimix due to nitrogen narcosis. However, it is believed that reduction of the nitrogen partial pressure to 12 to 14% will still reduce the HPNS but not result in any unnecessary narcosis. Experiments to confirm this are being conducted during 1975 at Duke University Medical Center.

Here then may be the solution to many of the problems which have limited diving depth in the past decade and is likely to be an area of increasing research interest in the years ahead.

REFERENCES

BACHRACH, A. J. & BENNETT, P. B. (1973) Tremor in diving. *Aerospace Med.* **44**, 613–625.

BENNETT, P. B. (1965) *Psychometric Impairment in Men Breathing Oxygen–Helium at Increased Pressures.* Medical Research Council, RN Personnel Research Committee, Underwater Physiology Sub-Committee, Report No. 251.

BENNETT, P. B. (1967) Performance impairment in deep diving due to nitrogen, helium, neon and oxygen. In *Proc. 3rd Symp. Underwater Physiology.* Ed. C. J. Lambertsen. pp. 327–340. Baltimore: Williams and Wilkins.

BENNETT, P. B. & DOSSETT, A. N. (1967) *Undesirable Effects of Oxygen–Helium Breathing at Great Depths.* Medical Research Council, RN Personnel Research Committee, Underwater Physiology Sub-committee, Report No. 260.

BENNETT, P. B. & DOSSETT, A. N. (1973) Alterations in EEG frequencies in animals exposed to 700 ft. and 4000 ft. *Aerospace Med.* **44**, 239–244.

BENNETT, P. B. & GRAY, S. P. (1971) Changes in human urine and blood chemistry during a simulated oxygen–helium dive to 1500 ft. *Aerospace Med.* **42**, 868–874.

BENNETT, P. B. & TOWSE, E. J. (1971a) The High Pressure Nervous Syndrome during a simulated oxygen–helium dive to 1500 ft. *Electroenceph. clin. Neurophysiol.* **31**, 383–393.

BENNETT, P. B. & TOWSE, E. J. (1971b) Performance efficiency of men breathing oxygen–helium at depths between 100 feet and 1500 feet. *Aerospace Med.* **42**, 1147–1156.

BENNETT, P. B. & TOWSE, E. J. (1972) *Electroencephalogram, Tremors and Mental Performance During Exposure to Air or Oxygen–Helium at 100 ft., 200 ft. and 300 ft.* RN Physiological Laboratory, Alverstoke, Report 3/72. Ministry of Defence (Navy).

BENNETT, P. B., PAPAHADJOPOULOS, D. & BANGHAM, A. D. (1967) The effect of raised pressures of inert gases on phospholipid model membranes. *Life Sci.* **6**, 2527–2533.

BENNETT, P. B., BLENKARN, G. D., ROBY, J. & YOUNGBLOOD, D. (1974) Suppression of the high pressure nervous syndrome in human deep dives by He–N_2–O_2. *Undersea Biomed. Res.* **1**, 221–237.

BENNETT, P. B., MORRISON, J. B., BARNARD, E. E. P. & EATON, J. (1971) *Experimental Observations on Men at Pressures between 4 bars (100 ft.) and 47 bars (1500 ft.)* RN Physiological Laboratory, Alverstoke, Report 1/71. pp. 1–137. Ministry of Defence (Navy).

BIERSNER, R. J. & CAMERON, B. J. (1970) Memory impairment during a deep helium dive. *Aerospace Med.* **41**, 658–661.

BRAUER, R. W. (1968) Seeking man's depth level. *Ocean Industry* **3**, 28–33.

BRAUER, R. W., WAY, R. O., JORDAN, M. R. & PARRISH, D. E. (1971) Experimental studies on the High Pressure Nervous Syndrome in various mammalian species. In *Proc. 4th Symp. Underwater Physiology.* Ed. C. J. Lambertsen. pp. 487–500. New York: Academic Press.

BÜHLMANN, A. A., MATTHYS, H., OVERRATH, G., BENNETT, P. B., ELLIOTT, D. H. & GRAY, S. P. (1970) Saturation exposures of 31 ats in an oxygen–helium atmosphere with excursions to 36 ats. *Aerospace Med.* **41**, 394–402.

CABARROU, P., HARTMANN, H., WEINER, K. H., ALINAT, P. & FUST, H. D. (1966) Introduction de la physiologie de 'Homo Aquaticus'. *Presse Méd.* **74**, 2771–2773.

CARPENTER, F. G. (1953) Anesthetic action of inert and unreactive gases on intact animals and isolated tissues. *Am. J. Physiol.* **178**, 505–509.

CHOUTEAU, J., OCANA DE SENTUARY, J. & PIRONTI, L. (1971) *Theoretical, Experimental and Comparative Study of Compression During Emergency and Saturation Dives to Great Depths.* Report No. 1/71. Centre d'Études Marines Avancées, Marseille.

FRUCTUS, X. R. (Ed.) (1972) Down below the great depths. In *Proc. 3rd International Conference on Hyperbaric and Underwater Physiology.* pp. 13–22. Paris: Doin.

FRUCTUS, X. R. & CHARPY, J. P. (1972) *Étude psychometrique de 2 sujets lors d'une plongée fictive jusqu'à 52·42 ATA.* Bulletin Medsubhyp, Service D'Hyperbare, Hôpital Salvator, Marseille. Report No. 7. October.

FRUCTUS, X. R., AGARATE, C. & SICARDI, F. (1975) Postponing the High Pressure Nervous Syndrome (HPNS) down to 500 m and deeper. In *Underwater Physiology. Vth. Symp. Underwater Physiology.* Ed. C. J. Lambertsen. Bethesda: Fedn Am. Socs exp. Biol.

FRUCTUS, X. R., BRAUER, R. W. & NAQUET, R. (1971) Physiological effects observed in the course of simulated deep chamber dives to a maximum of 36·5 atm in helium–oxygen atm. In *Proc. 4th Symp. Underwater Physiology.* Ed. C. J. Lambertsen. pp. 545–550. New York: Academic Press.

HAMILTON, R. W., MACINNIS, J. B., NOBLE, A. D. & SCHREINER, H. R. (1966) *Saturation Diving at 650 ft*. Technical Memorandum B1 411 Ocean Systems Inc., New York.

HILLS, B. A. (1911) Gas-induced osmosis as a factor influencing the distribution of body water. *Clin. Sci.* **40**, 175–191.

HUNTER, W. L. & BENNETT, P. B. (1974) The causes, mechanisms and prevention of the high pressure nervous syndrome. *Undersea Biomed. Res.* **1**, 1–28.

KELLY, J. S., BURCH, P. G., BRADLEY, M. E. & CAMPBELL, D. E. (1968) Visual function in divers at 15 to 26 atmospheres pressure. *Milit. Med.* **133**, 827–829.

KYLSTRA, J. A., LONGMUIR, I. S. & GRACE, M. (1968) Dysbarism: a study of gas osmosis. *Science, N.Y.* **161**, 289.

LAMBERTSEN, C. J. (Ed.) (1975) Collaborative investigation of limits of human tolerance to pressurization with helium, neon and nitrogen. Simulation of density equivalent to helium–oxygen respiration at depths to 2000, 3000, 4000, and 5000 ft. of sea water. In *Underwater Physiology*. *Vth Symp. Underwater Physiology*. Bethesda: Fedn Am. Socs exp. Biol.

LEVER, M. J., MILLER, K. W., PATON, W. D. M. & SMITH, E. B. (1971) Pressure reversal of anesthesia. *Nature, Lond.* **231**, 368–371.

MORRISON, J. B. & FLORIO, J. T. (1971) Respiratory function during a simulated dive to 1500 ft. *J. appl. Physiol.* **30**, 724–732.

OVERFELD, E. M., SALTZMAN, H. A., KYLSTRA, J. A. & SALZANO, J. V. (1969) Respiratory gas exchange in normal men breathing 0·9% oxygen in helium at 31·3 ats. *J. appl. Physiol.* **27**, 471–475.

PROCTOR, L. D., CAREY, C. R., LEE, R. M., SCHAEFER, K. E. & VAN DEN ENDE, H. (1971) Electroencephalographic changes during saturation excursion dives to a simulated seawater depth of 1000 feet. *Aerospace Med.* **43**, 867–877.

SALZANO, J., RAUSCH, D. C. & SALTZMAN, H. A. (1970) Cardio-respiratory responses to exercise at a simulated seawater depth of 1000 ft. *J. appl. Physiol.* **28**, 34–41.

SCHAEFER, K. E., CAREY, C. R. & DOUGHERTY, J. H. (1970) Pulmonary gas exchange and urinary electrolyte excretion during saturation–excursion diving to pressures equivalent to 800 and 1000 feet of seawater. *Aerospace Med.* **41**, 856–864.

SMITH, E. B. (1969) The role of exotic gases in the study of narcosis. In *The Physiology and Medicine of Diving and Compressed Air Work*. (First Edition). Ed. P. B. Bennett and D. H. Elliot. pp. 183–192. London: Baillière, Tindall & Cassell.

SUMMITT, J. K., KELLY, J. S., HERRON, J. M. & SALTZMAN, H. A. (1971) 1000-foot helium saturation exposure. In *Proc. 4th Symp. Underwater Physiology*. Ed. C. J. Lambertsen. pp. 519–527. New York: Academic Press.

VIGREUX, J. (1970) *Contribution to the Study of the Neurological and Mental Reactions of the Organism of the Higher Mammal to Gaseous Mixtures Under Pressure*. MD Thesis. Toulouse University.

WALDVOGEL, W. & BÜHLMANN, A. A. (1968) Man's reaction to long-lasting overpressure exposure: Examination of the saturated organism at a helium pressure of 21–22 ats. *Helv. med. Acta*, **34**, 130–150.

WEYBREW, B. B. & PARKER, J. W. (1968) *Performance Effects of Increased Ambient Pressure. I. Helium–oxygen saturation and excursion dive to a simulated depth of 900 ft*. Report 556, USN Submarine Medical Center, Groton, Connecticut.

ZALTSMAN, G. L. (1961) *Physiological Principles of a Sojourn of a Human in Conditions of Raised Pressure of the Gaseous Medium*. Leningrad. English translation, Foreign Technology Division, Wright-Patterson Air Force Base, Ohio, AD 655 360, 1967.

ZALTSMAN, G. L. (Ed.) (1968) *Hyperbaric Epilepsy and Narcosis (Neurophysiological Studies)* pp. 1–265. Leningrad: Sechenov Institute of Evolutionary Physiology and Biochemistry, USSR Academy of Sciences.

15

Underwater Performance

A. J. BACHRACH

The major purpose for placing a diver in the water is to accomplish some sort of useful work such as exploration, salvage, or marine biology. Understandably, in view of the serious physiological problems encountered in diving, the emphasis has largely been on getting the diver safely to the work site and back, rather than on the work itself. As Bennett (1965) observed:

> For too long a period of time one considered the safety of the ascent as the major problem in diving. Although it is undeniable that an appropriately adjusted decompression is of vital necessity, it should not be forgotten that this constitutes wasted effort if man, working under pressure, is not in perfect physical and mental condition.

It is perhaps for this reason that research emphasis in recent years has broadened from respiratory physiology and decompression to central nervous system dysfunction (particularly the high pressure nervous syndrome [HPNS]) (Hunter & Bennett 1974), and how the diver performs once he is established under pressure at the work site.

Excellent reviews of underwater performance may be found in Shilling and Werts (in press), Adolfson and Berghage (1974) and Bennett (Chapters 12 and 14 in this volume). Rather than review a large number of specific studies, this chapter will concentrate on methodological considerations in the planning and execution of research basic to the assessment of diver performance.

CONTRADICTORY RESULTS, DIFFERENT TESTS, AND THE NEED FOR STANDARDIZATION

There are still myriads of unsolved problems in diver performance and efficiency. Many of these derive from the conditions of underwater and hyperbaric experiments themselves; many also are part of the general problem of assessing human performance accurately and quantitatively, particularly under stress. That such problems are not unique to the underwater environment is illustrated by a quotation from Theologus et al. (1973):

Examination of the literature on environmental stressors and their effects upon performance reveals a number of problems impeding the development of a systematic body of knowledge and the application of that knowledge. Within any particular study, environmental stressor variables and performance measures may be defined precisely, and employed effectively. However, it is often impossible to relate them systematically to different variables from other studies. Various researchers have employed different measures of performance, different methods of testing and different data analysis techniques. Descriptive data relating to the values and ranges of environmental stressors employed, the intervals of exposure, and the characteristics of subjects indicate considerable variation from study to study. Until the relationships among these and similar components are established systematically, development of a cohesive body of knowledge may be impossible.

A similar observation regarding stress was made

by Tune (1964) who studied the effects of high altitude on performance and found reported results either to be contradictory across studies or reported with insufficient details to permit conclusive inference. In particular, techniques varied to the degree where Tune noted, 'It is impossible to compare the performance of *S*s [subjects] in these studies because of lack of standardization of the techniques used'.

Comments by Bennett at a Workshop on The Development of Standardized Assessment of Underwater Performance (Bennett 1974) support the existence of this problem in underwater research. Bennett reported that approximately 50 tests have been used under varying circumstances for hyperbaric and underwater research. These included standard tests such as mental arithmetic and short-term memory measures, as well as tests without clear face validity, often made up on the spot, and applied without norms or reliability indicators.

It is interesting to note that even in cases of standardized tests in use for many years caution is necessary. For example, criticisms of the structure and validity of the Purdue Pegboard, an old standby since the mid-1940s, appear in Ghiselli (1949), Harrell (1949), Packard (1949) and Warren (1959).

The problems of standardization are even more acute in the underwater environment for many standardized tests cannot be easily transferred from a 1 ATA dry situation to a pressurized dry or wet condition. In a recent dive, for example, Miller, Bachrach and Walsh (in preparation) reported on the use of several tests in the water at depths to 250 ft (8·6 ATA) out of a habitat. A standardized vigilance task (Kennedy 1971a) using an auditory signal was unusable at depth because the diver's exhalation noise obscured the stimulus. Systematic exploration of available and constructed tasks under identical conditions, controlled for subject homogeneity and environmental similarity, is needed.

PERFORMANCE ASSESSMENT

A major objective of performance assessment is to determine whether the output of the performing subject is degraded from some standard, normal condition. The first priority is to determine the parameters to be studied. In underwater performance the first step is to determine what the diver does, how to assess what he does to determine decrement, and to establish possible causes of such decrement.

The types of work a diver actually does in the water have been outlined by Liffick (1971) as salvage, rescue, search and recovery, inspection and repair, construction and maintenance, tactical diving missions, and science support. In addition, the diver performs visual surveillance, navigates, retrieves and processes information, engages in decision making, and performs useful work. This list, while abstract to a large degree, could subsume most of the specific tasks a diver performs, employing tools and his own sensory apparatus.

What an operator does in complex systems is detailed by Christensen and Mills (1967) and might be applied to the underwater field to illuminate specific behaviors. For example, in the activity of searching for and receiving information the specific behaviors are: 'detects, inspects, observes, reads, receives, scans, and surveys' (Table 15.1). This scheme was devised to describe aviator behaviors, but its applicability to diver performance is obviously relevant.

How to assess what the diver does to establish base-lines and to determine possible decrement requires a definition of terms (Bachrach 1974) so that reported results can be accurately compared. Bachrach states:

For example, *dysfunction* is a general term indicating a breakdown in normal performance. *Decrement* is defined as a transitory state, a decline that is potentially reversible; so, one may talk about a decrement from a normal baseline indicating some *deterioration*, which is impairment (also transitory), a process of change worsening from a baseline. *Deficiency* is a lack of a particular function, while *deficit* is a loss, presumably irreversible. Thus, . . . one can talk about a baseline with a hearing decrement or impairment, which is transitory, to be reversed upon return to the surface or other change. Deterioration is the specific process by which the change or decrement occurs, and deficit is the irreversible loss that may occur as a result of the environmental conditions that impose the deterioration and decrement.

TABLE 15.1

Classification of behaviors*

Processes	Activities	Specific behaviors
1. Perceptual processes	(a) Searching for and receiving information	Detects Inspects Observes Reads Receives Scans Surveys
	(b) Identifying objects, actions, events	Discriminates Identifies Locates
2. Mediational processes	(a) Information processing	Categorizes Calculates Codes Computes Interpolates Itemizes Tabulates Translates
	(b) Problem solving and decision making	Analyses Calculates Chooses Compares Computes Estimates Plans
3. Communication processes		Advises Answers Communicates Directs Indicates Informs Instructs Requests Transmits
4. Motor processes	(a) Simple/discrete	Activates Closes Connects Disconnects Joins Moves Sets
	(b) Complex/continuous	Adjusts Aligns Regulates Synchronizes Tracks

* Modified from Christensen and Mills (1967), as adapted from Berliner, Angell, and Shearer (1964).

Basic to the assessment of a diver's performance is the inference of cause of decrement. If decrement is measured and determined to exist, what is the source of the change? There are three levels of approach in an experimental methodology. The first is to determine whether or not the phenomenon exists, then to determine its magnitude, and finally, to infer the cause of any change in its existence and magnitude. In this latter approach it is necessary to determine the functional relationship among events—under what specific conditions does the event occur? Emphasis has been on developing the techniques to measure actual change. For, given a quantification of performance differences, it is then possible to associate changes with such factors as environmental conditions, breathing mixes, diver motivation, and states of physiological stress. The three most likely influences upon diver performance, then, would include the breathing mix (e.g. helium v. hyperbaric air); hydrostatic pressure itself; and diver condition.

In shallow dives, hyperbaric air with increased nitrogen effects and hydrostatic pressure seem to be implicated as causes of decrement, and the changes appear mostly in the intellectual-cognitive area. In deep dives, there appears to be an excitation of the central nervous system, so the causes of decrement would be more neuro-anatomical and neurophysiological. Hunter and Bennett (1974) stressed the necessity for differentiating between the high pressure nervous syndrome as manifested during compression, and hydrostatic pressure alone. They suggest the terms *compression syndrome* and *hydrostatic pressure syndrome* may be more meaningful as a differentiation. The compression syndrome is largely characterized by symptoms such as tremor, changes in the electroencephalogram (particularly increasing theta, 4 to 8 Hz [c/s]) somnolence or loss of vigilance, and neuromuscular incoordination (e.g. loss of balance). Compression rate has been implicated as a cause of tremor by research such as that of Dossett and Hempleman (1972), who found that in rats compressed at three atmospheres a minute, tremors appeared at 1200 to 1400 ft (37·3 to 43·4 ATA); whereas, rats compressed at 0·3 atmospheres a minute did not tremble until 3500 ft (108 ATA). Fructus and Agarate (1971)

noted that tremors appear to be highly susceptible to compression rate. Slower compression rates, particularly at deeper depths, seem to diminish some of the syndrome symptomatology.

The breathing mix is also implicated in neurophysiological changes at depth. While the terms *helium tremor* and *compression tremor* have largely fallen into disuse, there have been some indications that the breathing mix may markedly affect such neurophysiological change. For example, in a recent series of dives, Bennett et al. (1974) report that the addition of nitrogen (18% at 1000 ft [31·3 ATA], 25% at 720 ft [22·8 ATA]) in a trimix of helium, oxygen, and nitrogen damps out high pressure syndome symtomatology with reduced tremor and improved performance.

The choice of tests for different kinds of dives has stabilized over the years into using measures that appear to be most sensitive to the particular situation. For example, in shallow dives (less than 200 ft [7·1 ATA]) cognitive tests (most frequently computational or arithmetic tests) are usually administered to divers under conditions of hyperbaric air, while central nervous system status tests (psychomotor and perceptual-sensory) are most often administered to subjects on deeper dives (below 600 ft [19·2 ATA]), where physiological concerns tend to override psychological assessment. Experience (Biersner 1971) has shown that neuromuscular motor performance is most affected by deep dives, while cognitive, intellectual performance is less affected. Very much the opposite is true in hyperbaric air where factors (presumably related to nitrogen narcosis) degrade cognitive functions more than psychomotor skills.

Biersner (1971) indicates that it 'is generally agreed that motor coordination shows the greatest decline under high pressures, whereas cognitive and intellectual functions undergo only small transitory changes. It is unclear, however, whether the impaired motor performance is related to hypercapnia, compression rate, temperature, or psychological stress, or to some combination of these factors'.

The types of measures to assess performance decrement suggested by Kennedy (1971b) may be divided into two basic elements—*central nervous system* (CNS) *status*, and *systems output*. The research strategy to assess CNS integrity employs

such measurement techniques as electroenceph-
alography (EEG), tremor measurements, vestibular tests, and statometry (standing steadiness).
The rationale behind assessing CNS status that is
if nerve pathways and the central nervous system
are degraded by environmental factors such as
pressure or breathing gases, the degradation will
impair performance. Hence, measurement of
tremor has been accomplished in a number of
dives to assess tremor as a CNS change and as
part of the high pressure nervous syndrome, which
could impair performance at depth.

The rationale for the systems approach, in
which the output of the operator is studied,
generally employs real-world work. As an example
of the systems output approach Kennedy (1971b)
notes:

> . . . it may take far longer for a free-swimming
> diver breathing air to disarm a torpedo in murky
> water at 100 ft than it takes him under ideal
> conditions. However, one does not know how
> much of this additional time is due to one or all
> of the following: (a) the conduction medium
> (murky water) degrades seeing, (b) the friction
> of the water impedes muscular responses, or (c) the
> hyperbaria and/or time at depth adversely affects
> the CNS in some way.

Thus, there may be interactions of all of these
factors, with muscular performance, vision, and
CNS integrity affected. Real-world tasks generally
measure immediate systems output, and are
exemplified by an underwater assembly task such
as the UCLA pipe puzzle (Weltman et al. 1971),
and complex underwater assembly tasks
(MacInnis 1971). It is clear that there is no firm
dichotomy between CNS status and system output tests. The overlap is real, but it is useful to
consider the emphasis of each.

Factor analysis of performance

A factor analysis of performance involves breaking down basic abilities and responses of the
operator to task components and overall task
time. Fleishman (1964), a pioneer in the factor
analysis of performance, found that less than a
dozen measurably distinct factors (or basic
abilities) were being assessed by large numbers of
tests. From such research of basic abilities have
come four broad categories of human performance

(which have some overlap) under the rubrics of
cognitive, perceptual-sensory, psychomotor, and
physical proficiency. Examples of cognitive tests
are memory span, conceptual reasoning, and
associative memory; examples of perceptual-
sensory tests are perceptual speed and spatial
orientation. Examples of psychomotor tests have
been given (Theologus et al. 1973) as visual
reaction time, manual dexterity, and arm–hand
steadiness. Evans and Consolazio (1967) studied
three types of *physical proficiency,* described as
explosive strength, dynamic strength, and stam-
ina. There seems to be some general agreement
on the types of tests that are used among researchers who approach human performance
assessment from the factor analytic standpoint.

Several models have been proposed to approach
the measurement of human performance and the
interaction of the environmental factors upon it.
(Table 15.2). Models, such as that of Fleishman
(1964, 1967), have identified a set of abilities to
measure by specific individual tasks. For example,
Poston, Osburn, and Sheer (1967) analysed
individual performance abilities in a task battery
composed of 18 psychomotor tests grouped into
five major ability categories:

1. Fine manipulation.
2. Gross positioning and movement.
3. System equalization.
4. Perception and cognition.
5. Reaction time.

Research factored out six relatively independent
psychomotor dimensions identified as

1. Reaction time.
2. Finger dexterity.
3. Arm–hand steadiness.
4. Wrist–finger speed.
5. Response orientation.
6. Control precision.

Another system to measure human mental and
perceptual motor functions at pressures equivalent to a depth of 1000 ft of seawater is reported
by Reilly and Cameron (1968). This system, known
as SINDBAD I (Systematic Investigation of
Diver Behaviour at Depth) is based on a primary
abilities and related performance measure
rationale to be applied to diver activities. The

TABLE 15.2

Historical steps in the development of a perceptual-motor taxonomy*

Buxton (1938)	Seashore (1951)	Fleishman (1954)	Fleishman (1960)
1. Fine manipulative performance	1. Speed of single reaction	1. Reaction time	1. Reaction time
2. Spatial perception	2. Spatial relations	2. Spatial relations	2. Response orientation
3. Steadiness	3. Steadiness	3. Arm–hand steadiness	3. Arm–hand steadiness
4. Speed	4. Finger–hand speed in restricted oscillatory movement	4. Finger dexterity or fine dexterity	4. Finger dexterity
5. Motor learning	5. Forearm and hand speed in oscillatory movement of moderate extent	5. Wrist–finger speed	5. Wrist–finger speed
6. Gross manipulative performance	6. Unidentifiable or residual	6. Rate of arm movement	6. Speed of arm movement
		7. Aiming or controlled manual movement	7. Aiming
		8. Manual dexterity	8. Manual dexterity
		9. Psychomotor speed	9. Rate control
		10. Psychomotor coordination	10. Multiple limb coordination
		11. Postural discrimination	11. Control precision

* Courtesy of T. E. Berghage.

system was designed for either wet or dry simulation in the environmental chambers of the US Navy Experimental Diving Unit. Twenty-six specific tests have been programmed ranging from simple reaction time to manual tracking and from monitoring a simple panel display to solving involved mental arithmetic problems. The system is automated, with remote administration and scoring of the tasks, and is designed to provide a standardized assessment of diver performance within the basic abilities framework.

The first systematic investigation of SINDBAD tests (Bain & Berghage 1974) presented the baseline results and analysis of SINDBAD data gathered at the Experimental Diving Unit. These investigators selected 22 of the 26 tests in the SINDBAD battery to administer in a dry hyperbaric chamber at surface pressure. The major subject population was constituted of 27 first class divers.

Factor analysis results show that each measure was unique and the expected redundancy among the 26 SINDBAD tests did not appear. Examples of the factors that were studied and the tests representing these factors are manual dexterity (tested by wrench and cylinder coordination), reaction time (tested by visual reaction time), response orientation (tested by choice reaction time), perceptual speed (tested by number comparison), and time sharing (tested by tracking and monitoring). A description of the tests appears in Bain and Berghage (1974).

A factor analytic approach may be helpful in pointing out task elements that have sometimes been obscured in the measures that have been characteristically used in underwater performance assessment. For example, Baddeley (1966) and Kiessling and Maag (1962) both report measuring manual dexterity. An analysis of the tasks, however, shows that Baddeley, using a nut and bolt assembly, was indeed measuring manual dexterity defined as arm–hand performance under speed conditions, while Kiessling and Maag were measuring finger dexterity (a fine coordination) by placing pegs in the Purdue Pegboard.

One of the problems in measuring performance (and particularly performance degradation) is that performance does not always 'fall off' in a simple linear fashion. Assuming that a diver may have input overload from environmental factors and task requirements, Fitts and Posner (1967), drawing on a model from Miller (1964), suggest that an individual may adapt to input overload conditions by several types of performance alteration. He may, for example, work faster and let errors increase, make less carefully considered decisions, and respond without considering all the information available to him. A related process is to disregard or filter out part of the incoming information.

The process may be selective, and may improve performance by disregarding less important problems at hand or decisions to be made—it becomes a judgmental analysis of priorities. Another mechanism referred to as queuing can be applied, where input messages and other work are allowed to wait in line for action. This, again, is judgment —to decide that a number of tasks cannot be done simultaneously, and to assign priorities to ones that will be done first, and in sequence. Does the diver, for example, assess priorities by concentrating on one task at a time and queuing the remainder, or does he effectively handle simultaneous, divided-attention, time-sharing tasks? Superimposed upon these questions, are there possible alterations in judgment and decision making, perhaps occasioned by inert gas narcosis? This approach may provide a model upon which to develop a finer grain analysis of the processes subsumed under degradation.

Correlation with physiology

Another approach to performance assessment has been to correlate basic performance functions and the effects of environmental conditions by studying them in the context of physiological change (Teichner & Olson 1971). In this approach, Teichner and Olson (1971) have noted that the environment does not always degrade performance (and, the degradation is not always in a simple linear fashion). As Teichner and Olson observed:

> . . . the most frequent environmental data that have been obtained have been concerned with physiological effects rather than effects on performance. To take maximum advantage of the available information, it is necessary to develop relationships between performance and physio-

logical data and then to use these to predict the effects of the environment on performance for conditions where physiological but not performance data, are available.

This approach to the assessment of performance is particularly pertinent to a diving population where measures of a physiological nature such as tremor, heart rate, and oxygen consumption may frequently be obtained in normal diving operations. There are two fundamental approaches to physiological monitoring: direct measurement of the diver himself by electrode implacement as, for example, heart rate (Weltman et al. 1971); or indirect monitoring of the dive by such devices as the GE hard-wire diver monitor, where levels of oxygen in the equipment can be measured. Telemetry of diver physiology has been accomplished by Kanwisher, Lawson, and Strauss (1974) and Bachrach and Egstrom (1974) using the same apparatus.

Specific measures of physiological change related in particular to central nervous system activity have been based on the hypothesis that CNS activity, as a change induced by environmental events such as pressure and gas on the diver, can indicate impending dysfunctioning in physiological and behavioral performance. The major CNS activities measured in deep dives have been muscle tremor (Bachrach, Thorne & Conda 1971; Bennett & Towse 1971b; Bachrach & Bennett 1973a, Bachrach & Bennett 1973b; Thorne, Findling & Bachrach 1974); electro-encephalographic changes (EEG) (Serbanescu & Naquet 1969; Bennett & Towse 1971a; Naitoh, Johnson & Austin 1971; Proctor et al. 1972; Bachrach & Bennett 1973b; Wilcox & Russo 1974). Labyrinthine and vestibular effects have also been viewed as a serious problem in deep diving (Edmonds et al. 1973; Coles 1973; Braithwaite, Berghage & Crothers 1974; Kennedy 1974). Research on vestibular system response at 49·5 ATA has been reported by Braithwaite, Berghage and Crothers (1974), who found in a 1600 ft (49·5 ATA) chamber dive that standing steadiness was significantly altered from surface values, with performance on both the balance rail and stato-meter (a balance board) showing striking deterioration. Here, again, is an example of a physiological response (Adolfson, Goldberg & Berghage 1972;

Braithwaite, Berghage & Crothers 1974) from which performance decrement may be inferred.

Teichner and Olson (1971) comment on the environment having a direct effect on motor activity and upon sense organ functioning. They give as examples increased tremor during vibration and decreased thermal sensitivity of the skin during exposure to cold. They indicate that such direct effects will alter performance and need to be given specific consideration, although it cannot be assumed that these effects will always degrade performance—it is possible for a human to alter his response to achieve the same performance results. This altered response has been noted in many ways. For example, Zaltsman (1961) measured tremor in deep diving in a chamber and found that by motivation, or by what he calls 'force of will', a diver could overcome physiological tremor and proceed with work.

Another aspect presented by Teichner and Olson (1971) is that some physiological parameters do cross a number of environments—for example, hypoxia occurs in many stressful, unusual environments. They note, 'Even though not all environments have the same critical physiological effects, they may have similar activation effects'. They further note that such effects may be correlated with change in respiration rate, heart rate, oxygen consumption, arterial oxygen saturation, and blood flow. If such similarities and cross-environmental changes are true, these are variables to which performance should be related and with which CNS variables should be related.

FACTORS AFFECTING HUMAN PERFORMANCE

Types of stress

Let us consider performance as a dependent variable, affected and effected by many events, some objectively measurable (current, temperature) and some not (motivation, anxiety). First, performance must not be considered an 'either-or' phenomenon (i.e. we must not assume that degrading environmental conditions always effect performance decrement). Broadbent (1963), for example, demonstrated that combined effects of different stresses (noise, high temperature, and

sleeplessness) could be additive, independent of each other, or partially cancel each other. Wilkinson (1967) demonstrated that stresses may influence the working efficiency of man, though whether they will improve his performance or impair it depends largely on the nature and the degree of the stress and on the task he is performing. For example, Wilkinson found that alcohol and anoxia combine to produce high levels of impairment, while Corcoran (1962) found that combined stresses (such as lack of sleep and loud noise—similar to Broadbent's) may impair efficiency independently, but when combined may produce no additive adverse effect. As we have seen, Teichner and Olson (1971) express the opinion that a changed environment does not always degrade performance—a person frequently alters his performance to achieve the same result. Certainly a diver in a high turbidity environment is expected to be flexible and modify his work methods.

An example of a stress effect that could be expected to degrade performance, but did not, is found in a report by Frankenhaeuser, Graff-Lonnevig and Hesser (1960). These investigators compared performance on a mirror-drawing test and a reaction time task in subjects breathing pure oxygen at 3 ATA with the same tasks and same subjects breathing air at 1 ATA. No decrement in performance was found under elevated pressure, even in one subject whose performance on mirror drawing was not affected up to the point where he began to convulse from oxygen. Berkun et al. (1962) showed that subjects' belief in the authenticity of the stress was a crucial factor. Field-stressed subjects showed higher response than laboratory subjects. This obviously relates to chamber versus open-sea research dives and the perception by the subjects of the stress situation. One may speculate about individual susceptibilities to such stressors and the lack of sensitivity of some tests to detect impending dysfunction.

Baddeley (1967), specifically approaching the problem of interaction of stresses on diver performance, reports on three experiments. In Experiment I, Baddeley (1966) tested a group of experimental divers performing a manual dexterity task (transferring nuts and bolts from one end of a screwplate to the other) on dry land, and at 10 ft and 100 ft in water at sea. Another group of experienced divers was tested at equivalent pressures in a dry hyperbaric chamber. Results showed a decrement in performance of 5·5% in the chamber at depth.

The open-sea condition showed a marked drop in efficiency (28%) when the task was performed underwater, and an effect of depth (19·8%) significantly greater than the chamber decrement. Baddeley notes, '. . . the impairment at depth underwater is considerably greater than would be expected from a simple addition of the effect of working underwater and of working at pressure'.

Experiment II (Baddeley & Flemming 1967) compared the efficiency of divers breathing air or a 75% He, 25% O_2 mixture on a screwplate task at depths of 5 ft and 200 ft. They also tested divers in a dry pressure chamber at the same depths breathing the helium–oxygen mixture. Baddeley's conclusion was that 'Both the open-sea conditions showed a considerable impairment of efficiency at depth, and although this is somewhat less marked on oxygen–helium the degree of impairment is still considerably greater than would be expected from the dry chamber test where the decrease in efficiency though significant is small'.

In Experiment III (Baddeley et al. 1968), divers were tested with a screwplate and two other tasks at depths of 5 ft and 100 ft in an open-sea inlet. The 'exaggerated fall in efficiency previously observed at depth was not occurring', and therefore a larger sampling of 18 divers was tested twice at each depth. The results showed that working underwater evoked an impairment identical to that seen in Experiment I (28%); working at depth in water showed the same impairment as the group in Experiment I (19·8%); but working in a dry pressure chamber had not evoked the effect of diving stress shown in the water. Baddeley's inference is that Experiment III, done close to shore next to a quay, placed divers in relatively shallow, clear water, while the previous experiments were done in the open sea from a boat moored at sea, with reduced visibility—an experience that Baddeley states 'seemed to generate considerable anxiety, especially since the divers in both studies were working at a greater depth than was usual for

them'. He infers three states of stress interaction: the diver is at pressure, underwater, and anxious. Baddeley's final suggestion, based on an analysis of the interactions is that the major stress-induced decrement is one of an interaction between inert gas narcosis and anxiety exacerbated by degrading conditions of cold and reduced visibility.

Anxiety itself, as a possible interfering variable, needs further analysis. Certainly, apprehension in divers has been shown to have a marked effect on performance (Weltman & Egstrom 1966; Bachrach 1970; Egstrom & Bachrach 1971). The important aspect of Baddeley's experiments (aside from the problem of interference as to degrading stress effects) is that they are among the rare experiments in which simulated pressure and open-sea conditions were compared.

To return to apprehension and anxiety, the former as a physiological sign was inferred by Bachrach and Bennett (1973b) from measures accomplished on a deep chamber dive at Duke University, with divers breathing helium–oxygen and resting at 870 ft (27·4 ATA) (saturated) just prior to compression to 1000 ft (31·3 ATA). Two of three divers tested on a force-transducer tremor device showed pathological tremor (in a 3 to 5 Hz range), which disappeared, their tremor pattern returning to normal as they reached 31·3 ATA. Inasmuch as this could not have been a pure pressure or gas phenomenon, these investigators infer real physiological response to the stress of awaiting compression to 1000 ft (31·3 ATA). As far back as 1906, Hill and Greenwood, in studies in a chamber to a total of 7 ATA concluded that it is probable 'That the subjective effects of increased pressure, apart from voice changes and lip anaesthesia, depend upon psychical conditions such as anxiety and excitement'. But anxiety is always an inferential explanation. It is important to concentrate on objective measures of change, keeping inference to a second order.

Theologus et al. (1973) have observed that research on a large diversity of stress has repeatedly shown differential effects for different aspects of performance. They cite the work of Gorham and Orr (1957, 1958) on effects of experimentally induced stress (fear) on components of a complex skill. Gorham and Orr found that performance on perceptual-vigilance and numerical ability components (cognitive and perceptual skills) deteriorated; whereas motor coordination and response orientation components were maintained during the stress (the latter were in the psychomotor skill range).

Biersner (1971) has noted in regard to psychological stress and anxiety that such stress increases during the initial phase of a hazardous dive, but tends to decline noticeably during the period of maximum threat.

Kiessling and Maag (1962) felt that the degree of decrement encountered was in direct relationship to the complexity of the task and added '. . . the neural structures which support reasoning and immediate memory show greater functional impairment than do those supporting simple motor coordination and choice reactions'. While the 'neural structure' explanation is largely inferential, Kiessling and Maag do demonstrate differences in performance, noting that these differences in performance efficiency '. . . between various tasks help to account for contradictions in other research investigations which indicate little or no performance decrement at depths exceeding 150 to 250 ft' (5·5 to 8·6 ATA). This statement included the work by Miles and Mackay (1959) who used arithmetic and memory tests to study divers in water at pressures ranging from 100 (4 ATA) to 180 ft (6·5 ATA) and found no decrement. Kiessling and Maag's observation that the presence or absence of performance impairment is to a great extent a function of the performance measure that is used seems apt. When no effects are discovered, it is necessary to ask whether the measure itself is insensitive to change or whether the environmental conditions interacting with individual performance produced no effects.

Effects of various gases

Hamilton (1975) used a battery of tests to measure 'fine and gross coordination, manual dexterity and the use of tools, cognitive ability, reaction time, time and force estimation' among other parameters. He found that on a dive to 1200 ft (37 ATA) in a dry pressure chamber, subjects' scores did not change while breathing either helium or neon, but most were affected in a detrimental fashion by nitrogen, which suggests there may be some sensitivity of these measures to certain gas mixtures.

Thomas et al. (1975) trained animals to emit complex timing and counting behaviors under the discrimination of external stimulus control. The animals then performed at varying depths to 250 ft (8·6 ATA) breathing a 80% He, 20% O_2 mixture, compressed air, and a crude neon mixture. Response rates for performance were less disrupted under helium–oxygen than compressed air, although decrements in performance were observed in the latter. Unlike Hamilton's results, crude neon affected a specific type of performance, that of timing behavior, with estimates of time lengthened. High rates of responding generally decreased under hyperbaric exposure, while low rates of responding increased. These investigators report similar effects on human subjects in preliminary dives.

Effects of equipment

Imbert, Chouteau, and Alinat (1968) discuss 'the constraints resulting from the equipment and safety requirements' as one of the three types of factors related to human performance impairment during the course of a dive. In their report on psychometric and ergonomic methods they concentrate on such areas as neuromuscular functioning and narcosis; they stress psychometric measures of performance, but do not discuss the effect of equipment and safety requirements on human performance although they consider it one of three major factors. This neglect of equipment impact on human performance in diving has been marked in many areas.

As Bachrach and Egstrom (1974) observed, there has been little systematic human engineering of diving equipment, and, indeed, the diver is implicitly or explicitly expected to compensate for possible shortcomings in equipment. Only recently have there been beginnings of systematic studies of static anthropometry in diving, focusing on size and dimension of divers (Beatty, Berghage & Chandler 1971; Beatty & Berghage 1972). Dynamic anthropometry, dealing with functional movements, particularly range of motion as it affects the performance of the diver in hard-hat systems, is reported in a study by Bachrach, Egstrom, and Blackmun (in press) in which a biomechanical analysis was made comparing the standard hard-hat suit Mark V with the US Navy prototype Mark XII. Using 14 biomechanical measurements believed to be critical in work in the hard-hat rigs, these investigators compared flexibility in the Mark V and Mark XII with swim-suit base-lines. Assuming that range of motion is limited by internal mechanical stops (how far can a movement go and what is its limit), joints were measured to determine the external mechanical limitations of the diving suits. The more flexible Mark XII suit

was found to be superior in most respects in performing the range-of-movement tasks.

In addition to the biomechanical analysis of the two systems, physiological monitoring of heart rate was accomplished while the divers were in the water off a ship in 60 ft of water performing a series of tasks using tools, the Enerpac (a cutting device), a self-contained load-handling pontoon (Conda & Armstrong 1973), and the UCLA pipe puzzle (Weltman et al. 1971). A detailed report of all of the experiments in the technical evaluation appears in Armstrong et al. (1974). Fig. 15.1, from a related study (Bachrach & Egstrom 1974), is an example of the heart rate

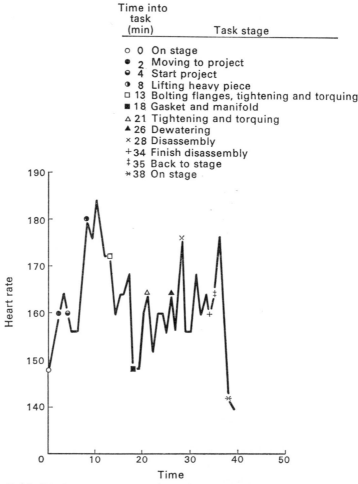

Subj. #1—Pipe puzzle MKV, HeO$_2$ Mode breathing air

Fig. 15.1. Heart rate measured in the Mark V diving dress

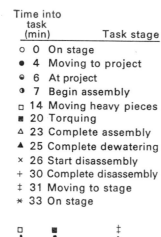

Time into task (min)		Task stage
○	0	On stage
●	4	Moving to project
◑	6	At project
◔	7	Begin assembly
□	14	Moving heavy pieces
■	20	Torquing
△	23	Complete assembly
▲	25	Complete dewatering
×	26	Start disassembly
+	30	Complete disassembly
‡	31	Moving to stage
✳	33	On stage

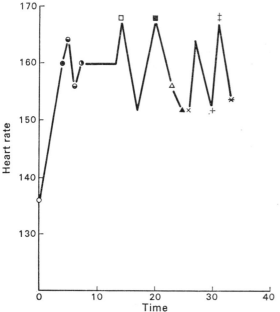

Subj.#1 –Pipe puzzle MK XIII, HeO$_2$ Mode breathing air

Fig. 15.2. Heart rate measured in the Mark XII diving dress

of a diver wearing the Mark V suit and working the UCLA pipe puzzle. The diver's heart rate peaked at 184 beats/min in the Mark V, while in the Mark XII (Fig. 15.2) his highest rate was 168 beats/min, suggesting more diver effort was required when working in the Mark V canvas dress. The diver's resting heart rate was approximately 80 beats/min on board the ship.

Bachrach and Egstrom (1974), reporting on human engineering considerations in the evaluation of diving equipment, observed that bio-

mechanical movements are relatively straightforward, and may be measured with a reasonable degree of accuracy. Less straightforward, however, are the differences resulting from the limitations imposed by an individual diver's strength and endurance. They state, 'A diver in one set of equipment might be required to work harder to overcome the equipment restrictions even though the flexibility of both sets might be similar'. Thus, diver strength and endurance are important variables in underwater performance that should be monitored as is a specific work methodology to accomplish a task. Bachrach and Egstrom further recommended that comparisons of equipment and work should include the monitoring of physiological parameters such as heart rate, which 'is essentially linear with increased oxygen consumption and workload'. Teichner and Olsen (1971) noted that operators do develop different ways of approaching the same task, and Bachrach and Egstrom believe it is possible that a diver can 'become proficient and effective in completing a task even though he may be utilizing a relatively inefficient methodology'. This raises the question of what demands this makes on the diver's overall efficiency over periods of time.

The impact of equipment on performance of underwater breathing apparatus has also been discussed by Bradley (1970), who sees in certain types of breathing apparatus restrictions upon respiration and work. Such considerations need more thorough and systematic investigation than has been accomplished in the past. They are definitely significant aspects of underwater performance.

Training

Another facet of the relationship of equipment to performance is the specific training in the use of the equipment and the task itself. Weltman et al. (1971) detail an experiment on a specific underwater assembly task, the UCLA pipe puzzle. The question asked was whether any differences in performing a complex underwater task could be determined between divers who were trained in the task on dry land and divers who were trained to do the task underwater. The results clearly indicated a superiority of the water-trained divers over those trained on dry land—even with the advantages in the latter condition of more direct contact with the training personnel and immediate corrective feedback. The mean total completion time for the water-trained teams was 25% faster. The results of this experiment suggest that not only are the movements different in the water, but also that performance, and accordingly, performance assessment, must be different in the water. Movements are different in a relatively weightless, tractionless, viscous medium.

The study by Weltman et al. (1971) underscores this variable. They recommend that when an individual poses the question of how well is the diver doing under specific conditions, the corollary would be 'compared to what?' This suggests that the comparison should be how well the job can be accomplished under ideal diving conditions (clear, low-current comfortable water, with a minimum of protective gear) so that the comparison of diving conditions and diving work would be against ideal diving circumstances, not a dry land or pressure chamber base-line.

Practice effects and learning

Another source of variance derives from practice effects. It is well known in performance assessment that improvement with practice will occur on many tasks so that a test performed during initial runs will not be functionally the same test after the individual has been exposed to it for a number of times. For this reason different forms of tests that are supposedly equivalent have been developed, but, in general, the effects of practice are always there. Crossman (1959) has found that even after thousands of trials, there is still a possibility of improvement. Baddeley (1967) discusses practice and transfer effects in relationship to diving performance assessment. He notes, 'It may . . . be possible to learn ways of coping with a particular task while suffering from narcosis, and since these may be quite irrelevant to performance at normal pressure, no amount of training before the experiment will eliminate practice effects on being required to perform the task under the new conditions'. This is reminiscent of Teichner and Olson's (1971) observation that people under environmental stress may find other ways of performing the same task. Baddeley et al. (1968) showed that test sub-jects at 1 and 4 ATA on both cognitive and manual dexterity tasks showed improvement on the second day of testing over the performance on the first day, suggesting some learning and practice effects were involved.

The logistics of deep diving in themselves militate against normal experimental design, as, for example, Baddeley (1967) observes in commenting on an experiment by Adolfson (1967):

> . . . in an otherwise excellent study of performance at pressures ranging from 1 to 13 atmospheres (0 to 130 m), since his subjects apparently all began with low pressures and worked systematically up to 13 kg/cm^2 (atmospheres absolute) followed by a final test at 1 kg/cm^2. This is not on the whole a good strategy since the effects of practice, fatigue, and depth are inextricably confounded, making interpretation very difficult. The result in Adolfson's case seems to have been a loss in test sensitivity since he finds atypically small performance decrements even at relatively high pressures. It is interesting to note that the only task to show effects at depths less than 60 m in Adolfson's study was mental arithmetic, the one test on which he attempted to take account of practice effects.

Thus we note that ideal experimental design is difficult under diving conditions. Perhaps the optimal way to reverse pressure effects that account for performance changes would be to test from surface to deep pressure with sequential assessment, and to use not only a surface control for base-line (with all the problems attendant upon it), but also to start at about 300 ft (10 ATA) and work up. It is manifestly impossible to begin an experiment at 300 ft without all of the influences of such factors as compression rate and gas effects; therefore, one experimental logistic is denied to the experimenter. Control groups with a large series of subjects are also denied to the experimenter, with most deep dives restricted to low numbers of subjects. For example, research in the University of Pennsylvania dive reported by Hamilton (1972) and Thorne, Findling and Bachrach (1974) was restricted to intensive study of two subjects (hardly a parametric population), as was Bennett (1970a, b) in the RNPL 1500 ft (46·4 ATA) chamber dive.

To return to problems of practice effects and

their influence on performance assessment, suppose it were possible to have one group of subjects tested under shallow conditions first and deep conditions second, with another group of subjects tested under deep conditions first and shallow conditions second. Of this procedure, Baddeley asks whether one can assume that practice effects will not be a problem and responds, ' Alas no. Such a conclusion will only be justified if the practice effects are symmetrical, that is if doing the task at the surface will affect performance at pressure just as much as practice at pressure will influence subsequent performance on the surface'. This condition is not unique to diving performance assessment, but is a factor in all performance research. More detailed consideration of practice effects may be found in Baddeley (1967), as well as comments by Poulton, Catton and Carpenter (1964) and Poulton and Freeman (1966). Practice effects are another source of variance (perhaps not entirely controllable) that should be remembered in diving performance assessment.

Adaptation

Braithwaite, Berghage and Crothers (1974) underscore an important physiological event— adaptation to environmental factors with improvement in performance over time. Adaptation to environmental effects such as pressure and gas have been reported in animal research by Walsh (1974), Walsh and Bachrach (1971), and Walsh and Bachrach (1974); and in human research by such authorities as Miles (1969), and Shilling and Willgrube (1937). Physiological changes inherent in adapting to presumably degrading environmental effects constitute an important aspect of performance assessment inferred from physiological events and are a crucial research area.

PERFORMANCE EVALUATION CONSIDERATIONS

Subject variability

The number of subjects generally available in deep diving makes the normal experimental design difficult, if not impossible, to accomplish. For meaningful confidence levels in statistical analysis of data, the larger the number in general

the more comfortable the experimenter can be in assuming that his results are not due to chance, but are, indeed, a function of the experimental variable. Bennett (1966), discussing subject variability, observed:

> The degree of motivation between different individuals participating in psychometric tests is a variable factor which is also difficult to control and the extent of learning and acclimatization to the effects of pressure are conditions which are often ignored. Effective control of the subjects, which have varied between trained and inexperienced divers, officers and men of the armed forces, medical students and the experimenters themselves is commonly ignored in spite of the knowledge that work, fatigue, apprehension and alcohol affect the severity of the narcosis. This is often because the psychometric tests are *ad hoc* investigations in experiments primarily designed to provide physiological information.

There are several exceptionally important points in that brief paragraph of Bennett's. Subject variability as a function of motivation is something that is true, to be sure, in all human assessment. It is a known variable that the individual brings into an experiment that which is not entirely under the control of the experimenter. Diver experience is also a major factor in subject variability. Shilling and Willgrube (1937) observed that in studying the effects of increased pressure '. . . increased experience materially lessens the subjective effect of pressure . . .'. They also state that 'men with high mental ability do not fail as quickly under pressure as do those with low mental ability'. Age is still another subject variable that is not controlled or even reported in virtually all diving experiments, as Bachrach and Kennedy (1975) note. Age variables are rarely given.

A dramatic example of the variability noted above can be seen by comparing four of the most quoted experiments on the effects of increased pressure on psychometric performance: Shilling and Willgrube (1937), Case and Haldane (1941), Kiessling and Maag (1962), and Frankenhaeuser, Graff-Lonnevig and Hesser (1963). All of these were well-designed experiments with a general goal of studying the effects of increased pressure on psychomotor functions and behaviors during nitrogen narcosis (among other variables). The

tests used in Shilling and Willgrube were arithmetic (addition, multiplication, subtraction, and
division), number cancellation, and a light-to-
touch reaction time (a simple reaction time). The
subjects were 46 officers and men of the Deep Sea
Diving School and the Experimental Diving Unit.

In the Frankenhaeuser, Graff-Lonnevig and
Hesser study, there were 12 subjects ranging
in age from 19 to 39 years, including 1 female
technician, 2 professional male divers, and 8 male
medical students of whom 2 were amateur divers.
Three psychomotor tasks were given, i.e. choice
reaction time, mirror drawing, and a simple
visual reaction time. In the Kiessling and Maag
experiment there were 10 subjects, of whom 2
were senior medical students, 8 were experienced
divers, and 1 was a medical officer. The age range
was not given. The tests used were a choice
reaction time, finger dexterity (modified Purdue
Pegboard), and a conceptual reasoning test.

In the Case and Haldane experiment (1941),
there was a series of studies involving a total of
17 subjects (including the authors) of which 15
were male and 2 were female. The age range was
from 23 to 47 years. The subject variability is
illustrated by this statement describing the
subjects: 'The majority are English, but two are
Irish, one Spanish, one Czech, and one German.
Their occupations had varied from prime minister
to tailor, and loader for a transport company. The
majority are, however, university graduates'.
That is a charming illustration of subject variability of experienced and inexperienced diving
subjects. (The tests used in the Case and Haldane
experiments consisted of a manual dexterity test
[R–V], a ball-bearing test in which steel ball-
bearings were dropped into three holes [in reality
a finger dexterity measure], and a four-figure
multiplication test [e.g. 9746×4956]).

Davis et al. (1972) described the subjects of
their 1969–70 experiments as '...16 male
students (mainly medical students), aged 20 to 28
years, with previous diving experience ranging
from nil to eight years'. Looking at the general
design of the Davis experiments, the subjects are
obviously varied.

Considering the variability in subjects and the
many factors known to affect human performance,
it is not surprising to find discrepancies across

reported experiments. More stringent control of
the homogeneity of subjects, their ages, skills, and
diving training must be exercised.

Task variability

Another major factor that must be considered in
the comparison of research results is the variation
in the tasks themselves.

To return specifically to reaction time experiments, let us begin with Shilling and Willgrube
(1937) who had in their simple light-to-touch
reaction time experiment a subject in the chamber
who 'watched an electric light bulb situated in
an eye port. When the light was turned on, the
subject pressed a telegraph key'. The light was on
and off at intervals during a 2-min run.

In the Frankenhaeuser, Graff-Lonnevig and
Hesser experiments (1960, 1963) there were two
reaction time tasks—one was a four-choice visual
reaction time in which the subject was seated
before a panel on which appeared a triangle of
three coloured neon signal bulbs, red below green,
and yellow to the left of the two others. The
subject's task was to respond rapidly by closing
one of two telegraph keys in the following pattern:
(1) red light, press left-hand key; (2) green light,
press right-hand key; (3) red and yellow lights
simultaneously, press right-hand key; (4) green
and yellow lights simultaneously, press left-hand
key. The second task involving simple visual
reaction time was the same as the four-choice
visual task, but only the yellow light appeared;
the subject was to respond as rapidly as possible,
pressing one key. The scores were the means of
40 reaction times recorded within each 2-min
period. On the four-choice reaction time task, the
scores were for each test trial of 40 responses—
after one 10-sec period with three stimuli there
was a 5-sec pause.

The Kiessling and Maag (1962) vigilance task
of the choice reaction time consisted of a panel of
two lights—a red on the left and a green on the
right, with two hand switches. When a light
appeared, the subject was to respond with the
hand switch on the appropriate side, which would
extinguish the stimulus light on that particular
side. The light stimuli were released without prior
warning at random intervals varying from 3 to
13 sec.

Choice reaction time, as considered by Teichner and Krebs (1974) is far from the simple coordination function it has been assumed to be. Teichner and Krebs isolate the relative temporal contributions to choice reaction time into four stages of information processing, which they identify as stimulus coding, stimulus-stimulus translation, stimulus response translation, and response selection. The choice reaction time, as an information processing procedure, further illuminates the problems inherent in comparing the four-choice reaction time of Frankenhaeuser, Graff-Lonnevig and Hesser (1963) with that of Kiessling and Maag (1962), where stimulus presentation and response selection were entirely different in complexity. Teichner (1974) has also observed that elements as basic as stimulus duration and stimulus intensity seem not to be covered in many of the choice reaction and simple reaction time experiments. As noted above, the electric light bulb used by Shilling and Willgrube (1937) is nowhere near the same type of stimulus that the red neon bulbs used in the Frankenhaeuser, Graff-Lonnevig and Hesser experiments represented.

Bennett (1966) commented on this series of experiments:

> The degree of impairment (in Frankenhaeuser, Graff-Lonnevig, and Hesser 1963) at 5 atmospheres absolute (130 feet) is similar to that reported by Case and Haldane (1941) but considerably less than that found by Shilling and Willgrube (1937) and Kiessling and Maag (1962). The reasons for the discrepancy are not clear. Hesser (1963) suggests that the reason could be the presence of small quantities of carbon dioxide in the pressure chamber in the latter two experiments or differences in individual susceptibility. Whatever the reason, the results do illustrate the difficulty of obtaining repeatable objective measurements of performance impairment due to increased pressure of air.

Is it not more reasonable to assume that possible or observed discrepancies in the results are due to subject and task variability, rather than small quantities of carbon dioxide? Certainly subject and task variability appear to be a more economical explanation of psychomotor task differences on performance.

Control of variability

So far discussion has focused on factors affecting human performance and has considered in some detail problems of variability between subjects and tasks. Inherent in any experimental design is the necessity for control of variables. Thus, the use of the hyperbaric chamber to model the pressure of the open-sea environment has been accepted as a necessary type of control. Bachrach (1972) referring to Egon Brunswik's (1952) representative design described the ideal experiment as one that has a minimum of artificiality and a maximum of control. As the experimenter gets closer to the real world, the loss of control becomes greater.

The goal of minimal artificiality and optimal control is addressed by Chapanis (1967), who observed:

> . . . laboratory experiments try to get the maximum precision possible by controlling extraneous variables and by a variety of design stratagems, all of which are aimed at reducing the amount of error variability. By minimizing unaccounted-for variability a laboratory experiment maximizes the chances of revealing a statistically significant outcome. And therein, of course, lies the power of the laboratory experiment. Unfortunately, this very power of a laboratory experiment constitutes its major weakness. Behavior in the real-world is subject to all sorts of uncontrolled variability.

An example of real-world loss of control occurred in an experiment reported by Armstrong et al. (1974). A performance assessment of a tool task in open water was in several cases impossible to complete inasmuch as the required decompression time and getting organized at the work site left little time for performance assessment. This problem of bottom-time availability in open water is part of the real-world loss of control not present under the more artificial circumstances of the pressure chamber.

GENERALIZATION OF RESULTS

The elements common to both the simulated environment of the chamber and the open sea are pressure and breathing mixtures. The physiological effects of gas and pressure, then, may be measured as may effects of pressure on such events as nitrogen narcosis. However, unless some simulation of real-world problems such as turbidity and cold can be achieved (perhaps in a wet pot—which would be another type of simulator), real-world characteristics are not present. Weltman et al. (1971) stated that the proper standard for comparison of performance is not from dry land or hyperbaric chamber to open sea, but from one water situation to another. They recommend that base-line behaviors be measured in ideal water conditions of warmth and clarity, and then comparisons of performance degradation may be made upon water base-lines, not land or simulated pressure base-lines.

What we may derive from the above discussion is perhaps a formulation of the obvious. One cannot directly compare open-sea and hyperbaric chamber conditions, nor (as we have seen from Baddeley) can we necessarily compare open-sea conditions from a boat moored far from land with open-sea conditions next to a pier, with different water conditions, and the psychological effects of presumed security.

Baddeley (1966) tested the influence of depth on the manual dexterity of free divers both in the open sea and hyperbaric chamber and compared the work of Kiessling and Maag (1962) with his own experiments. He describes Kiessling and Maag's experiment as 'Probably the only reasonably detailed study of manual dexterity at pressure . . .'. Here again, is a problem of variability. Kiessling and Maag found very little dexterity decrement in their subjects at 100 ft (4 ATA) in a dry pressure chamber, using a Purdue Pegboard. Baddeley (1966) found marked manual dexterity decrement in subjects at the same depth in open water, using a screwplate test with nuts and bolts. It is not enough to compare the conditions of open sea and dry chamber—these are admittedly two different conditions—and two different tests, the Purdue Pegboard and the screwplate. It is also imperative to note that while Baddeley compares the two as tests of manual dexterity, the factor analysis of human performance clearly shows that such a fine coordination test as the Purdue Pegboard is really a finger dexterity exercise, while manual dexterity is a factor reserved for arm and hand—a coordination more gross than the finger dexterity of the Pegboard. Accordingly,

the screwplate task, using wider movements, does not measure the same type of dexterity that the Purdue Pegboard represents. Again, we not only have two different conditions, we have two different tests and two different groups of subjects. It is inaccurate to compare the results of the two experiments.

Sometimes the same task is not considered to be equivalent. A very important methodological note regarding the land–sea comparisons of Baddeley's data on screwplate assembly is underscored in a comment by Davis et al. (1972), who observe '. . . Baddeley's screwplate test, which did not stand on a firm base, was much more difficult to handle under water than on dry land'. (The divers in the Davis et al. experiment worked at a bench top; Baddeley's divers did not.) In effect it was not the same task.

The Davis et al. (1972) report on the screwplate test demonstrates that the same task under two different conditions (land and open sea) cannot be considered to be equivalent unless its administration is standardized—the results between the two cannot be compared. The specificity of the tasks is obviously crucial.

Animal to man

Added to the concerns of generalizing data from chamber to open sea, and from different open-sea circumstances to others, is the problem of generalizing from animal experimentation to human application. Much valuable information comes from carefully controlled animal experiments that could not be done with humans. An example of animal work providing application to human diving comes from the area of neurophysiological research. One of the most frequently observed behaviors in research on the high pressure nervous syndrome is referred to as microsleep (loss of vigilance or somnolence). Microsleep indicates a depression of CNS activity which appears as divers go deeper in chamber dives; it follows indicators of excitation of the nervous system, such as tremor and EEG changes. Animals have shown hyperexcitability to the point of seizures (Brauer, Jordan & Way 1968). The pattern has been a suggested depression of the neocortex, with a hyperexcitability in the subcortical, more 'primitive' areas. In humans, electroencephalograms have been taken using surface electrodes, which give cortical tracings; in animals deep electrodes have been implanted, which give deep recordings on the electro-encephalogram. Chang-Chun (1960) implanted cats and rabbits and compressed them to 10 ATA; he found changes in cerebellar and subcortical ganglia rather than cortical changes. Thus, the changes in the EEG from the human subjects reflect only a part of the potential effects of hydrostatic pressure and compression.

On an even more fundamental level, Friess, Jefferson, and Durant (1971), working with a rat phrenic nerve-diaphragm preparation, analysed effects of varying nitrogen–helium partial pressure ratios under hyperbaric conditions. The response studied was a twitch in the neuromuscular pre-paration. Effects of excitation by helium on the preparation were determined under different con-ditions and suggest applications to the heliox diver 'if the human phrenic nerve-diaphragm complex exhibits an He:N_2 sensitivity compar-able to that of the rat'. These studies also have possible application to the previously noted re-search by Bennett et al. (1974) on trimix diving with increased nitrogen partial pressures.

Animal work provides leads to potential future research with humans, but, more importantly, indicates what may be occurring during pressur-ization of human and animal subjects. For example, a study in which essentially the same techniques were used on animal and human subjects was reported by Thomas et al. (1972). Timing behavior was studied in both rats and humans breathing different gas mixtures to 250 ft (8·6 ATA). The results were similar in both species.

Acknowledgements

The manuscript review and suggestions of Lieut.-Cdr. T. E. Berghage are warmly acknow-ledged, as is the editorial assistance of Ms Mary M. Matzen and patient typing of the manuscript by Ms Judy A. Shafer.

REFERENCES

ADOLFSON, J. (1967) *Human Performance and Behaviour in Hyperbaric Environments*. Stockholm: Almqvist and Wiksell. (Cited in Baddeley 1967, p. 65.)

ADOLFSON, J. & BERGHAGE, T. E. (1974) *Perception and Performance Underwater*. New York: John Wiley.

ADOLFSON, J., GOLDBERG, L. & BERGHAGE, T. (1972) Effects of increased ambient air pressures on standing steadiness in man. *Aerospace Med.* **43**, 520–524.

ARMSTRONG, F. W., BACHRACH, A. J., CONDA, K. J., HOLIMAN, M. J. & EGSTROM, G. H. (1974) *Comparative Human Factors Analysis of the U.S. Navy Mark V and Mark XII Dive Systems*. Bethesda, Md.: US Naval Medical Research Institute.

BACHRACH, A. J. (1970) Diving behavior. In *Human Performance in Scuba Diving*, pp. 119–138. Chicago, Ill.: Tho Athletic Institute.

BACHRACH, A. J. (1972) *Psychological Research: An Introduction*. 3rd edition. New York: Random House.

BACHRACH, A. J. (1974) *Early Indicators of Behavioral and Physiological Dysfunctioning in Deep Dives*. Ed. A. J. Bachrach, p. 3. Report of the Third Undersea Medical Society Workshop. Bethesda, Md.: Undersea Medical Society.

BACHRACH, A. J. & BENNETT, P. B. (1973a) Tremor in diving. *Aerospace Med.* **44**, 613–623.

BACHRACH, A. J. & BENNETT, P. B. (1973b) The high pressure nervous syndrome during human deep saturation and excursion diving. *Försvarsmedicin* **9**, 490–495.

BACHRACH, A. J. & EGSTROM, G. H. (1974) Human engineering considerations in the evaluation of diving equipment. *The Working Diver—1974*. Columbus, Ohio: Battelle.

BACHRACH, A. J. & KENNEDY, R. S. (1975) *Psychophysiological Performance Testing under Water and Pressure: Problems and Prospects*. Bethesda, Md.: US Naval Medical Research Institute. (In press.)

BACHRACH, A. J., EGSTROM, G. H. & BLACKMUN, S. M. (in press) Biomechanical analysis of the U.S. Navy Mark V and XII diving systems. *Hum. Factors*.

BACHRACH, A. J., THORNE, D. R. & CONDA, K. J. (1971) Measurement of tremor in the Makai 250-foot saturation dive. *Aerospace Med.* **42**, 856–860.

BADDELEY, A. D. (1966) Influence of depth on the manual dexterity of free divers: a comparison between open sea and pressure chamber testing. *J. appl. Psychol.* **50**, 81–85.

BADDELEY, A. D. (1967) Diver performance and the interaction of stresses. *Underwat. Ass. Rep.* **2**, 35–38.

BADDELEY, A. D. & FLEMMING, N. C. (1967) The efficiency of divers breathing oxy-helium. *Ergonomics* **10**, 311–319.

BADDELEY, A. D., deFIGUEREDO, J. W., HAWKSWELL-CURTIS, J. W., & WILLIAMS, A. N. (1968) Nitrogen narcosis and performance underwater. *Ergonomics* **11**, 157–164.

BAIN, E. C., III, & BERGHAGE, T. E. (1974) *Evaluation of Sindbad Tests*. Report 4-74, US Navy Experimental Diving Unit, Washington, D.C.

BEATTY, H. T. & BERGHAGE, T. E. (1972) *Diver Anthropometrics*. EDU Report 10–72, US Navy Experimental Diving Unit, Washington, D.C.

BEATTY, H. T., BERGHAGE, T. E. & CHANDLER, D. R. (1971) *Preliminary Survey of Diver Anthropometrics*. Report NED-URR-7-71, US Navy Experimental Diving Unit, Washington, D.C. AD 729664.

BENNETT, P. B. (1965) Narcosis due to helium and air at pressure between 2 and 15·2 ats and the effects of such gases on oxygen toxicity. In *Proc. Symp. on Human Performance Capabilities in Undersea Operations*, Panama City, Fla., 1965. (Unpublished).

BENNETT, P. B. (1966) *The Aetiology of Compressed Air Intoxication and Inert Gas Narcosis*. London: Pergamon Press.

BENNETT, P. B. (1970a) *Interim Report on Some Physiological Studies during a 1500-ft Simulated Dive*. Report IR 1-70, Royal Naval Physiological Laboratory, Alverstoke, England.

BENNETT, P. B. (1970b) Neurophysiological, psychological, biochemical, and other studies. In *Experimental Observations on Men at Pressures between 4 bars (100 ft) and 47 Bars (1500 ft)*, pp. 60–113. Report 1-71, Royal Naval Physiological Laboratory, Alverstoke, England.

BENNETT, P. B. (1974) Systems of underwater performance assessment. In *The Development of Standardized Assessment of Underwater Performance*. Ed. A. J. Bachrach. Report of the Fourth Undersea Medical Society Workshop. Bethesda, Md.: Undersea Medical Society.

BENNETT, P. B. & TOWSE, E. J. (1971a) The high pressure nervous syndrome during a simulated oxygen–helium dive at 1500 ft. *Electroenceph. clin. Neurophysiol.* **31**, 383–393.

BENNETT, P. B. & TOWSE, E. J. (1971b) Performance efficiency of men breathing oxygen–helium at depths between 100 ft and 1500 ft. *Aerospace Med.* **42**, 1147–1156.

BENNETT, P. B., BLENKARN, G. D., ROBY, J. & YOUNGBLOOD, D. (1974) Suppression of the high pressure nervous syndrome (HPNS) in human dives to 720 ft and 1000 ft. by use of $N_2/He/O_2$. *Undersea Biomed. Res.* **1**, 221–237.

BERKUN, M. M., BIALEK, H. M., KERN, R. P. & YAGI, K. (1962) Experimental studies of psychological stress in man. *Psychol. Mongr.* **76**, No. 534.

BERLINER, C., ANGELL, D. & SHEARER, J. W. (1964) Behaviors, measures and instruments for performance evaluation in simulated environments. Paper presented at the Symposium and Workshop on the Quantification on Human Performance. Albuquerque, 17–19 August.

BIERSNER, R. J. (1971) Human performance at great depths. In *Underwater Physiology. Proc. 4th Symp. Underwater Physiology*. Ed. C. J. Lambertsen. pp. 479–485. New York: Academic Press.

BRADLEY, M. E. (1970) The interaction of stresses in diving and adaptation of these stresses. In *Human Performance and Scuba Diving*, pp. 63–69. Chicago, Ill.: The Athletic Institute.

BRAITHWAITE, W., BERGHAGE, T. E. & CROTHERS, J. (1974) Postural equilibrium and vestibular response at 49·5 ATA. Undersea Medical Society Annual Scientific Meeting (Abstracts), Washington, D.C., 10–11 May, 1974. *Undersea Biomed. Res.* **1**, A11.

BRAUER, R. W., JORDAN, M. R. & WAY, R. O. (1968) Modification of the conclusive seizure phase of the high pressure excitability syndrome in mice. *Fedn Proc. Fedn Am. Socs exp. Biol.* **27**, 284.

BROADBENT, D. E. (1963) Differences and interactions between stresses. *Q. Jl exp. Psychol.* **15**, 205–211.

BRUNSWIK, E. (1952) The conceptual framework of psychology. *Int. Encyl. Unified Sci.* **6**, 659–751.

BUXTON, C. (1968) The application of multiple factorial methods to the study of motor abilities. *Psychometrika* **3**, 85–93.

CASE, E. M. & HALDANE, J. B. S. (1941) Human physiology under high pressure. 1. Effects of nitrogen, carbon dioxide and cold. *J. Hyg. (Camb.)* **41**, 225–249.

CHANG-CHUN (1960) Comparative study of the action of oxygen, nitrogen, and helium on the central nervous system of the organism at raised pressure. (Dissertation.) Cited in Zaltsman (1961).

CHAPANIS, A. (1967) The relevance of laboratory studies to practical situations. *Ergonomics* **10**, 557–577.

CHRISTENSEN, J. M. & MILLS, R. G. (1967) What does the operator do in complex systems? *Hum. Factors* **9**, 329–340.

COLES, R. R. A. (1973) Labyrinthine disorders in British Navy diving. *Försvarsmedicin* **9**, 428–433.

CONDA, K. J. & ARMSTRONG, F. W. (1973) *A Self-contained Load-handling Pontoon*. Bethesda, Md.: Naval Medical Research Institute.

CORCORAN, D. W. J. (1962) Noise and loss of sleep. *Q. Jl exp. Psychol.* **14**, 178–182.

CROSSMAN, E. R. F. W. (1959) A theory of the acquisition of speed skill. *Ergonomics* **2**, 153–166.

DAVIS, F. M., OSBORNE, J. P., BADDELEY, A. D. & GRAHAM, I. M. F. (1972) Diver performance: Nitrogen narcosis and anxiety. *Aerospace Med.* **43**, 1079–1082.

DOSSETT, A. N. & HEMPLEMAN, H. V. (1972) Importance for mammals of rate of compression. *Symp. Soc. exp. Biol.* **26**, 355–361.

EDMONDS, C., FREEMAN, R., THOMAS, R., TONKIN, J. & BLACKWOOD, F. A. (1973) *Otological Aspects of Diving*. Glebe, New South Wales: Australasian Medical Publishing Co.

EGSTROM, G. H. & BACHRACH, A. J. (1971) Diver panic. *Skin Diver* **20**, 36–37, 54–57.

EVANS, W. O. & CONSOLAZIO, F. C. (1967) Effects of high altitude on performance of three different types of work. *Percept. Mot. Skills Res.* **25**, 41–50.

FITTS, P. M. & POSNER, M. I. (1967) *Human performance*. Belmont, Calif.: Brooks-Cole.

FLEISHMAN, E. A. (1954) Dimensional analysis of psychomotor abilities. *J. exp. Psychol.* **48**, 437.

FLEISHMAN, E. A. (1960) Psychomotor tests in drug research. In *Drugs and Behavior*. Ed. Uhr & Miller. New York: John Wiley.

FLEISHMAN, E. A. (1964) *The Structure and Measurement of Physical Fitness*. Englewood Cliffs, N.J.: Prentice-Hall.

FLEISHMAN, E. A. (1967) Performance assessment based on an empirically derived task taxonomy. *Hum. Factors* **9**, 349–366.

FRANKENHAEUSER, M., GRAFF-LONNEVIG, M. V. & HESSER, C. M. (1960) Psychomotor performance in man as affected by high oxygen pressure (3 atmospheres). *Acta physiol. Scand.* **50**, 1–7.

FRANKENHAEUSER, M., GRAFF-LONNEVIG, M. V. & HESSER, C. M. (1963) Effects on psychomotor functions of different nitrogen–oxygen gas mixtures at increased ambient pressures. *Acta physiol. Scand.* **59**, 400–409.

FRIESS, S. L., JEFFERSON, T. A. & DURANT, R. C. (1971) Viability of neuromuscular tissues in hyperbaric gaseous environments containing variable N_2:He content ratios. *Toxic. appl. Pharmac.* **20**, 1–13.

FRUCTUS, X. & AGARATE, C. (1971) The high pressure nervous syndrome. *Medna Sport.* **24**, 272–278.

GHISSELLI, E. E. (1949) Review of the Purdue Pegboard. In *The Third Mental Measurements Yearbook.* Ed. O. K. Buros. p. 666. Highland Park, N.J.: The Gryphon Press.

GORHAM, W. A. & ORR, D. B. (1957) *Research on Behavior Impairment due to Stress.* Report AIR-B-14-57-IR-64 American Institute of Research, Silver Spring, Md.

GORHAM, W. A. & ORR, D. B. (1958) *Research on Behavior Impairment due to Stress: Experiments in Impairment Reduction.* Report AIR-B14-58-FR-189, American Institute of Research, Silver Spring, Md.

HAMILTON, R. W. Jr. (1975) Psychomotor performance in normoxic neon and helium at 37 atmospheres. In *Underwater Physiology. Vth Symp. Underwater Physiology.* Ed. C. J. Lambertsen. Bethesda: Fedn Am. Socs exp. Biol.

HARRELL, T. W. (1949) Review of the Purdue Pegboard. In *The Third Mental Measurements Yearbook.* Ed. O. K. Buros. pp. 666–667. Highland Park, N.J.: The Gryphon Press.

HESSER, C. M. (1963) Measurement of inert gas narcosis in man. In *Proc. 2nd Symp. Underwater Physiology.* Ed. C. J. Lambertsen & L. J. Greenbaum. Washington, D.C.: Natl Acad. Sci.-Natl Res. Council. (Publ. 1181.)

HILL, L. & GREENWOOD, M. (1906) The influence of increased barometric pressure on man. *Proc. R. Soc.* **77B**, 442–453.

HUNTER, W. L., Jr. & BENNETT, P. B. (1974) The causes, mechanisms and prevention of the high pressure nervous syndrome. *Undersea Biomed. Res.* **1**, 1–28.

IMBERT, G., CHOUTEAU, J. & ALINAT, J. (1968) Sur l'utilisation des methodes psychometriques et ergonomiques en physiologie hyperbare (On the utilization of psychometric methods and ergonomic methods in hyperbaric physiology.) *Proceedings of the Physiology Studies No. 3/68.* C. E. M. A. Marseille. Engl. transl. by S. Savage, NAVSHIPS Transl. No. 1262. Scientific Documentation Division, (205), Naval Ships Systems Command, Washington, D.C.

KANWISHER, J., LAWSON, K. & STRAUSS, R. (1974) Acoustic telemetry from human divers. *Undersea Biomed. Res.* **1**, A11.

KENNEDY, R. S. (1971a) A comparison of performance on visual and auditory monitoring tasks. *Hum. Factors* **13**, 93–97.

KENNEDY, R. S. (1971b) Performance assessments in exotic environments: a flexible economical and standardized vigilance test, p. 2. Presented at the Fifteenth Annual Human Factors Society Meeting, 18–21 October, 1971, New York.

KENNEDY, R. S. (1974) General history of vestibular disorders of diving. *Undersea Biomed. Res.* **1**, 73–82.

KIESSLING, R. J. & MAAG, C. H. (1962) Performance impairment as a function of nitrogen narcosis. *J. appl. Psychol.* **46**, 91–95.

LIFFICK, G. L. (1971) Hydraulic tools and equipment for underwater salvage. In *Marine Technology Society 7th Annual Conference* (Preprints), August 1971, Washington, D.C. pp. 307–328. Published by the Society.

MacINNIS, J. (1971) Performance aspects of an open sea saturation exposure at 615 feet. In *Underwater physiology. Proc. 4th Symp. Underwater Physiology.* Ed. C. J. Lambertsen. New York: Academic Press.

MILES, S. (1969) *Underwater Medicine.* Philadelphia: Lippincott.

MILES, S. & MACKAY, D. E. (1959) *The Nitrogen Narcosis Hazard and the Self-Contained Diver.* Medical Research Council, RN Personnel Research Committee, Report.

MILLER, J. G. (1964) Adjusting to overloads of information. In *Disorders of Communication.* Ed. D. McK. Rioch & E. A. Weinstein. *Res. Publ. Ass. res. nerv. ment. Dis.* **42**, 87–100.

MILLER, J. W., BACHRACH, A. J. & WALSH, J. M. (in preparation) Open sea narcosis assessment at depths up to 250 feet.

NAITOH, P., JOHNSON, L. C. & AUSTIN, M. (1971) Aquanaut sleep patterns during Tektite I: A 60-day habitation under hyperbaric nitrogen saturation. *Aerospace Med.* **42**, 69–77.

PACKARD, A. G. (1949) Review of the Purdue Pegboard. In *The Third Mental Measurements Yearbook.* Ed. O. K. Buros. p. 667. Highland Park, N.J.: The Gryphon Press.

POSTON, R., OSBURN, H. G. & SHEER, D. E. (1967) *Factor Analytic Evaluation of the Biotechnology Perceptual-Motor Performance Console (Model 365).* Contract 3200-3103-02, Department of Psychology, University of Houston, Texas.

POULTON, E. C. & FREEMAN, P. P. (1966) Unwanted asymmetrical transfer effects with balanced experimental designs. *Psychol. Bull.* **66**, 1–8.

POULTON, E. C., CATTON, M. J. & CARPENTER, A. (1964) Efficiency at sorting cards in compressed air. *Br. J. ind. Med.* **21**, 242–245.

PROCTOR, L. D., CAREY, C. R., LEE, R. M., SCHAEFER, K. E. & VAN DEN ENDE, H. (1972) Electroencephalographic changes during saturation-excursion dives to a simulated seawater depth of 1000 feet. *Aerospace Med.* **43**, 867–877.

REILLY, R. E. & CAMERON, B. J. (1968) *An Integrated Measurement System for the Study of Human Performance in an Underwater Environment. The Sindbad System.* Contract N00014-67-C-0410. BioTechnology, Inc., Falls Church, Va.

SEASHORE, R. H. (1951) Work and motor performance. In Handbook of Experimental Psychology. Ed. S. S. Stevens, pp. 1342–1362, New York: John Wiley.

SERBANESCU, T. F. & NAQUET, F. (1969) Study of the EEG of sleep under prolonged increase of pressure (The Operation 'Ludeon II'). *Electroenceph. clin. Neurophysiol.* **26**, 639. (Abstr.)

SHILLING, C. W. & WERTS, M. (Eds) (in press) *Underwater Bioengineering Handbook.* New York: Plenum.

SHILLING, C. W. & WILLGRUBE, W. W. (1937) Quantitative study of mental and neuromuscular reactions as influenced by increased air pressure. *Nav. med. Bull.* **35**, 373–380.

TEICHNER, W. H. (1974) In *The Development of Standardized Assessment of Underwater Performance.* Ed. A. J. Bachrach. Report of the Fourth Undersea Medical Society Workshop. Bethesda, Md.: Undersea Medical Society.

TEICHNER, W. H. & KREBS, M. J. (1974) Laws of visual choice reaction time. *Psychol Rev.* **81**, 75–98.

TEICHNER, W. H. & OLSON, D. E. (1971) A preliminary theory of the effects of task and environmental factors on human performance. *Hum. Factors* **13**, 295–344.

THEOLOGUS, G. C., WHEATON, G. R., MIRABELLA, A., BRAHLEK, R. E. & FLEISHMAN, E. A. (1973) *Development of a Standardized Battery of Performance Tests for the Assessment of Noise Stress Effects*, p. 2. NASA Report CR-2149, Washington, D.C.

THOMAS, J. R., WALSH, J. M., BACHRACH, A. J. & THORNE, D. R. (1975) Differential behavioral effects of nitrogen, helium, and neon at increased pressures. In *Underwater Physiology. Vth Symp. Underwater Physiology.* Ed. C. J. Lambertsen. Bethesda: Fedn Am. Socs exp. Biol.

THORNE, D. R., FINDLING, A. & BACHRACH, A. J. (1974) Muscle tremors under helium, neon, nitrogen, and nitrous oxide at 1 to 37 atmospheres. *J. appl. Physiol.* **37**, 875–879.

TUNE, G. S. (1964) Psychological effects of hypoxia: A review of certain literature from the period 1950 to 1963. *Percept. Mot. Skills Res.* **19**, 551–562. (Cited in Theologus et al. 1973, p. 560.)

WALSH, J. M. (1974) Parameters of behavioral adaptation to nitrogen narcosis. Undersea Medical Society Annual Scientific Meeting (Abstracts), Washington, D.C. 10–11 May, 1974. *Underwater Biomed. Res.* **1**, A28.

WALSH, J. M. & BACHRACH, A. J. (1971) *Timing Behavior in the Assessment of Adaptation to Nitrogen Narcosis.* Bethesda, Md.: US Naval Medical Research Institute.

WALSH, J. M. & BACHRACH, A. J. (1974) Adaptation to nitrogen narcosis manifested by timing behavior in the rat. *J. comp. Physiol. Psychol.* **86**, 883–889.

WARREN, N. D. (1959). Review of the Purdue Pegboard. In *The Fifth Mental Measurement Yearbook.* Ed. O. K. Buros. pp. 873–874. Highland Park, N.J.: The Gryphon Press.

WELTMAN, G. & EGSTROM, G. H. (1966) Perceptual narrowing in novice divers. *Hum. Factors* **8**, 499–506.

WELTMAN, G., EGSTROM, G. H., WILLIS, M. A. & CUCCARO, W. (1971) *Underwater Work Measurement Techniques: Final Report.* UCLA-ENG-7140. BioTechnology Laboratory, University of California at Los Angeles. AD 734014.

WILCOX, R. & RUSSO, F. (1974) Sleep and the helium barrier. *Proc. 14th Annual Meeting, Association for the Psychophysiological Study of Sleep*, 5–8 May, Jackson Hole, Wyo. (Abstracts.)

WILKINSON, R. T. (1967) Effects of environmental stress upon performance. In *Environmental and Human Factors in Engineering.* Ed. E. J. Richards & M. J. B. Shelton. London: John Wiley.

ZALTSMAN, G. L. (1961) *Physiological Principles of a Sojourn of a Human in Conditions of Raised Pressure of the Gaseous Medium.* Leningrad. English translation, Foreign Technology Division, Wright-Patterson Air Force Base, Ohio. AD 655 360, 1967.

16

Cold Exposure

P. WEBB

Since ocean waters are generally cold, as are most rivers and lakes, diving is a cold activity. Below 1000 m (100·4 ATA) water temperature is close to 0°C, but nearer the surface where men go diving, air warms the water according to latitude and climate. Surface water near the equator approaches 30°C, but at the poles it is near 0°C. A typical temperature at a depth of 200 m (21 ATA) would be 20°C near the equator and 1°C in high latitudes, while at 500 m (50·6 ATA) the corresponding values would be 11°C and 4°C. But typical patterns are modified by upwelling of cold waters on western continental coastlines and by major currents like the Kuroshio current and the Gulf Stream. Divers work where they must, whatever the water temperature, for offshore oil is found in the North Sea as well as in the Gulf of Mexico.

During World War II, a great deal of attention was paid to exposure to cold water because of the numerous ship sinkings. Keatinge (1969) summarized these experiences and described the physiology and treatment of immersion hypothermia. But the diver's regular and voluntary exposure to cold water seldom produces serious hypothermia. Nevertheless, he is often uncomfortably cold, and sometimes in danger from it.

It is quite possible that a number of unexplained diving accidents, even in relatively shallow water, have been caused by hypothermia. In the present era of deeper and deeper dives and of saturation diving, the effects of cold may become critical. Men diving under these conditions are remote from topside help. Furthermore, men may be expected to dive more than once a day from an undersea habitat or diving bell, so that repetitive dives carry a possible thermal penalty just as they carry a penalty for decompression sickness. And in deep diving operations the magnitude of heat transfer between the dense gas and the body surface, and the increased heat loss from breathing dense gas, add to the problem of preserving body heat.

The physiology of cold exposure is authoritatively presented elsewhere, as in Burton and Edholm (1955) and in Carlson and Hsieh (1965). This chapter will not review the general subject, but will proceed directly to the relevant topics, namely: heat loss in cold water, tolerance limits in cold, respiratory heat loss, the medical condition of hypothermia, rewarming, the limiting effects of being cold, thermal protection of divers, and the curious energy drain of living in comfortable hyperbaric environments.

HEAT LOSS IN COLD WATER

One must first understand the basic mechanics of heat transfer in order to analytically discuss the problem of heat loss from a diver submerged in cold water. Heat transfer, a form of energy transport, occurs whenever a temperature gradient

$$\left(\frac{\Delta T}{L} = \frac{T_1 - T_2}{L} \right)$$

exists within a system; or when two systems at different temperatures are so positioned that there is thermal energy transfer over a linear distance

(L) from the system of higher temperature (T_1) to that of the lower temperature (T_2). The principle that heat flows only from a region of higher temperature to a region of lower temperature is in accordance with the second law of thermodynamics.

There are three distinct modes of heat transmission that are recognized in the study of classical heat transfer: conduction, convection and radiation. In various complex types of heat transmission one mode may dominate the other two, in which case accurate engineering approximations of the heat transmission phenomena may be conducted by analyzing only the dominant mode of heat transmission.

Conduction. Conduction heat transfer is flow of heat from a region of higher temperature to a region of lower temperature within a medium, or between two media of different temperatures that are in physical contact. The thermal energy is considered to flow by direct molecular communication without appreciable displacement of the molecules in the medium.

Convection. Heat flow by convection is usually the dominating mode of heat transmission between the surface of a solid and a fluid (liquid or gas) or between two fluids in motion. The exact process of heat transmission by convection is performed in several steps. In the case of a solid body at a higher temperature than the surrounding fluid, initially the heat will flow by conduction from the solid to the thin layer of fluid that is in direct contact with the solid. This transmitted energy increases the internal energy and temperature of the fluid particles in the thin layer. These fluid particles are then transported to a region of lower temperature where they mix with cooler fluid particles. They are replaced by particles from, and at the same temperature as, the colder surroundings. The warmer fluid particles of the mixture then transfer thermal energy to the cooler ones by means of conduction. The mode of fluid particle transport from the thin layer next to the conducting solid is a function of the flow characteristics of the fluid in which the solid is submerged. For this reason, the study of convection heat transfer is closely linked to the study of the associated fluid mechanics. Convective heat transfer characteristics vary considerably between the laminar and turbulent flow conditions of the surrounding fluid.

Radiation. Radiation is the process of energy transmission between two bodies at different temperatures across an intervening space, even when this space is a vacuum. The radiant heat transmission usually occurs in the form of electromagnetic waves over a range of frequencies and wavelengths. The characteristics of the radiant heat emission are a function of the temperature, material and surface of the emitting and absorbing body. The radiation phenomena include the radiation and transmission of light, but the most significant heat transmission occurs at different wavelengths of the electromagnetic wave spectrum.

A more detailed explanation of the basic mechanics, and their associated equations, may be found in Kreith (1973).

The difference between a water medium and an ordinary air medium, thermally speaking, is the difference in the rates at which the two conduct heat from the body surface. Water at 25°C feels cold, while air at the same temperature feels neutral. This is because the specific heat of water is 1000 times as great, and the heat conduction of water is 25 times greater than that of air. For water to feel neither cold nor hot, it must be at 32 or 33°C, and for an unclothed man to stay comfortable in water for many hours the temperature must be 34 to 36°C. Most people can swim comfortably in water temperatures of 24 to 28°, but to rest for long in water at the same temperature makes you feel cold, and shivering begins in 15 or 20 min.

For an immersed nude diver the heat loss or transfer process can be imagined as a two part phenomena. First, heat is transferred from the core of the body to the skin by conduction of heat through the body tissue. Then this same heat is transferred from the skin to the water by means of convection. This process is analogous to a simple direct current (dc) electrical circuit where the temperatures at different points are similar to the analogous voltage potentials; and the flow of the heat is similar to the flow of the current in the dc circuit. The unit resistances of the body to heat transfer by conduction and by convection are expressed as the inverse of the tissue thermal

T_c = body core temperature, T_s = skin temperature, T_w = water temperature, I = electrical current, R = resistance, V = voltage, and q = heat.

conductance (K), and the inverse of the skin–water film conductance (h_w), respectively.

Thermal conductance (K) is defined as the heat flow per unit area per unit time per unit degree temperature differential $W/m^2 - °C$. Thermal conductance of an immersed body is more suitable to physiological observations and calculations than is the similar thermal conductivity, (k), which is defined as heat flow over a unit path length per unit area per unit time per unit degree temperature differential $W - m/m^2 - °C$. This is because it is extremely difficult to measure the actual conduction path length in a physiological specimen for use in calculating heat flow with the thermal conductivity (k).

When a nude or underprotected person is submerged in cold water, a definite sequence of events follows. First, the cold water causes a drop in skin temperature which produces vasoconstriction in the cutaneous circulation; this makes the skin temperature drop even faster because it is no longer being warmed from underneath. Peripheral and shell insulation is increased by decreasing the blood flow (and direct peripheral tissue heat input) between the body core and the surface. This cold-induced vasoconstriction provides a variable resistance, or insulation, in the body shell that is a function of the peripheral blood flow rate. The end of this sequence is reached when skin temperature approaches water temperature. Heat from the warm tissues in the centre of the body continues to pass by direct conduction toward the surface, aided by whatever circulation there is from the deeper structures. In a resting man, the cooled shell becomes larger and larger and the relatively warm and stable

core becomes smaller and smaller. A further response is an increase in heat production, which is soon detected as visible shivering, but preceded by an increase in muscle tension. If heat conservation through vasoconstriction and increased heat production from shivering are not sufficient to produce a thermal balance, the end result is a fall in core temperature, leading to hypothermia.

Further analysis of this sequence of events leads to greater complexity. Cutaneous vasoconstriction varies from one part of the body to another. In response to a strong cold stimulus, vasoconstriction is quite complete on the hands and feet, somewhat less on the arms and legs, possibly less on the torso, while on the head there is no significant vasoconstriction. Furthermore, there is a genuine difference in the rates of heat loss between thin and fat persons, since subcutaneous fat acts as a layer of insulation when the circulation to the skin has been shut off. Heat loss after full vasoconstriction depends on the thermal conductivity of different kinds of tissue, which has been determined, but it is extremely hard to apply such numbers to the real geometry of a man. Rather than determining heat loss from the sum of tissue conductivities, physiologists usually consider the man as a whole, and describe conductance values for the overall rate of heat loss from man to water. This kind of measurement gives values for skin-to-water heat transfer coefficients, but there is disagreement amongst values obtained in different laboratories.

Heat transfer from skin to water

Idealistically, heat flows from the body core through the tissues to the skin, and then this same quantity of heat flows from the skin into the surrounding water. This heat flow is analogous to the current flowing in the series electrical circuit previously discussed. The highly variable tissue thermal conductance makes it difficult to analyse the mean rate of heat transfer through the body. However, the rate of convective heat loss from the skin to the surrounding water is considerably easier to analyse due to stability of the skin–water film conductance, and the ease in determining the mean skin temperature. This concept of analysis is acceptable since the heat transferred by conduction through the tissues is equal to that transferred by convection into the water.

Heat flows from a warmer to a colder body at a rate proportional to the temperature difference between the two multiplied by a transfer coefficient. Whether this is mostly conductive or convective heat transfer is perhaps academic. Bullard and Rapp (1970) argue that the majority of heat transfer is conductive, but most workers are content with a single transfer coefficient that combines the conductive and convective elements together. This coefficient appears in the following equation:

$$H_w = h_w(\bar{T}_s - T_w) \qquad (1)$$

where H_w is the heat transfer rate in watts per square metres (W/m²); h_w is the skin–water film heat transfer coefficient in $W/m^2 - °C$; $\bar{T}_s$ is mean skin temperature; and T_w is water temperature. The value for h_w can be arrived at analytically, or by the use of a suitable physical model, such as a heated manikin placed in cold water, or from human experimental data. If the coefficient is known, heat loss can be predicted accurately. But there are problems with each of the methods used. Examples of all three will be discussed.

In their analysis, Bullard and Rapp (1970) and Rapp (1971) assume that the man is a single cylinder over which water moves in a forced parallel laminar flow, and, further, that the heat production exactly equals the heat loss to the water, so that there is no storage. Using values for tissue conductance from the literature, these authors estimated a skin-to-water temperature gradient of 0·45°C differential (ΔT) in a state of thermal equilibrium. The value for the conductive

portion of the heat transfer coefficient is small and steady at 11 W/m² − °C, while the convective portion varies as a direct function of water velocity. In still water the combined value is 105 W/m² − °C, increasing nearly linearly to 411 W/m² − °C at a water speed of 0·5 m/sec.

A good example of the second method of analysis is that of Witherspoon, Goldman and Breckenridge (1971), who measured heat loss from a heated copper manikin in water moving at several velocities. They obtained a curvilinear function of heat transfer versus water speed. Their values between 0 and 0·5 m/sec are similar to those of Bullard and Rapp, as shown in Fig. 16.1.

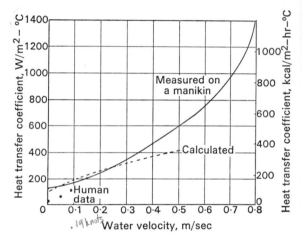

FIG. 16.1. The combined convective and conductive heat transfer coefficient from skin to water (h_w). The human data points are from Boutelier (1973) and Boutelier, Timbal and Colin (1968); the calculated curve from Rapp (1970); and the manikin results from Witherspoon, Goldman and Breckenridge (1971)

Unfortunately, neither the analytical model nor the physical model includes effects for vasoconstriction, heat exchange between arteries and veins in the limbs, change in body heat stores, or from the irregular deformable surface of a human. On the other hand, human data is notoriously variable, and the sources of variability are not always known. In nearly every case the apparent value for h_w is lower than that predicted by the analytical or physical model. Human data points are also shown in Fig. 16.1.

A thorough study of human subjects is that by

Boutelier (1973). The water velocity through the bath was approximately 0·1 m/sec without a man in it, but the relative velocity between water and man was assumed to be something less than 0·1 m/sec. At a neutral water temperature between 32·5 and 33·5°C, h_w was 62 ± 2 W/m² − °C. At lower water temperatures, the value became increasingly large, with the highest value being 105 ± 4 W/m² − °C.

We assume that skin temperature becomes very nearly equal to water temperature, yet the value for the transfer coefficient h_w is greatly influenced by the true temperature difference between skin and water. For example, if a subject in thermal balance is lying in cool water and producing 100 W/m² of heat, and the temperature difference between skin and water is 1°C, then the value for h_w is 100. If, however, the temperature difference is 0·5°C, the value for h_w would be 200.

Boutelier (1973), using carefully selected measuring techniques, showed that the difference between mean skin temperature and water temperature varied with the water temperature. With neutral water temperature the difference was approximately 0·6°C, and as the water became colder the difference increased to about 1·3°C. There was a scatter of about 0·2°C between subjects in the near neutral temperature, and of about 0·5°C in the colder water. Furthermore, local skin-to-water temperature differentials (ΔT) varied with body site. The variability was least at neutral water temperature and greatest in the colder water temperatures.

Thus with the present state of our knowledge of the correct values for the transfer coefficient between skin and water, it seems unlikely that one can reliably predict rates of heat loss even for the unclothed man, much less for a clothed diver.

Vasoconstriction

Cold water exposure immediately increases the rate of heat loss from the skin, which causes a decrease in skin temperature. The physiological response to this is vasoconstriction in the cutaneous blood vessels, which causes the skin temperature to fall even faster. The result is conservation of heat, because as skin temperature goes lower and lower and approaches the temperature of the water, the temperature differentials (ΔT) be-

tween skin and water are less, therefore heat flow is less. This is a major and important physiological response to cold exposure.

Vasoconstriction is mediated by sympathetic nerves which release norepinephrine; there is also a direct effect of cold on the superficial blood vessels which is probably as important as the effect of the sympathetic nerves. Skin blood flow and muscle blood flow are separately controlled, but if the muscle in the forearm, for example, is at rest, the decreased blood flow to the skin is matched by a decreased blood flow in the muscle. Keatinge (1969) cites data for blood flow in the entire forearm, that is, both skin and muscle, where the blood flow for the whole varies from 0·5 ml/100 ml of tissue/min to 17·6 ml/100 ml of tissue/min when fully vasodilated. Fig. 16.2 sum-

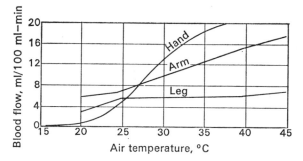

FIG. 16.2. The change in blood flows in hand, arm, and leg when subjects are exposed to ambient conditions from cool to warm (after Carlson & Hsieh 1965)

marizes the data from several studies, and shows that the hand behaves differently from the arm, and the arm differently from the leg. Maximum vasoconstriction, resulting in minimum tissue conductance and maximum insulation, occurs at skin temperatures less than 30°C (Bullard & Rapp 1970).

There is one major modifier of the vasoconstrictive response in a given site, and that is the general thermal state of the subjects. Carlson and Hsieh (1965) show that the logarithm of blood flow is directly related to the temperature of the hand, but that bood flow is generally lower at any hand (skin) temperature when the subject is staying in a cold room than when he is in a comfortable or warm room.

There is no direct data for cutaneous circulation in either the torso or the head because such measurements are made with occlusion plethysmography, a technique which can only be applied to a limb. But there is evidence that the torso and the head differ quite remarkably from the limbs. When limbs have started to cool and vasoconstriction becomes established, the heat loss from these parts becomes rather small. However, the trunk continues to lose considerable heat, if for no other reason than that despite cutaneous vasoconstriction there is blood flow in major organs near the surface, like the liver. Keatinge (1969) cites measurements from heat flow discs on the torso which support this notion. What is not clear is whether there is significant vasoconstriction in the skin blood vessels of the trunk, or whether they constrict less than those in the limbs.

The head is a special example of an area with high heat loss despite strong surface cooling. There are no vasoconstrictor fibers to the vessels of the scalp, and they seem to be slow in responding to the direct effect of cooling. This phenomenon of high heat loss despite strong cooling was first described by Froese and Burton (1957) and verified by Nunneley, Troutman and Webb (1971) and by Schvartz (1970). A practical implication of this is that an underwater swimmer moving headfirst through the water should carefully insulate the top of his head.

An additional heat conservation takes place in the limbs from a process originally described by Bazett et al. (1948). Once the superficial veins of an arm or a leg stop returning blood because of surface vasoconstriction, the entire venous return from the arm or leg takes place in the deeper veins which run adjacent to the arteries supplying blood to that limb. Thus a situation is set up for a countercurrent heat exchange, in which the warm outflowing blood in the artery loses heat to the cold blood coming back in the adjacent veins. Arterial blood temperature can be as low as 21°C in the radial artery at the wrist.

The limbs of the severely cold exposed man get colder and colder, and the cold is not simply superficial but reaches deeper structures like muscle and bone. At the same time the central masses of his head and trunk stay warm, despite deep chilling in the limbs. Thus a low tempera-ture shell can be distinguished from the higher temperature core. This is a thermal distinction; the idea is that the major heat loss in the beginning of cold exposure takes place in the shell, and that the shell expands at the expense of the core where temperatures are relatively constant (Carlson & Hsieh 1965). But it must be noted that the skeletal muscles involved in swimming and other underwater activities are located largely in the limbs and in the superficial part of the torso, so these muscle masses are part of the shell. The skeletal muscles are, of course, the site of added heat, both from working and from shivering and, since they are located closer to the surface than the central organs of the body, the heat loss rate from them is relatively high.

There is one further phenomenon to be described, something usually called cold-induced vasodilation (CIVD). This phenomenon has intrigued physiologists since it was first described by Sir Thomas Lewis more than 40 years ago. We now know that it is particularly evident in hands, to some degree in the feet, and much less elsewhere in the body. A hand which has been immersed in cold water (5°C or less) cools exponentially toward the water temperature, but after some minutes there is an increase in hand temperature and an increase in hand blood flow. This increase is followed by a subsequent decrease and later by another increase, in a cyclic fashion. The time for a full cycle is usually between 15 and 30 min. Keatinge (1969) explains CIVD on the basis of local paralysis of smooth muscle, which occurs after the muscle in the wall of the blood vessels reaches 10°C. When the smooth muscle is paralysed by cold it will not respond to the norepinephrine being released by the vasoconstrictor nerves, so the vessels relax and open up again. Flow then returns, which warms up the smooth muscle and it is then able to respond once again to the still present vasoconstrictor stimuli. The problem from cold-induced vasodilation is that even in well-insulated obese men the overall heat loss in cold water increases significantly. Cannon and Keatinge (1960) showed that with cold-induced vasodilation indicated by increasing blood flow, the rectal temperature fell with the same cyclic pattern. However, Bullard and Rapp (1970) have suggested that it may be difficult to distinguish the effect of recurrent bouts of shivering from that of vasodilation, since both occur at the same time and both mechanisms increase heat loss. That is, shivering increases the relative motion of the water next to the skin, and increases convective heat transfer from the skin.

The overall loss of heat from the body is definitely reduced by cutaneous vasoconstriction, and this reduced heat loss is evident in a decrease of the tissue conductance; but tissue conductance is further modified by the quantity of subcutaneous fat in each subject, which is the next topic for discussion.

Subcutaneous fat

Once cutaneous vasoconstriction is well established, body heat loss is mainly by direct conduction through the tissue. A significant layer of subcutaneous fat helps, since the thermal conductivity of fat is about half that of muscle. Thermal conductivities for various tissues are given in Table 16.1.

How much help is subcutaneous fat? A dramatic example was described by Pugh and Edholm (1955). A professional channel swimmer swam a 10-mile race in Lake Windermere, England, staying in the water for about 6 hours. The water temperature was 16°C. A tall thin man, who was not a professional swimmer, swam in the same lake at the same water temperature and was in desperate trouble after a little more than an hour. After 15 min he began to shiver, and his muscles became weaker and weaker. His rectal temperature dropped steadily, and after 80 min he had to be helped from the water. Both of these men were later studied at rest in a water bath at the same temperature of 16°C. Again, the thin man lost heat faster. Comparisons of the rectal temperatures of the two men for the two situations are shown in Fig. 16.3. In Fig. 16.4 is shown an approximate silhouette of the two men, with the body fat layers somewhat exaggerated but with the data for skinfold thicknesses shown numerically with each figure. This subcutaneous fat layer was the obvious difference between the two men. Another factor was that the professional channel swimmer had trained himself to maintain a high level of metabolic heat production for many hours at a time.

TABLE 16.1

Thermal conductivities of body tissues and other substances, expressed as heat conducted (kcal/hr) through a 1 cm thick slab 1 m square, per degree of temperature gradient

	Thermal conductivity kcal-cm/m²-hr-°C	Source
Skin	27·7	Lipkin & Hardy (1954)
Fat	14·4	Henriques & Moritz (1947)
	15·8	Bullard & Rapp (1970)
	17·3	Hatfield & Pugh (1951)
	17·6	Hardy & Soderstrom (1938)
	18·6	Lipkin & Hardy (1954)
Muscle	33·1	Hatfield & Pugh (1951)
	34·9	Bullard & Rapp (1970)
	35·2	Lipkin & Hardy (1954)
	39·6	Henriques & Moritz (1947)
Water	52	Bullard & Rapp (1970)
Rubber	16	Beckman (1963)
Rubberized cloth	16	Beckman (1963)
Wool	8	Beckman (1963)
Foamed neoprene	4·6	Beckman (1963)
Still air	2·3	Beckman (1963)

Further evidence of the protective value of subcutaneous fat layers is shown in the study of Hanna and Hong (1972), in which they determined the lowest water temperature an individual could tolerate without shivering over a 3-hour exposure, that temperature being termed the 'critical water temperature'. They found that the thicker the subcutaneous fat layer the lower the critical water temperature. There was also a difference between scuba divers who were accustomed to swimming in cool water and control subjects, the scuba divers having a lower critical water temperature for a given subcutaneous fat thickness. These data are shown in Fig. 16.5.

In a study of the fall in rectal temperature in 10 men who were immersed in stirred water at 15°C, Keatinge (1969) showed that the men with the

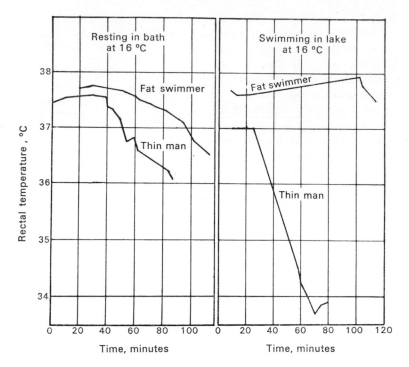

FIG. 16.3. The contrast between a fat distance swimmer and a thin man, in terms of the falls in their rectal temperatures while resting in a 16°C water bath or swimming in a lake in 16°C water. The thin man reached tolerance in both cases; the distance swimmer maintained body temperature while swimming, and managed nearly two hours at rest without serious discomfort (after Pugh & Edholm 1955)

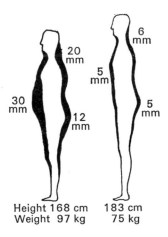

FIG. 16.4. Silhouettes of the fat distance swimmer and the thin man of Fig. 16.3, with the thickness of their skinfolds indicated numerically in mm. Heights are to scale, but skinfold thicknesses have been exaggerated (after Pugh & Edholm, 1955)

thicker skinfolds had a lesser fall. Similarly, Sloan and Keatinge (1973) observed in boys and girls who were training for competitive swimming that the fall in body temperature varied inversely with skinfold fat layer. Along the same lines, Carlson et al. (1958) measured the apparent body insulation for subjects in a bath calorimeter and found that insulation increased as percentage of body fat increased.

Body heat loss; conductance

Having described what is known about the transfer coefficients between skin and water at various water velocities, the conservation of heat by cutaneous vasoconstriction, and the value of subcutaneous fat as insulation, we can now consider the rates and quantities of body heat loss in experimental determinations. Nearly all such experiments are made with nude subjects,

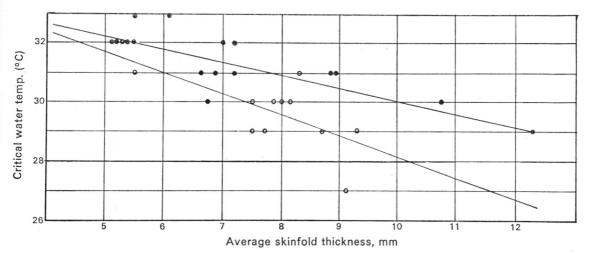

FIG. 16.5. Critical water temperatures (the lowest water temperature endured for 3 hours without shivering) for divers (open circles and lower line) and control subjects (solid circles and upper line) versus the average skinfold thickness measured at nine sites (after Hanna & Hong 1972)

and most with men immersed to the neck in water.

To start, neutral water temperature is that temperature where body heat loss exactly matches heat production from metabolism, and no change in body temperature occurs. This is not the same as critical water temperature, referred to earlier, in which a person can stay for 3 hours without shivering; in those experiments of Hanna and Hong (1972), there was a drop in rectal temperature of about 1°C. One definition for neutrality during immersion at rest was given by Boutelier (1973); a resting subject must show a basal metabolic heat production, a constant rectal temperature in the neighbourhood of 36·7 to 36·8°C and a mean skin temperature of $34 \pm 0·1$°C. In 10 subjects, he found that the thermally neutral water temperature at rest was between 33 and 34°C. A slightly higher temperature, 35°C, was given by Craig and Dvorak (1968); their criterion was that the ear canal temperature showed no change over a 60-min exposure.

When subjects exercise, the neutral water temperature is lower since the heat production is higher. At 2·5 times resting metabolism (mean oxygen consumption of 0·7 L/min), Craig and Dvorak (1968) found the neutral water temperature to be 32°C, and for a working level of 3 to 3·4 times resting (mean oxygen consumption of

0·92 L/min) the neutral water temperature was 26°C.

Exposure to neutral water temperature involves loss of heat from the body, but that loss is no greater than the heat produced by the body; thus there is little change in body heat stores. In cold water exposures that are below the neutral temperature, there is negative heat storage. The proper way to determine how much negative heat storage occurs is with a direct calorimeter, but it is also possible to attempt to determine negative storage by the change in various body temperatures multiplied by the body masses they represent and the specific heat of the body. That procedure involves a number of assumptions and is thereby somewhat questionable.

The net rate of loss of body heat is not linear with time, rather it is apparently exponential. Just as the drop in skin temperature on first exposure to cold water is essentially exponential, with the major drop occurring in the first few minutes, so Craig and Dvorak (1975) have shown that in a bath calorimeter the rate of heat loss is greatest in the beginning and decreases with time. They found that when subjects were exposed to 24°C water they lost on the average about 180 kcal in 1 hour, 40% of it in the first 10 min, 60% of it in the first 20 min. The high initial rate of cooling represents loss of heat from the shell of the body.

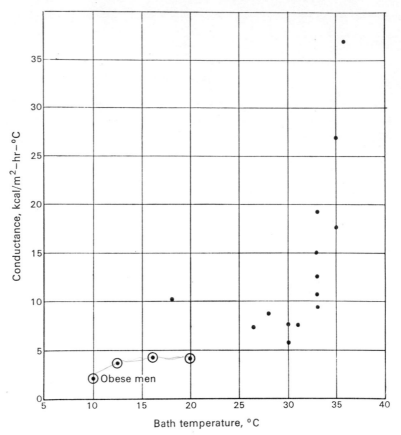

F I G . 16.6. Conductance values for resting men immersed to the neck at
various bath temperatures. Note the four low values for obese men who
can achieve an apparent steady state in lower bath temperatures than
non-obese men. (Based on data of Burton & Bazett, 1936; Carlson et al.
1958; Cannon & Keatinge, 1960; Rennie et al. 1962a and b; Boutelier,
Timbal & Colin 1968; Boutelier, 1973)

As the superficial tissues approach water temperature, the rate of heat loss from them decreases
since the temperature difference (ΔT) between
the skin and surrounding water becomes smaller.

With bath temperatures in the range of 24 to
34°C, a number of investigators have shown that
after the initial period of rapid cooling a quasi-
steady state occurs in which, with full vasoconstriction, skin temperatures and rectal
temperatures are nearly steady, and an apparent
balance exists between heat produced and heat
lost. It is during these quasi-steady state conditions that values for whole body conductance have
been measured.

The method for calculating whole body conductance during cold water exposure is as follows:

$$k = \frac{M - H_{\mathrm{resp}} \pm S}{(T_{\mathrm{c}} - \bar{T}_{\mathrm{s}})A_{\mathrm{b}}} \qquad (2)$$

where k is tissue thermal conductance in kcal/
m²-hr-°C; M is metabolic heat production in
kcal/hr; H_{resp} is respiratory heat loss in kcal/hr;
S is storage of heat in the body in kcals; T_{c} is core
temperature; $\bar{T}_{\mathrm{s}}$ is skin temperature; and A_{b} is
the body surface area. The range of values found
for k is seen in Fig. 16.6. Notice that bath temperatures for studies with non-obese men are from
26 to 36°C, except for one value at 18°C. Values
for obese men are shown with bath temperatures
between 10 and 20°C.

The values for whole body conductance in neutral to warm water are from 15 to 35 kcal/m²-hr-°C, while conductance values for cooler water, which causes vasoconstriction, are between 5 and 15 kcal/m²-hr-°C. Taking a typical value for k of 7·5 at a water temperature of 30°C, one can estimate body heat loss as follows: if the skin temperature is 30·6°C, the core is 37°C, then the temperature differential (ΔT) is 6·4°C; assuming a surface area of 1·8 m², the value for heat loss is $7·5 \times 6·4 \times 1·8 = 86·4$ kcal/hr. (To convert to watts, multiply by 1·16 or 100·2 W.)

Shivering

Shivering is a regulatory response which increases heat production by increasing the activity of skeletal muscle. During exposure to cold water, resting levels of heat production may increase by two to five times. Thus oxygen consumption can rise to over 1 L/min, which means a heat production of more than 200 kcal/hr. More typically, a resting heat production of 40–60 kcal/m²-hr will rise to 100 to 150 kcal/m²-hr. Specific experimental data of this sort can be found in Boutelier (1973), Carlson et al. (1958), Craig and Dvorak (1968), Kang et al. (1965) and Keatinge (1969).

Do muscular work and swimming prevent the increment in heat production caused by shivering? A clear answer has been furnished by Nielsen (1973), who studied swimmers with oxygen consumptions of from 1 to 2 L/min from the swimming alone. The men swam in water temperatures between 20 and 36°C, and were visibly shivering at the lower temperatures despite vigorous swimming. The incremental increase in metabolic rate was definite: for each °C decrease in skin temperature (water temperature), there was an increase in heat production of 12 kcal/hr. Similarly, Nadel et al. (1974) reported shivering and increased oxygen consumption during swimming at submaximal effort in water temperatures of 18 and 26°C.

Tolerance limits

A rectal temperature of 35°C is a mandatory low limit for cold exposure since, beyond this, serious problems from hypothermia begin. The thin subject in Pugh and Edholm's study (1955) was incapacitated when his rectal temperature had fallen to 34°C. It is certainly no coincidence that the Korean diving women, who have built up a wealth of human experience over a period of 2000 years, leave the water when they have learned that they must, and this happens when their rectal temperature is 35°C (Kang et al. 1965).

Beckman and Reeves (1966) found that in a water temperature of 24°C, 24 men exposed nude were able to tolerate an average of 8·1 hours of exposure. More than half of the men had to stop because of painful spasms and cramps in large muscle groups. Two of the 24 men had to stop because their rectal temperature had reached 35°C; several others stopped because of low blood sugar and the symptoms associated with it. The authors concluded that the several reasons for termination were related to excessive body heat loss.

Well-motivated laboratory subjects will stay in cold water beyond the initial cold shock and beyond the time when hands and feet become painfully cold. Behnke and Yaglou (1951) reported on three heroic subjects who were immersed nude in a cold bath with ice floating in it and having a temperature of 5°C. The men were able to endure this for almost an hour. Internal temperatures measured in the mouth, rectum, and stomach fell slowly to 36°C, while skin temperatures dropped rapidly and stayed between 6 and 8°C.

It would be satisfying to be able to specify physiological tolerance in terms of body heat loss. The best experimental data are those of Craig and Dvorak (1975), who exposed 10 nearly nude subjects to 24°C water in a bath calorimeter. The experiments lasted for 60 min and the subjects were acutely uncomfortable and shivering for most of the time. The average fall in the temperature of the ear canal was 0·37°C, and the average fall in skin temperature was 7·9°C. These exposures were not tolerance-limited, but the subjects would not have willingly endured much more. The mean value for heat loss in all 10 subjects was 183 kcal in the 1 hour of exposure. One particular subject showed a heat loss of 226 kcal in the 1-hour exposure. In a second experiment, he wore a foamed neoprene wetsuit in 24°C water, stayed for 2 hours, and had a heat loss of 276 kcal. Despite the higher heat loss, this man was more comfortable in the wetsuit, shivered hardly at all, and showed the same 0·2°C change in ear canal temperature as he had in the 1-hour exposure without protection.

Additional calorimetric data were obtained in three subjects studied by Webb (1973) during exposures to water temperatures of 5, 10, and 15°C; the men were wearing lightweight rubber diving suits and swimming underwater against a fixed load. The dives lasted from 45 to 60 min, when the men had reached a voluntary limit of endurance for the cold exposure. After emerging from the cold water, their body heat content was restored with a liquid tubing suit operated as a direct calorimeter. They were rewarmed until a normal state of heat balance was reached, in which the heat produced was matched by the heat lost from the body surface. The amount of heat required to rewarm to this condition was believed to match the heat lost during the cold water exposure. For one subject the mean value for heat lost in the three exposures was 183 kcal; for another, 202 kcal; and for the third, 242 kcal. At the end of the cold underwater swims, rectal and esophageal temperatures were between 36 and 36·5°C, while skin temperatures of hands and feet had dropped to within 3°C of the water temperature.

These laboratory experiences begin to define physiological endpoints in terms of body heat loss, falls in internal temperature, and skin temperature. But there are other endpoints which are harder to define. Performance becomes impaired when hands become cold and numb, and when muscular power decreases from cold. These effects are independent of major loss of body heat, and low core temperature.

Men who are accustomed to diving are accustomed to being cold, and they stop when they become seriously fatigued. Fatigue is very likely related to being cold. A diver will stop when he becomes unable to carry out the tasks he has been assigned. The old hands at diving have probably learned, like the Korean ama, just when to stop. Perhaps they have experienced the insidious effects of developing hypothermia, and have nearly had serious accidents. The reverse is likely to be true: that those men who ignore these symptoms do not become old hands in the underwater world.

Adaptation

Hibernators show a clear adaptive pattern to cold exposure, and many animals increase their heat production when chronically exposed to low air temperatures. Diving mammals (seals, whales, porpoises) shut off peripheral circulation completely and rely on thick subcutaneous fat layers to conserve heat.

Although man evidently does not develop strong adaptive responses, there are several studies which do suggest a mild adaptation to chronic cold water exposure. In their extensive study of the Korean ama, Hong (1965) and Rennie (1965) have shown that thermal conductance in a given water temperature is lower for diving women than for non-diving Korean women, even though the subcutaneous fat thickness is no different. In other words, the diving women, who are daily exposed to cold water, have apparently learned to restrict their cutaneous circulation better. At the same time, the diving women show a higher resting metabolic rate, and there is some suggestion that this is like the non-shivering thermogenesis observed in animals.

Evidence of short-term adaptation was reported by Skreslet and Aarefjord (1968). There appeared to be an improved vasoconstriction, i.e. reduced thermal conductance of the tissue, during a standardized exposure in a cold bath, over a period of 45 days during which the 3 subjects were regularly exposed to cold water while scuba diving in the sub-Arctic. Hanna and Hong (1972) observed lower critical water temperatures for the same skinfold thickness in scuba divers when compared to control subjects (see Fig. 16.5).

RESPIRATORY HEAT LOSS

In diving, loss of heat from the respiratory tract is a major threat to maintaining body heat content, although at 1 ATA respiratory heat loss is usually no more than about 10% of metabolic heat production even in very cold air. Respiratory heat loss is treated separately from the loss of heat from the body surface because none of the thermoregulatory responses affect it, and because the loss of heat is from the core, i.e. from the central blood stream.

A major function of the upper respiratory tract is air conditioning. Incoming air is usually cooler than body temperature (37°C), and nearly always drier than air saturated at body temperature. It has long been established that in sea level conditions the incoming air is warmed and moistened to reach 37°C and 47 mm Hg vapour pressure (saturation vapour pressure at 37°C) along the first 10 to 15 cm of the upper tract.

The greater the quantity of air breathed, the greater the respiratory heat loss. Thus respiratory heat loss is virtually a constant fraction of metabolism because of the near linear relationship between respiratory minute volume and oxygen consumption. Respiratory heat loss also increases as the inspired air is drier. The evaporation of water from the lining of the upper tract requires energy for the latent heat of vaporization, and the drier the incoming gas the more water must be added to saturate it. At 1 ATA, the evaporative component is the major component of respiratory heat loss. Respiratory heat loss increases slightly with colder incoming air, since convective heat transfer is a direct function of the temperature difference between inspired air and body temperature. If the air were exhaled at 37°C and saturated, it would be a simple matter to calculate respiratory heat loss. However, this is not the case.

There is a conservation of heat by the simple process of heat exchange between the warm moist air leaving the deeper portions of the respiratory tract and the previously cooled lining of the upper tract. Thus in a normal room temperature, exhaled air is close to 34°C and saturated at that temperature, having a vapour pressure of 40 mm Hg. As inhaled air is colder and drier, the cooling of the upper tract is greater and the heat conservation is also greater. None of this is of any great consequence in the heat economy of the body under sea level conditions, since the respiratory component of body heat loss is only about 10%.

However, the situation changes in diving because the gas breathed at pressures equal to the surrounding hydrostatic pressure is dense and

has a high heat capacity. At depth, convection becomes the dominant component of respiratory heat loss. One can calculate the respiratory heat loss if the magnitude of the heat conservation mechanism is known, which involves being able to predict expiratory gas temperature from the inspiratory gas temperature.

Expired gas temperature

Experimental data on the expired gas temperature as a function of inspired air temperature under hyperbaric conditions have been reported by Goodman et al. (1971), Hoke et al. (1975), Varène et al. (1973), and Webb and Annis (1966). The several findings are summarized in the predictive equation:

$$T_{ex} = 24 + 0.32 T_{in} \qquad (3)$$

where T_{ex} is expired gas temperature in °C and T_{in} is inspired gas temperature in °C. This predictive equation is valid for pressures between 1 and 31 ATA when the inspired gas is dry (Varène et al. 1973), and an almost identical equation was derived by Braithwaite (1972) from the data of Goodman et al. (1971).

Calculation of respiratory heat loss

The calculation of respiratory heat loss depends upon the quantity of gas exchanged, the density and the specific heat of the gas, the temperature difference between inspired and expired gas, plus the difference in the water content of inspired and expired air times the latent heat of vaporization. Since its effect is small, it is permissible to neglect the evaporative term. Thus one may use the following:

$$RHL = \dot{V}_E \times \rho C_p (T_{in} - T_{ex}) \qquad (4)$$

where RHL is respiratory heat loss in kcal/min; $\dot{V}_E$ is respiratory minute volume in L/min (BPTS); ρ is gas density in g/L; C_p is the specific heat of the gas in kcal/g. To change the answer from kcal/min to watts, multiply the answer by 69.733.

To compute the density and specific heat of the gas mixture breathed, first determine by analysis the components of the gas mixture, then proportion the effect of each component (helium, oxygen, etc.) by multiplying specific heat and density of each by its mol fraction in the mixture (Hoke et al. 1975; Webb & Annis 1966). Specific heat does not vary significantly with pressure, but density varies directly with pressure and with absolute temperature.

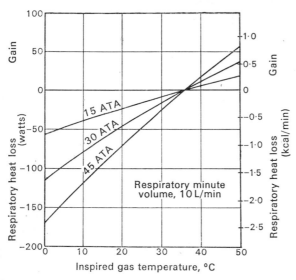

FIG. 16.7. Respiratory heat loss or gain breathing normoxic helium–oxygen at the three pressures shown, for a resting man breathing 10 L/min. For 20 L/min, multiply by 2; for 30, by 3, etc.

Fig. 16.7 illustrates the use of equations 3 and 4 in calculating the respiratory heat loss for normoxic helium–oxygen mixtures at 15, 30, and 45 ATA. Only one respiratory minute volume is shown on the graph, 10 L/min, which is typical for a resting man. If the respiratory minute volume were 20, the values for respiratory heat loss would be exactly double those shown in Fig. 16.7. Also in Fig. 16.7 is shown respiratory heat gain if the breathing gas mixture is warmer than 37°C, for there have been suggestions that respiratory heating could be used to rewarm a chilled diver and the magnitude of such warming is evident from Fig. 16.7.

Since a resting man generates heat at the rate of about 100 watts, notice that at 30 ATA breathing gas with a temperature of 4°C means that all of a diver's metabolic heat would be leaving via the respiratory tract no matter what is done to protect his body surface. And further, since respiratory minute volume increases in direct proportion to increasing metabolism (oxygen consumption), exercising would not help, for heat loss would still equal heat production.

Effects of breathing cold hyperbaric gas

The most serious effect of breathing unheated gas at depth, where the respiratory equipment a diver wears in the water takes on the temperature of the water, is a serious drain of body heat. In the experiments reported by Hoke et al. (1975), subjects were living under saturation diving conditions in comfortably warm heliox at a pressure equivalent of 250 m (25·8 ATA). The men were given cold gas to breathe via a mouthpiece. It was fascinating to see a man in a warm, 30°C environment breathing 5°C gas while pedalling a bicycle and after 15 or 20 min shivering violently. Some subjects were so cold they could not complete the scheduled work. Core temperatures fell without any decrease in surface temperature.

Another distressing effect of breathing cold gas is the stimulation of a copious secretion of liquid and mucus in the respiratory tract, enough to foul the mouthpiece and in some cases cause choking and gagging. Goodman et al. (1971) and Hoke et al. (1975) commented on the seriousness of this problem, and postulated that divers operating in cold water at great depth would have trouble from this effect alone. The amount of secretion seemed to be more than could be explained by condensation of water in the exhaled gas.

A third effect of breathing cold gas has been postulated. The high heat capacity of hyperbaric gases most likely means that the penetration of cold gas into the respiratory tract is considerably deeper than occurs at sea level. During air breathing at 1 ATA, penetration of cold gas is no greater than 10 or 15 cm. During hyperbaric breathing, it seems likely that cold gas penetrates beyond the trachea and into the branching of the bronchi. Such cooling may cause unusual physiological responses such as bronchial constriction. Gas temperature also affects flow and the work of breathing, and gaseous diffusion as well. So it will not be enough to simply know the overall heat exchange. We need direct experimental evidence of the depth to which cold gas penetrates.

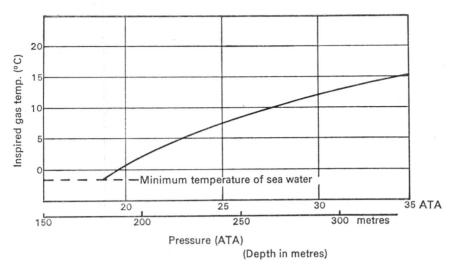

FIG. 16.8. A recommended minimum safe temperature for breathing hyperbaric gas as a function of the pressure (depth) shown (after Braithwaite 1972)

Heating the respiratory gas

The obvious solution to the problem of hyperbaric respiratory heat loss is to heat the gas in the breathing apparatus. If possible the gas should be heated to between 30 and 35°C, with warmer temperatures at greater depths. If this is not possible, it would be wise to heed Braithwaite (1972), who calculated minimum safe inspired gas temperatures for various depths in terms of the hazard from rapid body heat loss and also from copious mucus secretions. He recommended the minimum temperatures shown in Fig. 16.8, but stated clearly that higher temperatures would be desirable whenever possible.

HYPOTHERMIA AND REWARMING

Hypothermia exists when enough body heat has been lost so that the rectal temperature is below 35°C and symptoms begin to appear, symptoms like mental confusion, lethargy, poor speech articulation, hallucinations, decreased sensation, and impaired motor function. Such symptoms must not be allowed to develop in a diver, for such a man is losing control and on the verge of making some fatal mistake. The onset of hypothermia is often insidious, somewhat like the symptoms of hypoxia in aviators. For this reason it would be easy for even experienced divers to drift into dangerous hypothermia without struggling to get out of the situation.

Hypothermia is a grave medical condition. It happens to people accidentally immersed in cold water, to elderly persons living alone in meagrely heated houses, to someone who has fallen asleep outdoors after a night of heavy drinking, to accident victims, and to hikers and climbers who have become exhausted. Profound hypothermia, in which the rectal temperature is 32°C, produces a patient who is barely conscious, who will not respond to painful stimuli, has a very slow heart beat and possibly cardiac irregularities. In very profound hypothermia, the patient is often mistaken for dead. If the core temperature reaches 30°C the patient is in profound coma, he is cold to the touch, and his skin is pale and of greyish colour. The neck and extremities resist bending; no peripheral pulse can be found; there appears to be no breathing, and pupillary reflexes are absent. Laboratory findings include: hypotension; cardiac irregularities, typically atrial fibrillation and a J wave associated with the QRS complex; metabolic acidosis producing a low blood pH, especially in cases where hypothermia follows exhaustion and prolonged shivering; low blood CO_2 content; and a high blood sugar.

The treatment of hypothermia is rewarming.

There are two approaches to rewarming, fast and slow, but only one of them makes sense in the context of diving operations. Rapid rewarming is used in situations where the hypothermia has developed rapidly, meaning in a period of 1 to 3 hours; slow rewarming is used when hypothermia has developed slowly and there is a sizable component of fatigue and serious electrolyte imbalance. In diving and other cold water exposures, hypothermia is presumed to have developed rapidly and therefore rapid rewarming should be started without delay.

Rapid rewarming is achieved by putting the hypothermic patient into a tub of well-stirred hot water in order to restore body heat content as quickly as possible. Similar results should be achievable with the water-heated suits which are being used more and more in diving today. Even more rapid rewarming could be achieved by peritoneal dialysis with warm saline, or with an extracorporeal blood circuit which passes blood through a heat exchanger. These methods are intellectually attractive but of little use in the remote locations where diving operations usually take place. It would be inexcusable to delay treatment of hypothermia while a patient was evacuated to a competent medical facility for such elaborate measures.

The hot bath should be maintained at a temperature of between 40 and 42°C and the water should be stirred briskly in order to achieve best heat transfer to the cold skin. Rectal temperatures should be read frequently, and when the rectal temperature has been brought up to 36°C the patient can be removed from the tub. His own metabolic heat should be sufficient to complete the rewarming.

As the rectal temperature is monitored from the outset of rewarming, there is almost invariably an initial drop before the rise begins. This after-drop is a matter of concern only if the initial rectal temperature is below 32°C, because below this level cardiac irregularities become more frequent, and there is danger of sending the heart into ventricular fibrillation as cold blood returns from the body shell. However, it is unlikely that a diver would be rescued in such profound hypothermia.

In the milder stages of hypothermia, when the patient is rational and able to cooperate the hot tub treatment is unnecessary and a more conservative approach is recommended. This consists of a hot shower (which does more for the spirits than it does for restoring body heat), warm dry clothing, and hot liquids to drink. Alcohol should be avoided in the beginning because it causes peripheral vasodilation. One should be aware that it takes many hours for even mild hypothermia to be overcome by the slow accumulation of metabolic heat.

When is body heat restored? According to some recent work, body heat is reliably restored when normal thermoregulation via vasomotor control in the skin has reappeared (Webb 1973). However, this may be difficult to recognize. A practical rule is that heat has been surely restored if rewarming is continued to the point of early sweating, which probably represents some degree of overwarming. Thus a cooperating subject could be given warm clothing, hot drinks, and made to exercise until he became warm enough to sweat.

The important thing is that rewarming must be complete before any further diving is done. Unless heat has surely been restored, a second dive means that the tolerance time for a given cold exposure is reduced. Eventually, we may need repetitive dive tables for cold exposure just as we have them for absorption and release of inert gas.

EFFECTS OF COLD

Surely the most serious effect of cold is the lethal diving accident caused by progressive hypothermia, but such deaths are not reported as being caused by cold. Rawlins and Tauber (1971), however, mentioned cold as a major contributing factor in the death of a diver who had already made one dive, become very cold, had not had an opportunity to rewarm properly, and had started the second dive, which lasted only a few minutes. This was an illustration of the danger of a repeat dive without adequate restoration of heat lost in the first dive. It is quite possible that when diving physicians and dive supervisors become conscious of the insidious yet serious character of cold exposure many diving accidents will become identified as being caused by cold.

There are two other effects of cold to be considered, the probable relationship between cold exposure and decompression sickness, and the effect of cold upon human performance.

Decompression sickness

A full discussion of decompression sickness is given in a later chapter, but cold as a contributing factor has been implicated preliminarily. It is reasonable to suppose that since the elimination of inert gas is aided by high tissue perfusion, the reduced circulation in skin, subcutaneous fat, and deeper substance of arms and legs delays the release of dissolved inert gas.

Hempleman (1967) has shown an increased incidence of bubble formation in rats who were exposed to cold and then subjected to a standard compression-decompression procedure. Balldin (1973) has shown that men eliminate dissolved nitrogen more rapidly while breathing oxygen if they are immersed in warm water (37°C). Carrying this one step further, he showed that men who had breathed oxygen for 25 min at 1 ATA while in warm water had a lower incidence of bends when exposed to 0·2 ATA (155 mm Hg) in an altitude chamber than if they had breathed oxygen for 25 min sitting in a neutral air temperature of 28°C.

Quite probably, a diver who starts his dive being relatively warm absorbs and distributes the inert gas of the breathing mixture at depth while his circulation is still good, but then if he is cold exposed, his peripheral circulation decreases, and during decompression this reduced circulation is a handicap. The solution is to keep the diver warm throughout the dive, or at least to make sure he is warm during his decompression period.

Performance

A diver is already hampered by protective clothing and by the buoyancy and high viscosity of the water medium. His performance can only be worsened by the effects of cold. Manual manipulations are often critical, and the hands are the hardest part of the body to keep warm. Nearly everyone who has lived in a cold climate has experienced the numbness and loss of dexterity from cold hands. Objective data on decreased tactile sensitivity are provided by Bowen (1968),

Provins and Morton (1960) and Stang and Weiner (1970). The kinesthetic sense is also decreased in cold hands. Then, when the arms and hands are cold, muscle strength decreases, and manual dexterity is further worsened, as shown by a poorer ability to manipulate tools and small parts (Beckman 1963; Provins & Clarke 1960; Stang & Weiner 1970; Vaughan & Andersen 1973).

Among the more general effects of cold exposure are that it has been shown to cause poor tracking proficiency and increased reaction time (Provins & Clarke 1960). Bowen (1968) showed that it took longer for a group of divers to assemble a structure underwater if the water was cold, and he speculated that slowing of job performance might be the result of an impaired time sense in cold water.

Continued cold exposure causes a gradual decrement in cognitive tasks such as navigation, signal detection, and problem solving. Among the several explanations offered are distraction, which produces an initial decrement (Bowen 1968; Stang and Weiner 1970; Vaughan and Andersen 1973); increasing discomfort, which causes a gradual decrement (Vaughan and Andersen 1973); and a dysfunction which accounts for failures in response and occasional misses in response or problem solving (Bowen 1968; Vaughan & Andersen 1973).

This brief review of the effects of cold on diver performance does not do justice to the importance of the matter. Divers themselves, and diving supervisors, must be continually concerned, and further studies are surely warranted.

THERMAL PROTECTION

To prevent the serious effects of cold exposure, the diver may use an insulating garment to reduce body heat loss, or he may wear an insulating garment plus supplemental heating. Since such garments are not yet perfected for all diving conditions, it is hard to disagree with Rawlins and Tauber (1971), who urged that there be a sufficient technological effort so that the thermal problems of the diver could be circumvented. There are a number of difficulties to overcome. For one thing, insulation that works well near the surface becomes compressed and loses its insulating quality at depth; for another, hands and feet are difficult to insulate, especially since a diver's hands must be relatively unencumbered. Electrically heated suits are at present far from perfect, and hot water heating works best when the diver is operating close to a fixed support station.

Insulation in clothing increases in direct proportion to the thickness of the clothing layers and in inverse proportion to the density of the material used. The traditional diving dress of heavy rubberized canvas can be worn with sufficient woollen underclothing to keep a man warm enough to do the job in many circumstances. Breathing gas in the suit prevents total compression of the garment layers and thus preserves insulation. But if no gas is added to equalize the hydrostatic pressure around the man, the compression of the layers of insulation reduces insulation to a third or less of its value in air (Goldman et al. 1966).

A familiar form of insulation in diving garments is the closed cell foamed neoprene used in a skin diver's wetsuit. When the diver is operating in relatively shallow water, this provides excellent insulation even if the water is extremely cold, as it is under the arctic ice. Better than the wetsuit for divers working in the cold air and cold water in arctic and sub-arctic areas is the foamed neoprene dry suit made with waterproof zippers (MacInnis 1972). Unfortunately, the closed cell neoprene foam becomes compressed so that beyond 15 or 20 m the insulating quality decreases rapidly. Specific data on compression and loss of insulating value are supplied in the reports of Barthélémy (1970), Beckman (1967) and Rawlins and Tauber (1971). A solution to this problem is to use an open cell foam, and to enclose this inside a gas-retaining shell, so that breathing gas can be added to maintain suit pressure equal to hydrostatic pressure as the diver descends (Barthélémy 1970). Another solution would be to make a suit of an insulation which does not compress with hydrostatic pressure; a few such materials exist, but no practical diving suit has yet been made from them.

Supplemental heating can overcome the deficiencies of insulation. The amount of heat required will vary with the water temperature, the work level, and the efficiency of insulation at a given depth. Beckman (1967) estimated that 500 W was a reasonable requirement for supplemental heating for a competent foamed neoprene wetsuit in very cold water. Rawlins and Tauber (1971), estimating needs for deeper dives, assumed higher heat loss with constant volume dry suits or re-expanded foamed neoprene suits, and also included respiratory heat loss if the breathing gas were not heated; their estimates of supplemental heating came to 1500 to 3000 W. But how is that heat to be delivered?

One method is by using a suit of underwear containing electrical resistance wires. But after intensive development by several firms, a fully reliable electrically heated suit has not appeared. The problems come from broken wires, breaks at the electrical connectors, short circuits which make hot spots that cause skin burns, and the almost inevitable leakage of water to the electrical conductors with potential shock hazard to the diver.

Another means of delivering the heat is via hot water. Two styles of suit have emerged, the liquid tubing suit and the free flooded suit. Tubing suits were first developed in the aerospace field; several designs and uses of these garments have been reviewed by Nunneley (1970). So far the tubing suits have found only occasional application in the diving field.

Free flooded suits have been successfully used to prolong working dives at depths to 100 m and in water temperatures down to 4°C (Long 1972). The diver is connected by a hose to a hot water boiler on the surface, and 10 to 15 L/min of hot water are pumped down to him. The hot water is distributed inside a standard diver's dress by means of hoses and allowed to escape around the face and hands. In a slightly different version, the diver wears a foamed neoprene wetsuit in which distribution tubes are located, and water floods through the layer between the suit and the skin, exiting at any available opening. The diver can adjust the flow of water and to some degree the water temperature. These suits are wasteful of energy, which is no serious matter usually, but there are greater problems as the distance between the diver and the hot water source increases. On the other hand, in the liquid tubing suit the warm water could be recirculated and a small electrically powered heater and pump could be part of the diver's equipment; a relatively small cable would be needed to connect him to the power source.

Heating of the respiratory gases is necessary in dives beyond 200 m. This has been accomplished both with an electric heater and with a hot water loop running through a heat exchanger in the respiratory assembly.

What applies to the diver in the water also applies to the diving bell or transfer capsule which moves him to and from great depth. These vehicles should be insulated and heated in order that high convective and respiratory heat losses do not occur in the hyperbaric environment (Rawlins & Tauber 1971; Riegel & Glasgow 1970).

COMFORT AND THERMAL DRAIN IN HYPERBARIC ENVIRONMENTS

In saturation diving, men spend days and weeks in hyperbaric gaseous environments, usually normoxic helium–oxygen mixtures, which have unusual thermal characteristics. The environment is highly convective (Raymond et al. 1968) and conductive because of the increased density of the gas and (in the case of helium) the high thermal conductivity. The man becomes tightly coupled to the environment, as evidenced by a much smaller than usual temperature differential (ΔT) between the gas and the skin (Webb 1970). The hyperbaric gas also hampers evaporative heat loss, and there is decreased gaseous diffusion and slow mixing (Puglia & Webb 1974). The unusual character of this environment is revealed in two ways, the temperatures that men find comfortable, and the evidence of an energetic imbalance despite comfortably warm temperatures.

Comfort temperatures in hyperbaric gases are shown in Table 16.2, which lists the temperatures chosen by men staying for some days in normoxic helium–oxygen mixtures in the range of pressures from 1·5 to 37·4 ATA. The table makes it clear that the higher the pressure, the warmer the gas must be for comfort. Also, at the lower pressures the width of the temperature band which is

TABLE 16.2

Comfort temperatures for normoxic helium–oxygen mixtures as a function of pressure

Gas pressure (ATA)	Gas temperature (°C)	Source
1·5	28·7	Varène et al. (1975)
2·3	29·6	Varène et al. (1975)
4·4	30·0	Varène et al. (1975)
7·2	29·0	Raymond et al. (1968)
8·4	30·7	Varène et al. (1975)
13·1	28·5–31·5	Puglia & Webb (1974)
14·6	28·9	Raymond et al. (1968)
16·1	29	Moore et al. (1975)
16·1	31·8	Varène et al. (1975)
22·2	29·0–31·5	Puglia & Webb (1974)
28·3	30·0–32·0	Puglia & Webb (1974)
30·8	32·4	Varène et al. (1975)
37·4	32·5–33·5	Puglia & Webb (1974)

comfortable is greater than at the higher pressures. At 2·2 ATA, subjects easily tolerate a variation in temperature of $\pm 2°C$, but at 30 ATA the comfort band is only $\pm 0·5°C$.

Cold exposure in a hyperbaric environment was the unusual experience of the men in a saturation dive in Hawaiian waters. During 5 days at 16·7 ATA, the habitat temperature was kept between 22 and 25°C and the men were constantly cold, a situation which kept them stressed and severely limited their diving operations (Pegg 1971).

The narrowness of the comfort band is emphasized by the observation that the temperature chosen by the occupants of a hyperbaric chamber is correct for lightly clothed men who are mildly active, but it is too cold for the same men when asleep. Apparently obligatory heat loss is too high for a man with the low metabolic rate of sleep. Extra blankets or extra heat are required in the bunk areas.

An oft-repeated observation on weight loss leads to the hypothesis that comfortable hyperbaric environments represent a thermal drain. Nearly everyone in a saturation dive loses weight despite eating large amounts of food. This experience is summarized in Table 16.3. In most cases the weight losses are too high to be explained simply by a fluid shift, and after the dive is over, the weight is regained slowly over a period of many days.

TABLE 16.3

Body weight loss in ocean and dry chamber saturation dives (Webb 1975)

	Gaseous environment	Mean weight loss (kg)	Food intake (kcal/day)	No. of subjects	Duration at depth (days)	total dive (days)
Tektite I (Caribbean)	Air, 2·15 ATA	1·6	'adequate'	4	60	
Tektite II (Caribbean)	Air, 2·3 ATA	2·0	>3500	53	14–21	
Helgoland (North Sea)	Air, 3·3 ATA	3–5	6000	9	10	
Genesis E (dry chamber)	HeO_2, 7 ATA	0·6	4200	3	12	
Sealab II (Bermuda)	HeN_2O_2, 7·2 ATA	2	>4000 (est)	28	15	
Univ. Hawaii (dry chamber)	HeO_2, 16·1 ATA	0·6	>4000	6	2	9
Aegir (Hawaii)	HeO_2, 16·6 ATA	2·9	ad lib	6	6	14
US Navy-EDU (dry chamber)	HeO_2, 19·2 ATA	1·2	ad lib	7	8	16
Univ. Penn., 1971 (dry chamber)	HeO_2, 37 ATA	4	3510	4	6	21

The explanation of the weight loss is not yet clear. There is no definitive evidence that oxygen consumption is high, as Varène et al. (1975) show, but oxygen consumption data taken so far are episodic short-term measurements. The fluid balance theory is at least a partial explanation, which Moore et al. (1975) link to the possibility that the hyperbaric environment acts like a mild cold exposure, causing a cold diuresis. Puglia and Webb (1975) estimated that, if the weight loss is from caloric imbalance, men who lived at 37 ATA and ate 3500 calories per day were in a caloric deficit of 1400 kcal/day. A careful caloric balance study has not yet been done; there is always the possibility that the food eaten is not properly absorbed or metabolized.

The rates of weight loss observed are not alarming, and in the saturation dives to date the effect would hardly be considered debilitating. However, the problem is intriguing, and its solution may have some influence on the logistics of saturation dives in the ocean. Incidentally, the weight loss figures for saturation dives in the open ocean are generally higher because the subjects not only stay in the habitat but also venture forth, usually more than once a day, into the cold surrounding water.

If the hyperbaric environment does, in fact, represent a thermal drain, then it is a poor environment in which to rewarm. Saturation dives in the ocean are for the purpose of allowing men to go out and work at great depth, and until we have perfected thermal protection so that the men do not lose heat, the matter of rewarming when they return will need careful attention.

REFERENCES

BALLDIN, U. I. (1973) The preventive effect of denitrogenation during warm water immersion on decompression sickness in man. *Försvarsmedicin* **9**, 239–243.

BARTHÉLÉMY, L. (1970) Déperdition calorique et protection thermique du plongeur. *Le Travail Humain.* **33**, 195–216.

BAZETT, H. C., LOVE, L., NEWTON, M., EISENBERG, L., DAY, R. & FORSTER, R. (1948) Temperature changes in blood flowing in arteries and veins in man. *J. appl. Physiol.* **1**, 3–19.

BECKMAN, E. L. (1963) Thermal protection during immersion in cold water. In *Proc. 2nd Symp. Underwater Physiology.* Ed. C. J. Lambertsen and L. J. Greenbaum Jr. pp. 247–266. Washington, D.C.: Natl. Acad. Sci.–Natl. Res. Council. (Publ. 1181.)

BECKMAN, E. L. (1967) Thermal protective suits for underwater swimmers. *Milit. Med.* **132**, 195–209.
BECKMAN, E. L. & REEVES, E. (1966) Physiological implications as to survival during immersion in water at 75°F. *Aerospace Med.* **37**, 1136–1142.
BEHNKE, A. R. & YAGLOU, C. P. (1951) Physiological responses of men to chilling in ice water and to slow and fast rewarming. *J. appl. Physiol.* **3**, 591–602.
BOUTELIER, C. (1973) *Échanges thermiques du corps humain dans l'eau.* Thesis. University of Lille.
BOUTELIER, C., TIMBAL, J. & COLIN, J. (1968) Conductance thermique des tissus périphériques du corps humain plongé dans l'eau froide. *J. Physiol., Paris* **60**, 223–224.
BOWEN, H. M. (1968) Diver performance and the effects of cold. *Hum. Factors* **10**, 445–463.
BRAITHWAITE, W. R. (1972) *The Calculation of Minimum Safe Inspired Gas Temperature Limits for Deep Diving.* Report 12–72, US Navy Experimental Diving Unit, Washington, D.C.
BULLARD, R. W. & RAPP, G. M. (1970) Problems of body heat loss in water immersion. *Aerospace Med.* **41**, 1269–1277.
BURTON, A. C. & BAZETT, H. C. (1936) A study of the average temperature of the tissues, of the exchanges of heat and vasomotor responses in man by means of a bath calorimeter. *Am. J. Physiol.* **117**, 36–54.
BURTON, A. C. & EDHOLM, O. G. (1955) *Man in a Cold Environment.* London: Edward Arnold.
CANNON, P. & KEATINGE, W. R. (1960) The metabolic rate and heat loss of fat and thin men in heat balance in cold and warm water. *J. Physiol., Lond.* **154**, 329–344.
CARLSON, L. D. & HSIEH, A. C. L. (1965) Cold. In *The Physiology of Human Survival.* Ed. O. G. Edholm, & A. L. Bachrach, pp. 15–51. London: Academic Press.
CARLSON, L. D., HSIEH, A. C. L., FULLINGTON, F. & ELSNER, R. W. (1958) Immersion in cold water and body tissue insulation. *J. Aviat. Med.* **29**, 145–152.
CRAIG, A. B., Jr. & DVORAK, M. (1968) Thermal regulation of man exercising during water immersion. *J. appl. Physiol.* **25**, 28–35.
CRAIG, A. B. Jr. & DVORAK, M. (1975) Heat exchanges between man and the water environment. In *Underwater Physiology. Vth Symp. Underwater Physiology.* Ed. C. J. Lambertsen. Bethesda: Fedn Am. Socs exp. Biol.
FROESE, G. & BURTON, A. C. (1957) Heat losses from the human head. *J. appl. Physiol.* **10**, 235–241.
GOLDMAN, R. F., BRECKENRIDGE, J. R., REEVES, E. & BECKMAN, E. L. (1966) 'Wet' vs. 'dry' suit approaches to water immersion protective clothing. *Aerospace Med.* **37**, 485–487.
GOODMAN, M. W., SMITH, N. E., COLSTON, J. W., & RICH, E. L. (1971) *Hyperbaric respiratory heat loss study.* Final report, Contract N00014-71-C-0099, Office of Naval Research, Washington, D.C.
HANNA, J. M. & HONG, S. K. (1972) Critical water temperature and effective insulation in scuba divers in Hawaii. *J. appl. Physiol.* **33**, 770–773.
HARDY, J. D. & SODERSTROM, G. F. (1938) Heat loss from the nude body and peripheral blood flow at temperatures of 22°C to 35°C. *J. Nutr.* **16**, 493–510.
HATFIELD, H. S. & PUGH, L. G. C. (1951) Thermal conductivity of human fat and muscle. *Nature, Lond.* **168**, 918–919.
HEMPLEMAN, H. V. (1967) Cited by Elliott, D. H. In *The Physiology and Medicine of Diving and Compressed Air Work.* First Edition. Ed. P. B. Bennett and D. H. Elliott. London: Ballière, Tindall and Cassell.
HENRIQUES, F. C. Jr. & MORITZ, A. R. (1947) Studies of thermal injury: conduction of heat to and through skin and temperatures attained therein; theoretical and experimental investigation. *Am. J. Pathol.* **23**, 531–549.
HOKE, B., JACKSON, D. L., ALEXANDER, J. M. & FLYNN, E. T. (1975) Respiratory heat loss and pulmonary function during cold gas breathing at high pressures. In *Underwater Physiology. Vth Symp. Underwater Physiology.* Ed. C. J. Lambertsen. Bethesda: Fedn Am. Socs exp. Biol.
HONG, S. K. (1965) Heat exchange and basal metabolism of Ama. In *Physiology of Breath-Hold Diving and the Ama of Japan.* Ed. H. Rahn and T. Yokoyama. pp. 303–314. (Publ. 1341). Washington, D.C.: Natl. Acad. Sci.
KANG, D. H., KIM, P. K., KANG, B. S., SONG, S. H. & HONG, S. K. (1965) Energy metabolism and body temperature of the ama. *J. appl. Physiol.* **20**, 46–50.
KEATINGE, W. R. (1969) *Survival in Cold Water.* Oxford: Blackwell.
KREITH, F. (1973) *Principles of Heat Transfer.* Intext Educational: New York and London.
LIPKIN, M. & HARDY, J. D. (1954) Measurement of some thermal properties of human tissues. *J. appl. Physiol.* **7**, 212–217.
LONG, R. W. (1972) Hot water diving—state of the art. In *Proc. Symposium The Working Diver.* pp. 239–248. Washington, D.C.: Marine Technology Society.
MACINNES, J. B. (1972) Arctic diving and the problems of performance. In *Proc. Symposium The Working Diver.* pp. 159–172. Washington, D.C.: Marine Technology Society.
MOORE, T. O., MORLOCK, J. F., LALLY, D. A., & HONG, S. K. (1975) Thermal cost of saturation diving: respiratory and whole body heat loss at 16·1 ATA. In *Underwater Physiology. Vth Symp. Underwater Physiology.* Ed. C. J. Lambertsen. Bethesda: Fedn Am. Socs exp. Biol.
NADEL, E. R., HOLMER, I., BERGH, U., ÅSTRAND, P.-O. & STOLWIJK, J. A. J. (1974) Energy exchanges of swimming man. *J. appl. Physiol.* **36**, 465–471.
NIELSEN, B. (1973) Metabolic reactions to cold during swimming at different speeds. Paper given at the International Ergonomics Conference, Strasbourg.
NUNNELEY, S. A. (1970) Water cooled garments: a review. *Space Life Sciences* **2**, 335–360.
NUNNELEY, S. A., TROUTMAN, S. J., Jr. & WEBB, P. (1971) Head cooling in work and heat stress. *Aerospace Med.* **42**, 64–68.
PEGG, J. (1971) Five hundred sixteen ft. (16·6 ATA) five-day ocean saturation dive using a mobile habitat. *Aerospace Med.* **42**, 1257–1262.
PROVINS, K. A. & CLARKE, R. S. (1960) The effect of cold on manual performance. *J. occup. Med.* **2**, 169–176.
PROVINS, K. A. & MORTON, R. (1960) Tactile discrimination and skin temperature. *J. appl. Physiol.* **15**, 155–160.
PUGH, L. G. C. & EDHOLM, O. G. (1955) The physiology of channel swimmers. *Lancet*, **2**, 761–768.
PUGLIA, C. & WEBB, P. (1974) Thermal and metabolic effects of a comfortable hyperbaric helium environment. (In preparation.)

RAPP, G. M. (1970) Convection coefficients of man in a forensic area of thermal physiology: heat transfer in under-water exercise. *J. Physiol., Paris* **63**, 392–396.

RAWLINS, J. S. P. & TAUBER, J. F. (1971) Thermal balance at depth. In *Underwater Physiology. Proc. 4th Symp. Underwater Physiology*. Ed. C. J. Lambertsen. pp. 435–442. New York: Academic Press.

RAYMOND, L. W., BELL, W. H., BONDI, K. R. & LINDBERG, C. R. (1968) Body temperature and metabolism in hyperbaric helium atmospheres. *J. appl. Physiol.* **24**, 678–684.

RENNIE, D. W. (1965) Thermal insulation of Korean diving women and non-divers in water. In *Physiology of Breath-Hold Diving and the Ama of Japan*. Ed. H. Rahn and T. Yokoyama. pp. 315–324. (Publ. 1341.) Washington, D.C.: Natl. Acad. Sci.

RENNIE, D. W., COVINO, B. G., BLAIR, M. R. & RODAHL, K. (1962a) Physical regulation of temperature in Eskimos. *J. appl. Physiol.* **17**, 326–332.

RENNIE, D. W., COVINO, B. G., HOWELL, B. J., SONG, S. H., KANG, B. S. & HONG, S. K. (1962b) Physical insulation of Korean diving women. *J. appl. Physiol.* **17**, 961–966.

RIEGEL, P. S. & GLASGOW, J. S. (1970) Experimental determination of heat requirements for the Mark I PTC. In *Proc. Symposium Equipment for the Working Diver*, pp. 119–130. Washington, D.C.: Marine Technology Society.

SHVARTZ, E. (1970) Effect of a cooling hood on physiological responses to work in a hot environment. *J. appl. Physiol.* **29**, 36–39.

SKRESLET, S. & AAREFJORD, F. (1968) Acclimatization to cold in man induced by frequent scuba diving in cold water. *J. appl. Physiol.* **24**, 177–181.

SLOAN, R. E. G. & KEATINGE, W. R. (1973) Cooling rates of young people swimming in cold water. *J. appl. Physiol.* **35**, 371–375.

STANG, P. R. & WEINER, E. L. (1970) Diver performance in cold water. *Hum. Factors*, **12**, 391–399.

VARÈNE, P., TIMBAL, J., VIEILLEFOND, H., GUÉNARD, H. & L'HUILLIER, J. (1975) Energetic balance of man in simulated dive from 1·5 to 31 ATA. In *Underwater Physiology. Vth Symp. Underwater Physiology*. Ed. C. J. Lambertsen. Bethesda: Fedn Am. Socs exp. Biol.

VARÈNE, P., VIEILLEFOND, H., GUÉNARD, H., L'HUILLIER, H., PEYROT, H., TIMBAL, J. & CHARGÉ, C. (1973) *Échanges thermiques par convection respiratoire au niveau de la mer et en plongée*. Study No. 998, Centre d'Essais en Vol., Bretigny.

VAUGHAN, W. S. Jr. & ANDERSEN, B. G. (1973) *Effects of Long-duration Cold Exposure on Performance of Tasks in Naval Inshore Warfare Operations*. Technical report, Contract N00014-72-C-0309, Office of Naval Research, Washington, D.C.

WEBB, P. (1970) Body heat loss in undersea gaseous environments. *Aerospace Med.* **41**, 1282–1288.

WEBB, P. (1973) Rewarming after diving in cold water. *Aerospace Med.* **44**, 1152–1157.

WEBB, P. (1975) Thermal stress in undersea activity. In *Underwater Physiology. Vth Symp. Underwater Physiology*. Ed. C. J. Lambertsen. Bethesda: Fedn Am. Socs exp. Biol.

WEBB, P. & ANNIS, J. F. (1966) *Respiratory Heat Loss with High Density Gas Mixtures*. Final Report, Contract Nonr 4965(00), Office of Naval Research, Washington, D.C.

WITHERSPOON, J. M., GOLDMAN, R. F., & BRECKENRIDGE, J. R. (1971) Heat transfer coefficients of humans in cold water. *J. Physiol., Paris*, **63**, 459–462.

17

Decompression Theory: American Practice

R. D. WORKMAN and R. C. BORNMANN

The object of decompression research is the development of ascent procedures which are feasible in diving operations and which will not permit formation of inert gas bubbles in the tissues of the diver. Exposure to the oxygen content of the breathing mixture must not induce manifestations of acute or chronic toxicity. The choice of the inert gas component is limited by breathing resistance induced by density, tissue solubility and manifestations of narcosis affecting performance of the diver.

Operational considerations dictate that the diver must be returned to the surface in all sea states and water temperature conditions in the minimum time consistent with the avoidance of all possible risk of decompression sickness. Logistics of gas handling aboard ship restrict the number of different breathing mixtures that may be employed to hasten the elimination of inert gas from the tissues of the diver. A further constraint is imposed by the fire hazard associated with use of high oxygen tensions in the pressure chamber breathing atmosphere.

All these and other limiting factors must be considered in developing safe, efficient decompression procedures. The most crucial, and still controversial, aspect of decompression is the mathematical treatment of inert gas transport in the body tissues. This must meet two key criteria: it must be capable of dealing adequately with the limitations imposed by operational diving and it must permit the extraction of information from diving experience that is of predictive value to increase the probability of successful decompres-

sion under diving conditions in which parameters of pressure exposure, time and composition of the breathing mixture have been changed.

The mathematical models of inert gas transport and bubble formation in use today, and developed through years of experience in diving, differ mainly in their interpretation of three basic concepts. These are (1) the nature of the rate-limiting process in inert gas transport; (2) the character of the body tissues as this affects gas transport; and (3) the process of gas phase separation leading to formation of gas bubbles in body fluids and tissues, and thus to decompression sickness.

EARLY DEVELOPMENT OF DECOMPRESSION PROCEDURES IN THE US NAVY

The history of use and development of decompression procedures by the US Navy relates primarily to the decompression schedules developed for the use of the Royal Navy by J. S. Haldane and co-workers (Boycott, Damant & Haldane 1908) and submitted in the *Report to the Admiralty of the Deep-water Diving Committee* (Hamilton et al. 1907). These schedules provided stage decompression of the diver breathing air for diving depths to 204 ft (7·2 ATA). It is certain that the Haldane Tables, as they became known, were soon thereafter introduced into use by divers of the US Navy by French, who received diving training in the Royal Navy and by Stillson who directed the first experimental diving studies of the US Navy at the Brooklyn Navy Yard (Stillson 1915).

Experience in air diving at greater depths than provided by the Haldane Tables was begun under direction of French and Stillson, and culminated in a number of successful dives at a depth of 304 ft (10·4 ATA) during the salvage operation of the F-4 off Honolulu in 1915 (French 1916). Publication of schedules to provide for deeper air dives for use by the Royal Navy followed the work of Damant in 1933 (Davis 1962). Uniformly safe decompression from depths of 204 to 304 ft (7·2 to 10·4 ATA) required use of oxygen decompression from a stage depth of 60 ft (2·8 ATA) to the surface in the Davis submersible decompression chamber, which the diver entered for decompression following his depth exposure.

The Haldane Tables of the Royal Navy remained in use by the US Navy until revised decompression schedules were developed and tested by the US Navy Experimental Diving Unit in Washington D.C. in 1937. These schedules, as well as those for helium–oxygen diving developed at that time, employed the basic concepts and calculation procedures developed by Haldane. The primary difference was in the use of varying supersaturation criteria for the various half-time tissues controlling the ascent rather than the 2 to 1 ratio employed by Haldane for each tissue considered. (All ratios calculated using absolute pressures.)

Subsequent decompression studies used to develop repetitive decompression schedules for air and helium diving, surface decompression, and exceptional exposure schedules have all employed the basic Haldane concepts, with modifications considered necessary in refinement of the method to meet the varying requirements of far greater complexity than for air dives of limited depth and exposure time to which the original effort had been directed.

It is appropriate at this point to explore the Haldane theory of inert gas exchange in tissues and control of supersaturation of inert gas in tissue fluids so that symptoms of decompression sickness related to bubble formation do not occur. The various modifications that have been made to the basic method employed in developing the different decompression procedures for

mixed gas and repetitive diving will then be discussed.

DEVELOPMENT OF THE HALDANE METHOD OF DECOMPRESSION

The first systematic study of decompression requirements following exposure of animals and men to increased ambient pressure of air was reported by Boycott, Damant and Haldane (1908). As a result of numerous pressure exposures of small animals, goats and man, a rational basis for calculation of decompression schedules was derived. The basic tenets of their procedure, which has become known as the 'Haldane Method' relate to the estimation of the percentage of complete saturation or desaturation of the body tissues with nitrogen during any pressure exposure time-course, and the pressure of excess nitrogen in the body tissues related to hydrostatic pressure which is permissible without symptoms of decompression sickness occurring during or following the reduction of pressure to the surface (1 ATA).

The processes of saturation and desaturation with nitrogen were considered in the following manner. The blood passing through the lungs of a man breathing compressed air becomes instantly saturated with nitrogen at the existing partial pressure in the air. When this blood reaches the systemic capillaries, most of the excess nitrogen will diffuse out into the body tissues, and the blood will return to the lungs for a fresh charge. The process is repeated until all tissues are equilibrated with nitrogen at the same partial pressure as the air breathed. Since the blood supply to different parts of the body varies greatly, as does the capacity for dissolving nitrogen, it can be seen that the time taken for different parts of the body to become saturated with nitrogen will also vary.

Haldane and his associates (Boycott, Damant & Haldane 1908) estimated that the whole body of a man weighing 70 kg will take up about 1 L of nitrogen per atmosphere of excess air pressure, about 70% more nitrogen than an equal amount of blood would dissolve. With the weight of blood in man equal to 6·5% of the body weight, the amount of nitrogen held in solution in the completely saturated body tissues would be about

$170\% \div 6\cdot5\%$, or 26 times as great as the amount held in the blood alone. If the composition of the body were the same throughout, and the blood evenly distributed to all tissues, the body would receive in one round of circulation following sudden exposure to increased air pressure, one twenty-sixth of the nitrogen acquired at complete saturation. Each successive round of circulation would add one twenty-sixth of the remaining excess of nitrogen. The body tissues would be half-saturated in less than 20 rounds of circulation, or about 10 minutes, and equilibration would be complete in about an hour. The process of tissue saturation would follow an exponential curve for a specific tissue site, but it was not considered that this rate of saturation and desaturation would apply to the body as a whole. Actually, the rate of saturation would vary widely in different parts of the body, but for any particular part the rate of saturation and desaturation would follow a curve of this form, the circulation rate remaining constant (Fig. 17.1).

The variable time-course of nitrogen uptake for various parts of the body, relating to the different tissue perfusion rates with blood and capacities for dissolving nitrogen, was simulated by use of a geometrical series of discrete hypothetical half-time tissues (5, 10, 20, 40 and 75 min) to represent the spectrum of inert gas exchange rates of the whole body.

In decompression studies with goats, differences in respiratory exchange and cardiac output related to man were considered to be two-thirds greater for the goat per kg of body weight by direct measurements. Thus, a time of 3 hours was thought to be required for complete saturation of goats, while 5 hours was considered the requirement for man. The 75-min half-time used in their calculation of decompression would represent 7·5 hours time to 98·5% saturation. It appears that an attempt was made toward conservatism in that more time might be required for equilibration with nitrogen in some subjects. This rule was indicated to be adequate for 'obviating the risk of serious symptoms while at the same time reducing the chance of bends to a minimum' in the short dives at depths to 200 ft (7·1 ATA) typical of their day (Boycott, Damant & Haldane 1908).

In defining the time required for complete equilibration to the inert gas partial pressure of exposure depth, pressure exposure time was varied

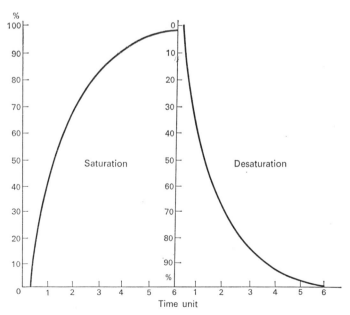

FIG. 17.1. Tissue saturation and desaturation curves. Time unit is equivalent to the specific half-time tissue considered

in animal experiments, the pressure and decompression time remaining constant. It is not evident from the data reported that equilibrium time was defined for man, as most exposures were not sufficiently long. This has become apparent in the inadequacy of schedules for longer dives derived by this method to provide safe decompression until half-times of 120 to 240 min were used.

Of equal importance to the method of estimating uptake and elimination of nitrogen is the concept of stage decompression developed from these studies. This procedure makes the fullest use of the permissible difference between nitrogen pressure in the tissues and blood to hasten the elimination of nitrogen from the body tissues. The limit applied to reduction of hydrostatic pressure was to never allow the computed nitrogen pressure in the tissues to be more than twice the ambient pressure. This 2 to 1 ratio actually assumed equilibration of the tissues to the ambient pressure of the depth exposure, rather than the nitrogen partial pressure. The absolute pressure of the maximum depth was then halved to determine the first decompression stop depth. A special case was assumed for air, for with its 79% nitrogen content the actual ratio of nitrogen pressure upon equilibration to ambient pressure would be

$$\frac{2}{1} \text{ATA} \times 0.79 = \frac{1.58}{1} \text{ATA}$$

It is true that this ignores the presence of oxygen in the breathing mixture as a factor in bubble formation. Extensive diving with nitrogen and helium mixture enriched with oxygen in excess of 21% in air has confirmed the absence of significant effect of oxygen as a part of the total pressure in decompression. It appears that if sufficient time is permitted for excess oxygen in tissues to be metabolized during reduction of pressure, decompression sickness due to oxygen supersaturation in tissues is unlikely to occur.

Decompression schedules for men based on the 2 to 1 ratio concept have, however, not provided adequate decompression for longer and deeper exposures. Haldane himself discussed this in his book *Respiration* (Haldane & Priestley 1935) by stating that for air dives exceeding 165 ft (6 ATA) some reduction of this ratio was required.

FURTHER STUDIES TO DEFINE SUPERSATURATION LIMITS IN DECOMPRESSION

Hawkins, Shilling and Hansen (1935) felt that the ratio of 2 to 1 was too conservative for fast tissues and not conservative enough for slow tissues. On the basis of an analysis of 2143 dives to depths between 100 and 200 ft (4·0 and 7·0 ATA) they determined more appropriate safe ratios for tissues of given desaturation half-times (Table 17.1). For calculation of decompression schedules

TABLE 17.1

Half-time for tissue desaturation (min)	Safe ratio
5	5·5 : 1
10	4·5 : 1
20	3·2 : 1
40	2·4 : 1
75	1·8 : 1 to 2·0 : 1

they ignored the 5- and 10-min tissues and used a ratio of 2·8 : 1 for the 20-min tissue, and 2·0 : 1 for the 40- and 75-min tissues. This modification made possible more efficient decompression in that deeper water stops than necessary are avoided and the fullest use is made of the permissible difference in pressure to hasten elimination of nitrogen from the body tissues.

Yarbrough (1937) calculated and tested revised US Navy Standard Air Decompression Tables by controlling only the 20-, 40- and 75-min tissues. The tissue ratios for the 5- and 10-min tissues appeared to be so high that they were not normally brought into control. The pattern of ratio reduction was somewhat irregular but the values were applied to fit empirical results (Table 17.2). Test of schedules calculated by the

TABLE 17.2

Half-time for tissue desaturation (min)	Safe ratio
20	2·45 : 1 to 2·8 : 1
40	1·75 : 1 to 2·0 : 1
75	1·75 : 1 to 2·0 : 1

three-tissue method indicated that the ratios had to be reduced to the lower values after prolonged exposure at greater depths. This requirement reflected increased rates of equilibration with nitrogen during exercise performed by the divers in tests of the schedules, whereas the tests carried out by Hawkins, Shilling and Hansen (1935) were at rest or with little exercise.

Further extensive evaluation of these decompression schedules was carried out by Van Der Aue, Brinton and Kellar (1945) in tests of surface decompression using air. They reported that 24% of 81 subjects developed symptoms of decompression sickness when standard decompression was used for working dives of long duration.

They further analysed available data to find logical values for tissue ratios. As a result of calculation and extensive testing of a series of surface decompression schedules using oxygen (Van Der Aue 1951) it was found that tissue ratios must be reduced considerably for all components in longer, deeper dives (2·2:1 to 2·0:1), that the fast tissues sometimes control deep stops even with high tissue ratios and that the surfacing ratios could be increased (Table 17.3).

TABLE 17.3

Half-time for tissue desaturation (min)	Safe ratio
5	3·8:1
10	3·4:1
20	2·8:1
40	2·27:1
75	2·06:1
120	2·00:1

Tissue ratios used to determine safety during the brief surface interval before recompression to 40 ft (2·2 ATA) with oxygen breathing are shown in Table 17.4.

Reduction of tissue ratios from values permissible upon surfacing to control supersaturation at decompression stops appears to be essential for calculations of safe decompression schedules by the Haldane method (Behnke 1947; Van Der Aue et al. 1951). There are several mathematical

TABLE 17.4

Half-time for tissue desaturation (min)	Safe ratio
20	3·54:1
40	3·54:1
75	2·94:1
120	2·60:1

physical evaluations to support this concept. Bateman (1951) derived a mathematical relationship between 'decompression ratio for symptom threshold' and 'body saturation with air before decompression'. Basically it results in a smooth reduction of tissue ratio with increased pressure. Piccard (1941) discussed the mathematical probability of a reduction in allowable supersaturation as the total mass of dissolved gas increases with increasing pressure. Russian studies have attempted to analyse permissible supersaturation ratios for air, helium–oxygen and helium–nitrogen–oxygen mixtures in diving (Brestkin 1965; Aleksandrov & Brestkin 1965; Brestkin, Gramenitskii & Sidorov 1965; Zal'tsman & Zinov'eva 1965). The permissible supersaturation value of the body with nitrogen following 6-hour air exposure of divers at 1 ATA and 7 ATA decreased from a ratio of 1·72:1 at 1 ATA to 1·3:1 at 7 ATA. For helium–oxygen mixtures breathed during dives at 3·25 ATA, a value of 2·66:1 was obtained, as compared with 2·4:1 at 2·95 ATA for air after 6-hour exposures under pressure.

Brestkin (1965) has attempted to analyse the changing critical ratio, initial gas tension/final absolute pressure (Po/P), of helium, nitrogen and carbon dioxide in water, with the production of visible bubbles as an endpoint. With an increase in gas tension, the critical ratio decreases as tension of gas increases up to 20 ATS and remains constant for further increases for helium and nitrogen. The absolute value for the critical ratio, as well as the magnitude of decrease with pressure, is greater for nitrogen than for helium. The pressure-dependent function of the critical ratio is explained by Laplacian surface tension and radius factors. The significance of these studies to operational diving has also been discussed with emphasis on the difference between physical and physiological systems (Zal'tsman & Zinov'eva 1965).

Calculation of revised US Navy Standard Air Decompression Schedules using a tenth-power relationship between tissue ratio at the surface (1 ATA) and at the depth of the decompression stop, with surfacing ratios and permissible depth ratios indicated by Van Der Aue et al. (1951), was reported by Des Granges (1956). The equation used to project the tissues ratios at depth, as developed by Dwyer (1956), is as follows:

$$M = 33 \left(\frac{rs}{rd}\right)^{10} + rd - 1$$

where M = maximum safe tissue pressure of nitrogen in feet of seawater absolute, rs = surfacing ratio in ATA, and rd = depth ratio at decompression stop in ATA.

Decompression schedules for air dives to a depth of 190 ft (6·8 ATA) were developed and tested at the US Navy Experimental Diving Unit, becoming available for fleet use in 1960. A review (Doll 1965) of decompression sickness resulting from use of these schedules over a two-year period reported an incidence of 0·69% as compared to 1·1% when using the schedules developed by Yarbrough (1937).

The current air decompression schedules (*US Navy Diving Manual 1974*) provide more adequately for scuba diving operations, in that depth increments of 10 ft and exposure time increments of 5 to 10 min are available for use. A 60 ft/min rate of ascent to the first decompression stop or to the surface permits ascent at an easy swim rate, where the 25 ft/min ascent rate of the previous air decompression schedules are considered too slow.

DEVELOPMENT OF REPETITIVE DIVE SCHEDULES FOR AIR DIVING

Operational use of scuba requires that many dives to various depths be performed over a period of hours. Thus, once the revised Standard Air Decompression Tables were developed, it became a necessity to devise a repetitive dive procedure employing them for use with scuba. After any

dive in which compressed air is breathed, variable and diminishing amounts of residual nitrogen remain in the body tissues of the diver for periods of 24 hours or more. This partial saturation will shorten the exposure time permitted for any subsequent repetitive dive deeper than 33 ft (2 ATA). The longer and deeper the first dive, the greater is the amount of residual tissue nitrogen remaining to obligate decompression for subsequent dives. Under such circumstances, the no-decompression depth-time allowances can no longer be employed with safety.

The many possible combinations of depth and exposure time of dives were grouped according to the initial surfacing tissue tension of nitrogen. It was then possible to determine the amount that the diver had desaturated during his surface time interval before diving again. It was then determined how many minutes it would require, at the depth of any subsequent dive, to equilibrate to the condition with which descent commenced. This permits addition of that time obligation to the actual exposure time to obtain an adequate decompression schedule from the Standard Air Decompression Table of the *US Navy Diving Manual*.

This procedure was implemented by assigning a letter group obligation in 2-ft increments to nitrogen supersaturation in the 120-min half-time tissue upon surfacing from any pressure exposure permitted from 0 ft (1 ATA) to 33 ft (2 ATA). Each dive schedule upon surfacing was then assigned a tissue group obligation from A through O, each of which represents 2 ft of inert gas in excess of 0 ft (1 ATA). Dive schedules requiring no decompression were also assigned letter group obligations on this basis. A surface interval credit table was then developed in hours and minutes required to lose tissue nitrogen and thus decrease obligation for decompression time of subsequent dives.

Equivalent depth-time exposures in terms of the same repetitive letter group obligations were developed in a repetitive dive timetable. Thus, following the surface interval, obligation to exposure time at various depths could be related to accumulated decompression obligation for subsequent dives. The Repetitive Dive Decompression Tables reported by Des Granges (1957) and detailed in the *US Navy Diving Manual* (NAVSHIPS 0994–001–9010, 1974), have been used safely and effectively to make thousands of repetitive dives breathing air since official approval for use by fleet divers in 1960.

Air decompression schedules for exceptional exposures

The revised Standard Air Decompression Table (Des Granges 1957) was developed to provide safe decompression for dives up to 190 ft (6·7 ATA) for 60 min. Dives between 200 and 300 ft (7·1 and 10·1 ATA) were tested and reported as a part of that study, but were included in a second report (Workman 1957) as the second half of the Revised Tables for exceptional exposures. It was considered that air dives to greater depths than 190 ft (7·6 ATA) for 60 min would not be a part of routine diving practice and should be in a separate table of dives for longer and deeper exposures.

An Air Saturation Decompression Table to provide for the emergency situation of the trapped diver whose exposure exceeded that of the Standard Air Decompression Table had been developed previously on the basis of the Haldane method in which the 75-min half-time tissue was controlled on a constant 2 to 1 ratio of absolute pressure. Though this Table had been in the *US Navy Diving Manual* for years, there was little information on the safety in its use following prolonged exposure to compressed air. Following the extensive testing of decompression schedules reported by Des Granges (1957), it became recognized that marked reduction in ratios for slower tissues than 75 min was required at decompression stops in the water and upon surfacing. An attempt was made to develop and test schedules to provide safe decompression from deeper and longer air dives (Workman 1957).

The tenth-power reduction of depth ratios reported by Dwyer (1956), used to calculate the revised Standard Air Decompression Tables (Des Granges 1957), was used initially to develop decompression schedules to be tested for air dives of 140 ft (5·25 ATA) for 90- to 360-min exposures. This type of supersaturation control, and several other empirical approaches, proved inadequate until applied to half-time tissues of 120, 160 and 240 min. Review of a series of air exposures evaluated by Van der Aue (1945, unpublished) of 12 hours at 99 ft (4 ATA), followed by 12 to 24 hours at 33 ft (2 ATA), showed that a 2 to 1 ratio was unsafe upon surfacing and that half-time tissues of 240 min required control in decompression.

Using an empirical reduction of tissue ratio for the 40-, 80-, 120-, 160- and 240-min half-time tissues based on safe values at 33 ft (2 ATA), decompression schedules were developed to provide for air exposures of 40 ft (2·2 ATA) to 140 ft (5·25 ATA) for 12 hours, 170 ft (6·15 ATA) for 8 hours, 200 ft (7 ATA) for 6 hours, 250 ft (8·6 ATA) for 4 hours and 300 ft (10 ATA) for 3 hours. Test of these schedules was only possible for 140 ft (5·25 ATA) for 6 hours and 300 ft (10 ATA) for 1 hour in which the results were sufficiently good to warrant promulgation for use on an emergency basis.

STUDIES OF THE RATE-LIMITING PROCESS IN INERT GAS TRANSPORT

While the use of 160- and 240-min half-time compartments in control of air decompression has been questioned (Behnke 1967; Hempleman 1967), Jones (1950), in one very fully studied case, demonstrated a nitrogen elimination rate constant ($K_5 = 0.0025$) equivalent to 277-min half-time. Recent studies in dogs show that 80 to 90% of the total nitrogen is stored in slow compartments perfused by 10 to 15% of the cardiac output and has a time constant of 150 to 250 min (Farhi, Homma & Berger 1962). It is also considered a distinct possibility that whole body nitrogen elimination studies, performed by analysis of nitrogen in exhaled gas during oxygen breathing may be quite limited in determination of the trace amounts of nitrogen in mixed venous blood returned to the lungs from poorly perfused tissue depots. Thus the slowest rate constants for inert gas elimination would never be defined by this method.

In carefully performed determinations of the bends threshold depth for large dogs (48 to 82 lb) exposed to air for 7, 12, 18 and 24 hours followed by direct ascent to surface (1 ATA), Reeves and

Beckman (1966) reported that the bends threshold was consistently reproducible for each individual animal, that the range of threshold depth varied between animals from 57 ft (2·7 ATA) and 86 ft (3·6 ATA) and that the threshold depth was less following durations of pressure exposure of 18 and 24 hours than at 7 hours' exposure. It would appear that equilibration with the nitrogen pressure in air was not achieved following 7 hours' exposure, and that the additional nitrogen taken up by body tissues following 18- to 24-hour exposures resulted in decompression sickness being manifest in these animals when exposed at the same depth as for 7 hours. Since it is considered that animals with less body mass have a greater rate of tissue perfusion with blood than man (Kindwall 1962), equilibration time of 18 hours for large dogs would predict even longer equilibration time for man. In these studies, equivalence of rate of gas uptake and elimination is not in question since ascent was made directly to surface (1 ATA) where the animals were observed for onset of decompression sickness. This was readily evident when it occurred and was promptly resolved with recompression of the animal such that endpoint criteria were decisively demonstrated.

DEVELOPMENT OF HELIUM–OXYGEN DECOMPRESSION SCHEDULES FOR DEEP DIVING

Initial interest in the use of helium–oxygen mixtures in diving originated in a series of letters by Elihu Thomson to W. R. Watson of the General Electric Laboratories in which it was suggested that helium be used in caisson and diving work (Roth 1967). Its use was to avoid the limit set on diving depth by the supposed unavailability of oxygen from compressed air at great depths. The idea was based on 'the principle of superior rapidity of diffusion of the low density gas' (Thomson 1927). Shortly thereafter, the eminent physical chemist J. H. Hildebrand suggested to Sayers and Yant of the Bureau of Mines that the lesser coefficient of solubility of helium than nitrogen would make it of use in preventing caisson disease, Sayers and Yant (1925, 1926) performed experiments using helium–

oxygen mixtures with guinea pigs to show decompression advantage over compressed air and suggested that helium be tried in human dives. End (1937) reported on the use of helium in human diving with decompression time as low as one twenty-third of that predicted by the air schedules used at that time.

Behnke and Yarbrough (1938) reported their experience with helium in diving operations in which it was used primarily to avoid the narcotic effects of nitrogen at depths as great as 300 ft (10 ATA). They suggested that the lower oil/water solubility ratio of helium should decrease decompression sickness as well as nitrogen narcosis. In their studies it was reported that there was a distinct absence of severe symptoms of decompression sickness in divers who experienced bends. No cases of unconsciousness or paralysis were reported and itching and skin rash occurred without other sequelae. This compared to air diving in which neurocirculatory collapse and paralysis occurred. Pains which occurred following helium dives were promptly relieved by recompression, whereas pain tended to persist following equivalent air dives. Behnke postulated that when helium–oxygen mixtures were breathed in diving, the controlling tissues during decompression are those which are rapidly saturated and desaturated, whereas with nitrogen the slow or fatty tissues controlled.

Behnke and Willmon (1941) compared the saturation–desaturation curves for nitrogen and helium. The helium capacity of the body was found to be $8·0 \pm 1·3$ cm^3/kg of body weight when the tissues are in equilibrium with a helium alveolar pressure of 1 ATA. This value is about 40% of the total nitrogen absorbed under these conditions. However, helium–oxygen saturation periods of only 3·5 hours were used which may not have been sufficiently long to establish equilibrium of body tissues with alveolar helium partial pressure. They also found that the time required to eliminate absorbed helium is 50% of the time required for nitrogen elimination. This period for helium elimination was decreased by half with exercise.

Exposure time at depth is an important factor in predicting decompression hazard. The total amount of gas dissolved in the body tissues at depth is determined by the saturation-time relationship implied by desaturation curves for nitrogen and helium. Behnke (1947) in analysing this, suggested that 75% of the total body nitrogen is eliminated from the body tissues of lean men in about 2 hours. Following exposure at the usual diving depths, this rapidly exchanging nitrogen is eliminated without causing symptoms. It is the small amount of nitrogen dissolved in fatty tissues that requires many hours for elimination. Behnke demonstrated that, for a subject breathing air at 90 ft (3·7 ATA) for 9 hours, about 12 hours of decompression were required. If helium–oxygen mixtures were used instead of air no more than 79 min of oxygen-breathing decompression were required after all durations of exposure to this depth up to 9 hours.

If lipid substances are responsible for the prolongation of nitrogen absorption and elimination, helium, possessing a lesser solubility coefficient in slowly perfusing fatty tissue, should be eliminated in a shorter period of time. We have seen that total body nitrogen elimination curves have been interpreted to demonstrate slow compartments of 150 to 280 min half-time. Comparable total body helium elimination curves have been published by Jones (1950), Behnke and Willmon (1941) and Duffner and Snider (1958). These studies report the slowest compartment to be 70, 115 and 95 min half-time, respectively. The studies of Duffner and Snider followed 12-hour exposures at depths to 50 ft (2·5 ATA), whereas the other two studies were conducted following much shorter exposures. It would appear that half-time tissues at least as slow as 115 min would require control in calculation of helium–oxygen dives. Comparing the accepted values of the partition coefficient (water/tissue) for nitrogen as a_1 and helium as a_2, where $a_1 = 1/5·2$ and $a_2 = 1/1·7$, then $a_1/a_2 = 1/3$. This means that the very slow fat compartment seen when breathing nitrogen will be altered when breathing helium to a tissue with a half-time three times smaller. Taking 280 min as an upper range for the half-time on nitrogen, one would expect the corresponding half-time on helium to be approximately 100 min, which is very close to that derived by the studies discussed previously. The effective satura-

tion time for helium would then be of the order of 10 to 12 hours.

If the error of analysis for helium is comparable to nitrogen, the lesser quantity of helium eliminated in alveolar gas should cause the elimination curve to approach an asymptote sooner than for nitrogen, thus giving the impression that helium had all been eliminated from the body tissues when it had not. Thus, there is a possibility for somewhat slower half-time tissues to exist for helium than determined in whole body elimination studies by the alveolar gas analysis method.

The first helium–oxygen decompression schedules developed for use of operational fleet divers were reported by Momsen and Wheland (1939). These schedules were subsequently revised by Molumphy (1950) by reducing the depth of oxygen breathing stops during decompression from 60 ft (2·8 ATA) and 50 ft (2·5 ATA) to 50 ft (2·5 ATA) and 40 ft (2·2 ATA).

The method used to calculate these schedules was basically that developed by Haldane with certain modifications required for the helium–oxygen diving equipment and mixtures to be used at great depths. These modifications are as follows:

1. The partial pressure of helium in the mixture breathed at the depth of the dive was used to compute schedules from 60 ft (2·8 ATA) to 410 ft (12·4 ATA) in 10-ft increments.

2. Exposure time on each partial pressure schedule was provided in 10- to 20-min increments from 10 to 240 min.

3. The minimum oxygen percentage permitted was 16%, with all calculations made on an 86% helium–14% oxygen mixture to allow for oxygen use by the diver in a recirculating system.

4. All dives were calculated for twice the exposure time of the schedule to allow for increased helium uptake by body tissues during exercise on working dives.

5. Half-time tissues were considered in arithmetical progression, i.e. 5, 10, 20, 30, 40, 50, 60 and 70 min.

6. A ratio of 1·7 to 1 of tissue helium pressure to absolute pressure of the decompression stop depth was used to control the limit of supersaturation. This is equivalent to a 2·15 to 1 ratio of absolute pressure of the exposure depth to

absolute pressure of the decompression stop as used by Haldane where air is considered 100% nitrogen. It was not stated in the report how the 1·7 to 1 ratio was derived, but its value of 56 to 33 ft absolute coincides with the minimum safe surfacing value determined by Duffner and Snider (1958) following 12-hour exposures at 37 ft (2·12 ATA) while breathing an 80% helium–20% oxygen mixture.

7. Divers breathed 100% oxygen at decompression stops at 60 ft (2·8 ATA) and 50 ft (2·5 ATA) to complete decompression, following which they surfaced directly. The oxygen was considered to contain 20% helium or to be 80% efficient.

8. A method of surface decompression was developed by which divers breathed oxygen at 50 ft (2·5 ATA) for time equal to the oxygen period at 60 ft (2·8 ATA) before surfacing directly, to be recompressed again within 5 min to 50 ft (2·5 ATA) to complete the full scheduled oxygen breathing time at that depth in the deck pressure chamber.

9. Rate of ascent to the first water stop and between water stops varied from 10 to 75 ft/min, increasing with depth and oxygen percentage in the breathing mixture. Ascent time for all except the initial ascent to the first stop was included in the decompression time of the subsequent stop.

10. Repetitive diving was not allowed for a period of 12 hours after surfacing from a dive.

The first operational use of the helium–oxygen tables for deep diving was reported by Behnke and Willmon (1939) during salvage operations on the submarine *Squalus*. A review of incidence of decompression sickness in use of these helium–oxygen schedules (Doll 1965) reported 6 cases in 721 dives, an incidence of 0·83%.

Molumphy (1950) reported results of 49 dives at greater depth than the published schedules performed at the US Navy Experimental Diving Unit. Dives of 10-min exposure were made to depths of 495 ft (16 ATA) and 561 ft (18 ATA) with freedom from symptoms. A number of attempts were made to perform working dives at 495 ft (16 ATA) for 20-min exposures, with bends resulting in 12 of 26 dives, though the supersaturation ratio controlling decompression was reduced to 1·5 to 1 from 1·7 to 1, and half-time

tissues to 100 min were considered. Symptoms occurred at decompression stops as deep as 110 ft, as an indication of the relative inadequacy of the decompression. As a matter of interest, two 10-min dives to 485 ft (15·7 ATA) were made in the open sea off Key West and a 500-ft (16·2 ATA) dive was made off Panama in 1949 without incident.

Use of helium–oxygen in mixed gas scuba

Further study of helium–oxygen decompression was undertaken by Duffner, Snyder and Smith (1959) in a task to develop schedules for use of helium–oxygen mixtures in semi-closed mixed gas scuba. It was considered desirable to avoid risk of carbon dioxide retention, oxygen toxicity and narcosis at depth by substituting a less dense breathing mixture for nitrogen–oxygen, in current use by operational swimmers at that time. A minimal decompression curve for dives in which 80% helium–20% oxygen was breathed by subjects was established during 109 test dive schedules at various depth-time exposures. Seventy-eight dive schedules employing decompression were tested to determine adequacy of decompression predicted by a calculation procedure developed by Rashbass (1955). This procedure considered only one critical hypothetical tissue in which inert gas diffuses slowly across a tissue slab linearly rather than by perfusion or transcapillary radial diffusion. The structure and inert gas equilibration characteristics were made consistent with well-established ascent schedules in diving. The time course of the quantity of nitrogen or helium in the tissue following a step function in the blood gas tension at a time when the tissue and blood are in equilibrium was analysed by Hill's (1928) solution of the Fick equation. In contrast to a limiting supersaturation ratio of the Haldane approach, the Rashbass method used a finite tissue pressure head of inert gas (ΔP) exceeding ambient pressure as critical. This was fixed at 30 ft (0·9 ATA) of water for nitrogen by Rashbass, and 37 ft (1·12 ATA) of water for helium by Duffner.

The minimal decompression curve for 80% helium–20% oxygen was projected as a function of pressure (P) and the square root of time (t) at depth ($Pt^{1/2}$ = constant). Comparison of safe minimal decompression dives for helium–oxygen show a significantly longer exposure time permitted at all depths tested than for comparable air dives. Similar to air diving practice, a 60 ft/min ascent rate was found safe for both minimal dives and decompression dives.

Workman and Reynolds (1965) evaluated the complete log of all dives performed in the study by Duffner, Snyder and Smith (1959) and determined that decompression prediction by the calculation method of Duffner, modified from Rashbass (1955), was not adequate for longer exposures. This, and the necessity to develop a repetitive dive method for helium–oxygen dives which had been done successfully for air dives by the modified Haldane method (Des Granges 1957), encouraged them to utilize this method of calculation. Recalculation of existing safe dive schedules permitted determination of permissible surfacing tissue tension values for minimal and decompression dives (Table 17.5). It will be noted that the

TABLE 17.5

Half-time for tissue desaturation (min)	Safe ratio	Safe $He + N_2$ tissue tension (ft)
5	3·50	116
10	2·80	92
20	2·24	74
40	1·88	62
80	1·70	56
120	1·60	53

ratio, and its statement in feet of seawater tissue tension of helium and nitrogen residual in tissues, differs from the ratio used by Haldane for air diving in which total pressure of the exposure was considered to be with 100% nitrogen. In the helium–oxygen schedules of Momsen and Wheland (1939) and Molumphy (1950), the helium pressure of the inspired mixture was used in calculation, as well as 26 ft (0·79 ATA) of nitrogen to which the tissues were equilibrated on air prior to the helium dive. In calculation of the helium–oxygen schedules for mixed gas diving, it was determined that the sum of the gas exchange gradients for helium and nitrogen during uptake

and elimination was equal to that when only one inert gas was considered. This would be the worst case that could occur, even though the anatomical tissue sites represented by the same theoretical half-time tissue differ for helium and nitrogen.

The surfacing ratios of helium and nitrogen were not projected to depth as constant ratios (Po/P), but rather as a constant value of tissue tension exceeding ambient or hydrostatic pressure by the following equation:

$$Po - P = \text{constant}$$

where Po = tissue tension of $He + N_2$ (feet, seawater), and P = hydrostatic pressure (feet, seawater). The values for control of supersaturation at decompression stops are shown in Table 17.6.

TABLE 17.6

Half-time for tissue desaturation (min)	$Po - P$ (ATS)	$Po - P$ (ft seawater)
5	2·50	83
10	1·80	59
20	1·24	41
40	0·88	29
80	0·70	23
120	0·60	20

The $Po - P = K$ control for each half-time tissue was used when it became apparent that somewhat deeper decompression stops were required for helium dives than air dives, after the tenth-power air controls of supersaturation had been employed with little success.

Once single dive decompression schedules were proved adequate for dives in a range of 50 ft (2·5 ATA) for 200 min, to 200 ft (7 ATA) for 30 min with a 75% helium to 25% oxygen breathing mixture, a repetitive dive format identical to that developed for air dives was constructed. Twenty-seven series of three repetitive dives per series were evaluated to test all possible variables of shallow, medium and deep depth and short, medium and long exposure time and surface interval time. These dive series were made up to avoid duplication of depth and exposure time, to permit testing as many different individual dive schedules as possible throughout the test series.

Uniformly safe results of these tests confirmed the prediction of safe decompression from repetitive dives when helium–oxygen was breathed, a matter which had no prior verification.

A method utilizing oxygen decompression at 30 ft (1·9 ATA) and 20 ft (1·6 ATA) depth water stops was also provided as optional for both single and repetitive dives to decrease decompression time and provide maximum freedom from symptoms of decompression sickness. More than 400 single and repetitive open-sea dives at depths to 200 ft (7 ATA) have been performed without decompression sickness or oxygen toxicity occurring during use by operational diving personnel.

DECOMPRESSION AFTER SATURATION DIVING

For project Sealab of the US Navy and Operation Genesis which preceded it, the Experimental Diving Unit was asked to formulate and test decompression schedules from exposures of several days duration at 100 ft (4 ATA), 200 ft (7 ATA), 300 ft (10 ATA) and 450 ft (14·6 ATA). Operation Genesis was a series of laboratory investigations by Bond (1963, 1964) to test methods and procedures for saturation diving prior to placing human divers on the sea bottom to operate from an undersea station, the Sealab operations of 1964 and 1965.

The inert gas of the breathing mixture used in these studies was principally helium. The oxygen partial pressure was carefully controlled between 0·2 and 0·5 ATA to avoid manifestation of long-term pulmonary oxygen toxicity.

As the duration of pressure exposure increases, the obligated decompression increases since a greater amount of inert gas dissolves in the more slowly desaturating tissues. An advantage is offered through the application of saturation diving in that after some finite period of time the body tissues become completely equilibrated with inert gas in the atmosphere at the pressure of the exposure. The decompression obligation is limited to that amount. Further exposure should result in no increase in decompression requirement and the ratio of dive time to decompression time becomes more favourable. Since even the slowest equilibrating tissues are saturated with inert gas

at the exposure depth, decompression will be regulated by the rate at which these tissues eliminate the inert gas. Therefore the technique of a uniform rate of ascent appears to be most appropriate for decompression from saturation exposures.

Schreiner and Kelley (1967) have provided an excellent review of the mathematical and theoretical aspects of linear ascent of saturation and non-saturation exposures. Their approach is that of Haldane inert gas exchange concepts, but with the extent of tissue supersaturation with inert gas as a function of ambient pressure and the rate constant of gas exchange as described by Workman (1965).

$$\sum \pi \leq M \text{ (ATA)}$$
$$M = f(D \text{ ATA}, K)$$

where $\sum \pi$ = sum of partial pressure of dissolved inert gas in tissue, M = permissible inert gas partial pressure as supersaturation criteria, K = specific time constant of inert gas exchange in tissue = $\ln 2/t_{1/2}$, $t_{1/2}$ = half-time and D = seawater depth. The rate at which inert gas is taken up or released by a given half-time tissue is proportional to the difference between the ambient inert gas partial pressure and the partial pressure of the same inert gas dissolved in a given tissue. Thus

$$\frac{d\pi}{dt} = K(P - \pi)$$

with the boundary condition $t = 0$, $\pi = \pi_0$, where P = partial pressure of inspired inert gas and t = time (min). In the special case of saturation diving with helium–oxygen with P_{O_2} = constant

$$M = H + \Delta P \ \Delta P_{240} = \text{constant}$$

where H = absolute hydrostatic pressure, ΔP = excess supersaturation pressure of inert gas dissolved in tissue = $(\pi - H)$, and 240 = minutes of half-time tissue.

$$P = D + A - P_{O_2}$$

where A = atmospheric sea level pressure (1 ATA) and $D = \pi - \Delta P - A$. Then

$$P = \pi - \Delta P - P_{O_2}$$
$$(\Delta P + P_{O_2}) = (P - \pi) = \text{constant}$$

$$\frac{d\pi}{dt} = K(\pi - \Delta P - Po_2 - \pi)$$

$$= -K(\Delta P + Po_2)$$

Thus, when a constant Po_2 and a constant ΔP are specified for a given theoretical half-time tissue, it follows that the driving force for gas exchange $(P - \pi)$ is also constant. In this case the ascent function must be linear. The ascent rate must be such that 1 ft of inert gas will desaturate from the 240-min half-time tissue during the time required to decrease ambient pressure by 1 ft.

$$\frac{d\pi}{dt} = -\frac{0.693}{240H}(20 + 10) = \frac{11.6 \text{ min}}{1 \text{ ft}}$$

$0.693 = \ln 2$, $K = 0.693/t_{1/2}$, $\Delta P = 20$ ft seawater, $Po_2 = 0.3$ ATA $= 10$ ft seawater. Therefore, about 12 min are required to ascend 1 ft of seawater depth when the 240-min half-time tissue controls the helium elimination at a permissible supersaturation (ΔP) of 20 ft seawater pressure of helium.

A series of 24-hour exposures dives at 200 ft (7 ATA), 300 ft (10 ATA) and 400 ft (13 ATA) with subjects breathing a helium–oxygen atmosphere in a dry chamber, with Po_2 maintained at 0.5 ATA, was made to determine subject performance and adequacy of decompression. It was assumed initially that a limiting 180-min half-time tissue would provide conservative decompression and that a 150-min half-time might be the slowest to be considered. Three subjects were decompressed without symptoms following a 12-day exposure at 200 ft (7 ATA) at a constant rate of 8.25 min/ft seawater depth.

During the decompression from the first exposure of two subjects to 300 ft (10 ATA) for 24 hours, one diver noted onset of pain in one knee at 75 ft (3.28 ATA) with use of the 8.25 min/ft ascent rate. Recompression was effective in resolving symptoms and he was brought to the surface safely at the twice slower rate of 16.5 min/ft.

It was now considered necessary to control half-time tissues as slow as 240 min, since the 180-min half-time control proved unsafe for this subject. With a constant Po_2 of 0.5 ATA maintained in the helium–oxygen atmosphere and a ΔP supersaturation of 20 ft (0.6 ATA), the constant rate of ascent required would be 11 min/ft.

Another pair of divers completed a similar exposure to 300 ft (10 ATA) and were decompressed without incident at this rate. A third pair of divers were exposed for 24 hours to a pressure of 400 ft (13 ATA) and similarly decompressed without incident (Bornmann 1967).

The method of continuous ascent at a constant rate was used to decompress four divers in Sealab I following a 12-day exposure at 193 ft (6.9 ATA) without incident. In the Sealab II operation at 204 ft (7.2 ATA), 28 successful decompressions were made at a constant rate of 10 min/ft of ascent. The length of the dives was 2 weeks, except for one subject who stayed at depth for 4 weeks. One diver who celebrated his fiftieth birthday during the dive developed knee pain at 35 ft (2.1 ATA) which was treated successfully by recompression, oxygen breathing and slower ascent to the surface.

In preparatory dives for Sealab III at the Experimental Diving Unit, teams of 4 men on each dive have been exposed up to 72 hours at depths to 450 ft (14.6 ATA), during which they have completed excursion dives from 450 ft (14.6 ATA) to 600 ft (19.2 ATA) to perform useful work for 1 hour, with direct return to 450 ft (14.6 ATA) without incident. These simulated dives in the wet–dry pressure complex have demonstrated the feasibility of divers working down to the depth of the continental shelf limits from an underwater station at 450 ft (14.6 ATA).

During these deeper saturation dives with rapid compression to depth, joint pain has been noticed in all subjects within several hours after reaching maximum depth of 200 ft (7 ATA) or more. Linear compression at a rate of 1.5 min/ft was instituted to permit hydrostatic pressure distribution in semi-rigid tissues such as cartilage, in which it has been hypothesized that shearing forces were developed by rapid compression, and maintained for sufficient time to induce tissue injury in painful joints. By this means symptoms incidental to compression have been largely avoided. This avoidance of tissue injury is felt to be important to provide safe decompression for these divers.

In these dives, a Po_2 of 0.3 ATS has been maintained in the chamber atmosphere to reduce risk of pulmonary oxygen effects and of combustion hazard. Therefore, it was necessary to reduce the ascent rate to 12·5 min/ft depth decrease. As this rate did not provide freedom from symptoms in some subjects, a rate of 15 min/ft and stages of 4 hours at depth changes of 100 ft (3 ATA) up to 150 ft (5·55 ATA) and at 50-ft stages to the surface were instituted. This was an attempt to interrupt the excess supersaturation time-dependent probability function in bubble formation. It is apparent that supersaturation of tissues with inert gas is maintained for much longer periods of time during ascent from deeper dives.

EXCURSION DIVING FROM SATURATION EXPOSURES AT DEPTH

Through use of submersible decompression chambers (SDC), it has become possible for the diver to be placed at the underwater site to carry out productive work for a period of hours, and then be returned to a deck decompression chamber (DDC) for final decompression. Series of work dives may be carried out by teams of divers from a saturation depth in the DDC, being transferred to and from the work site by the SDC. Decompression is then required only upon completion of the work period. The development of saturation diving techniques has naturally led to a consideration of the advantage of 'excursion diving' from these deeper platforms. It is not a completely new concept, however, since normal diving from sea level has also been excursion diving from a saturation exposure to nitrogen–oxygen at a pressure of one atmosphere. If one calculates decompression by the method used in the US Navy (Workman 1965) it can be shown (Figs 17.2 and 17.3) that the allowable inert gas oversaturation, which is the limiting element for these excursions, becomes greater as depth increases. Therefore, the magnitude of dives permitted from a saturation exposure at depth becomes greater and greater compared to excursion dives from the surface. This was first demonstrated (Larsen & Mazzone 1967) in a study prior to Sealab II to establish safe depth-time limits for air excursions from an air saturation dive at 35 ft (2·1 ATA). Other work using helium–oxygen mixtures soon followed (Krasberg 1966; Hamilton, Fructus & Fructus 1968; Schreiner & Kelley 1970).

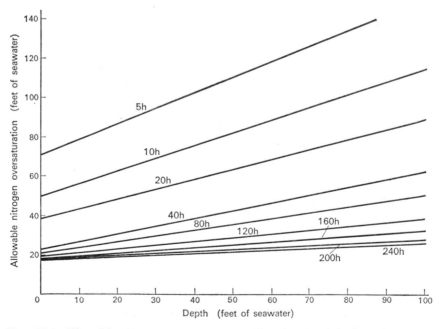

FIG. 17.2. Allowable nitrogen oversaturation related to depth in feet of seawater for half-time tissues (*h*) from 5 through 240 min.

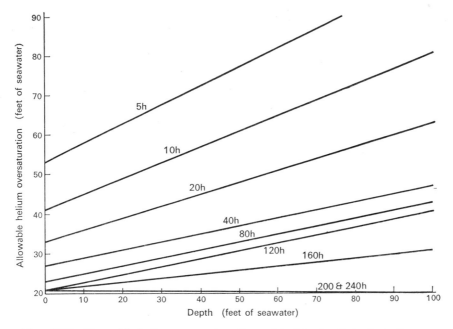

FIG. 17.3. Allowable helium oversaturation related to depth in feet of sea-water for half-time tissues (*h*) from 5 through 240 min.

TABLE 17.7

No-decompression limit table, repetitive group designation table, and repetitive excursion timetable for excursions from a saturation exposure at a depth between 150 ft and 300 ft of seawater gauge depth

Depth of excursion from saturation exposure	No-decompression limits (min)	Repetitive group designation					
		A	B	C	D	E	F
Plus 25 feet		60	150	300	600		
50	270	30	60	100	150	210	270
75	150	20	40	65	90	120	150
100	60	10	20	30	40	50	60

In 1969 the US Navy carried out a year-long test of tables for no-decompression helium–oxygen excursions from helium–oxygen saturation dives (Bornmann 1970). In the program at the Experimental Diving Unit 1126 individual repetitive dives were made without incident and three tables (Tables 17.7, 17.8 and 17.9) were approved for service use in accordance with the instructions given in Appendix I of that report. The tables are similar in format and use to the other repetitive diving tables of the US Navy.

Basic calculations in the design of these tables were made in accordance with the method of Workman. These are summarized in Fig. 17.4, where it can be seen that the limiting elements were considered to be the 20- and 40- as well as the 200-min half-time tissue. The surprising absence of any difficulty with the excursions during the testing period does suggest that some safety and conservatism was embodied in the limits chosen. The criterion for adequacy was the absence of symptoms of decompression sickness during the

TABLE 17.8

No-decompression limit table, repetitive group designation table, and repetitive excursion timetable for excursions from a saturation exposure at a depth between 300 ft and 600 ft of seawater gauge depth

Depth of excursion from saturation exposure	No-decompression limits (min)	Repetitive group designation					
		A	B	C	D	E	F
Plus 25 feet	—	60	150	300	600		
50	270	30	60	100	150	210	270
75	150	20	40	65	90	120	150
100	100	15	30	45	60	80	100
125	75	10	20	30	45	60	75
150	60	10	20	30	40	50	60

TABLE 17.9

Habitat interval credit table for saturation exposure at a depth between 150 ft and 600 ft of seawater gauge depth

Repetitive group at the beginning of the habitat interval (from previous excursion)	Repetitive group at the end of the habitat interval (before repetitive excursion)					
	F	E	D	C	B	A
F	to 1:00	2:30	4:00	6:30	12:00	24:00
E		1:30	3:00	5:30	10:00	24:00
D			2:00	4:00	8:00	24:00
C				2:30	6:30	24:00
B					4:00	24:00
A						24:00

24-hour period following the excursion. Some difficulty was encountered in subsequent decompression from the saturation exposure, as will be described later, and it is possible that this was related to the earlier situation of repetitive excursion diving. Barnard (1971) in an unpublished investigation at the Royal Naval Physiological Laboratory at Alverstoke studied a profile of decompression from helium–oxygen saturation dives which utilized a combination of 24-hour stage stops and fairly rapid intervening ascents. It is interesting to note that initial ascents of considerable magnitude could be made without incident, but these did seem to be associated with difficulty following other ascents later in the decompression. Still, a relatively minor adjustment of the M values permitted at depth would allow for a 50% increase of excursion time in the American tables, and a follow-on

program of testing was planned by the Experimental Diving Unit for the spring of 1974 to investigate this possibility. That experience will be analysed and the results inserted, as corrections if necessary, into the M value matrix.

A considerable amount of work, sponsored chiefly by the US Navy and the National Oceanic and Atmospheric Administration (NOAA), has been conducted to study excursions from saturation dives between 30 and 100 ft (1·9 and 4·0 ATA) using compressed air or nitrogen–oxygen atmosphere (Hamilton et al. 1973; Adams 1974). Due to the complexity and cost of maintaining a closed-chamber environment of helium–oxygen mixture, shallow saturation diving using a gaseous atmosphere obtained from air could be accomplished considerably more easily and more cheaply. It has been postulated also that in caisson operations to depths greater than 75 feet

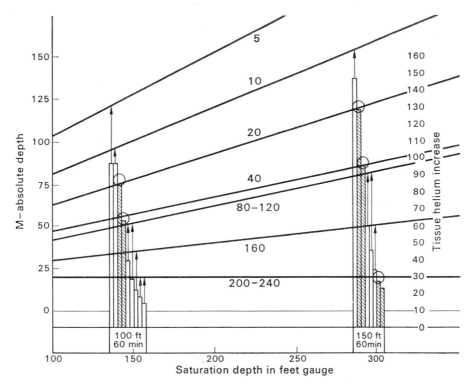

FIG. 17.4. Use of display of M values in relation to depth as a means of estimating the shallowest saturation exposure possible for certain no-decompression excursions

(3·3 ATA) there is considerable advantage in economy as well as in safety to the use of a saturation-excursion technique. An increasing amount of evidence indicates that the incidence of aseptic bone necrosis of compressed air work is related more to the adequacy and frequency of decompressions than to any other factor. A short, safe ascent from the pressure of the working face to an air saturation exposure at 35 to 50 feet (2·1 to 2·5 ATA) would permit more working time per shift. The major decompression from that level to the surface might require several days to complete but would need to be undergone only once or twice per month. If the frequency of aseptic bone necrosis in the workers was reduced by this technique, that factor alone would compensate for the increased capital investment required.

Evidence from one NOAA-sponsored study (Hamilton et al. 1973) indicates that nitrogen narcosis in an air excursion dive from a nitrogen saturation base at 100 ft (4 ATA) is not as incapacitating as in deep air dives to the equivalent depth from the surface. That project and a related Navy one (Adams 1974) tested limits also for 'negative' excursion dives, i.e. excursions upward in depth to pressures less than that of the saturation exposure.

The statement has been made that dives to depths greater than 1000 ft (31 ATA) can be more easily reached as excursions from helium saturation exposures near 800 ft (25·2 ATA) as a base depth. However, where the main focus of the intermediate depth studies mentioned has been to delineate the limits for decompression under the conditions tested, much more understanding is required of the effect of pressure per se and pressure rate changes at great depths on the cerebrospinal and cardiovascular responses of the human diver before such deep excursion operations can be routinely and safely executed.

Contrary to expectations, the saturation decompression procedures developed for the Sealab program did not work as well as had been hoped in the Experimental Diving Unit program of saturation-excursion table testing. It was not certain that the prior period of extensive excursion pressure changes was the cause of the difficulties encountered, most of which appeared between 50 ft (2·5 ATA) and the surface. However, it was felt that further slowing of the rate of ascent throughout the entire decompression was not the optimum correction. A continuous, long-term exposure to sustained inert gas over-pressures within the body seems to be qualitatively different from the usual situation in stage decompression where tissue gas levels are raised initially and then fall off over the period of the stop. A uniform daily schedule was tested in which the rate of ascent is determined by the depth, with slowing as the diver approaches the surface, but the ascent itself is done in a continuous fashion in two separate 8-hour periods separated by a 2-hour stage stop in the afternoon and a 6-hour overnight 'sleep' stop. Although the new method did not completely eliminate decompression sickness in this Navy series, it sharply decreased its incidence and the few cases seen were 'pain only bends', easily treated by a short return to higher pressure. More study is required to compare the results of European methods of saturation decompression which bring the diver out in roughly one half of the time used in American practice.

DEEPER WORKING DIVES WITH HELIUM–OXYGEN

Working dives with 15 min actual time at depth have been completed successfully for depths from 300 ft (10 ATA) to 600 ft (19·2 ATA) in the Experimental Diving Unit wet–dry pressure facilities using helium–oxygen breathing mixtures at depth and nitrogen–oxygen or helium–nitrogen–oxygen mixtures for decompression (Fig. 17.5). Both stage and linear ascent decompression at a varying rate have been used successfully (Workman 1967).

It was decided that working dives of 1 and 2 hours would be needed to accomplish work which would require a considerable number of shorter dives to complete. The considerable amount of inert gas taken up in slowly equilibrating tissues

during such long pressure exposures obligates a prolonged decompression which is only possible through use of the SDC-DDC technique to remove the diver from the water.

For simplicity, an air atmosphere has been used in the decompression chamber, with divers continuing to breathe a helium–oxygen mixture supplied by demand regulators and masks in the chamber until a depth of 100 ft (4 ATA) is reached. Air breathing is then begun to aid helium elimination, supplemented by intermittent oxygen breathing at depths less than 40 ft (2·2 ATA) to increase elimination of both nitrogen and helium from body tissues.

Working dives of 2 hours' duration have been accomplished by this technique to depths through 300 ft (10 ATA) (Figs. 17.3 and 17.6) and for 1 hour to 450 ft (14·6 ATA). While 15 hours' ascent time is required after 2-hour working dives at 300 ft (10 ATA) and 22 hours' after 1 hour at 450 ft (14·6 ATA) it is considered that the ratio of productive work to decompression time is more favourable for such dives than those with shorter bottom time.

DECOMPRESSION WITH HELIUM–NITROGEN–OXYGEN MIXTURES WITH CONSTANT Po_2 MIXED GAS SCUBA

In addition to work with deeper diving systems, a considerable number of dives have been made to evaluate a closed circuit constant Po_2 mixed gas scuba. Working dives of a range from 300 ft (10 ATA) for 20 min to 70 ft (3·12 ATA) for 220 min have been made to demonstrate depth and duration capabilities. Separate inert gas supply for helium and nitrogen permit switching of the inert gas fraction of the mixture during the dive and decompression.

A series of minimal decompression dives, and those of duration permitted by 15-min decompression time, using helium–nitrogen inert gas mixture with Po_2 of 1·3 to 1·6 ATS have been evaluated at the Experimental Diving Unit. Significant extension of dive duration has been observed with this procedure over that possible with helium–oxygen used in semi-closed mixed gas scuba (Workman 1967) (Table 17.10). The

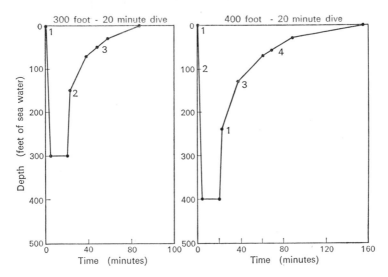

FIG. 17.5. Helium–oxygen dive schedules with continuous ascent decompression for 20-min exposure at 300 and 400 ft seawater depth

Breathing mixtures at 300 ft: (1) 80% helium, 20% oxygen; (2) 60% nitrogen, 40% oxygen; (3) 100% oxygen; and at 400 ft: (1) 37% nitrogen, 37% helium; 26% oxygen; (2) 85% helium, 15% oxygen; (3) 30% nitrogen, 30% helium, 40% oxygen; (4) 100% oxygen.

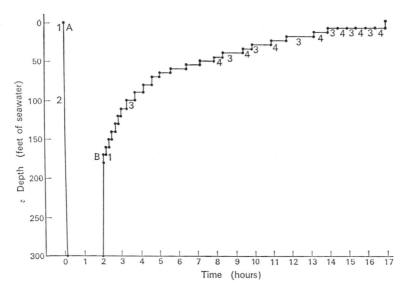

FIG. 17.6. 300-ft, 2-hour helium–oxygen dive with decompression on air and oxygen

Breathing mixtures: (1) 80% helium, 20% oxygen; (2) 90% helium, 10% oxygen; (3) air; (4) 100% oxygen. (A) Wet chamber; (B) dry chamber.

TABLE 17.10

Comparison of dives on He–O$_2$ and N$_2$–He–O$_2$ with no decompression and with 15 minutes' decompression

Depth (ft)	Bottom time (min) 75–25% helium–oxygen			Bottom time (min) Nitrogen–helium–oxygen		
	(A)	(B)	(C)	(D)	(E)	(F)
70	85	100	115	240	—	—
80	60	70	80	140	—	—
90	45	60	70	70	130	—
100	35	45	50	50	100	—
110	30	40	50	40 ↑	70	—
120	25	35	40	35 ↓	60	—
130	20	30	35	30	45	—
140	15	25	30	25	40	—
150	15	25	25	20	—	40
160	10	15	20	15	—	30
170	10	12	20	12	—	25
180	5	10	15	10	—	20
190	—	10	10	9	—	17
200	—	8	—	8	—	15

(Annotations in column D: rows 90–110 marked "1·3 ATS Po$_2$"; rows 120–140 marked "1·6 ATS Po$_2$".)

(A) No decompression. (B) 15 min decompression. (C) 15 min oxygen decompression. (D) No decompression—1·3 to 1·6 ATS Po$_2$. (E) 15 min decompression—1·3 ATS Po$_2$. (F) 15 min decompression—1·6 ATS Po$_2$.

mechanism to explain this difference may relate to varying inert gas distribution in body tissues in accordance with solubilities of the gases, as described by Bjurstedt and Severin (1948), and nucleation and bubble growth characteristics differing with tensions of several inert gases in solution in body tissues.

RATIONALE FOR MODIFICATIONS MADE TO THE HALDANE METHOD OF DECOMPRESSION CALCULATION IN THE US NAVY

Subsequent experiments on uptake and elimination of nitrogen and helium by Shaw et al. (1935) and Behnke, Thomson and Shaw (1935) have yielded quantitative data to validate the gas exchange processes indicated by Boycott, Damant and Haldane (1908). From data obtained in a series of studies on dogs and human subjects they concluded that nitrogen absorption is proportional to the partial pressure of nitrogen in the lungs, that with the same pressure gradient the rate of nitrogen absorption is equal to the rate of

elimination, and that the time for complete nitrogen elimination, and percentage rate of nitrogen elimination for corresponding periods of time, are the same irrespective of the quantity of nitrogen absorbed by the body.

Forster (1964) concluded on the basis of theoretical calculation that nitrogen in the alveolus would achieve 99% equilibration with alveolar capillary blood in 0·01 sec, and thus have plenty of time to equilibrate completely in transit time through the capillary. He also concluded from a mathematical evaluation of inert gas transport in resting muscle by radial diffusion from a capillary that the half-time for equilibration would be 54·7 sec. Thus, an inert gas will only equilibrate between capillary blood and the surrounding tissue in one transit time in tissues with a high capillary density, but it appears likely that equilibration will not occur in tissues with a lower capillary density. The time constant (K) for exchange of inert gas in the tissue is equal to the volume of blood flow per minute per volume of tissue multiplied by the ratio of solubility of the inert gas in blood to the solubility in tissue. This is the same rate constant for inert gas exchange derived by Jones (1950) in elimination studies of gases with molecular weight varying from helium through xenon. Forster (1964) further states that lack of equilibration between venous blood and tissue would produce an apparent change in the rate constant, which could not be distinguished from a real change in volume of blood per volume of tissue or the ratio of blood to tissue solubilities without additional information not presently available for inert gases.

It is recognized that inert gas uptake in body tissues during exercise will be far greater than during rest due to increased cardiac output, tissue perfusion and decreased intercapillary diffusion distance. For resting muscle, capillary blood flow may vary by a factor of 25 from the exercise state. Tissues with even less vascularity, as connective tissue and cartilage, may have even less blood perfusion and limit greatly the inert gas exchange rate, though inert gas solubility in these tissues is less than for body fat.

Determination of safe supersaturation limits for working dives with direct return to 1 ATA does provide, in some measure, for the difference in inert gas exchange between exercise and rest. However, as the depth of the dive increases, the inert gas exchange gradient between blood and tissues becomes greater than for the minimal decompression dives for which surfacing super-saturation limits are derived, to magnify the error in predicted inert gas uptake. It appears that for dives in excess of 200 ft (7 ATA) some factor must be multiplied by the time interval of exposure to provide for the additional inert gas uptake with exercise. A factor of 1·5 provides well for many dives tested, though a factor of 2·0 was used in calculation of helium–oxygen schedules in the present *US Navy Diving Manual*. Further studies will be required to define this factor of difference to provide for safe decom-pression.

Several studies of effects of oxygen breathing at increased pressure have demonstrated a reduction in the volume of blood perfusing organs and extremities. This effect is both Po_2 and time dependent. Blood flow reduction of 25% has been shown in the lower extremity of men breathing oxygen at 2 ATA Po_2 (Bird & Telfer 1965). Time for equivalent tissue perfusion of blood for inert gas elimination would be increased 133%. This, however, does not allow for increase in inter-capillary diffusion distances, as discussed earlier, in slowing gas exchange in all body tissues. Use of intermittent air and oxygen breathing during decompression may take advantage of increased perfusion of tissues with reduction of the inspired Po_2. In any event, the efficiency of inert gas elimination during oxygen breathing is diminished to less than predicted on the basis of the gradient between the inert gas tension in arterial blood and tissue as a result of decreased tissue perfusion.

The necessity to consider larger values of tissue half-time to calculate decompression for both helium and nitrogen dives has been discussed previously. The inadequacy of methods used to study inert gas elimination has also been described. Recent studies by Groom and Farhi (1967) in which nitrogen elimination from large dogs surrounded by an oxygen atmosphere permitted precise definition of rate constants of the slowest tissue components, reported half-times as slow as 190 min. Thus, the range of half-time tissues considered appropriate for man in decompression calculations for air dives relates well to these studies on animals of lesser body mass.

The depth and half-time dependence of the supersaturation criteria have been discussed earlier in some detail as this varies from the original theory of Haldane. Further definition of the mechanism of pressure and time-concen-tration dependence of nucleation and bubble growth is required in living animal preparations to extend the information available to permit calculation of more efficient, safe decompression.

APPENDIX: COMPUTATIONS FOR DECOMPRESSION

The conventional Haldane method of decompres-sion rests on the assumption that the time-rate of change (dP/dt) of the inert gas tissue tension (P) is proportional to the difference between the inspired partial pressure of the inert gas (P_I) and the instantaneous value of P.
Thus

$$\frac{dP}{dt} = K(P_I - P) \tag{1}$$

If P_I is constant from time zero ($t = 0$), and if P_0 is the inert gas tension at $t = 0$, then the inert gas tissue tension (P) at time t can be determined as a function of P_I, P_0 and t. Upon separation of the variables of equation (1) and the insertion of limits,

$$\int_{P_0}^{P} \frac{dP}{(P_I - P)} = \int_0^t K \, dt$$

The solution of this equation is

$$\ln (P_I - P) \Big|_{P_0}^{P} = -Kt \tag{2}$$

or

$$P_I - P = (P_I - P_0) \, e^{-Kt}$$

Subtraction of P_0 from both sides and rearrangement of terms lead to the desired expression

$$P = P_0 + (P_I - P_0)(l - e^{-Kt}) \tag{3}$$

During decompression, P_I is reduced in steps at intervals intended to effect rapid but safe elimination of the inert gas absorbed in the tissues (P). The time for ($P_I - P$) to decrease to one half its value imme-diately after a reduction of P_I is called the half-time ($t_{1/2}$). This time is characteristic of the partic-ular tissue and inert gas involved, but it is inde-pendent of the actual values of P_I and P within the range of pressures for which equation (1) is valid. Then from equation (2)

$$\ln \frac{P_{\mathrm{I}} - P t_{1/2}}{P_{\mathrm{I}} - P_0} = \ln \tfrac{1}{2} = -K t_{1/2}$$

and

$$K = \frac{\ln 2}{t_{1/2}} = \frac{0 \cdot 693}{t_{1/2}} \qquad (4)$$

Then the exponent in equation (3) can be expressed as

$$-\frac{0 \cdot 693 t}{t_{1/2}}$$

The acceptance of equation (1) requires the further assumption that inert gas is uniformly distributed throughout the tissue represented by $t_{1/2}$ at all times. Jones (1950) used radioactive tracers to examine the distribution of inert gas in tissues. Roughton (1952) examined the relationship among the tissue half-times, the coaxial diffusion cylinder of the capillary, and the diffusion coefficients of inert gases in tissues. It was concluded from this study that the inert gas diffuses immediately and uniformly throughout the tissues. Two concepts are presently employed in determining critical supersaturation values. The supersaturation ratio is the sum of dissolved gas tension ($\sum P_{\mathrm{I}}$) to ambient or hydro-static pressure (H_{p}):

$$\sum_{i=0}^{n} \sum P_{\mathrm{I}} / H_{\mathrm{p}}$$

The supersaturation gradient (ΔP) is the difference between the sum of the dissolved gas tissue tension ($\sum P_{\mathrm{I}}$) and the hydrostatic pressure:

$$\Delta P = \sum_{i=0}^{n} \sum P_{\mathrm{I}} - H_{\mathrm{p}}$$

where n is the number of gases with significant partial pressures within the tissue of concern ($t_{1/2}$). ΔP may vary as a function of the rate constant (K) and with water depth (D).

That is

$$\Delta P = f(D \, \mathrm{ATA}, K)$$
$$\Delta P = \Delta P_s t g D$$

where g = rate of change of P as function of depth, and P_s = P at surface (1 ATA).

REFERENCES

ADAMS, G. M. (1974) Shallow Habitat Air Dive: *1–30 Days at a Simulated Depth of 50 Feet of Seawater with Excursions between 5 and 235 Feet.* NMSMRL Report No. 775, US Naval Submarine Medical Research Laboratory.

ALEKSANDROV, A. I. & BRESTKIN, A. P. (1965) The permissible supersaturation coefficients in human beings breathing air and a helium–oxygen mixture. *The Effects of the Gas Medium and Pressure on Body Functions.* Ed. M. P. Brestkin. pp. 5–9, Collection No. 3, NASA-TT-F-358, Washington, D.C.

BARNARD, E. E. P. (1971) Institute of Naval Medicine, Gosport, UK. Personal communication.

BATEMAN, J. B. (1951) Part I. Review of data on value of pre-oxygenation in prevention of decompression sickness. In *Decompression Sickness.* Ed. J. F. Fulton, pp. 242–321. Philadelphia: W. B. Saunders.

BEHNKE, A. R. (1947) *A Review of Physiological and Clinical Data Pertaining to Decompression Sickness.* Proj. X-443, Report No. 4, Naval Medical Research Institute, Bethesda, Maryland.

BEHNKE, A. R. (1967) The isobaric (oxygen window) principle of decompression. *Transactions of the Third Annual Conference of the Marine Technology Society,* pp. 213–228. Washington: Marine Technology Society.

BEHNKE, A. R., THOMSON, R. M. & SHAW, L. A. (1935) The rate of elimination of dissolved nitrogen in man in relation to the fat and water content of the body. *Am. J. Physiol.* **114,** 137–146.

BEHNKE, A. R. & WILLMON, T. L. (1939) USS *Squalus.* Medical aspects of the rescue and salvage operations and the use of oxygen in deep-sea diving. *Nav. med. Bull.* **37,** 629–640.

BEHNKE, A. R. & WILLMON, T. L. (1941) Cutaneous diffusion of helium in relation to peripheral blood flow and absorption of atmospheric nitrogen through the skin. *Am. J. Physiol.* **131,** 627–632.

BEHNKE, A. R. & YARBROUGH, O. D. (1938) Physiologic studies of helium. *Nav. med. Bull.* **36,** 542–558.

BIRD, A. D. & TELFER, A. B. M. (1965) The effect of increased oxygen tension on peripheral blood flow. *Hyperbaric oxygenation. Proceedings of The Second International Congress.* Ed. I. M. C. A. Ledingham. pp. 424–430. Edinburgh: Livingstone.

BJURSTEDT, H. & SEVERIN, G. (1948) The prevention of decompression sickness and nitrogen narcosis by the use of hydrogen as a substitute for nitrogen (the Arne Zetterstrom method for deep diving). *Milit. Surg.* **103,** 107–116.

BOND, G. F. (1963) A new under-sea capability. *Navy Technical Forum* NAVEXOS P-2193. Fall 1963, pp. 1–10 (Confidential).

BOND, G. F. (1964) New developments in high pressure living. *Archs envir. Hlth* **9,** 310–314.

BORNMANN, R. C. (1967) Decompression after saturation diving. In *Proc. 3rd Symp. Underwater Physiology.* Ed. C. J. Lambertsen. pp. 109–121. Baltimore: Williams & Wilkins.

BORNMANN, R. C. (1970) *Decompression Schedule Development for Repetitive Saturation-excursion Helium–oxygen Diving.* Research Report 1–70, Deep Submergence Systems Project Office, Chevy Chase, Maryland.

BOYCOTT, A. E., DAMANT, G. C. C. & HALDANE, J. S. (1908) The prevention of compressed air illness. *J. Hyg., Camb.* **8,** 342–443.

BRESTKIN, A. P. (1965) Relationship between the supersaturation coefficient of gas–liquid systems and the tension of dissolved gas. In *The Effect of the Gas Medium and Pressure on Body Functions.* Ed. M. P. Brestkin. pp. 10–17, Collection No. 3, NASA-TT-F-358, Washington, D.C.

BRESTKIN, A. P., GRAMENITSKII, P. M. & SIDOROV, N. YA. (1965) Study of the safe supersaturation of the body with indifferent gases at different pressures. In *The Effect of the Gas Medium and Pressure on Body Functions*. Ed. M. P. Brestkin. pp. 18–27, Collection No. 3, NASA-TT-F-358, Washington, D.C.

DAVIS, R. H. (1962) *Deep Diving and Submarine Operations*, pp. 7–9. London: St. Catherine Press.

DES GRANGES, M. (1956) *Standard Air Decompression Tables*. Research report 5–57, US Navy Experimental Diving Unit, Washington, D.C.

DES GRANGES, M. (1957) *Repetitive Diving Decompression Tables*. Research report 6–57, US Navy Experimental Diving Unit, Washington, D.C.

DOLL, R. E. (1965) *Decompression Sickness among U.S. Navy Operational Divers: an Estimate of Incidence using Air Decompression Tables*. Research report 4–64, US Navy Experimental Diving Unit, Washington, D.C.

DUFFNER, G. J. & SNIDER, H. H. (1958) *Effects of Exposing Men to Compressed Air and Helium–oxygen Mixtures for 12 Hours at Pressures 2–2·6 Atmospheres*. Research report 1–59, US Navy Experimental Diving Unit, Washington, D.C.

DUFFNER, G. J., SNYDER, J. F. & SMITH, L. L. (1959) *Adaptation of Helium–oxygen to Mixed Gas Scuba*. Research report 3–59, US Navy Experimental Diving Unit, Washington, D.C.

DWYER, J. V. (1956) *Calculation of Repetitive Diving Decompression Tables*. Research report 1–57, US Navy Experimental Diving Unit, Washington, D.C.

END, E. (1937) Rapid decompression following inhalation of helium–oxygen mixtures under pressure. *Am. J. Physiol.* **120**, 712–718.

FARHI, L. E., HOMMA, T., BERGER, D. (1962) Tissue N_2 washout in the whole animal and in individual organs. *Physiologist* **5(3)**, 138.

FORSTER, R. E. (1964) Diffusion of gases. In *Handbook of Physiology, Sec. 3, Respiration:* Vol. I. Ed. W. O. Fenn & H. Rahn. pp. 839–872. Washington: American Physiological Soc.

FRENCH, G. R. W. (1916) Diving operations in connection with the salvage of the USS F-4. *Nav. med. Bull.* **10**, 74–91.

GROOM, A. C. & FARHI, L. E. (1967) Cutaneous diffusion of atmospheric N_2 during N_2 washout in the dog. *J. appl. Physiol.* **22**, 740–745.

HALDANE, J. S. & PRIESTLEY, J. G. (1935) *Respiration*, 2nd edn. New Haven: Yale University Press.

HAMILTON, R. W., FRUCTUS, P. & FRUCTUS, X. R. (1968) *Physiological Surveillance and Performance Tests During a Seven Day Exposure at 9·5 Atmospheres*. Presented to the 24th International Congress of Physiological Sciences, Washington, D.C.

HAMILTON, F. T., BACON, R. H., HALDANE, J. S. & LEES, E. (1907) *Report to the Admiralty of the Deep-Water Diving Committee*. London: H.M. Stationery Office.

HAMILTON, R. W., KENYON, D. J., FREITAG, M. & SCHREINER, H. R. (1973) *NOAA OPS I and II; Formulation of Excursion Procedures for Shallow Undersea Habitats*. Technical Memorandum UCRI-731, Union Carbide Corporation, New York.

HAWKINS, J. A., SHILLING, C. S. & HANSEN, R. A. (1935) A suggested change in calculating decompression tables for diving. *Bull.* **33**, 327–338.

HEMPLEMAN, H. V. (1967) Decompression procedures for deep, open sea operations. In *Proc. 3rd Symp. Underwater Physiology*. Ed. C. J. Lambertsen. pp. 255–266. Baltimore: Williams & Wilkins.

HILL, A. V. (1928) The diffusion of oxygen and lactic acid through tissues. *Proc. R. Soc. Biol.* **104**, 39–96.

JONES, H. B. (1950) Respiratory System: nitrogen elimination. *Medical Physics*, Vol. II. Ed. O. Glasser. pp. 855–871. Chicago: Year Book Publishers.

KINDWALL, E. P. (1962) Metabolic rate and animal size correlated with decompression sickness. *Am. J. Physiol.* **203** (2), 385–388.

KRASBERG, A. R. (1966) Saturation diving techniques. In *Proc. Fourth Int. Congress Biometeorology*. Rutgers Univ., New Brunswick, New Jersey.

LARSEN, R. T. & MAZZONE, W. F. (1967) Excursion diving from saturation exposures at depth. In *Proc. 3rd Symp. Underwater Physiology*. Ed. C. J. Lambertsen. pp. 241–254. Baltimore: Williams & Wilkins.

MOLUMPHY, C. G. (1950a) *Computation of Helium–oxygen Decompression Tables*. Research report 7–50. US Navy Experimental Diving Unit, Washington, D.C.

MOLUMPHY, C. G. (1950b) *Evaluation of Newly Computed Helium–oxygen Decompression Tables at Depths Greater than Provided for in Published Tables*. Research report 9–50. US Navy Experimental Diving Unit, Washington, D.C.

MOMSEN, C. B. & WHELAND, K. R. (1939) *Report on use of Helium–oxygen Mixtures for Diving*. (Revised 1942). US Navy Experimental Diving Unit, Washington, D.C.

PICCARD, J. (1941) Aero-emphysema and the birth of gas bubbles. *Proc. Mayo Clin.* **16**, 700–704.

RASHBASS, C. (1955) *Investigation into the Decompression Tables*. Report. Medical Research Council, RN Personnel Research Committee, U.P.S. 151, London.

REEVES, E. & BECKMAN, E. L. (1966) *The Incidence of Decompression Sickness in Dogs Following 7, 12, 18 and 24 hour Saturation Dives with 'No-stop' Decompression*, Report No. 4, Naval Medical Research Institute, Bethesda, Maryland.

ROTH, E. M. (1967) *Space Cabin Atmospheres. Part III. Physiological Factors of Inert Gases*. NASA SP-117, Washington: Office of Technology Utilization. Natl Aeron. Space Admin.

ROUGHTON, F. J. W. (1952) Diffusion and chemical reaction velocity in cylindrical and spherical systems of physiological interest. *Proc. R. Soc. B*, **140**, 203–229.

SAYERS, R. R. & YANT, W. P. (1926) The value of helium–oxygen atmosphere in diving and caisson operations. *Anesth. Analg.* **5**, 127–138.

SAYERS, R. R., YANT, W. P. & HILDEBRAND, J. (1925) *Possibilities in the Use of Helium–oxygen Mixtures as a Mitigation of Caisson Disease*. Report of Invest. No. 2670. US Dept. of Interior.

SCHREINER, H. R. & KELLEY, P. L. (1967) Computation methods for decompression from deep dives. In *Proc. 3rd Symp. Underwater Physiology*. Ed. C. J. Lambertsen. pp. 277–299. Baltimore: Williams & Wilkins.

SCHREINER, H. R. & KELLEY, P. L. (1970) Decompression Schedules for Saturation-excursion Dives. *Aerospace Med.* **51**, 491–494.

SHAW, L. A., BEHNKE, A. R., MESSER, A. C., THOMSON, R. M. & MOTLEY, E. P. (1935) The equilibrium time of the gaseous nitrogen in the dog's body following changes of nitrogen tension in the lungs. *Am. J. Physiol.* **112**, 545.

STILLSON, G. D. (1915) *Report on Deep Diving Tests.* p. 252. Bureau of Construction and Repair, Navy Dept. Washington, D.C.: US Gov. Printing Office.

THOMSON, E. (1927) Helium in deep diving. *Science, N.Y.* **65**, 36–38.

US Navy Diving Manual (NAVSHIPS 0994–001–9010). (Revised 1974.) Navy Dept. Washington, D.C.: US Gov. Printing Office.

VAN DER AUE, O. E., BRINTON, E. S. & KELLAR, R. J. (1945) *Surface Decompression, Derivation and Testing of Decompression Tables with Safety Limits for Certain Depths and Exposures.* Research project X-476, Research report I. US Navy Experimental Diving Unit, Washington, D.C.

VAN DER AUE, O. E., KELLAR, R. J., BRINTON, E. S., BARRON, G., GILLIAM, H. D. & JONES, R. J. (1951) *Calculation and Testing of Decompression Tables for Air Dives Employing the Procedure of Surface Decompression and the Use of Oxygen.* Research report 1. US Navy Experimental Diving Unit, Washington, D.C.

WORKMAN, R. D. (1957) *Calculations of Air Saturation Decompression Tables.* Research report 11–57. US Navy Experimental Diving Unit, Washington, D.C.

WORKMAN, R. D. (1965) *Calculation of Decompression Schedules for Nitrogen–oxygen and Helium–oxygen Dives.* Research report 6–65. US Navy Experimental Diving Unit, Washington, D.C.

WORKMAN, R. D. (1967) Underwater research interests of the US Navy. In *Proc. 3rd Symp. Underwater Physiology,* Ed. C. J. Lambertsen. pp. 4–15. Baltimore: Williams & Wilkins.

WORKMAN, R. D. & REYNOLDS, J. L. (1965) *Adaptation of Helium–oxygen to Mixed Gas Scuba.* Research report 1–65. US Navy Experimental Diving Unit, Washington, D.C.

YARBROUGH, O. D. (1937) *Calculation of Decompression Tables.* Research report. US Naval Experimental Diving Unit. Washington, D.C.

ZAL'TSMAN, G. L. & ZINOV'EVA, I. D. (1965) Comparative determinations of the permissible supersaturation value of the human body with indifferent gases under different conditions. In *The Effect of the Gas Medium and Pressure on Body Functions.* Ed. M. P. Brestkin. pp. 28–33. Collection No. 3, NASA-TT-F-358, Washington, D.C.

18

Decompression Theory: British Practice

H. V. HEMPLEMAN

The complexities of physics and physiology involved in the aetiology of decompression sickness are so great that attempts to formulate detailed quantitative analyses of the phenomena will only succeed by a happy accident. The size, shape and location of the bubble, or bubbles, in mild decompression sickness are still matters for conjecture. Even were such necessary variables clearly defined, the physics of initiation and growth of the gaseous emboli would require a knowledge of nucleation phenomena and bubble growth in biological media which certainly does not exist. Added to these difficulties is the further one of the collection of reliable data. Given these circumstances it is first necessary to examine the generally accepted facts that have arisen from various sources. Hopefully, these data will lead to the establishment of a set of ideas which can be used to calculate decompression procedures in a wide variety of conditions.

BASIC DECOMPRESSION DATA

Decompression sickness can manifest itself in a number of different ways, varying in severity from mild skin itching and rashes to death. The most commonly observed mild form of decompression sickness is a pain felt in or around a joint, and is commonly termed 'the bends'. It has been established that if attacks of the bends can be avoided, then the more serious forms of decompression sickness become extremely rare events. It is proposed, therefore, to examine principally the factors which evoke this form of mild decompression sickness.

Careful records have been kept of all cases of decompression sickness occurring in the United Kingdom at any major compressed air undertakings. It has been established that if men work for periods of time varying between 8 and 12 hours in compressed air at pressures less than 14 psi gauge (31 ft; 1·95 ATA), and are then decompressed back to atmospheric pressure in not less than 2 min, then decompression sickness requiring therapeutic recompression is rare (less than 0·2% of man-decompressions). Data for exposures to compressed air for periods of time longer than 12 hours are very inadequate. Such evidence as has been accumulated is summarized in a report by Hamilton et al. (1973). It would seem that there is some lowering of the decompression threshold pressure from the value of 14 psi gauge (31 ft; 1·95 ATA), to 12 psi gauge (27 ft; 1·8 ATA). This lowering of the threshold no doubt reflects the fact that the tissues of the body take longer than 12 hours to saturate fully with nitrogen gas, or it may also indicate that some form of physiological adaptation to high pressure is not complete in 12 hours. Similar threshold pressure data are available from the use of oxy-helium mixtures (Duffner & Snyder 1958; Hempleman 1967) and although once again there is a paucity of suitable data, it is possible to make two gross statements from the evidence available. First, the threshold value for no-decompression stoppages breathing oxy-helium is significantly greater than that for air, certainly exceeding 33 ft (2 ATA), and more likely to be in the region of 36 ft (2·1 ATA) for the more sensitive individuals. Secondly, there would not appear to be a great deal of difference between the threshold performance after only 6 hours on oxy-helium as compared with 24 hours on the same mixture. This is in marked contrast to the findings just noted above on air. There are a few experiments using oxygen–argon breathing mixtures (Hempleman 1967) and these would indicate that the threshold pressure on argon is noticeably lower than that on nitrogen. Thus there would seem to be a progressive lowering of the bend threshold pressure when transferring from helium to nitrogen to argon. This could be related to their respective solubilities or diffusion coefficient or some such similar properties, but the evidence available is far too slight to enable any definitive analysis.

A considerable volume of evidence exists defining the bend threshold for subatmospheric excursions (Fryer 1969). It would seem that nearly all normal men can sustain rapid decompression to 0·5 ATA without ill effects. This threshold value may be compared with the value noted above for compressed air from which two points become obvious. First, whatever is provoking decompression sickness it is not described by a constant partial pressure drop nor, secondly, can it be described by a constant pressure ratio. The precise way in which the permitted threshold pressure drop varies with the absolute pressure of the dive has never been properly established. There are, however, some helpful qualitative observations. Most decompression procedures for compressed air workers in use today consist of a fast phase followed by one or more slower phases. The pressure dividing the fast and slow phases of the decompression used to be based upon the Haldane ratio principle. This created a large number of bends, particularly for pressures in excess of 3 ATA. The State of New York Regulations (1922), which specify a rapid pressure drop to half gauge pressure, were very successful in reducing the number of cases of bends, as was the introduction of an intermediate stage by Catton (1967). These observations imply the necessity of a diminution of the permitted decompression ratio with pressure.

Barnard (1975) completed a fundamental set of exposures to oxy-helium breathing and defined the relationship between permitted pressure changes and the absolute pressure. As with air, so with oxy-helium, it was not possible to describe the change in threshold performance in a simple manner, e.g. constant ratio, or constant pressure difference. However, with deference to the original Haldane concept, it must be noted that the data conform more nearly to a constant ratio than they do to a constant pressure difference. For example, 24 hours exposure at a depth of 69 m (7·8 ATA) can be safely followed by rapid ascent to 47 m (5·7 ATA) giving a decompression ratio of approximately 1·4 and a pressure difference of 22 m (3·2 ATA), whereas rapid decompression following 24 hours at 24 m (3·4 ATA) can only be safely followed by ascent to 10 m (2 ATA), giving a decompression ratio of 1·7 and a pressure difference of 14 m (1·4 ATS).

Nearly all cases of bends are preceded by a latent period during which the diver or compressed air worker is generally unaware of any untoward signs or symptoms. This period of virtually trouble-free waiting, prior to the onset of bends, can vary from a few minutes to several hours and the explanation normally advanced is that silent bubbles are generated during the decompression, and that some time is needed for the growth of these small silent bubbles into large painful ones. This explanation may be an over-simplification, as has been pointed out by Hills (1966) and Hempleman (1975), who both draw attention to the possibilities of coalescence or interdiffusion between bubbles as contributory or even dominant factors.

Whenever marginal cases of decompression sickness are promptly treated by recompression then the pain symptoms are nearly always relieved immediately. If the bends pains are not treated promptly then a chronic condition develops which may not respond to recompression and indeed it is not unknown for such cases actually to become worse upon recompression. Just as the evidence of waiting prior to the onset of bends is considered indicative of bubble growth, so the effectiveness of the recompression in removing the pain symptoms in bends is considered as further evidence that separated gas is responsible for this form of decompression sickness. These deductions are further supported by direct evidence of the presence of bubbles by several workers using ultrasonic techniques (Rubissow & Mackay 1971; Smith & Spencer 1970). Nevertheless, despite this unanimity of views regarding the causative agent in bends, there are some well-established observations regarding sensitivity to bends pain which render quantitative explanations very difficult. Barnard (1967), for example, described several cases of decompression sickness developing at pressures of about 100 ft (4 ATA) where pains could be relieved or exacerbated by pressure changes of only the order of 1 ft (0·03 ATS). The effectiveness of such small pressure changes at such comparatively high total pressures implies a very sensitive mechanism for the provocation and relief of bends pain.

Anyone who has taken part in experimental diving realizes that a dive can result in a persistent low level pain ('niggle') in a joint, and that such a niggle can cause intermittent trouble over a period of 2 or 3 days. An exaggerated example is provided by the Ocean Systems diver who was still sensitive to flight in an unpressurized aircraft several days after completion of his saturation helium dive (Hamilton et al. 1966). It is inferred from such observations that there is a tissue-bubble complex formed as a result of diving and that the physics of this new situation is not representative of the physics of the tissue when the bubble is not occluding the circulation. Once this concept of a tissue-bubble complex is accepted, then grave doubts arise about whether or not such complexes are, to a lesser degree, also influencing the whole decompression problem.

In a double approach to this problem, the present author considered that he had succeeded in showing that in normal diving procedures the rate of acquisition of gas was not the same as the rate of loss of gas. It is necessary to emphasize the phrase 'in normal diving procedures', where large initial pressure changes are involved. It may be possible by such techniques as are advocated by Behnke (1967) and Hills (1966) to avoid the formation of a gas phase. These unequal rates of uptake and elimination of gas were demonstrated by the following experiments.

First it was shown in a population of goats that the time required to equilibrate all relevant body tissues to a constant raised pressure of air was of

the order of 6 hours (Hempleman 1967). Secondly, it was shown that if goats were exposed for 6 hours to a pressure of air P_1 and then rapidly decompressed in 150 sec to pressure P_2 where a threshold bend is obtained, then the ratio (r) P_1/P_2 is virtually constant over a large range of P_1 values, but for lower P_1 values r increases noticeably (Hempleman 1967). If it is true that uptake of gas by all relevant tissues is the same as the release of gas, then the following experimental sequence should be quite trouble-free.

1. Expose for 6 hours to pressure P_1.
2. Decompress rapidly to P_2, such that no decompression sickness occurs.
3. Wait 6 hours at P_2 to equilibrate all the tissues to the new pressure level.
4. Decompress to P_3 such that

$$\frac{P_1}{P_2} = r = \frac{P_2}{P_3}.$$

It is found experimentally that procedure (4) is unsafe if the value of r is near to the critical threshold value and the conclusion reached is that the 6-hour period at pressure P_2 does not permit ascent to pressure P_3 because some change has taken place as a result of the first pressure drop from P_1 to P_2. Presumably this change is concerned with the appearance of silent bubbles and these interfere with tissue gas exchange.

Proof that a physical change in the body has occurred as a result of decompression is not given by the above experiments. The results could have been obtained from a change in physiological responses caused by, for instance, breathing raised pressures of air for such prolonged periods. In order to attempt to investigate the physics and physiology of this situation, a second entirely different series of experiments was performed. In outline these experiments were as follows. First, the decompression sickness threshold pressures were obtained for several animals. They were rapidly compressed to pressure P for a time t. At the end of time t they were decompressed back to atmospheric pressure in 150 sec. Certain fixed values of t were selected and the P values were obtained which gave mild threshold bends on return to atmospheric pressure.

Assume now that there exists a set of tissues with half-times of 5, 10, 20, 40, and 80 min. The choice of these particular tissues is purely arbitrary but this does not affect the validity of the subsequent reasoning. It is now possible, as a result of performing a range of exposure times, to assign permitted ratios to each of these hypothetical tissues for each of the animals. As the threshold 'bends' are all obtained at atmospheric pressure the possibility of altered physiological factors interfering with the experimental results is eliminated.

Following this series of experiments, a third series was performed using the same animals in order to compare each animal with itself. In the third series each individual experiment consisted of a double exposure to pressure of 25-min duration, with a surface interval of 90 min between them. For the first 25-min exposure, the animal was compressed rapidly to pressure P_1 which was a pressure exactly 10 ft (0·3 ATS) less than the threshold bend pressure for that particular animal and for that particular exposure time. The animal was then decompressed back to atmospheric pressure in 150 sec and left at atmospheric pressure for 90 min. There was no risk of decompression sickness from this procedure because, as mentioned, the animal had been exposed to a pressure well below the 'bend' threshold value for this particular duration of exposure. Nevertheless, a large amount of dissolved gas had been acquired in the body tissues as a result. During the 90-min wait at atmospheric pressure all tissues are losing this excess dissolved gas, and it is a simple calculation to follow this process using the Haldane-like tissues with their appropriate exponential time course.

The second exposure consisted, as before, of a rapid pressurization to some pressure P_2 and stay at this pressure for 25 min, followed by decompression back to atmospheric pressure. P_2 is the pressure at which a threshold 'bend' just occurs when the animal returns to atmospheric pressure for the second time. It is now quite easy to calculate the excess gas present in the various tissues at the time of reaching atmospheric pressure following this double pressure excursion. The 'bend' threshold values for the various tissues for the single and double dives can now be compared as in Table 18.1 where goat 34 is given as a typical example of this experimental series. Here the 5-min tissue had shown in the dive (A) of 25 min to 130 ft

(4·9 ATA) that it was capable of performing a decompression ratio of 4·81 on return to atmospheric pressure. Anything less than a 4·81 ratio should not affect this tissue, as these values represent its threshold performance. Examination of the double dive data reveals that this particular tissue only performed a 4·08 ratio drop. This difference is very great and must mean that the 5-min tissue played no part whatsoever in the bend produced by the double dive.

In a similar manner, all other proposed tissue half-times can be eliminated.

Six other goats were used in these experiments. Each tissue half-time on every goat showed disparities similar to the example given above. Thus it is quite impossible to use the same reasoning for the uptake of the gas as for the elimination. It is suggested that a tissue-bubble complex is formed during decompression. The sole question remaining is whether such a complex situation forms from every decompression, or whether there are ways of avoiding this.

The findings just discussed refer, of course, to individual animal results. Even if it were possible to avoid the formation of a tissue-bubble complex during the course of a decompression it would still be necessary, for practical purposes, to regard the rate of acquisition of gas as being faster than the rate of elimination of dissolved gas. This arises from the following elementary considerations. In any population there will be those subjects who absorb gas rather more rapidly than others, and there will also be those who eliminate gas more slowly. In order, therefore, to deal adequately with a population of animals or men it will be necessary to introduce unequal rates of uptake and elimination of inert gas in order to cover adequately the envelope of the behaviour of the whole group.

Whenever men are exposed regularly to hyperbaric conditions they seem to develop a marked resistance to attacks of bends in many cases. This effect is particularly noticeable in caisson and tunnel workers (Golding et al. 1960). This form of adaptation or acclimatization to hyperbaric exposures can be seen to occur both when breathing compressed air or oxy-helium mixtures. It is by no means certain that all forms of diving exposures will lead to adaptation.

TABLE 18.1

Examples of bend threshold experiments

Goat no.	Dive no.	Time (in min)	Gauge depth reading ft	Tissue half-times (min) — Total air pressure ft (abs)					Tissue half-times (min) — Tissue ratios					Remarks
				5	10	20	40	80	5	10	20	40	80	
33	A	25	145	173·2	152·5	117·0	83·9	61·2	5·249	4·620	3·545	2·540	1·855	Bend
	B	50	120	153·0	149·0	132·0	102·5	75·1	4·636	4·515	4·000	3·106	2·276	Bend
	C	90	100	133·0	133·0	128·6	112·0	87·1	4·030	4·030	3·879	3·394	2·639	Bend
	D	25	135	163·5	144·2	111·2	80·4	59·2	4·956	4·370	3·370	2·437	1·794	No bend
		80 min on surface +	135	163·5	144·2	113·2	88·1	69·8	4·956	4·370	3·430	2·670	2·115	Bend
	E	360	60	93·0	93·0	93·0	93·0	90·4	2·818	2·818	2·818	2·818	2·740	No bend
Maximum attained in single dives				173·2	152·5	132·0	112·0	90·4	5·249	4·620	4·000	3·394	2·740	
Maximum attained in double dives				163·5	144·2	113·2	88·1	69·8	4·956	4·370	3·430	2·670	2·115	
Difference				−9·7	−8·3	−18·8	−23·9	−20·6	−0·293	−0·250	−0·570	−0·724	−0·625	
34	A	25	130	158·7	140·1	108·3	78·6	58·3	4·809	4·246	3·282	2·382	1·767	Bend
	B	50	95	128·0	124·9	111·3	88·0	66·3	3·878	3·785	3·372	2·667	2·010	Bend
	C	90	85	118·0	118·0	114·3	100·2	79·0	3·576	3·576	3·463	3·036	2·394	Bend
	D	25	120	149·0	132·0	102·5	75·1	56·3	4·515	4·000	3·106	2·276	1·706	No bend
		80 min on surface +	120	134·5	119·5	95·6	76·7	62·8	4·076	3·622	2·897	2·324	1·903	Bend
	E	360	45	78·0	78·0	78·0	78·0	76·0	2·364	2·364	2·364	2·364	2·303	No bend
Maximum attained in single dives				158·7	140·1	114·3	100·2	79·0	4·809	4·246	3·463	3·036	2·394	
Maximum attained in double dives				134·5	119·5	95·6	76·7	62·8	4·076	3·622	2·897	2·324	1·903	
Difference				−24·2	−20·6	−18·7	−23·5	−16·2	−0·733	−0·624	−0·566	−0·712	−0·491	

The simplest form of non-saturation diving occurs when the diver exposes himself to raised pressure and then without any decompression stoppages returns to atmospheric pressure. Such dives are called 'no-stop dives'. Two groups of workers have attempted to define with controlled experimentation the no-stop diving limit (Hawkins, Shilling & Hanson 1935; Albano 1960). Unfortunately, however, in the light of modern knowledge these attempts can be seen to represent only rough estimates of the normal diving population. No account could be taken of acclimatization or adaptation to regular diving during the experimental series. It is likely, therefore, that the more sensitive results were obtained from the shallow diving data and that as the experiments continued with greater and greater depths the men became more and more resistant. Furthermore, these two sets of results available in the literature are considerably at variance with one another. In these circumstances the results from experiments using large animals are the only available indicators of human performance.

Hempleman (1963) completed a large series of no-stop dives using goats as the experimental subjects and his data will first be used as indicators of possible human performance. It was observed that if the median average value of the no-stop bend threshold pressure was multiplied by the square root of the exposure time to pressure then a constant value was obtained, which remained similar in value until the time of exposure exceeded about 100 min. To find such a simple relationship is extremely encouraging and it is now necessary to enquire whether such a relationship will apply to the human situation.

In view of the conflicting experimental results available, one may resort to the findings from many hundreds of thousands of field trial exposures using the US Navy Air Diving Tables. For a dive to 100 ft the no-stop duration is given as 25 min, yielding a $P\sqrt{t}$ value of $100\sqrt{25}=500$. Reference to the 50 ft no-stop dive durations shows a value of 100 min and for this dive $P\sqrt{t}=50\sqrt{100}=500$. In fact, without elaborating further examples, the relationship $P\sqrt{t}=500$ quite satisfactorily describes the no-stop diving curve as currently used in the US Navy, for all values of t

less than 2 hours. For values of t greater than 2 hours it is clear that this relationship becomes increasingly less accurate. Taken to the opposite extreme of the time scale, this relationship predicts that a dive to 500 ft (16 ATA) which was just safe would be of 1 min duration. Reference to experience with submarine escape by the buoyant ascent method using air as the breathing medium will confirm this prediction.

There is such a dearth of statistically valid information using oxy-helium for no-stop diving that it is not possible to test this simple relationship on another gas mixture. In any case, due to the rate with which helium will equilibrate in body tissues, the relationship would only hold for some 30 to 40 min.

It is relevant to note that there are several other forms of mathematical analysis which can be used to fit the no-stop data on both air and helium with an accuracy quite adequate for the available data. The most used of these is an extension of the Haldane multi-exponential analysis which was so successfully exploited by Dwyer (1956) in his calculations for the current US Navy Air Diving Tables. There is no particular merit in any form of mathematical analysis except in so far as it leads to a simple, elegant, and versatile way of encompassing the known facts and accurately predicting some new ones, and also whether it leads to some insight into the aetiology of the particular form of decompression sickness.

It has been known for some years (Donald 1956), that oxygen can play a role in the onset of limb bends, and a recent study by Eaton and Hempleman (1973) confirms and extends some of these findings using both oxygen–nitrogen and oxygen–helium breathing mixtures. Making allowances in the calculations for the presence of high partial pressures of oxygen in brief non-saturation dives is difficult and will almost certainly, in the present state of knowledge, have to be done somewhat arbitrarily.

Saturation, or steady state diving presents in many ways a much simpler problem than discussed previously. Nevertheless, not a great deal of systematic work has been performed using steady state or saturation diving techniques. The reason is not far to seek, and concerns the fact that the collection of data is extremely time consuming and often hazardous. Sometimes attempts are made to avoid the time-consuming work required to define the rate of saturation of the body with inert gases. This was done, for example, in certain preliminary experiments to the Tektite project, where a method was evolved to achieve total saturation in reduced time in the slowest tissues. For the purpose of this experimentation it was assumed that doubling the desired nitrogen partial pressure gradient will produce the required saturation of the slowest (360 min) tissues within 1 tissue half-time (Edel 1971a). One has the utmost sympathy with attempts to reduce the tedium necessary for defining saturation exposure requirements, but unfortunately any short-cut does need a theoretical basis and, when assumptions of a theoretical nature become necessary, the objective validity of the experiment is immediately endangered. In the complex situation pertaining in diving experiments there seem to be no short-cuts available.

From the point of view of defining the boundary conditions of the decompression sickness problem the most useful experiments are those where the appearance or non-appearance of decompression sickness is used to assess the limits of any experimental procedures. Using these criteria the following two facts emerge. First, as the diving becomes deeper, and particularly at depths greater than around 200 m (21 ATA), there is a change in the nature of the decompression sickness which presents itself from minimal provocation. At lower depths if one exceeds certain rates of pressure decrease, or perhaps takes too great a pressure change on the Haldane-like stage decompression procedure, then the first presenting form of decompression sickness is nearly always a mild limb pain. At greater depths this does not seem to hold true and the new first presenting form of decompression sickness is generally concerned with the vestibular apparatus, or the hearing. Hills (1971) has already drawn attention to the fact that certain pressure-time courses, when breathing air, predispose the subjects to present CNS symptoms rather than simple limb bends. Thus the assumption often made by decompression calculators that if one avoids mild limb pains then one will also avoid nearly all other more serious forms of decompression sickness, is in need of some modifica-

tion depending upon the type of diving envisaged. Secondly, decompression from saturation or steady state exposures is very sensitive to the partial pressure of oxygen being breathed by the subject. Partial pressures of oxygen not exceeding 0·22 bar will not allow trouble-free decompression procedures from depths greater than about 120 m (13 ATA) however long those procedures. Changing the oxygen partial pressure to that used by the US Navy, namely 0·3 to 0·35 bar oxygen partial pressure, will give somewhat more satisfactory results but still yields far too many cases of mild bends, particularly when decompressing from depths in excess of about 150 m (16 ATA). Changing to 0·4 bar oxygen partial pressure transforms the nature of the diving and yields trouble-free diving in subjects certainly for all depths down to 250 m (25·8 ATA) when using decompressions of the more conservative type, as adopted by the US Navy. When employing even high partial pressures of oxygen it should be noted that Bühlmann completed a number of successful dives at the Royal Naval Physiological Laboratory, Alverstoke, with comparatively short decompression times, from depths as great as 300 m (1000 ft; 31 ATA). In support of a relationship between oxygen partial pressure and total exposure pressure is the work of Berghage, Conda and Armstrong (1973). Whilst acknowledging that their results were obtained using small animals as experimental subjects and that it is unwise to transfer such results 'in toto' to the human situation, there is nevertheless a strong indication that, in this particular case, the human and small animal results have a large measure of qualitative agreement.

Although divers can be satisfactorily protected from attacks of acute decompression sickness, and can be given effective therapy for these disorders, providing treatment is prompt, it is unfortunate that a number of cases of dysbaric osteonecrosis do nevertheless seem to occur. Fortunately, the vast majority of these osteonecrotic lesions are asymptomatic but the avoidance of these bone changes is of prime concern to anyone concerned with decompression procedures. The months which must elapse before detection of the lesions and the difficulty of obtaining sufficient reliable 'follow-up' data, over a period of several years, are proving formidable barriers to progressing towards an understanding of this disorder.

One or two facts are, however, quite clear. Osteonecrosis can follow from only a single exposure to raised air pressure (Swain 1942), although, not unexpectedly, the chance of developing a lesion is related to the number of entries into hyperbaric conditions (Walder 1970). Some men who have had several attacks of mild decompression sickness are quite free from osteonecrotic lesions, whereas others who have had no overt attacks of bends nevertheless develop bone lesions.

A great mass of data is available concerning the non-appearance of decompression sickness, for instance in excursion diving from saturation or steady state conditions (Bornmann 1971). Whilst such facts are unhelpful for defining the boundaries of the decompression problem they do form a gross first-order test of any quantitative ideas.

A summary of the diving data

A general summary of the major points which have just been outlined will now be given prior to an attempt to see whether one can make a quantitative analysis.

1. There are many forms of decompression sickness. The simplifying assumption will be made that if mild bends pains can be avoided then all more serious forms of decompression sickness will become extremely rare. It is noted that there are some exceptions to this general rule, particularly when deep oxy-helium dives are being undertaken.

2. Following prolonged exposure to pressure it is observed that the bend threshold is greater when breathing helium–oxygen than nitrogen–oxygen (air) and greater again than argon–oxygen.

3. Prolonged exposures to pressure, followed by rapid decompression to a new just-safe level are feasible up to great pressures, at least 350 m (36 ATA). The relationship between the pressure of exposure and the pressure to which one decompresses just safely is not a simple one.

4. In most cases of mild bends there is a trouble-free waiting period prior to the onset of bends which can vary from a few minutes to several hours.

5. All mild bends cases will resolve if treated promptly by recompression.

6. In a population there are people who absorb gas rapidly on compression and there are those who eliminate gas more slowly on decompression. There is thus an asymmetry in the uptake and elimination of inert gas when viewing the population as a whole during the compression and decompression phases of a dive. Equally it has been established that using normal diving procedures there appears to be an asymmetry between the uptake and elimination of gases during compression and decompression procedures even for the individual.

7. Certain forms of diving can lead to adaptation or acclimatization which increases the resistance of the divers to attacks of mild decompression sickness.

8. The no-stop dive data using air as a breathing medium can be simply explained on a $P\sqrt{t}$ relationship providing t does not exceed about 100 min.

9. The outcome of decompression from a saturation or steady state dive, is very sensitive to the oxygen partial pressure being breathed. This sensitivity is also related to the pressure of the dive.

10. Osteonecrosis occurs as a result of hyperbaric exposures in a small proportion of men. Men without any history of overt attacks of the bends can, nevertheless, show osteonecrotic lesions; conversely, men who have had numerous attacks of the bends are sometimes quite free from any such bone disorders.

11. A mass of 'safe' diving data is available and useful as a gross preliminary test of ideas, e.g. excursion dives, surface decompression, etc.

A PHYSICAL MODEL FOR CALCULATION PURPOSES

All systems of calculation seem to have only one point of common agreement, namely that a bubble (or separated gas) is the primary aetiological agent causing limb bends. The following further hypotheses regarding the formation of the gas phase are quite tenable in the present state of knowledge, and it would be an unprofitable exercise to defend one rather than another.

1. A gas nucleus is always present, either in a 'crack', or due to tribonucleation phenomena, or

perhaps vortices in the heart. No decompression can, therefore, be undertaken following a dive according to this hypothesis without a gas phase being present in the tissues or circulation.

2. There is a small pressure drop permissible without gas formation due to the partial unsaturation of tissues caused largely by the oxygen content of the gas being breathed. Thus, provided the decompression is kept within certain limits it is possible to avoid forming a gas phase in the body, and this should lead to a much safer decompression.

3. There is a permissible decompression ratio. Anything less than this permitted decompression ratio has a vanishingly small risk of causing decompression sickness. Any greater ratio has a near certainty of causing decompression sickness. Most decompression schedules in use today depend upon this idea.

Coupled with these three concepts are two major dichotomies of view: namely that bubbles are intravascular or that bubbles are extravascular— and there are sub-divisions of these opinions.

4. The relevant bubbles are intravascular.

(a) The intravascular bubbles are first formed in the arterial circulation.

(b) The intravascular bubbles are first formed in the venous circulation.

5. The relevant bubbles are extravascular.

(a) The extravascular bubbles are formed in interstitial fluid.

(b) The extravascular bubbles are formed in intracellular material.

Added to these various aetiological pathways are two other possibilities:

6. The rate of elimination of dissolved gas from the relevant tissue is largely dependent upon the circulation.

7. The rate of elimination of the dissolved gas from the relevant tissue is largely dependent upon the rate of diffusion of the dissolved gas through the tissue spaces.

There are several paths through the hypotheses mentioned above and these represent only the initial difficulties for anyone attempting a physical picture of events leading to an attack of the bends. Many divergent views are held by highly intelligent and well-informed workers in this field. This serves to illustrate the fact that if anyone found an accurate physicomathematical analysis, it would be an astonishing piece of good fortune. What has happened in the history of the development of attempts to formulate a theoretical structure from which to calculate decompression procedures is that certain basic facts have been used as a reasonable foundation for an approach, and this approach has then been tested in areas of diving not covered by the original observations. The approach has been seen to be only partially successful and has been modified in the light of the new evidence and the cycle of refinement started again. When firm theoretical concepts are eventually established by these methods it will be possible to re-examine the plethora of possibilities regarding the aetiology of decompression sickness. Meantime, hopefully someone will develop a technique, e.g. ultra-sound, which will unequivocally establish where the symptomatic bubble is, and then accurately monitor its growth and resolution, in a large variety of differing circumstances.

The point to be made is that a precise knowledge of the aetiology of the bends is not a necessary prerequisite for successful decompression table calculations. The basic diving data must, of course, be incorporated into any system of calculation which is employed, but a knowledge of the underlying physiology involved can largely be ignored. The author would now like to advance the following scheme for calculating decompression procedures which has met with considerable success and is sufficiently versatile in overall concept to allow further modifications with the advance of more reliable data. There are two principal assumptions and the quantitative aspects of these assumptions will first be described as they relate to the calculation of air decompression procedures. In the first assumption it is considered that if after a long period at P_1 a man is to be decompressed rapidly to some lower pressure P_2, then the permitted decompression ratio $P_1/P_2 = r$ varies with P_1 in the following manner.

$$\frac{P_1}{P_2} = r = \frac{27 \cdot 5714}{P_1 + 12 \cdot 407}$$

where the pressure is measured in bar (ATA approx.).

Thus as P_1 increases, the permissible pressure ratio r decreases according to the above relationship. This expression attempts to cover quantitatively the well-established observations described previously. It predicts that after very long exposures to compressed air at an absolute pressure of 1·92 bar, rapid decompression to an absolute pressure of 1 bar can be undertaken without any ill effects. In the light of the latest evidence from the Tektite exposures, this value of 1·92 may be slightly too high. There must be diminution in the permitted ratio as the pressure increases. For man the problem is open to some doubt as to how much diminution is necessary, because there is a lack of appropriately controlled experimentation, but with animals the matter is beyond dispute and a cut-back in this ratio with increase of pressure is easily and quantitatively demonstrable. It is estimated by analogy from large animal experiments that for man the permitted ratio will change approximately from 1·9 to 1·6 over the range of gauge pressures of 0·96 bar to 3·4 bar. Once again it must be noted that this is just an estimate from animal work and it may be necessary to consider even more cut-back in the permitted decompression ratios as experience dictates. The second assumption concerns the observation that the shape of the pressure time curve for the onset of decompression sickness seems to be the same as that of the curve for the uptake of nitrogen by the whole body, and this in turn is the same shape as a curve describing the quantity of gas diffusing into a slab of material when only one of the faces is exposed to the pressure of gas. Thus there is an exact and well-known physical analogy to describe the uptake of gas curve, or the acquisition of danger curve. The particular equation being used is:

fractional saturation

$$= 1 - \frac{8}{\pi^2} \left\{ e^{-Kt} + \frac{1}{9}\,e^{-9Kt} + \frac{1}{25}\,e^{-25Kt} + \cdots \right\}$$

where $K = D\pi^2/4b^2$, $D =$ diffusion coefficient, and $b =$ thickness of the slab exposed on one side.

This is a solution to Fick's law

$$-\frac{dc}{dt} = D\,\frac{d^2c}{dx^2}$$

where c is the gas concentration (or partial pressure (at some distance x inside the slab, for the particular conditions of thickness b, the slab being initially free of nitrogen and then having one face suddenly exposed at time $t = 0$ to a fixed raised pressure of nitrogen or other gas.

This equation has been put into a computer for the particular value of $K = 0·007928$, which value gives a 30% saturation after 22 min and was considered to be the most realistic fixed point on which to base the shape of this curve. Using this K value implies that in about 9 hours the body is 99% desaturated with gas. This order of time may not be enough in the light of new facts and the K value may need adjusting in the not too distant future from the value which has just been given. As will become apparent in the discussion which follows, the success of these systems of calculation is such that, for the moment at any rate, drastic changes are not warranted.

Bearing in mind that decompression tables are meant to protect the more sensitive men in a large population of healthy divers, the following scheme was evolved. It was assumed that the rate of uptake of gas is 1·5 times faster than the rate of elimination. That the uptake of gas and the elimination of it by a group of healthy men will not be symmetrical is beyond dispute but the assessment of the factor as being 1·5 is, of course, just an estimate and like several other of the previous estimates may need modification in the light of experience.

As an example of the type of calculation involved let it be supposed that one has to decompress a tunnel worker who has been exposed to a gauge pressure of 50 psi, i.e. 3·4 bars for 30 min. In view of the fact that the bar seems to be becoming accepted as a major international pressure unit this will be used throughout in the calculation but, of course, the principle is exactly the same whether feet, metres of seawater or psi gauge are involved.

After 30 min the worker's body is 42·9% saturated, this value being obtained by reference to the basic equation, and thus the quantity of gas in the relevant tissue(s) (or slab analogy) is the same as if he had been at a gauge pressure of 1·46 (i.e. 3·4 times 42·9%) bar for an indefinitely long period. The permitted ratio which can be used with this quantity of gas is obtained from assumption

(1), given above, and is 1·85. Hence the first stage of the decompression is at an absolute pressure of 2·46 divided by 1·85 = 1·3 bar or a gauge pressure of 0·3 bar. For a safe decompression, therefore, the fast phase should end at a gauge pressure of 0·3 bar. It is convenient to place the decompression stages at 0·2 bar intervals and in this case would mean stopping the fast phase at a gauge pressure of 0·4 bar. The calculation continues as follows. The exposure to a gauge pressure of 3·4 bar for 30 min followed by a rapid drop in pressure to a gauge pressure of 0·4 bar may be regarded as equivalent to adding together two exposures, one of which carried on indefinitely absorbing gas at a gauge pressure of 3·4 bar, followed after 30 min by a negative exposure of 3·4 minus 0·4, i.e. gauge pressure of 3·0 bar, which also carried on indefinitely. Ultimately the two curves would become asymptotic and the gas left in the body would be at a gauge pressure of 0·4 bar; but it is only necessary to wait long enough to make the next pressure drop to a gauge pressure of 0·2 bar. At a gauge pressure of 0·2 bar, the permitted excess gas pressure is easily calculated from assumption (1), as 1·26 bar. The superimposition of the ingoing and outgoing curves is continued until it can be seen that an excess gas pressure of 1·26 bar is left. At this point a drop to a gauge pressure of 0·2 bar is permitted. The duration of this stage is calculated by superimposing a pressure drop of 0·2 bar (negative) curve on the existing two curves. The calculation is continued in this simple manner until it is safe to reach atmospheric pressure with an excess gas pressure of 0·92 bar remaining. It must be borne in mind when doing these decompression calculations that the fast graph is used for estimating gas uptake and that at the moment of decompression there is a discontinuity when the slow elimination graph is employed.

All of this simple but somewhat tedious mathematical analysis is best left to the computer. Merely by the insertion of appropriate factors it is possible to calculate quite easily any decompression procedure in any units. Accordingly a set of decompression procedures for use by caisson workers has been in use since 1966 with pounds per square inch as principal units of pressure, whereas since 1968 Air Diving Tables using feet of seawater with the final stop placed at 20 ft (1·6 ATA) have been under active testing. More recently in 1972, as a result of experience with these 1968 Air Diving Tables, a revised metric version, using 5 m (0·5 ATS) increments of depth for decompression stages has been calculated and issued for use.

The decompression ratios estimated from assumption (1) are based on experiments using air as the breathing medium, and consequently in the calculations air was regarded as a single gas. This did not lead to a sufficient cut-back in the permitted decompression ratio and an allowance in the calculations is now made for high oxygen partial pressures. Whenever the partial pressure of oxygen in air (or mixture) exceeds 0·6 bar then it is considered that significant amounts of dissolved oxygen are present in the tissues and that there is an increased decompression risk. This is estimated by adding 25% to the dive depth, and proceeding with the calculations as just outlined using assumption (1). An oxygen first stop depth is thus obtained, and 5 min is spent at this depth to allow for metabolic usage of the excess dissolved oxygen gas. Following this 'oxygen stop' the calculations proceed as outlined above.

Calculation of oxy-helium tables follows exactly the same principles but the real difficulty with these calculations is that assumption (1), concerning the permitted ratios to be used at varying depths, is only obtainable after considerable diving experience and such experience has not yet been gained. Consequently, as with the air diving, the relationship between permitted ratio and dive pressure is somewhat uncertain.

TESTING DECOMPRESSION SCHEDULES

One can examine the literature of compressed air diving and caisson work and read such statements as 'only 10 cases of bends occurred from 10,000 exposures, giving an incidence of 0·1%'. Such statements unaccompanied by a proper further analysis are valueless and misleading. In the first place the nature of the exposures to pressure should be clearly stated. For example, 10 exposures to 30 psi gauge (67 ft; 3 ATA) followed by 10 bends and then 9990 trouble-free exposures to

12 psi gauge (27 ft; 1·8 ATA) would give the results quoted above, but there is very obviously
something amiss with the first decompression procedure despite the very low overall figure. For
diving tables and sometimes for decompression
meters, great claims are made with regard to
success in protecting the diver from mild decompression sickness. Almost invariably the type of
diving which forms the basis for these claims is
very largely of the no-stop variety. Dives such as
15 min at 90 ft (3·7 ATA) or 40 min at 60 ft
(2·8 ATA) dominate the statistics with thousands
of results whereas exposures of 1 hour duration at
160 ft (5·8 ATA), where the adequacy of the decompression procedures is really revealed, represent a minute proportion of the overall numbers.

Assessing decompression procedures from field
trial results is an extremely difficult problem. Very
rarely in practical circumstances does a diver proceed exactly to the limits of a particular decompression profile. It would be rare to find a diver
exactly at 100 ft, for example, for exactly 20 min
and decompressing exactly along the procedures
laid down for this particular dive by any recommended decompression schedule. Thus the adequacy of the decompression routines is never properly evaluated in actual diving circumstances. It
is also well known that divers add on safety factors
in both time and depth in areas of the decompression tables which they have discovered from actual
practice are not offering them adequate security.
Now whilst this is a readily understandable and
indeed quite sensible practice for the working
diver, it is not conducive to reliable statistical
evidence for analysis by those principally concerned with assembling objective data.

Bearing these points in mind, it is now necessary
to examine how the tables based upon the above
calculations have fared when put to stringent controlled testing. With regard to air diving, using
the 1968 calculations whereby the diver was decompressed in 10 ft (0·3 ATS) increments except
for the final stage which was placed at 20 ft
(1·6 ATA), the following has now emerged. Both
Royal Navy and Royal Canadian Navy divers
were tested for 1 hour at 160 ft (5·8 ATA) on the
Air Tables issued either by the US Navy or the
Royal Navy, and a disappointingly high percentage of bends were obtained on both these air

diving schedules. Following these trials, the 1968
Air Diving Procedures were tested by RN divers
and there were no cases of decompression sickness
either in the laboratory dry chamber tests or in the
subsequent wet tests in the laboratory and in the
open sea. Random trials have since continued over
a period of 4 years using acclimatized and un-
acclimatized personnel for the tests, and there has
been an increase in confidence that these particular profiles represent a distinct advance on the
currently available Air Diving Tables. However,
when dives of the order of 1 hour at 200 ft (7 ATA)
were performed at sea on 10 different men, there
were no cases of bends, but subsequent testing in
the dry chambers in the laboratory yielded one or
two 'niggles' and one mild bend, which occurred
upon surfacing. This is an indication that once
again these ideas have an area of usefulness but
that when pushed to extremes they will not offer
adequate protection for the diver. From a practical standpoint, this limitation is of no great
moment because a survey of all diving activity
showed that only extremely rarely were such
dives as 1 hour at 200 ft (7 ATA) ever undertaken
and indeed 200 ft is now being regarded as beyond
the suitable limit for air diving due to the increased respiratory problems encountered at this
depth when attempting heavy exercise. A small
modification was, nevertheless, made to the 1968
tables before issuing the metricized version in
1972 and this was an acknowledgement of the
fact that the no-stop curve calculated for the 1968
tables was somewhat overconservative. For example, the no-stop dive at 100 ft (30 m; 4 ATA)
was given as 15 min and this can be seen to contrast quite markedly with the 25 min given in the
USN no-stop dive for this depth. Consequently, a
change was made to bring the no-stop diving
limits close to the RN diving table limits, as at
present published in the *RN Diving Manual* and,
for example, at 100 ft (30 m; 4 ATA) this would be
20 min. Other than this minor modification dictated by experience, the 1972 calculations are on
exactly similar lines to the 1968 tables.

Regarding the applicability of these calculations
to caisson work, there is little doubt that they represent a good step forward and that the bends
percentages over most of the pressure–time combinations encountered in tunnel and caisson work

have been lowered. Nevertheless, there are clear indications that if the working pressure is sufficiently great and the exposure time sufficiently long then these ideas are inadequate to offer satisfactory protection to the tunnel worker. By 'unsatisfactory protection' is meant a bends percentage not in excess of 2·0%. It is difficult to assess the true reason for the inadequacies which appear, but undoubtedly working for several hours at pressures of 3 ATA or more exposes men's lungs to raised pressures of oxygen which may have some effect upon the subsequent decompression, although, as noted earlier, it is also probable that the K value being used for the elimination of nitrogen is too large and is leading to the view that nitrogen is eliminated from the body rather more rapidly than turns out to be the case in a proportion of the population.

With regard to the incidence of dysbaric osteonecrosis it can be said that after 7 years, and 42 000 entries into compressed air at pressures in excess of 14 psi gauge (1·9 ATA), using these decompression procedures there have been no cases of this disorder of sufficient severity to warrant surgical intervention. Whilst this is, of course, very encouraging, it will be some years yet before one can declare unequivocally whether serious forms of dysbaric osteonecrosis are non-existent using these tables. It is somewhat unfortunate that similar large-scale systematic observations are not available from prolonged and exclusive use of other air decompression tables, as it would then be possible to make objective statements regarding the effectiveness of various pressure-time courses. The incidence of dysbaric osteonecrosis has now become one of the major measures of the effectiveness of decompression tables.

Regarding helium diving, all schedules for short-term diving down to 500 ft (16 ATA) depth for 15 min duration have been given very thorough laboratory and seagoing tests. Once again it is clear that a steady inadequacy is apparent as the dives progress to greater depths. For example, a typical set of recent tests show 0 bends from 98 dives at 200 ft (7 ATA), 2 mild bends from 115 dives at 300 ft (10 ATA) and 4 mild bends from 22 dives at 450 ft (14·6 ATA). The original tests, performed to establish these schedules as suitable, gave 0 bends at either 300 ft or 500 ft

(10 or 16 ATA). It is now apparent, however, that for these early tests the divers had been diving regularly and were indubitably fully 'acclimatized' or 'adapted' to helium diving of this short-duration type. Furthermore, the tests were conducted in the obvious manner, by commencing at the shallow depth and gradually working deeper. This meant that fully 'worked up' men were tried on the more difficult 450 and 500 ft (14·6 and 16 ATA) schedules. Modifications are now in hand to make the deep schedules more suitable for general diver use. Nevertheless even these deep schedules offer a very good security to the diver at very considerable depths, and the worst result from their use seems to be a mild limb pain occurring at, or close to, surface pressure.

AETIOLOGY OF 'THE BENDS'

It is possible, by observing the various decompression schedules which have been used with varying success to decompress divers and caisson workers, to reach preliminary ideas on the aetiology of the bends.

If one examines the no-stop air or oxy-helium diving curves, the following gross fact becomes apparent. Short dives can be performed safely at great depths and long-duration dives can only be performed safely at shallow depths. There arises, therefore, the idea that a quantity of gas is involved in the provocation of limb bend pains. This idea has received considerable support from some very pertinent experiments by Hills (1970) who concludes, 'It is far more likely that the quantity of gas separating from solution determines the imminence of decompression sickness rather than its mere presence as determined by a critical limit to supersaturation'.

It is well known that very serious neurological signs and symptoms can sometimes be presented as a result of decompression, and yet when prompt recompression is given there is generally complete and dramatic relief. As Barnard (1965) pointed out, such remarkable reversibility can only occur if the nervous tissue is substantially undamaged during the course of the attack. If bubbles formed extravascularly in the cell substance then the mechanical damage from the presence of these bubbles necessary to produce a hemiplegia, for example, would be severe, and would hardly be rapidly reversible. However, if one assumes that the bubbles are intravascular, then partial occlusion of the circulation could cause widespread depression of activity which is quite rapidly reversible if not maintained over too long a period. The same argument can be advanced for the milder form of decompression sickness, namely limb pains (bends), which is often accompanied by neurological signs such as diminished reflexes (Barnard 1965), and all such signs are removed completely by recompression.

Following prolonged exposure to compressed air, workers can be decompressed along one of two quite different types of pressure-time profiles in use today. These two different decompression procedures are illustrated by considering the Washington State Regulations and the Blackpool Tables as used in the United Kingdom. The former set of schedules use a continuous decompression procedure and the latter use the more conventional Haldane stage decompression procedure. If these two time courses are compared it can be seen that they are quite dissimilar. The important point to be noticed from the results of operating these two quite dissimilar routines is that from a decompression sickness point of view the outcome is very similar. Here are two totally dissimilar pressure-time courses offering good protection from attacks of limb pains.

The same diversity of decompression paths is becoming apparent when considering decompression from long exposures to raised pressures of oxy-helium. Prolonged excursions from saturation or steady state pressure are now an everyday occurrence and it is clear that large sudden pressure changes are feasible even at depths as great as 300 m (31 ATA; Bühlmann et al. 1970). The systematic experiments of Barnard (1975), already referred to in the text, further illustrate that decompression can be successfully undertaken employing the classic Haldane stage method. Thus, as with air, so with oxy-helium, the time course offered to the diver for his protection can vary quite markedly and yet still be successful. Originally the findings of Barnard (1974) on stage decompression from saturation/steady state dives were considered to have demonstrated that this stage method was only useful at pressures of 100 m (11 ATA) or less.

It has since been realized that the partial pressure of oxygen used (0·22 bar) will not allow successful decompression, on other quite different pressure-time courses at pressures in excess of about 120 m. There is a synergistic effect between oxygen partial pressure and absolute pressure, which has been mentioned previously.

The matter may be restated as follows. If a diver is exposed to a pressure P_1 and then wishes to decompress himself to a lower pressure P_2, the possibilities ahead of him are as follows. If P_2 can be reached in a short period of time without causing decompression sickness, then clearly this is the most economical path. If P_2 cannot be reached without provoking decompression sickness then two major possibilities present themselves for his consideration. First, he can decompress rapidly to some intermediate pressure, P_3, such that the sudden change from pressure P_1 to P_3 does not provoke decompression sickness, but he will now have to stay at pressure P_3 until such time as he can make the next large move towards pressure P_2. Alternatively, he may attempt to decompress himself quite slowly from P_1 in order to stay away from provocation of bends as much as possible. He will thus spend time travelling from P_1 to P_3, which could have been achieved on the previous system much more speedily. However, the hope is that through spending this extra time, and being more conservative, he will have a safer and possibly speedier decompression. There are practical and theoretical advantages in both systems of decompression and experience dictates which to choose for certain circumstances. For example, no-stop diving is a discontinuous or stage system of decompression, but no-one would be foolish enough to suggest that this form of diving should be abandoned in order to avoid formation of some, perhaps even non-existent, silent bubbles. Whereas at great depths on oxy-helium mixtures, there is a distinct risk that sudden large changes in pressure may provoke rather more serious forms of decompression sickness than mild limb pains. Consequently, there is an understandable reluctance to employ this form of pressure-time profile at great depths. From a practical standpoint the fact that one can decompress quite safely from both saturation or non-saturation dives using stages in much the same order of time, or in many cases much less time than by any other system, means that the relevant tissues behave 'as if' supersaturation was possible.

In actual fact of course, bubbles may be present in the relevant tissues, but perhaps due to their position in the blood vessel, or to the little understood growth patterns of very small bubbles, it may be that no serious interference with tissue gas exchange takes place until quite a substantial pressure change occurs. This problem was also answered in a different manner in Chapter 11 of the first edition of this book by Behnke, who said:

(1) A metastable condition of gas transport probably did not extend through successive decrement of pressure.

(2) What appeared to be a condition of supersaturation was a reflection of tolerance of the vascular system to bubble accumulation.

However, use of the phrase 'What appeared to be a condition of supersaturation' concedes the practical fact that one can consider decompression 'as if' supersaturation did exist. Nevertheless, the experiments of Hills (1970) prevent anyone supposing that there are fixed supersaturation limits, as proposed by Haldane and used in modified form by most groups since. This idea, and the numerous variations of it, must now be considered inadequate. In support of the Hills findings the author must mention that the last stop on the air diving tables, calculated as outlined above, was at 20 ft (1·6 ATA) and not the usual 10 ft (1·3 ATA), and this departure from normal practice has been highly successful.

'De-canting' and 'surface decompression' procedures have been practised with complete safety for many years. If one decompresses to atmospheric pressure following an exposure to pressure which will obviously lead to decompression sickness, there is nevertheless a 'safe period' at atmospheric pressure before the onset of trouble, and it was discovered by Edel (1971b) that for the Tektite I depth levels a 15-min surface interval could be safely tolerated.

If one examines the idea of Hills (1970) that in the 'worst possible case' all excess inert gas is released at once upon decompression, then clearly the critical volume which causes decompression sickness is not immediately effective in causing

symptoms. One must invoke the further idea that this volume of gas takes time to re-arrange itself, via coalescence, into a pain-provoking shape. As mentioned above, from many thousands of observations with surface decompression procedures, and the onset of mild bends from other forms of diving it is possible to state that the chances of such coalescence occurring on surfacing, i.e. instantaneous or 'worst possible' coalescence, are negligible and to be realistic one must introduce a mechanism offering a very low probability at zero time. Thus one is forced to accept a probability/time function for coalescence.

This causes re-examination of the statistical aspects of bubble formation, leading to the original idea of phase equilibration, and limited supersaturation.

Given infinite time, a gas-saturated solution will spontaneously form a gas nucleus. In a reasonable period of time, say 1 hour, the probability of this event occurring is so small as to be unworthy of consideration. If the solution is decompressed, and a state of supersaturation supervenes then it is obvious that the probability of bubble formation is dependent upon two variables, the degree of supersaturation and the total time involved at that level of supersaturation. It may be objected at this point that mechanical factors such as tribonucleation, muscle contraction etc. will invalidate this probability concept, but if one once invokes such precipitating factors then for the 'worst possible' case one must abandon inherent unsaturation, oxygen window, etc., because if these mechanical factors are stressing the solutions and causing cavitation, they can cause bubble formation even in undersaturated solutions. Thus, if one ignores mechanical factors, the limited supersaturation and the phase equilibration theories, although apparently at variance, do in fact converge when it is realized that the level of sustained supersaturation is a critical variable. A complex set of functions describing the probability of nucleation for various levels of supersaturation from zero time to infinity, are necessary. Simple phase equilibration takes the probability after infinite time, i.e. 1·0. whereas simple supersaturation theory takes the probability after a very short time; both views are therefore extremes of a much more complicated situation. The enormity of the computational task confronting the schedule calculator is now becoming very apparent.

Finally, it is possible to explain the fact qualitatively in a very different way. It may be supposed that bubbles are always present regardless of the nature of the decompression. Dissolved gas in the tissue(s) has two paths for elimination during decompression, first via the blood stream and secondly into the bubble, and the bubble itself is subject to expansion according to Boyle's Law. Thus three factors are determining the outcome of the pressure-time profile. The prospects of rendering this model quantitative are indeed daunting, especially when the difficulties of understanding the growth of small bubbles are appreciated.

Regarding the site of origin of these bubbles, one must agree with Behnke (1971) that the evidence is heavily in favour of it being intravascular. Furthermore, bubbles are almost certainly first found in the arterial circulation, as various observers over many years attest, e.g. Wagner (1945), Lever et al. (1966), Hempleman (1968) and Buckles (1968).

Bubbles in the arterial circulation would be thrust into the capillary bed and, if large enough, would cause blockage, whereas such bubbles generated on the venous side would be prone to being dislodged by the blood flow. Bubbles occluding the arterial side of the tissue circulation would not grow against the arterial pressure, but they would extend down the pressure gradient into the venous side and it is this apparent venous occlusion accompanied by bubble generation which can be mistaken for true venous origin and blockage.

Further evidence that the arterial vessels are implicated as sources of 'separated gas' is gleaned from the observations that when dead animals, with no circulation, are given exposures to high pressures of air or other gases the bubbles seen upon decompression are always in the arterial system (Hempleman 1968; Smit-Sivertsen 1975).

CONCLUSION

Bearing in mind the complexity of events leading to 'bends' pains it is astonishing to find that simple calculations, such as those described earlier, can lead to quite successful practical procedures over quite a wide range of pressures and times. All current theories have incorrect or grossly oversimplified underlying assumptions, and a good deal of further experimentation is needed to reduce the extent of our ignorance.

Although attention has largely been directed towards avoidance of the 'bends' it must be re-emphasised that avoidance of bone damage is equally, if not more, important.

REFERENCES

ALBANO, G. (1960) Études sur la decompression chez l'homme. Les valeurs critiques du gradient de pression à la remonte sans paliers. *1st Int. Conf. Sub-Aquatic Med.*, Cannes, 15–19 June.

BARNARD, E. E. P. (1965) Methods used in the treatment of decompression sickness. *Le pétrole et la mer*, Section IV, No. 411.

BARNARD, E. E. P. (1967) The treatment of decompression sickness developing at extreme pressures. In *Proc. 3rd Symp. Underwater Physiology*. Ed. C. J. Lambertsen. Baltimore: Williams & Wilkins.

BARNARD, E. E. P. (1975) Fundamental studies in decompression from steady state exposures. In *Underwater Physiology. Vth Symp. Underwater Physiology*. Bethesda: Fedn Am. Socs exp. Biol.

BEHNKE, A. R. (1967) The isobaric (oxygen window) principle of decompression. In *The New Thrust Seaward. Trans. 3rd a. Conf. and Exib.* Washington: Marine Technology Society.

BEHNKE, A. R. (1971) Decompression sickness; advances and interpretations. *Aerospace Med.* **42**, 255–267.

BERHAGE, T. E., CONDA, K. J. & ARMSTRONG, F. W. (1973) *The Synergistic Effect of Pressure and Oxygen and its Relationship to Decompression Sickness in Mice.* Research report 22–73, Navy Experimental Diving Unit, Washington, D.C.

BORNMANN, R. C. (1971) Helium–oxygen saturation-excursion diving for US Navy. In *Underwater Physiology. Proc. 4th Symp. Underwater Physiology*. Ed. C. J. Lambertsen. pp. 529–536. New York: Academic Press.

BUCKLES, R. G. (1968) The physics of bubble formation and growth. *Aerospace Med.* **39**, 1062–1069.

BÜHLMANN, A. A., MATTHYS, H., OVERRATH, G., BENNETT, P. B., ELLIOTT, D. H. & GRAY, S. P. (1970) Saturation exposures at 31 ata in an oxygen–helium atmosphere with excursions to 36 ata. *Aerospace Med.* **40**, 394–402.

CATTON, M. J. (1967) Prevention of Decompression Sickness by Special Procedures. In *Decompression of Compressed Air Workers in Civil Engineering*. Proc. of International Working Party, CIBA Foundation, London, 1965. Ed. R. I. McCallum. Newcastle-upon-Tyne: Oriel Press.

DONALD, K. W. (1955) Oxygen bends. *J. appl. Physiol.* **7**, 639–644.

DUFFNER, C. J. & SNYDER, H. H. (1958) *Effects of Exposing Men to Compressed Air and Helium–oxygen Mixtures for*

12 Hours at Pressure of 2–2:6 Atmospheres. Research Report 1–59. US Navy Experimental Diving Unit, Washington, D.C.

DWYER, J. V. (1956) *Calculation of Repetitive Diving Decompression Tables.* Research Report 1–57. US Navy Experimental Diving Unit, Washington, D.C.

EATON, W. J. & HEMPLEMAN, H. V. (1973) *The Role of Oxygen in the Aetiology of Acute Decompression Sickness.* Report 12/73. R.N. Physiological Laboratory, Alverstoke.

EDEL, P. O. (1971a) *Experiments to Determine Decompression Tables for the Tektite II 100 fsw Mission.* Report for NASA Contract No. 14-01-0001-1384. Houston: J and J Marine Diving Co.

EDEL, P. O. (1971b) Delineation of emergency surface decompression and treatment procedures for project Tektite aquanauts. *Aerospace Med.* **42**, 616–621.

FRYER, D. I. (1969) *Sub-Atmospheric Decompression Sickness in Man.* Technivision Services: Slough.

GOLDING, F. C., GRIFFITHS, P. D., HEMPLEMAN, H. V., PATON, W. D. M. & WALDER, D. N. (1960) Decompression sickness during construction of the Dartford Tunnel. *Br. J. ind. Med.* **17**, 167–180.

HAMILTON, R. W., KENYON, D. J., FREITAG, N. & SCHREINER, H. R. (1973) *Formulation of Excursion Procedures for Shallow Undersea Habitats.* Final Report to the Office of Manned Undersea Science and Technology NOAA Contract 2-35479, Union Carbide Corporation, New York.

HAMILTON, R. W., MacINNIS, J. B., NOBLE, A. D. & SCHREINER, H. R. (1966) *Saturation Diving at 650 feet.* Ocean Systems Technical Memorandum B-411. Tonawanda, New York.

HAWKINS, J. A., SHILLING, C. W. & HANSON, R. A. (1935) A suggested change in calculating decompression tables for diving. *Nav. med Bull.* **33**, 327–338.

HEMPLEMAN, H. V. (1963) Tissue Inert Gas Exchange and Decompression Sickness. In *Proc. 2nd Symp. Underwater Physiology.* Ed. C. J. Lambertsen and L. J. Greenbaum, Jr. pp. 6–13. Natl Acad Sci-Natl Res. Council. Washington, D.C.

HEMPLEMAN, H. V. (1967) Decompression procedures for deep, open sea operations. In *Proc. 3rd Symp. Underwater Physiology.* Ed. C. J. Lambertsen. Baltimore: Williams & Wilkins.

HEMPLEMAN, H. V. (1968) Bubble formation and decompression sickness. *Rev. Physiol. Sub-Aq. Med Hyperbare* **1**, 181–183.

HEMPLEMAN, H. V. (1975) In *Underwater Physiology. Vth Symp. Underwater Physiology.* Bethesda: Fedn Am. Socs exp. Biol.

HILLS, B. (1966) *A Thermo-dynamic and Kinetic Approach to Decompression Sickness.* Adelaide: Libraries Board of S. Australia.

HILLS, B. A. (1970) Limited supersaturation versus phase equilibration in predicting the occurrence of decompression sickness. *Clin. Sci.* **38**, 251–267.

HILLS, B.A. (1971) Decompression sickness: a fundamental study of 'surface excursion' diving and the selection of limb bends versus CNS symptoms. *Aerospace Med.* **42**, 833–836.

LEVER, M. J., MILLER, K. W., PATON, W. D. M. & SMITH, E. B. (1966) Experiments on the genisis of bubbles as a result of rapid decompression. *J. Physiol. Lond.* **184**, 964–969.

RUBISSOW, G. J. & MACKAY, R. S. (1971) Ultra-sonic imaging of in vivo bubbles in decompression sickness. *Ultrasonics* **9**, 225–234.

SMITH, K. H. & SPENCER, M. P. (1970) Doppler indices of decompression sickness: Their evaluation and use. *Aerospace Med.* **41**, 1396–1400.

SMIT-SIVERTSEN, J. (1975) In *Underwater Physiology. Vth Symp. Underwater Physiology.* Bethesda: Fedn Am. Socs exp. Biol.

State of New York Regulations (1922) *State of New York Industrial Code Bulletin 22–23A,* 1 May 1922.

SWAIN, V. A. J. (1942) Caisson disease (compressed air illness) of bone with a report of a case. *Br. J. Surg.* **29**, 365–370.

WAGNER, C. E. (1945) Observations of gas bubbles in peal vessels of cats following rapid decompression from high atmospheres. *J. Neurophysiol.* **8**, 29–32.

WALDER, D. N. (1970) In *Proc. 4th Int. Congr. Hyperbaric Medicine.* Sapporo, Japan, September 1969, pp. 83–88. Baltimore: Williams & Wilkins.

19

Decompression Theory: Swiss Practice

A. A. BÜHLMANN

In 1959 a young Swiss, Hannes Keller, confronted the world with the problems of deep diving. At that time little progress was being made in developing deep diving techniques by the leading maritime countries such as England, France and the USA. There was no Swiss Decompression Theory and no tradition to restrict the approach. Such lack of experience favours the development of a simple working hypothesis.

DEVELOPMENT OF THE METHOD OF 'MIXED GAS DECOMPRESSION'

The newcomer to this field of research had five facts to work from:

1. Reasonably safe decompression tables existed for air diving to depths as far as 200 ft (7 ATA).

2. Inert gases were known to have cerebral effects, which varied between individuals. An accepted figure for P_{N_2} tolerance was 5 to 6 ATS.

3. The greater gas density at depth increased the breathing resistance, particularly where turbulent flow existed in valves and air passages.

4. The possibility of shortening decompression time by breathing a high P_{O_2} was limited by the toxic effects of hyperoxia.

5. The observation that longer decompression was necessary to avoid troubles after oxyhelium dives with short bottom time than with equivalent air dives.

These facts suggested that the saturation of some tissues occurred faster with helium than with nitrogen. The assumption of different saturation speeds implied a possibility of shortening decompression time by combining advantageously a sequence of inert gases such as helium, nitrogen, hydrogen, neon and argon with a high partial pressure of oxygen. In theory it seemed clear that a change of inert gas from helium to nitrogen during decompression, would hasten the elimination of helium because the helium pressure gradient between blood and tissue is increased, while at the same time the intake of nitrogen would occur more slowly.

The special features of the pilot experiments in deep diving were:

Slow compression, breathing 100% oxygen, from 1·0 to 2·5 ATA.

Fast compression at a rate of 2 to 3 ATS/min to total pressure.

Change from helium to nitrogen during decompression.

Continuous decompression to maintain a high pressure gradient of inert gas between tissues and blood.

Premixed gases breathed through a mouthpiece from either open circuit or semi-closed apparatus.

Assumptions made in calculating saturation and desaturation with different inert gases

Saturation and desaturation follow an exponential curve. A spectrum of various half-times can be used to calculate the equalization of the partial

TABLE 19.1

Molecular weights and solubility coefficients of various gases at 37° to 38°C (FASEB 1971)

	H_2	He	Ne	N_2	Ar	O_2
Molecular weight	2·016	4·003	20·183	28·016	39·948	32·00
Solubility, ml/ml at 760 mm Hg, 37°C						
Water	0·0166	0·0086	0·0096	0·0123	0·028	0·0239
Whole blood	0·0149	0·0088	0·0093	0·0130	0·026	0·0223
Olive oil	0·0484	0·0159	0·0199	0·0670	0·148	0·1120

TABLE 19.2

Relationship of solubility coefficients

	N_2/H_2	N_2/He	N_2/Ne	N_2/Ar	H_2/He
Whole blood and watery tissues	0·872	1·477	1·398	0·500	1·693
Pure fat as oil	1·384	4·214	3·367	0·453	3·044

pressures of inspired inert gas and of inert gas dissolved in the tissues. In 1959 the conventional air tables were based on a maximum half-time for nitrogen of about 4 hours.

For a study of inert gas exchange it was important to determine the different saturation speeds for individual gases. It was easy to explain the different half-times for the same gas by differences in the perfusion rates for the tissues. For a constant perfusion rate, the saturation speed depends mainly on the physicochemical properties of the inert gases. A difference in the saturation speed could be the result of different solubility coefficients in fatty and watery tissues; or different speeds of pressure equalization, related to the molecular weight of the inert gases.

Tables 19.1 and 19.2 give the molecular weights, the solubility factors in whole blood, water and olive oil, and the relationship between the solubility coefficients.

The different solubilities imply considerable variation in the masses of the dissolved gases for full saturation of all tissues. This is of significance for their toxic effects as well as for decompression.

In decompression sickness, the available mass of gas controls both volume and surface area of

bubbles formed; this in turn determines the degree of tissue deformation. The size of the bubbles also depends on the gas volume due to the diffusion of oxygen, carbon dioxide and other inert gases. In this connection helium is preferable to hydrogen as a light gas, while as a heavy gas nitrogen is preferable to argon. Neon would be just as suitable as helium. The great variation in the solubility ratios of these gases in oil and water (Table 19.3) influences the speed of saturation during compression, bottom time and decompression. The partition coefficient is practically identical for nitrogen and argon. For hydrogen the coefficient is smaller than either of these two gases but larger than the values for helium and neon.

Because of these ratios, the rate of saturation of helium in purely fat tissue is approximately three times faster than nitrogen. This would apply to subcutaneous fat. The equalization of pressure for hydrogen in a fatty tissue is, however, only 1·8 times faster than nitrogen. There are no significant differences between helium and neon, or between nitrogen and argon. For very fatty tissues, hydrogen with a slightly slower saturation speed would have certain advantages over helium.

As far as the speed of equalization of pressures

TABLE 19.3

Partition coefficients at 37° to 38°C oil/water

	H_2 2·921	He 1·849	Ne 2·073	N_2 5·460	Ar 5·286	O_2 4·694
Relationship	N_2/H_2 1·869	N_2/He 2·953	N_2/Ne 2·634	N_2/Ar 1·033	H_2/He 1·580	

TABLE 19.4

Square roots of molecular weights

	H_2 1·420	He 2·001	Ne 4·492	N_2 5·293	Ar 6·320	O_2 5·657
Relationship	N_2/H_2 3·728	N_2/He 2·646	N_2/Ne 1·178	N_2/Ar 0·837	H_2/He 0·710	

in watery tissues is concerned, the different solu-bility coefficients of these inert gases in oil and water are not important. With virtually equal solubility in blood and tissue, the conditions corre-spond to a diffusion-limited system. This would be the case for very poorly perfused and capillarized tissues with relatively long diffusion routes. Under these conditions the rate of pressure equalization depends on diffusion, which is governed by the molecular weight of the gases. The saturation speeds of two gases are in inverse proportion to the square root of their molecular weights (Table 19.4). Thus, for watery tissues, saturation and desatura-tion will occur approximately 3·7 times faster with hydrogen than with nitrogen. Helium will be about 2·6 times faster than nitrogen and no signi-ficant differences may be expected between neon, nitrogen and argon. It may be concluded that a practical advantage in the use of different inert gases could be obtained by using helium and nitrogen but that no such advantage could be expected from the use of neon or argon. *The gases suitable for multiple inert gas decompression are, therefore, reduced to helium and nitrogen.* In re-viewing these theoretical assumptions it can now be said that the conclusions have been substanti-ated. The tests with argon, neon and hydrogen, which were carried out in the early part of the

programme, did not suggest any advantage in using them for decompression after deep diving.

The hypothesis for calculation of decompression in 1960 was reduced to this simple model:

For the same inert gas, different half-times were related to the perfusion rates of the tissues.

For a tissue with a given perfusion rate, the ratio of half-times for different inert gases is equal to the square root of their molecular weights.

The same supersaturation factors for different inert gases are based only on the ratio between the inert gas pressure in the tissue and the total ambient pressure.

The partial pressures of the different inert gases in the same tissue must be added together. It would be wrong to attempt a decompression where the supersaturation factor was not exceeded for each gas individually.

Using this working hypothesis some deep diving experiments were devised and performed in the wet chamber facilities of the French Navy in Toulon (GERS) and of the US Navy in Washing-ton (EDU) during 1960/61 (Table 19.5).

The financial support of the US Navy enabled the development and improvement of the method of 'mixed gas decompression' and it was shown

TABLE 19.5

Pilot experiments with H. Keller

Date	ATA	Bottom time	Decom-pression (min)	Location
4.11.60	26·0	c. 10 sec	47	GERS
25.4.61	31·0	c. 10 sec	31	GERS
26.4.61	22·5	10 min*	140	GERS
10.5.61	22·5	10 min*	135	EDU

* With physical work.

that this method is also valid for longer bottom times and for different divers.

EXPERIMENTS IN 1962 SPONSORED BY THE US NAVY

All the decompressions to be described, with the exception of the 26·0 and 31·0 ATA experiments (see Table 19.6), were carried out successfully by

TABLE 19.6

Mixed gas decompression after helium dives

ATA	Bottom time (min)	Decom-pression (min)	Decom-pressions (number)	Different subjects
5·0	120	20	7	7
10·0–11·0	60*	105–125	9	9
16·0	30	220	6	6
21·0	20*	230	5	5
26·0	10	270	2	2
31·0	5*	270	4	2

* Carried out in the pressure chamber, and also with swimming excursions in the sea (Keller & Bühlmann 1965).

at least four different divers without serious symptoms of oxygen poisoning or decompression sickness. Like the pilot experiments mentioned earlier, these tests were carried out with pre-mixed gases and an open circuit or semi-closed breathing system. The inert gas change takes place immediately using this technique. Further, the short decompression time after short exposures permits the change from helium to nitrogen to be combined with a high oxygen concentration. If oxygen is given through a mouthpiece, the concentration can be increased to 100% without any great risk,

provided the decompression is performed in a pressure chamber filled with air. Decompression took place continuously in all these experiments.

In Fig. 19.1 is illustrated the possibility of shortening decompression time by changing the inert gas from helium to nitrogen on the bottom. The exposure is 120 mins at 130 ft (5 ATA). The P_{O_2} amounts to 2 ATS during the exposure and the decompression. The change of inert gas from helium to nitrogen takes place during the dive at 130 ft (5 ATA). Nitrogen can be breathed without trouble at this depth and the change permits the elimination of helium. The P_{N_2} of a tissue with, say, a 50-min half-time, decreases during the helium phase of the exposure from 0·8 ATS to approximately 0·3 ATS; it then increases during the nitrogen phase to 1·65 ATS. The P_{He} in the corresponding tissue with a helium half-time of 20 min increases to 2·7 ATS during the first phase and decreases again to approximately 0·4 ATS during the nitrogen phase. This results in a P_{inert} total of only 2 ATS. By breathing oxygen for 15 min, the P_{He} and P_{N_2} are decreased till the critical value for surfacing is reached (total $P_{inert} = 1·6$ ATS).

If the experiment were to be performed with 60% nitrogen as the sole inert gas, a P_{N_2} of approximately 2·6 ATS would occur in the same tissue after 120 min. This pressure would only decrease to the critical value after breathing pure oxygen for 40 min. Thus the change of inert gas on the bottom results in a saving of 25 min in decompression time.

If, however, the diver breathes 60% helium during the whole exposure, the 20-min tissue is almost saturated after 120 min; this, together with the remaining N_2, would result in a P_{inert} total of some 3·2 ATS in the tissue. In this case breathing oxygen for 25 min from 50 ft to the surface would be sufficient to decrease the P_{inert} total to 1·6 ATS.

If a mixture of 40% oxygen, 44% helium and 16% nitrogen were to be breathed during the first phase (thus maintaining the P_{N_2} constant at 0·8 ATS) the decompression using 100% oxygen between 50 ft (2·5 ATA) and the surface would take 20 min. The total decompression time would then be nearly as short as the experiment illustrated.

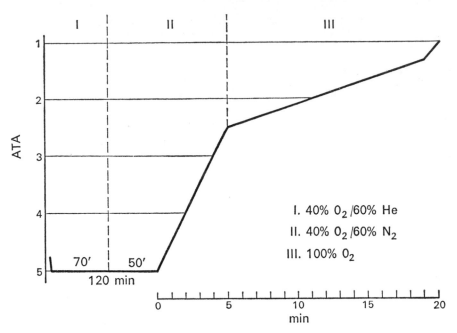

F IG. 19.1. Bottom time 120 min at 130 ft (5 ATA) with 40% oxygen, 60% helium (P_{He} = 3 ATS). Inert gas change from helium to nitrogen after 70 min. Decompression time 20 min with inhalation of 100% oxygen from 50 ft to surface (2·5 to 1·0 ATA)

The differences in decompression time described above show that the change of inert gas from helium to nitrogen, after exposures at shallow depth, is only an advantage in shortening decompression time for bottom times up to about 120 min. For longer exposures and at greater depths, the inert gas change can take place only during the decompression and is moved more and more towards the final phase as these features of the dive increase.

Fig. 19.2 shows two possible ways of decompressing after an exposure of 60 min at 330 ft (11 ATA). The P_{O_2} amounts to 1·65 ATS during the period at depth and also increases to more than 2 ATS for a short time during decompression. In version (a) the diver breathes air between 200 and 115 ft (7 and 4·5 ATA), 50% oxygen and 50% nitrogen between 115 and 50 ft (4·5 and 2·5 ATA) and thereafter 100% oxygen. In version (b) there is no phase of breathing pure oxygen and the total decompression time is 385 min, whereas it was only 105 min in version (a).

Fig. 19.3 gives an example of a short decom-

pression for a 30-min exposure at 500 ft (16 ATA). The P_{O_2} is 2·4 to 2·5 ATS and the nitrogen concentration of the breathing mixture is increased in the early decompression phases.

Decompressions using the same gas mixtures but with lower oxygen concentration at full pressure, have been performed after bottom times of 20 min at 660 ft (21 ATA), 10 min at 825 ft (26 ATA) and 5 min at 1000 ft (31 ATA). For further details see Figs 19.4 and 19.5.

By the end of these tests, which finished in December 1962 off San Diego, USA, the following conclusions could be drawn:

It is possible to undertake deep diving in the ocean and permit work on the Continental Shelf.

The bottom times necessary for work require many hours of decompression. It is difficult for divers to use breathing apparatus for these periods so an underwater pressure chamber becomes essential for deep diving.

Long bottom and decompression times cause the slow tissues, such as bones and joints, to

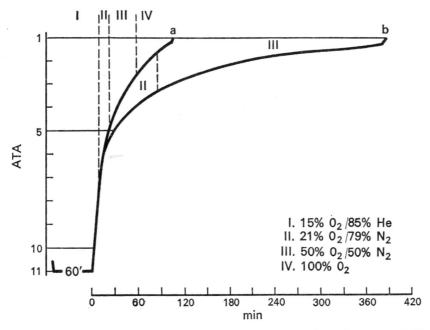

FIG. 19.2. Bottom time 60 min at 330 ft (11 ATA) with 15% oxygen, 85% helium ($P_{He} = 9 \cdot 35$ ATS). Version (a)—inert gas change from helium to nitrogen with different oxygen partial pressures and 100% oxygen at pressures less than 50 ft (2·5 ATA). Total decompression time 105 min. Version (b)—air breathing from 120 to 35 ft (6 to 2·5 ATA) following 50% oxygen/50% nitrogen. Total decompression time 385 min

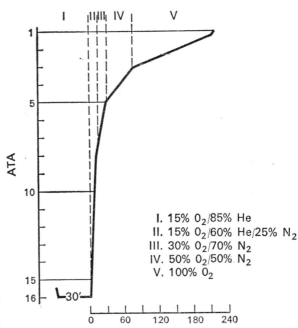

FIG. 19.3. Bottom time 30 min at 500 ft (16 ATA) with 15% oxygen, 85% helium ($P_{He} = 13 \cdot 6$ ATS). Adding stepwise oxygen and nitrogen. 100% oxygen below 2·5 ATA. Total decompression time 220 min

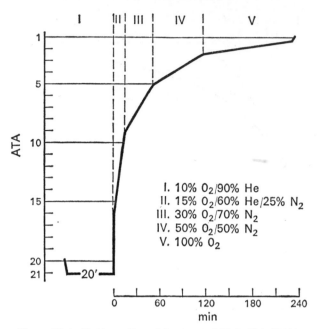

FIG. 19.4. Bottom time 20 min at 660 ft (21 ATA) with 10% oxygen, 90% helium ($P_{He} = 18 \cdot 9$ ATS). Stepwise increase of oxygen to 100%. From 500 to 260 ft (16 to 9 ATA) helium as well as nitrogen in the gas mixture, thereafter nitrogen only. Total decompression time 230 min

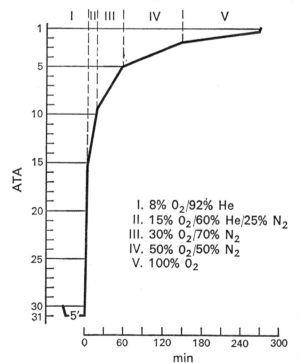

FIG. 19.5. Bottom time 5 min at 1000 ft (31 ATA) with 8% oxygen, 92% helium ($P_{He} = 28 \cdot 5$ ATS). Carried out in the pressure chamber and in water. Identical procedure as in Fig. 19.4. Total decompression time 270 min

become saturated. These are the tissues that control the rate of decompression.

It would be impossible to develop decompression tables, which would be reasonably safe for professional divers, without a study of saturation dives.

FUNDAMENTAL RESEARCH AND PROLONGED EXPERIMENTS AS A BASIS FOR DETERMINING DECOMPRESSION TABLES 1964 TO 1972

The general features of the trials were as follows:

Compression rate 1·0 to 1·5 ATS/min.

Chamber initially filled with air and pressurized with helium and pure oxygen, thus maintaining a constant P_{N_2} of 0·8 ATS. Change from helium to nitrogen as the inert gas by flushing the chamber with air.

Independent analysis of oxygen, helium, nitrogen and carbon dioxide.

Due allowance for the contamination of oxy-helium atmosphere by nitrogen in calculating decompression.

Limiting the use of breathing apparatus, with prepared gas mixtures, to excursions in the water.

Measured physical work during bottom time.

Continuous decompression to first stop and thereafter decompression in steps.

These conditions could only be achieved with a fully equipped system of high pressure chambers as was available in Zürich after 1964.

Half-time spectrum for helium and nitrogen

In order to calculate the decompression for long exposures and to determine the optimum time for changing inert gases, it is essential to know the half-time of the slowest tissues. Assuming that the same half-times are valid for saturation and desaturation, the longest half-times were determined by finding the minimum decompression time, breathing pure oxygen, after prolonged periods at 100 ft (4 ATA) during which either 20% oxygen, 80% helium or 20% oxygen, 80% nitrogen was used (Bühlmann, Frey & Keller 1967). No bends occur after an exposure to a P_{He} of 3·2 ATS (Fig. 19.6), provided that decompression is based on the longest half-time of 160 to 180 min. In

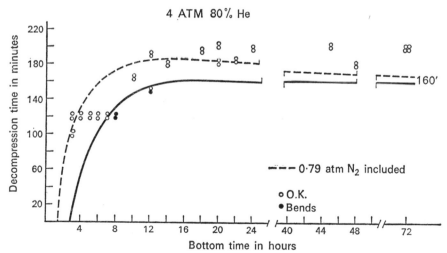

Fig. 19.6. The results of 40 experiments are presented. Bottom times with 80% helium, 20% oxygen at 100 ft (4 ATA) varied from 3 to 72 hours (abscissa). Decompression times breathing 100% oxygen are given in minutes on the ordinate. The line in dashes represents the minimum decompression times for a half-time of 160 min starting with a normal P_{N_2} of 0·8 ATS in the tissues. This P_{N_2} in the tissues decreases with a half-time of 420 min during exposure on the bottom. The unbroken line represents the true minimum decompression time for a half-time of 160 min in the absence of nitrogen throughout the entire experiment

these experiments the initial P_{N_2} of 0·8 ATS was allowed for, and a ratio between the total partial pressure of inert gases and the ambient pressure on the surface of 1·55 to 1·60 was used in calculation. After an exposure of 24 hours 99% saturation is reached; beyond this, as can be seen in Fig. 19.6, no longer time for decompression is required whatever the bottom time.

The corresponding experiments with air indicated that 64 to 72 hours were required for complete saturation and the longest half-time for nitrogen is about 480 min. This difference between helium and nitrogen is in agreement with the theoretical predictions for a 'diffusion-limited' system with equal solubility in blood and tissue and for a delayed saturation and desaturation of very fatty tissues due to the different partition coefficients of the gases. However, these experiments are only representative of the slowest tissue. They do not answer the question whether the varying saturation rates of helium and nitrogen are due to their different solubility rates in blood and fat tissues or to their different molecular weights.

As the tissues in ligaments, joint capsules and menisci are mainly water, the predilection of the bends for knee and ankle joints with either helium or nitrogen suggests that a 'diffusion-limited' system is involved.

Because of the results of the saturation experiments at 100 ft (4 ATA) (see Fig. 19.7) and successful decompressions after short exposures at high pressure, we assume *that saturation and de-*

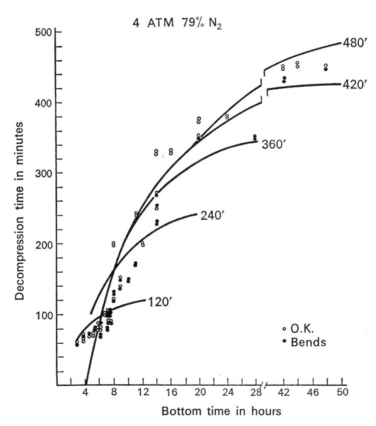

FIG. 19.7. The results of 80 experiments are presented. Bottom times with compressed air at 100 ft (4 ATA) varied from 3 to 48 hours (abscissa). Decompression times breathing 100% oxygen are given in minutes on the ordinate. The lines represent the minimum decompression times for half-times of 120 to 480 min calculated with a surfacing ratio of 1·6 to 1·0

saturation in all tissues is 2·6 times faster with helium than with nitrogen.

If we suppose the half-time to be determined mainly by the perfusion of the different tissues, it can be expected that any change of half-time will depend on physical work, particularly for the slow tissues. It is probable that during sleep, with a reduction of cardiac output, the longest half-times will increase. When saturation with helium, on the basis of a longest half-time of 180 min, involves decompression lasting many hours or even days we allow maximum half-times of 240 min for helium and 635 min for nitrogen in calculating the actual decompression. This method of allowing for the effect of physical work applies only to saturation dives. More specific account must be taken of physical work in determining the decompression for intervention dives with bottom times between 30 and 60 min.

The influence of physical work on decompression

The effect of physical work on decompression was examined by determining the minimum decompression time for simulated oxy-helium dives by 82 different subjects (Schibli & Bühlmann 1972). Details of the experimental conditions are summarized in Table 19.7.

The descent times of 7 min for the 4·5 ATA tests and 12 min for the 10 ATA tests, were not included in the bottom times.

The P_{N_2} remained constant at 0·8 ATS during descent and time on bottom. The subjects performed work on a bicycle ergometer with a load of 80W (490 m-kg/min) before the experiments and during time on the bottom. Each subject worked 15 min/hour on the bottom. The average pulse rate increased from 60 to 100. During decompression the same form of bicycling was done, starting below 2·5 ATA breathing pure oxygen.

A simple oxygen decompression was used for the 4·5 ATA experiments. Mixed gas decompression was used for the 10 ATA experiments; air was breathed between 6·0 and 4·0 ATA, 50% oxygen, 50% nitrogen between 4·0 and 2·0 ATA and 100% oxygen between 2·0 and 1·0 ATA.

Minimum decompression times were established, first without work on the bottom and secondly with work on the bottom. If bends occurred in muscles or joints during or after decompression, then the decompression was recalculated and increased for the next experimental run.

After 180 min at 4·5 ATA the minimum decompression time without work was 150 min and with work it was 180 min (Fig. 19.8).

The minimum decompression time without work after 60 min at 10 ATA was 250 min. If work was performed this minimum decompression without symptoms increased to 360 min (Fig. 19.9). This decompression time after work is approximately equal to the decompression computed for a 90-min bottom time at 10 ATA without work.

For the longer period of 120 min bottom time at 10 ATA the minimum decompression time was 475 min without work and 565 min with work on the bottom (Fig. 19.10).

These results demonstrate clearly that the minimum decompression time must be longer after a dive with work than after a similar dive without work. These differences in decompression decrease with longer bottom time. The results can be interpreted as an increased perfusion with work in the muscles, joints and skin, whereas the perfusion of

TABLE 19.7

Experimental conditions

ATA	Bottom time (min)	Breathing gas on bottom (%)			Tests without work	Tests with work	Tests with work on bottom and decompressing	Total
		O_2	He	N_2				
4·5	180	11	71	18	12	25	18	76
10·0	60	10	82	8	15	39	22	42
10·0	120	10	82	8	15	27	—	55
					42	91	40	173

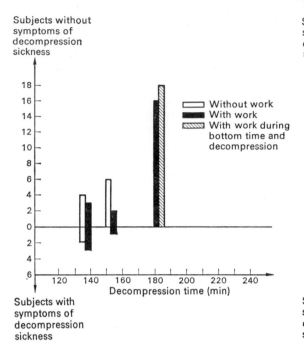

FIG. 19.8. The results of 55 decompressions are presented. 180-min bottom time at 115 ft (4·5 ATA) breathing 11% oxygen, 71% helium, 18% nitrogen. Number of subjects without and with symptoms of insufficient decompression shown as function of decompression time, for cases without work (white), with work at bottom (black), and with work at bottom as well as during decompression (hatched)

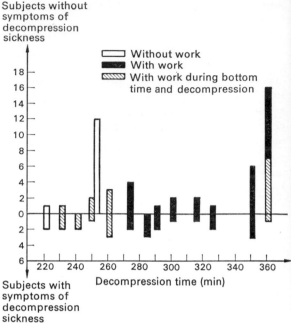

FIG. 19.9. The results of 76 decompressions are presented. 60-min bottom time at 300 ft (10 ATA) breathing 10% oxygen, 82% helium, 8% nitrogen. (For explanations see Fig. 19.8)

TABLE 19.8

Adaptation of half-times for dives with physical work

He *half-time* (*min*)	*Virtual bottom time as a percentage of real bottom time*
105	120
120	120
150	135
180	135
210	145
240	145

the central nervous system is practically constant. Accordingly, the first phase of decompression, which is limited by the fast tissues, is equal whether or not work is performed. The second phase, however, must be prolonged when work takes place on the bottom, since the slow tissues, which are more fully saturated than without work, now control the rate of ascent. To take account of these considerations decompression after work is computed using *virtual bottom times* for tissues with helium half-times of 105 to 240 min (Table 19.8).

Theoretically it might be assumed that work during decompression will shorten the decompression time as a result of the increased blood flow in the slow tissues of the extremities. This question cannot be resolved from these experiments but it is unlikely, since the decompression time is too long for continuous work. However, no symptoms of insufficient decompression were provoked by

bicycling during decompression. There may be some benefit in intermittent work during decompression as it counteracts the reduced circulation caused by high oxygen partial pressure.

Summarizing, it may be said that the effect of physical work in increasing the saturation of the inert gas has to be taken into account for calculating the decompression after short-duration dives. The use of *virtual bottom times* in doing this has the advantage that the spectrum of half-times and

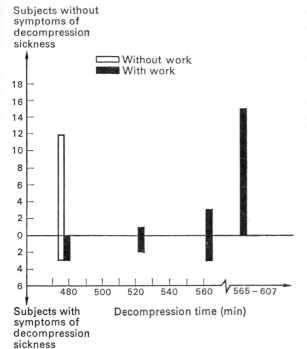

FIG. 19.10. The results of 42 decompressions are presented. 120-min bottom time at 300 ft (10 ATA) breathing 10% oxygen, 82% helium, 8% nitrogen. (For explanations see Fig. 19.8)

the supersaturation factors are constant for all dives.

Tolerable supersaturation factors

It has been learned by experience that Haldane's supersaturation factor of 1·6 is tolerated by the slow tissues during the surfacing phase. Fast tissues can take a higher factor, near 2·0, without provoking symptoms. Deep diving experience demonstrates that the supersaturation factors have to be drastically reduced for all tissues. There is no theoretical concept to account for this phenomenon. In practice, the factors for different half-times are reduced in relation to the total partial pressure of inert gas. Present experience concerning tolerable supersaturation factors is given in Fig. 19.11. The factors for the slow tissues are well confirmed by saturation experiments up to 31 ATA. The curve for helium half-times of 45 to 90 min is the result of the analysis of so-called vertigo bends during decompression after experiments between 5·0 and 31·0 ATA (Bühlmann & Gehring 1975). No troubles of this kind occurred using supersaturation factors in accordance with this curve. The factors for tissues with helium half-times of 5 to 10 min are estimated and not confirmed by decompression incidents.

Prolonged exposures and saturation experiments

The saturation experiments were conducted on the same basis as those at 100 ft (4 ATA). Details of the experiments are summarized in Table 19.9.

Some of these dives formed part of the 1966 'Capshell' trials in the Mediterranean, which were organized by Cdr J. R. Carr, RN (retd).

Decompression after deep dives lasting for some hours and for full saturation was simplified by putting oxygen, helium and air directly into the pressure chambers. The Po_2 averaged less than 1·0 ATS, with a short and transient increase above

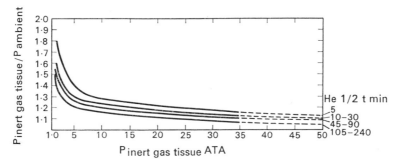

FIG. 19.11. Tolerated supersaturation (ordinate) for tissues with different helium half-times depending on the total inert gas pressure in the respective tissues (abscissa). A helium half-time of 240 min corresponds to a nitrogen half-time of 635 min

TABLE 19.9

Mixed gas decompression after long and saturation
dives at 4 to 31 ATA with oxy-helium

ATA	Bottom time (hours)	Decom- pression (hours)	Decom- pressions (number)	Different subjects
4	72*	6	4	4
11	6	22	6	5
16	6	40	6	5
23	6*	52	22	12
23	2 × 6†	60	6	5
23	68 & 78	62, 64, 68	7	5
31	2	50	2	2
31	3	58	2	2
31	4	64	2	2
31	81	88	3	3
(51	80	156		)

* Carried out in the pressure chamber, and also with swimming excursions in the sea.
† Carried out as a repetitive dive for 6 and 4 to 6 hours within
48 hours, partly in the water.

2·0 ATS when using a 50% oxygen, 50% nitrogen
mixture. In all these experiments there was a comfortable temperature, practically no CO_2 and a

relative humidity of 70 to 90% in the chambers.
The contamination of oxy-nitrogen mixtures with
helium was measured and taken into consideration when calculating the effective pressure
gradient for helium. The effects of venous admixture was estimated by reducing the calculated
helium elimination by 10% during the first decompression stop and again for one stop after
changing from helium to nitrogen. Decompression
was carried out in steps, varying between 15 and
120 min. A supersaturation factor of approximately 1·5 was used for the final step when returning to atmospheric pressure.

The decompression procedures in our prolonged
experiments were identical once the same total
inert gas pressure of helium and nitrogen was
reached in the tissues with a helium half-time of
180 to 240 min (Bühlmann 1971).

In Fig. 19.12 is shown the decompression profile
of the saturation dive at 31 ATA performed 3–
10 February 1969 in the Deep Trials Unit of the
Royal Navy at Alverstoke. On the first day the
three divers made an excursion to 36·0 ATA for
1 hour. During the second and third days they

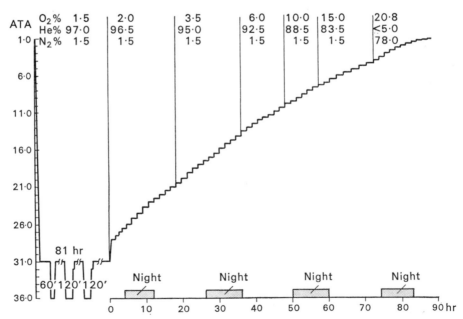

FIG. 19.12. Decompression after saturation at 1000 ft (31 ATA) with 97% helium.
During the first, second, and third days, excursions were made to 1150 ft (36 ATA)
utilizing the same breathing mixture. Stepwise increase of oxygen to 15%. Change
to air breathing at 100 ft (4 ATA). Total decompression time 88 hours

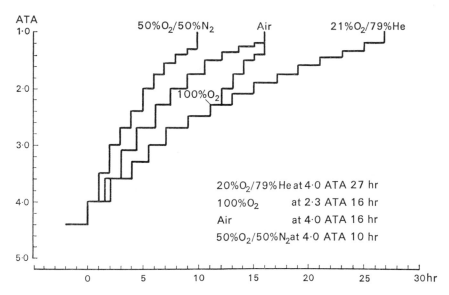

FIG. 19.13. Final decompression below 100 ft (4 ATA) after saturation and long-duration diving with oxygen–helium mixtures using the same principles of calculation: 10 hours with 50% oxygen, 50% nitrogen below 75 to 100 ft (3·3 to 4·0 ATA); 16 hours with air below 100 ft (4 ATA); 27 hours with 21% oxygen, 79% helium (not performed); and 16 hours with 100% oxygen below 45 ft (2·4 ATA) (not performed)

made excursions of 2 hours to 36·0 ATA, with swimming and physical work in the wet compartment.

Decompression from 36·0 to 31·0 ATA in 20 and 30 min respectively occurred without incident. The total decompression time, scheduled for 88 hours, was trouble free except for one diver who had knee pains in the final stages and had to be separated from the others for short treatment. Unlike the other two, who were in diving practice, this subject had made his previous dive 12 months before the saturation experiment.

The three saturation dives at 23·0 ATA, which were performed by 5 different subjects (2 made two dives each), passed off without any symptoms of insufficient decompression.

It is interesting to compare different theoretical versions of the final states of decompression below 4·0 ATA (Fig. 19.13).

Final decompression would take 27 hours breathing 21% oxygen, 79% helium, against 16 hours using air, and 10 hours using 50% oxygen, 50% nitrogen, if the same factors are used in the calculations. While the gain in changing inert gas in the final stage (below 4·0 ATA) is not so very large, it is sufficient to be of value in practice. Experience with the two versions of the final decompression is given in Table 19.10.

The frequency of minor bends, some of which disappear without treatment, is not high but it shows that the decompression is near the limit. If these results are compared with the much longer procedures of American, British and French methods, this technique of calculating decompression is no less safe and is certainly more economical in time.

The saturation dives at 23·0 ATA and 31·0 ATA confirmed the assumption of a longest helium half-time of 240 min and a longest nitrogen half-time of 635 min in calculating decompressions which last for days.

Deep diving with mixed inert gases

Contrary to the expectation of some authors, mainly in America, the technique of saturation diving has had limited practical application. However, only 7 years after the pilot experiments, short-duration diving using oxy-helium has become

TABLE 19.10

Final decompression stage after prolonged deep dives

Breathing gas	Decompressions (number)	Minor bends (number)	Subjects (number)
A. 50% O_2/50% N_2 below 3·3 to 4·0 ATA	16	1	8
B. Air below 4·0 ATA	6	1	4
	22	2	12*

* 8 different subjects.

Dives—Repetitive dive within 24 hours with total bottom time of 8 to 12 hours at 23·0 ATA; saturation at 23·0 ATA; bottom times of 2 to 4 hours at 31·0 ATA; saturation at 31·0 ATA.

TABLE 19.11

30 min bottom time at 500 ft (16·0 ATA)

	Breathing mixture 6·0 to 16·0 ATA O_2	He	N_2	Breathing mixture during decompression	Decompression time (min)
Version a	6	89	5	20% O_2 below 6 ATA 100% O_2 below 2 ATA	1010
Version b	6	89	5	air below 6 ATA 100% O_2 below 2 ATA	645
Version c^1	6	70	24	air below 6 ATA 100% O_2 below 2 ATA	580
Version c^2	6	70	24	air below 6 ATA and up to surface	850

Version a: descent time 15 min, compression with oxygen–helium. Version b: compression with air to 6·0 ATA.

Version c^1 and version c^2 mixture is 3 parts air, 7 parts helium. Allowance is made in the calculations for a contamination of 2 to 4% helium when air is breathed.

routine work for a large number of professional divers in water depths between 300 and 600 ft (10 and 19 ATA) with bottom times chiefly between 15 and 45 min.

This leads to the questions whether the consumption of helium, which is very expensive in Europe, can be reduced and whether decompression times can be shortened, by using oxygen–helium–nitrogen breathing mixtures.

From the practical point of view it is desirable that the mixtures should be prepared by using air and pure helium.

Tables 19.11 and 19.12 show that a small shortening of decompression time is possible, using identical values for descent time, oxygen concentration on bottom, supersaturation factors and corrections for physical work.

TABLE 19.12

P_{inert} in the slowest tissues at the end of decompression

	He	N_2
Version a	1·19	0·32
Version b	0·61	0·90
Version c^1	0·50	0·01
Version c^2	0·25	1·26

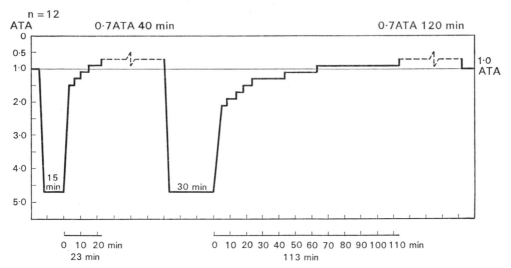

FIG. 19.14. Decompression after air diving in altitude. Simulated repetitive dive at 0·7 ATA altitude (10 000 ft; 3000 m). 15-min bottom time at 133 ft (4·7 ATA). Decompression time 23 min breathing air. 40-min interval at 0·7 ATA. Second dive with 30-min bottom time. Decompression time 113 min. Last step but one at 1·1 ATA, last step at 0·9 ATA. 120-min interval at 0·7 ATA

AIR DIVING AT HIGH ALTITUDES

Although at high altitude the P_{N_2} in the body is lower at a given depth than it would be at this depth at sea level, the ratio between P_{N_2} at depth and P ambient at surface is greater. If the same supersaturation factors are used for diving at high altitude, it is necessary to modify decompression tables that are valid for sea level. Hitherto there have been no tested decompression tables for diving at high altitude. In Switzerland, diving in mountain lakes is important both for sports divers and for the Swiss Army. We have calculated decompression tables for use at heights of 2500 ft (750 m) up to 10 000 ft (3000 m), which are based on the supersaturation factors quoted in Fig. 19.11, the effective P_{N_2} and the ambient pressure. These were tested by simulated dives at 0·7 ATA (10 000 ft; 3000 m) and by real dives at 4000 ft (1250 m; 0·85 ATA).

In order to allow greater safety it was supposed that the diver reached the mountain lake by helicopter within a few minutes, before his body could become adapted to the lower pressure. Thus the calculations were made for an initial P_{N_2} of 0·8 ATS in all tissues. Furthermore the supersaturation factor on surfacing was chosen to allow for a further reduction of pressure, which might be brought about by travelling by plane or car to a higher place after the dive. Repetitive diving is needed by sport and military divers and so a high proportion of simulated and real dives were undertaken as repetitive dives with a surface interval of 10 to 15 min (Fig. 19.14). At this point additional tissues with nitrogen half-times up to 200 min were considered. After the simulated dives the subjects remained at 0·7 ATA for 120 to 180 min after surfacing so that any delayed symptoms of decompression sickness would not be suppressed by returning to normal atmospheric pressure. Physical work on the bicycle ergometer was undertaken during the tests. The same final steps, at 13 ft (4 m) and 7 ft (2 m), are used in decompression after all high altitude dives.

These experiments, which were free of symptoms due to insufficient decompression, have shown that calculations, based on our simple working hypothesis for deep diving, also give satisfactory results for diving at high altitudes (Bühlmann, Schibli & Gehring 1973).

SUMMARY

No theory has been developed to describe uptake and elimination of inert gases and their

TABLE 19.13

106 simulated dives at 0·7 ATA

Depth (ATA)	Bottom time (min)	Decompression (min)	Interval at 0·7 ATA after dive (min)	Number of subjects
5·2	30	105	180	12
4·2	60	158	120	12
4·2	120	376	120	˙12
4·7	25	60	45	11
3·7*	17	42	180	3
3·7*	22	52	120	8
4·7	15	23	40	12
4·7*	30	113	120	12
4·7	20	25	45	12
4·7*	25	113	120	12
				106 (50 different subjects)

* Repetitive dives.

TABLE 19.14

222 real dives at 4000 ft altitude (0·85 ATA), water temperature 10 to 16°C

Depth (ATA)	Bottom time (min)	Decompression (min)	Interval at 0·85 ATA after dive	Number of subjects
3·85	15	17	20 to 24 hours	14
3·85	15	12	20 to 24 hours	28
2·35	15	3	45 min	20
2·65*	15	15	20 to 24 hours	20
2·85	10	3	10 min	70
2·35*	15	13	20 to 24 hours	70
				222 (112 different subjects)

* Repetitive dives.

behaviour in the human body during pressure changes. The 'Swiss Decompression Theory' is only a method of calculating saturation and desaturation in a way which permits safe decompression. The use of different inert gases, such as helium and nitrogen, to shorten decompression is a characteristic of this method.

The calculation is based on the following principles:

Saturation and desaturation are treated as an equalization of pressure throughout the body.

Different half-times for the same inert gas are interpreted as the result of different perfusion rates in the tissues, which vary with the haemodynamic condition.

The ratio of half-times between nitrogen and helium is 2·646 for a given perfusion rate (diffusion-limited system).

A spectrum of half-times of 2 to 240 min is employed for helium with a corresponding one of 5·3 to 635 min for nitrogen.

Supersaturation factors ($P_{\text{inert total}}/P_{\text{ambient}}$)

decrease with increasing P_{inert} total and also with longer half-times. They have to be determined experimentally.

The faster saturation of slow tissues, which are sensitive to bends, during muscular work is allowed for by introducing '*virtual bottom time*'.

This method of calculation applies, without any special adaptation, to:

Simulated and real dives.

Air diving at sea level and at high altitudes, where the ambient pressure is reduced.

Saturation diving in conventional depths using air or oxy-helium.

Deep diving to 31 ATA for all exposures, from short periods up to full saturation.

Exposures using mixtures of different inert gases at the same time.

Change of inert gas during decompression.

Use of pure oxygen as breathing gas to shorten the final stages of decompression.

REFERENCES

BÜHLMANN, A. A. (1971) Decompression in saturation diving. In *Underwater Physiology. Proc. 4th Symp. Underwater Physiology*. p. 221. New York and London: Academic Press.

BÜHLMANN, A. A. & GEHRING, H. (1975) Inner ear disorders as a result of inadequate decompression, so-called vertigo bends. In *Underwater Physiology. Vth Symp. Underwater Physiology*. Ed. C. J. Lambertsen. Bethesda: Fedn Am. Socs exp. Biol.

BÜHLMANN, A. A., FREY, P. & KELLER, H. (1967) Saturation and desaturation with nitrogen and helium at 4 ATA. *J. appl. Physiol.* **23**, 458.

BÜHLMANN, A. A., SCHIBLI, R. A. & GEHRING, H. (1973) Experimentelle Untersuchingen über die Dekompression nach Tauchgängen in Bergseen bei vermindertem Luftdruck. *Schweitz. med. Wschr.* **103**, 378.

BÜHLMANN, A. A., ZIEGLER, W. H. & MÜLLER, J. (1970) Catecholamine excretion and plasma corticosteroids during deep diving breathing oxygen–helium mixtures. In *Proc. Third int. Conf. hyperbaric and Underwater Physiology*, June 1970, Marseille. p. 69. Paris: Doin.

FASEB (1971) *Respiration and Circulation*. Bethesda, Md.: Federation of American Societies of Experimental Biology.

KELLER, H. & BÜHLMANN, A. A. (1965) Deep diving and short decompression by breathing mixed gases. *J. appl. Physiol.* **20**, 1267.

SCHIBLI, R. A. & BÜHLMANN, A. A. (1972) The influence of physical work upon decompression time after simulated oxy-helium dives. *Helv. med. Acta* **36**, 327.

WALDVOGEL, W. & BÜHLMANN, A. A. (1968) Man's reaction to long-lasting overpressure exposure. Examination of the saturated organism at a helium pressure of 21–22 ATA. *Helv. med. Acta* **34**, 130.

20

Biophysical Aspects of Decompression

B. A. HILLS

The decompression syndrome involves mechanisms which are undoubtedly more complex than were envisaged even a decade ago. Interest has now arisen in the biochemical and haematological aspects. In this chapter, however, only the biophysical approaches will be considered since these are still more likely to provide any fundamental basis generally adopted for designing safe diving tables.

The present wide diversity of approaches indicates that there are probably an infinite number of computational routines for safely decompressing a subject following just one particular hyperbaric exposure. If the truly optimal procedure is to be found other than by trial and error, it is therefore necessary to determine the true model. At least each feature established adds a further constraint to the present proliferation of calculation methods.

Vital issues

There are many interesting physical and physiological questions in hyperbaria to which one would like to know the answers, but there are a few which cannot be avoided. Answers must be found, or assumed, for each of these vital issues before any comprehensive mathematical model can be put forward on fundamental grounds for deriving safe decompression schedules. These are:

1. The number of tissue types which can give rise to marginal bends, since this determines the number of independent conditions to be satisfied and hence the number of separate equations to be used in calculating a format.

2. Whether there is a critical limit to the degree of supersupersaturation of a tissue by a gas, and thus whether the separation of the gas phase from solution can occur in the vital tissue(s) during any asymptomatic decompression. This is a rather more specific statement of the old issue concerning 'silent bubbles' (Behnke 1951), the term 'bubble' being avoided here since it tends to suggest a particular geometric form for the separated gas. This issue is the most important since it determines the driving force for tissue desaturation *during* decompression.

3. The kinetics for separation of the gas phase from solution once it is nucleated; is the onset of symptoms determined by the rate of transfer of gas to the gaseous phase or by coalescence or both?

4. Whether the rate-limiting process for the transfer of gas *in solution* is blood perfusion, bulk diffusion, membrane permeation or a combination thereof. This determines the nature of the time function to be used in the computation of tables.

A critical analysis is therefore needed of the evidence considered relevant to each of these vital issues.

SITE AND MECHANISM OF DECOMPRESSION SICKNESS

Number of tissue types involved

To establish the features of the true mathematical model for calculating diving tables, we are concerned with avoiding any discomfort to the diver and must therefore consider the *marginal* case where decompression has caused some critical insult to one or more 'sensitive' tissues. If these vary in function, they are also likely to do so in both the nature of their reaction and their time response to the exposure. Hence, for a multi-tissue system, we could reasonably expect a correlation between the time-course of the dive and the type of symptom observed. However, this does not appear to be the case, although one exception is sometimes quoted. This concerns a propensity for pain to occur in the lower limbs of caisson workers (Golding et al. 1960; Rose 1962) as opposed to the upper limbs of divers (Rivera 1964; Slark 1962), but may still involve *one* tissue type.

It can be argued that the similarity of Type I symptoms arises since the most sensitive tissue has one anatomical identity, but is kinetically heterogeneous, so that a wide spectrum of response times needs to be considered, as in the original Haldane calculation method (Boycott, Damant & Haldane 1908). However, it is then difficult to envisage the physical basis for a parallel spectrum of degrees of critical insult needed to explain the varying ratio (or M value) required by subsequent workers (Workman 1965; Schreiner 1968) in order to force a better fit of the Haldane model to practical data.

Experimental approaches

It is particularly difficult to design an experiment to differentiate conclusively between the involvement of one or more tissues in Type I decompression sickness (DCS). However, an ingenious attempt by Rashbass (1954) invoked the relationship between equivalent combinations of pressures (P_1 and P_2) of two consecutive exposures, each of constant duration. It can be shown by a simple mathematical argument, which does not require any specific transport model to be assumed, that the linear relationship actually found by Rashbass provides strong evidence of the involvement of no more than one tissue type. Subsequent repetition of this experiment by Hempleman (1957) essentially confirmed these findings except in the region where $P_1 \gg P_2$. Deviation in this particular region can easily be explained by the lower driving force for tissue gas transfer arising from gas phase formation during the second exposure (P_2) due to the large decompression

(P_1-P_2) immediately preceding it. This concept is discussed in detail later.

It can also be argued that if one tissue supersedes another as the closest to its respective threshold for provoking marginal symptoms, there should be a transition point in the parameters defining safe decompression limits. Selecting exposure pressure and time as the two parameters most interdependent in determining the imminence of symptoms, no such transition point (kink) could be detected in any bounce dive curves. Data examined include the no-stop decompressions of Duffner, Van der Aue and Behnke (1946) for oxy-helium mixtures, Van der Aue et al. (1951), Albano (1962) and many goat curves obtained in the author's laboratory for air diving.

Yet another feature in favour of the one-tissue concept is the ability to express the empirical time function depicted by the bounce dive curve (Hills 1969b) by a single bulk diffusion equation (see Fig. 20.8).

Although the evidence is far from adequate for any conclusion, it would tend to favour a one-tissue model for Type I DCS as classified by the MRC Decompression Panel.

Other symptoms

Although Type II DCS obviously represents different physiological manifestations to Type I, there is the mathematical problem of deciding whether they represent a further development of the same basic mechanism or whether they are derived in a different tissue or from a different form of insult to the body. CNS symptoms can invariably be produced by extreme decompressions from exposures well beyond the safe limits such as the bounce dive curve for no-stop decompression. Usually Type I symptoms develop first, so that it would be convenient to dismiss Type II from our modelling considerations as not representative of a marginal case.

However, a method has now been found for producing Type II DCS as *marginal symptoms* by interposing an upward excursion between the exposure and a regular decompression (Hills 1972a) This technique is illustrated in Fig. 20.1, and now provides a convenient model for studying the treatment of CNS symptoms, in goats at least. The particular case when the upward excursion

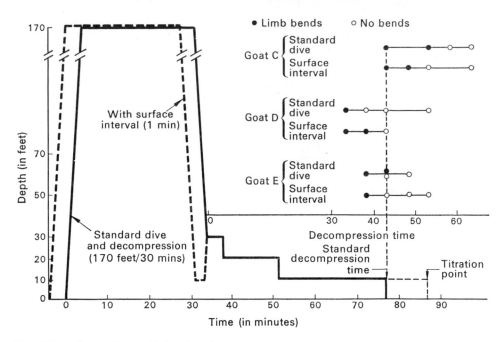

FIG. 20.1. Comparison of 'titrations' of the standard US Navy decompression table for an exposure of 30 min at 170 ft, both with and without an 'upward excursion', depicted as a stop at 10 ft in this particular case (after Hills 1971d)

pressure coincides with normal atmospheric represents the popular naval practice of 'surface decompression' or 'decanting'. However, for normal diving, decompression schedules which eliminate Type I DCS are likely to avoid all but the most minimal of Type II, but this reasoning should not be extrapolated from prevention to treatment, particularly for a CNS manifestation.

This is certainly not the case for dysbaric osteonecrosis which may not result from inadequate decompression or even from decompression per se (Hills 1970a). This major worry to the designer of diving tables is discussed in detail later. However, in the absence of more specific knowledge, his essential task is still the estimation of the imminence of limb pain.

MECHANISM OF 'LIMB BENDS'

The concept that the pain is ischemic in origin has been dismissed by Ferris and Engel (1951) for numerous clinical and physiological reasons, which they list.

More likely, perhaps, are the implications derived from the simple experiments of Inman and Saunders (Inman & Saunders 1944; Saunders & Inman 1943). When they injected Ringer's solution through fine hypodermic needles into various tissues, they found that there was a well-defined pressure threshold for inducing pain. This pressure differential was about 15 cm water gauge (0·015 ATS) irrespective of the fluid flow required to maintain it. Related to decompression, this indicates that the pressure differential between the separated gas phase and tissue (δ) which can bend, or otherwise distort, a nerve ending can do so without effect until it reaches a pain-provoking threshold corresponding to a critical pressure differential (δ'), i.e. bends pain occurs if:

$$\delta > \delta' \simeq 15 \text{ cm w.g.} = 11 \text{ mm Hg} \qquad (1)$$

This simple mechanical concept has been adopted by Nims (1951) and Hills (1966) for their very different approaches in relating the critical degree of embolism to parameters of the hyperbaric exposure.

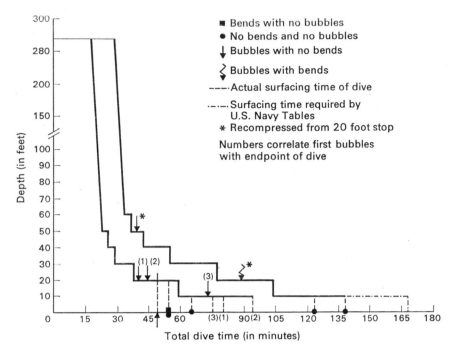

■ Bends with no bubbles
● No bends and no bubbles
↓ Bubbles with no bends
⌇ Bubbles with bends
---- Actual surfacing time of dive
·—·—· Surfacing time required by
        U.S. Navy Tables
∗ Recompressed from 20 foot stop

Numbers correlate first bubbles
with endpoint of dive

FIG. 20.2. Two standard US Navy decompressions showing the points at which
bubbles were first heard and whether symptoms occurred (after Vann et al. 1973)

Intravascular versus extravascular site

Ferris and Engel (1951) list the clinical and physiological evidence on this issue, all of which tends to favour extravascular sites for the gas giving rise to 'limb bends'. Their chief point is that extreme recompression should reduce any gas emboli to a size at which they could be expected to pass through the capillary bed if they were intravascular, so that symptoms would not be expected to re-occur in the same sites as they are found to do upon subsequent decompression (Blankenhorn et al. 1942).

It is also difficult to cavitate blood *de novo* (Harvey 1951) so that, overall, it means that intravascular bubbles are probably derived from gas initially deposited from solution in extravascular sites, vascular lesions having been first demonstrated after decompression by Chase (1934) and Tureen and Devine (1936). The likely origin of circulating bubbles would then be tissues with a predominance of lipid in which nitrogen is 5 times more soluble than in water. This implied tissue disruption by gas is compatible with the appear-ance of fat emboli (Shim, Patterson & Kendall 1967) and the remains of endothelial cells (Philp, Inwood & Warren 1972) in the circulating blood upon decompression.

Along this line of reasoning, intravascular bubbles therefore have little meaning in determining the imminence of 'limb bends', as several surveys of different decompressions with ultrasonic Doppler detectors have shown (Spencer & Campbell 1968; Evans, Barnard & Walder 1971; Vann et al. 1973 [see Fig. 20.2]).

This then raises the question of where to look for the relevant gas and, therefore, what is the anatomical identity of the tissue type responsible for marginal limb bends?

Identification of critical tissue

Pathological investigations have, on the whole, yielded surprisingly little information pertinent to establishing the true tissue model (Haymaker 1957), except to eliminate liver, heart and skeletal muscle from the list of possibilities as bubble-free after decompression. Previous discussions (Ferris

& Engel 1951) point to a well-innervated pre-dominantly aqueous tissue occurring around joints and associated with the locomotor system, but not muscle. This suggests a connective tissue.

Hence it is interesting that Gersh, Hawkinson and Rathbun 1944) found that the incidence of 'bends' in small animals offered a better correlation with the gas content of excised tendon than with that of any other tissue. Other parameters which yield values compatible with tendon include the bulk modulus (Hills 1966), the ratio of 'elastic' to 'plastic' components for its load bearing, and the time for passive relaxation of the 'plastic' fraction (Hills 1969c) as a mechanical interpretation of known acclimatization (Walder 1966). These determinations of mechanical aspects were all based upon equation (1) in which the gas pressure differential (δ) can be related to the modulus (K) and the volume of gas (v) congregated in unit volume of tissue as:

$$\delta = Kv \qquad (2)$$

This expression is compatible with the linear increase in susceptibility with age described by Gray (1951), since the elastic modulus K is known to increase with age in most tissues, particularly the aorta (Hallock & Benson 1937). Thus the subject should be able to tolerate a lesser degree of embolism (v) as aging increases K, provided his pain threshold for δ remains the same.

However, this raises the next vital issue concerning whether 'limb bends' are, in fact, determined by a critical degree of embolism or by critical supersaturation.

PHASE CONDITIONS DURING DECOMPRESSION

Significance of this issue

An essential feature of all calculation methods is a critical condition to apply to the time response to determine whether a 'trigger point' has been reached for either the formation of the gas phase or the precipitation of a state which will lead to symptoms. In the case of the Haldane calculation method, and its many empirical modifications (Workman 1965; Schreiner 1968), these conditions are assumed to coincide since the same time functions are used to describe gas elimination during

decompression as were employed to estimate gas uptake at pressure. This 'mathematical symmetry' is only valid provided the physics of the system is unaltered and, hence, all tissue gas has remained *in true physical solution*. If the gas phase *is* present, then not only is it inadequate just to change a time constant, but the popular exponential is no longer the appropriate function.

The conventional 'symmetrical' approach is only valid if there is a metastable limit to the saturation of a solution beyond equilibrium, a concept originally proposed for crystallization studies by Ostwald, a contemporary of Haldane.

Metastable limit versus random nucleation

A survey of the disciplines in the physical sciences where suppressed transformation occurs has shown that the concept of the metastable limit has been replaced by theories based upon random nucleation, with a finite probability for any condition in excess of equilibrium.

In justifying limited supersaturation, most proponents of theories of decompression sickness tend to quote values for the degree of supersaturation obtained by decompressing liquids in vitro. These are often designated 'tensile strengths', the values of which have been obtained under both static and dynamic conditions by a wide variety of methods. These are listed in Table 20.1.

The variation of values quoted in Table 20.1 needs no comment. Moreover, typical values (Table 20.2) for small animals indicate that cavitation is equally random in vivo.

Hydrophobic interfaces

It would seem most significant that bubbles formed by simple decompression in vitro almost invariably appear at the walls of the container (Wismer 1922). Moreover Harvey (1951) commented that nucleation is more profuse when the solid surface is hydrophobic.

This has also been found to hold at the liquid–liquid interface, which is significant since fat is fluid at body temperatures. A study of 580 decompressions of a hydrophobic fluid in contact with various aqueous fluids (Hills 1967d) has shown that cavitation is random and, when it occurs, invariably does so at the interface, ap-

TABLE 20.1

Recorded tensile strengths' of various liquids

Tensile strength (ATS)	Liquid	Reference	Method
300	Water	Bethelot (1850)*	Static
4·8	Water	Reynolds (1870)	Dynamic
30	Water	Meyer (1911)	Static
40	Ether	Meyer (1911)	Static
150	Water	Dixon (1914)	Static
207	Cell sap	Dixon (1914)	Static
2·38	Water	Vincent (1941)	Static
2·94	Mineral oil	Vincent (1941)	Static
2·9–114	Mineral oil	Vincent (1941)	Static
100–1000	Water	Harvey (1944)	Static
0·8	Water	Dean (1944)	Dynamic
100–200	Water	Pease & Blinks (1947)	Static
280	Water (10°C)	Briggs (1947)	Dynamic
20	Water	Willard (1953)	Ultrasonic
200	Water	Galloway (1954)	Ultrasonic
140	Benzene	Galloway (1954)	Ultrasonic

* Quoted and checked by Meyer and Dixon using the same method.

TABLE 20.2

Bubbles observed in resting cats

Time at pressure (P_1)	Initial pressure (P_1) (ATA)	Final pressure (P_2) (ATA)	Number of cats in trial	Number displaying bubbles
∞	1	0·14	37	4
∞	1		11	1 + 2 ?
	3·5	1	18	9
	3·14	1	10	7
	2·64	0·14	10	4
2 to 5 hours	3	1	12	3
	2·5	1	6	0
	2·0	1	5	0
	9	2	10	4
	6·8	2–3	8	0

This table gives a summary of data from Harvey et al. (1944) and McElroy et al. (1944).

parently with no significant metastable limit (Fig. 20.3).

Direct searches in intact tissue

The development of ultrasonic techniques for detection of the gas phase is described in another chapter (22), but those approaches invoking the Doppler principle seem to be emerging as the most successful. As stated earlier, these instruments often detect intravascular bubbles during asymp-

tomatic decompressions using naval tables based upon the supersaturation concept—sometimes as early as the 50 ft stop (2·5 ATA; Fig. 20.2). However, in all fairness to the Haldane calculation method, one has no idea whether these *intravascular* bubbles detected are related to the state of the critical tissue in any way.

If the gas responsible for marginal DCS is deposited in extravascular sites or is lodged in capillaries as effectively extravascular, then we

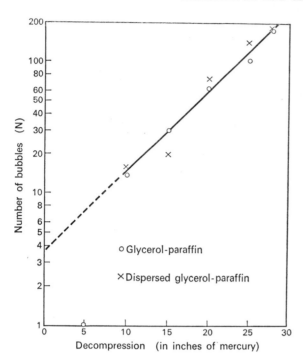

FIG. 20.3. The frequency of bubble formation at a hydrophobic-hydrophilic phase boundary in twenty runs for each extent of decompression (ΔP) from atmospheric

than the value of 307 mm Hg corresponding to 7550 m which is the minimum bends altitude for the most susceptible individuals (Gray 1944), and certainly much closer to the value of 497 mm Hg calculated as the pressure for phase equilibration on the basis of equation (6) (Hills 1966). Thus the X-ray data would certainly favour the concept of gas separation occurring closer to the saturation point than to any predicted on the basis of critical supersaturation.

Conductance measurements

Electrical resistance of tissue has been monitored during decompression (Hills 1971c) since it is a parameter which can be measured very accurately and should be sensitive to both intravascular and extravascular gas, particularly if deposited in a finely dispersed state at lipid-aqueous boundaries. The results (Fig. 20.4) show a clear transition point upon decompression from ambient pressure, i.e. a point of sudden increase in the resistance between electrodes deposited subcutaneously across a rat tail. These points occurred for decompressions from normal atmospheric pressure of only 96, 127 or 145 mm Hg depending upon whether the animal had been breathing 80% He, N_2 or N_2O mixed with 20% O_2. There was little doubt that the changes were caused by the gas phase since the resistance increased more rapidly the greater the solubility of the inert gas present and the effect was reversed by recompression. Each transition point occurred when the extent of decompression was slightly greater than the inherent gas unsaturation arising in tissue by virtue of metabolism (see equation (6) and Fig. 20.6), whether the latter is predicted theoretically or measured experimentally (Hills & LeMessurier, 1969). This implies that the gas phase was first formed for a decompression much closer to the pressure for saturation than to any which could have been predicted by any ratio used in diving tables to describe a hypothetical limit to supersaturation.

However, it may be argued that the gas monitored was an artefact produced when a hydrophobic interface was introduced in the form of an electrode. Recent development of an electrodeless device (Searle & Hills 1975), based on the principle of the inductive conductivity meter, essentially

would need to seek other means of detection for answering this vital supersaturation issue. Other methods which have been used include conductance measurements, X-rays (Webb et al. 1943; Blankenhorn & Ferris 1944; Thomas & Williams 1944), monitoring cerebrospinal fluid volume, and the density measurements of Gersh, Hawkinson and Rathbun (1944) already discussed when implicating tendon as a likely critical tissue for limb bends. Details of the X-ray studies are given elsewhere, but two points require mention here:

Repetition of this work with modern X-ray equipment at Duke University, North Carolina, has essentially confirmed these early findings, but the nature of the streaking along tendon or muscle bundles becomes less regular with time or exercise, indicating coalescence.

Ryder et al. (1945) found the first indications of this 'streaking' to occur at an altitude of about 3950 m, i.e. an absolute pressure of about 483 mm Hg. This pressure is considerably higher

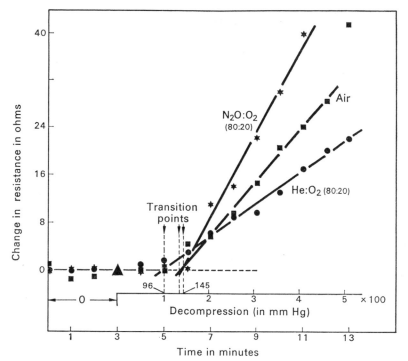

F IG. 20.4. The change in the electrical resistance across the tails of rats
that had been breathing mixtures of 80% He–20% O_2, 80% N_2O–20%
O_2 or air at normal pressure for 6 hours before death immediately followed
by decompression (after Hills 1971c)

confirms these earlier findings. This device also
appears most promising for further development
into a non-invasive means of detecting that first
onset of the separation of the gas phase from solution in divers.

Even though the rat tail used in these experiments is largely tendon, it can easily be argued
that none of the direct approaches need have been
detecting the gaseous phase relevant to Type I
DCS. However, before discussing the indirect
approaches which have been developed to try to
overcome this objection, it might be as well to
consider the importance of the presence of the
gaseous phase in influencing gas elimination *during* decompression.

Driving force during decompression

Let us consider a tissue zone in which gas has
been deposited from solution (Fig. 20.5). It has
been shown from studies of the composition of gas
pockets in animals (Campbell 1924; Van Liew et al.

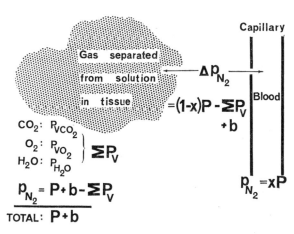

F IG. 20.5. Illustrating the driving force (ΔP_{N_2}) for
the elimination from tissue of the nitrogen in gas
separated from solution (equation 6). Absolute pressure of this gas is $(P+b)$ where b is a small factor
allowing for surface tension and tissue distensibility
(equation 4), while x is the wet volume fraction of inspired nitrogen

1965) that the partial pressures of CO_2 and O_2 in those pockets rapidly revert to near-venous values following any change in external pressure. Since gas separated from solution must be in mechanical equilibrium with its surroundings, the partial pressure of nitrogen (P'_{N_2}) can be deduced by difference as:

$$P'_{N_2} = P - P_v O_2 - P_v CO_2 - P_w + b = P + c \quad (3)$$

where b is a small term to allow for tissue compliance (δ) and curvature (radius $-r_b$) of the gas–tissue interface (tension $-\gamma$) i.e.

$$b = \delta + 2\gamma/r_b = c + P_v O_2 + P_v CO_2 + P_w \quad (4)$$

At the adjacent capillary, the nitrogen tension (P_{N_2}) will be given by:

$$P_{N_2} = (P - P_w) F_{I_{N2}} \quad (5)$$

where $F_{I_{N2}}$ is the volume fraction of nitrogen in inspired air on a dry gas basis.

Hence we can derive the driving force (ΔP_{N_2}) for nitrogen transfer from the gaseous phase to the capillary simply by subtracting equations (3) and (5), and eliminating b, when:

$$\Delta P_{N_2} = P'_{N_2} - P_{N_2} = P(1 - F_{I_{N2}}) + c' \quad (6)$$

where

$$c' = c - P_w . F_{I_{N2}} \quad (7)$$

For the comparison with the conventional supersaturation approach, if the nitrogen had remained in solution it would have a tension P''_{N_2}, say, higher than P'_{N_2}, and given by:

$$\Delta P''_{N_2} = P''_{N_2} - P_{N_2} = P''_{N_2} - (P - P_w) F_{I_{N2}} \quad (8)$$

Below convulsive limits of oxygen, $P_v O_2$ is approximately independent of pressure and hence so is c'—the term: $b - P_v O_2 - P_v CO_2 - P_w(1 - F_{I_{N2}})$. Thus the very important feature emerging from equation (6) is that ΔP_{N_2} *increases* with P since $F_{I_{N2}}$ must be less than 1. This suggests a *greater* driving force for resolution of separated gas provided the *gas phase is present*.

Equation (6) emphasizes the importance of knowing whether the gas phase is present since, if it is not, then it is better to decompress further and so obtain a greater driving force for nitrogen elimination intended by the first long 'pull' to-

wards the surface in Haldane-type schedules ($\Delta P''_{N_2}$ increases with *decreased P* in equation (7)). However, once the gas phase forms, further decompression is the worst action possible since one is now not only forming more gas, but is reducing the driving force for its elimination according to equation (6), since ΔP_{N_2} is now *decreasing as P decreases*.

Equation (6) also expresses quantitatively the known benefit of oxygen treatment, where a decrease in $F_{I_{N2}}$ increases ΔP_{N_2}.

Proof of the validity of equation (6) in vivo has been provided by considering what would happen if the separated gas in Fig. 20.5 were now encased in a rigid yet permeable capsule. As steady state conditions were reached, a partial vacuum would develop by virtue of the *inherent unsaturation*—a concept depicted in Fig. 20.6. This has been found to vary with change of $F_{I_{N2}}$ and absolute pressure (P) exactly as predicted for ΔP_{N_2} in equation (6) (Hills & LeMessurier 1969). If the walls of the capsule were suddenly removed, there would be a sudden increase in total pressure of the contained gas. The O_2, CO_2 and water vapour would adjust rapidly to new venous values leaving an increase in the P_{N_2} equal to the inherent unsaturation whose characteristics can thus be taken as those of ΔP_{N_2} in equation (6).

Hence, in any calculation, it is vital to know when the gas phase is first formed.

To avoid the major objection to the direct methods described earlier for determining this point, it is necessary to ensure that one is dealing with the tissue type(s) responsible for marginal symptoms. One means of guaranteeing this condition is to use the occurrence of symptoms as the outward indication of the methods employed to differentiate between the possible thermodynamic states of the critical tissue(s).

Indirect methods

Hempleman (1960) performed a number of double exposures upon goats, 'titrating' the pressure of the second exposure to a bends point. By varying time intervals, he was able to show that gas elimination from the critical tissue(s) was slower than uptake for the corresponding pressure differences. This would indicate a basic asymmetry between uptake and elimination indicative

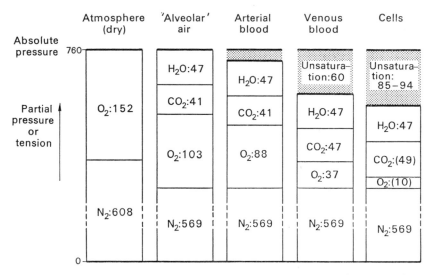

FIG. 20.6. Typical partial pressures of the respiratory gases and their tensions in solution (in mm Hg) for a day when the absolute atmospheric pressure is 760 mm Hg. The deficit in the total represented by the shaded areas represents the inherent unsaturation (after Hills 1974)

of asymptomatic gas in the critical tissue, such as a switch from equation (8) to (6).

A somewhat similar experiment has been performed recently in which the interval between two fixed exposures to pressure was changed (Griffiths et al., 1971). They found that the bends incidence in small animals increased as the interval increased—which they conclude is the opposite to the trend predicted by the critical supersaturation concept.

An experiment to determine the state of the tissue has exploited the difference between equations (6) and (8) (Hills 1968, 1970b). Goats were given an exposure to compressed air (60 min at 160 ft; 53 m) followed by a standard US Naval decompression calculated by conventional methods based upon the concept of critical supersaturation (Workman 1965). Total decompression time was then 'titrated' for each animal by cutting back upon the time spent at the last (10 ft) stop until bends occurred. When these 'titrations' were repeated upon the same animals, using the same procedure apart from carrying on at the 20 ft stop and 'surfacing' directly from this pressure, it was found that less total decompression time was needed for each goat. This indicates more effective elimination of gas at 20 ft than at 10 ft and is con-

sistent with equation (6) where (ΔP_{N_2}) increases with P. It is directly opposed to equation (8) by which the reverse should hold and must therefore add strong support for the presence of the gas phase in the critical tissue(s).

Taking a different approach, it was found that in 3 goats which had just completed marginally safe decompressions, symptoms could not be induced by exposure of their limbs to high intensity ultrasound (Hills 1970b). This indicates that their critical tissues were already equilibrated or that any increase in the number of equilibrated regions did not increase the local volume of separated gas per unit volume of nucleated tissue. These results are hard to reconcile with a metastable limit to supersaturation.

Conclusion

With so much evidence from both direct and indirect approaches to this problem, there is now little doubt that, during an asymptomatic dive, there can be not only intravascular bubbles, but the gas phase present in the critical tissue for limb bends. Moreover, it would appear that the gas phase starts to form soon after the position of phase equilibrium is exceeded. Thus, for calculation purposes, it remains a purely academic question whether there is a negligible decompression threshold to nucleation in vivo (Hills 1966) or there are always macronuclei present under ambient conditions (Evans and Walder 1969) when they could be stabilized by shear forces of the type which have been used to predict bubble stabilization in isotropic media (Gent and Tompkins 1969). The evidence on this vital issue has been reviewed more recently (Hills 1970c).

GROWTH OR COALESCENCE

While the above conclusion would eliminate conventional calculation methods based upon critical supersaturation, it raises the question of whether the period between initiation of the gas phase and the onset of symptoms has any significant influence upon the incidence. This poses the further question concerning whether the rate of onset of marginal symptoms is determined by the rate of transfer of gas to the gaseous phase from solution, i.e. growth, or by the coalescence or congregation of separated gas into a bubble of critical size. Theories for the former argument have been put forward by Nims (1951), while Bateman (1951) includes further nucleation upon a semi-empirical basis and Albano (1962) allows for the presence of nuclei. However, when expressing their driving force for N_2 elimination mathematically, these approaches do not allow for the desaturation of tissue which bubble growth must cause. This does not invalidate the growth-rate-limiting concept in which interest has recently been revived by Griffiths et al. (1971), but leaves a need for a comprehensive analytical treatment.

The second approach (Hills 1966) largely avoids these kinetic aspects by considering only the 'worst possible case' or those few regions where nucleation is so profuse as to permit total local desaturation within a few minutes. This gas then coalesces. It has been claimed that the random onset time of symptoms is more compatible with the random nature of coalescence than with any time course based upon continuous growth.

Before developing this zero supersaturation approach further, it is necessary to have a physical model for gas transfer in the absence of the gas phase.

TRANSPORT

When a subject starts breathing a different inert gas, its macro-distribution over the body must be effected by the circulation, while beyond the capillaries it must then proceed by diffusion.

Conventional approach

The physiological literature in general favours blood perfusion as the rate-limiting process (Kety 1951; Jones 1951). However, there is at least one disquieting fact which forces one to question what would otherwise be a simple model giving a single exponential function for each tissue, a form which has proven so easy to handle in the Haldane calculation method, yet tends to be retained in subsequent approaches largely for its mathematical simplicity.

Helium versus nitrogen

Hempleman (1967) has indicated, that for corresponding partial pressures of inert gas, the air and oxygen–helium 'bounce dive' curves intersect for both goats and men. For long exposure times, greater pressures can be tolerated when the inert gas is helium than when it is nitrogen. This is compatible with the lower solubility of helium in tissue, whether aqueous or lipid. However, for exposure times of less than 20 min, resulting in a predecompression state further from saturation, and hence emphasizing the kinetics, the same subject can be exposed to a greater pressure upon air than He:O_2. This can easily be explained on the basis of the slower diffusion of nitrogen, where Graham's Law would predict a ratio of coefficients (He:N_2) of 2·65:1 which would override the solubility effect over this range. Hempleman points out that a similar ratio (3:1) of time constants can be predicted on the basis of the perfusion-limiting model, but only if the faster tissue were lipid—a most unlikely situation.

The perfusion/diffusion confusion

Observations such as these have led the author to search back into the vast physiological literature based upon this assumption to see why blood perfusion was accepted as the rate-limiting process in the first place. This has led to a long and critical

TABLE 20.3

Analysis of inert gas elimination from man (data from Jones 1951)

Gas	Method of enumeration of Jones					Time constants in order of extraction				
	k_1	k_2	k_3	k_4	k_5	k_1	k_2	k_3	k_4	k_5
N₂	0·46	0·087*	0·024†	0·0047‡		0·0047‡	0·024†	0·087*	0·46	—
Xe	0·35	0·987	0·024	0·0038	0·0008	0·0008	0·0038	0·024	0·087	0·35
He	0·50	0·084	0·024	—	—	0·024	0·084	0·50	—	—
Ratio (N₂/Xe)	1·32	1·00	1·00	1·24	—	5·87	6·32	3·62	5·29	—
Ratio (He/N₂)	1·09	0·97	1·00	—	—	5·11	3·50	5·74	—	—

Nitrogen values given by Behnke (1951) are: * $0·085$ min⁻¹, † $0·019$ min⁻¹, ‡ $0·0054$ min⁻¹.

review (Hills 1970d) from which several broad conclusions have been made:

1. The data is difficult to interpret on the basis of models advocating either simple homogeneous perfusion or simple linear diffusion in a homogeneous medium.

2. It is necessary to postulate that both of these processes are rate controlling or that diffusion occurs in a heterogeneous medium or that perfusion is heterogeneous. This involves either much more rigorous mathematical application of simple physical principles in the first two cases or postulating more complex physiological mechanisms to overcome the inadequacy of simple equations relevant to the last case, the latter proving more popular.

3. Most evidence is equally compatible with either heterogeneous perfusion or diffusion in a heterogeneous medium. A typical example often quoted in favour of perfusion limitation is the data of Jones (1951) who has argued that if blood perfusion is rate limiting, then all inert gases should have much the same time constants for gas elimination from aqueous tissues. When he extracts from two to four time constants (k) each by backward projection for He, N₂, Kr and Xe, he arranges them in a table such as shown on the left-hand side of Table 20.3. These do indeed tend to agree as laid out in this arbitrary manner.

However, when enumerated according to their order of extraction, these values offer a better correlation on a diffusion-controlling basis (Table 20.3, right-hand side).

Despite the ambiguity of interpretation of most data, there are a few points which afford a better chance to differentiate.

Critical experiments

From the vast mass of material, the following critical points have been selected.

During uptake, the highest inert gas tension must be the arterial value and the lowest must be mean tissue, with venous somewhere in between. Kety and Schmidt (1945) argue that if perfusion is rate limiting, the venous tension will approach mean tissue tension, while if diffusion is rate limiting, venous will approach arterial. They perform a series of experiments in which they estimate mean tissue values by arteriovenous differences to find that they approximate to venous values, implicating a perfusion controlling system. However, if allowance is made in the integration for the time for encumbent blood to be displaced, then the venous and mean tissue values no longer coincide. What is more disturbing are the values for blood perfusion which one derives from the time constants in Kety and Schmidt's experiments. These differ by factors of as much as 2 from the values derived independently from a–v differences, but in such a direction as to be compatible with a significant controlling influence exerted by diffusion (Hills, 1970d; Table 20.4).

Kety (1951), Cavert and Lifson (1958), Forster (1964) and Roughton (1952), using the same radial diffusion equation, have calculated that mean extravascular tissue tension should attain 95 to 99% of the asymptotic value within 1 to 5 sec of a 'step' change in the blood tension of that gas. Thus they dismiss diffusion as an insignificant factor in controlling blood–tissue gas exchange. However, to describe this *transient* situation, they use *overall* tissue values of 10^{-5} cm² sec⁻¹ for the diffusion coefficient, as determined by a *steady*

TABLE 20.4

Comparison of cerebral blood flow ($\dot{Q}$) determined from the same experiments for the uptake of nitrous oxide by brain and calculated: (I) from the time constant, (II) by arteriovenous difference, and (III) by direct measurement (data from Kety & Schmidt 1945)

Time constant in min^{-1}	Tissue: blood partition ($1/\lambda$)	Cerebral blood flow ($\dot{Q}$) in ml/(g tissue min)		
		(I) $1/\lambda$ (perfusion controlling)	(II) by a–v balance	(III) by direct measurement
0·182	1·3	0·24	0·36	0·37
0·198	1·6	0·32	0·35	0·42
0·102	1·0	0·10	0·22	0·17
0·154	1·4	0·22	0·42	0·46
0·287	1·3	0·38	0·62	0·60
0·089	1·3	0·12	0·30	0·31
0·266	1·4	0·37	0·36	0·38
0·230	1·5	0·34	0·66	0·76
0·138	1·2	0·17	0·34	0·32

state method and therefore only acceptable in this context if tissue is uniform.

Determinations of diffusion coefficients in cytoplasm by truly *transient* methods have given very much lower values of $1·5 \times 10^{-8}$ to $5·0 \times 10^{-10}$ for water (Dick 1959), 3×10^{-8} to 3×10^{-10} for 10 polar solutes (Fenichel & Horowitz 1963) and $2·3 \times 10^{-10}$ cm^2 sec^{-1} for certain gases (Hills 1967a). Recalculation of tissue saturation times using these values indicates much slower diffusion and hence a much greater diffusion limitation.

Rigorous mathematical analyses show that it is easier to differentiate between perfusion and diffusion as the rate-limiting process for small time intervals, but these, unfortunately, represent the range of greatest uncertainty in the practical data. Over the well-defined 'asymptotic' region (large time values) the respective time functions become similar, yet still tend to indicate bulk diffusion as the relevant mode of uptake, yielding diffusion coefficients within the range of 'transient' values quoted above (Hennessy 1971).

Very recent studies of the separation of multiple inert gases from solution in tissue (Hills 1975) have indicated that the empirical time functions, $\Phi(t)$ by analysis of practical data using equation (12), are almost identical for nitrogen and helium uptake in man. This would provide strong support for a perfusion-limited system if it were not for the equally close agreement which both functions show for the $\sqrt{t}$ relationship of

Hempleman (1952)—the ultimate approximation of all models for bulk diffusion (Hills 1966). These apparently conflicting observations have been interpreted on the basis of bulk diffusion of gas through capillary bundles of alternating patency; this model gives the $\sqrt{t}$ effect.

THERMODYNAMIC (ZERO SUPERSATURATION) APPROACH

The foregoing reasoning leads to some fairly definite conclusions to some of the *vital issues*, while upon others such as the perfusion/diffusion controversy the answers are less obvious. This type of analysis of the evidence available led to a new quantitative approach to Type I DCS which was termed 'Thermodynamic' (Hills 1966), although it could have been more appropriately named 'Zero Supersaturation' to emphasize the major issue on which it diverged totally from conventional approaches at that time. On several points it is compatible with the 'Oxygen Window' concept developed more qualitatively and quite independently by Behnke (1967).

Features

The salient features of the thermodynamic approach may be listed as follows:

1. It involves only one critical tissue type for Type I DCS.

2. Nucleation of the gas phase in this critical

tissue upon decompression is presumed to be as random as found in tissues of known identity and in the multi-phase systems investigated in vitro, both in decompression threshold and in spacial distribution.

3. The relevant sites to be considered in estimating the imminence of decompression sickness are taken as the 'worst possible'. These are the few micro-regions, or may be only one in many million possibilities, where caviatation has occurred (a) soon after equilibrium conditions have been exceeded, and (b) in such profusion that any local supersaturation is soon dissipated by virtue of the short diffusion paths for the excess gas in reaching the nearest nucleus, i.e. excess gas is 'dumped'.

These conditions define the 'worst possible' since they represent not only the maximum volume of gas separating from solution per unit volume of tissue (v in equation 2), but the minimum driving force for its elimination via the circulation once formed (equation 6).

4. The phase equilibration (growth of gas phase) of these profusely nucleated micro-regions is considered to occur within a few minutes of a change of pressure. Fortunately this avoids the insuperable mathematical complexity introduced by superimposing slow growth of nuclei upon their pattern of random distribution.

5. This gas separated from solution will then tend to coalesce, or to congregate by other means, until its local displacement of tissue bends or otherwise distorts a nerve ending beyond its pain-provoking threshold. Physically, this can be regarded as a concentration of mechanical stress (δ) until it exceeds the critical value (δ') as expressed by equation (1).

6. When the gaseous phase has formed, the driving force for its elimination via the circulation is provided by the *inherent unsaturation* alone (equation 6).

Quantitative description of general case

The bends-provoking stress (δ) is difficult to measure but, fortunately, it can be eliminated from equation (1) and (2) to give the critical condition for bends as:

$$v > \delta'/K \qquad (9)$$

where the total volume of all separated gases per unit volume of tissue (v) can be related to the

nitrogen separated from solution in the gaseous phase from a simple balance for this gas in tissue as:

$$vP'_{N_2} = \underset{\text{(separated)}}{S(P_0 - P_w)F_{I_{N2}}} + \underset{\text{(uptake)}}{G_u} - \underset{\substack{\text{(elimi-}\\\text{nated)}}}{G_e} - \underset{\substack{\text{(remaining}\\\text{in solution)}}}{SP'_{N_2}} \quad (10)$$

where S is the solubility of nitrogen, $F_{I_{N2}}$ is its inspired fraction and G_e is the nitrogen eliminated during gradual decompression, while the nitrogen taken up at the 'bottom' pressure (P_b) is given by the time function, $\Phi(t)$, such that:

$$G_u = S(P_b - P_0)F_{I_{N2}} \cdot \Phi(\tau) \qquad (11)$$

where τ is the 'bottom' time.

Elimination of G_u, P'_{N_2} and v from equations (3), (9) and (10) gives the general condition for the occurrence of a limb bend as:

$$\frac{[P_0 - P_w + (P_b - P_0) \cdot \Phi(\tau)]F_{I_{N2}} - (G_e/S) - P - c}{(P + c)}$$
$$> \frac{\delta'}{KS} = f \quad (12)$$

where f is the critical volume fraction and, if pressures are given in units of atmospheres, S is then the Bunsen coefficient for nitrogen. c is given by equation (4).

Assessment

In qualitative terms, this comprehensive expression (equation 13) can be seen to predict a greater likelihood of bends for a greater 'bottom' pressure ($P_b \uparrow$), greater decompression ($P \downarrow$), a longer exposure time ($\tau \uparrow$), more nitrogen in the $O_2:N_2$ breathing mixture ($F_{I_{N2}} \uparrow$), less decompression time ($G_e \downarrow$), a more soluble inert gas ($S \uparrow$) or a less compliant critical tissue ($K \uparrow$).

Quantitatively, this expression can offer a reason why a decompression ratio would appear to hold—at least, for the particular conditions of the experiments (Boycott & Damant 1908) which led to the introduction of this concept by Haldane, viz. saturation exposure, $\Phi(\tau) = 1$, followed by no-stop decompression ($G_e = o$), when equation (12) gives:

$$P_b = P(f+1)F_{I_{N2}} + c' \qquad (13)$$

Where f is a constant for a particular individual and c'' is a small constant (relative to diving values for P_b), given by:

$$c'' = c(f+1)/F_{I_{N2}} + P_w \qquad (14)$$

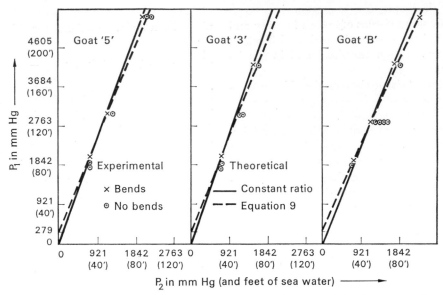

FIG. 20.7. Data from Hempleman (1957) for the outcome of the decompression of goats from an effective steady state at P_1 to a lower absolute pressure (P_2). It can be seen that the broken line (equation 13), based upon the total volume of separated gas offers a slightly better separation of 'bends' from 'no bends' points than a simple ratio as depicted by the full line

Thus equation (13) represents a linear relationship between P_b and P offering a slightly better correlation than the ratio for experimental data (Hempleman 1957) extending the test to higher pressures (Fig. 20.7 where $P_1 = P_b$ and $P_2 = P$). For these higher exposure pressures (P_b), c'' becomes negligible, when its omission from equation (13) gives an apparent ratio of $(f+1)/F_{\mathrm{IN_2}}$.

This omission cannot be made for aerial decompression when c' is now appreciable relative to the absolute pressure. Equation (13) can now be used to correlate aerial data with underwater to give the same values of f for pilots and divers of corresponding sensitivity to decompression, taking $c = 74$ mm Hg and $b = 200$ mm Hg (Hills 1969a). This includes a comparison of helium and nitrogen data for which the critical values of f are found to lie in the ratio of their solubilities (S) as predicted by equation (12).

General analysis

The test of this expression has been extended from these special yet important cases to an analysis of the bends incidence in 10 sets of exposures, each followed by a conventional decompression. It has offered a better prediction (Hills 1966) than the supersaturation ratio concept on which those trials were designed. This analysis departed markedly from Haldanian traditions by recognizing the presence of the gas phase following the typical long initial 'pull' to the surface and, moreover, refuting any connection between the gas elimination (G_e) and the uptake function $\Phi(t)$. Rather, G_e was taken as increasing linearly with ambient pressure (P) on the basis of the inherent unsaturation. ($G_e \propto \Delta P_{\mathrm{N_2}}$ in equation 6).

However, before extending the thermodynamic approach from a general analysis of dives irrespective of their design to decompression optimization, it is first necessary to consider the transport model in more detail.

The transport model

Most approaches are synthetic in so far as they select one or more time functions for gas *uptake*, each with suitably chosen constants, and then use the same function to describe *elimination*. Others modify those constants empirically to allow for some degree of asymmetry of gas transfer between exposure and decompression.

A different approach is the analytical one. This avoids uncertainties in mathematical symmetry by considering no-stop decompressions only ($G_e = 0$) and then invoking the comprehensive (equation 12) to derive the true uptake function, $\Phi(t)$. This has been done (Hills 1969b) and effectively assumes that the critical tissue contains the same quantity of gas at the start of decompression from all exposures described by the bounce dive curve. The analytical uptake function can then be compared with those derived by mathematical expressions describing blood perfusion limitation, diffusion into a flat slab and radial diffusion from

a cylindrical capillary. It can be seen in Fig. 20.8 that no equation fits exactly, indicating that gas transfer is probably limited by both diffusion and the circulation as discussed earlier. However, by far the closest fit is afforded by a model representing radial diffusion from a capillary of radius (a) and intercapillary distance ($2b$), when:

$$\Phi(t) = 1 - \frac{4}{(b/a)^2 - 1}$$
$$\times \sum_{0}^{\infty} \frac{e^{-\alpha_n{}^2 Dt}}{(a\alpha_n)^2 \{[J_0(a\alpha_n)/J_1(b\alpha_n)]^2 - 1\}} \quad (15)$$

where D is the diffusion coefficient and α_n is the nth root, real and positive, of the equation:

$$J_0(a\alpha_n) \cdot Y_1(b\alpha_n) = Y_0(a\alpha_n) \cdot J_1(b\alpha_n)$$

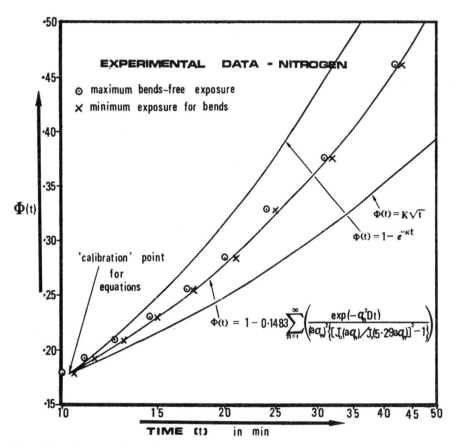

FIG. 20.8. A comparison of the uptake function for nitrogen, $\Phi(t)$, determined by applying equation (12) to the comprehensive bounce dive data of Albano (1962), with various theoretical functions. In descending order, those represent blood perfusion, radial bulk diffusion and linear diffusion, with one point being sacrificed as a 'calibration' to determine the one constant required by each model (after Hills 1969b)

J and Y represent Bessel and Neumann functions as defined by Watson (1944).

The above expression for $\Phi(t)$ can easily be derived from equations given in standard mathematical texts describing the inert gas tension (p) at a radial location (r) at time (t) following a sudden change from O to P_1 within the capillary $(r < a)$ as:

$$\frac{p}{P_1} = 1 - \pi$$
$$\times \sum_0^\infty \frac{[J_0(r\alpha_n) Y_0(a\alpha_n) - Y_0(r\alpha_n) J_0(a\alpha_n)]\, e^{-\alpha_n^2 Dt}}{[J_0(a\alpha_n)/J_1(b\alpha_n)]^2 - 1} \tag{16}$$

Optimization

Whatever model or approach one adopts, optimization of a decompression profile amounts to selecting the pressure at each moment at which the driving force for inert gas elimination is a maximum. If the gas phase is not present, then this is the lowest pressure before it forms (equation 8) while, if it *is* present, then the optimal is the highest pressure at which the gas phase exists (equation 6). These coincide with each other only at the position of thermodynamic equilibrium on the 'Zero Supersaturation' approach and thus represent the ideal situation to try to follow.

Even though a subject may have reached a steady state condition after prolonged exposure to pressure, he must always be significantly undersaturated for the reasons given earlier. He can thus be rapidly decompressed by his *inherent unsaturation* before any point in his critical tissue need be saturated in the true thermodynamic sense. Upon reaching this new ambient pressure, the unsaturation will re-establish itself in capillary blood in accordance with this new value of P in equation (6) and more inert gas will tend to be eliminated under the newly established gradient. This will decrease the peak gas tension and change its location, both of which can then be calculated to determine the next pressure to which the system can be moved to re-establish a point of phase equilibrium.

If the computation is correct, then no gas phase should have formed, so that the same time function can be used to describe inert gas elimination as uptake, i.e. successive steps described by equation (16) can be superposed to obtain the distribution of inert gas at any time.

In superposing the effects of successive changes of pressure, these are only additive for linear time functions, such as the simple exponential as used in the Haldane approach. In the above case of radial diffusion Hennessy has derived the expression (17) to describe the tension (p) at a general location (r) after a switch to a capillary tension (P_1) following any previous history resulting in a general distribution $h(r)$ at zero time.

$$\frac{p}{P_1} = P_1 + \pi$$
$$\times \sum_1^\infty \frac{[J_0(r\alpha_n)\cdot Y_0(a\alpha_n) - Y_0(r\alpha_n)\cdot J_0(a\alpha_n)]\, e^{-\alpha_n^2 Dt}}{\{[J_0(a\alpha_n)/J_1(b\alpha_n)]^2 - 1\}}$$
$$\times \int_a^b \frac{\pi}{2}\cdot \alpha_n^2 x [h(x) - P_1]$$
$$\times [J_0(x\alpha_n)\cdot Y_0(a\alpha_n) - Y_0(x\alpha_n)\cdot J_0(a\alpha_n)]\, \mathrm{d}x \tag{17}$$

This integral has offered no problem when computed by J. Moore at the Texas A & M Computing Center, using Legendre quadrature.

The computation routine therefore consists of the following steps:

1. Very rapid decompression from the exposure pressure by the inherent unsaturation at P_b (equation 6).

2. Determination of the radial distribution of gas.

3. Find the location and then the height of the peak (equation 16).

4. Adjust the absolute pressure to coincide with this peak (see Fig. 20.10d).

5. Calculate the blood gas tension and repeat steps 2 to 4.

6. Continue this routine until a pressure is reached at which one can surface directly and purposely form the gas phase, but to just below the pain-provoking dimensions.

This type of computation is very tedious since a new term is superposed with each change of pressure, 1-min intervals proving convenient on a digital computer. However this complexity has been avoided until recently by the use of an analogue.

Decompression analogues

The exact similarity in mathematical descriptions of diffusion and thermal conduction has led

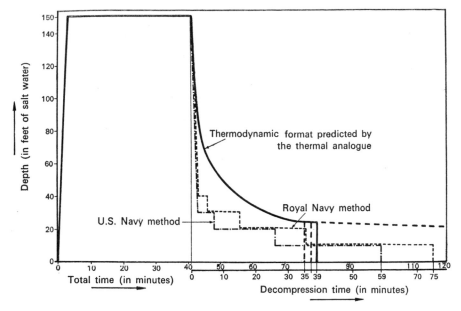

FIG. 20.9. The optimal deployment of decompression time as indicated by a thermal analogue based upon the zero supersaturation concept. Total decompression times indicated were those found by experimental 'titration' of large goats

to a thermal analogue to simulate the radial diffusion model (Hills 1967b). This has given the format shown in Fig. 20.9 which, when tested upon goats, showed an appreciable saving in total decompression time compared with the similar titration of the same animals upon the corresponding US Navy profiles.

It is particularly interesting to see the resemblance between this type of format and the purely empirical decompressions devised at the expense of many lives by Okinawan pearl divers operating in Australian coastal waters (LeMessurier & Hills 1965). These men also show substantial savings in total decompression time and feature both the same propensity for deep stops at the start of decompression and immediate surfacing upon reaching 22 to 35 feet. In terms of numbers of dives, the experience of these pearl divers must far outweigh that of all the navies combined.

However, the thermal analogue has the great disadvantage that it cannot allow for formation of the gaseous phase in tissue, a shortcoming also common to meters based upon the principle of critical supersaturation. These include the single air chamber fitted with a porous resistance plug

made by S.O.S. (Italian patent 624174), the Canadian multi-chamber/orifice meter (Stubbs & Kidd 1965), the recent chamber/membrane meter (Borom & Johnson 1973) and several electrical analogues (Wittenborn 1963). All of these are essentially based upon equation (7) with no mechanism for reverting to equation (6) if the gas phase forms. Moreover, even if each were correct in the condition imposed for determining separation of the gas phase from solution, then any unheeded violation would cause the meter to register less gas remaining in the tissue and hence indicate even faster decompression—so exacerbating the initial error.

General analogue

An attempt to overcome these shortcomings has been made (Hills 1967c) by permitting each chamber of a 27-compartment pneumatic analogue to expand wherever the simulated total gas tension exceeds the absolute pressure $(P+b)$. Thus the driving force is reduced in accordance with equation (6) (Fig. 20.10) while the total expansion must be proportional to the volume of tissue gas since Boyle's Law is applied automatically

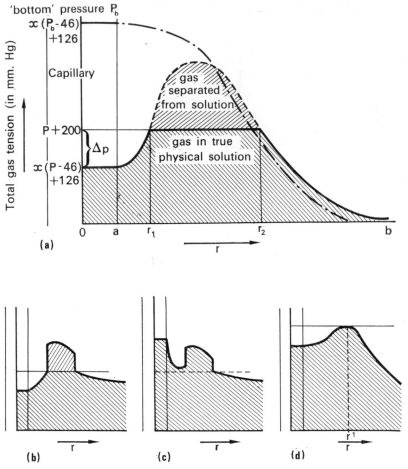

FIG. 20.10. Radial tension and separated gas distributions illustrated for phase equilibration at various stages of decompression and recompression. The inherent unsaturation (ΔP) is shown as the driving force for diffusion (1) —·—·— before decompression, and (2) ———— immediately after decompression to pressure, P

(Fig. 20.11). While this very large analogue (Fig. 20.12) has correlated the incidence of bends from decompressions based upon very different approaches, it has now been reduced to a small liquid-filled 6-chamber version for use as a meter (Hills 1973a) for optimizing on the zero super-saturation principle and capable of rescheduling following a diver mistake and gas phase formation.

OTHER BIOPHYSICAL ASPECTS

There are a number of interesting biophysical phenomena which have been reported recently.

These include several facets of dysbaric osteo-necrosis, gas-induced osmosis, collision fission of microbubbles and counter-diffusion supersatura-tion. The latter is an ingenious concept (Graves et al. 1973) which is described in another chapter (21) and could well explain hyperbaric urticaria (no-decompression skin bends), as observed by Blenkarn et al. (1971).

Collision fission of bubbles

Recent experiments in the author's laboratory have shown that microbubbles formed by air in-jection (Fig. 20.13) into human plasma in vitro

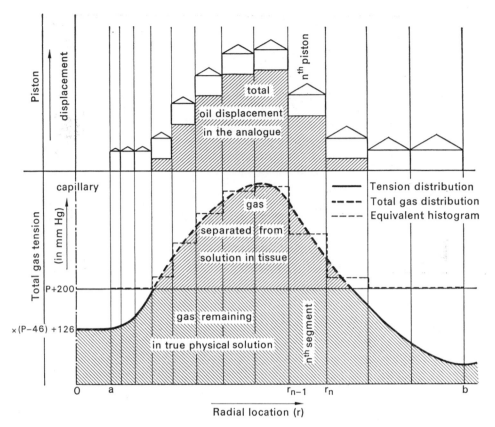

FIG. 20.11. Each radial segment around a cylindrical capillary is represented by a chamber of fixed minimum volume (see Fig. 20.12) but sealed by a moveable piston to ensure that its internal pressure does not exceed ambient. This simulates the 'cut-off' in driving force for gas elimination imposed by phase separation, limiting it to the inherent unsaturation (equation 6). Since Boyle's Law is applied to chamber gas, the piston displacements represent a histogram of the volume distribution of separated gas illustrated in Fig. 20.10

burst into many small bubbles upon collision. It is surprising that this only occurs if the diameter of the progenitors is less than 200 to 250 μm, while their size seems to have a negligible effect upon that of the progeny (about 40 to 50 μm diameter). This phenomenon could represent a protective mechanism of the body in minimizing the pathological effects of air emboli by reducing their size, although increasing their number.

It was found that the progeny of collisions would dissolve, even in air-saturated fluids, so supersaturating plasma!

Gas-induced osmosis

It has been demonstrated, by a transient technique, that nitrous oxide can induce osmosis across a synthetic membrane specifically formulated to be impermeable to that gas relative to water (Kylstra, Longmuir & Grace 1968). Moreover, it has now been shown that the phenomenon applies to biological membranes, since several gases have been shown to induce osmosis across various excised tissue sections under steady state conditions and in vivo (Hills 1971a). More significant to diving, perhaps, is the observation that nitrogen can 'pull' water away from helium if high pressure is used to emphasize the physical differences in these gases (Hills 1971b).

In any hyperbaric exposure this phenomenon has two potential components: a transient

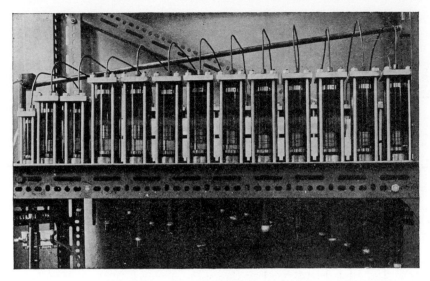

FIG. 20.12. A pneumatic analogue capable of simulating radial diffusion and the phase change indicated in Figs 20.9 and 20.10. The instrument has been used to analyse data irrespective of the rationale underlying the decompression design

contributed by the inert gas until it equilibrates throughout the tissue (see Fig. 20.14) and a change in the steady state effect of the permanent gradients of the metabolic gases, O_2 and CO_2. The former offers a convenient explanation for the time-dependent aspects of hyperbaric arthralgia, the high pressure nervous syndrome, minor changes in narcosis, vestibular problems, etc.

The steady state contributions suggest a possible involvement of osmosis in neurological oxygen toxicity (Hills 1972c) while it has implications in pulmonary O_2 poisoning, i.e. the effect of Lorraine Smith [1902]. This is based upon the observation that a lung selectively ventilated with 80% N_2O +20% O_2 accumulates more extravascular fluid than a control ventilated with air in the same animal (Hills 1972a).

Longmuir and Grace (1969) have shown transient changes in the volume of red cells when suddenly exposed to nitrous oxide solutions, the effect indicating an osmotic mechanism. The subject of gas-induced osmosis has been recently reviewed (Hills 1972b) with the conclusion that the osmotic potency of gases is simply an extrapolation from those of non-volatile solutes (Fig. 20.15).

Dysbaric osteonecrosis

The thermodynamic approach to decompression sickness would seem particularly compatible with the clinical data which shows no correlation between the incidence of bends and bone lesions in non-experimental divers and caisson workers, in so far as its calculation method predicts the formation of the gaseous phase, and hence 'silent bubbles', in the bends-free diver. It should thus be possible to avoid these 'silent bubbles' to which bone lesions are widely attributed (James 1945; McCallum & Walder 1966) by continuing the gradual ascent to the surface without the 'drop out' from 25 ft (1·7 ATA) now advocated. Support for this approach was provided by Doppler monitoring (Vann et al. 1973) when it was found that intravascular bubbles were not detected upon 'thermodynamic' profiles until the 'drop out' (Fig. 20.16).

However, if silent bubbles, thrombi or fat emboli were responsible for dysbaric osteonecrosis, one could expect a much shorter time course for the disease than the clinical evidence seems to indicate. This is discussed in detail in another chapter (27) but, if these doubts are well founded,

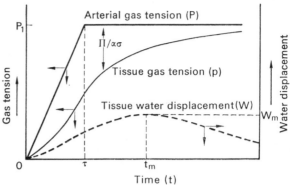

FIG. 20.14. The predicted transient displacement of fluid induced osmotically across a blood–tissue barrier by compression, at a uniform rate, to a 'bottom' pressure which is then held constant

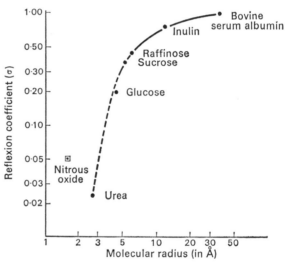

FIG. 20.15. The osmotic potency of a gas (nitrous oxide) is shown to be roughly predictable from an extrapolation of data for non-volatile solutes on the basis of the reflexion coefficient (σ). This is proportional to the number of solute molecules which are reflected rather than transmitted upon collision with the membrane.

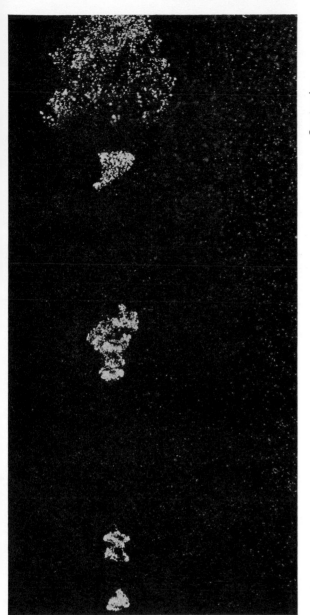

FIG. 20.13. The disintegration of successive complexes, each formed by the collision of two microbubbles of less than 200 μm diameter in plasma (from Hills 1974)

then it would appear that a much more subtle form of insult to the bone occurs upon hyperbaric exposure, to become manifest much later as the ischemia leading to necrosis. A process which could continue slowly with no further exposure is the deposition of bone mineral in unwanted sites due to the known permanent supersaturation of hydroxyapatite in body fluids. This has led to two mechanisms to be proposed for dysbaric osteonecrosis based upon uncontrolled mineral precipation. Sobell (1971) has shown changes in colla-

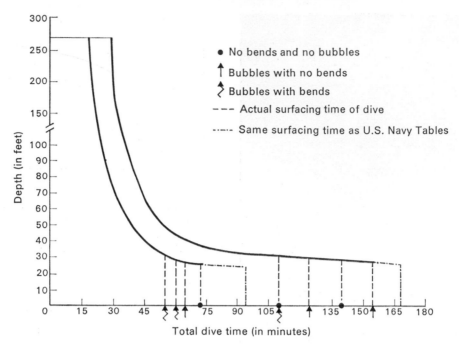

F IG. 20.16. Two decompressions optimized on the 'thermodynamic' principle, showing that bubbles were not detected by a Doppler ultrasonic meter until after the final 'drop out' from about 25 ft (1·7 ATA) (after Vann et al. 1973)

gen following quite small increases in inspired oxygen partial pressure, implicating that these sites of chemical cross-linking could be more inducive to mineral precipitation. Hills (1970a; 1972b) has shown that bones are good osmometers and that articular cartilage is an effective osmotic membrane for gases. Thus, if the ions do not move as easily as the water, there could be further local supersaturation resulting in spontaneous formation of nuclei, whose growth to sizes of clinical significance could take months or years. This hypothesis (Hills 1970a) would implicate any rapid change of pressure—either rapid decompression to the first stop or compression!

REFERENCES

ALBANO, G. (1960) *Études sur la decompression chez l'homme*. Premier Colloque de Medecine Subaquatique, Cannes.

ALBANO, G. (1962) *Medna Sport* **2**, 57.

BATEMAN, J. B. (1951) Review of data on value of preoxygenation in prevention of decompression sickness. In *Decompression Sickness*. Ed. J. F. Fulton. p. 242. Philadelphia: Saunders.

BEHNKE, A. R. (1951) Decompression sickness following exposure to high pressures. In *Decompression Sickness*. Ed. J. F. Fulton. pp. 53–89. Philadelphia: Saunders.

BEHNKE, A. R. (1967) The isobaric (oxygen window) principle of decompression. In *Trans. Third Annual Conference of the Marine Technol. Society*, pp. 213–228. Washington, D.C.: Marine Technology Society.

BLANKENHORN, M. A. & FERRIS, E. B. (1944) The nature of aviators bends. *Trans. Ass. Am. Physiol.* **58**, 86–91.

BLANKENHORN, M. A., FERRIS, E. B., ROMANO, J., RYDER, H. W., ENGEL, G. L., WEBB, J. P., SAFER, I. A. & STEVENS, C. D. (1942) *Decompression Sickness: (Exploratory Study)*. Report 6. U.S. Natl Res. Council, Comm. Aviat. Med., Washington, D.C.

BLENKARN, G. D., AQUADRO, C., HILLS, B. A., SALTZMAN, H. A. & KYLSTRA, J. A. (1971) Urticaria following sequential breathing of various inert gases at 7 ATA: a possible manifestation of gas-induced osmosis. *Aerospace Med.* **42**, 141–146.

BOROM, M. R. & JOHNSON, L. A. (1973) *A Decompression Meter for Scuba Diving Utilizing Semipermeable Membranes*. Report 73 CRD 729. New York: General Electric Co.

BOYCOTT, A. E. & DAMANT, C. C. (1908) Experiments on the influence of fatness on susceptibility to caisson disease. *J. Hyg., Camb.*, **8**, 445–456.

BOYCOTT, A. E., DAMANT, C. C. & HALDANE, J. S. (1908) The prevention of compressed-air illness. *J. Hyg., Camb.* **8**, 342–443.

BRIGGS, L. (1947) Possible explanation of Brigg's limiting negative pressure data. *J. appl. Physics*, **23**, 931–935.

CAMPBELL, J. A. (1924) Changes in the tension of carbon dioxide and oxygen injected under the skin and into the abdominal cavities. *J. Physiol., Lond.* **59**, 1–6.

CHASE, W. H. (1934) Anatomical and experimental observations on air embolism. *Surg. Gynec. Obstet.*, **56**, 569–577.

DEAN, R. B. (1944) The formation of bubbles. *J. appl. Physics* **15**, 446–449.

DICK, D. A. T. (1959) The rate of diffusion of water in the protoplasm of living cells. *Exp. Cell. Res.* **17**, 5–12.

DIXON, H. H. (1914) *Transpiration and the Ascent of Sap in Trees*. London: Macmillan.

DUFFNER, G. J., VAN DER AUE, O. E. & BEHNKE, A. R. (1946) *The Treatment of Decompression Sickness*. Research report 3. Project X. 443. US Navy Experimental Diving Unit, Washington, D.C.

EVANS, A. & WALDER, D. N. (1969) Significance of gas macronuclei in the aetiology of decompression sickness. *Nature, Lond.* **222**, 251–252.

EVANS, A., BARNARD, E. E. P. & WALDER, D. N. (1971) Detection of gas bubbles in man at decompression. *Aerospace Med.* **43**, 1095–1096.

FENICHEL, I. R. & HOROWITZ, S. B. (1963) The transport of non-electrolytes in muscle as a diffusional process in cytoplasm. *Acta physiol. scand.* **60**, suppl. 221, 1–63.

FERRIS, E. B. & ENGEL, G. L. (1951) The clinical nature of high altitude decompression sickness. In *Decompression Sickness*. Ed. J. F. Fulton. pp. 4–52. Philadelphia: Saunders.

FORSTER, R. E. (1964) Diffusion factors in gases and liquids. In *The Uptake and Distribution of Anesthetic Agents*. Ed. E. M. Papper and R. J. Kitz. pp. 20–29. New York: McGraw-Hill.

GALLOWAY, W. (1954) *J. acous. Soc. Am.* **26**, 849.

GENT, A. N. & TOMPKINS, D. A. (1969) Nucleation and growth of gas bubbles in elastomers. *J. appl. Physics*, **40**, 2520–2525.

GERSH, I., HAWKINSON, G. E. & RATHBUN, E. M. (1944) Tissue and vascular bubbles after decompression from high pressure atmospheres, correlation of specific gravity with morphological changes. *J. Cell comp. Physiol.* **24**, 35–70.

GOLDING, F. C., GRIFFITHS, P. D., HEMPLEMAN, H. V., PATON, W. D. M. & WALDER, D. N. (1960) Decompression sickness during construction of the Dartford Tunnel. *Br. J. indust. Med.* **17**, 167–180.

GRAVES, D. J., IDICULA, J., LAMBERTSEN, C. J. & QUINN, J. A. (1973) Bubble formation resulting from counterdiffusion supersaturation: a possible explanation for isobaric inert gas 'urticaria' and vertigo. *Physics Med. Biol.*, **18**, 256–264.

GRAY, J. S. (1944) *Aeroembolism Induced by Exercise in Cadets at 23,000 Feet*. US Natl Res. Council, Comm. Aviat. Med. report 260, Washington, D.C.

GRAY, J. S. (1951) Constitutional factors affecting susceptibility to decompression sickness. In *Decompression Sickness*. Ed. J. F. Fulton. pp. 182–191. Philadelphia: Saunders.

GRIFFITHS, H. B., MILLER, K. W., PATON, W. D. M. & SMITH, E. B. (1971) On the role of separated gas in decompression sickness. *Proc. R. Soc. B* **178**, 389–406.

HALLOCK, P. & BENSON, I. C. (1937) Studies on the elastic properties of human aorta. *J. clin. Invest.* **16**, 595.

HARVEY, E. N. (1945) Decompression sickness and bubble formation in blood and tissues. *Bull. N.Y. Acad. Med.* **21**, 505–536.

HARVEY, E. N. (1951) Physical factors in bubble formation. In *Decompression Sickness*. Ed. J. F. Fulton. pp. 90–114. Philadelphia: Saunders.

HARVEY, E. N., McELROY, W. D., WHITELEY, A. H., WARREN, G. H. & PEASE, D. C. (1944a) Bubble formation in animals. III. An analysis of gas tension and hydrostatic pressure in rats. *J. Cell comp. Physiol.* **24**, 117–132.

HARVEY, E. N., WHITELEY, A. H., McELROY, W. D., PEASE, D. C. & BARNES, D. K. (1944b) Bubble formation in animals. II. Gas nuclei and their distribution in blood and tissues. *J. Cell comp. Physiol.* **24**, 23–34.

HARVEY, E. N., BARNES, D. K., McELROY, W. D., WHITELEY, A. H., PEASE, D. C. & COOPER, K. W. (1944c) Bubble formation in animals. I. Physical factors. *J. Cell comp. Physiol.* **24**, 1–22.

HAYMAKER, W. (1957) Decompression sickness, etiology and pathogenesis. In *Handbuch der Speziellen Pathologischen Anatomie und Histologie*. Ed. A. Lubarsh, F. Henke & R. Rossle. pp. 1600–1675. Berlin: Springer-Verlag.

HEMPLEMAN, H. V. (1952) *Investigation into the Decompression Tables. III. A New Theoretical Basis for the Calculation of Decompression Tables*. Medical Research Council, RN Personnel Research Committee Report. U.P.S. 131, London.

HEMPLEMAN, H. V. (1957) *Investigation into the Decompression Tables, Further Basic Facts*. Medical Research Council, RN Personnel Research Committee Report. U.P.S. 168, London.

HEMPLEMAN, H. V. (1960) *The Unequal Rates of Uptake and Elimination of Tissue Nitrogen in Diving Procedures*. Medical Research Council, RN Personnel Research Committee Report. U.P.S. 195, London.

HEMPLEMAN, H. V. (1961) *Investigations into the Decompression Tables. An Extension of the Experimental Findings of Report V of this Series*. Medical Research Council, RN Personnel Research Committee Report U.P.S. 202, London.

HEMPLEMAN, H. V. (1967) Decompression procedures for deep, open sea operations. In *Proc. 3rd Symp. Underwater Physiology*. Ed. C. J. Lambertsen. pp. 255–266. Baltimore: Williams & Wilkins.

HENNESSY, T. R. (1971) Inert gas diffusion in heterogeneous tissue. I: without perfusion. *Bull. Math. Biophys.*, **33**, 235–248.

HILLS, B. A. (1966) *A Thermodynamic and Kinetic Approach to Decompression Sickness*. Adelaide: Libraries Board of S. Australia.

HILLS, B. A. (1967a) Diffusion versus blood perfusion in limiting the rate of uptake of inert non-polar gases by skeletal rabbit muscle. *Clin. Sci.* **33**, 67–87.

HILLS, B. A. (1967b) A thermal analogue for the optimal decompression of divers. *Physics Med. Biol.* **12**, 437–454.

HILLS, B. A. (1967c) A pneumatic analogue for predicting the occurrence of decompression sickness. *Med. biol. Engng* **5**, 421–432.

HILLS, B. A. (1967d) Decompression sickness: a study of cavitation at the liquid–liquid interface. *Aerospace Med.* **38**, 814–7.

HILLS, B. A. (1968) Relevant phase conditions for predicting occurrence of decompression sickness. *J. appl. Physiol.* **25**, 310–315.

HILLS, B. A. (1969a) A quantitative correlation of conditions for the occurrence of decompression sickness for aerial and underwater exposures. *Rev. subaqua. Physiol.* **1**, 249–254.

HILLS, B. A. (1969b) The time course for the uptake of inert gases by the tissue type responsible for marginal symptoms of decompression sickness. *Rev. subaqua. Physiol.*, **1**, 255–261.

HILLS, B. A. (1969c) Acclimatization to decompression sickness: a study of passive relaxation in several tissues. *Clin. Sci.* **37**, 109–124.

HILLS, B. A. (1970a) Gas-induced osmosis as an aetiologic agent for inert gas narcosis, gouty arthritis and aseptic bone necrosis induced by exposure to compressed air. *Rev. subaqua. Physiol. hyperbar. Med.* **2**, 3–7.

HILLS, B. A. (1970b) Limited supersaturation versus phase equilibration in predicting the occurrence of decompression sickness. *Clin. Sci.* **38**, 251–267.

HILLS, B. A. (1970c) Vital issues in computing decompression schedules from fundamentals. I. Critical supersaturation versus phase equilibration. *Int. J. Bioclim. Biomet.* **14**, 111–131.

HILLS, B. A. (1970d) Vital issues in computing decompression schedules from fundamentals. II. Diffusion versus blood perfusion in controlling blood: tissue exchange. *Int. J. Bioclim. Biomet.* **14**, 323–342.

HILLS, B. A. (1971a) Gas-induced osmosis as a factor influencing the distribution of body water. *Clin. Sci.* **40**, 175–191.

HILLS, B. A. (1971b) Osmosis induced by nitrogen. *Aerospace Med.* **42**, 664–666.

HILLS, B. A. (1971c) Concepts of inert gas exchange in tissue during decompression. In *Underwater Physiology. Proc. 4th Symp. Underwater Physiology.* Ed. C. J. Lambertsen. pp. 115–122. New York: Academic Press.

HILLS, B. A. (1971d) Decompression sickness: a fundamental study of 'surface excursion' diving and the selection of limb bends versus C.N.S. symptoms. *Aerospace Med.* **42**, 833–836.

HILLS, B. A. (1972a) Gas-induced osmosis in the lung. *J. appl. Physiol.*, **33**, 126–129.

HILLS, B. A. (1972b) Clinical implications of gas-induced osmosis. *Archs intern. Med.* **129**, 356–362.

HILLS, B. A. (1973a) *Decompression meter.* Brit. pat. 50003/72.

HILLS, B. A. (1973b) Chemical facilitation of thermal conduction in physiological systems. *Science, N.Y.* **182**, 823–825.

HILLS, B. A. (1974) Air embolism: fission of microbubbles upon collision in plasma. *Clin. Sci. Molec. Biol.* **46**. (In press.)

HILLS, B. A. (1975) Decompression after inspiring various inert gases simultaneously or sequentially. RNPL report. (In press.)

HILLS, B. A. & LeMESSURIER, D. H. (1969) Unsaturation in living tissue relative to the pressure and composition of inhaled gas and its significance in decompression theory. *Clin. Sci.* **36**, 185–195.

INMAN, V. T. & SAUNDERS, J. B. (1944) Referred pain from skeletal structures. *J. nerv. ment. Dis.* **99**, 660–667.

JAMES, C. C. M. (1945) Late bone lesions in caisson disease. Three cases in submarine personnel. *Lancet* **2**, 6.

JONES, H. B. (1951) Gas exchange and blood-tissue perfusion factors in various body tissues. In *Decompression Sickness.* Ed. J. F. Fulton. pp. 278–321. Philadelphia: Saunders.

KETY, S. S. (1951) Theory and applications of exchange of inert gases at lungs and tissue. *Pharmac. Rev.* **3**, 1–41.

KETY, S. S. & SCHMIDT, C. F. (1945) The determination of cerebral blood flow in man by the use of nitrous oxide in low concentrations. *Am. J. Physiol.*, **143**, 53–56.

KYLSTRA, J. A., LONGMUIR, I. S. and GRACE, M. (1968) Dysbarism: a study of gas osmosis. *Science, N.Y.* **161**, 289.

LeMESSURIER, D. H. & HILLS, B. A. (1965) Decompression sickness: a thermodynamic hypothesis arising from a study of Torres Strait diving techniques. *Hvalråd. Skr.* **48**, 54–84.

LONGMUIR, I. S. & GRACE, M. (1969) Physiological effect of the osmotic pressure of dissolved gas. *Fedn Proc. Fedn Am. Socs exp. Biol.* **28**, 720.

McCALLUM, R. I. & WALDER, D. N. (1966) Bone lesions in compressed air workers. *J. Bone Jt Surg.* **488**, 207–235.

McELROY, W. D., WHITELEY, A. H., WARREN, G. H. & HARVEY, E. N. (1944a) Bubble formation in animals. IV. The relative importance of CO_2 concentration and mechanical tension during muscle contraction. *J. Cell. comp. Physiol.* **24**, 133–146.

McELROY, W. D., WHITELEY, A. H., COOPER, K. W., PEASE, D. C., WARREN, G. H. & HARVEY, E. N. (1944b) Bubble formation in animals. VI. Physiological factors: the role of circulation and respiration. *J. Cell. comp. Physiol.* **24**, 273–290.

MEYER, J. (1911) *Z. Electrochem.* **17**, 743.

NIMS, L. F. (1951) Environmental factors affecting decompression sickness: a physical theory of decompression sickness. In *Decompression Sickness.* Ed. J. F. Fulton. pp. 192–222. Philadelphia: Saunders.

PEASE, D. C. & BLINKS, L. R. (1947) Cavitation from solid surfaces in the absence of gas nuclei. *J. phys. Chem., Ithaca* **51**, 556–567.

PHILP, R. B., INWOOD, M. J. & WARREN, B. A. (1972) Interactions between gas bubbles and components of the blood: implications in decompression sickness. *Aerospace Med.* **43**, 946–953.

RASHBASS, C. (1954) *Investigation into the Decompression Tables: a Consideration of Basic Theories of Decompression Sickness.* Medical Research Council, R.N. Personnel Research Committee Report. U.P.S. 139, London.

REYNOLDS, O. (1878) *Mem. Manch. Lit. Phil. Soc.* **17**, 159.

RIVERA, J. C. (1964) Decompression sickness among divers: an analysis of 935 cases. *Milit. Med.* **129**, 314–334.

ROSE, R. J. (1962) *Survey of Work in Compressed-air During the Construction of the Auckland Harbour Bridge.* Special report No. 6, Medical Statistics Branch, Wellington: N.Z. Dept. of Health.

ROUGHTON, J. F. W. (1952) Diffusion and chemical reaction velocity in cylindrical and spherical systems of physiological interest. *Proc. R. Soc. B* **140**, 203–221.

RYDER, H. W., STEVENS, C. D., WEBB, J. P. & BLANKENHORN, M. A. (1945) *The Measurement of Decompression Sickness.* US Natl Res. Council. Comm. Aviat. Med. Report 412, Washington, D.C.

SAUNDERS, J. B. & INMAN, V. T. (1943) *Preliminary Observations on the Qualitative and Quantitative Characteristics of Pain Elicited by Stimulation of Somatic Structures.* Unpublished results quoted by Nims (1951).

SCHREINER, H. R. (1968) Safe ascent after deep dives. *Rev. subaqua. Physiol.* **1**, 28–37.

SEARLE, J. R. & HILLS, B. A. (1975) Development of an electrodeless conductivity instrument for the detection of the gas phase in tissue. In *Underwater Physiology. Vth Symp. Underwater Physiology.* Ed. C. J. Lambertsen. Bethesda: Fedn Am. Socs exp. Biol.

SHIM, S. S., PATTERSON, F. P. & KENDALL, M. J. (1967) Hyperbaric chamber and decompression sickness. *Canad. med. Ass. J.* **97**, 1263–1272.

SLARK, A. G. (1962) *Treatment of 127 Cases of Decompression Sickness.* Medical Research Council, RN Personnel Research Committee Report 63/1030, London.

SOBELL, H. (1971) *Effect of Hyperbaric Oxygen–nitrogen Mixtures.* O.N.R. Program on Underwater Physiology Report ACR-175. Arlington: US Navy.

SPENCER, M. P. & CAMPBELL, S. D. (1968) Development of bubbles in venous and arterial blood during hyperbaric decompression. *Bull. Mason Clin.* **22**, 26–32.

STUBBS, R. A. & KIDD, D. J. (1965) *A Pneumatic Analogue Decompression Computer.* Inst. Aviat. Med. Report 65-RD-1. Toronto: Canadian Forces Medical Service.

THOMAS, S. & WILLIAMS, O. L. (1944) *High Altitude Joint Pains: their Radiographic Aspects.* US Natl Res. Council Comm. Aviat. Med. Report 395, Washington, D.C.

TUREEN, L. L. & DEVINE, J. B. (1936) The pathology of air embolism. *J. Mo. Med. Ass.* **33**, 141–4.

VAN DER AUE, O. E., KELLER, R. J., BRINTON, E. S., GILLIAM, H. D. & JONES, R. J. (1951) *Calculation and Testing of Decompression Tables for Air Dives.* EDU report MM 002.007, Washington: US Navy.

VAN LIEW, H. D., BISHOP, B. P., WALDER, D. & RAHN, H. (1965) Effects of compression on composition and absorption of tissue gas pockets. *J. appl. Physiol.,* **20**, 927–933.

VANN, R. D., WIDELL, P. J., YOUNGBLOOD, D. A. & HILLS, B. A. (1973) Decompressions of widely differing profile monitored by the ultrasonic bubble detector. In *Proc. Symp. Blood Bubble Detection,* Seattle.

VINCENT, R. S. (1941) Measurement of tension in liquids by means of a metal bellows. *Proc. physics. Soc.* **53**, 126–129.

WALDER, D. N. (1966) Adaptation to decompression sickness in caisson work. In *Biometeorology,* Vol. II. Ed. S. W. Tromp & W. H. Weihe. pp. 350–359. Oxford: Pergamon.

WATSON, G. N. (1944) *Theory of Bessel Functions,* 2nd ed. Cambridge: Cambridge University Press.

WEBB, J. P., RYDER, H. W., ENGEL, G. L., ROMANO, J., BLANKENHORN, M. A. & FERRIS, E. B. (1943) *The Effect on Susceptibility to Decompression Sickness of Preflight Oxygen Inhalation at Rest as Compared to O_2 Inhalation During Strenuous Exercise.* US Natl Res. Council, Comm. Aviat. Med. Report 134, Washington, D.C.

WILLARD, G. (1953) Ultrasonically induced cavitation in water. *J. acoust. Soc. Am.* **25**, 669–686.

WISMER, K. (1922) Supersaturated solutions of gases. *Trans. R. Soc. Canad.* **16**, 217–227.

WITTENBORN, A. F. (1963) An analytical development of a decompression computer. In Proc. 2nd Symp. Underwater Physiology. Ed. C. J. Lambertsen & L. J. Greenbaum. pp. 82–90. Washington D.C.: Natl Acad. Sci.

WORKMAN, R. D. (1965) *Calculation of Decompression Schedules for Nitrogen–oxygen and Helium–oxygen Dives.* US Navy Experimental Diving Unit Report 6–65, Washington, D.C.

21

Early Quantitative Studies of Gas Dynamics in Decompression

A. R. BEHNKE

The potential value of quantitative assessment of gas transport has long been appreciated in diving but investigations have been limited in scope and content. Decompression following conventional diving, despite the elaborate mathematical models and sophisticated analysis discussed in previous chapters, has been unsatisfactory and, on occasion, assuredly not safe for any diver. Particularly disturbing is the high incidence of decompression sickness (DCS) occurring under pressure in helium–oxygen diving. Saturation diving has been attended with less difficulty but the prolonged schedules are largely the result of trial and error.

In this section a review of some quantitative studies should serve as an introduction to a systematic program essential in future diving physiology.

INERT GAS TRANSPORT

Many of the handicaps which confronted earlier investigators such as tedious methodology in gas analysis and inability to quantify total body water and fat, which are the chief solvents of inert gases, no longer exist. Helium, for example, can be measured to one part in a million by means of the thermal conductivity cell, and nitrogen can be measured continuously during the course of breathing with the mass spectrometer. With reference to body composition, investigations during the past 25 years have yielded the in vivo content of fat, total body water, blood, potassium and other electrolytes. With knowledge of the solutes of inert gases and total amount of absorption by the body, together with utilization of radioisotopes as part of the newer spectrum of gasometry, essential problems in decompression can be resolved. Models of excellence in recent studies are reports by Groom, Morin and Farhi (1967) and Groom and Farhi (1967). Yet this type of investigation is singularly isolated and discontinuous.

A challenging problem is quantitation of the correct half-time of transport of N_2 and helium following equilibration with body tissues. There is currently a fourfold discrepancy between empirical observations and measurements (admittedly incomplete) of desaturation half-times of the slowest tissue in air (480 min compared with 80 to 150 min) and 240 min compared with 60 min in an helium–oxygen atmosphere (Bühlmann, Frey & Keller 1967). Part of the discrepancy arising from these carefully executed and systematic tests, is that the slowest tissue was subjected to an oversaturation ratio of 1·6 to 1. The decompression procedure was therefore not isobaric, and with evolution of bubbles in early stages, time of decompression may well be prolonged. The decompressions may well represent quasi-therapy.

Nitrogen uptake and elimination in the dog

During the period 1932 to 1935, Shaw et al. designed a closed system of 100 L volume to measure N_2 desaturation (or subsequent uptake following

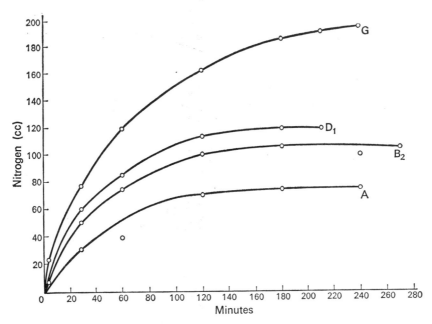

FIG. 21.1. Nitrogen recovery from four anesthetized dogs placed in a closed oxygen (99%) system for periods up to 280 min at 1 ATA. At the end of this period nitrogen elimination is not complete in dog (G) which was old and fat (after Shaw et al. 1935)

initial desaturation) in anesthetized dogs immersed in pure oxygen. Rinsing of the system and the time required for decompression from higher pressures precluded recovery of N_2 during the initial period of 7 to 8 min. The final concentration of N_2 in the system was usually not less than 98·5%. A high degree of analytical accuracy (±1 part/100,000) was obtained by reduction of large samples following absorption of oxygen, to the 0·25 ml or 0·5 ml calibration of the Van Slyke chamber. The range of variation in control tests was usually within 3 ml. Typical desaturation curves (Fig. 21.1) exhibit individual variation attributed to size, age and fatness. In lean dogs nitrogen recovery approached an endpoint after 3 to 4 hours, in contrast with elimination of nitrogen from a fat dog (G, upper curve on Fig. 21.1). These experiments served to confirm data in goat experiments concerning desaturation time and the importance of fat as a nitrogen reservoir (Boycott & Damant 1908; Boycott, Damant & Haldane 1908). By contrast, in systematic determinations of bends threshold depths for large dogs (48 to 82 lb) exposed in compressed air up to 24 hours followed

by rapid 'no-decompression' to 1 ATA, Reeves and Beckman (1966) observed that threshold depth was less following the prolonged exposures than it was up to 7 hours. Either equilibration with nitrogen in compressed air was not attained at the end of 7 hours, or prolonged exposures were conducive to bends independent of the nitrogen content of the dog, at least as measured grossly.

Other curves (Fig. 21.2) revealed noteworthy findings. Thus, during the course of cumulative nitrogen clearance (with the exception of the first 7 min) from tissues of the same dog (D) on different days at 1 and 4 ATA, there was no 'break' or departure from normal (1 ATA) in the nitrogen curves, 4 to 1 ATA. Also, the desaturation curve following partial equilibration is not the reverse of the saturation curve. Thus, following nitrogen clearance at 1 ATA (Fig. 21.2), dog D breathed air for 67 min, and then was cleared of nitrogen (curve B). Following nitrogen clearance after saturation (4-hour exposure) at 4 ATA (curve C), dog D was re-exposed to 4 ATA for 67 min. Nitrogen clearance following abrupt decompression to 1 ATA is represented by curve D.

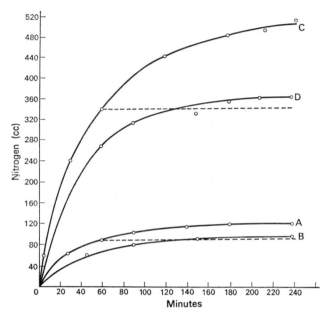

FIG. 21.2. Saturation time compared with desaturation time for anesthetized dog (D). Nitrogen eliminated during the first 7 min (lung rinsing) was not measured. Curve A: N_2 desaturation at 1 ATA; the dog then breathed air for 67 min (1 ATA) followed by N_2 recovery (curve B). Curve C: N_2 desaturation following N_2 equilibration at 4 ATA. The 'N$_2$-free' dog then breathed air at 4 ATA for 67 min; curve D represents recovery of the N_2 absorbed during the previous 67-min exposure

In an effort to change the shape of the nitrogen recovery curve, say from exponential decay to linear declivity, it was not possible to decompress from higher pressures after long exposures. Either the dog lived and the curve was 'normal' following the sharp drop from higher pressure (i.e. similar to clearance at 1 ATA in the absence of hyperbaric exposure), or the dog succumbed from fulminating gas embolization.

Analysis of the carcass of dog D yielded the following values: weight, 12·23 kg; fat, 1·89 kg; water, 7·23 kg; and dry solids, 3·12 kg. The total body N_2 and component N_2 (Table 21.1) are compared with measured and calculated N_2 during time periods 0 to 7, 8 to 20, and 21 to 180 min. The calculations derive from the equation:

$$\text{Total } N_2 \text{ at time } (t) = \text{Water } N_2(1 - e^{-kt})$$
$$+ \text{Fat } N_2(1 - e^{-kt})$$
$$= 65 \text{ ml} + 102 \text{ ml}$$

Half-time $(T_{1/2})$ fat from the experimental N_2

curve (see Fig. 21.1) is 30 min ($k = 0·023$, and 6 time units [TU] = 180 min). Subtraction of calculated fat N_2 from N_2 measured during the period 21 to 180 min (i.e. $85 - 64 = 21$ ml) represents clearance of water N_2 for this period, and by difference (total water $N_2 - 21$), 44 ml of water N_2 was eliminated from 0 to 21 min.

Measured and calculated N_2 clearances are within the range of analytical error but the N_2 recovery data and computed values from carcass analysis are widely divergent from empirical observations of the time required for N_2 equilibration which is greatly in excess of 180 min (6 TU or 98·4% desaturation).

Uptake of radioactive krypton

Regional studies—uptake in the hand. In 1941, Professor Hildebrand who pioneered the application of helium in diving, initiated a cooperative effort by the Donner Laboratory of Medical

TABLE 21.1

Measured N_2 elimination and calculated N_2 content of fluids and fat derived from carcass analysis of dog (D) following multiple tests (Figs 21.1 and 21.2)

Carcass analysis (kg)		N_2 content (ml)	$T_{1/2}$* (min)	6 TU (min)	k
Weight	12·23	—			
Fat	1·89	102	30	180	0·023
Water	7·23	65	12	72	0·058
Solids	3·11	—	—	—	—

		Nitrogen elimination		
Period (min)	Measured (ml)	Calculated (ml)		
		Water N_2	Fat N_2	Total
0–7		22	15	37
8–20	39	22	23	45
21–180	85	21	64	85

* Half-time ($T_{1/2}$) is exponential 50% saturation or desaturation (1 time unit, TU); 6 TU = 98·4% uptake or desaturation; k is the rate constant = $0·693/T_{1/2}$ where 0·693 is ln 2.

Physics and the US Navy Experimental Diving Unit to detect and follow the course of intravascular bubbles by use of radioisotopes. Impressive at that time was the air transport of radioactive krypton ($T_{1/2}$ = 36 hours) from California to Washington, D.C. and the subsequent implementation by Dr. Hardin Jones of an inhalation-scanning technique. Although the initial objective of in vivo bubble detection was not realized, it was possible nevertheless to monitor radioactive uptake and elimination of krypton not only in the body as a whole but in regional areas as the forearm and hand as well (Jones 1951). Notable in one series of tests was the accelerated uptake of krypton following release of previously occluded blood supply to the arm for a period of 10 min (Fig. 21.3). The area between curves A and B presumably reflects the relative size of the hyperaemic capillary bed. This type of response may be operative in the remarkable acclimatization associated with repeated exposures in compressed air.

This digression to a discussion of krypton kinetics is apropos of a better definition of the manner of inert gas clearance following *partial saturation* of the body. Use of a radioisotope as a tracer

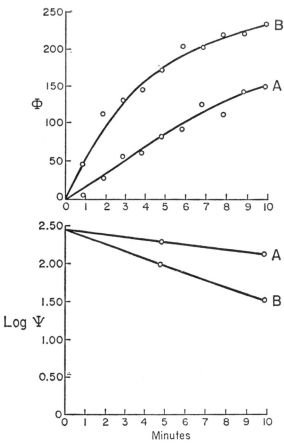

FIG. 21.3. Absorption of inhaled radioactive krypton tracer by the tissues of the shielded hand and forearm. Curve A (upper diagram) depicts absorption of gas by the resting individual. Curve B depicts the absorption of krypton following occlusion of blood supply to the arm for a period of 10 min. Inhalation of krypton began at the end of the occlusive period. Lower diagram shows a semi-logarithmic plot of the upper curves. (Based on the technique of Jones, Hamilton & Lawrence at the Experimental Diving Unit, Washington, D.C., 1942)

affords a refined technique to demonstrate transport of small amounts of gas to or from tissues.

Desaturation time following inhalation of radioactive krypton. A paramount consideration in decompression is the length of time required for complete desaturation following fractional periods of uptake of inert gas. In the studies of Tobias et al. (1949) it was found that an uptake of krypton during a 20-min period of inhalation required more than 100 min for elimination, whereas inhalation of krypton over a much longer period (117 min) required only slightly longer time (about 120 min) for krypton clearance. However, the shape of the desaturation curves is different for relatively short compared with long exposures.

Tobias et al. (1949) were able to distinguish between 'three distinctly different reservoirs' containing inert gas. The filling of these three reservoirs appeared to be somewhat independent, each characterized by a time-rate constant within a definite range. It is noteworthy that the three half-time values for the respective components are nearly identical both for short and long periods of krypton inhalation. Thus, following a 20-min period of krypton inhalation, the half-times are 6, 39 and 310 min respectively for the three components. Following an inhalation period of 117 min, half-time desaturation values are 6, 41 and 310 min for the respective components. These findings are in accordance with results of N_2 elimination from the dog, and helium recovery from man, namely that the tension of inert gas in various tissues of the body (excluding the bone marrow and perhaps the white matter of the spinal cord) tends toward perfusion–diffusion equalization at a pressure commensurate with the previous level of partial saturation. In a general way, the partial saturation level regulates volume of gas in tissues (i.e. gas content) but not time rate of tissue clearance.

'*Bends' retardation of krypton elimination at simulated altitude.* In the dog experiments it was not possible to demonstrate any change in the shape of the N_2 elimination curves following abrupt reduction of pressure from several hyperbaric levels presumably sufficient to induce gas phase separation ('silent' bubbles) in the blood stream. Reference will be made in a subsequent paragraph to less effective N_2 elimination during oxygen inhalation at simulated altitudes above 20 000 ft (0·46 ATA), compared with N_2 elimination at ground level (1 ATA) and this was cited as possible retardation of blood flow by 'silent' bubbles. Unequivocal evidence of an altered condition of the blood, and decompression sickness associated with retardation of krypton elimination (Fig. 21.4) is provided by the experiments of Tobias et al. (1949). It is observed that there was a slowing of the rate of krypton desaturation at

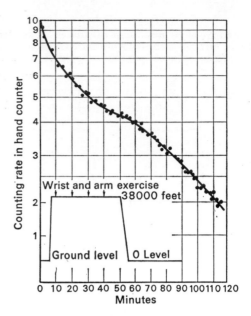

FIG. 21.4. Demonstration of retardation of krypton elimination in the hand during a 1-hour stay at a simulated altitude of 38 000 ft (0·204 ATA) associated with incapacitating bends. On recompression to ground level (1 ATA) pre-recovery rate was restored (after Tobias et al. 1949)

simulated altitude during the time when the subject had incapacitating pain in his knee, shoulder, elbow and wrist. After recompression to ground level the rate of krypton clearance returned to the pre-incapacitation level. Three out of five subjects who remained free from bends at 35 000 ft (0·24 ATA) did not show an altitude-induced change in their krypton curves. One subject, susceptible to bends on previous exposures to altitude, showed a definite slowing of krypton elimination during an altitude test in which he experienced no pain. This retardation could be attributed to the presence of 'silent' bubbles.

Partial saturation relative to diver decompressions and N_2 transport

In 1934, Kagiyama showed that divers could ascend progressively from deeper depths without decompression, provided that exposure time was shortened. Thus a dive could be made to 82 ft (3·5 ATA) for 30 min followed by rapid ascent to the surface, and likewise to a depth of 164 ft (6·0 ATA) for a stay of 15 min without subsequent decompression stops. In submarine escape tests Shilling and Hawkins (1936) compiled a remarkable series of rapid ascents in the pressurized wet chamber. A large number of simulated escapes (2140) were made with a Momsen lung using air or oxygen from depths of 100 to 200 ft (4 to 7 ATA) with a graded exposure time at each depth until bends supervened. It was found safe under these 'adaptive' conditions to remain 37 min at 100 ft, 18 min at 150 ft and 14 min at 185 ft (6·6 ATA), in no-stop ascents. Incredibly, men of the Royal Navy have made no-stop air-breathing submarine escapes in the open sea from 600 ft (19·9 ATA) with a compression time of 20 sec and decompression of 1 min.

The safe exposure time at depth followed by minimal (no-stop) decompression may be computed from the N_2 elimination curve for the body as a whole (Behnke 1937). The body appears to tolerate a constant volume of excess inert gas for a one-cycle, no-stop decompression, such that the depth times volume relationship is remarkably constant.

N_2 *transport at different pressure levels following relatively short exposures.* If P_{N_2} tends to equalize by perfusion–diffusion throughout the 'body core' during the course of partial saturation in compressed air, then subsequently, recovery of N_2

during oxygen inhalation should be independent of depth. Preliminary tests supported in part this concept. For example, the quantity of N_2 recovered following a 75-min exposure in compressed air at 100 ft (4 ATA), tended to be the same at the 20, 50, and 100 ft level (Table 21.2). On the other hand, N_2 recovery at 1 ATA following a 2-min decompression from 100 ft (4 ATA) was in two tests strikingly less than it was at higher pressure levels. Early conclusions in regard to partial saturation and N_2 equilibration, possibly naïve in oversimplification, nevertheless are correct in orientation. 'With the exception of tissues with a high fat content (fat deposits, bone marrow and spinal cord) the division of the body into tissues which saturate or desaturate at different rates is largely arbitrary, and the body can be regarded essentially as a unit' (Behnke 1937). An application of this concept in formulation of surface-depth and return decompression is illustrated in Fig. 21.5.

Analysis of nitrogen elimination in man

In man the first measurements of N_2 recovery during the course of oxygen inhalation, were reported in 1913 by Bornstein in studies of cardiac output. It was not until 1931 that Campbell and Hill, employing a modification of the Bornstein method, found that approximately 200 to 300 ml

TABLE 21.2

Nitrogen recovery from a diver exposed to a simulated depth of 100 ft for 75 min compared with nitrogen recovery following an exposure of 30 min at 100 ft. Pure oxygen was inhaled throughout the recovery period

Exposure		Stop		Tests	Nitrogen recovery ml		
(min)	(ft)	(ft)	(ATA)		3 to 30 min at stop	33 to 90 min 0 ft (1 ATA)	Total
75	100	20	1·43	1	1478	834	2312
75	100	50	2·52	2	1533	957	2590
75	100	100	4·0	2	1415	739	2154
30	100	44	2·33	1	1343	548	1891
30	100	50	2·52	1	1312	565	1877
30	100	66	3·0	1	1341	522	1863
30	100	0*	1	1	626	401	1027
30	100	0	1	1	1191	499	1690
30	100	0	1	1	892	856	1748
30	100	0	1	1	1147	511	1658

* 2 min decompression from 100 to 0 ft in the 4 tests.
Data from Willmon and Behnke (1941).

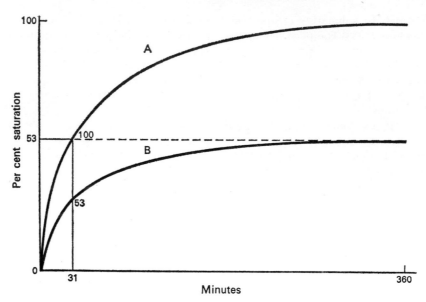

FIG. 21.5. After a dive of 31 min at 100 ft (4 ATA), the body as a whole of
this lean diver is 53% saturated as shown on curve A. Equivalent depth is
53 ft and gauge pressure can be reduced to this level. Curve B represents the
probable course of N_2 elimination if oxygen were inhaled at the 40 ft level
(Behnke 1937)

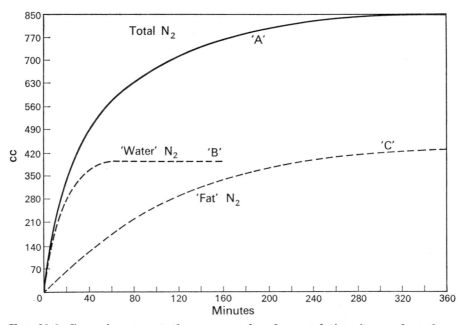

FIG. 21.6. Curve A represents the average values for cumulative nitrogen from three
lean men (average weight 64 kg) who breathed oxygen at atmospheric pressure in a
helmet system. 'Water' N_2 (B) and 'fat' N_2 (C) are exponential curves with half-
times of 7 and 82 min respectively. Nitrogen recovered during the first 5 min (rinsing period) would add a third (faster) half-time component, while progressive fat
loading would add a fourth or possibly a fifth half-time component (Behnke 1937)

of nitrogen, about 25 to 33% of the estimated total content in a lean man, were eliminated during the first 9 min of oxygen breathing. Subsequent experiments have confirmed and extended these findings in some degree (Shaw et al. 1935; Behnke et al. 1935; Willmon & Behnke 1941; Stevens et al. 1947; Jones 1950; Boothby, Luft & Benson 1951; Kety 1951; Lundin 1953, 1960).

The amount of N_2 recovered per minute diminishes during the course of oxygen inhalation from an initial calculated 50 ml/min ($P_{N_2} = 573$ mm Hg) to less than 0·1 ml/min from lean men at the end of 9 hours. At this time diffusion of N_2 through the skin (body, except head surrounded by air) accounts for the greater part of the N_2 recovered; the remainder diffuses into the closed system through the spirometer water seal and other gas-permeable components. The curve depicting cumulative N_2 recovery (Fig. 21.6) was dichotomized, as outlined previously for the dog, into the exponential components comprising the chief body solutes for N_2 in a 64-kg 'composite' diver.

Total N_2 (6 hours)	= Water N_2 +	Fat N_2
850 ml (6 hours)	= 392	458
Exponential rate		
constant (k)	= 0·098	0·0085
Half-time ($T_{1/2}$) in min =	7	82
% desaturation		
(6 hours)	= complete	$\approx$ 95

Assessment of body fat and water was not possible at the time; N_2 in the initial period of 6 min was calculated, and the desaturation time of fat (95% in 6 hours) could not be firmly established.

Logarithmic analysis of a similar curve without reference to water and fat solvents, yielded three components:

Total N_2 (at time, t)

$$= 172\,e^{-0·13t} + 353\,e^{-0·028t} + 255\,e^{-0·0079t}$$

The extensive measurements of Jones (1950), over usually not more than several hours, were resolved in one extended experiment into five components referrable to tissues with different rates of blood flow. However, diffusion plays an important role (Hills 1966). Haber (1951) stated that it is hazardous to infer that the exponential components derived from an accurate fit of data are representative of such entities as blood, muscle and fat. He added, 'Furthermore an exponential equation is so flexible that a variable number of constants can be found to fit the data without being representative of the actual physical mechanisms involved.' Haber pointed out the value of recording minute-to-minute quantities of exhaled N_2 as a prerequisite in the calculation of the rate constants. This objective has been realized in part by radioisotopic analysis of Jones (1950), and advanced by Lundin (1960) as a result of development of a highly sensitive N_2 meter.

Lundin's N_2 elimination measurements

In his 1953 paper, Lundin reported cumulative measurements of N_2 from subjects who breathed oxygen in a closed system. He characterized N_2 clearance as a three-stage exponential process:

1. A rapid phase with an elimination half-time of about 1·5 min.
2. A slower phase with a half-time of 12 to 13 min.
3. A slow phase with a half-time of about 100 to 200 min.

From the analysis of Jones (1950) it is reasonable that the first phase corresponds to the N_2 from highly vascular tissue such as liver, brain, heart, intestines, and other organ systems, the middle phase mainly from muscle (and skin), and the slowest from fat. In Lundin's 1960 paper, N_2 elimination was assessed, not in a closed system by cumulative increments, but by an original technique of measurement of end-tidal volume concentrations of N_2 by the sensitive meter previously mentioned. This technique, although not productive of absolute amounts of N_2 eliminated, satisfies Haber's criterion for accurate measurement of rate of N_2 elimination by multiple recordings at short intervals.

In the recording of data, N_2-metered readings in arbitrary units (every 60 sec for the first 20 min, then every 5 min) were plotted on a logarithmic scale against time. N_2 clearance was not measured during the first 6 to 8 min (lung rinsing period during normal breathing) and experiments were terminated at the end of 4 hours (Fig. 21.7). It is this type of technique and newer knowledge of body composition which should provide a firm basis for future studies of gas transport. In the meantime it seems worthwhile to recast earlier work into a newer mold.

Lundin's analysis of N_2 elimination

The exponential N_2 decay curve (Fig. 21.7) can be resolved into two linear components, one relatively rapid (interpreted as N_2 elimination from muscles, chiefly), the other, a slow component indicative of N_2 clearance from fat (Table 21.3). The arbitrary units referrable to N_2 recovered can

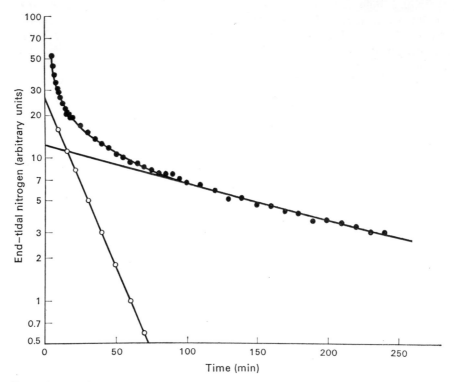

FIG. 21.7. Nitrogen elimination curve, semi-log scale. The end-tidal N_2 (ordinate) is recorded in arbitrary units. (Reproduced from Lundin 1960 by permission of the Editor, *Journal of Physiology, London*)

TABLE 21.3

Semi-logarithmic N_2 clearance from 'muscle' (II) and 'fat' (III) components of the body and the respective k constants during the course of 4-hour end-tidal volume measurements of metered N_2

Subject	Age (years)	Weight (kg)	Height (cm)	'Muscle'*			'Fat'*		
				k	$T_{1/2}$ (min)	N_2	k	$T_{1/2}$ (min)	N_2
1	33	79	182	0·055	12·6	500	0·0059	117	2050
2	28	59	165	0·061	11·4	460	0·0048	144	2670
3	45	80	183	0·051	13·6	588	0·0047	147	2870
4	16	60	163	0·050	13·9	234	0·0051	136	1570
5	16	53	163	0·046	15·1	520	0·0079	88	900
6	22	60	176	0·051	13·6	490	0·0059	117	1290

* N_2 elimination is expressed in arbitrary units relative to the readings of the nitrogen meter. Data from Lundin (1960).

be converted into absolute values derived from indirect estimates of muscle (M) and fat (F) as projected by Lundin.

If body weight $(W) - F \times 0.50 = M$ (1)

and if $FN_2 = 6MN_2,$ $\text{Fat} = \dfrac{N_2 F}{6 N_2 M} \times M$ (2)

Substituting arbitrary units from Table 21.2 in (2), then it follows for Subject 1 that $F = 0.684\,M$ and from (1), that $\text{Fat} = 0.684\,(W - F) \times 0.50 = 20.1$ kg. For Subject 2, $\text{Fat} = 19.2$ kg, and for Subject 3, 23·2 kg.

The correctness of these estimates of body fat derived from logarithmic linear conversions of N_2 clearance data, was confirmed by densitometry (underwater weighing) where densitometric fat was determined as 20·8, 18·7, and 22·8 kg for Subjects 1, 2, and 3 respectively. In order to complete Lundin's novel analysis by addition to categories II and III (Table 21.3), the initial most rapidly desaturating tissues (i.e. in missing category I), it is necessary to outline a practical method for valid assessment of body fat.

QUANTITATIVE APPRAISAL OF BODY FAT RELATIVE TO N_2 TRANSPORT

Reference data

In 1939, following rescue and salvage operations in connection with the USS *Squalus* disaster (Behnke & Willmon 1939), there was renewed interest in a practical method to assess fat in US Navy divers who were then engaged in test dives to 500 ft (15·2 ATA). Since volume displacement of a submarine and buoyancy were matters of daily discussion, serendipity led to the determination of body volume in diving tanks (Fig. 21.8) and the Archimedean parameter of density as a 'third dimension' of the body in addition to weight and stature (Behnke, Feen & Welham 1942). This elementary procedure in discriminate hands has become standard for accurate assessment of body fat (Behnke & Wilmore 1974). If immersion water temperature is 31 to 32°C, then

$$\% \text{ Body fat} = \frac{1.000 - \text{sp. gr. (body)}}{0.002}$$

or, in densitometric units:

$$\% \text{ Body fat} = \frac{495.0}{\text{d (body)}} - 450.0$$

This is Siri's equation (Siri 1961).

Hundreds of densitometric determinations on young adult males define gross composition of a *reference man* in terms of fat, and with normal hydration, total body water. In the reference man (Table 21.4), fat in adipose tissue is 8 kg, lean body weight is body weight less adipose tissue fat. Fat-free weight is lean body weight less 'essential' fat in lipid-rich tissue as bone marrow and the nervous system. An estimate of 'essential' fat is 2 kg (3% lean body weight), not large, but an entity which merits careful scrutiny in pathology of bone and spinal cord. Total body water is 72%

TABLE 21.4

Gross body composition data of a *reference man* in relation to the inert gas content of body fluid and fat solvents

Reference man

Age, 20 to 24 years; weight, 70 kg; stature, 174 cm	
Fat in adipose tissue (AT)	8 kg
Lean body weight (LBW)	62 kg
'Essential' organ, marrow fat	2 kg
Fat-free weight	60 kg
Total body water (TBW), 72% LBW	44·6 kg

Solubility data (P_{N_2}, $P_{He} = 570$ mm Hg; 37°C)

N_2 in tissue fluids	9 ml/kg
N_2 in fat	54 ml/kg
He in tissue fluids	5·9 ml/kg
He in fat	12·2 ml/kg

Variation of parameters*

	-2σ	-1σ	M	$+1\sigma$	$+2\sigma$
LBW (kg)	47·2	54·6	62	68·4	75·8
TBW (kg)	29·3	39·3	44·6	49·2	54·6
Fluid N_2 (ml)	264	354	401	443	491
Fluid He (ml)	172	230	261	288	319

AT fat (kg)	Very lean	Ref. man	+	+ +	+ + +
	4	8	12	16	20
N_2 content (ml)	216	432	648	864	1080
He content (ml)	48	97	145	194	242

* Calculated from representative coefficients of variation of lean and total body weights of 12% (range 10 to 14%).

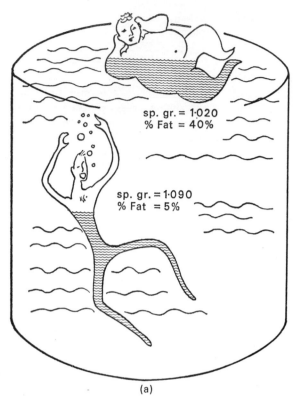

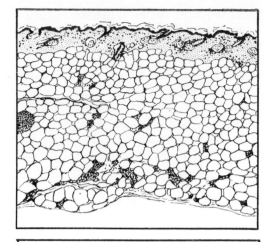

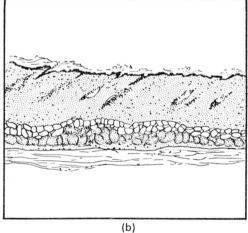

Fig. 21.8 (a) The technique of underwater weighing referrable in principle to Archimedes provides an accurate assessment of body fat which is inversely proportional to net body fat sp. gr. (water temp. 31 to 32°C)

Fig. 21.8 (b) The panniculus adiposus of fat in lean mice is analogous to the variation in fat content of the diver's tela subcutanea (after Hausberger 1957)

(range 68 to 76%) of lean body weight, and in the animal carcass, 73% of fat-free weight.

The following solubility values, derived from Bunsen coefficients (37 to 38°C) are not rigidly established but suffice for this analysis.

	Water	Oil
N_2	0·013	0·065
He	0·0085	0·015
He/N_2	64·5%	23·1%

Gas solubility in tissue fluid (water) requires a correction for dissolved solutes. With reference to N_2 (solubility 0·975 vol %, P_N = 570 mm Hg) the correction derived from urine analysis (to be discussed subsequently) is,

$$0·975 - \frac{\text{sp. gr. (fluids)} - 1·0}{0·2} = 0·90$$

(sp. gr. [fluids] 1·015)

Updating this type of analysis is the authoritative investigation of Klocke and Rahn (1961).

In Table 21.4, fat has been converted to kg by multiplying volume by 0·90 (d fat 0·90) to obtain a rounded value of 6 as the ratio in Lundin's analysis of fat to fluid nitrogen. The Gausserian distribution of lean body weight and total body weight relates to a coefficient of variation of 12% (range 10 to 14%), and includes about 95% of mean values of lean body weight and total body weight for young adult males whose stature (h) is 174 cm, and for different statures, mean lean body weight = 0·204 h^2 (h in decimeters). The range of values for adipose tissue fat are projected as 4 kg (very lean), 8 kg (reference diver), and 4(+), 8(++), and 12(+++) of excess fatness.

Effect of increased fatness on N_2 transport

If 12 kg of fat accumulate during the course of hypertrophy of adipose tissue (i.e. without hyperplasia or additional blood supply), weight (reference man) is increased from 70 to 82 kg and total body fat from 11·4 to 24·4%. The following range of estimates pertain to the time course of N_2 desaturation of the *excess* plus reference fat (12+8 kg) compared with reference fat (which includes, in category III, 'essential' fat and water).

	N_2 content	k	$T_{1/2}$ (min)	Cumulative N_2 (ml)				
				6	30	60	90	6 TU*
min								
Reference fat	542	0·0082	85	26	118	210	282	533
(1) + 12 kg	1190	0·0048	143	35	159	300	421	1171
(2) + 12 kg	1190	0·0037	187	26	138	238	339	1171

* 6 TU (reference fat) 510 min, excess fat (1) 864 min, excess fat (2) 1122 min.

The tabular values pertaining to (1) approximate Lundin's half-times for the slowest tissue in his moderately fat subjects, and were calculated from the ratio,

$$\frac{(1190)^{2/3}}{(542)^{2/3}} \times 85 \text{ min}$$

where 542 ml is the N_2 content of category III (reference man) and 85 min is half-time. The values (2) are calculated as an increase in half-time proportional to N_2 content of fat (reference man). The challenging aspect of N_2 measurements of young men of variable fatness (assessed by underwater weighing) is the insight afforded into the relative role of diffusion compared with perfusion. Impressive in earlier but incomplete studies was the unusually large amount of N_2 recovered in the first 2 hours which was well in excess of the quantity calculated for perfusion-limited adipose tissue. Measurements currently should be carried out, preferably over a period of 24 hours, starting at 1 ATA and continuing the N_2 recovery in an altitude chamber at 0·25 ATA. In such tests it is necessary to circumvent diffusion of N_2 through the skin.

In Table 21·5, three tissue categories are projected for the reference man and the amounts of water and fat in each category are derived from reliable source data. The blood supply in the resting state (not given in Table 21.5) is about 4 L for category I, 1·2 L for category II, and 0·5 L for category III. It is apparent that the disparity between the distribution of blood flow and tissue mass in category III severely impairs the transport of lipophilic gases such as nitrogen.

The k values and half-times $T_{1/2}$ for category II are from Lundin's data; for category III, from earlier measurements of N_2 elimination in lean men (Behnke 1937); and for category I, from an estimate of N_2 clearance from highly vascularized tissue. If the lungs are rinsed free of N_2 within 45 sec, N_2 from category I can be quantified.

Application of 3-component analysis to Lundin's data

The partition of N_2 dissolved in fluid and fat into three categories has been applied to four of Lundin's subjects (Table 21.6). Total body water referrable to tissue content is allocated to I (27%), II (62%) and III (11%) categories. Essential fat (in organs) approximated as 1% of lean body weight is in category I, and bone marrow fat (2% lean body weight) is in category III which also harbours all of the adipose tissue fat. The N_2 clearance half-times are 5 min (I) and 14 min (II) since the range of variation appears to be narrow for these largely aqueous categories. In III, the half-times are those derived from logarithmic analysis.

The principles underlying this analysis are applicable to techniques of N_2 measurement in which appreciable time (5 to 7 min) elapses for clearance of lung nitrogen, and in which estimates of body fat and the rate constants are derived from logarithmic analysis. Densitometric quantification of body fat provides a check on the logarithmic derivation as well as an accurate estimate of total

TABLE 21.5

Nitrogen solvents, content, and transport in three categories of tissues referrable to a young, lean, adult male

Entity	Reference man	Tissue category			
		I Organs Viscera	II Muscle Skin Spinal cord Nerves	III Bone*	Adipose tissue
Weight (kg)	70				
Fluids (kg)	44·6	12	27·6	3	2
(%)	72	27	62	11	
Fat:					
Essential (kg)	2·0	0·4	0·4	1·2	—
Adipose tissue (kg)	8·0	—	—	—	8·0
Nitrogen (ml)					
Fluids	401	108	248	27	18
Fat:					
Essential	109	22	22	65	—
Adipose tissue	432	—	—	—	432
Total N$_2$	942	130	270	542	

Cumulative N$_2$ transport (ml)		Category		
		I	II	III
Time period (min)	Total			
6	169	73	70	26
30	454	128	208	118
60	597	130	257	210
90	679	130	267	282
510 (6 TU)	933	130	270	533
$T_{1/2}$ (min)		5	14	85
k		0·14	0·05	0·0082

* N$_2$ clearance of bone marrow not known; tentatively projected to have a half-time of 85 min.

TABLE 21.6

Partition of body N$_2$ into aqueous and lipid solvents and assignment of the aliquots to tissue categories I, II and III for four subjects in Table 21.3

Subject	Lean body weight (kg)	Fat*			Total body water (kg)	Category N$_2$† (ml)					Category $T_{1/2}$ (min)		
		Adipose tissue	Essential O	B		I		II	III		I	II	III
						w	f	w	w	f			
1	58·2	20·8	0·58	1·16	41·9	102	31	234	42	1186	5	14	117
2	40·3	18·7	0·40	0·81	29·0	70	22	162	29	1054	5	14	144
3	57·2	22·8	0·57	1·14	41·2	100	31	230	41	1293	5	14	147
4	46·4	6·7	0·46	0·93	33·4	81	25	187	33	412	5	14	88

* Adipose tissue lipid and 'essential' organ (O) and marrow (B) fat.
† Category N$_2$ allocated to aqueous (w) and lipid (f) solvents.

N_2 content and subsequent allocation to fluid and fat. Determination only of end-tidal N_2 at small intervals greatly simplifies the technique and should provide the missing data pertaining to prolonged N_2 recovery.

CUTANEOUS DIFFUSION OF INERT GASES

Until the last decade practically no attention was focused on a factor which during the course of prolonged decompression from saturation dives may play an appreciable role. Earlier tests in man indicated that about 10% of the body's store of helium diffused through the skin per hour when oxygen was inhaled and the body immersed in helium. The technique employed at the time permitted measurement of inward (skin to lungs) or outward (lungs to skin) transport of helium. The data in Table 21.7 show a three- to four-fold increase in transport of helium at elevated ambient temperature (Fig. 21.9).

With regard to N_2, cutaneous diffusion through the dog's tissues will replace the entire N_2 store every 24 hours (Groom & Farhi 1967). In a representative test the half-time of the slowest wash-out compartment of the dog surrounded by air was 332 min in contrast to 117 min with the dog immersed in oxygen. Open skin incisions greatly augment the diffusion of helium into tissues. During the course of N_2 clearance tests conducted at the Harvard School of Public Health (1932 to 1935), oxygen was inhaled by the anesthetized dog through a tracheal cannula. Not more than 4 hours (in later experiments) were required to reduce N_2 recovery from the lungs to 3 ml/hour. However, in earlier tests, about 10 ml of N_2 per hour were recovered in the reservoir spirometer for periods of at least 14 hours (Fig. 2.10). 'What appeared to be spontaneous generation of N_2 in the dog's body was found to be diffusion of N_2 from air into tissues through two incisions, one made for the tracheal cannula, and the other over

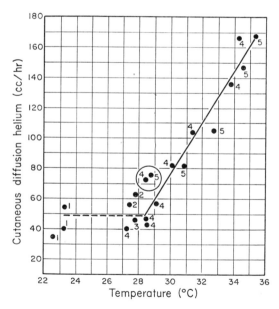

FIG. 21.9. Cutaneous diffusion of helium in relation to temperature, measured as ml (cc/hr) of helium recovered from the lungs per hour when the body (head out) is immersed in helium ($P_{He} = 700$ mm Hg). Numbers 1 to 5 refer to different subjects. The encircled values were obtained after the previously heated ambient helium had been cooled to 29°C (from Behnke & Willmon 1941)

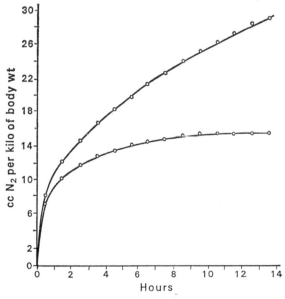

FIG. 21.10. The upper curve represents the elimination of N_2 via the lungs of anesthetized dogs with open incisions over the trachea and femoral artery of one leg. The lower curve represents the elimination of N_2 under the same conditions with the exception that the incisions were closed by suture. The area between the curves reflects the quantity of N_2 diffusing from ambient air into the dog's tissues through the incisions (data from Behnke & Shaw 1934)

TABLE 21.7

Cutaneous diffusion of helium in relation to skin temperature

Subject	Body in helium*		Body in air†	
	Skin T (°C)	Helium‡	Skin T (°C)	Helium‡
1	37·7	104	37·2	61
2	37·8	57	36·9	54
3	38·2	107	36·9	109
4	37·2	93	37·1	100
Average		90		81
1	35·0	23		
2	34·6	16		
3	34·2	20		
4	33·8	27		
Average		21·5		

* Body in a gas-tight bag (head out connected to spirometer system).
† Body in a gas-tight bag (subject breathed an helium–oxygen mixture).
‡ ml of He/m²/hour, computed for $P_{He} = 760$ mm Hg. When body was in helium, helium was recovered from the lungs; when the body was in air, helium was recovered from the bag system.

the femoral artery to record blood pressure. Closure of the incisions rendered N_2 elimination complete in the expected 4 to 5 hours and concluded the attempt to measure the N_2 of the atmosphere through the tissues of the dog.'

In a human test, N_2 clearance from tissues of a 70-kg diver was reduced to a level of 47 ml/hour which represented N_2 diffusion into the spirometer system and through the skin immersed in air. The replacement of air by oxygen around the body skin surface brought about a reduction of inward diffusion from 47 to 24 ml/hour (Behnke & Willmon 1941).

a factor of three or more (diffusion and perfusion are complementary in this phenomenon). Diffusivity of helium in oil is 3 times greater than that of N_2, and more than 2·5 times greater in water. These values are well in excess of the general relationship postulated for diffusion of gases in tissue, namely,

$$\frac{\dot{V}_{He}}{\dot{V}_N} = \frac{soln./\sqrt{mol.\ wt.}}{soln./\sqrt{mol.\ wt.}} = 1·73$$

Systematic investigation of cutaneous gas diffusion merits prosecution for several reasons. The perceptive and in-depth demonstration that

Nitrogen recovery from the lungs relative to ambient gas

Subject 1	Air				Oxygen				Air
Hours of test	7·5	8·5	9·5		11	12	13	14	15
N_2 recovery (ml)	53	52	47		46	33	34	24	48

Subject 2	Oxygen					Air	
Hours of test	9·5	11	12	13	14	15	16
N_2 recovery (ml)	55	49	47	46	41	60	67

These preliminary tests were terminated by military exigency but it appeared that in contrast with diffusion of helium, the quantity of N_2 diffusing percutaneously into the circulation was less by

bubble formation can occur in tissues by 'counter-diffusion' at fixed ambient pressure (Graves et al. 1975) serves to explain the intense itching and skin rash which supervened when a switch was made to air at hyperbaric pressure and the body surface was immersed in helium. The practice of substitution of air for helium–oxygen mixture during decompression was routine at the Experimental Diving Unit during the 1938–1941 test period. Pruritus, macular skin lesions and delayed onset of 'diver's fatigue' were attributed to bubbles in subcutaneous vessels as a result of abridged decompression, and notably following chilling of the skin. Hypothermic circulatory stasis served to explain the adverse phenomena. Since the changeover from inhalation of helium–oxygen to air was gradual, it is not likely that the counter-diffusion phenomenon compounded the decompression problem. On the other hand, the importance of the phenomenon during decompression diving has been demonstrated under certain conditions.

Investigation of cutaneous diffusion is essential in assessment of the feasibility of head-out immersion in water to eliminate inward diffusion through the skin during decompression in helium atmospheres as well as for body temperature control. Immersion to the neck in water not only serves to circumvent inward percutaneous diffusion of helium and to regulate body temperature, but also to enhance inert gas transport (Balldin & Lundgren 1972). The final consideration is that the challenging problems outlined are amenable to ready solution by current refinements in gas analysis, in temperature control, in measurements of blood flow and tissue diffusion, and by fabrication of 'lung-body' collection systems impervious to gas diffusion and accurately calibrated as to volume.

INERT GAS CONTENT OF URINE

Leonard Hill (1912) analysed urine of divers to ascertain N_2 equilibration time with kidney tissue. Behnke and Yarbrough (1938–39) and subsequently, Van Der Aue, Brinton and Kellar (1945) analysed inert gas content of urine before and following dives in wet and dry chambers. The objective was to provide a simple and practical test presumptive of gas held in supersaturation or in bubbles circulating in blood. In recent years procedures directed to analyses of inert gas content of urine and blood, relative to alveolar concentrations of P_{N_2} have been refined in elegant tests of

Klocke and Rahn (1961) and Farhi, Edwards and Homma (1963). The earlier unpublished studies did not lead to an unequivocal prognosis of dysbarism but the techniques with subsequent refinement appear to have wide application in current decompression procedure.

Underlying methodology is a comparison of urinary P_{N_2} (without loss of inert gas) with that of an aliquot of urine equilibrated with room air at 38°C. A condition of equilibrium through the media of arterial blood and kidneys is presumed to exist between gas tension in urine, lungs, venous blood and tissues at constant barometric pressure. There is temporary disequilibria when a diver is compressed or decompressed; re-establishment of gaseous equilibrium between P_{N_2} in urine and alveolar air presumably will be delayed by phase separation of gas in circulating blood.

In initial procedures, urine from divers who breathed a helium–oxygen mixture under pressure, and subsequently air during decompression, was collected before a dive (control sample), immediately after surfacing, and then at hourly intervals until normal gaseous equilibria prevailed. Large samples of urine were analysed by extraction of gases in the Van Slyke chamber and after chemical absorption of oxygen and carbon dioxide the inert residual was assessed for nitrogen, and helium, if present.

Analytical data

In 76 analyses, the N_2 content of bladder urine ($P_{N_2} = 570$ mm Hg) averaged 0·015 vol. % higher than the gas content of urine equilibrated at 38°C by bubbling air slowly through the sample ($P_{N_2} = 563$ mm Hg). The greatest difference was 0·039 vol. %; in eight analyses urine N_2 was slightly lower (from 0·006 to 0·016 vol. %) than that of the equilibrated sample.

Inert gas content of equilibrated samples of urine was inversely proportional to specific gravity (i.e., 'salt' lowering effect on solubility) and a correction was made previously applied to N_2 solubility in body fluids.

N_2 content of urine (570 mm Hg, 38°C) in vol. % corrected for sp. gr. is:

$$0·975 - \frac{\text{sp. gr. urine} - 1·0}{0·2}$$

TABLE 21.8

Results of analysis of inert gas (I) and carbon dioxide (free and combined) in the urine of an 'alkalinized' and an 'acidified' diver in dry chamber tests to 100 ft 4·03 ATA)*

Time	Sample	Urine‡ (ml)	Sp. gr.	Sample (I) (vol.%)	Equilibrated (vol.%)	Excess (vol.%)§	CO_2 (vol.%)
Diver 'alkalinized'†							
0800	control	405	1·022	0·901	0·862	0·039	57·5
0850	surface	30	1·023	1·865	(0·860)¶	1·005	110·0
0950	1 hour	50	1·025	1·251	(0·850)	0·401	104·0
1050	2 hour	80	1·016	0·971	0·893	0·078	105·0
1150	3 hour	180	1·006	0·979	0·960	0·019	94·4
Diver 'acidified'							
0715	control	75	1·019	0·916	0·914	0·002	4·1
0850	surface	130	1·015	1·810	(0·90)	0·910	6·0
0950	1 hour	165	1·016	1·220	(0·895)	0·325	2·8
1050	2 hour	80	1·014	0·996	0·916	0·080	3·5
1150	3 hour	245	1·005	0·986	0·952	0·034	3·8

* 2 min compression, 28 min on bottom, 2 min decompression.
† 'Alkalinized', a total of 60 g $NaHCO_3$ in divided doses preceding day and morning of dive; 'acidified' with ammonium mandelate on day preceding and morning of dive.
‡ Fluid intake: 250 ml water at 0800, 0900, 1000, and 1100.
§ Sample (I)—equilibrated aliquot with air at 1 ATA = Excess inert.
¶ In parentheses: calculated vol. % from sp. gr. (see text).

TABLE 21.9

Inert (I) gas content of urine in relation to forced fluid intake during the period of air compression in a dry chamber at 2 ATA, and during the post-decompression period

Time period (min)	Fluid intake	Urine voided (ml)	sp. gr.	Vol. % inert
Pre-compression	—	55	1·022	0·865
Compression				
30	250	275	1·016	1·471
60	250	275	1·005	1·917
90	250	605	1·001	1·965
120	250	600	1·001	1·972
150	250	365	1·001	—
180	—	460	1·001	1·948
	1250	2580		
Post-decompression				
30	250	260	1·003	1·550
70	250	75	1·011	1·052
90	250	175	1·003	1·005
120	250	370	1·004	0·997
150	250	100	1·006	0·968
180	250	275	1·001	0·979
210	—	125	1·001	0·968
	1500	1380		

Thus for every 0·002 'units' of sp. gr., N_2 solubility is lowered by 0·001 vol. %. Pertinent is the finding that no substances, except ethanol, will give false positive values of inert gas content of urine. Van Der Aue, Brinton & Keller (1945) found in analysis of urine of divers with 'hangovers' that ethanol vapour rendered invalid assessment of inert gas. On the other hand, such measures as high degree of acidification or alkalinization of divers failed to influence residual urinary gas content (Table 21.8).

The N_2 content of urine was determined relative to time periods following compression to 15 psi gauge (2 ATA) and subsequently after rapid decompression to normal pressure (Table 21.9).

Approximately 90 min were required both after compression and decompression to attain N_2 equilibrium in voided and equilibrated samples. During the compression period in this particular test, the quantity of urine excreted was strikingly in excess of the forced fluid intake.

In the initial tests (not confirmed by Van Der Aue, Brinton & Kellar 1945) the elevated N_2 content of urine voided during the second hour post dive, appeared to have prognostic import as to bends occurrence. Although higher N_2 values compared with equilibrated samples were frequently associated with subsequent onset of bends (Table 21.10), inhalation of oxygen during the decompression period tended to clear the

TABLE 21.10

Excess inert gas in urine in the second hour sample following long exposures in compressed air. Group A was decompressed in two min; Group B received extended air decompression; and Group C was given relatively short oxygen decompression at the 60 ft (2·82 ATA) level

Divers	Depth (ft)	Duration (hrs)	Excess N_2* 2-hour sample (vol. %)	Decompression sickness
Group A				
1	38	12	0·127	yes
2	38	12	0·124	yes
3	38	24	0·143	yes
4	38	9	0·061	yes
5	38	9	0·039	yes
6	30	12	0·047	no
7	30	12·5	0·010	no
8	30	12	− 0·006	no
9	30	18	0·047	no
Group B				
1	60	6	0·020	no
2	90	6	0·038	no
3	90	6	0·005	no
4	90	6	0·022	yes (12-hour delay)
5	90	9	0·047	yes
Group C†				
1	60	6	0·000	no
2	60	12	0·012	yes
3	60	12	0·005	yes
4	60	12	0·002	yes
5	60	12	0·015	yes

* N_2 in 2-hour sample less N_2 in sample equilibrated with room air.
† Oxygen decompression at 60 ft level, then 5 min to 1 ATA followed by air inhalation 2 hours.

urine of N_2 and (although air was breathed at normal pressure for a 2-hour period) to mask any prognostic implications.

Rapid diffusion of helium

In one diver unusually resistant to bends, high values of urinary inert gas persisted through the second and third hours post dive. Helium was detected in these samples as well as in venous blood. This is the only instance in numerous helium–oxygen dives featured by air decompression in which helium could be detected in the 2-hour urine sample. Helium was usually present however, in the immediate post-dive (surface) sample.

During decompression when air was inhaled in place of the helium–oxygen mixture, there was reason to believe that helium diffused out of the bladder urine, notably if the bladder were distended. In a test designed to quantify helium loss from retained bladder urine, it was found that over a period of 3 hours, 1·63 vol. % helium dissolved in isotonic saline and introduced into the bladder, was reduced to 0·07 vol. %. Making allowance for dilution of helium by urine secreted into the bladder during the 3-hour period, it was computed that nine-tenths of the helium initially present had diffused through the bladder wall.

Abnormal urinary secretion during deeper helium dives

As much as a liter of urine was secreted during the course of wet tank helium dives (350 to 400 ft, 11·6 to 13·1 ATA) of 20 min bottom time followed by 220 min decompression. In 12 dives to 300 ft (10 ATA) of 20 min duration followed by 86 min decompression, the following urinary volumes were recorded.

Surface	1 hour	2 hours
610	114	182

The surface sample had been retained during the dive and decompression for 106 min; the average per hour during this period was 345 ml. Prior to the 1- and 2-hour samples, 250 ml of fluid was ingested.

Urinary volumes and inert gas content are recorded for a 500 ft (16·2 ATA) wet chamber dive (Table 21.11). Diver was in helmet and conventional diving dress, tightly laced around the lower extremities with snugly fitting lead belt around the waist. On bottom he breathed 85% helium, 15% oxygen for 12 min; during decompression there was a switch to air at 210 ft (7·4 ATA). The diuresis has a substantial explanation in the hydrostatic pressure gradient acting on the tightly laced lower extremities and body trunk distal to the weighted belt. The effect of this gradient is engorgement of intrathoracic circulation comparable to that in head-out immersion in water extensively investigated in connection with space flight. This redistribution of blood volume is similar to that of continuous negative pressure breathing. As in any procedure which causes engorgement of intrathoracic circulation, diuresis follows. The phenomenon has been interpreted as

TABLE 21.11

Volumes of urine excreted and inert (I) gas content prior to and following a 500 ft (16·2 ATA) wet chamber dive of 12 min bottom time followed by air decompression from 210 ft (7·36 ATA)

Time	Sample	Urine* (ml)	Sp. gr.	Sample (I) (vol. %)	Equilibrated (vol. %)	Excess† (vol. %)	CO_2‡ (vol. %)
0820	Control	40	1·019	0·890	0·898	− 0·008	4·2
1310	Surface	1040	1·005	1·643	0·967	0·686	23·4
1410	1 hour	100	1·013	1·259	0·927	0·332	10·0
1510	2 hour	45	1·019	0·998	0·897	0·101	4·2
1600	3 hour	30	—	0·908	0·883	0·025	—

    * Fluids: 500 ml night prior to dive, 375 ml morning of dive, and 375 ml immediately following dive, then 250 ml each hour thereafter.
    † Excess inert gas = Sample (I) less equilibrated aliquot with air (1 ATA).
    ‡ Free (dissolved) and combined CO_2 liberated from urinary base.

an expression of volume regulation by stimulation of receptors in the intrathoracic circulation (Gauer, Henry & Behn 1970). Hormonal changes as well as suppression of plasma renin activity and aldosterone excretion are observed in water-to-the-neck immersion (Epstein, Duncan & Fishman 1972).

In 1945, at the instigation of Captain Van Der Aue, Dr. Gregory Pincus reported surprisingly low values of ketosteroids in urine from divers engaged in saturation dives at times which were attended by a high incidence of decompression sickness. The need for follow-up of these incomplete studies is apparent.

EMPIRICAL CONCEPTS RELEVANT TO CURRENT DECOMPRESSION PRACTICE

Asymptomatic ('silent') bubbles

The Doppler ultrasonic technique (Mackay & Rubissow 1971; Spencer, Johanson & Campbell 1975) in support of previous observations and sur-

mise, detects bubbles in the circulation which do not give rise to decompression sickness. In altitude chamber tests at the Experimental Diving Unit (1939 to 1940) oxygen inhalation above 20 000 ft (0·46 ATA) afforded less protection against dysbarism than pre-oxygenation at 1 ATA. A debilitating fatigue, often delayed until return to ground level, frequently supervened during several hours' exposure at 20 000 to 25 000 ft (0·46 to 0·37 ATA) in the absence of pre-oxygenation at normal pressure (1 ATA). This altitude 'gray' zone was designated as one productive of 'silent' bubbles (Behnke 1942). The concept may be considered with reference to events depicted in Fig. 21.11 which shows that out of 39 divers in an older age group, only one was able to remain at 38 500 ft (0·2 ATA) for 4 hours in the absence of pre-oxygenation (1 ATA). It is inferred that those divers who developed decompression sickness after varying intervals at altitude, had circulating bubbles prior to onset of symptoms. All of the divers, except one who had 4 hours of pre-oxygenation (1 ATA), were able to remain symptom-free at altitude for at least 4 hours, and several subjects

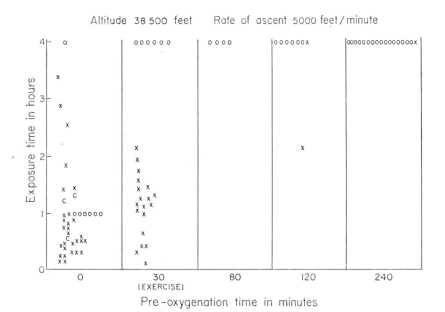

FIG. 21.11. The relationship between pre-oxygenation time (1 ATA) and duration of stay at simulated altitude of 38 500 ft (0·2 ATA) for periods up to 4 hours. Incidence of bends (X) of chokes (c) and of tolerance (O) relate closely to degree of N_2 clearance prior to ascent. One diver with an old injury (leg) was susceptible to bends despite 4 hours of pre-oxygenation

(not divers) were in good condition for at least 1·5 hours at 48 000 to 52 000 ft (0·13 to 0·10 ATA).

In submarine escape training during the course of successive exposures to 100 ft (4 ATA) followed by 30 sec ascent to the surface, the first ascent may be symptom-free, the second accompanied by delayed fatigue, while the third ascent may be followed by frank bends and other involvement. In test dives presumptive evidence of graded separation of gas from solution is afforded by the systematic work dives followed by limited oxygen 'surface decompression' conducted by Van Der

Aue et al. (1951). The gradation of reactions varies from no symptoms, to fatigue, itch, fatigue and itch, and mild decompression sickness (Table 21.12). These responses followed the systematic shortening of oxygen recompression time (i.e. following the short surface interval) of divers who engaged in heavy work at depth. A special contribution of this solid investigation is the greater susceptibility to bends brought about by a heavy work load and presumably related to the excess CO_2 which augmented latent bubble size. The results are similar to the thoroughly established

TABLE 21.12

Reactions attending the systematic shortening of oxygen recompression time of divers who engaged in heavy work at a depth of 100 ft (4 ATA) and were then bought rapidly to the surface*

Number of dives	Time at depth (min)	Water stops (min)	Recomp. oxygen 2·21 ATA	Reactions				
				None	Fatigue	Itch	F & I†	Bends
4	26	0	0	4	—	—	—	—
4	28	0	0	1	3	—	—	—
4	30	0	0	2	2	—	—	—
4	40	0	0	1	1	1	1	—
4	50	0	10	4	—	—	—	—
8	60	0	33	5	3	—	—	—
4	60	0	26	—	2	—	2	—
4	60	0	20	1	2	1	—	—
4	60	0	15	4	—	—	—	—
4	60	0	9	1	—	2	1	—
4	60	0	7	2	1	—	1	—
4	60	0	5	1	—	1	—	2
8	75	0	19	6	1	1	—	—
4	75	0	16	3	—	—	—	1
4	75	0	13	2	—	1	—	1
4	75	0	11	1	—	—	—	3
8	85	0	51	8	—	—	—	—
4	85	0	25	3	—	1	—	—
4	85	0	19	2	1	—	—	1
4	85	0	16	1	—	—	—	3
4	100	0	35	4	—	—	—	—
4	120	0	47	3	—	—	—	1
4	120	3 (at 30 ft)	50	3	1	—	—	—
4	120	3 (at 30 ft)	41	1	—	—	—	3

* Rate of ascent, 25 ft/min; at surface for 3·5 min; time elapsed between bottom depth and chamber recompression was 10 min.
† F & I (fatigue and itch). Note: Bends were usually mild and did not require recompression.
Data from Van Der Aue, Brinton and Kellar (1945) and Van Der Aue et al. (1951).

increase in decompression sickness incident to exercise at altitude. Fit divers with a lower respiratory quotient ($RQ = 1·2$) would be less susceptible than unfit divers with a work RQ of 1·4 or higher. A rest period following heavy work should be enforced prior to decompression to permit elimination of excess CO_2 which otherwise complicates the transport of inert gas.

During the latent period prior to onset of decompression sickness in man, bubbles in the circulation can now be identified by the Doppler technique. In the rapidly decompressed dog, these presymptomatic bubbles are observed in rapid circulatory transit. More amenable to confirmation is the observation that during the oxygen recompression period (to +30 psi gauge; 3 ATA) visible bubbles in blood vessels vanish and cardinal signs of decompression sickness are reversed (tachypnea, bradycardia, rise in pulmonic and fall in peripheral arterial pressures), only to reappear when pressure is prematurely reduced to 1 ATA (Behnke et al. 1936).

With reference again to Van Der Aue's tests, surface decompression was attended by a high incidence of fatigue and other mild impediments which usually did not require treatment. The remarkable ability of aqueous tissues to contain, at least initially, high pressures of N_2 without symptoms during the early stages of decompression, is probably responsible for the long-standing error of decompressing divers and caisson workers too rapidly in the early stages of decompression. The venerable postulate that bubbles form as soon as a condition of supersaturation is initiated supported the conclusion that supersaturation ratios were probably indices of permissible embolization. It may well be that the separation of gas from solution and consequent retardation of tissue perfusion may explain the empiricism underlying the prolonged desaturation time of 'the slowest tissue' postulated both for air and helium–oxygen dives. In effect decompression tables for subsaturation dives are treatment tables. Yet there is no proof that, in the absence of symptoms, phase separation of gas (silent bubbles) impairs normal circulation and thus nitrogen transport in tissues.

Decompression experience in earlier chamber tests

Decompressions according to Haldane's stage method following extended exposures in compressed air of 3 to 4 hours' duration (45 psi gauge, 4 ATA) were frequently complicated by bends at the Harvard School of Public Health during the period 1932 to 1935. In 1934, a bend was recorded by an engineer at a level of 3 psi gauge during the course of stage decompression following an exposure of 99 hours at 30 psi gauge (3 ATA). The initial drop in pressure, according to a conservative schedule at the time, was from 30 to 15 psi gauge and some 7 hours were taken to arrive at the 3 psi gauge level. This unfavorable experience stimulated physiologic investigation at Harvard and served to emphasize the need for decompression studies following saturation exposures. Such tests were conducted at the Experimental Diving Unit during the period 1940 to 1945. These tests in compressed air served to establish a depth (dry) of 33 ft (2 ATA) as limiting for a saturation exposure (12 hours) followed by no-decompression stoppages. Exposures of longer duration were only occasionally complicated by tolerated bends which did not require recompression. Of special interest was the role apparently of the small quantity of N_2 (which could not be measured at the time) absorbed after 6 hours relative to occurrence of bends. At depths deeper than 33 ft (2 ATA) the attempt was made to decompress on oxygen at a single level (60 ft; 2·82 ATA) which would assure isobaric transport of N_2 at an optimal level (Table 21.13). Despite this precaution, bends occurred frequently and it was clearly evident that the time allocated for oxygen inhalation (calculated to permit a surfacing ratio of N_2 of about 1·6 to 1) was inadequate.

The isobaric (oxygen window) principle of decompression

In any gas mixture there is a certain percentage of oxygen compatible with well being. During the course of blood perfusion of tissues, oxygen is unloaded in different quantities to the various tissues. The result of this transfer of oxygen is that the blood can transport an equivalent amount of inert gas from tissues to lungs. During the late Thirties, Momsen (1939) and his group at the EDU referred to the 'space' available for transport of inert gas in solution as the 'partial pressure vacancy'.

TABLE 21.13

Saturation air dives in the dry or wet tank

No. tests	ATA	ft	Exposure time (hours)	Decompression		Outcome*
				Depth stop (ft)	Time (min)	
4 Resting	2·00	33	12	—	—	NS
4 Work	2·00	33	12	—	—	NS
4 Resting	2·00	33	24	—	—	NS
8 Resting	2·00	33	36			2(X) 6 NS
4 Resting	2·06	35	12	—	—	1(O) 3 NS
4 Work	2·06	35	12	—	—	NS
14 Resting	2·21	40	12	—	—	4(O) 9 NS
14 Work	2·21	40	12	—	—	5(O) 4 NS 5(X)
1 Resting	2·82	60	12	60 oxygen	63	(X)
1 Resting	2·82	60	12	60 oxygen	69	(X)
1 Resting	2·82	60	12	60 oxygen	80	(X)
1 Resting	2·82	60	12	60 oxygen	92	(X)
1 Resting	3·82	90	6	40 oxygen	111	NS
1 Resting	3·82	90	6	40 oxygen	111	(X)
4 Resting	4·00	99	6	33 air	12 hours	1(X) 3(NS)
2 Resting	4·00	99	9	33 air	12 hours	1(X) 1(O)
2 Resting	4·00	99	9	33 air	18 hours	NS
2 Resting	4·00	99	12	33 air	24 hours	1(X) 1(O)

* NS = No symptoms; (X) = Bends; (O) = Mild bends, no recompression.
Data from Behnke (1940) and Van Der Aue (1945).

At normal pressure during inhalation of air, the partial pressure of oxygen in the arterial blood falls to about 40 mm Hg on the average in capillaries. If Pa_{O2} is elevated to 287 mm Hg, there is a subsequent decrease in the capillaries to about 50 mm Hg, only 10 mm higher than the previous level. Noteworthy is the possibility of an increase of Pa_{O2} to about 1500 mm Hg without incurring a rise of more than several hundred mm of oxygen pressure in the capillaries. Since oxygen becomes abruptly toxic above the level of 2 ATA for work or sustained inhalation, there is a physiologic limit to the size of the *oxygen window*.

In non-saturation diving the isobaric principle is compromised between the ideal 'bubble-free' decompression and a relatively abridged schedule based on empiricism and dictated by expediency. This limitation did not preclude helium–oxygen dives in the open sea to depths greater than 500 ft (16·2 ATA) in the earlier era but the exposures were short and generally limited to accomplishment of a single task, previously well rehearsed on the surface. With standard oxygen decompression at essentially two stops, 50 and 40 ft (2·25 and 2·21 ATA), as it was during the salvage operations to raise the USS *Squalus*, then out of hundreds of dives there were only occasional cases of decompression sickness, and minimal, if any, residual disability.

Current calculations pertaining to decompression following helium–oxygen saturation dives postulate a half-time for the slowest desaturating tissue of at least 240 min, which is greatly in excess of measurements, admittedly incomplete, made in a previous era and of deductions referrable to helium solubility in fluid and fat. Thus if

π is the pressure of helium in the 'slowest' tissue ($T_{1/2}=240$ min), ΔP permissible supersaturation in ft of seawater, and P_{O_2} the *oxygen window*, then the rate of clearance of the slowest tissue is

$$\frac{\mathrm{d}\pi}{\mathrm{d}t} = -\frac{0{\cdot}693}{240}\,T_{1/2}\cdot(20+10) = \frac{11{\cdot}6\ \text{min}}{1\ \text{ft}}$$

If, however, ΔP is non-existent or a mathematical strategem, and if we consider only oxygen exchange (i.e. 10 ft equiv.), half-time for the slowest tissue becomes 80 min. To complete the analysis of isobaric transport, consider,

	Gas tensions	*Gas tensions*
	LUNGS	TISSUES-CAPILLARIES
Helium	2000	2230
Oxygen	287	50
CO_2	40	47
H_2O vapor	47	47
	2374 mm	2374 mm

Isobaric decomposition can now progress uniformly at a rate of 1 ft every 11·5 min and concomitantly there is an isobaric tension decrease of helium of 230 mm Hg during the course of each foot of ascent.

REFERENCES

BALLDIN, U. I. & LUNDGREN, C. E. G. (1972) Effects of immersion with the head above water on tissue nitrogen elimination in man. *Aerospace Med.* **43**, 1101–1108.

BEHNKE, A. R. (1937) The application of measurements of nitrogen elimination to the problem of decompressing divers. *Nav. med. Bull.* **35**, 219–240.

BEHNKE, A. R. (1942) Investigations concerned with problems of high altitude flying and deep diving; application of certain findings pertaining to physical fitness and to the general military service. *Milit. Surg.* **90**, 9–28.

BEHNKE, A. R. (1967) The isobaric (oxygen window) principle of decompression. In *The New Thrust Seaward. Trans. Third Marine Technology Soc. Conf.* 5–7 June, San Diego. Washington, D.C.: Marine Technology Soc.

BEHNKE, A. R. & WILLMON, T. L. (1939) USS *Squalus:* Medical aspects of the rescue and salvage operations and the use of oxygen in deep-sea diving. *Nav. Med. Bull.* **37**, 629–640.

BEHNKE, A. R. & WILLMON, T. L. (1941) Cutaneous diffusion of helium in relation to peripheral blood flow and the absorption of atmospheric nitrogen through the skin. *Am. J. Physiol.* **131**, 627–632.

BEHNKE, A. R. & WILMORE, J. H. (1974) *Evaluation and Regulation of Body Build and Composition.* New Jersey: Prentice-Hall.

BEHNKE, A. R., & YARBROUGH, O. D. (1938–39) Unpublished data in Momsen (1939).

BEHNKE, A. R., FEEN, B. J. & WELHAM, W. C. (1942) The specific gravity of healthy men. *J. Am. med. Ass.* **118**, 495–498.

BEHNKE, A. R., SHAW, L. A., MESSER, A. C., THOMSON, R. M. & MOTLEY, E. P. (1935) The rate of elimination of dissolved nitrogen in man in relation to the fat and water content of the body. *Am. J. Physiol.* **114**, 137–146.

BEHNKE, A. R., SHAW, L. A., MESSER, A. C., THOMSON, R. M. & MOTLEY, E. P. (1936) The circulatory and respiratory disturbances of acute compressed air illness and the administration of oxygen as a therapeutic measure. *Am. J. Physiol.* **114**, 526–533.

BOOTHBY, W. M., LUFT, U. C. & BENSON, O. O. (1951) *Gaseous Nitrogen Elimination.* Proj. no. 21-53 003, Report 1, USAF School of Aviation Medicine, Randolph Field, Texas.

BORNSTEIN, A. (1913) Weitere untersuchungen über Herzschlagvolumen. *Z. exp Path. Ther.* **14**, 135–150.

BOYCOTT, A. E. & DAMANT, G. C. C. (1908) Experiments on the influence of fatness on susceptibility to caisson disease. *J. Hyg., Camb.* **8**, 445–456.

BOYCOTT, A. E., DAMANT, G. C. C. & HALDANE, J. B. (1908) The prevention of compressed air illness. *J. Hyg., Camb.* **8**, 342–343.

BÜHLMANN, A. A., FREY, P. & KELLER, H. (1967) Saturation and desaturation with N_2 and He at 4 atm. *J. appl. Physiol.* **23**, 458–462.

CAMPBELL, J. A. & HILL, L. (1931) Concerning the amount of nitrogen gas in the tissues and its removal by breathing almost pure oxygen. *J. Physiol., Lond.* **71**, 309–322.

EPSTEIN, M., DUNCAN, D. C. & FISHMAN, L. M. (1972) Characterization of the natriuresis caused in normal man by immersion in water. *Clin. Sci.* **43**, 275–287.

FARHI, L. E., EDWARDS, W. T. & HOMMA, T. (1963) Determination of dissolved N_2 in blood by gas chromatography and (a–A) N_2 difference. *J. appl. Physiol.* **18**, 97–106.

GAUER, O. H., HENRY, J. P. & BEHN, C. (1970) The regulation of extracellular fluid volume. *A. Rev. Physiol.* **32**, 547–595.

GRAVES, D. J., IDICULA, J., LAMBERTSEN, C. J. & QUINN, J. A. (1975) Bubble formation resulting from counter-diffusion supersaturation: a possible explanation for 'inert gas urticaria' and vertigo. In *Underwater Physiology. Vth Symp. Underwater Physiology.* Ed. C. J. Lambertsen. Bethesda: Fedn Am. Socs exp. Biol.

GROOM, A. C. & FARHI, L. E. (1967) Cutaneous diffusion of atmospheric N_2 during N_2 washout in the dog. *J. appl. Physiol.* **22**, 740–745.

GROOM, A. C., MORIN, R. & FARHI, L. E. (1967) Determination of dissolved N_2 in blood and investigation of N_2 washout from the body. *J. appl. Physiol.* **23**, 706–712.

HABER, H. (1951) Appendix in USAF Report by Boothby, Luft & Benson (1951).

HAUSBERGER, F. X. (1957) Composition of adipose tissue in several forms of obesity. *Anat. Rec.* **127**, 305.

HILL, L. (1912) *Caisson Sickness and the Physiology of Work in Compressed Air*. London: Edward Arnold.

HILLS, B. A. (1966) *A Thermodynamic and Kinetic Approach to Decompression Sickness*. Thesis. Adelaide: Libraries Board, S. Australia.

JONES, H. F. (1950) Respiratory system: Nitrogen elimination. In *Medical Physics*. Vol. 2. Ed. O. Glasser. Chicago: Year Book Publishers.

JONES, H. F. (1951) Molecular exchange and blood perfusion through tissue regions. In *Advances in Biology and Medical Physics*. Ed. J. Lawrence. New York: Academic Press.

KAGIYAMA, S. (1934). Studies on prevention of caisson disease. *J. Kumamoto med. Soc.* **10**, 562–564.

KLOCKE, F. J. & RAHN, H. (1961) A method for determining inert gas ('N$_2$') solubility in urine. *J. clin. Invest.* **40**, 279–285.

KETY, S. (1951) The theory and applications of the exchange of inert gas at the lungs and tissues. *Pharmac. Rev.* **3**, 1–41.

LUNDIN, G. (1953) Nitrogen elimination during oxygen breathing. *Acta physiol. scand.* **30**, Suppl. 111, 130–143.

LUNDIN, G. (1960) Nitrogen elimination from the tissues during oxygen breathing and its relationship to fat: muscle ratio and the localization of bends. *J. Physiol., Lond.* **152**, 167–175.

MACKAY, R. S. & RUBISSOW, G. (1971) Detection of bubbles in tissues and blood. In *Underwater Physiology. Proc. 4th Symp. Underwater Physiology.* Ed. C. J. Lambertsen. New York: Academic Press.

MOMSEN, C. B. (1939) *The Use of Helium–oxygen Mixtures for Diving* (revised Oct. 1948) Report Experimental Diving Unit, Navy Yard, Washington, D.C.

REEVES, E. & BECKMAN, E. L. (1966) *The Incidence of Decompression Sickness in Dogs following 7, 12, 18, & 24 hour Saturation Dives with 'No-Stop' Decompression*, Report No. 4, Naval Medical Research Institute, Bethesda, Maryland.

SHAW, L. A., BEHNKE, A. R., MESSER, A. C., THOMSON, R. M. & MOTLEY, E. P. (1935) The equilibrium time of the gaseous nitrogen in the dog's body following changes in nitrogen tension in the lungs. *Am. J. Physiol.* **112**, 545–553.

SHILLING, C. W. & HAWKINS, J. A. (1936) The hazard of caisson disease in individual submarine escape. *Nav. med. Bull.* **34**, 47–52.

SIRI, W. E. (1961) Body composition from fluid spaces and density, analysis of methods. In *Techniques for Measuring Body Composition*. Ed. J. Brožek & A. Henschel, p.230. Washington, D.C.: Natl Acad. Sci.-Natl Res. Council.

SPENCER, M. P., JOHANSON, D. C. & CAMPBELL, S. D. (1972) Safe decompression with the Doppler ultrasonic blood bubble detector. In *Underwater Physiology. Vth Symp. Underwater Physiology.* Ed. C. J. Lambertsen. Bethesda: Fedn Am. Socs exp. Biol.

STEVENS, F. D., RYDER, H. W., FERRIS, E. B., JR. & INATOME, M. (1947) The rate of nitrogen elimination from the body through the lungs. *J. Aviat. Med.* **18**, 111–133.

TOBIAS, C. A., JONES, H. B., LAWRENCE, J. H. & HAMILTON, J. G. (1949) The uptake and elimination of Krypton and other inert gases by the human body. *J. clin. Invest.* **28**, 1375–1385.

VAN DER AUE, O. E., BRINTON, E. S. & KELLAR, R. J. (1945a) *Variations of the Inert Gas Content of the Urine under der Increased Barometric Pressure and their Prognostic Value in the Occurrence of Compressed Air Illness*. Report No. 4, Project X-476 (Sub. No. 98) Experimental Diving Unit, Washington, D.C.

VAN DER AUE, O. E., BRINTON, E. S. & KELLAR, R. J. (1945b) *Surface Decompression, Derivation and Testing of Decompression Tables with Safety Limits for Certain Depths and Exposures*. Research project X-476, Research report 1, Experimental Diving Unit, Washington, D.C.

VAN DER AUE, O. E., KELLAR, R. J., BRINTON, E. S., BARRON, G., GILLIAM, H. D. & JONES, R. J. (1951) *Calculation and Testing of Decompression Tables for Air Dives Employing the Procedure of Surface Decompression and the Use of Oxygen*. Research report 1. Experimental Diving Unit, Washington, D.C.

WILLMON, T. L. & BEHNKE, A. R. (1941) Nitrogen elimination and oxygen absorption at high barometric pressures. *Am. J. Physiol.* **131**, 633–638.

22

Ultrasonic Surveillance of Decompression

A. EVANS

For centuries man has made use of electromagnetic radiation, or rather those radiations with wavelengths in the range 0·4 to 0·7 μm which we know as visible light, for diagnostic purposes. One of the earliest applications to the study of decompression was reported by the Hon. Robert Boyle in what must be one of the most widely quoted papers of the seventeenth century (Boyle 1670). However, except in unusual structures such as the hamster's cheek pouch (Buckles 1968) or the web of the frog's foot (Hill & Macleod 1903), relatively little has been learned from observation of the intact animal. Much greater insight in the search for gas bubbles is gained by dissection, though major problems then arise such as gas which was not previously there but which enters through the cut surfaces.

The useful portion of the electromagnetic spectrum was greatly extended in 1895 by Becquerel's discovery of X-rays, which are of smaller wavelength and much greater penetrating power than visible light. Almost from that time, the shadowgraphs of the human body made with these rays have become invaluable as diagnostic aids. Unfortunately the effect of a small gas bubble upon an X-ray beam is very small, though Ferris and Engel (1951) discussed reports of changes detected by X-radiography near the joints of fliers undergoing simulated high altitude flight. The recent introduction of the 'microfocal' X-ray tube has considerably improved the resolution of small structures, though the detection of single gas bubbles is still very difficult.

More recently, the even more energetic gamma (γ) rays emitted by certain radioactive substances have been used with considerable success to obtain information from the intact body, and the way in which radio strontium and fluorine are distributed in the region of the lesions seen in caisson disease of bone may well prove to be a valuable adjunct to radiology in the study of this condition. Cockett, Swanson and Kado (1969) have demonstrated, by means of the distribution of a radioisotope, ischaemia thought to be due to pulmonary emboli in animals following decompression. Unfortunately, even if a suitable radioisotope were to become available, the lateral resolution in the scanning equipment which is used at present is insufficient to pick out a single bubble of separated radioactive gas.

Some indirect methods for detecting the separation of free gas have been described. For example, there are ECG changes reported by Wilton-Davies (1970), indications with an electromagnetic blood flow meter (Spencer & Campbell 1968) and inductance conductivity (Hills, Chapter 20 in this volume). However, in order to pinpoint the position of a bubble within a muscle, or to detect a single bubble in the intact circulation, ultrasonic surveillance has been a method of much contemporary interest.

It appears that four distinct effects have been used so far in the search for free gas at decompression by means of ultrasound with varying degrees of success. These are:

1. The attenuation of a beam of sound waves on passing through a relevant region. Either stationary or moving bubbles should be detected.

2. The distortion introduced into a sound beam as it traverses a tissue containing bubbles. Either stationary or moving bubbles would be effective.

3. The B scan technique. This is widely used to visualize internal structures in medical ultrasonics and has been used also to seek bubble echoes. Either stationary or very slowly moving bubbles should be detected in this way.

4. The ultrasonic Doppler detector. This is widely used to detect fetal heart movements and blood flow and has been used to search for bubbles moving in the cardiovascular system.

Two of these techniques depend on reflection of sound by the bubbles and so the orientation of the transducer can give a good guide to their position. The other two, although giving less precise positional information, are potentially more sensitive and so should indicate the presence of smaller bubbles.

Those techniques which depend on the attenuation will be considered first, followed by the related distortion technique and, finally, the techniques which depend on reflection, including the highly successful Doppler method. Before attempting to describe any technique in detail, however, it seems appropriate to review some basic properties of ultrasonic waves and their interaction with their medium, and to discuss briefly the heart of any ultrasonic system, the transducer.

SOME PROPERTIES OF SOUND WAVES

Sound

In some respects sound waves are very similar to light waves, the properties of which are widely known. Thus they are sinusoidal disturbances which travel in straight lines at a well-defined speed, with a known wavelength, and can be reflected, refracted and absorbed. In other respects, however, there are differences, perhaps the most important being that as they are waves of compression and rarefaction passing through a material they cannot traverse a vacuum. Sound waves travel well through gases, most solids and many liquids, so transmission within the body normally presents little problem.

Sound waves in fluids also differ from light waves in that the wave motion in sound is along the direction of travel. This means that there can be no acoustic equivalent of polarized light, which consists of aligned transverse waves and which is used to reveal interesting aspects of biological specimens.

A further discrepancy, well known to observers of thunderstorms, is that sound travels much more slowly than light. Although the velocity of light is about 300 million m/sec, sound energy only travels at a few thousand m/sec. This is quite fast enough for most diagnostic applications, though it can be a limitation to at least one of the latest techniques, pulsed Doppler.

As sound is an oscillation of the material through which it passes, it may be anticipated that its velocity is determined by the elastic properties (represented by the bulk modulus E) and the inertia (represented by the density ρ of the material through which it travels. The relationship is:

$$C^2 = E/\rho$$

where C is the velocity. The velocity of sound in some materials commonly encountered in medical ultrasonics are given in Table 22.1.

The basic characteristic of a sound wave is the frequency which remains essentially constant, even though the wavelength may change on passing through materials with various velocities of propagation. Sound waves can be generated over a very wide range of frequencies, from below 1 to at least 10^9 cycles/sec (hertz [Hz]). The higher frequencies are quoted in kilohertz (kHz, 10^3 cycles/sec) and megahertz (MHz, 10^6 cycles/sec).

The sonic spectrum is conventionally broken down into three ranges. The human ear can detect sounds in the range from about 50 Hz to about 20 kHz, the audio range. Sounds of lower frequency are termed 'Infrasound' and waves of frequency in excess of 20 kHz are termed 'Ultrasound'. The experiments described in this review employ ultrasound of frequencies in the range 50 kHz to 15 MHz.

The length of one wave (λ) associated with a given frequency (f) is determined by the velocity:

$$f\lambda = C$$

This applies to any wave motion. The very small

TABLE 22.1

Values for the velocity of sound (C) and the specific acoustic impedance (Z) of some substances

Material	C (m/sec)	Z (g/cm² sec)
Air	330	43
Hydrogen	1300	11
Helium	970	17
Neon	435	39
Water	1490	$1 \cdot 5 \times 10^5$
Glycerine	1910	$2 \cdot 4 \times 10^5$
Castor oil	1500	$1 \cdot 4 \times 10^5$
Aluminium	6400	17×10^5
Brass	4250	36×10^5
Steel	6000	47×10^5
Barium titanate	5000	27×10^5
Quartz	5700	15×10^5
Polymethylmethacrylate	2700	$3 \cdot 2 \times 10^5$
Epoxy resin adhesive	—	$3 \cdot 0 \times 10^5$
Muscular human tissue	1540	$1 \cdot 63 \times 10^5$
Dog brain	1515	$1 \cdot 56 \times 10^5$
Blood	1570	$1 \cdot 61 \times 10^5$
Bone (skull)	4080	$7 \cdot 8 \ \times 10^5$

velocity of sound, when compared with electromagnetic radiation, means that the wavelengths are much smaller. The range of frequencies commonly used in ultrasonic diagnosis is broadly the same as those of the 'medium wave' radio transmissions, for which the wavelengths are some hundreds of metres. However, ultrasonic waves of these frequencies have wavelenths of the order of a millimetre. Knowledge of the wavelength is important when considering the possible resolution of any technique.

It would not be possible to extract any useful information by passing sound beams into the body if they passed through unchanged. Several changes can occur, the most important being reflection and absorption. Other changes, such as the selective change in velocity, are much more difficult to detect, and so are of less value in the study of internal structure and function.

As with light, reflection occurs when the sound encounters an interface between two media. The relevant property of each medium is the product of the velocity (C) and the density (ρ) which is known as the specific acoustic impedance (Z).

The proportion of sound energy which is reflected when a sound wave travelling in a medium with acoustic impedance Z_1 is normally incident on a plane interface with another medium of acoustic impedance Z_2 depends on the extent by which Z_1 and Z_2 differ. The ratio of intensities of reflected wave to incident wave is found to be

$$\left(\frac{Z_1 - Z_2}{Z_1 + Z_2}\right)^2, \quad \text{and the remainder or} \quad \frac{4Z_1 Z_2}{(Z_1 + Z_2)^2}$$

is the proportion of the incident wave which continues into the second medium.

Approximate values of Z for some common materials are also given in Table 22.1. It will be seen that the values for many soft tissues are similar, though the variations are sufficient to give the excellent ultrasonic sections obtained in obstetrics. Water differs slightly from these and more so from bone, but the most striking change is in the values for the gases. It may be clearly seen that ultrasound, incident on a gross tissue–gas interface, will be almost totally reflected.

However, even if attention is restricted to a single medium, sound waves do not proceed with the same intensity indefinitely. If they come from a point source, emitting in all directions, the intensity will decrease as the square of the distance. In order to counteract this, an attempt is made, described below, to confine the energy as far as possible to only one direction of propagation.

Nevertheless, even with a highly collimated beam, the intensity decreases with distance travelled. For water this attenuation is quite low, and so long-distance SONAR is possible even though the attenuation in some other fluids can be very high. This absorption, which is associated with the imperfect elasticity of the medium, is found, for many pure fluids, to increase as the square of the frequency. The attenuation in biological tissues also rises with increasing frequency and this factor may limit the highest frequency which can be used. High frequencies are of course desirable because of the associated small wavelength and hence fine resolution.

If gas bubbles appear in the path of a sound beam, the apparent attenuation must become larger than before. Gross bubbles will reflect some of the energy, so that the emergent beam is selectively weakened. However, even bubbles which are small compared with the wavelength can have an important effect. Such a bubble will 'see' the passage of a sound wave as a sinusoidal variation in the local hydrostatic pressure, and the gas inside will respond by periodic contraction and expansion. The pulsating bubble boundary will in turn re-radiate sound energy in all directions, and this scattered sound is removed from the incident beam. This effect occurs for bubbles of any size (if the radius is much less than λ) though it is most marked at a certain frequency for any given radius. This resonant frequency is given approximately by Minnaert's relation

$$f_0 r = 328$$

where f_0 is in hertz and r is in centimetres. Further damping by pulsating bubbles is due to the thermal lag between the compression and rarefaction phases of the gas within the bubble, and by the viscosity of the surrounding liquid. The whole problem is discussed in some detail by Devlin (1959).

The introduction of a free gas phase into the path of an ultrasonic wave can therefore result in a considerable attenuation of that wave. Several investigators have taken advantage of this effect in the search for bubbles at decompression.

Safety

Although ultrasonic techniques were for a long time considered to be a completely safe diagnostic aid, in recent years there has been some concern that the radiation of sound waves into the body may lead to some irreversible changes. In fact most of the May 1972 issue of the *British Journal of Radiology*, **45**, was devoted to this subject. The principal object for concern has been the very young fetus, where any interference with cell division may have profound consequences. The important criterion here is the intensity, or power transmitted per unit area of the beam, as this determines the particle displacement and possible destructive effect of the wave. The intensities encountered in the devices which have been applied to man are of the order of 10 mW/cm². For comparison most investigators report no cellular damage at continuous power levels up to 14 W/cm², or pulsed sound with peak power levels up to 150 W/cm², though Macintosh and Davey (1972)

alone suggest chromosome alterations with a Doptone at power levels as low as 8 mW/cm². It is probably safe to assume that, in a healthy adult, no ill effects will result from the intermittent application of the devices currently in use.

A related consideration which is peculiar to the surveillance of potentially supersaturated mammals, including man, is the possibility of ultrasonically induced cavitation (Hempleman 1971). It has been known for a long time that if sufficiently high intensities of sound energy are directed into water, bubbles may form even in the absence of dissolved gas. As the very interesting problems of bubble formation and growth are outside the scope of this review, perhaps it will be sufficient to say that cavitation was detected by a very sensitive method in saturated tap water (known to contain gas micronuclei) at a frequency of 1 MHz and an intensity about 20 W/cm² (Coakley 1971). As this is a factor of 10^3 higher than the values presently used for monitoring, it would seem safe to assume that there will be no appreciably increased risk of bubble formation with the power levels now in use.

Although absolute values for acoustic intensity are rarely encountered other than in safety considerations, it is often necessary to compare intensities. As the useful range is so wide, a logarithmic scale is employed so that equal intensity ratios occupy the same interval on the scale. The unit is the decibel, which is defined as 10 times the common logarithm of the ratio of intensities, or $dB = 10 \log_{10} (I_1/I_2)$. Thus a ratio of 10:1 is written as 10 dB, 1000:1 as 30 dB, and so on; the table of logarithms shows that 2:1 is about 3 dB and 4:1 is about 6 dB. The advantage of the logarithmic scale is that successive attenuations may be combined merely by adding: thus a reduction to 1% (20 dB) followed by a further reduction to one-half (3 dB) gives an overall reduction of 23 dB.

Transducers

The device which overcomes the transition between the mechanical energy of the ultrasonic wave and the electrical energy of the associated circuitry is an electromechanical transducer. The active element of any transducer is made of a material which changes in length in response to an electrical signal, and will also generate an electrical response to an impressed mechanical distortion.

As will be shown later, the dimensions of such a transducer follow the wavelength of the sound. Although a large loudspeaker is required to cope adequately with the lower notes of the audio frequency range, at ultrasonic frequencies a small element is sufficient. The traditional material for this element was crystalline quartz, cut in a special way. However, as these were costly and required a driving signal of some hundreds of volts, there was no reluctance to adopt the artificial 'crystals' when these became available. The majority of modern transducers are made of the new ceramic materials, which are based on lead zirconate titanate, and which may be moulded into any desired size and shape, including focusing bowls. They are polarized by cooling through the Curie point in a strong electric field, generated between silver electrodes deposited on the faces; thereafter they behave in the same way as quartz, though requiring the application of only a few tens of volts for satisfactory operation.

The transducer elements which are encountered in medical ultrasonics tend to be thin discs, with each face coated with silver. Thin wires are soldered to the faces so that a signal can be applied from the driving circuit, normally via a coaxial cable. If a sinusoidal voltage is applied, the thickness of the disc will change in sympathy and sound waves will radiate from each face. This occurs to some extent at any frequency, though transducers are normally driven at or near their resonant frequency. At resonance, the sound waves build up by reflection at the faces within the 'crystal' to give a much larger response for a given applied voltage. This resonance frequency is determined by the sound velocity in the ceramic, and the thickness of the disc. Therefore, such 'crystals' are always sold of a thickness appropriate to the required operating frequency.

A free 'crystal' operated in this way is in fact a mechanical resonator rather like an organ pipe, and it is a known property of resonators that the useful frequency range is inversely proportional to the damping, or losses. Thus, a free transducer element will only respond adequately to quite a narrow band of frequencies. This may be perfectly satisfactory in a Doppler system where the range is small, but in a pulse echo system it is necessary for the transducer to cope with a considerable range of frequencies in order to generate a pulse of useful shape. To achieve this, one side of the 'crystal' is damped by a large block of sound-absorbent material, for example tungsten powder in an epoxy resin adhesive (Fig. 22.1). This gives

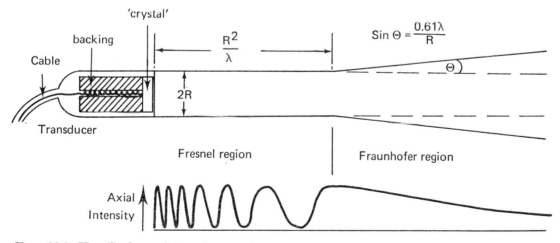

FIG. 22.1. Heavily damped transducer and typical sound field. The Freznel region is that just in front of the transducer where interference between the sound emitted from various parts of the transducer results in wide fluctuations in intensity. The Fraunhofer region is that in which intensity decreases uniformly. It is in the form of a cone gradually diverging with a half angle θ, where $\sin \theta = 0.61 \ \lambda/R$.

the larger, heavier transducer which is associated with obstetric B scanning equipment.

All transducer elements are normally mounted in some sort of case for protection. If the transducer is to be exposed to raised pressure, it is a sensible precaution to drill a hole through the casing to any air space within. It is also inadvisable to subject transducers to rapid decompression. They should be decompressed as carefully as men.

In order to achieve a relatively narrow, non-divergent beam a transducer of large diameter compared with the sound wavelength is required.

The transducer must not just radiate aimlessly into water. It must pass sound into and possibly receive sound back from living tissues. If it is implanted, tissue fluid will ensure adequate coupling. If not, it is insufficient just to press the transducer against the skin. It is possible to achieve good coupling by filling the intervening space with a fluid which has an acoustic impedance similar to that of the joined surfaces. It can be shown that if the thickness of the film is much less than the wavelength (which is easy to achieve at the lower ultrasonic frequencies) the presence of the coupling medium can be ignored and the surfaces behave as if they were in intimate contact. Olive oil, special coupling gels, or a water bath, are common coupling materials.

ABSORPTION

As suggested above, the introduction of free gas bubbles into a previously homogeneous medium

will lead to a reduction in the intensity of any sound waves passing through. The effect will be most marked if there are bubbles of resonant size present, though bubbles of any size will be effective in abstracting energy from the forward beam. If the bubbles grow to such a size that their dimensions become comparable with the acoustic wavelength, reflection will occur and give an even greater attenuation.

It is helpful first to consider the wavelengths and dimensions of resonant bubbles associated with the ultrasonic frequencies which have been used in monitoring decompression. Some values are given in Table 22.2. The wavelength is that associated with sound transmission at the mean velocity for human tissue of 1540 m/sec, and the resonant frequency for an air-bubble in water at atmospheric pressure is after Minnaert (1933). The remaining columns represent an attempt to estimate the resonant size for an air bubble surrounded by tissue, using the modification of Minnaert's formula suggested by Andreeva (1964) to account for the acoustic behaviour of the swimbladders of fish. In addition to the value for atmospheric pressure, which should apply after decompression is complete, values are also quoted for pressures of 3 ATA and 10 ATA which might apply during a decompression.

Although the figures in the last three columns are no more than estimates, the table does show the orders of magnitude involved. Sound wavelengths are of millimetre size, whereas the diameters of resonant bubbles are measured in micrometres. It is also clear that the technique

TABLE 22.2

Wavelengths and dimensions of resonant bubbles associated with ultrasonic frequencies used in monitoring decompression

Frequency	Tissue wavelength (mm)	Radius of resonant bubble (μm)			
		Minnaert	Tissue 1 ATA	Tissue 3 ATA	Tissue 10 ATA
100 kHz	15.4	33	64	79	117
200 kHz	7·7	16	32	40	59
500 kHz	3·1	6·6	13	16	24
1 MHz	1·54	3·3	6·4	7·9	11·7
2 MHz	0·77	1·6	3·2	4·0	5·9
5 MHz	0·31	0·66	1·3	1·6	2·4
10 MHz	0·15	0·33	0·64	0·79	1·17

will be less sensitive at pressure during the decompression, particularly as any detected bubble should grow even more when the pressure is finally released.

Unfortunately, it has not been possible to apply the very sensitive reverberant sphere absorption technique of Iyengar and Richardson (1958) to biological specimens, though Walder's application of the pulse echo technique described by Turner (1961) will be discussed later.

Ultrasonic attenuation during decompression

The first investigation to use ultrasonic attenuation for monitoring decompression appears to have been carried out in Canada in 1963 under the direction of Stubbs and Kidd (Huntec 1964). Two quartz crystal transducers of 2 MHz resonant frequency were mounted on opposite sides of the specimen. Pulsed ultrasound of frequency 50 to 230 kHz generated by one transducer traversed the specimen to the receiving transducer, from which the signal was amplified and displayed on an oscilloscope, and also recorded using a servo-system.

A test at 100 kHz showed that a stream of air bubbles in water issuing from a small glass orifice (mean diameter ~ 0.67 mm) gave an attenuation of about 6·6 dB in the signal. These bubbles were too small to reflect significantly, and yet led to a fourfold decrease in the signal even though each bubble was 1000 times the volume required for resonance. In further tests, at several frequencies, it was shown that subatmospheric decompression of tap water led to attenuations of 10 dB or more.

Trials were then carried out using this absorbtion technique to try to detect decompression-induced bubbles, by means of changes in the transmission of ultrasound through a segment of forearm and wrist. Two 2 MHz barium titanate transducers were fitted with cones so that they acted as point sources. The waveform of the received signal was somewhat complex, due to the possibility of transmission of other than longitudinal waves in the bone. Tests carried out to determine the influence of isobaric muscular movement resulted in fluctuations of the order of 2 dB.

Subatmospheric decompression to a simulated altitude of 37 000 ft at a rate of 10 000 ft/min led,

in some runs, to more than twice this attenuation (with a change in waveform of the received signal) but in the small number of tests reported this sign was not clearly associated with the onset of symptoms. However, it was suggested that the method was feasible, though the limitations of muscular movement made it of uncertain routine value.

In a later publication, Kidd (1969) mentioned that the technique was still used and that attenuations of 7 dB were seen prior to reported symptoms of bends in hyperbaric decompression, though changes of 3 to 5 dB were commonly seen in their absence.

The principle of detecting the attenuation of the signal between two transducers strapped to the arm of a man was also used by Manley (1969). This instrument, which was constructed for trials at the RN Physiological Laboratory, Alverstoke, worked at 50 to 80 kHz, and the received signal was amplified and displayed on an oscilloscope. It is stated that 'bubbles were detected' though the influence of muscular movement was again noted. In the same paper, Manley describes a device for detecting air emboli in blood in an extracorporeal circulation, by means of the attenuation of either 43 or 130 kHz beams passing through a special chamber in the circuit. Considerable attenuation was recorded.

The most recent exponent of this method is Powell (1972a) who uses an instrument which transmits pulses of energy at 5·7 MHz between a pair of transducers through the tissue under investigation. The power level is of the order of 1 to 5 mW/cm². The system enables a continuous record of signal attenuation in dB to be extracted, so that it can for example be plotted against pressure on an X-Y recorder. The feet and thigh muscles of rats have been surveyed. The system is insensitive to pressure per se within 2 to 3 dB, though after hyperbaric exposure to 6 ATA attenuations have been recorded at decompression, which increase with the length of the exposure and have been as great as 25 dB. A sudden increase in attenuation often preceded the death of the animal, though recompression results in an increase in signal to the pre-decompression level. These results are essentially similar to those which obtained with the back peak technique described later. Subsequently Powell (1973) has given a brief report of the first application of the technique to man. The sound beam was directed through the calf muscle of a subject undergoing simulated saturation diving experiments. The dives were symptom-free, and no excess attenuation was noted.

Acoustic optical imaging

One of the most ingenious techniques which has emerged is that of Buckles and Knox (1969) who used acoustic optical imaging to give a visual indication of variations in intensity across a plane acoustic beam. The idea of an ultrasonic camera is not new, and in fact Smyth and Sayers (1959) suggested that their instrument might have medical uses. Buckles and Knox made use of the technique of Korpel (1966) to obtain an optical image of the residual intensity of a plane acoustic beam, of frequency 8·5 MHz, propagated from a quartz transducer in a water bath through the hind leg of an anaesthetized hamster. A converging beam of monochromatic light from a laser crosses the acoustic beam, and is diffracted in such a way that an optical image of the sound beam can be obtained. Unfortunately this image is demagnified by a factor equal to the ratio of the wavelengths of the light and the sound, which in this case is $3·6 \times 10^{-3}$, so it is necessary to resort to microscopy to see and photograph the image.

It was used to monitor the development of bubbles in an animal's legs after a rapid decompression from an exposure of 200 psi (15 ATA) of air for 30 min. Undoubted increases in absorption, probably due to profuse bubble formation, were seen in both experiments reported, in which the animals died. The authors suggest a theoretical limit of resolution of 0·7 mm, though they say that the presence of smaller bubbles was detected.

If the apparatus were to be used inside a hyperbaric chamber it would clearly be of value to observe massive bubble formation following severe decompressions, though it is not certain that it would be possible to detect the marginal bubble formation which would be tolerated by man.

Back peak system

The other absorption technique which has been studied at some length is the back peak system

(Walder 1967; Walder, Evans & Hempleman 1968). Although a considerable time was occupied in assessing this method both at Newcastle and at the RN Physiological Laboratory, there are only the above two brief reports in the literature.

The principle relies on a short pulse of sound energy being transmitted by a single, highly damped transducer through the specimen. At the far side it is reflected, by means of a suitable interface, and then the pulse once more traverses the specimen and is detected by the same transducer. The size of the received pulse, which we call the back peak, is initially determined by the reflection coefficient of the far interface. However, if this remains constant, any variations seen in the height of this pulse must be due to attenuation within the specimen.

The basic instrument used was a Smith–Kline Eskoline 20, which operates at a frequency of 2·25 MHz and gives a conventional A scan display on an oscilloscope, so that the size of the back peak can be monitored. Earlier experiments were carried out by measurement and by photographic recording of the oscilloscope trace. The instrument was subsequently modified in such a way that the back peak could be selected electronically and a signal proportional to its area recorded, together with chamber pressure, on a continuous chart.

As the apparatus was used with small animals, a transducer 7 mm in diameter was used, and held to the appropriate body segment by means of a clip. The transducer was coupled to the skin, though the far side was left dry to ensure that the pulse was adequately reflected. Most experiments were with guinea pigs, using a fold of back skin, the thigh muscle or an ear lobe.

In any of these positions there has been, repeatedly, a clear response to severe decompression. For example, after an exposure to 80 psi (6·3 ATA) for 60 min and a 2-min decompression, the back peak disappears normally after an interval of about 2 min. This corresponds to an excess attenuation of at least 10 dB, and probably 20 dB. However, the peak may be restored to its previous level by recompression to the original pressure, which strongly suggests that the effect is due to gas bubbles as anticipated. A typical sequence of photographs is given by Walder, Evans and Hempleman (1968).

The performance with marginal exposures is less convincing, although reversible reductions in back peak height have been observed with less severe decompressions. One possible difficulty with this technique, in its original form, is that the skinfold is compressed somewhat in order to retain the clip and this may have interfered with the circulation of blood. However, similar results were obtained on muscle, where no great pressure is necessary. The fact that the observed response is normally a sudden reduction in peak height some minutes after the decompression suggests that fully formed large gas masses are entering the region surveyed, probably via the circulation. The same may well apply to the experiments of Powell (1972a). In a few trials of this technique on man, in symptomless decompressions, no clear reduction in back peak height has been seen.

Occasionally a third peak has been seen midway between the main transmitted pulse and the back peak while monitoring a fold of skin. This is undoubtedly due to reflection from a sheet of interstitial gas. That this is not seen regularly lends support to the view that the usual attenuation is due to discrete small bubbles, probably within the circulation.

DISTORTION

A technique which is related to, though distinct from, the attenuation techniques depends upon the effect of the non-linear response which a medium with gas bubbles will have on a sinusoidal sonic waveform.

It is obvious that the introduction of a cloud of small bubbles into an otherwise pure fluid will increase its compressibility, and so will influence the velocity of sound waves. However, as a fixed mass of gas in a bubble will more readily expand under the negative pressure portions of an incident sinusoidal sound wave than it will compress under the positive portions, the wave emerges somewhat distorted. The best way to detect this distortion, and therefore the presence of bubbles, is to monitor the level of the harmonics at various multiples or sub-multiples of the frequency of the fundamental wave.

The idea that gas bubbles associated with decompression might be detected in this way was first suggested by Tucker and Welsby (1968). The authors refer to an internal memorandum (Welsby 1968) in which it is suggested that acoustic non-linearity might be applied to the problem of gas bubbles in man. The theory which had been outlined in an earlier memorandum (Welsby 1967) shows that if a plane acoustic wave passes through a homogeneous medium, the amplitude of the signal detected at twice the fundamental wave frequency rises very markedly if only a very small number of small gas bubbles are introduced. In fact, it is shown that it should be possible to detect 1 part in 10^8 by volume of free gas in this way.

Subsequently, with the cooperation of Dr Welsby, an evaluation of this technique was carried out at Newcastle. A schematic diagram of the apparatus used is shown in Fig. 22.2. A 160 kHz oscillator feeds via a filter to exclude any harmonic (320 kHz) signal to an undamped transmitting transducer, coupled to one side of the specimen. The sound signal passes through the specimen, and is detected at a second transducer. This signal is split; one connection is directly to one beam of a two-beam oscilloscope, and also to a recorder; the other portion passes to a filter to exclude the fundamental frequency (160 kHz) and then to an amplifier tuned to 320 kHz, the output from which passes to the other beam of the scope and another channel of the recorder.

As the amplitude of the harmonic signal is many orders of magnitude smaller than the fundamental, it is evident that the second filter must be exceptionally effective. In preliminary trials a wave analyser was used, though later the apparatus was simplified by using the filter shown in Fig. 22.3. This overcomes the difficulty experienced with normal L-C filters due to the finite resistance of the inductance, which limits the impedance presented by the filter at the required frequency. With the bridged-T arrangement (Welsby 1950) the variable resistance r may be adjusted to counteract R_L, so that the impedance is effectively infinite. In this way a harmonic signal free from fundamental distortion could be amplified for display and recording.

A swarm of small bubbles introduced into a container of water surveyed in this way led to a most impressive rise in the level of the harmonic

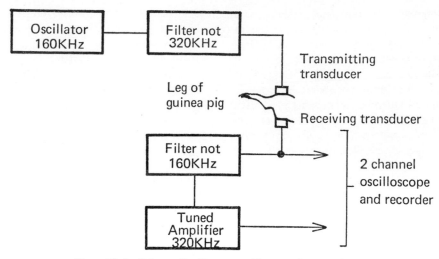

FIG. 22.2. Schematic diagram of harmonic experiment

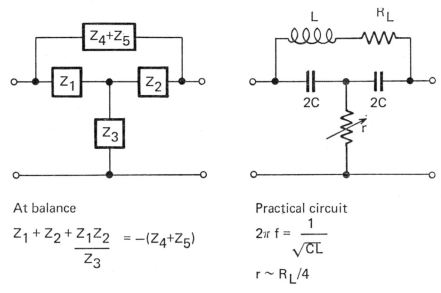

At balance

$$Z_1 + Z_2 + \frac{Z_1 Z_2}{Z_3} = -(Z_4 + Z_5)$$

Practical circuit

$$2\pi f = \frac{1}{\sqrt{CL}}$$

$$r \sim R_L/4$$

FIG. 22.3. The bridged-T filter (after Welsby 1950)

signal. Animal trials were then carried out on anaesthetized guinea pigs, which were also surveyed by other techniques so that a comparative study was possible.

Both transmitting and receiving transducers, which were about 7 mm in diameter had the same resonant frequency of about 160 kHz and were attached by a clip so that they rested lightly on the skin surface on opposite sides of the thigh muscle, to ensure a continuous acoustic path.

An effect which was noticed immediately was the large, apparently spontaneous, variation in the detected second harmonic signal strength while the animal was lying peacefully in the chamber at atmospheric pressure. These were probably due to instability or perhaps due to temperature variations, in the electronic circuitry. One great disadvantage of a very sharp 'notch' filter, two of which are incorporated in the apparatus, is the very small tolerance which they show for drift in frequency, and so a small change in either filter or the driver oscillator can lead to a completely misleading apparent increase in harmonic signal. In a subsidiary experiment it was shown that compressing the transducers did not have an important effect on their performance when connected to a Perspex block.

Some seven pressure excursions were completed, with the transducers across a fold of back skin in three cases. The results were not at all clear. In one case a spectacular increase in harmonic signal was recorded during the decompression, with no perceptible effect on the size of the back peak which was monitored at the same time. In order to try to reduce the influence of the filters, some later runs were carried out using transducers of 485 and 970 kHz resonant frequency, so that the harmonic should be preferentially detected by the receiver, though it was still very sensitive to the fundamental. However, the apparently random fluctuations which continued to influence the harmonic signal persisted throughout, and reluctantly the technique was abandoned.

Martin, Hudgens and Wonn (1973) of Westinghouse report preliminary tests of the distortion technique on man. A fundamental frequency of 115 kHz was used, with the beam usually directed across the muscles of the thigh or upper arm. The fundamental level was monitored using a shortwave radio receiver. US Navy oxygen recompression dives, mostly 100 ft for 110 min or 150 ft for 30 min, were simulated in a chamber with exercise at pressure.

They monitored 18 man-dives, and on five of these indications of single bubbles were seen as transients in the harmonic level. Three of these positive dives were symptom-free; itching was experienced on the other two.

One point is that the technique works best if the fundamental sound frequency is much lower than the resonant frequency of the bubbles, and so a lower fundamental frequency might be preferable. Also, it may be an advantage to study the sub-harmonic at half the fundamental frequency (Eller & Flynn 1969). The study of distortion is a potentially very sensitive technique, and it might well repay further investigation.

REFLECTION

Although, in theory, techniques based on reflection of sound energy should be less sensitive and only give an indication when considerable accumulations of separated gas have formed, in practice the reflection techniques seem to have been most successful. Two distinct approaches have been followed: the B scan technique, to give a visual indication of the position of intense reflectors, and the Doppler technique, which generates an audible signal from bubbles in the circulation.

It is interesting to consider first the size of bubble which we might expect to detect by means of reflected ultrasound. This problem has been analysed in some detail by Nishi (1972) who comes to the conclusion that the scattering cross-section (a guide to the fraction of an incident sound wave which will be reflected) decreases continuously as the radius is reduced. An air bubble in water does show a local peak response due to resonance, though due to the higher viscosity the same bubble in blood merely shows a slight change in gradient of the curve (Nishi & Livingstone 1973). For radii below about 1 μm the scattering cross-section falls off very rapidly, so that it is most improbable that bubbles smaller than this can be detected.

Experimental studies suggest that the limit may be rather higher than this. Patterson et al. (1972) were able to detect plastic microspheres of 40 μm radius easily with their 5 MHz apparatus, though spheres of 25 μm radius largely went undetected. The smallest bubbles mentioned by Nishi (1972) are of 50 μm radius, though Rubissow and Mackay (1971) state that their apparatus is capable of detecting single bubbles of 1 μm radius, Cathignol, Roche and Grivel (1973) working in vitro with a 5 MHz instrument were able to detect bubbles smaller than 20 μm radius, and Nishi and Livingstone (1973) suggest that they may have been able to detect silent bubbles of only 2·5 μm radius. It would thus appear that it should be easy to detect, by reflection of ultrasound, large separated gas masses, though bubbles less than 100 μm in diameter may prove to be more elusive.

Although the pulse echo technique has been extensively used for exploring mammalian internal structures since its introduction by Wild (1950), the first full description of its application to gas bubble detection seems to have been by Austen and Howry (1965) who used a commercial flaw detector to monitor the flow of blood through the external circuit in cardiopulmonary bypass. The technique has been employed for bubble detection in vivo by Mackay (1963, 1968), Mackay and Rubissow (1971) and Rubissow and Mackay (1971).

These authors use an automatic sector scanning system, with a frequency of 7·5 or 10 MHz and a pulse repetition rate of 1 or 3 kHz. The specimen (for example, the leg of a guinea pig) was immersed in water in the lower part of a compression chamber, and was irradiated by the transducer immersed in another water bath outside the chamber through a plastic window. The transducer was fitted with a lens to give a lateral resolution of 1·5 mm; the depth resolution is of the order of the wavelength. The returning signal is displayed as either a deflection-modulated or an intensity-modulated B scan on an oscilloscope, to give sections composed of 300 lines 10 times per second, which are photographed for permanency and comparison with subsequent images.

Representative sections of animals' legs are shown in both of the 1971 papers. The development of bubbles after severe decompressions is seen most clearly, and therapeutic recompression gives a spectacular decrease in abnormal echoes, over a period of 10 min. It was observed that on subsequent decompression, echoes tended to reappear at the same sites, implying that recompression had caused bubbles to shrink beyond the limit of resolution.

In the later report (Rubissow & Mackay 1971) the results of some trials on men are also included. The muscles of the arm and leg, and also the wrist and knee were surveyed using the B scan apparatus; a 10 MHz Doppler instrument was also directed towards superficial veins. Only 'safe' dives were attempted and no certain bubbles were identified using either technique.

The most extensive studies have been with the Doppler technique in various configurations. All techniques described so far respond to stationary gas inclusions, or to moving gas for the period when it is in the field of view. The Doppler system will only give an indication from moving structures and, as it is a reflection technique, it will in general only respond to the larger bubble. Never-

theless, this technique has been studied in several centres and it has been used to demonstrate bubbles in the circulation of man in the absence of any symptoms of decompression sickness.

The ultrasonic Doppler technique makes use of the change in frequency experienced by a sound wave when it is reflected from a moving interface. It can be shown that when a wave of frequency f encounters an interface with a component of velocity V in the direction of wave propagation, the reflected wave is shifted in frequency by an amount

$$\delta f = \frac{2V}{C} \cdot f$$

where C is the sonic velocity. In the Doppler instrument the returning signal is mixed with the incident frequency so that beats at the difference frequency result. These are amplified and, as they fall in the audio range are fed to a loudspeaker or headphones. Reflection from stationary structures gives no Doppler shift, and so no signal.

The original apparatus of Franklin, Schlegel and Rushmer (1961) was used to detect the flow of blood in the descending aorta of a dog. Two 5 MHz transducers were mounted at an angle of 45° on opposite sides of the vessel, to which they were coupled by water. With a rather high intensity of 2 W/cm², the flow of blood was detected, and it is suggested that the reflection might be from 'foreign particles such as small bubbles'.

A similar system, was used by Gillis, Peterson and Karagianes (1968) to detect bubbles following decompression in the vena cava of a pig. The transducer assembly (Fig. 22.4a) was implanted surgically to surround the vessel, and after the animal had recovered it received a simulated dive on a compression chamber at a pressure of 6·3 ATA for 60 min, followed by a decompression lasting 6 min. The first 'embolic event' was detected during the decompression, at about 4 ATA pressure, and subsequently they become so numerous that the flow signal was completely masked. However, after recompression to the original pressure for a further hour, these events had largely been eliminated.

At the same time Spencer and Campbell (1968) were using implanted Doppler transducers with

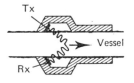

(a)

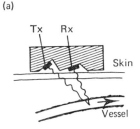

(b)

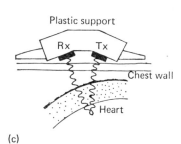

(c)

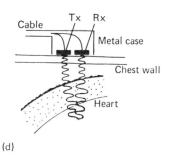

(d)

FIG. 22.4. Various Doppler transducer assemblies. (a) cuff type, crystals opposite (after Spencer et al. 1969). (b) transcutaneous type. (c) Seattle pre-cordial transducer (after Spencer & Clarke 1972). (d) Sonicaid transducer

sheep. They report the results of three exposures of 60 min to a pressure equivalent to 200 ft (7·1 ATA) seawater. Two animals were fitted with a transducer either around the descending aorta or around the vena cava, and the third animal was

fitted with both. In the first experiment the probe of an electromagnetic flowmeter was also attached to the aorta. A 4-min linear decompression was given, during the course of which bubbles were detected by means of abnormal flow sounds with the venous monitor at 96 and 83 ft (3·9 and 3·5 ATA). Arterial bubbles were not detected until after a period of 12 min at atmospheric pressure in the animal, both by the Doppler system and also by abnormal signals on the record from the electromagnetic flowmeter; the animal developed convulsions. The other arterial monitor gave an indication during the decompression, at 5 ft (1·15 ATA), again accompanied by convulsions. The abnormal signals were eliminated by recompression.

It is clear from these results that some abnormal flow sound can be detected by the Doppler cuff, and that venous abnormalities occur well in advance of arterial signals which are accompanied by obvious symptoms.

The normal flow signal, detected with any Doppler transducer in a blood vessel, is quite characteristic though it defies clear description. The pulse can be heard clearly in arteries. The venous sounds follow respiration. The new sounds associated with decompression are quite unmistakable by ear, and have variously been described as 'chirps', 'crackles', 'clicks' or 'plunks', and with many bubbles the sound grows to a roar.

The technique was further extended by Smith and Spencer (1970) who managed to operate simultaneously four implanted cuff-type transducers surrounding different vessels in a sheep. The basic electronics was the 10 MHz Parkes Model 803, with four receiving channels which together with voice, pressure and time marks were recorded on a seven-channel recorder. A period of 2 weeks was allowed for recovery following the surgical implantation.

Some 41 simulated dives were experienced by nine sheep monitored in this way. In every case where signs of decompression sickness were produced, advance warning was given by the Doppler transducers. The order in which bubbles were detected in the various vessels tended to be the same. First the anterior vena cava (at 2·6 ± 2 min), second the pulmonary artery (6·9 ± 4 min), third the posterior vena cava (9·5 ± 5·3 min) and finally the femoral vein. The times of appearance of the first indication seem to have been relatively insensitive to the pressure or duration of the hyperbaric exposure.

The authors recommend the pulmonary artery as the most suitable vessel for subsequent surveillance. Although it did not yield the earliest indication of circulating emboli, it does receive the efflux from all veins, and furthermore it should be possible to monitor it with an external transducer.

Spencer and Oyama (1971) subsequently used a cuff-type transducer implanted into sheep to study the fate of various gases injected into the venous system, and Cathignol, Roche and Grivel (1973) showed with a 5 MHz Doppler apparatus that it was possible to detect injected bubbles much less than a millimetre in diameter.

One great advantage of the cuff-type transducer implanted to surround a blood vessel is that it is held firmly in position, and movements of the host animal are unlikely to affect its performance. It might be interesting to use such a cuff, with transducer elements on opposite sides of the vessel in order to study the absorption or distortion characteristic of the flowing blood. This could reveal the presence of smaller bubbles than has been possible by the Doppler shift. The implanted Doppler is probably a technique which must be restricted to the experimental animal but the transcutaneous development is immediately applicable to man.

The first report of Doppler bubble detection with an external transducer (see Fig. 22.4b) is by Gillis, Karagianes and Peterson (1968). A dog, a pig and a goat were exposed to a pressure of 6·3 ATA for periods of 60, 30 and 40 min, and were decompressed linearly in 10, 12 and 7 min respectively. Bubbles were detected as abnormal flow sounds in the first two animals, during the decompression in superficial veins, and all three were found after return to atmospheric pressure to have numerous detectable venous bubbles.

Spencer et al. (1969) report seven human decompressions monitored with superficial Doppler apparatus and one in which the subject had a small catheter tip transducer passed via his superficial saphenous vein into his vena cava. All

exposures were according to the *US Navy Diving Manual*. Bubble sounds were later identified in the recorded signals from two of the experiments though the rest proved to be negative. Gillis, Karagianes and Peterson (1969) report three other simulated dives according to the US Naval Tables, none of which yielded bubble signals although one subject reported symptoms of bends. More recently Powell (1972b) has used a transcutaneous vascular Doppler system in the search for bubbles in decompressed rats, which were subsequently dissected for confirmation.

Before leaving vascular transducers, it is relevant to point out that the emboli detected in this way may not all be gas bubbles. Mason et al. (1971), who used a cuff-type transducer in a dog, report that 'simulated thrombotic emboli and fat emboli caused deflections on the embolus detector'. Subsequently Kelly, Dodi and Eisman (1972) used the superficial transducer of the Parkes Model 803 (10 MHz) to monitor the femoral veins of 23 dogs whose legs had been broken. Chirps attributable to fat emboli were detected in 21 of the dogs and also in 12 of 42 patients with symptoms of fat embolism who were studied in a similar way.

The final development of the Doppler technique is to use an external transducer to monitor not just one vein, but the entire systemic venous output by directing the sound beam towards the heart following Satomura (1957) and Abelson (1968). For detection of air in man this seems to have been the most popular technique yet described, though it was initially applied not for use in decompression studies but to detect surgical embolism.

Maroon et al. (1968) describe the use of an unspecified Doppler instrument placed over the heart of a dog to detect 0·12 ml of air injected into the vena cava. This compared very favourably with the minimum quantity of 15 ml which could be heard by stethoscope. Edmonds-Seal, Prys Roberts and Adams (1970) subsequently confirmed with dogs that the Doppler technique was more sensitive than any other, and Maroon, Edmonds-Seal and Campbell (1969) and Edmonds-Seal and Maroon (1969) describe the use of the 5 MHz or 2·25 MHz Doptone for the detection of air emboli in neurosurgical patients. Fry (1970) also demonstrated that it was possible to detect as little as 0·025 ml of injected air with the 2 MHz Sonicaid fetal heart detector probe, strapped over the heart on to the chest of a pig.

By this time Evans and Walder (1970) had shown that bubbles passing through the heart of a guinea pig during and after a severe decompression could easily be detected. A home-made miniature 2 MHz transducer was used with the Sonicaid instrument and it was found that the bubble signals (which rapidly disappeared on recompression) were largely in the range 1·5 to 2·0 kHz. Subsequent experiments using goats showed that a very satisfactory cardiac signal and bubble sounds following decompression could be detected using the normal probe supplied with the Sonicaid fetal heart detector (see Fig. 22.4d); this is a 25 mm diameter PZT5A disc (2·0 MHz resonant frequency) split along a diameter to give transmitting and receiving elements. Although the crystals are inclined at a small angle, there is no clearly defined 'focal region'. With large animals and man the bubble signals fall within the frequency range 600 to 800 Hz.

A brief description of the Seattle precordial monitor was given by Spencer, Simmons and Clarke (1971) and the instrument is described in full by Spencer and Clarke (1972). Two half-inch square crystals are mounted, with their axes making an angle of 26°, at the separation to give a non-critical 'focal depth' of about 5 cm from the crystal faces (see Fig. 22.4c). The unit has an operating frequency of 5 MHz, and there is an optional low-audio frequency attenuator. The audio signal is heard with headphones and the entire unit is battery-operated and so is also completely portable.

The unit was tested by injecting 4 ml of carbon dioxide into the feet of two men. After an interval of 8 seconds, bubbles were detected in the heart for 20 to 30 sec. Due to the higher operating frequency, bubble signals are described as 'chirps and squeaks' rather than the lower-frequency 'plops' which are found with the 2 MHz instrument.

Spencer and Clark (1972) used their monitor on two men undergoing a simulated dive of 200 ft (7·1 ATA) for 30 min on air, according to US Naval Tables. In one subject some bubbles were detected at the last stop, and their number in-

creased to a maximum between 1 and 3 hours after 'surfacing'. Bubble signals were still present 5 hours after the dive, though none were heard at 20 hours. The other subject remained bubble-free throughout. No symptoms were reported. Several of the Seattle instruments have now been constructed, and are being evaluated. Powell, Hamilton and Kenyon (1974) have used one with pigs after hyperbaric exposures on air, helium and neon. Some bubbles were detected in the absence of signs of decompression sickness, though as the dive profiles were rather severe many dives resulted in a continuous roar from the apparatus indicating a profusion of circulating bubbles. Although signs of decompression sickness were only seen in 40% of the air dives (which were to 130 ft for 30 min) with this indication, signs developed in 75% of the rare gas dives (which were to 400 ft for 18 min) with the roar. If such a low proportion of false positives can be attained reproducibly in man, the development of bubble-free, rather than symptom-free, decompression schedules might be feasible, at least for oxy-helium. In the United Kingdom the Sonicaid instrument has been in use for several years to monitor men undergoing simulated dives at the RN Physiological Laboratory (Evans, Barnard & Walder 1972). Recently the Sonicaid has also been used to monitor men simulating high altitude flight in a subatmospheric decompression chamber (Evans, Walder & MacMillan 1973). Although one subject remained at a pressure below the critical value corresponding to 18 000 ft altitude for more than 12 min, no clear bubble sounds were obtained. However, bubble sounds are regularly detected during and after hyperbaric decompression.

The principal difficulty with the cardiac Doppler technique at present is that a discerning ear is necessary to recognize the abnormal sounds. The reason for this may be seen from Fig. 22.5, which shows a crude spectral analysis of the Sonicaid heart sounds of a goat with and without decompression-induced bubbles. The bubbles were occurring regularly, though not continuously. It will be seen that the two signals differ by as much as 10 dB in the 600 to 800 Hz range of frequency, but that there is an immense amount of common background signal which in this context can be

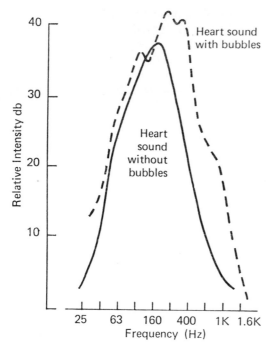

FIG. 22.5. Crude spectral distribution of Doppler heart sounds with and without bubbles

regarded as 'noise'. This results largely from moving structures which are of no interest, for example, the ventricular walls to which the transducer responds very well.

A possible improvement would be the use of the pulsed Doppler system, described by Wells (1969) and Baker (1970). In this the transmitted signal is interrupted to give long pulses, which then interact with moving structures in the same way as in the continuous system. As the transmitting transducer would be idle between pulses, it can be used to receive as well. By arranging that the receiver is only sensitive for suitable intervals it is possible to detect signals from only a known but adjustable range of depths within the specimen. It is here that the sonic velocity may be a limitation.

In this way it should be possible to record a signal only from the blood within the heart (Gramiak & Shah 1971) but reject the wall signals, and so give much more prominent bubble sounds which might be filterable to enable automatic detection.

A refinement suggested by Fish et al. (1972) is to incorporate the pulsed Doppler principle into a B scan display on which only moving structures appear. It may be possible in this way to see and perhaps count bubbles passing the heart, or in major vessels elsewhere. Another recent development (Kelsey 1970) which might be useful is the display of the intensity-modulated signal from a pulse-echo transducer sweeping slowly down an oscilloscope screen, or in a later development recording continuously on a UV chart recorder. If the heart is surveyed in this way the motion of the ventricular walls and valves is clearly seen and any bubble should appear conspicuously. Clearly there are several avenues still to be explored.

REFERENCES

ABELSON, M. (1968) Ultrasonic Doppler auscultation of the heart. J. Am. med. Ass. 204, 438–443.

ANDREEVA, I. B. (1964) Scattering of sound by air bladders of fish in deep sound-scattering ocean layers. Soviet Phys. Acoust. 10, 17–20.

AUSTEN, W. G. & HOWRY, D. H. (1965) Ultrasound as a method to detect bubbles or particulate matter in the arterial line during cardio-pulmonary bypass. J. Surg. Res. 5, 283–284.

BAKER, D. W. (1970) Pulsed ultrasonic Doppler blood-flow sensing. IEEE Sonics & Ultrasonics SU17, 170–185.

BOYLE, R. (1670) New pneumatical experiments about respiration. Phil. Trans. R. Soc. 5, 2044.

BUCKLES, R. G. (1968) The physics of bubble formation and growth. Aerospace Med. 39, 1062–1069.

BUCKLES, R. G. & KNOX, C. (1969) In vivo bubble detection by acoustic-optical imaging techniques. Nature, Lond. 222, 771–772.

CATHIGNOL, D., ROCHE, M. & GRIVEL, M. L. (1973) Formation des bulles intravasculaires: Détection ultrasonore par effet Doppler. Nouv. Presse Méd. 2, 117–118.

COAKLEY, W. T. (1971) Acoustic detection of single cavitation events in a focussed field in water at 1 MHz. J. acoust. Soc. Am. 49, 792–801.

COCKETT, A. T. K., SWANSON, L. E. & KADO, R. T. (1969) Location of pulmonary emboli following decompression by radio-isotopic lung scanning. Revue Physiol. subaquat. Méd. hyperbare 1, 283–288.

DEVLIN, C. (1959) Survey of thermal, radiation and viscous damping of pulsating air bubbles in water. J. acoust. Soc. Am. 31, 1654–1667.

EDMONDS-SEAL, J. & MAROON, J. C. (1969) Detection of air embolus by Doppler ultrasonics. Proc. R. Soc. Med. 62, 30.

EDMONDS-SEAL, J., PRYS ROBERTS, C. & ADAMS, A. P. (1970) Transcutaneous Doppler ultrasonic flow detectors for diagnosis of air embolism. Proc. R. Soc. Med. 63, 831–832.

ELLER, A. & FLYNN, H. G. (1969) Generation of subharmonics of order one-half by bubbles in a sound field. *J. acoust. Soc. Am.* **46**, 722–727.

EVANS, A. & WALDER, D. N. (1970) Detection of circulating bubbles in the intact mammal. *Ultrasonics* **8**, 216–217.

EVANS, A., BARNARD, E. E. P. & WALDER, D. N. (1972). Detection of gas bubbles in man at decompression. *Aerospace Med.* **43**, 1095–1096.

EVANS, A., WALDER, D. N. & MACMILLAN, A. J. F. (1973) Ultrasonic surveillance of subatmospheric decompression. *Nature, Lond.* **246**, 522–523.

FERRIS, E. B. & ENGEL, G. L. (1951) The clinical nature of high altitude decompression sickness. In *Decompression Sickness*. Ed. J. F. Fulton. p. 31. Philadelphia: Saunders.

FISH, P. J., KAKKAR, V. V., CORRIGAN, T. & NICOLAIDES, A. N. (1972) Arteriography using ultrasound. *Lancet* **1**, 1269–1270.

FRANKLIN, D. L., SCHLEGEL, W. & RUSHMER, R. F. (1961) Blood flow measured by Doppler frequency shift of backscattered ultrasound. *Science, N.Y.* **134**, 564–565.

FRY, D. I. (1970) Ultrasonic monitoring for air embolism. *Anaesthesia* **25**, 144.

GILLIS, M. F., KARAGIANES, M. T. & PETERSON, P. L. (1968) Bends: detection of circulating gas emboli with external sensors. *Science, N.Y.* **161**, 579–580.

GILLIS, M. F., KARAGIANES, M. T. & PETERSON, P. L. (1969) Detection of gas emboli associated with decompression using the Doppler flowmeter. *J. occup. Med.* **11**, 245–247.

GILLIS, M. F., PETERSON, P. L. & KARAGIANES, M. T. (1968) In vivo detection of circulating gas emboli associated with decompression sickness using the Doppler flowmeter. *Nature, Lond.* **217**, 965–967.

GRAMIAK, R. & SHAH, P. M. (1971) Detection of intracardiac blood flow by pulsed echo ranging ultrasound. *Radiology* **100**, 415–418.

HEMPLEMAN, H. V. (1971) Discussion remarks. In *Underwater Physiology. Proc. 4th Symp. Underwater Physiology*. Ed. C. J. Lambertsen. p. 162. New York: Academic Press.

HILL, L. & MACLEOD, J. J. R. (1903) Caisson illness and divers' palsy. An experimental study. *J Hyg., Camb.* **3**, 401–445.

HUNTEC (1964) *Application of Ultrasonics to the Aetiology of Decompression Sickness: A Feasibility Study*. Parts 1 & 2. R. & D. Div., Huntec Ltd, Toronto.

IYENGAR, K. S. & RICHARDSON, E. G. (1958) Measurements on the air-nuclei in natural water which give rise to cavitation. *Br. J. appl. Phys.* **9**, 154–158.

KELLY, G. L., DODI, G. & EISMAN, B. (1972) Ultrasound detection of fat emboli. *Surgical Forum*, **XXIII**, 459–461.

KELSEY, C. A. (1970) A time–motion display method for A–scope ultrasonic units. *J. Ass. adv. med. Inst.* **4**, 165–166.

KIDD, D. J. (1969) Use of the pneumatic analogue computer for divers. In *The Physiology & Medicine of Diving & Compressed Air Work*. First Edition. Ed. P. B. Bennett & D. H. Elliott. pp. 386–413. London: Ballière, Tindall & Cassell.

KORPEL, A. (1966) Visualisation of the cross section of a sound beam by Bragg diffraction of light. *Appl. Phys. Letters* **9**, 425–427.

MACINTOSH, I. J. C. & DAVEY, D. A. (1972) Relationship between the intensity of ultrasound and induction of chromosome abberations. *Br. J. Radiol.* **45**, 320–327.

MACKAY, R. S. (1963) Discussion remark in *Proc. 2nd Symp. Underwater Physiology*. (Publ. 1181.) Ed. C. J. Lambertsen & L. J. Greenbaum. p. 41. Washington D.C.: Natl Acad. Sci.—Natl Res. Council.

MACKAY, R. S. (1968) Editorial comment in *Bioscience* **18**, 43.

MACKAY, R. S., & RUBISSOW, G. J. (1971) Detection of bubbles in tissues and blood. In *Underwater Physiology. Proc. 4th Symp. Underwater Physiology*. Ed. C. J. Lambertsen. pp. 151–160. New York: Academic Press.

MANLEY, D. M. J. P. (1969) Ultrasonic detection of gas bubbles in blood. *Ultrasonics* **7**, 102–105.

MAROON, J. C., EDMONDS-SEAL, J. & CAMPBELL, R. L. (1969) An ultrasonic method for detecting air embolism. *J. Neurosurg.* **31**, 196–201.

MAROON, J. C., GOODMAN, J. M., HORNER, T. G. & CAMPBELL, R. L. (1968) Detection of minute venous air emboli with ultrasound. *Surg. Gynec. Obstet.* **127**, 1236–1238.

MARTIN, F. E., HUDGENS, J. E. & WONN, J. E. (1973) *Manned Hyperbaric Demonstration of Incipient Bubble Detection using Nonlinear Ultrasonic Propagation*. ONR, Westinghouse Oceanic Division Report, 31 May.

MASON, W. VAN H., DAMON, E. G., DICKINSON, A. R. & NEVISON, T. O. (1971) Arterial gas emboli after blast injury. *Proc. Soc. exp. Biol. Med.* **136**, 1253–1255.

MINNAERT, M. (1933) On musical air bubbles and the sound of running water. *Phil. Mag.* (7th Ser.) **16**, 235–248.

NISHI, R. Y. (1972) Ultrasonic detection of bubbles with Doppler flow transducers. *Ultrasonics* **10**, 173–179.

NISHI, R. Y., & LIVINGSTONE, S. D. (1973) Intravascular changes associated with hyperbaric decompression: theoretical considerations using ultrasound. *Aerospace Med.* **44**, 179–183.

PATTERSON, R. H., KESSLER, J., BRENNAN, R. W. & TWICHELL, J. B. (1972) Ultrasonic detection of microemboli from artificial surfaces. *Bull. N.Y. Acad. Med.* **48**, 452–458.

POWELL, M. R. (1972a) Leg pain and gas bubbles in the rat following decompression from pressure: monitoring by ultrasound. *Aerospace Med.* **43**, 168–172.

POWELL, M. R. (1972b) Gas phase separation following decompression in asymptomatic rats: visual & ultrasonic monitoring. *Aerospace Med.* **43**, 1240–1244.

POWELL, M. R. (1973) In *NOAA OPS I and II: Formulation of Excursion Procedures for Shallow Undersea Habitats*. Ed. R. W. Hamilton, D. J. Kenyon, M. Freitag & H. R. Schreiner. UCRl-731, p. 126. Tarrytown, N.Y.: Union Carbide Corporation.

POWELL, M. R., HAMILTON, R. W. & KENYON, D. J. (1974) Comparison of helium, neon and neon–nitrogen mixtures for diving. *Undersea Biomed. Res.* **1**, A7.

RUBISSOW, G. J. & MACKAY, R. S. (1971) Ultrasonic imaging of in vivo bubbles in decompression sickness. *Ultrasonics* **9**, 225–234.

SATOMURA, S. (1957) Ultrasonic Doppler method for the inspection of cardiac functions. *J. acoust Soc. Am.* **29**, 1181–1185.

SMITH, K. H. & SPENCER, M. P. (1970) Doppler indices of decompression sickness: their evaluation and use. *Aerospace Med.* **41**, 1396–1400.

SMYTH, C. N. & SAYERS, J. F. (1959) Ultrasonic image camera. *Engineer, Lond.* **207**, 348–350.

SPENCER, M. P. & CAMPBELL, S. D. (1968) The development of bubbles in the venous and arterial blood during hyperbaric decompression. *Bull. Mason Clin.* **22**, 26–32.

SPENCER, M. P. & CLARKE, H. F. (1972) Precordial monitoring of pulmonary gas embolism and decompression bubbles. *Aerospace Med.* **43**, 762–767.

SPENCER, M. P. & OYAMA, Y. (1971) Pulmonary capacity for dissipation of venous gas emboli. *Aerospace Med.* **42**, 822–827.

SPENCER, M. P., SIMMONS, N. & CLARKE, H. P. (1971) A precordial transcutaneous cardiac output and aeroembolism monitor. *Fedn Proc. Fedn Am. Socs exp. Biol.* **30**, 703.

SPENCER, M. P., CAMPBELL, S. D., SEALEY, J. L., HENRY, F. C. & LINDBERGH, J. (1969) Experiments on decompression bubbles in the circulation using ultrasonic and electromagnetic flowmeters. *J. occup. Med.* **11**, 238–244.

TUCKER, D. G. & WELSBY, V. G. (1968) Ultrasonic monitoring of decompression. *Lancet* **1**, 1253.

TURNER, W. R. (1961) Microbubble persistence in fresh water. *J. acoust. Soc. Am.* **33**, 1223–1233.

WALDER, D. N. (1967) Ultrasonics in the detection of intravascular bubbles. *Can. med. Ass. J.* **96**, 1233–1234.

WALDER, D. N., EVANS, A. & HEMPLEMAN, H. V. (1968) Ultrasonic monitoring of decompression. *Lancet* **1**, 897–898.

WELLS, P. N. T. (1969) A range-gated ultrasonic Doppler system. *Med. biol. Engng.* **7**, 641–652.

WELSBY, V. G. (1950) *The Theory and Design of Inductance Coils.* p. 152, London: McDonald.

WELSBY, V. G. (1967) *Acoustic Non-linearity Due to Microbubbles in Water.* Dept. Memo No. 311. (Rev.) Department of Electronic & Electrical Engineering, University of Birmingham, England.

WELSBY, V. G. (1968) *Acoustic Detection of Gas Bubbles in the Bloodstream or Tissues.* Dept. Memo No. 359. Department of Electronic & Electrical Engineering, University of Birmingham, England.

WILD, J. J. (1950) The use of ultrasonic pulses for the measurement of biologic tissues and the detection of tissue density changes. *Surgery, St. Louis,* **27**, 183–188.

WILTON-DAVIES, C. C. (1970) *Computer-assisted Monitoring of ECG and Heart Sounds—1 Method.* Royal Naval Physiological Laboratory Report No. 7/70.

23

The Pathophysiology of Decompression Sickness

D. H. ELLIOTT & J. M. HALLENBECK

VALIDITY OF EXPERIMENTAL AND PATHOLOGICAL FINDINGS

A better understanding of the dynamic pathological processes of acute decompression sickness is essential if there is to be a rational basis for improved methods of prevention and treatment. It is the purpose of this brief review to reassess the available evidence relating to the course of events which may follow the formation of the hypothetical bubble.

Our knowledge of the pathology of decompression sickness in man is unavoidably scanty. We know that symptoms are preceded by a reduction of environmental pressure and, from the rapid response of most patients to treatment by recompression, deduce that bubbles are responsible. The illness itself is transient and any evidence from the post-mortem examination of fatal decompression sickness in animals and man must be qualified by the fact that it has been demonstrated that many bubbles are formed after death (Boycott, Damant & Haldane 1908), possibly accentuated by carbon dioxide accumulation (Harris et al. 1945a). Indeed the mere presence of bubbles in a body that has been exposed to raised environmental pressure requires careful interpretation since it has been shown by Hempleman (1968) that many bubbles are found in the bodies of animals not exposed to raised pressures till after death. Nevertheless examination of post-mortem material does demonstrate some ante-mortem changes that presumably can be attributed to the presence of bubbles.

Long before decompression became a hazard for man, bubbles had been seen in animals on decompression to the low pressures of simulated altitude (Boyle 1670a, b) and the consequences of bubbles in the cerebral circulation had been foreseen (Musschenbroek 1715). From the many early studies, which have been summarized and reviewed by Bert (1878) and Hill (1912), it is evident that bubbles may later be found in both the tissues and the blood vessels of animals decompressed from raised environmental pressures. Those found in the tissues were considered to have been formed there, whereas those found in the vessels could have originated in any part of the circulatory system or could be from the rupture of extravascular gas into the blood stream.

Since then it has been possible to consider with greater confidence the evidence for bubble formation during decompression sickness arising from in vivo studies in animals, particularly when interference with the tissues is kept to the minimum, and from post-mortem studies in which careful timing and techniques have reduced the chances of artefacts as far as possible (for instance, Gersh 1945; Lever et al. 1966; Spencer & Campbell 1968). More recently studies of decompression sickness have been concerned with the secondary changes induced by the presence of bubbles and such evidence will be reviewed in detail later in this chapter.

The pathology of decompression sickness resulting from exposure to ambient pressures less than 1 atmosphere absolute (1 bar; sea level) is relevant, but any indiscriminate transfer of findings from altitude to depth is unwise. Decompression to altitude increases the potential role of water vapour in bubble formation and growth, and also increases the significance of carbon dioxide which, as the pressure diminishes, remains at constant tension in the blood thus becoming an increasing proportion of the dissolved gases. Bubbles are evolved from a solution decompressed from atmospheric to a low ambient pressure less rapidly than from a solution decompressed from a raised pressure to atmospheric when the absolute ratio of pressure change in both instances is the same (Piccard 1941, 1944) and the differences between the clinical manifestations of decompression sickness in the diver and the aviator have been well described (Behnke & Stephenson 1942; Ferris & Engel 1951).

A similar reservation must be made when considering evidence from arterial and venous air embolism. While such findings are certainly relevant to the embolic hypotheses of decompression sickness, the presence of a potential supersaturation of dissolved gases in the tissues after decompression must modify any comparison of the effects of gaseous emboli in these different circumstances.

BUBBLE FORMATION

Decompression sickness is a result of a reduction of environmental pressure and is considered to be due to the formation of bubbles from gases dissolved in the tissues. A number of factors determine the quantity of gas dissolved in the tissues prior to the causative decompression. The primary factors are the depth and duration of the dive. The formation of bubbles is determined essentially by the rate of decompression of the individual from depth back to the surface. The principal factors are again pressure and time. As described in earlier chapters (17, 18, 19, 20 and 21), these are the parameters which basically determine the design of diving tables for the safe decompression of those at raised pressure and the prevention of decompression sickness. However,

the calculation of these tables is based on mathematical hypotheses which may estimate gas uptake in theoretical tissues, predict permissible supersaturations and may use functions derived from bubble regression curves, but which are not claimed to be truly analagous to physiological processes. The inestimable value of these tables has been to predict the decompression performance of the vast majority of workers in compressed air and divers with an outstanding measure of success. Nevertheless, with all such tables there remains a percentage (sometimes very small) of individuals who suffer from decompression sickness. Bert (1878) considered that one of the strangest features of decompression sickness was that if a group of men were decompressed together after the same exposure and most remained unaffected just one might become severely ill.

Thus in addition to the extrinsic factors imposed upon the individual there are the other factors which determine individual variability in susceptibility to decompression sickness. If the nucleation of the bubble is itself a random phenomenon (Hills 1966) this might account for some differences between individuals. The relevance of gas solubility and diffusion coefficients, tissue perfusion and the biophysics of bubble formation and growth are discussed elsewhere (Haldane & Priestly 1935; Behnke 1951; Harvey 1951; Hempleman 1963; Hills, 1966) and in previous chapters. Variability in susceptibility is also affected by those individual factors which probably influence the rate of inert gas uptake and elimination and the formation of bubbles: exercise at depth; exercise during the decompression; the quantities present of oxygen, carbon dioxide and contaminants such as the oxides of nitrogen; the obesity of the diver; his water balance, the ambient temperature both at depth and during the decompression; and the presence of any localized injury. The phenomenon of progressively greater tolerance to the effects of decompression has been described in man (Aldrich 1900; McWhorter 1910), even when the susceptible workers have been eliminated (Paton & Walder 1954), and has also been described in experimental animals (Aver'yanov 1965). This adaptation could also account for apparent variations in individual susceptibility to decompression sickness. If the outcome of these many factors is the formation of bubbles on decompression, then—in addition to variations in the amount and distribution of the bubbles formed—there is also potential variation in the response of the individual to these bubbles, response at the enzymatic and cellular level, as well as the possible response at higher levels such as the pain threshold. Thus the formation of bubbles in the tissues on decompression is an event which can lead to a number of different manifestations or which may remain asymptomatic.

Recently several laboratories using ultrasound have shown that bubbles exist in the circulation of apparently healthy individuals after decompressions which have caused no overt decompression sickness (Spencer & Oyama 1971; Spencer & Okino 1972; Evans, Barnard & Walder 1972). This finding confirms the hypothesis of the 'silent bubble' (Behnke 1945) and, together with evidence of the presence of silent bubbles from the double-dive experiments of Griffiths et al. (1971), also supports the view that tissues cannot retain a supersaturation of dissolved gas but that bubbles are formed on almost every decompression (Hills 1968). The role of the so-called silent bubble in the asymptomatic individual and also in an individual during the latent period before the onset of decompression illness is not yet fully understood, but as our knowledge increases it is probable that the pathophysiological significance of the 'silent' bubble will similarly increase.

Extravascular bubbles

Intracellular bubbles. The detection of intracellular bubbles is not easy. Certainly at postmortem fatty tissues commonly contain bubbles, more so in the less vascular abdominal fat than in the subcutaneous fat. After decompression of experimental animals gas bubbles were set free in the fat of tissue cells, disrupting them and causing related blood vessels to be filled with columns of bubbles (Hill 1912). A few intracellular bubbles have been described in the liver and larger numbers in the cord (Boycott, Damant & Haldane 1908; Boycott & Damant 1908).

A detailed study of the distribution of bubbles was undertaken in a series of experiments in which tissue, organ and whole-limb samples from freshly killed or live guinea pigs and rabbits were immersed in isopentane at $-150°C$ for a few seconds and then dried in a vacuum chamber at $-30°C$ prior to nitrocellulose infiltration (Gersh 1932). There is the reservation that this technique might produce bubbles as artefacts at sites where there had been no bubbles ante-mortem, but the absence of bubbles from these sites after lesser dive exposures suggests that the bubbles that are seen do at least identify potential bubble-producing areas. Minute bubbles were found as cell inclusions following simulated dives breathing different gases. The severity could be related to the fat solubility of the gas used, argon with 20% oxygen dives producing bubbles the same size as those produced by air dives, but twice as many (Gersh, Hawkinson & Jenney 1945). No extravascular bubbles were seen following exposures to simulated altitude, only intravascular ones—a finding that also followed the shallowest lethal dives (Gersh & Catchpole, 1946). After severe exposures to high pressures, bubbles were present in the extravascular tissues of bone marrow (Gersh 1945) and other fatty tissues such as the adrenal cortex and the myelin sheaths of nerves (Gersh & Hawkinson 1944). In fat tissue all gradations of bubble damage could be seen from minute bubbles within the fatty inclusions of cells to the gross gaseous distention and rupture of fat cells (Gersh, Hawkinson & Rathbun 1944). Cell rupture may cause local inflammation and haemorrhage and the release of gas bubbles and fatty emboli into the circulation (Hill 1912; Gersh & Hawkinson 1944; Haymaker 1957; Rait 1959) and the interstitial fluids.

Extracellular bubbles. On one occasion Boycott, Damant and Haldane (1908) found bubbles in the vitreous humour of the eye of a goat, though none in the aqueous humour. Similar observations have been made in man following oxy-nitrogen saturation dives (Beckman & Smith 1972). Bubbles have been seen in the anterior chamber of the eye by many including Harvey (1951) and Cockett, Nakamura and Franks (1965).

Extracellular bubbles have also been found in the synovial fluid, the amniotic fluid and the cerebrospinal fluid (Boycott, Damant & Haldane 1908; Harvey 1951).

If one accepts Guyton's view (1963) that interstitial fluid pressure averages 7 mm Hg below ambient, then, with the relatively high tissue tensions of dissolved gas which follow a dive, the formation of bubbles in the interstitial fluids of the body remains a significant possibility in spite of meagre supporting evidence. It is also probable that surface activity at the gas–fluid interface of the extracellular bubble can initiate secondary events such as those which will be discussed more fully in relation to intravascular and lymphatic bubbles.

Intravascular and lymphatic bubbles

The presence of bubbles in the blood vessels following relatively severe decompressions from raised pressures or to high altitude has been acknowledged since Hoppe-Selyer (1857). The observation that bubbles were more common in the veins was considered to be due to the lower pressure in veins than in arteries (Bert 1878). While early studies of intravascular bubbles (Behnke et al. 1936) suggested that the observed macroscopic bubbles represented a fairly late stage of severe decompression sickness, the concept of small 'silent bubbles', intravascular bubbles with no associated symptoms, was also proposed (Behnke 1945, 1955). Recent evidence from the use of ultrasonic bubble detectors implies that in fact gas embolism to the lungs is more common during decompression than had been thought previously. Such intravascular bubbles have been detected following asymptomatic decompressions and also in association with the peripheral musculoskeletal manifestations of decompression sickness in man (Spencer & Campbell 1968, 1974; Gillis, Karagianes & Peterson 1969; Evans, Barnard & Walder 1972).

There is no doubt that bubbles occur in the lymphatics (Boycott, Damant & Haldane 1908; Blinks, Twitty & Whitaker 1951; Lever 1967; Arturson & Grotte 1971). Such bubbles may be from the interstitial spaces or formed within the lymphatic vessels where pressure averages some 7 mm Hg below ambient (Guyton 1963).

The distribution of intravascular bubbles. In order to understand the apparent contradictions in the literature concerning the site of origin and the possible distribution of intravascular bubbles in decompression sickness, it is necessary to appreciate that not only are the various conclusions based on observations at different sites under dissimilar conditions but also that it has been shown that it is possible for bubbles or beads to pass through both systemic capillaries (Van Allen, Hrdina & Clark 1929; Emerson, Hempleman & Lentle 1967; Wells et al. 1971) and pulmonary capillaries (Prinzmetal et al. 1948; Tobin & Zariquiey 1953; Niden & Aviado 1956; Ring et al. 1961). Thus, for instance, while the first bubble at a particular site might be arterial, this observation may be only a consequence of the previous arrival of venous bubbles at the lung; and, similarly, a conclusion that intravenous bubbles represent an early phase in the development of decompression sickness is not incompatible with a hypothesis that intravascular bubbles originate in the lungs.

Following decompression from raised environmental pressure, intravascular bubbles have been seen first in the veins, particularly in the veins draining fatty tissues (Hill 1912; Gersh & Hawkinson 1944; Gersh, Hawkinson & Rathbun 1944). Bubbles may also be found in veins adjacent to fatty tissues but with which they have no anastomotic connections, for instance, in the abdominal wall overlying the pelvic fat (Lever 1967). However, post-mortem bubbles appear in the arteries only after decompressions which induce greater supersaturations of inert gas in the tissues than are required to produce bubbles in the veins (Harris et al. 1945b).

Muscular activity during decompression to altitude has produced bubbles in the veins of the active limb but none in the veins of the inactive limb (Whitaker et al. 1945). Ultrasound has demonstrated bubbles in the veins of a limb of a diver suffering from elbow pain due to decompression sickness, but none in the contralateral pain-free limb (Spencer & Campbell 1975).

Following decompression, arterial bubbles appeared before venous bubbles in cat cerebral vessels viewed through a Forbes window. Arterial bubbles were followed by a reduction of blood flow and a clumping of red cells with clear zones between the aggregations. Venous bubbles then appeared. The appearance of bubbles in the arteries before the veins after a severe decompression was also described in mice by Lever et al. 1966). There was a latent period of about 3 min before the sudden appearance in an abdominal skin flap of discrete bubbles passing rapidly through the arteries. The bubbles which lodged in the smaller arterial branches expanded in a retrograde direction to become columns of gas but no bubbles could be seen in the veins at this stage. Within 30 sec, bubbles appeared in the veins and enlarged rapidly so that most of the arteries and veins were soon filled with air, and blood remained in only some of the smaller veins. The arrival of arterial bubbles as the first observable event was noted at two other sites in these same animals, in the femoral and the mesenteric vessels.

The retrograde enlargement of an arterial bubble after embolism in a peripheral tissue may be responsible for the release of further small bubbles into other arteries by a process of budding off from the proximal end of the elongated primary bubble when it has extended back to the junction with another artery (Emerson, Hempleman & Lentle 1967). However, it should be noted that this conclusion is based on observations made during fulminant decompression sickness in small animals and may represent a mechanism found only when the circulation is failing.

The significance of the discrete arterial bubbles observed as the first event in certain sites (Lever et al. 1966) was studied further by Lever (1967). It was found that bubbles were seen after a latent period following decompression, first in the vena cava and particularly in the veins from the iliolumbar region and urogenital tract. These venous bubbles preceded the appearance of small arterial bubbles in the sites previously reported. In mild cases, the bubbles from the pelvic region were very few in number; the occasional bubbles moving slowly up the vena cava were often followed by a gasping respiration. Arterial bubbles were seen in less than 1% of the animals which recovered (Lever 1967).

In a number of studies on the sequence of events in acute decompression sickness viewing cuvettes have been placed in the femoral artery and vein (Leverett, Bitter & McIver 1963). On decompression of anaesthetized dogs from 60 min at 165 feet (6 ATA) to the surface in $2\frac{1}{2}$ minutes, bubbles were seen only in the venous cuvette. The animals remained at sea level for between 30 and 45 min during which they developed a shallow

respiration and a rapid rise of pulmonary artery pressure. It was not till the animals were further decompressed by exposure to altitude that bubbles were seen in the arterial cuvette. A similar sequence of events was observed by Gramenitskii and Savich (1965) using bubble traps inserted in the femoral vein and the carotid artery of dogs and rabbits. In animals exposed to 41 feet (2·25 ATA) for 6 hours venous but no arterial bubbles were seen. After exposure to 3 ATA, bubbles appeared in the venous trap after a latency of 5 to 8 min following rapid decompression. The venous foaming began to diminish after some 30 min and had gone by about 90 min. In three of five animals, all of which survived, some 10 to 20 bubbles appeared in the arterial trap but only at 10 to 12 min, i.e. some 5 min after the onset of venous bubbling. After decompression from even greater pressures (6 ATA) bubbles appeared in both venous and arterial traps; but if the animals were destined to survive, the appearance of further arterial bubbles ceased after some 12 to 20 min, even though venous bubbling continued vigourously. Similarly, McIver, Fife and Ikels (1965) reported that bubbles were always seen first in the venous viewing cuvette of dogs decompressed from nitrous oxide at raised environmental pressure.

The same sequence of events was found during the decompression of a sheep in which ultrasonic probes had been implanted on the inferior vena cava and the abdominal aorta (Spencer & Campbell 1968).

Studies of decompression bubbles in the microcirculation of the hamster cheek pouch have also confirmed that the first observed event in certain peripheral sites is the arrival of an embolic arterial bubble (Buckles 1968). The site of origin of the bubble is undetermined although its arrival after a rise of respiratory and heart rates suggested that it followed pulmonary bubble embolism. The cheek pouch preparation, mounted in a pressure chamber with controlled environmental conditions, can be observed microscopically and filmed with laser holography, thus allowing a more detailed study in vivo than was possible previously. Intravenous bubbles were seen in the cheek pouch only after the intra-arterial, but there were no intracapillary bubbles. It was observed that the venous bubbles entered the field of view in a retrograde manner after perfusion had been reduced by the arterial emboli. No bubbles were initiated within the field of view and no extravascular bubbles were seen.

From studies such as these emerges the possibility that Paul Bert (1878) was approaching the truth when he considered that most pulmonary vessels are blocked by bubbles and a few may pass through to become arterial emboli.

The site of origin of intravenous bubbles is still unknown. They may arise in the microvasculature or veins *de novo* or arrive there from some other site. While their origin could be extravascular it has also been postulated that they might arise in the turbulence of the left ventricle (Lever et al. 1966), or in the quiescent and poorly perfused portions of the lungs (Hempleman 1968). There is also the hypothesis (Walder 1969) that, possibly as a result of a ball-valve obstruction to one or more of the smaller airways by mucus, a localized barotrauma may occur during decompression causing small volumes of trapped pulmonary gas to be forced into the pulmonary capillaries. The subsequent showers of small gas bubbles might or might not cause lesions due to arterial embolism, but they would also have a potential for growth in the presence of excess tensions of dissolved gas while they pass through the tissues towards the systemic veins.

The direct effects of bubbles

Until recently, the mechanical effects of bubbles were considered to be primarily responsible for the pathology of decompression sickness. The bubble could be intravascular, causing obstruction of microvascular perfusion, local hypoxia, tissue damage and infarction; or it could be extravascular, causing tissue distortion or disruption. While there is no doubt that such effects can play a role in the development of decompression sickness, it is now recognized that bubbles can also produce a number of indirect effects which may be important in determining the course of the illness. A current research problem is that of determining the relative importance of the various pathological sequences that the bubble can initiate.

The surface activity of bubbles

It was considered by Harvey et al. (1944) that a layer of lipoprotein is formed at the fluid–gas interface of the bubble and that this would inhibit bubble growth and coalescence. The protein monolayer at such an interface would become denatured and thus this surface film would become relatively strong (Langmuir 1938; Malette, Fitzgerald & Eiseman 1960).

More recently, Lee et al. (1961) and Lee and Hairston (1971) have described a 40 to 100 Ångstrom layer of electrokinetic forces at the blood–gas interface that tends to orientate the exposed globular proteins such that their hydrophilic groups are in the blood while their non-polar groups protrude into the gaseous phase with a resultant disruption of the native secondary and tertiary configuration of the proteins. Since the biological specificity of function of globular proteins is related to their secondary and tertiary configuration, structural alteration of the protein molecules at the blood–gas interface also causes a functional alteration. Many of the denatured proteins are lyophobic, thus promoting the clumping of cells. In this way surface activity of bubbles can lead to platelet aggregation and clumping of red cells. In addition, lipoproteins can be denatured, causing them to release bound lipid that then coalesces into globules which can lodge in microvessels and obstruct nutrient blood flow. Some of the proteins altered at the gas–blood interface acquire enhanced biological activity. Activation of the Hageman factor by the direct action of bubbles has been demonstrated (Hallenbeck et al. 1973). Thus surface activity will begin a series of events leading to possible intravascular coagulation and activation of the complement system, kinins, and other smooth muscle activating factors (Ratnoff 1969).

Both increased and decreased enzyme activity can result from the interfacial exposure of globular proteins (Lee & Hairston 1971). Any process causing an extensive or indiscriminate alteration of enzymes could be very disruptive to the normal dynamic equilibrium of various enzyme systems. The haphazard disruption of kinin, complement, coagulation and fibrinolytic systems could be another factor in the individual variability of decompression sickness.

The surface activity of bubbles in acute decompression sickness is considered to lead a

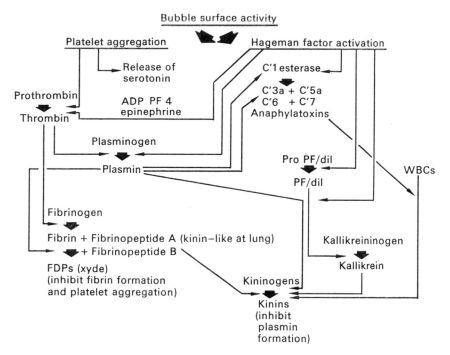

FIG. 23.1. Some pathways initiated by surface activity at the blood–bubble interface.

number of effects (Fig. 23.1) which include changes discussed below in the haemostatic mechanism, blood rheology, and the role of vaso-active substances.

INTRAVASCULAR EVENTS

Haematological effects

Many measurements have been made of the changes of various blood indices in relation to diving and decompression sickness. Some changes are initiated before decompression has begun, implying either some direct effect of pressure or an indirect effect by dissolved gases upon the body, but, while such changes may affect in some way the subsequent decompression performance, they are not considered further here as an integral part of decompression sickness.

The time course of acute decompression sickness is usually complete within hours of onset but it is worth considering some subtle and less rapid changes which occur after an apparently safe dive since they may have some relevance to the subse-

quent discussion of the pathology of the acute illness. Martin and Nichols (1972) estimated platelet levels daily before and after a compression chamber dive to 100 feet (30·5 m; 4 ATA) for 60 min with a 122-min decompression of established safety, and found a significant depression maximal on the third post-dive day. The fall was not apparent in a control group of naïve subjects who were not exposed to a change of environmental pressure during the simulated dive. Creatine phosphokinase, alkaline phosphatase, aspartate aminotransferase, cortisol and free fatty acids were also measured and showed changes suggesting an increased metabolic activity similar to that seen in a post-traumatic situation (Martin et al. 1975). No changes were found in prothrombin consumption index, fibrinogen or fibrin degradation products but there was an increase in euglobulin lysis activity in both dive and control groups indicating that this might be a psychosomatic response. Similar findings in swine have been reported by Stegall and Smith (1975) and the depression of platelets following a safe dive has been confirmed by Philp (1973). While changes which have a time course spread over several days are too slow to be a part of an acute illness which begins within hours if not minutes of surfacing, such changes may be relevant to the adaptation, or conversely the sensitization, of a diver to the effects of a further decompression undertaken before he has returned to his normal state.

A much more rapid fall in the number of circulating platelets has been reported in decompression sickness (Philp & Gowdey 1969; Sicardi 1970; Philp, Schacham & Gowdey 1971; Adebahr 1972; Philp et al. 1972; Stegall & Smith 1975). Using ^{51}Cr-tagged platelets in miniature swine Stegall, Smith and Hildibrandt (1973) showed that platelet survival time is markedly shortened in acute decompression sickness. The adherence of platelets to the gas–blood interface has been shown by both light microscopy (Adebahr 1971; Philp 1973) and electron microscopy (Philp, Inwood & Warren 1972). Transmitted electron microscopy revealed that there was a layer of densely packed platelets adhering to the bubble surface. In many instances large lipid particles were observed as well as a thin membrane around the bubble itself, a 200 Ångstrom electron dense layer thought to contain fibrinogen (Warren, Philp & Inwood 1973).

Platelet adherence, release and aggregation reactions

Platelets have three known primary functions (Salzman 1971); they participate in haemostasis, serve as vehicles for pharmacologically active agents and contribute to endothelial integrity.

The initial event in the process leading to platelet aggregation is adherence of platelets to a surface that has been conditioned by such adsorbed plasma proteins as fibrinogen and gamma globulin (Salzman 1971). Platelets adhere to subendothelial collagen or elastin and to many nonbiological surfaces including bubbles (Philp, Inwood & Warren 1972). Following adherence, platelets release from intracellular granules a number of pharmacologically active constituents such as serotonin, epinephrine, adenine nucleotides (ADP), calcium, potassium and a group of cationic proteins known collectively as platelet factor 4 (PF-4). PF-4 antagonizes the action of

heparin (Salzman 1972). Agents such as epinephrine, ADP, serotonin and thrombin, as well as surface adherence stimulate platelet release making the reaction self perpetuating and providing a pathway for interaction of platelets and plasma coagulation in haemostasis. There is also an alteration of the platelet membrane during this step which makes phospholipid (platelet factor 3) available for adsorption of plasma procoagulants thereby accelerating clotting (Salzman 1972). The release reaction of platelets is followed by aggregation of adjacent platelets to form a plug or thrombus (Salzman 1971). Platelet aggregation is associated with a reduction of platelet cyclic AMP, and agents that increase platelet cyclic AMP inhibit platelet aggregation (Zieve & Greenough 1969; Salzman 1972). Platelet aggregation is the initial event in arterial thrombosis and is a component of venous clotting (Mustard & Packham 1970).

INTRAVASCULAR COAGULATION

Disseminated intravascular coagulation may be defined as a generalized activation of the haemostatic mechanism by any of a variety of stimuli causing consumption of fibrinogen, platelets and sometimes various procoagulants with secondary activation of the fibrinolytic system. Whether the process remains clinically silent as a 'balanced consumption' tilts toward formation of stable clots in the microcirculation with tissue necrosis or tilts toward abnormal bleeding depends on the relative rates of thrombin elaboration and plasmin formation. A very lucid review of the subject is provided by Deykin (1970). Philp, Gowdey and Prasad (1967) suggested that intravascular bubbles might cause platelet aggregation and coalescence of plasma lipids which could lead to microvascular occlusion and contribute to the pathophysiology of decompression sickness. These suggestions arose from their experimental observations that severe bends in rats were accompanied by thrombocytopenia and reduced plasma lipids. The same laboratory has shown that artificially elevated platelet counts exacerbate decompression sickness (Philp & Gowdey 1969). Holland (1969) considered the relationship between decompression sickness and disseminated intravascular coagulation suggesting that this may occur in decompression sickness especially when complicated by shock. Sicardi (1970) also noted changes in platelets and coagulation factors during decompression sickness. The survival time of ^{125}I-labelled fibrinogen becomes markedly shortened following decompression sickness in miniature pigs (Smith et al. 1973). The in vitro demonstration that bubbling accelerates the clotting of whole blood and cell-free plasma (Hallenbeck et al. 1973) lends further support to the possibility that intravascular bubbling during decompression sickness could cause a generalized activation of the haemostatic mechanism. Indeed, reports abound of altered coagulation studies and changes in coagulation factors after extracorporeal circulation, a situation in which surface activity at the gas–blood interface is analogous to that in decompression sickness (Osborn et al. 1955; Penick et al. 1958; Nilsson and Swedberg 1959; Lee et al. 1961; Gans, Lillehei & Krivit 1961; Kevy et al. 1966). However, it should be stressed that the importance of intravascular coagulation in the pathology of decompression sickness remains to be evaluated.

Haemoconcentration and hypovolaemia

Haemoconcentration and shock have been recognized as complications of decompression sickness for some time, especially following altitude exposures (Brunner, Frick & Bühlmann 1964; Cockett & Nakamura 1964a, b; Fryer 1969). These were thought to be due to oedema caused by anoxic damage of the pulmonary capillaries (Masland 1948) or of all capillaries (Behnke et al. 1936). The shock has also been considered to be a result of cerebral fat embolism complicating decompression sickness (Haymaker 1957; Rait 1959). A supplementary or alternative hypothesis outlined below is that a localized increase of post-capillary viscosity due to bubble-induced cellular aggregation promotes transcapillary fluid loss. Haemoconcentration has amounted to as much as 45% in man (Cockett & Nakamura 1964b) and has also followed the introduction of large volumes of air into the circulation (Cooke 1962).

Cockett and Nakamura (1964a) documented hypovolaemia using ^{131}I-labelled plasma albumin

in anaesthetized dogs after decompression from 60 min at 165 feet (6 ATA). One hour later there was a 6 to 25% reduction and, 3 hours later, a 13 to 29% reduction of pre-dive plasma volumes. A similar study in dogs decompressed to 15 000 feet altitude (0·55 ATA) for 5 min and recompressed to ground level revealed a more than 30% reduction of plasma volume 5 hours later (Cockett, Nakamura & Franks 1965).

Labelled albumin may give a misleading picture of blood volume when there is also an increased permeability that permits albumin loss into the tissues. ^{51}Cr-tagged red cells serve as an indication that is confined to the intravascular space. These were combined with ^{125}I-labelled albumin in a study in which blood samples were taken at intervals following the single injection of the isotopes in order to detect deviations from the predicted concentration curve as a consequence of safe or hazardous dives (Hallenbeck et al. 1973).

In these studies safe and limb-bend provoking dives were not associated with plasma loss but paretic dives were accompanied by varying degrees of transcapillary isotonic plasma loss.

Rheological changes

On the basis of work by Swindle (1937) it was postulated that an aggregation of red blood cells was the primary cause of the manifestations of decompression sickness (End 1938) but no histological evidence to support this could be found by Catchpole and Gersh (1947). More recently the presence of red cell clumping in decompression sickness has been confirmed and has been related to concurrent rheological changes and increased blood viscosity (Wells et al. 1971). The interrelationships between blood rheology, flow resistance and transcapillary fluid movement have been reviewed by Chien (1969).

Anything which tends to lower flow velocity, such as the presence of myriads of intravascular bubbles, will also cause a higher viscosity in the post-capillary than in the pre-capillary segments because the shear rates are relatively low in the post-capillary segments. This rise in post-capillary viscosity causes an increase of flow resistance in these vessels thereby increasing capillary pressure and promoting transcapillary fluid loss (Fig. 23.2).

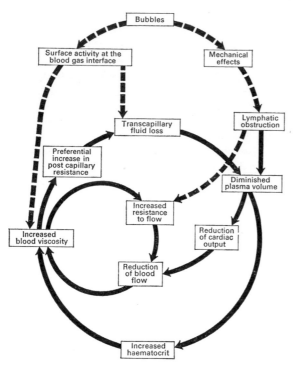

FIG. 23.2. Relationship between blood rheology, vascular resistance and transcapillary fluid shifts in decompression sickness.

Lipid emboli

The significance of the role of lipid emboli in acute decompression sickness has yet to be fully defined. The occasional finding of apparent bone marrow emboli in the lungs following decompression sickness (Clay 1963; Bennison, Catton & Fryer 1965; Cockett, Nakamura & Franks 1965) seems to support the hypothesis that expanding gas bubbles in the marrow can disrupt and dislodge bone marrow and fat cells with consequent intravasation of lipid and cell debris. It is also probable that another source of lipid emboli is the coalescence of plasma lipids into globules (Bergentz 1961; Sevitt 1962) after their release from lipoproteins which have been denatured at blood–gas interfaces (Lee et al. 1961). Indeed, lipid embolism may be the result of a change in the physical state of the blood associated with an activation of the haemostatic process (Bergentz 1968; Halleraker 1970).

Fat emboli have been found not only in the lungs but in the renal glomeruli of experimental animals (Clay 1963), in the choroid plexus of a compressed air worker (Bennison, Catton & Fryer 1965), and in the cerebral vessels of nine altitude fatalities, though none were noted in the cerebral vessels of three diving fatalities (Haymaker & Johnston 1955). Further cases of cerebral fat embolism after fatal exposure to altitude have been reported by Hickey and Stembridge (1958) and Odland (1959), and pulmonary fat embolism has been reported in two fatal cases of decompression sickness in compressed air workers (Fryer 1961). The amount of fat embolism found in such cases was insufficient to cause death (Fryer & Roxburgh 1965) but circulating fat may contribute to shock (Haymaker 1957; Rait 1959).

The possible role of lipid emboli in the aetiology of aseptic necrosis of bone, an occupational disease of divers and compressed air workers, is discussed elsewhere (Jones & Sakovich 1966).

Inflammatory and smooth muscle active amines, peptides and prostaglandins

Tissue damage due to direct mechanical effects of bubbles would be expected to cause the local release of mediators of inflammation. Bubble surface activity leads to platelet aggregation (Philp et al. 1972; Adebahr 1971) and during this process serotonin and epinephrine are released (Mustard & Packham 1970; Salzman 1972). Hageman factor activation by bubble surface activity has also been demonstrated (Hallenbeck et al. 1973) and this can lead to activation of the complement and kinin systems in addition to coagulation and fibrinolysis (Ratnoff 1969).

Chryssanthou et al. (1964) showed that bradykinin worsened decompression sickness in mice while such bradykinin antagonists as MA 1050 reduced mortality under the same experimental conditions. He and his co-workers isolated a smooth muscle activating factor (SMAF) that sensitized smooth muscle to the action of bradykinin, acetylcholine, serotonin and histamine as well as causing smooth muscle to contract and increasing capillary permeability (Chryssanthou et al. 1970). This substance was observed to increase in mouse lung during decompression sickness. Philp and Gowdey (1969) found that serotonin administration exacerbates decompression sickness in rats. However, Kindwall, Boreus and

Westerholm (1962) failed to detect changes in serotonin or histamine levels in various rat tissues following explosive decompression. They also found no mesenteric mast cell degranulation in these animals.

A great deal of basic investigative effort is required before the role of smooth muscle active substances in decompression sickness can be clearly defined. However, their *potential* contribution to the pathophysiology of the disease should be discussed. Serotonin, bradykinin and histamine are capable of provoking pain according to Armstrong et al. (1957). Majno and Palade (1961) and Majno, Palade and Shoefl (1961) have demonstrated that serotonin and histamine cause increased venular permeability to colloidal carbon by forming 1000 to 8000 Ångstrom interendothelial gaps. Kinins also increase capillary permeability (Spector 1958, Wilhelm 1962; Spector 1964) as do the complement anaphylatoxins, $C'3a$ and $C'5a$ (Kellermeyer & Graham 1968; Bruninga 1971). Thus these vasoactive substances may have a part in the plasma loss that accompanies severe decompression sickness. However, the permeability response in mildly injured vessels is biphasic. An early transient 30- to 60-min phase occurring in the venules is irrelevant to a much more important delayed and sustained phase which develops in the capillaries in response to an unknown mediator (Spector, Walters & Willoughby 1965; Wilhelm & Mason 1960). Histamine and serotonin and probably also the others are mediators of early permeability.

A number of studies suggest that various smooth muscle active substances may well participate in the pulmonary vascular and ventilatory changes that occur during decompression sickness. Serotonin, histamine and prostaglandins are inactivated as well as released by lung (Said 1968a; Lee 1971; Gruby et al. 1971). Said (1968b) has reviewed the capacity of lung to degrade and inactivate these smooth muscle active substances. Others have investigated their release by lung. Several authors have reported that autologous clot emboli in dogs caused serotonin release and consequent intrapulmonary venoconstriction (Yoshitake 1967; Daicoff et al. 1968). Alabaster and Bakhle (1970) found that histamine infusion in isolated rat and guinea pig lung caused a rise in perfusion pressure and release of serotonin, SRS-A, and prostaglandins. Palmer, Piper and Vane (1970a, b) reported that histamine, SRS-A, and prostaglandin release occurred when various particulates were embolized into perfused guinea pig lung. PGE_1 and PGE_2 were found by Lindsey and Wyllie (1970) in the effluent from perfused guinea pig lung after embolization with various particulates. These studies indicate that *embolized* lung can release vasoactive and smooth muscle active substances thereby increasing their concentration in blood. Histamine caused bronchospasm, increased airway pressure, decreased transmural capillary pressure and consequent increased pulmonary vascular resistance in an isolated lung preparation used by Kira and Rodbard (1971). The intrapulmonary venoconstriction due to serotonin has already been mentioned and this contributes to pulmonary artery pressure (PAP) rise (Yoshitake 1967; Daicoff et al. 1968). Said (1968a) noted that intravenous infusion of PGE_2 and PGF_2 caused a rise in PAP dogs. A rise in PAP contributes to the formation of pulmonary oedema (Szidon, Pietra & Fishman 1972). Pietra et al. (1971) documented an increased permeability of canine bronchial venules, but not pulmonary venules, after intravenous administration of histamine and bradykinin and this would also lead to an increase in pulmonary interstitial fluid. Such smooth muscle active substances as histamine, bradykinin and SRS-A cause bronchospasm and increased airflow resistance (Kellermeyer & Graham 1968; Orange & Austen 1969; Orange et al. 1971).

Thus there is ample indirect evidence to suggest that smooth muscle active substances are released both peripherally and from the lung during the course of acute decompression sickness and that these agents may well mediate to some extent pain, plasma loss, bronchospasm with increased airflow resistance, PAP rise and pulmonary oedema in various forms of the disease.

PULMONARY AND CARDIOVASCULAR EFFECTS

It was considered by Hoppe-Selyer (1857) that occlusion of the pulmonary capillaries by gases which had been set free in the circulation was a cause of death in acute decompression sickness. Also, as has been demonstrated by ultrasound (Spencer & Okino 1971; Evans, Barnard & Walder 1972; Spencer & Campbell 1975), it is probable that bubble emboli reach the lungs relatively harmlessly following decompression of many who remain symptom-free. With such a spectrum of effects it is tempting to postulate some dose-response relationship between the size and number of bubbles arriving at the lungs and the onset and severity of respiratory decompression sickness, even though there will be considerable variation between individuals in the nature of their response to these emboli.

Thus it is probable that bubbles arriving at the lungs, together with the products of their surface activity such as platelet and red cell aggregates, lipid emboli, vasoactive compounds and altered proteins, may cause a mechanical and reactive increase in pulmonary vascular resistance and release of local humoral agents (Chryssanthou et al. 1970) while the arriving bubbles will continue to have an indirect effect due to their surface activity.

In dogs decompressed from a 60 psi gauge (134 feet; 5 ATA) exposure for 90 min there is, after a latency of about 30 min, a rise in respiratory rate associated with the appearance of bubbles in cutaneous vessels (Behnke 1945). It was estimated by Bernthal, Horres and Taylor (1961) that not more than 10% of the pulmonary vascular bed was obstructed at the onset of increased frequency and decreased amplitude of breathing and therefore that it would be unlikely for any haemodynamic consequences of that obstruction to have caused the respiratory response. This is supported by the view of Binger, Brow and Branch (1924) that tachypnoea was a reflex response to a pulmonary arteriolar obstruction. The sudden respiratory gasp of an anaesthetised animal soon after the passage of an isolated bubble up the inferior vena cava (Lever 1967) also favours a mechanically induced reflex. The relative importance of the various causative factors of the tachypnoeic reflex in pulmonary embolism has been reviewed by Whitteridge (1950) and Marshall (1965).

The possible role of the lung in the production of severe decompression sickness is emphasized by the facts that serotonin, histamine and prostaglandins are released as well as inactivated by the lung (Said 1968a, b; Lee, 1971; Gruby et al. 1971). Indeed, embolization by various particulates has released serotonin, histamine, SRA-A and prostaglandins with an associated intrapulmonary venoconstriction and a rise of perfusion pressure (Daicoff et al. 1968; Alabaster & Bakhle 1970; Palmer, Piper & Vane 1970a, b) while PGE_1 and PGE_2 have been found in the effluent from embolized guinea pig lung (Lindsey & Wyllie 1970).

These smooth muscle active agents can cause a reactive increase in pulmonary vascular resistance, through a vasoconstriction mediated by locally released and blood-borne vasoactive substances. Smooth muscle active agents that provoke bronchospasm also cause an indirect reactive increase in pulmonary vascular resistance by decreasing transmural capillary pressure. In an isolated lung preparation, Kira and Rodbard (1971) showed that histamine caused bronchospasm, increased airway pressure, decreased transmural capillary pressure and consequently increased pulmonary vascular resistance. The serotonin-induced intrapulmonary venoconstriction contributes to a rise of pulmonary artery pressure (PAP). Infusion of PGE_2 and PGF_2 in dogs also caused a rise of PAP (Said 1968a). The combined effect of the mechanical and reactive increase of pulmonary vascular resistance leads to another significant effect, an interstitial pulmonary oedema (Szidon, Pietra & Fishman 1972). As in 'shock-lung', lysozome release from leucocytes may well contribute to pulmonary endothelial damage and interstitial oedema (Wilson 1972).

An increased permeability of canine bronchial venules after intravenous histamine and bradykinin also leads to an increase in pulmonary interstitial fluid (Pietra et al. 1971). The smooth muscle active substances also cause a bronchospasm and increased airflow resistance (Kellermeyer & Graham 1968; Orange & Austen 1969; Orange et al. 1971).

It seems probable that the response of the lungs to gas emboli will depend on the rate of arrival of the emboli. Thus a few bubbles may lose their gas by excretion through the lungs and the activation or release of the various smooth muscle active

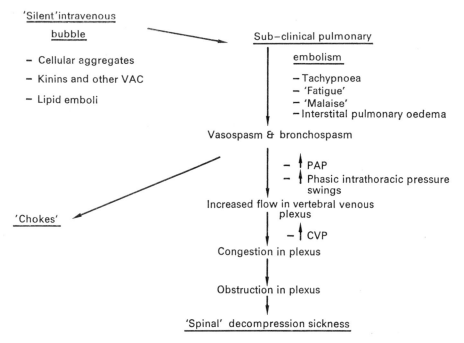

FIG. 23.3. The possible sequence of events leading from the intravenous bubble to respiratory and neurological decompression sickness

substances may cease. A few more bubbles may, by their mechanical and surface effects, cause some definite but asymptomatic change such as moderate tachypnoea with some interstitial pulmonary oedema. Yet more bubbles may lead to a rise of PAP, bronchospasm and, secondarily, a marked increase in the cyclic swings of intra-thoracic pressures with respiration.

The rise of pulmonary artery diastolic pressure (PADP) was associated with tachypnoea in decompression sickness in dogs and was reversed by recompression (McIver, Fife & Ikels 1965). When the bubbles were sufficient to cause an 'air-lock' in the right ventricle the decrease in cardiac output led to circulatory failure (Durant & Oppenheimer 1957). More recently, studies of PAP and right ventricular pressure (RVP) in dogs showed that these rose soon after ascent from 220 feet (7·7 ATA) for 40 min at the time that tachypnoea and bronchospasm became evident. Subsequently CVP and venous pressure at the confluence of sinuses rose, followed by a large rise of cerebro-spinal fluid pressure (CSFP) (Hallenbeck, Bove & Elliott 1975). The sequence of these events and

the associated change of blood flow in the epidural vertebral venous system (EVVS) will be discussed in relation to the onset of neurological decompression sickness (Fig. 23.3). Mean aortic pressure, as well as PAP, rose as the decompression sickness progressed. This was associated with a decrease in cardiac output and an increase in peripheral vascular resistance (Hallenbeck, Bove & Elliott 1975).

Similar changes have been noted in air embolism (Durant, Long & Oppenheimer 1947; Hallenbeck, Bove & Elliott 1975), and the observation by Durant and Oppenheimer (1957) that pain in the chest with an irritating cough was noted in some clinical cases of venous air embolism supports the analogy with pulmonary decompression sickness. However, Ferris and Engel (1951) postulated a lesion of the respiratory mucous membrane, similar to the cutaneous manifestations of decompression sickness, to account for the symptoms of 'chokes', a view supported by Fryer and Roxburgh (1965). Fryer (1969) maintained that in aviators, who show no evidence of pulmonary or venous congestion in altitude decompression sickness, the symptoms are not necessarily caused by embolic bubbles. On the other hand it is equally possible that some cutaneous manifestations of decompression sickness are themselves a reactive response to intravascular bubbles. It is relevant that pulmonary oedema and congestion are a consistent finding at post-mortem examination of altitude decompression sickness in man (Haymaker & Davison 1950; Haymaker 1957).

NEUROLOGICAL LESIONS

The distribution of neurological lesions in decompression sickness poses a fundamental problem. *A priori* several considerations favour the brain to be that portion of the central nervous system (CNS) to be predominantly affected by arterial emboli. In clinical embolic disorders such as subacute bacterial endocarditis, fat embolism or the presence of a mural thrombus in the left atrium, the brain is the principal target organ whereas arterial embolism of the spinal cord is extremely rare. For instance, in a series of 3737 autopsies at a hospital for neurological diseases there were only 11 cases of vascular disease of the cord and none were due to arterial emboli (Blackwood 1958). Indeed, a perusal of current textbooks of neuropathology shows that when describing arterial emboli most authors refer to the cord only because it is the site of some of the lesions of decompression sickness. Furthermore, it has been demonstrated experimentally that gas emboli are distributed with arterial flow according to their buoyancy (Van Allen, Hrdina & Clark 1929), a finding supported by the dominance of cerebral involvement in arterial air embolism complicating pulmonary barotrauma. Also, with the gross proportions of grey to white matter approximately the same in brain and cord, the brain constitutes some 98% of the mass of the human CNS (Truex & Carpenter 1969). Having some 75 to 85 more times the total blood flow of the cord (Kety 1960) the brain should accordingly receive proportionately more of any arterially distributed emboli.

Standing in stark contrast to the cerebral distribution of arterial emboli is the dominance of spinal cord lesions in the neurological manifestations of acute decompression sickness in man.

Besides a possibly greater lipid content (Brante 1949), the explanations for this can be related to the blood vessels of the cord. The findings of bubbles, inflammation and softening in the brain and spinal cord of laboratory animals and at post-mortem examination of human fatalities were reviewed in detail by many including Bert (1878), Heller, Mager & von Schrotter (1900), Hill (1912) and Haymaker (1957). Boycott, Damant and Haldane (1908) found extravascular bubbles in the CNS but considered the principal lesion to be due to arterial gas embolism. Small bubbles circulating slowly through white matter of the lower dorsal and upper lumbar segments of the spinal cord would quickly increase in size from gases dissolved in the surrounding tissues, lodge and produce infarction. They considered that at similar sites at other less affected parts of the cord, the collateral circulation would be more effective and, as in non-fatty tissues, infarction would not occur. This view of the embolic origin of cord lesions was supported by Behnke and Shaw (1937) who reported that neurological involvement was often preceded by respiratory disturbances and by Gersh and Catchpole (1951) who were unable to demonstrate histologically any extravascular bubbles in the cord. Gas bubbles could be demonstrated in the blood vessels of the cord and, in the peripheral nerves, gas bubbles could be seen, confined to the myelin sheath (Gersh, Hawkinson & Jenney 1945).

The hypothesis of Boycott, Damant and Haldane (1908) is supported by their observation that the arterial supply is relatively sparse especially in the deeper regions of the white matter of the cord (Boycott & Damant 1908) and by Kety (1960) who finds that the perfusion rate in the white matter of the cord is only some 60% of that in the white matter of the brain. However, an alternative hypothesis is based on the observation that the venous drainage of the spinal cord is into the epidural vertebral venous system (Batson 1940) in which flow is closely related to intrathoracic pressures.

It has been observed that decompression sickness is frequently associated with a period of respiratory embarrassment (Behnke & Shaw 1937). In a series of 24 cases of neurological decompression sickness, respiratory symptoms were recorded in 12; out of the 6 in whom the records describe separate times of onset there were 5 in whom the respiratory preceded the neurological symptoms (Elliott, Hallenbeck & Bove 1975).

The role of congestion in Batson's plexus and of arterial embolism were considered by Haymaker and Johnston (1955). Now, however, there is evidence that there is not merely a passive congestion of the vertebral venous system as a result of pulmonary vascular obstruction, but that there are localized areas of obstruction to venous drainage of the cord arising from the relationship between flow and the increased cyclic swings of intrathoracic pressure with respiration and also as an indirect result of the local effects of the surface activity of intravascular bubbles (Hallenbeck, Bove & Elliott 1975; Fig. 23.3).

Cinevenography of the vertebral venous plexus during pulmonary air embolism demonstrated a slowing of flow from the plexus during tachypnoea after an initial occasional slight increase. In one case a particulate contrast medium was seen to flow from the azygos vein into the vertebral venous system. Similar studies were undertaken in anaesthetized animals during the onset of acute neurological decompression sickness and showed changes from pre-dive flow patterns suggesting obstruction to flow of parts of the epidural vertebral venous plexus in the paretic dog.

Under similar conditions it was also found that, following the rise of PAP and RVP, there was a rise of CVP and pressure at the confluence of cerebral venous sinuses. This was accompanied by a marked rise of CSFP at which time the animals showed clear evidence of spinal cord dysfunction. After the signs of neurological decompression sickness had appeared the absence of normal manometric responses of cisternal fluid pressure to abdominal compression and lung inflation, which had been present before the dive, also suggested that, in the absence of a subarachnoid block, there was an obstruction to the vertebral venous system (Hallenbeck, Bove & Elliott 1975). Any tendency to stasis or congestion of a region of the EVVS will predispose that area to the formation and growth of bubbles, whether extravascular or intravascular, whether autochthonous or embolic, and lead to more platelet aggregation and further stasis. If stasis is maintained for roughly as long

as the silicone clotting time of the blood there will then be fibrin deposition (Botti & Ratnoff 1964). If an area of stasis or obstruction within the EVVS is situated near a critical radicular vein, the stage is set for further rheological disturbances leading to possible venous infarction.

The location of the lesions in these and similar studies as revealed macroscopically by intravital Evans Blue (Hallenbeck, Bove & Elliott 1975) was in close agreement with the location predicted by a preceding neurological examination. In 17 cases of paralytic decompression sickness, all had spinal cord involvement and 2 also had brain stem lesions. There was no brain involvement in these animals in which durations of exposure to depth had not approached saturation times. Venous congestion and blue staining by the albumin-bound dye were observed in paravertebral muscles of several dogs corresponding to the regions of spinal cord damage. Epidural and subarachnoid haemorrhages were also frequent. Residual thrombi within the epidural venous plexus and its tributaries were occasionally noted. In the cord, the infarcts were often grossly haemorrhagic and the white matter was principally affected. Together with the relative sparing of the grey matter these specimens formed a pathological picture typical of venous infarction of the CNS (Hensen & Parsons 1967). Examination by light and reflected electron microscopy confirmed the presence of intravenous pre-mortem thrombi in the cord and in the nerve roots where disruption of the myelin figures, possibly by extravascular gas, can also be seen (Elliott, Hallenbeck & Bove 1974).

Less frequently lesions of decompression sickness occur in other parts of the CNS. While a mechanism similar to that invoked for spinal cord lesions may be invoked for those seen in the brain stem, it remains possible that cerebral lesions, not common following dives of short duration, are a consequence of some other sequence of events in which the quantity of gas dissolved in the lipidrich tissues acquires greater significance.

The presence of areas of cerebral softening and of fluid-containing spaces as a frequent finding in the brains of compressed air workers has been reported by Roszaheygi (1959, 1967) though this has yet to be confirmed elsewhere. The lesions that may occur in the region of the inner ear require special mention and are described in Chapter 25.

MUSCULOSKELETAL EFFECTS

Perhaps the least known aspect of decompression sickness is the mechanism of the lesion which produces an acutely painful joint. This is in part because it is not accessible in man and is not reproducible in small animals. Goats show signs of joint pain incidental to experiments on decompression performance but, as far as is known, have not been sacrificed for examination during this relatively mild and easily reversible manifestation of the illness. Dogs also show similar signs but it is rare to be able to exclude some degree of neurological involvement in these animals either by clinical or by post-mortem examination.

Against any central mechanism for the origin of this pain is the observation by Spencer et al. (1969) of ultrasonically detected bubbles in the veins draining an affected elbow while none could be detected in the contralateral symptom-free limb. It was also observed that the local application of pressure equivalent to a descent of 10 000 ft has relieved the pain of limb bends induced at 35 000 ft altitude (Fryer 1969).

Theories concerning the site of bubble formation in limb bends have been discussed by Ferris & Engel (1951), Nims (1951) and Hills (1966, 1968), but the only histological studies have been on the joints of small animals after very rapid decompression (Gersh 1945). The only bubbles found were intravenous after brief exposures but, after more prolonged exposures, bubbles were seen in arteries, veins and sinusoids. Some Haversian systems were gas filled and there were some extravascular bubbles in the yellow marrow. Clay (1963) found disruption of the marrow and medullary haemorrhages in the femurs of a number of dogs exposed to a severe decompression. In the study by Gersh (1945) in guinea pigs there were, apart from some gas in one blood vessel in the capsule of the knee joint in one animal, no bubbles in the tissues of the joints, but numerous arteries and veins were gas filled in the vicinity of the long tendons near the ankle joint.

It is important to note that relatively large collections of free gas can be detected in human tissues both clinically and radiologically in persons who have no referable symptoms (Ferris & Engel 1951).

Aseptic necrosis of bone, an occupational hazard of work at raised environmental pressures, may be associated statistically with a history of decompression hazards (Walder 1970; Elliott 1971) but it is not necessarily a consequence of decompression sickness. It is discussed separately in Chapter 27.

CONCLUSION

Our knowledge of the dynamic processes which occur during decompression sickness is clearly far from complete. The evidence that does exist has been collected from many sources and it needs to be stressed that there are probably not only differences between different species but also that for each species there are probably several different forms of decompression sickness. Cases of decompression sickness are rarely confined to one clinical category but tend to spread to a lesser or greater degree throughout a range of possible manifestations. The final form of the illness is thus likely to be determined by many factors, both extrinsic—such as depth and duration of the dive, ambient temperature and decompression profile—and intrinsic—such as body weight and fat distribution, tissue perfusion rates and host response to bubbles. The focal point is now upon the surface activity at the blood–gas interface of the bubble, but it is not yet possible to assess the relative importance of these indirect surface effects vis-a-vis the direct mechanically obstructive effects of the bubble. Thus there are many possible pathophysiological pathways and one cannot predict the relative importance of each. Nevertheless it is encouraging that a logical and cohesive pattern is beginning to emerge.

REFERENCES

ADEBAHR, G. (1971) Zur frage der therapie bei Dekompressionkrankheit und bei Luftembolie. *Z. Rechtsmedizin* **68**, 225–238.

ADEBAHR, G. (1972) Morphologische Schokaquivalinte bei Luftembolie Taucherunfall und Decompressionskrankheit. *Beitr. gerichte. Med.* **29**, 87–91.

ALABASTER, V. A. & BAKHLE, Y. S. (1970) The release of biologically active substances from isolated lungs by 5-Hydroxytryptamine and Tryptamine. *Br. J. Pharmac.* **40**, 582–583.

ALDRICH, C. J. (1900) Compressed air illness; caisson disease. *Int. Clin.* (ser. 10) **2**, 73–78.

ARMSTRONG, D., JEPSOM, J. P., KEELE, C. A. & STEWART, J. W. (1957) Pain-producing substance in human inflammatory exudates and plasma. *J. Physiol, Lond.* **135**, 350–370.

ARTURSON, G. & GROTTE, G. (1971) Mechanism of edema formation in experimental decompression sickness. *Aerospace Med.* **42**, 58–61.

AVER'YANOV, V. A. (1965) Some conditions for the increase in body resistance to decompression disorders under the repeated effects of decompression. In *The Effect of the Gas Embolism and Pressures on Body Functions, III.* Ed. M. P. Brestkin. pp. 34–39. Washington D.C.: US Dept. of Commerce.

BATSON, O. V. (1940) The function of the vertebral veins and their role in the spread of metastasis. *Ann. Surgery* **112**, 138–149.

BECKMAN, E. L. & SMITH, E. M. (1972) Tektite II: Medical supervision of the scientists in the sea. *Tex. Rep. Biol. Med.* **30**, Suppl. 1–204.

BEHNKE, A. R. (1945) Decompression sickness incident to deep-sea diving and high-altitude ascent. *Medicine, Baltimore* **24**, 381–402.

BEHNKE, A. R. (1951) Decompression sickness following exposure to high pressures. In *Decompression Sickness.* Ed. J. F. Fulton. pp. 53–89. London: Saunders.

BEHNKE, A. R. (1955) Decompression sickness. *Milit. Med.* **117**, 257–271.

BEHNKE, A. R. & SHAW, L. A. (1937) The use of oxygen in the treatment of compressed-air illness. *Nav. med. Bull.* **35**, 61–73.

BEHNKE, A. R. & STEPHENSON, C. S. (1942) Applied physiology. *Am. Rev. Physiol.* **4**, 575–598.

BEHNKE, A. R., SHAW, L. A., MESSER, A. C., THOMSON, R. M. & MOTLEY, E. P. (1936) The circulatory and respiratory disturbances of acute compressed-air illness and the administration of oxygen as a therapeutic measure. *Am. J. Physiol.* **114**, 526–533.

BENNISON, W. H., CATTON, M. J. & FRYER, D. I. (1965) Fatal decompression sickness in a compressed-air worker. *J. Path. Bact.* **89**, 319–329.

BERGENTZ, S. E. (1961) Studies on the genesis of post-traumatic fat embolism. *Acta chir. scand.* Supplement 282.

BERGENTZ, S. E. (1968) Fat embolism. *Progr. Surg.* **6**, 85–120.

BERNTHAL, T., HORRES, A. D. & TAYLOR, J. T. (1961) Pulmonary vascular obstruction in graded tachypneagenic diffuse embolism. *Am. J. Physiol.* **200**, 279–286.

BERT, P. (1878) *La Pression Barometrique.* Paris: Masson. Translated by M. A. Hitchcock & F. A. Hitchcock (1943). Columbus: College Book Co.

BINGER, C. A., BROW, G. R. & BRANCH, A. (1924) Experimental studies on rapid breathing: tachypnoea dependent upon anoxaemia resulting from multiple emboli in the larger branches of the pulmonary artery. *J. clin. Invest.* **1**, 155–180.

BLACKWOOD, W. (1958) Discussion on vascular disease of the spinal cord. *Proc. R. Soc. Med.* **51**, 543–547.

BLINKS, L. A., TWITTY, V. C. & WHITAKER, D. M. (1951) Bubble formation in frogs and rats. In *Decompression Sickness.* Ed. J. F. Fulton. pp. 145–164. London: Saunders.

BOTTI, R. E. & RATNOFF, O. D. (1964) Studies on the pathogenesis of thrombosis; an experimental 'hypercoagulable' state induced by the intravenous injection of ellagic acid. *J. lab. clin. Med.* **64**, 385–398.

BOYCOTT, A. E. & DAMANT, G. C. C. (1908) Caisson disease: influence of fatness. *J. Hyg., Camb.* **8**, 445–456.

BOYCOTT, A. E., DAMANT, G. C. C. & HALDANE, J. S. (1908) Prevention of compressed air illness, *J. Hyg., Camb.* **8**, 342–443.

BOYLE, R. (1670a) New pneumatical observations about respiration. *Phil. Trans. R. Soc.* **5**, 2011–2031.

BOYLE, R. (1670b) Continuation of the observations concerning respiration. *Phil. Trans. R. Soc.* **5**, 2035–2056.

BRANTE, G. (1949) Studies on lipids in the nervous system with special reference to quantitative chemical determination and topical distribution. *Acta physiol. scand.* **18**, Supplement 63.

BRUNINGA, G. L. (1971) Complement—A review of the chemistry and reaction mechanisms. *Am. J. clin. Path.* **55**, 273–282.

BRUNNER, F. P., FRICK, P. G. & BÜHLMANN, A. A. (1964) Post-decompression shock due to extravasation of plasma. *Lancet* **1**, 1071–1073.

BUCKLES, R. G. (1968) The physics of formation and resolution of bubbles. *Aerospace Med.* **39**, 1062–1069.

CATCHPOLE, H. R. & GERSH, I. (1947) Pathogenetic factors and pathological consequences of decompression sickness. *Physiol. Rev.* **27**, 360–397.

CHIEN, S. (1969). Blood rheology and its relation to flow resistance and transcapillary exchange with special reference to shock. *Adv. Microcirc.* **2**, 89–103.

CHRYSSANTHOU, C., TEICHNER, F. & ANTOPOL, W. (1971) Studies on dysbarism IV. Production and prevention of decompression sickness in 'non-susceptible' animals. *Aerospace Med.* **42**, 864–867.

CHRYSSANTHOU, C., KALBERER, J., KOOPERSTEIN, S. & ANTOPOL, W. (1964) Studies on dysbarism II: Influence of Bradykinin and 'Bradykinin—antagonists' on decompression sickness in mice. *Aerospace Med.* **35**, 741–746.

CHRYSSANTHOU, C., TEICHNER, F., GOLDSTEIN, G., KALBERER, J. & ANTOPOL, W. (1970) Studies on dysbarism III: A smooth muscle-acting factor (SMAF) in mouse lungs and its increase in decompression sickness. *Aerospace Med.* **41**, 43–48.

CLAY, J. R. (1963) Histopathology of experimental decompression sickness. *Aerospace Med.* **34**, 1107–1110.

COCKETT, A. T. K. & NAKAMURA, R. M. (1964a) Newer concepts in the patho-physiology of experimental dysbarism—decompression sickness. *Am. Surg.* **30**, 447–451.

COCKETT, A. T. K. & NAKAMURA, R. M. (1964b) A new concept in the treatment of decompression sickness (dysbarism). *Lancet*, **1**, 1102.

COCKETT, A. T. K., NAKAMURA, R. M. & FRANKS, J. J. (1965) Recent findings in the pathogenesis of decompression sickness (dysbarism). *Surgery, St Louis* **58**, 384–389.

COOKE, J. (1962) Personal communication cited by Fryer, D. I. (1962) Observations concerning the mechanisms of sub-atmospheric decompression sickness. *Institute of Aviation Medicine Scientific Memorandum. No. 42.*

DAICOFF, G. R., CHAVEZ, F. R., ANTON, A. H., & SWENSON, E. W. (1968) Serotonin-induced pulmonary venous hypertension in pulmonary embolism. *J. thorac. cardiovasc. Surg.* **56**, 810–815.

DEYKIN, D. (1970) Clinical challenge of disseminated intravascular coagulation. *New Engl. J. Med.* **283**, 636–644.

DURANT, T. M. & OPPENHEIMER, M. J. (1957) Embolism due to air and other gases. *Med. Bull. M.B.I.* Dept. Med. & Surg. Veterans Admin. Wash.

DURANT, T. M., LONG, J. & OPPENHEIMER, M. J. (1947) Pulmonary (venous)-air embolism. *Am. Heart J.* **33**, 269–281.

ELLIOTT, D. H. (1971) The role of decompression inadequacy in aseptic bone necrosis of naval divers. *Proc. R. Soc. Med.* **69**, 1278–1280.

ELLIOTT, D. H., HALLENBECK, J. M. & BOVE, A. A. (1974) Acute decompression sickness. *Lancet* **2**, 1193–1199.

EMERSON, L. V., HEMPLEMAN, H. V. & LENTLE, R. G. (1967) The passage of gaseous emboli through the pulmonary circulation. *Resp. Physiol.* **3**, 312–319.

END, E. (1938) The use of new equipment and helium gas in a world record dive. *J. Indust. Hyg.* **20**, 511–520.

EVANS, A., BARNARD, E. E. P. & WALDER, D. N. (1972) Detection of gas bubbles in man at decompression. *Aerospace Med.* **43**, 1095–1096.

FERRIS, E. B. & ENGEL, G. L. (1951) The clinical nature of high altitude decompression sickness. In *Decompression Sickness, Caisson Sickness and Divers and Flier's Bends and Related Syndromes.* Ed. J. R. Fulton. pp. 514–552. Philadelphia: Saunders.

FRYER, D. I. (1961) Pathological findings in fatal sub-atmospheric decompression sickness. *Medicine Sci. Law* **2**, 110–123.

FRYER, D. I. (1969) *Sub-atmospheric Decompression Sickness in Man.* NATO AGARDograph 125.

FRYER, D. I. & ROXBURGH, H. L. (1965) Decompression sickness. In *Textbook of Aviation Physiology.* Ed. J. A. Gillies. pp. 122–151. Oxford: Pergamon.

GANS, H., LILLEHEI, C. W. & KRIVIT, W. (1961) Problems in haemostasis during open heart surgery: I. On the release of plasminogen activator. *Ann. Surg.* **154**, 915–924.

GERSH, I. (1932) The development of the Altmann freeze-drying method. *Anat. Rec.* **53**, 309–337.

GERSH, I. (1945) Gas bubbles in bone and associated structures, lung and spleen of guinea pigs decompressed rapidly from high-pressure atmospheres. *J. Cell. comp. Physiol.* **26**, 101–117.

GERSH, I. & CATCHPOLE, H. R. (1946) Appearance and distribution of gas bubbles in rabbits decompressed to altitude. *J. Cell comp. Physiol.* **28**, 253–270.

GERSH, I. & CATCHPOLE, H. R. (1951) Decompression sickness: physical factors and pathologic consequences. In *Decompression Sickness.* Ed. J. F. Fulton. pp. 165–181. London: Saunders.

GERSH, I. & HAWKINSON, G. E. (1944) *The Formation and Appearance of Tissue and Vascular Bubbles after Rapid Decompression of Guinea Pigs from High Pressure Atmospheres.* Research Project X-284. US Navy Medical Research Institute, Report No. 1.

GERSH, I., HAWKINSON, G. E. & JENNEY, E. H. (1945) Comparison of vascular and extravascular bubbles following decompression from high-pressure atmospheres of oxygen, helium–oxygen, argon–oxygen and air. *J. Cell. comp. Physiol.* **26**, 63–74.

GERSH, I., HAWKINSON, G. E. & RATHBUN, E. N. (1944) Tissue and vascular bubbles after decompression from high-pressure atmospheres—correlation of specific gravity with morphological changes. *J. Cell. comp. Physiol.* **24**, 35–61.

GILLIS, M. F., KARAGIANES, M. T. & PETERSON, P. L. (1969) Detection of gas emboli associated with decompression using the doppler flowmeter. *J. occup. Med.* **11**, 245–247.

GRAMENITSKII, P. M. & SAVICH, A. A. (1965) Results of experimental analysis of decompression air embolism. In *The Effect of Gas Embolism and Pressure on Body Functions, III.* Ed. M. P. Brestkin. pp. 47–56. Washington, D.C.: US Dept. of Commerce.

GRIFFITHS, H. B., MILLER, K. W., PATON, W. D. M. & SMITH, E. B. (1971) On the role of separated gas in decompression sickness. *Proc. R. Soc. B* **178**, 389–406.

GRUBY, L. A., ROWLANDS, C., VARLEY, B. Q. & WYLLIE, J. H. (1971) The fate of 5-Hydroxytryptamine in the lung. *Br. J. Surg.* **58**, 525–532.

GUYTON, A. C. (1963) Venous return. In *Handbook of Physiology*, Section 2: Circulation, vol. 2. Ed. W. F. Hamilton & P. Dow. pp. 1099–1133. Baltimore: Williams & Wilkins.

HALDANE, J. S. & PRIESTLEY, J. G. (1935) *Respiration.* Oxford: Clarendon Press.

HALLENBECK, J. M., BOVE, A. A. & ELLIOTT, D. H. (1975) Decompression sickness studies. In *Underwater Physiology. Vth Symp. Underwater Physiology.* Ed. C. J. Lambertsen. Bethesda: Fdn Am. Socs exp. Biol.

HALLENBECK, J. M., BOVE, A. A., MOQUIN, R. B. & ELLIOTT, D. H. (1973) Accelerated coagulation of whole blood and cell-free plasma by bubbling in vivo. *Aerospace Med.* **44**, 712–714.

HALLERAKER, B. (1970) Fat embolism and intravascular coagulation. *Acta path. microbiol. scand.* **78**, 432–436.

HARRIS, M., BERG, W. E., WHITAKER, D. M., TWITTY, V. C. & BLINKS, L. R. (1945a) Carbon dioxide as a facilitating agent in the initiation and growth of bubbles in animals decompressed to simulated altitudes. *J. gen. Physiol.* **28**, 225–240.

HARRIS, M., BERG, W. E., WHITAKER, D. M. & TWITTY, V. C. (1945b) The relation of exercise to bubble formation in animals decompressed to sea level from high barometric pressures. *J. gen. Physiol.* **28**, 241–251.

HARVEY, E. N. (1951) Physical factors in bubble formation. In *Decompression Sickness*. Ed. J. F. Fulton. pp. 90–144. London: Saunders.

HARVEY, E. N., BARNES, D. K., McELROY, W. D., WHITELEY, A. H., PEASE, D. C. & COOPER, K. W. (1944) Bubble formation in animals. I. Physical factors. *J. Cell. comp. Physiol.* **24**, 1–22.

HAYMAKER, W. (1957) Decompression sickness. In *Handbuch des Speziellen Pathologischen Anatomie und Histologie*. Ed. O. Lubarsch, F. Henke & R. Rossie. Vol. XIII, Pt. 1, pp. 1600–1672. Berlin: Springer-Verlag.

HAYMAKER, W. & DAVISON, C. (1950) Fatalities resulting from exposure to simulated high altitudes in decompression chambers. *J. Neuropath. exp. Neurol.* **9**, 29–59.

HAYMAKER, W. & JOHNSTON, A. D. (1955) Pathology of decompression sickness. A comparison of the lesion in airmen with those in caisson workers and divers. *Milit. Med.* **117**, 285–306.

HELLER, R., MAGER, W. & SCHROTTER, H. VON (1900) *Luftdrucker Krankungen mit Besonderer Berucksicktigung der Sogenannten Caisson Krankheit*. Wein: Alfred Holder.

HEMPLEMAN, H. V. (1963) Tissue inert gas exchange and decompression sickness. In *Proc. 2nd Symp. Underwater Physiology* (Publ. 1181.) Ed. C. J. Lambertsen & L. J. Greenbaum. pp. 6–13. Washington, D.C.: Natl Acad. Sci.-Natl Res. Council.

HEMPLEMAN, H. V. (1968) Bubble formation and decompression sickness. *Revue Physiol. Subaquatique* **1**, 181–183.

HEMPLEMAN, H. V. (1972) The site of origin of gaseous emboli produced by decompression from raised pressures of air and other gases. In *Proc. Third int. Conf. Hyperbaric and Underwater Physiology*. pp. 160–163. Doin: Paris.

HENSEN, R. A. & PARSONS, M. (1967) Ischemic lesions of the spinal cord: an illustrated review. *Q. Jl Med.* **36**, 205–222.

HICKEY, J. L. & STEMBRIDGE, V. A. (1958) Occurrence of pulmonary fat and tissue embolism in aircraft accident fatalities. *J. Aviat. Med.* **29**, 787–793.

HILL, L. (1912) *Caisson Sickness and the Physiology of Work in Compressed Air*. London: Arnold.

HILLS, B. A. (1966) *A Thermodynamic and Kinetic Approach to Decompression Sickness*. Adelaide: Libraries Board of S. Australia.

HILLS, B. A. (1968) Relevant phase conditions for predicting occurrence of decompression sickness. *J. appl. Physiol.* **25**, 310–315.

HOLLAND, J. A. (1969) *Discussion of Disseminated Intravascular Coagulation in Decompression Sickness*. US Navy. Sub-Med. Cen. Rep. 585.

HOPPE-SEYLER, F. (1857) Ueber den Einfluss, welchen der Wechsel des Lufdruckes auf das Blut ausubt. *Arch. Anat. Physiol.* **24**, 63–73.

JONES, P. J. & SAKOVICH, L. (1966) Fat embolism of bone. *J. Bone Jt Surg.* **48A**, 149–164.

KELLERMEYER, R. W. & GRAHAM, R. C. (1968) Kinins—possible physiologic and pathologic roles in man. *New Engl. J. Med.* **279**, 754–759, 802–807 & 859–866.

KETY, S. S. (1960) The cerebral circulation. In *Handbook of Physiology*, Section 1: Neurophysiology. Ed. J. Field, H. W. Magoun & V. E. Hall. pp. 1751–1960. Baltimore: Williams & Wilkins.

KEVY, S. V., GLICKMAN, R. M., BERNHARD, W. F., DIAMOND, L. K. & GROSS, R. E. (1966) The pathogenesis and control of the haemorrhagic defect in open heart surgery. *Surg. Gynec. Obstet.* **123**, 313–318.

KINDWALL, E. P., BOREUS, L. O. & WESTERHOLM, B. (1962) Failure to show change in rat tissue histamine and serotonin after rapid decompression. *Am. J. Physiol.* **203**, 389–390.

KIRA, S. & RODBARD, S. (1971) Effects of histamine and acetylcholine on the isolated perfused lung lobe. *Q. Jl exp. Physiol.* **56**, 1–11.

LANGMUIR, I. (1938) Discussion in *Cold Spring Harb. Symp. quant. Biol.* **6**, 136–137, 160–162.

LEE, J. B. (1971) Prostaglandins. *The Physiologist* **14**, 379–397.

LEE, W. H. & HAIRSTON, P. (1971) Structural effects on blood proteins at the gas–blood interface. *Fedn Proc. Fedn Am. Socs exp. Biol.* **30**, 1615–1620.

LEE, W. H., KRUMHAAR, D., FONKALSRUD, E. W., SCHJEIDE, C. A., & MALONFY, J. V. (1961) Denaturation of plasma proteins as a cause of morbidity and death after intracardiac operations. *Surgery* **50**, 29–39.

LEVER, M. J. (1967) Personal communication.

LEVER, M. J., MILLER, K. W., PATON, W. D. M. & SMITH, E. B. (1966) Experiments on the genesis of bubbles as a result of rapid decompression. *J. Physiol., Lond.* **184**, 964–969.

LEVERETT, S. D., BITTER, H. L. & McIVER, R. G. (1963) *Studies in Decompression Sickness: Circulatory and Respiratory Changes Associated with Decompression Sickness in Anaesthetized Dogs*. Report SAM-TDR-63.7. USAF School of Aerospace Medicine.

LINDSEY, H. E. & WYLLIE, J. H. (1970) Release of prostaglandins from embolized lungs. *Br. J. Surg.* **57**, 738–741.

MAJNO, G. & PALADE, G. E. (1961) Studies on inflammation I. The effect of Histamine and Serotonin on vascular permeability: an electron microscopic study. *J. biophys. biochem. Cytol.* **11**, 571–605.

MAJNO, G., PALADE, G. E. & SCHOEFL, B. I. (1961) Studies on inflammation II. The site of action of Histamine and Serotonin along the vascular tree: a topographic study. *J. biophys. biochem. Cytol.* **11**, 607–626.

MALETTE, W. G., FITZGERALD, J. B. & EISMAN, B. (1960) Aeroembolus: a protective substance. *Surg. Forum.* **11**, 155–156.

MARSHALL, R. (1965) *Pulmonary Embolism—Mechanisms and Managements*. Springfield: Thomas.

MARTIN, K. J. & NICHOLS, G. (1972) Observations on platelet changes in man, after simulated diving. *Aerospace Med.* **43**, 827–830.

MARTIN, K. H., CLARKSON, A. R., GRAY, S. P. & NICHOLS, G. (1975) The range of variation of selected blood constituents in different groups of men at high pressure. In *Underwater Physiology. Vth Symp. Underwater Physiology*. Ed. C. J. Lambertsen. Bethesda: Fedn Am. Socs exp. Biol.

MASLAND, R. L. (1948) Injury of the central nervous system resulting from decompression to simulated high altitudes. *Archs Neurol. Psychiat., Chicago* **59**, 445–456.

McIVER, R. G., FIFE, W. P. & IKELS, K. G. (1965) *Experimental Decompression Sickness from Hyperbaric Nitrous Oxide Anaesthesia*. Report SAM-TR-65-47. USAF School of Aerospace Medicine.

McWhorter, J. E. (1910) The etiological factors of compressed air illness. The gaseous content of tunnels: the occurrence of the disease in workers. *Am. J. med. Sci.* **139**, 373–383.

Musschenbroek, P. van (1715) *De Aeris Praesentis in Humoribus Animalibus.* Lugd. Bat.: Luchtmans.

Mustard, J. F. & Packham, M. A. (1970) Thromboembolism: a manifestation of the response of blood to injury. *Circulation* **42**, 1–21.

Niden, A. H. & Aviado, D. M. (1956) Effects of pulmonary embolism on the pulmonary circulation with special reference to arterio-venous shunts in the lung. *Circulation Res.* **4**, 67–73.

Nilsson, I. M. & Swedberg, J. (1959) Coagulation studies in cardiac surgery with extracorporeal circulation using a bubble oxygenater. *Acta chir. scand.* **117**, 47–54.

Nims, L. F. (1951) A physical theory of decompression sickness. Part I. Environmental factors affecting decompression sickness. In *Decompression Sickness.* Ed. J. F. Fulton. pp. 192–222. London: Saunders.

Odland, L. T. (1959) Fatal decompression sickness at an altitude of 22,000 feet. *Aerospace Med.* **30**, 840–846.

Orange, R. P. & Austen, K. F. (1969) Slow reacting substance of anaphlaxis. *Adv. Immunol.* **10**, 105–144.

Orange, R. P., Kaliner, M. A., Laria, P. J. & Austen, K. F. (1971) Immunological release of histamine and slow reacting substance of anaphlaxis from human lung. II. Influence of cellular levels of cyclic AMP. *Fedn Proc. Fedn Am. Socs exp. Biol.* **30**, 1725–1729.

Osborn, J. J., Mackenzie, R., Shaw, A., Perkins, H., Hurt, R. & Gerbode, F. (1955) Cause and prevention of haemorrhage following extracorporeal circulation. *Surg. Forum,* **6**, 96–100.

Palmer, M. A., Piper, P. J. & Vane, J. R. (1970a) The release of rabbit aorta contracting substance (RCS) from chopped lung and its antagonism by anti-inflammatory drugs. *Br. J. Pharmac. Chemother.* **40**, 581–582.

Palmer, M. A., Piper, P. J. & Vane, J. R. (1970b) Release of vasoactive substances from lungs by injection of particles. *Br. J. Pharmac. Chemother.* **40**, 547–548.

Paton, W. D. M. & Walder, D. N. (1954) *Compressed Air Illness.* Medical Research Council, Special Report 281, London.

Penick, G. D., Averette, H. E., Peters, R. M. & Brinkhous, K. M. (1958) The haemorrhagic syndrome complicating extracorporeal shunting of the blood: an experimental study of its pathogenesis. *Thromb. Diath. haemorrh.* **2**, 218–225.

Philp, R. B. (1973) Historical evolution of the blood–bubble interaction hypothesis in the pathogenesis of decompression sickness. In *Blood–Bubble Interaction in Decompression Sickness.* Ed. K. N. Ackles. pp. 5–16. DCIEM, Toronto. (In press.)

Philp, R. B. & Gowdey, C. W. (1969) Platelets as an etiological factor in experimental decompression sickness. *J. occup. Med.* **11**, 257–258.

Philp, R. B., Inwood, M. J. & Warren, B. A. (1972) Interactions between gas bubbles and components of the blood: implications and decompression sickness. *Aerospace Med.* **43** (9), 946–956.

Philp, R. B., Gowdey, C. W. & Prasad, M. (1967) Changes in blood lipid concentration and cell counts following decompression sickness in rats and the influence of dietary lipid. *Canad. J. Physiol. Pharmac.* **45**, 1047–1059.

Philp, R. B., Schacham, P. & Gowdey, C. W. (1971) Involvement of platelets and microthrombi in experimental decompression sickness: similarities with disseminated intravascular coagulation. *Aerospace Med.,* 494–502.

Philp, R. B., Ackles, K. N., Inwood, M. J., Livingstone, S. D., Achimastos, A., Binns-Smith, M. & Radomski, M. W. (1972) Changes in the haemostatic system and in blood and urine chemistry of human subjects following decompression from a hyperbaric environment. *Aerospace Med.* **43**, 498–505.

Pietra, G. G., Szidon, J. P., Leventhal, M. M. & Fishman, A. P. (1971) Histamine and interstitial pulmonary edema in the dog. *Circulation Res.* **29**, 323–337.

Piccard, J. (1941) Aeroemphysema and the birth of bubbles. *Proc. Mayo Clin.* **16**, 700–704.

Piccard, J. (1944) Aeroemphysema and caisson disease, a problem of colloid chemistry. In *Colloid Chemistry.* Ed. J. Alexander. pp. 1082–1094. New York: Reinhold.

Prinzmetal, M., Ornitz, E. M., Simkin, B. & Bergman, H. C. (1948) Arteriovenous anastamoses in liver, spleen and lung. *Am. J. Physiol.* **152**, 48–52.

Rait, W. L. (1959) The aetiology of post-decompression shock in aircrewmen. *U.S. arm. Forces med. J.* **10**, 790–804.

Ratnoff, O. D. (1969) Some relationships among haemostasis, fibrinolytic phenomena, immunity and the inflammatory response. *Adv. Immunol.* **10**, 145–227.

Ring, C. S., Blum, A. S., Kurbatov, T., Moss, W. G. & Smith, W. (1961) The size of microspheres passing through the pulmonary circuit in the dog. *Am. J. Physiol.* **200**, 1191–1196.

Rozahegyi, I. (1959) Late consequences of the neurological forms of decompression sickness. *Br. J. indust. Med.* **16**, 311–317.

Rozsahegyi, I. (1967) Neurological damage following decompression. In *Decompression of Compressed Air Workers in Civil Engineering.* pp. 127–137. Ed. R. I. McCallum. Edinburgh: Oriel.

Said, S. I. (1968a) Some respiratory effects of Prostaglandins E_2 and F_2. *Circulation Res.* **16**, 374.

Said, S. I. (1968b) The lung as a metabolic organ. *New Engl. J. Med.* **279**, 1330–1333.

Salzman, E. W. (1971) Role of platelets in blood–surface interactions. *Fedn Proc. Fedn Am. Socs exp. Biol.* **30**, 1503–1509.

Salzman, E. W. (1972) Cyclic AMP and platelet function. *New Engl. J. Med.* **286**, 358–363.

Sevitt, S. (1962) *Fat Embolism.* London: Butterworth.

Sicardi, F. (1970) La coagulation au cours de la plongée profonde. *Bull. Medsubhyp.* **4**, 15–16.

Smith, K. H., Stegall, P. J., Harker, L. A. & Slichter, S. J. (1973) Possible effects of bubble induced coagulation following decompression. In *Blood–Bubble Interaction in Decompression Sickness.* Ed. K. N. Ackles. pp. 260–267. DCIEM: Toronto. (In press.)

Spector, W. G. (1958) Substances which affect capillary permeability. *Pharmac. Rev.* **10**, 475–505.

Spector, W. G. (1964) Endogenous inflammatory mechanisms in the rat. In *International Symposium on Injury, Inflammation and Immunity.* Ed. L. Thomas, J. W. Uhr & L. H. Grant. pp. 178–182. Baltimore: Miles.

SPECTOR, W. G., WALTERS, M. & WILLOUGHBY, D. A. (1965) Venular and capillary permeability in thermal injury. *J. Path. Bact.* **90**, 635.

SPENCER, M. P. & CAMPBELL, S. D. (1968) Development of bubbles in venous and arterial blood during hyperbaric decompression. *Bull. Mason Clin.* **22**, 26–32.

SPENCER, M. P. & CAMPBELL, S. D. (1975) Decompression venous gas emboli. In *Underwater Physiology. Vth Symp. Underwater Physiology.* Ed. C. J. Lambertsen. Bethesda: Fedn Am. Socs exp. Biol.

SPENCER, M. P. & OKINO, H. (1972) Venous gas emboli following repeated breathold dives. *Fedn Proc. Fedn Am. Socs exp. Biol.* **31**, 355.

SPENCER, M. P. & OYAMA, Y. (1971) Pulmonary capacity for dissipation of venous gas emboli. *Aerospace Med.* 822–827.

SPENCER, M. P., CAMPBELL, S. D., SEALEY, J. L., HENRY, F. C. & LINDBERGH, J. (1969) Experiments on decompression bubbles in the circulation using ultrasonic and electromagnetic flowmeters. *J. occup. Med.* **11**, 238–244.

STEGALL, P. J. & SMITH, K. H. (1975) The etiology and pathogenesis of decompression sickness: radiologic, haematologic and histologic studies in miniature swine. In *Underwater Physiology. Vth Symp. Underwater Physiology.* Ed. C. J. Lambertsen. Bethesda: Fedn Am. Socs exp. Biol.

STEGALL, P., SMITH, K. H. & HILDIBRANDT, J. (1973) Selective platelet destruction and dysbaric osteonecrosis in miniature pigs after decompression. *Fedn Proc. Fedn Am. Socs exp. Biol.* **32**, 335.

SWINDLE, P. F. (1937) Occlusion of blood vessels by agglutinated red cells, mainly as seen in tadpoles and very young kangaroos. *Am. J. Physiol.* **120**, 59–74.

SZIDON, J. P., PIETRA, G. G. & FISHMAN, A. P. (1972) The alveolar-capillary membrane and pulmonary edema. *New Engl. J. Med.* **286**, 1200–1204.

TOBIN, C. E. & ZARIQUIEY, M. O. (1953) Some observations on the blood supply of the human lung. *Med. Radiogr. Photogr.* **29**, 9–21.

TRUEX, R. C. & CARPENTER, M. B. (1969) Origin and composition of the nervous system. *In Human Neuroanatomy.* Baltimore: Williams & Wilkins.

VAN ALLEN, C. M., HRDINA, L. S. & CLARK, J. (1929) Air embolism from the pulmonary vein. *Archs Surg., Chicago* **19**, 567–599.

WALDER, D. N. (1969) The prevention of decompression sickness in compressed air workers. In *The Physiology and Medicine of Diving and Compressed Air Work.* 1st Edition. Ed. P. B. Bennett & D. H. Elliott. pp. 437–450. London: Ballière, Tindall & Cassell.

WALDER, D. N. (1970) Caisson disease of bone in Great Britain. In *Proceedings of the Fourth International Congress on Hyperbaric Medicine.* Ed. J. Wada & T. Iwa. pp. 83–88. Tokyo: Shoin.

WARREN, B. A., PHILP, R. B. & INWOOD, M. J. (1973) The ultrastructural morphology of air embolism: platelet adhesion to the interface and endothelial damage. *Br. J. exp. Path.* **54**, 163–172.

WELLS, C. H., BOND, T. R., GUEST, M. M. & BARNHART, C. C. (1971) Rheologic impairment of the microcirculation during decompression sickness. *Microvasc. Res.* **3**, 162–169.

WHITAKER, D. M., BLINKS, L. A., BERG, W. E., TWITTY, V. C. & HARRIS, M. (1945) Muscular activity and bubble formation in animals decompressed to simulated altitude. *J. gen. Physiol.* **28**, 213–223.

WHITTERIDGE, D. (1950) Multiple embolism of lung and rapid shallow breathing. *Physiol. Rev.* **30**, 475–486.

WILHELM, D. L. (1962) The mediation of increased vascular permeability in inflammation. *Pharmac. Rev.* **14**, 251–280.

WILHELM, D. L. & MASON, B. (1960) Vascular permeability changes in inflammation. *Br. J. exp. Path.* **41**, 487–506.

WILSON, J. W. (1972) Leukocyte sequestration and morphologic augmentation in the pulmonary network following haemorrhagic shock and related forms of stress. *Adv. Microcirc.* **4**, 197–232.

YOSHITAKE, K. (1967) Pathophysiological significances of serotonin in pulmonary circulation. *Jap. Circul. J.* **31**, 853–871.

ZIEVE, P. D. & GREENOUGH III, W. B. (1969) *Biochem biophys. Res. Commun.* **35**, 462–466.

24

The Prevention of Decompression Sickness

D. N. WALDER

Decompression tables

Susceptibility to decompression sickness varies from man to man even in so-called fit individuals. Two compressed air workers on the same shift, or two divers carrying out the same dive simultaneously may fare quite differently—one completing his task without the slightest hint of trouble, and the other suffering an attack of decompression sickness. A decompression procedure which would be absolutely safe for all would have to be very long, since it would probably have to avoid all but very modest degrees of supersaturation of the tissues or perhaps any degree of supersaturation at all (Hills 1966).

It is for this reason that decompression tables which give less than 100% safety to those who use them are still regarded as satisfactory. In this matter Hills (1968) claims that the Weibull function provides a particularly good mathematical expression to describe the distribution of men in relation to their susceptibility to decompression sickness and thus allows the adaption of schedules of known efficacy for, say, a 2% bend rate. Of course the Weibull function tells us nothing about the sources of difference in susceptibility. The acceptance of even a 98% level of safety allows a considerable reduction in decompression time.

An important fact in decompression table development has been the tendency for decompression schedules to be adequate when tested under laboratory conditions, but not adequate when used on compressed air sites or at sea. It is

therefore essential to test tables properly in the field. Fortunately, it has become possible in recent years to gain practical experience with tables for compressed air work by actual observation and recording of the experiences at compressed air contracts (Decompression Sickness Panel [MRC] 1974). In the case of diving tables, however, the number of divers involved is severely limited and extensive testing would be a slow procedure, even if every diver cooperated.

Unfortunately, at the moment exact records are not generally kept by divers or their employers and so this vital source of information is denied us. Without the controlled feed-back from practical diving those who calculate decompression tables will continue to exercise their ingenuity without any objective measure of their success.

Until recently the onset of decompression sickness was taken as the sole criterion of an inadequate decompression, whereas we now know that there are other possible ill effects. For instance in 1966 it became obvious that in spite of apparent adherence to the accepted decompression tables damage to the bones was occurring (Decompression Sickness Panel [MRC] 1966). More recently evidence has accumulated to suggest that subtle biochemical effects may also be occurring on decompression which hitherto have passed unnoticed (Martin 1973). The significance of these latter changes is at present difficult to assess. It is therefore most important to understand to the full the implications for the body of decompression and to learn how the ill effects can best be avoided.

Returning however to the usual parameter of decompression table effectiveness, namely the decompression sickness rate, the following points must be made:

1. Although there is little difficulty in recognizing that a man has a definite Type I attack of decompression sickness, mild attacks, often referred to as 'niggles' because they are irritating but not painful, sometimes give rise to uncertainty. Any man who reports with symptoms after decompression should always be regarded as a case of decompression sickness and recompressed. Relief of the symptoms by recompression will confirm the diagnosis of decompression sickness.

2. The symptoms of Type II decompression sickness are also generally easy to recognize but care must be taken not to miss the case with unusual features such as nausea, vomiting or vestibular disturbance. They must all be treated and counted.

Oxygen decompression

For many years it has been recognized that oxygen breathing during decompression has some advantages in that, for instance, it hastens the elimination of nitrogen from the body (Ham & Hill 1905–6). In diving, the use of oxygen during decompression is firmly established but until recently it has not been used in civil engineering compressed air work (Wunsche, Fust & Pressel 1967). It is still not used in Great Britain, mainly because of its potential toxicity and fire hazard. The safe use necessitates a degree of discipline not usually found amongst compressed air workers. Obviously every man must wear his oxygen mask in a proper manner and the decompression chamber must be ventilated in such a way that no build-up of oxygen concentration can occur. The heightened fire risk would mean that all combustible materials and possible sources of ignition would have to be eliminated from the locks. In Japan where oxygen breathing during the decompression of compressed air workers has been tried, there has already been a disastrous fire involving the death of several men (Nashimoto 1967).

GENERAL FACTORS

Climatic conditions

Suggestions that local climatic conditions can influence the bends incidence seem to be without foundation. Caisson workers will often suggest that local weather conditions influence their susceptibility to decompression sickness—damp weather and frosty conditions both being blamed for increases in susceptibility. Paton and Walder (1954) compared the data supplied by an H.M. Meteorological Office five miles from a Compressed Air Contract with the bends incidence and were unable to discover any important correlation between the bends rate and any of the weekly averages of rainfall, sunshine, humidity, wind velocity, barometric pressure and maximum or minimum temperature.

The climatic environment of the tunnel itself has also been blamed for influencing the bends rate, but in fact this remains remarkably stable. The constancy of the temperature results from the depth of the tunnel below the surface and the consequent insulating effect of the surrounding ground. The constancy of the relative humidity is due to the fact that the ground surrounding all compressed air workings is water logged. In the case of divers there seems to be a well-recognized increased risk of decompression sickness when operating in cold water.

Exercise during decompression

The rate at which nitrogen is cleared from the tissues must be at least partly dependent on the blood supply and therefore an active man could be expected to desaturate his tissues during decompression more quickly than an inactive man. Exercise during decompression might therefore reduce the risk of decompression sickness; in fact the reverse is true. Exercise during decompression leads to a higher bends incidence than inactivity (Van der Aue, Kellar & Brinton 1949). A possible explanation is that exercise results in the nucleation of gas micronuclei or perhaps in the expansion of pre-existing gas pockets by producing a local rise of the partial pressure of CO_2 (Harvey et al. 1944), or in the mechanical development of localized sites of low pressure.

Hypoxia

It is generally believed that limb pains are commoner following circumstances in which hypoxia has been present (Fryer 1969). This, however, was not the finding of Motley, Chinn and Odell (1945) who studied aviators undergoing decompression tests. In their experience those men who had been hypoxic during the decompression suffered less severe pains than the others. More recently Yunkin (1970) has shown that, at least for mice, susceptibility is at its lowest in those which are most resistant to hypoxia.

Carbon dioxide

Harvey et al. (1944) pointed out that bubbles passing through tissues with a high partial pressure of CO_2 should grow rapidly and therefore an excess of CO_2 should promote the onset of decompression sickness.

Hodes and Larrabee (1945) showed that a high level of CO_2 in the blood of aviators can contribute to the genesis of decompression sickness, but the evidence that it does so in compressed air workers and divers is more equivocal. When, for expediency, a very small man-lock has been used to decompress the compressed air workers at the end of a shift, high levels of CO_2 have accumulated. Lewis and Paton (1957) reported CO_2 levels at one contract as high as the surface equivalent of $2 \cdot 63\%$ atmosphere, 18 min after the start of a decompression, and they believed that it was a factor contributing to the high incidence of decompression sickness (4%) recorded on that contract. There is no clear evidence that this effect has been observed in divers.

The quality of the air in tunnels and caissons

A matter which so far does not seem to have been systematically investigated is the influence which oil contamination of the compressed air supply may have on the incidence of bends. Scrubbers are normally included in the air line to remove as much oil as possible from the compressed air supply to the tunnel, but their efficiency is not always high. It is just possible that the inhalation of oil droplets could result in obstruction of the airways in the lungs, causing air trapping which might be a hazard. The problem is under investigation.

An interesting observation that Type II decompression sickness appears to be more common amongst welders than other tunnel workers (Paton & Walder 1954) could be linked with the bronchoconstrictor effects and consequent air trapping in the lungs of inhaling nitrogen dioxide produced during some types of welding. Measurements of nitrogen dioxide general levels in tunnels have not shown any excessively high concentration, but there remains the possibility of local high concentrations close to the work.

The nature of the work

If the work of a compressed air worker or diver was such that it required excessive exercise of a particular group of muscles or put a strain on to a particular joint, then any subsequent bend might be associated with those muscles or that joint. Investigations of the relationship between the various jobs carried out by compressed air workers and the site of their subsequent bend does not, however, show any obvious link. Face workers in a shield may work all day in a squatting situation and put great strain on their hips but they seem to get no more bends in their legs than caulkers who make particular use of their shoulder muscles. Paton and Walder (1954) found no significant difference between the susceptibility to, or site of, bends for groups of men with different occupations.

Recent injuries

Perhaps one of the most striking features of decompression sickness, even in a susceptible person, is the apparently random nature of its site of occurrence. One precipitating factor which has often been suggested is injury. It is, however, not easy to obtain factual data on such matters since tunnel workers do a rough job and there are few who cannot recall some blow or strain to the site of a subsequent bend. Yet the idea that limb bends occur at the site of an injury could have some theoretical foundation. It could be suggested that an impact might result in cavitation (of the tissues) with the formation of gas pockets which might increase in size during decompression to stretch the tissues and give rise to pain. Gray (1951) suggests that there is no positive correlation between old injuries and the incidence of bends, although when they occur they do tend to localize in a region which has been subjected to a recent minor injury (Thompson et al. 1944)

INDIVIDUAL FACTORS

The assessment of individual susceptibility to decompression sickness *before* exposure to pressure has not so far proved to be possible, but the search for the critical factors which determine susceptibility continues. One difficulty hampering investigation is that susceptibility varies from day to day under the same condition even after 'acclimatization' has occurred.

Age

Older men tend to be more susceptible to decompression sickness than younger men. This is well documented for aviators (Gersh & Catchpole 1951). Paton and Walder (1954) have shown that after the age of 40 the bends rate for compressed air workers rises steeply, and that the older the man starting compressed-air work, the sooner he will suffer from a bend.

For US Navy divers Wise (1963) was unable to discover any relationship between age and the susceptibility to decompression sickness. It must be remembered, however, that Navy divers are rarely over the age of 40. Summitt, Berghage and Every (1971) found that the older the diver, the more unlikely it is that he will obtain complete relief from bends symptoms on recompression, and the more likely that he will suffer a recurrence of symptoms on subsequent decompression. It is therefore clear that older men should, for their own safety, be excluded from hyperbaric exposure.

Obesity

It is tempting to try to explain the relationship between age and the susceptibility of compressed air workers to bends by suggesting that older men are fatter. The evidence for a relationship between fatness and susceptibility to bends has come mainly from animal experiments which show that fat animals are more susceptible to decompression sickness than thin ones. It is well known (Vernon 1907) that nitrogen is more soluble in fat than in water, but the suggestion that fat has a poor blood supply is not well authenticated.

Efforts to relate the obesity of compressed air workers to their susceptibility to decompression sickness has been attempted only recently. Weight is a poor index of body fat so in the observations carried out on the compressed air workers at the Tyne Tunnel fatness was estimated by the use of Harpenden skin calipers. The results (Decompression Sickness Panel [MRC] 1968) indicate a statistically significant relationship between skin-fold thickness and susceptibility, although this relationship is not sufficiently specific to permit skin-fold measurements to be used in predetermining the suitability of an individual for compressed air work.

Somatotype

Perhaps insufficient attention has been paid to the question of the ideal build for a compressed air worker or diver. Clearly he should be muscular to perform the arduous tasks which, especially in an emergency, he is sometimes called upon to carry out. Since fatness is related to the susceptibility to decompression sickness he must not be too fat, but on the other hand, in the case of divers, a layer of fat constitutes a most important protection from cold (Baker & Daniels 1955; Pugh & Edholm 1955; Keatinge 1972). There must be some optimum somatotype.

In the case of tunnel workers it has been suggested (P. D. Griffiths, personal communication) that 'barrel chested, short necked men' do poorly in air. Although a somatotyping survey of compressed air workers is now underway, so far we have no objective proof of this hypothesis. Wise made an attempt in 1963 to estimate body build using the Sheldon Index and found that there was a statistically significant relationship between this index and the susceptibility of divers to bends.

The analysis of properly made photographic records of divers for subsequent anthropometric measurement and somatotyping might lead to an excellent method of selecting the most suitable men to start a career in diving.

Acclimatization

An interesting observation is that men can acclimatize to working in compressed air. Daily exposures of a group of men to a compressed air environment leads to a progressive reduction in the incidence of bends following decompression until a minimum rate indicating full acclimatization is reached. The bends rate decreases initially with a half-time of about 7 ± 4 days (Paton & Walder 1954; Walder 1966).

Intervals away from compressed air work lead to a gradual loss of acclimatization, and increase in the rate of decompression sickness until by about the tenth day all acclimatization is lost.

Acclimatization to one working pressure does not give protection for a higher pressure. These effects have also been seen amongst divers who may become resistant to decompression sickness when performing long shallow dives, but who may lose this resistance when they change to short deep dives. Acclimatization then is specific for one pressure or depth and further acclimatization is required if the pressure or depth is increased.

It is tempting to suggest that acclimatization is due to a family of gas micronuclei normally present in the body which in some way is gradually depleted by a series of compressions and decompressions. The number of gas micronuclei available to lead to the symptoms of decompression sickness would then be reduced after repeated exposures to compressed air, thus explaining the decreasing bends rate. It can be further argued that gas micronuclei can reaccumulate in the absence of exposures to compression and decompression. It would also be necessary to assume that there are various families of gas micronuclei, each family requiring compression to or decompression from a different working pressure or depth to be eliminated.

Surface tension and fluid balance

Whatever the origin of bubbles in the body, one of the factors which will affect their life and fate is the surface tension of the fluid in which they are present. It has been claimed that a relationship exists between the static surface tension of the blood serum and the bends susceptibility of aviators. Men with a high surface tension are less susceptible to bends than those with a low surface tension (Walder 1948). The surface tension will affect the rate of growth of bubbles as well as the force required to move a bubble along a vessel which it is obstructing. It will also determine the critical size beneath which the bubble will spon-

taneously collapse. Aviators who drank a lot of water so that their serum surface tension was raised were found to be less susceptible to bends (Walder 1948). Warwick (1943) had also found a significant relationship between the fluid intake of aviators and their susceptibility to bends. Therefore the fluid intake of compressed air workers and divers may influence their susceptibility to bends.

It is very difficult to be sure about what compressed air workers drink, though it usually consists of both aqueous and alcoholic beverages. The details of a man's alcohol intake tend to be coloured by circumstances: if the individual wishes to impress he says it is high, but if he suspects some censure from authority then he says it is low. This is unfortunate since alcohol has the opposite effect to water on serum surface tension. Clearly, however, alcoholic beverages should be discouraged immediately before starting work in compressed air or diving; alcohol in tunnels is already prohibited by regulation in some countries.

Diurnal variation

The body undergoes many diurnal rhythms which might have an effect on the factors important in the aetiology of decompression sickness. In many compressed air contracts it is usual to work three shifts in 24 hours and consequently this affords an opportunity to see if there is any diurnal variation in bends rate. In fact the bends incidence on the back shift (3.00 p.m. to 11.00 p.m.) is greater than on the other two (11.00 p.m. to 7.00 a.m. and 7.00 a.m. to 3.00 p.m.) (Griffiths 1960).

Air trapping

A possible source of gas micronuclei during decompression is the lungs, where there exists an enormous air–blood interface separated by a thin endothelium. The fact that gas can be introduced into the circulation from the lungs at decompression was demonstrated by Malhotra and Wright (1960) in their experiments on animals to demonstrate the dangers of a closed glottis during submarine escape ascents. In these circumstances the volume of air which can be injected into the circulation is large and the resulting condition has been called aeroembolism. In these cases the tissues are not normally supersaturated with gas.

Such a condition, when it follows a prolonged exposure to high pressure and results in the formation of a whole mass of growing bubbles within the circulation, should then be called decompression sickness. In the past it has been the practice to use the term aeroembolism for those conditions which result from air which has entered the circulation from without. This distinction is unsatisfactory because in our present state of knowledge, it is difficult to be sure if bubbles have formed spontaneously within the circulation, or have been initiated by air from tears in the walls of the lung.

Individual decompression

A sensible approach to the elimination of decompression sickness, in all its forms, would be to monitor each man individually and to tailor the decompression to his requirements. If it were possible to detect bubbles before they gave rise to symptoms, the rate of decompression could then be adjusted accordingly.

Recently, several attempts have been made to detect bubbles within the living body by ultrasonic techniques, with a considerable degree of success. This subject is discussed at length in Chapter 22, where it is shown that free gas bubbles have regularly been detected without accompanying symptoms of decompression sickness. If this apparatus can be refined to the stage where each diver or compressed air worker can monitor his own progress throughout a decompression, a useful reduction in the incidence of decompression sickness may well result.

Such approaches to this problem at the moment seem to offer more hope in the control of decompression sickness than the design of blanket tables calculated from data which are subject to all the uncontrollable variables inherent in every biological experiment.

MEDICAL FITNESS

The medical examination of compressed air workers and divers

Clearly there are many risks associated with working in a hyperbaric environment and these must be borne in mind when considering the medical examination of men seeking to be accepted as fit for this type of work. At present the Factories Act in Great Britain requires both compressed air workers and divers covered by that Act to be certified fit for that employment by an appointed doctor. In contrast it is voluntarily becoming established that commercial divers undertaking diving in the North Sea in connection with the oil industry and who are at present outside the Factories Act require a detailed and stringent medical examination such as specified in *The Principles of Safe Diving Practice* (CIRIA 1972).

One important justification for this more stringent attitude towards the deep diver is economic. The investment both in terms of training and back-up equipment is extremely large, and failure at the end of training or on the job due to a medical disability would be an expensive error. Whilst admitting that there is some sense in accepting two medical standards for divers, it is nevertheless a fact that, with the enormous expansion in deep sea diving that is currently taking place, it is quite possible for a shallow water diver to be called upon, and to be tempted, without having been subjected to the more extensive medical examination, to undertake deep diving. On balance, therefore, it is surely wise to ensure that anyone who wishes to take up diving as a career must be given a comprehensive medical examination before he starts.

Another reason for a thorough medical examination at the beginning of any period of employment is to define exactly the man's physical state so that any disabilities which develop subsequently can be judged in the light of this. It is therefore important that the results of medical examinations, including radiographs, should be properly recorded and stored at some central place.

The British Medical Research Council Decompression Sickness Panel has designed a proforma on which the results of the medical examination of commercial divers can be recorded. A facsimile of this is published in *The Principles of Safe Diving Practice* (CIRIA 1972) and is reproduced at the end of this chapter. The results of these examinations are being kept in the MRC

Decompression Sickness Central Registry, Newcastle upon Tyne. They are of particular value when a series of annual examinations can be compared, for then it is possible to see if the medical fitness of an individual is being maintained or is deteriorating, and also to study what is happening to the group as a whole.

Disqualifying conditions

The conditions which disqualify a man for compressed air work and diving are:

1. Chronic catarrh of upper air passages, in particular recurrent sinus infection
2. Perforated eardrum, chronic otitis media or mastoid operation
3. Inability to 'clear the ears' via the Eustachian tubes
4. Any chronic lung disease, past or present, bronchial asthma or history of pneumothorax
5. Heart disease, essential hypertension
6. Epilepsy, severe head injury, cranial surgery, disease of the central nervous system
7. Severe hearing or visual defects
8. Excessive obesity
9. Diabetes
10. Psychiatric disorder
11. Gross abnormalities of the renal tract
12. The inability to communicate freely by voice (e.g. stammering)
13. Peptic ulcer
14. Hernia
15. Chronic diarrhoea
16. Sickle cell trait
17. Some skin diseases.

The psyche

It is important that a man who is psychologically unfit for diving should be excluded from the start. It is doubtful whether any special psychological aptitude tests are justified. A doctor who is experienced in the problems of divers and diving should be able to assess the state of mind of the prospective diver during the course of the general medical examination. The man's motivation is important. Diving naturally attracts the buccaneering type but this in itself is insufficient. There must be an underlying desire to be a professional and to do a job well. It is essential that this is matched by intelligence and the ability to

make reasoned judgements when under stress.

Evidence of worry about personal or home affairs or recent emotional upsets must always be regarded as potentially dangerous. Any preoccupation with worries unrelated to the work in hand will distract the diver from those details of preparation and execution which make him safe and efficient.

Age

In Great Britain the minimum age for starting to dive professionally and for working in compressed air is 18. To start a career in professional diving after the age of 30 is probably unrealistic. Although there can be no hard and fast rule, 45 is probably a critical time when very careful consideration should be given to allowing a diver to continue without limitation. Many men by this age will no longer be able to withstand the rigours of deep diving because of minor physical deterioration, and, if they are to continue, some curb on their activity may be required.

Much more important than setting a specific age limit is the ability to detect deterioration in the physical condition by comparison of annual medical examinations held over the years.

Body build

Neither height nor weight are important in themselves but must be considered in conjunction with each other, with past observation, and with other measurements.

Excessive weight associated with increasing total body fat as measured with the skin-fold calipers, would of course have to be carefully investigated.

A guide to the maximum weight for a given height is given in Table 24.1 but this is only valid if there is a proper proportion between height, weight and build of the individual. This is difficult to define at the moment, and there is a need for more exact information on the ideal somatotype for diving. Properly taken and recorded somatotype measurements and photographs would be most helpful for future study.

Skin-fold test

One of the simplest methods of assessing the total body fat is to measure the thickness of a fold

TABLE 24.1

Assessment of body build by maximum allowable weight for height

Height (in)	Maximum weight (lb)
64	164
65	169
66	174
67	179
68	184
69	189
70	194
71	199
72	205
73	211
74	218
75	224
76	230
77	236
78	242

From the *Manual of the Medical Dept. US Navy*, Washington, D.C. US Government Printing Office Sec. 15–30 C.

of skin over the mid-triceps area. The left arm should be used and the measurement made with a Harpenden skin-fold caliper (Edwards et al. 1955) when the arm is hanging relaxed. A reading below 15 mm is considered to be satisfactory. A greater reading suggests that the man is unusually fat.

Vision

A minimum of 20/30 vision in each eye corrected to 20/20 is desirable. This is not for underwater work but in connection with seeing danger signals in the diving area on the surface. Colour vision is also necessary for surface safety.

Teeth

Oral infections must be treated before acceptance on general hygiene grounds. All fillings must be sound and unaffected by changes in ambient pressure. Mal-occlusion, partial or total dentures are acceptable only if a mouthpiece can be properly maintained in position (without dentures).

Ears

Ears must be free from infection. Normal auditory acuity is desirable. The subject must be able to compensate easily for ambient pressure changes via the Eustachian tubes.

Recently it has been suggested that diving results in damage to the cochlea. The evidence for this is not yet absolutely convincing although Zannini, Odaglia and Sperati (1975) have claimed a high incidence of loss of hearing acuity amongst divers. In order to collect some firm evidence for or against this, audiograms should be carried out during the diver's first medical examination and the results deposited with some central authority (e.g. in Great Britain with the MRC Decompression Sickness Central Registry) and then reviewed in due course.

Sinuses

There should be no chronic sinus infection and the subject must be able to ventilate his sinuses freely during changes in ambient pressure.

Nose

There must be no obstruction to breathing, though septal deviation is not in itself a bar if ventilation is free.

Respiratory function

Physical examination must show the lungs to be normal. Respiratory function is particularly important for two reasons. First the diver must be able to breathe from apparatus without discomfort or embarrassment for prolonged periods. Secondly, even temporary airways obstruction, for instance from an upper respiratory infection, can lead to trapping of gas in the lungs during decompression and thus to aeroembolism or Type II decompression sickness.

Tests for respiratory function are useful in that they give an objective measurement which can be recorded numerically. Convenient measurements are of the forced expiratory ventilation in 1·0 sec (FEV_1) and the forced vital capacity (expiratory) (FVC) which can be estimated simultaneously with a spirograph. For interpretation of the results it is convenient to determine the percentage forced expiratory volume which is $100 \times FEV_1/FVC$. Normal values are given in Table 24.2.

In Great Britain, under the Factories Act, a chest X-ray is mandatory on the first examination of a diver, but not for a compressed air worker. It is at the discretion of the medical officer thereafter. In addition to gross pulmonary abnormalities the presence of bullae or cysts must be looked

TABLE 24.2

Assessment of respiratory function by the percentage forced expiratory volume

Age (years)	$100 \times FEV_1/FVC$
18–19	82·0
20–29	80·0
30–34	78·0
35–39	77·0
40–44	75·5
45–49	74·5

Data from Cara, L.M. & Martin, L.C. (1964)
In *L'exploration fonctionelle pulmonaire*. Ed.
H. Denolin et al. p. 112. Paris: Flammarion.

for in the radiograph and the man declared unfit for diving if they are present.

Cardiovascular system, including blood

The cardiovascular system must be without significant abnormality as determined by physical examination.

A persistently high resting pulse rate (above 100) should disqualify.

The blood pressure should not exceed 140 mm Hg systolic pressure, or 90 mm Hg diastolic pressure. Even if a subject has a higher blood pressure on first examination and it can be brought below the critical level by resting, the possibility that he has an excitable temperament should also be considered. Arrhythmias (except of sinus type), or evidence of atherosclerosis, should disqualify.

Varicose veins and haemorrhoids only disqualify if in danger of bleeding or being traumatized.

An electrocardiogram must be carried out both with the subject at rest and after the exercise test (see below). Abnormalities seen at rest or only after exercise will disqualify.

The blood should be examined for evidence of anaemia and, where the possibility exists, for evidence of abnormal haemoglobins including sickle cell trait. The presence of the latter disqualifies.

Gastro-intestinal system

Conditions resulting in chronic diarrhoea are obviously disqualifying. A history of peptic ulceration in the past will necessitate a gastro-

scopic examination in order to be certain that the lesion is healed before passing a man as fit to dive. Perforation or bleeding of an ulcer could be a very serious matter during a saturation dive or even when a diver is on the surface but far from a hospital. Surgical treatment within a few hours may be essential to save life.

A hernia will have to be satisfactorily repaired before a man can be certified as fit for compressed air work or diving.

Genito-urinary system

Chronic or recurrent disease (e.g. renal stones) disqualifies. The urine should be tested for albumin, sugar, blood and ketones.

Central nervous system (CNS)

In view of the fact that Type II decompression sickness may affect the CNS it is important to make a detailed examination of the cranial nerves, sensation over the trunk and limbs, tone and power of the limbs, reflexes and cerebellar function. Minor abnormalities even if not disabling must be noted. This prevents ambiguities when assessing the effectiveness of treatment for a spinal bend and also prevents unjust claims being made for residual effects of attacks of decompression sickness which were in fact present before the incident.

Locomotor system

Tests of joint mobility should be carried out. A full range of pain-free movements should be possible in all joints.

Skin

Acute or chronic skin disease may be infective or offensive if clothing has to be shared. It may be exacerbated by saturation diving.

SPECIAL TESTS

Oxygen toxicity

As high partial pressures of oxygen may be used in the respiratory gases in various diving situations, it would be advantageous if those men who are liable to convulse under these circumstances could be excluded. Various tests to detect sensitivity to oxygen have been devised and some are currently being used. The US Navy test of susceptibility to oxygen is as follows: the candidate has to breathe oxygen without untoward effect at a pressure of 60 ft (2·8 ATA) for a period of 30 min.

Unfortunately, it is doubtful whether much reliance can be placed on such tests because of the variability of oxygen sensitivity in man from day to day. Whereas a man may pass without difficulty an oxygen test on one day, it is quite possible for him to convulse at the same partial pressure of oxygen a day or two later.

Nitrogen narcosis

In some countries it has been the custom to test for undue sensitivity to nitrogen by exposing the candidate to air to 250 ft (80 m; 8·6 ATA) for 10 min. Since, in the interests of good diving practice, it is best that depth when breathing air be limited to 165 ft (50 m; 6 ATA), the test does not seem to be necessary.

Exercise tolerance

One test which is not only useful to the doctor but which also seems to catch the imagination of the divers is an Exercise Tolerance Test. They look upon this as a challenge which they can understand and they usually take a great pride in performing the test properly. There are many such tests and it would be an improvement if one particular test could be universally adopted. At present there has been little opportunity for international agreement on this subject.

Rather than specifying in detail how the test should be performed perhaps the solution lies in arranging for the subject to perform work at a given rate for a given time and then to record the pulse rate over some predetermined period. The method used to make the subject perform work is really immaterial and the apparatus used can be complex and expensive like an electromagnetically braked bicycle or ergometer or simple and cheap like a foot stool of specified height on which the subject steps up and down.

One such test is the Harvard Step Test (Brouha 1943). This consists in having the subject step up and down a 20 inch platform 30 times/min for 5 min unless he stops from exhaustion

before then. The pulse is then counted from 1 to $1\frac{1}{2}$, 2 to $2\frac{1}{2}$ and 3 to $3\frac{1}{2}$ min after the work stops. The score is obtained by dividing the duration of the exercise by the sum of pulses in recovery according to the formula:

$$\text{Index} = \frac{\text{Duration of exercise in sec} \times 100}{2 \times \text{sum of pulse counts in recovery}}$$

The meaning of the figures thus obtained is as shown in Table 24.3.

TABLE 24.3

Assessment of physical condition by the Harvard Step Test

Index	Physical condition
Below 55	poor
55–64	low average
65–79	high average
80–89	good
above 90	excellent

Carotid sinus syncope test

A simple and effective method of excluding those with an excessively sensitive carotid sinus reflex is to have the subject lie down and then press on the carotid sinus of *one* side whilst counting the radial pulse rate. A slowing of the pulse rate to less than 55 beats per minute should be taken as an indication of excessive sensitivity and the man disqualified. The test should then be repeated on the other side.

X-ray examination of bones

As discussed in Chapter 27 men who are regularly employed in compressed air work or who are regularly employed in deep diving should have their major joints X-rayed annually.

Recording and data analysis

Because of the many variables involved it has been in the past extremely difficult to obtain an accurate picture of the morbidity and mortality resulting from compressed air work and diving. This problem is aggravated by the fact that both compressed air workers and divers are peripatetic and this makes medical follow-up difficult.

In recent years the Medical Research Council Decompression Sickness Panel has had considerable success from studying the medical examination records and X-ray films of compressed air workers and divers at its Registry in Newcastle. For instance the regular medical examination carried out on any one diver over the years, wherever they have taken place, can be compared one with another and signs of physical deterioration readily detected. The development of bone lesions can be monitored so that immediately a suspected lesion becomes certain the diver can be warned. Not only is this of benefit to the individual, but is also of tremendous advantage to research workers. By studying the radiographs of whole groups of men they will be able to detect trends and relationships which will result in knowledge that before long may become of great importance to the compressed air workers and divers.

Ideally, as well as medical information, the details of each dive undertaken by each man should be collected. In the case of decompression sickness or other incident, full details must be recorded.

The problem of supplying information to a central bank when secret decompression tables are involved is well recognized, but there should be no objection to referring to such a table by a code number. Several data banks are now operating in the USA though it will be some time before any conclusions can be drawn.

CIRIA UNDERWATER ENGINEERING GROUP **Medical examination of commercial divers**

Set No

Book No

Full name _____ Date of birth _____

Address _____

1. How long have you been diving _____ Max. depth _____ Max. duration at that depth _____

2. Where were you trained as a diver _____

3. Are you being treated by a doctor at present _____

4. Are you having injections, medicines or tablets _____

5. Are you subject to colds _____

6. Are you ever seasick _____

7. Have you ever had any of the following:

Tuberculosis _____	Pneumonia _____	Bronchitis _____
Asthma _____	Hay fever _____	Spitting of blood _____
Nose bleeding _____	Sinusitis _____	Ear discharge _____
Rheumatic fever _____	Heart disease _____	High blood pressure _____
Digestive troubles _____	Gastric or duodenal ulcers _____	
Nervous breakdown _____	Fits _____	Recurrent headaches _____
Typhoid _____	Dysentery _____	Malaria _____
Other fever _____		
Serious injuries _____	Concussion _____	Operation _____
Anaesthetic _____		

Decompression sickness ('Bends', 'Chokes', or 'Staggers' etc.) _____

Damaged ear drums _____ Other diving 'accident' _____

8. Is there epilepsy, mental disease, tuberculosis or asthma in your family _____

9. Give your previous occupations and duration _____

10. Give dates of last inoculations:

Typhoid _____	Tetanus _____	B.C.G. _____	Smallpox _____
Polio _____	Cholera _____	Typhus _____	Yellow fever _____

11. Has your chest been x-rayed _____ When _____

12. Have your bones and joints been x-rayed _____ When _____

I declare the above answers to be true

Signed _____ Date _____

CIRIA UNDERWATER ENGINEERING GROUP **Medical examination of commercial divers**

Section 2   To be completed by the Medical Officer

Diver's Full Name _____   Diver's Date of Birth _____

Address _____

Height _____   Weight _____   Is he obese _____

Ext. Aud. Meatus _____   Right _____   Left _____

Are the ear drums healthy _____   Right _____   Left _____

Valsalva test _____   Right _____   Left _____

Any evidence of chronic upper respiratory tract infection _____

Are teeth and gums in good condition _____   Dentures _____

Any abnormality of the sinuses _____

Is the trachea central _____

Are respiratory movements normal _____

Does physical examination of the lungs reveal any abnormality _____

Is the apex beat in the normal position _____

Are the heart sounds normal _____   Blood pressure _____   Resting pulse rate _____

Does abdominal palpation reveal any abnormality _____

Any evidence of hernia _____   Haemorrhoids _____   Varicose veins _____

Is the skin healthy _____   Any identifying features, scars or tattoos _____

Are the cranial nerves normal   I _____   II _____   III _____   IV _____   V _____   VI _____
                                VII _____   VIII _____   IX _____   X _____   XI _____   XII _____

Is the tone and power of the limbs normal and equal _____

Are the reflexes normal :

Right :   Tri _____   Bi _____   Sup _____   K.J. _____   A.J. _____   Plantar _____

Left :   Tri _____   Bi _____   Sup _____   K.J. _____   A.J. _____   Plantar _____

Abdominal _____

Sensation to pinprick _____   Light touch _____   Temperature _____

Is proprioception normal _____   Is Rombergism present _____   Any evidence of cerebellar dysfunction _____

Special
Examination.
Distant vision without glasses _____   Right _____   Left _____

Distant vision with glasses _____   Right _____   Left _____

Colour vision _____   Visual fields _____   Right _____   Left _____

Audiometry _____   Right _____   Left _____

Exercise tolerance test :   Type used _____

Result _____

Is ECG normal after exercise _____

Urine _____   Albumin _____   Sugar _____   Blood _____   Ketones _____

Haematocrit _____

Skinfold thickness test _____   FEV₁ _____   FVC _____   FEV₁/FVC _____

Report on full plate chest radiograph _____   Date _____

Report on radiographs of major joints _____   Date _____

_____

Is the candidate free from physical defect and disease _____   Has he the physique for prolonged exertion _____

Particulars of any physical or psychological abnormalities detected : _____

In your opinion is the candidate fit to discharge the duties of a deep sea diver, an occupation which demands the highest physical and psychological standards together with a highly developed sense of responsibility and self reliance _____

Is he fit for service in a tropical climate _____

Name and address of medical examiner _____

Signature _____   Qualifications _____

See memorandum   Date _____

REFERENCES

BAKER, P. T. & DANIELS, F. (1955) Relationship between skin fold thickness and body cooling for 2 hours at 15°C. *J. appl. Physiol.* **8**, 409–416.

BROUHA, L. (1943) The step test: A simple method of measuring physical fitness for muscular work in young men. *Res. Q. Am. Ass. Hlth phys. Educ.* **14**, 31–35.

CIRIA (1972) *The Principles of Safe Diving Practice.* Construction Industry Research and Information Association Underwater Engineering Group. Report No. UR2.

DECOMPRESSION SICKNESS PANEL (MRC) (1974) *Experience with a New Decompression Table for Work in Compressed Air.* Construction Industry Research and Information Association. Technical Note 59.

DECOMPRESSION SICKNESS PANEL (MRC) (1966) Bone lesions in compressed air workers. *J. Bone Jt Surg.* **48B**, 207–235.

DECOMPRESSION SICKNESS PANEL (MRC) (1968) Decompression sickness and aseptic necrosis of bone. *Br. J. indust. Med.* **28**, 1–21.

EDWARDS, D. A. W., HEALY, M. J. R., TANNER, J. M. & WHITEHOUSE, R. H. (1955) Design and accuracy of calipers for measuring subcutaneous tissue thickness. *Br. J. Nutr.* **9**, 133–143.

FRYER, D. I. (1969) *Subatmospheric Decompression Sickness in Man.* NATO AGARDograph 125.

GERSH, I. & CATCHPOLE, H. R. (1951) Decompression sickness, physical factors and pathological consequences. In *Decompression Sickness.* Ed. J. F. Fulton. pp. 165–181. London: Saunders.

GRAY, J. S. (1951) Constitutional factors affecting susceptibility to decompression sickness. In *Decompression Sickness.* Ed. J. F. Fulton. pp. 182–191. London: Saunders.

GRIFFITHS, P. D. (1960) *Compressed Air Disease. A Clinical Review of Cases and Treatment.* M.D. Thesis, University of Cambridge.

HAM, C. & HILL, L. (1905–6) Oxygen inhalation as a means to prevent caisson and diver's sickness. *J. Physiol., Lond.* **33**, VII.

HARVEY, E. N., BARNES, D. K., McELROY, W. D., WHITELEY, A. H., PLEASE, D. C. & COOPER, K. W. (1944) Bubble formation in animals I: Physical factors. *J. Cell comp. Physiol.* **24**, 1–22.

HILLS, B. A. (1966) *A Thermodynamic and Kinetic approach to Decompression Sickness.* Adelaide: Libraries Board of S. Australia.

HILLS, B. A. (1968) The variation in susceptibility to decompression sickness. *Int. J. Bioclim. Biomet.* **12**, 343–449.

HODES, R. & LARRABEE, M. G. (1945) *The Relation between Alveolar Carbon Dioxide Tension and Susceptibility to Decompression Sickness.* US National Research Council CAM Report No. 448.

KEATINGE, W. R. (1972) Cold immersion and swimming. *Jl R. nav. med. Serv.* **58**, 171–176.

LEWIS, H. E. & PATON, W. D. M. (1957) Decompression sickness during the sinking of a caisson. *Br. J. indust. Med.* **14**, 5–12.

MALHOTRA, M. S. & WRIGHT, H. C. (1960) Arterial embolism during decompression under water and its prevention. *J. Physiol., Lond.* **151**, 32P.

MARTIN, K. J. (1973) *Serum Ceatinine Phosphokinase in Man during Diving Training.* Royal Naval Physiological Laboratory Report 4–73.

MOTLEY, H. L., CHINN, H. I. & ODELL, F. A. (1945) Studies on bends. *J. Aviat. Med.* **16**, 210–234.

NASHIMOTO, I. (1967) The use of oxygen during decompression of caisson workers. In *Decompression of Compressed Air Workers in Civil Engineering.* Ed. R. I. McCallum. Newcastle upon Tyne: Oriel Press.

PATON, W. D. M. & WALDER, D. N. (1954) *Compressed Air Illness.* Special Report Medical Research Council No. 281. London: HMSO.

PUGH, L. G. C. & EDHOLM, O. G. (1955) The physiology of channel swimmers. *Lancet* **2**, 761–768.

SUMMITT, J. K., BERGHAGE, T. E. & EVERY, M. G. (1971) *Review and Analysis of Cases of Decompression Sickness Occurring under Pressure.* US Navy Experimental Diving Unit, Research Report 12–71.

THOMPSON, J. W., STEWART, C. B., WARWICK, O. H., BATEMAN, G. L., MILNE, D. J. & GRAY, D. E. (1944) Flying Personnel Medical Section Report D–3 to the National Research Council, Canada.

VAN DER AUE, O. E., KELLAR, R. J. & BRINTON, E. S. (1949) *The Effect of Exercise during Decompression from Increased Barometric Pressures on the Incidence of Decompression Sickness in Man.* US Navy Experimental Diving Unit Research Report No. 8–49.

VERNON, H. M. (1907) The solubility of air in fat and its relation to caisson disease. *Proc. R. Soc. B.* **79**, 366–371.

WALDER, D. N. (1948) Serum surface tension and its relation to the decompression sickness of aviators. *J. Physiol., Lond.* **107**, 43P.

WALDER, D. N. (1963) A probable explanation for some cases of severe decompression sickness in compressed air workers. In *The Regulation of Human Respiration.* Ed. D. J. C. Cunningham & B. B. Lloyd. Oxford: Blackwell.

WALDER, D. N. (1966) Adaptation to decompression sickness in caisson work. In *Proceedings 3rd International Biometerology Congress.* Oxford: Pergamon.

WARWICK, O. H. (1943) *Further Studies on the Relationship of Fluid Intake and Output to the Incidence of Decompression Sickness.* Report by the Flying personnel medical section No. 1, 'Y' Depot RCAF Halifax, to the National Research Council of Canada.

WISE, D. A. (1963) *The Constitutional Factors in Decompression Sickness.* US Navy Experimental Diving Unit. Research Report 2–63.

WUNSCHE, O., FUST, H. D. & PRESSEL, G. (1967) *The Use of Oxygen Breathing for Decompression of Compressed Air Workers at Brunsbüttelkoog.* Dtsch. Luft. Raumfahrt, Report 67–47.

YUNKIN, I. P. (1970) Correlation of animal resistance to hypoxia and caisson disease. *Patol. Fiziol. eksp. Terap.* **14**, 71–73.

ZANNINI, D., ODAGLIA, G. & SPERATI, G. (1975) Audiographic changes in professional divers. In *Underwater Physiology Vth Symp. Underwater Physiology.* Ed. C. J. Lambertsen. Bethesda: Fedn Am. Socs exp. Biol.

25

Decompression Disorders in Divers

D. J. KIDD & D. H. ELLIOTT

The decompression disorders of divers include both decompression sickness and pulmonary barotrauma. Dysbarism is a term that has been used for decompression sickness alone but, from its derivation, it is best reserved for use when a single word is required to describe all the decompression disorders. The term 'aeroembolism' has acquired ambiguity from having been used for air embolism and, by other authors, for aviators' decompression sickness, and its use should therefore be avoided.

Decompression sickness is considered to be that illness following a reduction of environmental pressure which is sufficient to cause a pathological response to the formation or growth of bubbles from gases dissolved in the tissues. There are some differences in the decompression sickness syndrome which may be related to the nature of the precipitating decompression and it is therefore reasonable to use terms such as 'caisson disease' and 'aviators' decompression sickness' if it is intended to confine comment to a specific occupational group.

The term 'bends' is commonly used but needs to be defined with care. It was originally coined by the caisson workers of St Louis to describe the various limb pains, paralyses and cramps that they encountered but, after about 1870, it came to be used for limb pain in the absence of any sign of central nervous system dysfunction (Fryer 1969). More recently the term has come to be used much more loosely by some authors and has included, for instance, the death of small animals after decompression. Some qualification is thus needed

each time that the term is introduced and it is generally considered that it should be confined to the musculoskeletal type of decompression sickness, preferably in the hyphenated form 'limb-bends'.

The other major decompression disorder is pulmonary barotrauma; the term 'burst lung' is used often to describe this pathological entity. This is mechanical damage of the lungs as a direct result of the expansion of intrapulmonary gases during decompression. Decompression barotrauma can also occur in other gas-containing cavities such as the sinuses. Expansion of the gases in the lungs can lead to several serious consequences: pneumothorax, mediastinal emphysema, and arterial gas embolism. It is important at this stage to emphasize a difference between the bubbles of arterial embolism, in which the gas comes from the lungs and when there may be no significant quantities of gas dissolved in the tissues, and the bubbles of decompression sickness, in which the gases have arisen from gases dissolved in the body tissues.

DECOMPRESSION SICKNESS

CAUSES

The failure of the currently accepted prophylactic decompression schedules to prevent symptoms of decompression sickness may be due to one of the following factors.

1. *An error in decompression theory.* The theoretical basis for the decompression table (pressure/

time profile) being followed may be incorrect. Since there is still significant divergence of opinion concerning the factors which determine the precise ascent profile to be followed after any given exposure, it is likely that all current prophylactic tables are no more than general approximations to the truth, offering less than 100% probability of success.

2. *An error in decompression practice.* By intent or accident a suitable decompression profile may not be followed.

3. *An anomalous response of the individual.* A departure from normal tolerance may arise from additional stress factors such as heavy exercise, fatigue, anxiety and hypoglycaemia.

The magnitude of the exposure to pressure is not a reliable guide with which to assess the severity of a case of decompression sickness (Lanphier 1966) and cases may follow what appear to be innocuous exposures well within accepted minimum decompression limits (Berghage 1966). The possible sequence of pathophysiological events leading to decompression sickness in an individual have been discussed in Chapter 23.

MANIFESTATIONS

The diversity of signs and symptoms in over 250 cases of decompression sickness and 25 cases of pulmonary barotrauma are described here from the files of one of the present authors (Kidd). For the most part the cases presented in the course of the large number of simulated and actual dives carried out during the evaluation and development of on-line pneumatic analogue decompression computers (Stubbs & Kidd 1966; Kidd, Stubbs & Weaver 1971). The dives provided a wide spectrum of pressure/time profiles. They were well controlled, supervision of personnel was close and reporting of all symptoms was encouraged, thus supporting the conclusion that the manifestations described are a fair indication of morbidity from diving. Also included are cases arising from operational diving in the Canadian Armed Forces and some 30 cases from commercial and sports diving.

Experience in the Royal Navy of decompression sickness following deep sea diving is also discussed but, as the manifestations following deep

oxygen–helium exposures appear to differ from those following shallow air dives, such cases have not been included in the statistical summaries.

Various attempts have been made to classify the forms and severity of decompression sickness, but the most simple and useful for prognosis or the management of treatment is a modification of that used by Golding et al. (1960) which has two main categories, Type I and Type II.

This classification is particularly useful to medical practitioners in forming the basis for case management. It is also useful when retrospective analyses are required on the relative success or otherwise of decompression schedules. However, it needs to be emphasized that the spectrum of decompression sickness is so broad that such a simplistic classification can be misleading. Since the 'minor' symptoms (Type I) may herald the onset of more serious ones (Type II)—indeed both types of manifestation may be present in the same individual in more than 30% of cases (Slark 1962)—there is a danger that the inexperienced practitioner may overlook the more subtle Type II manifestations in the presence of severe Type I pain, and give the patient a treatment inadequate for his more serious symptoms.

Type I

This includes those cases where pain is the *only* symptom and those exhibiting cutaneous or lymphatic involvement either alone or with joint pain. Those cases in which these manifestations are present but in which some more serious condition is also present are *not* to be included in this category.

Musculoskeletal decompression sickness. Pain is the commonest manifestation, 70% in this series (Table 25.1) compared with 72% reported by Behnke (1947) and 79% by Rivera (1964). It was first described by Triger (1845) in two compressed air workers. Table 25.1 shows that the upper limbs were affected some three times more often than the lower limbs, a similar distribution to that reported elsewhere in other compressed air divers (Slark 1962; Rivera 1964). In caisson workers whose durations under pressure are more prolonged the reverse finding has been reported, lower limb symptoms being three to four times as frequent as those in the upper limb (Golding et al.

TABLE 25.1

Type I manifestations of decompression sickness. Presenting symptoms may occur in more sites than one and in more than one category.

Site	Pain	Cutaneous	Lymphatic	Fatigue
Shoulder	55	25	—	—
Axilla	4	1	14	—
Arm	24	7	—	—
Elbow	28	1	4	—
Forearm	5	4	—	—
Wrist	12	—	—	—
Hand	11	2	—	—
Finger	8	—	—	—
Hip	10	—	—	—
Thigh	4	—	2	—
Knee	16	—	—	—
Shin	4	—	—	—
Ankle	7	—	—	—
Toe	1	—	—	—
Head	—*	—	2	—
Thorax	1†	6	2	—
Abdomen	—	7	2	—
Total	190	53	26	—‡
Percentage	70	20	10	

* Headache was not a presenting symptom and was rarely complained of.
† This was not a girdle pain presaging Type II illness.
‡ Fatigue was never a presenting symptom.

1960; Rose 1962), an observation also true of the symptoms following deep sea oxygen–helium diving. Almost any synovial joint can be the site of pain, only the sternoclavicular joint seeming to be spared. More than one anatomical site may be involved but rarely is the distribution bilaterally symmetrical.

Descriptions of the pain of the musculoskeletal decompression sickness vary widely; pain does not conform to familiar sensory images and localization may be difficult. Joint pains may begin with some numbness in the area (Klintsevich 1965) and an awareness that 'something is not right' (Behnke 1945). The onset of a limb bend is sometimes associated with the desire to move the affected joint as though to ease the discomfort and indeed this type of movement has also been observed minutes before the diver himself has noticed, let alone reported, the onset of the pain.

In most cases the patient can indicate the site of pain at first with some precision. This is usually, but by no means exclusively, near a synovial joint. As time progresses localization becomes more difficult, the pain may radiate or become more diffuse. While it is usually described as a dull throbbing, gradual in onset, progressive and shifting in character (Behnke 1945) it has also been described as steady, boring and not throbbing (Dewey 1962). The pain may be so minor that if it is reported at all the diver may describe it as a 'niggle' or it may be so severe as to be described as an 'intense rending' (Aldrich 1900). The pain may be transient, it may seemingly flit from one joint to another or it may persist in intensity. Some limitation of joint movement and guarding may be found; reflexes and motor tone are normal yet power may be considerably diminished by inhibition. Some reluctance to use or bear weight on the affected limb is noticeable and 'push-ups' or 'deep knee bends' are performed, if they are at all possible in severe or long-standing cases, in a grossly asymmetrical manner. Internal rotation of a shoulder, for example, may illustrate that a particular position may ameliorate the pain. In most cases in which more than an hour has elapsed since the onset of severe pain, pitting oedema over the original site can be demonstrated if carefully sought. In the large majority of cases, however, signs are absent and the diagnosis rests entirely on the symptoms.

Cutaneous decompression sickness. This may be considered as two presentations: transient pruritus and cutaneous circulatory manifestations.

1. *Transient pruritus.* The colloquial 'skin-bends', only too familiar to divers decompressing in a compression chamber, are a mild, multifocal and transient pruritus (Behnke 1951) particularly noticeable about the ears, wrists and hands. These are associated with the deep and middle phases of ascent from 'deep bounce' dives and rarely from long or shallow exposures. While these fleeting sensations are undoubtedly related to fast component of inert gas exchange, probably via the skin (Rashbass 1957), there appears to be no prognostic value in the appearance or non-appearance of this symptom of which no signs are visible. Unlike the focal circulatory manifestation, no treatment is indicated for this self-resolving condition.

2. *Cutaneous circulatory manifestations.* As indi-

cated in Table 25.1 about 20% of Type I symptoms come under this category. Skin manifestations are always preceded by intense itching localized in one or perhaps two areas asymmetrically distributed, most often about the shoulder girdle, lower thorax and abdomen. After a period varying from a minute to an hour during which the focal irritation persists, often with waxing intensity and radiation about the original site, a patchy cutaneous vasodilatation develops. If untreated, this may be followed by evidence of vascular stasis—central cyanotic areas giving a mottled appearance to the skin. The lesions blanch on pressure, are not tender to touch and no crepitus has been observed. There is no obvious relationship with peripheral nerve distribution. Recompression treatment is rapidly effective. If untreated the symptoms are reported to regress slowly over 2 to 3 days. The skin lesions may presage the later appearance of a pain type 'bend', or both types may appear simultaneously. They occasionally follow 'bounce' dives (for example, 250 ft (8·6 ATA) for an hour), but are more frequently associated with longer exposures to shallower depths; dives where the threshold for cavitation would clearly be dictated by an inert gas component having one of the slower time constants. Miles (1966) holds the opposite view that this type of injury follows most commonly after short deep dives and rarely after long shallow ones.

Lymphatic decompression sickness. About 10% of Type I cases have an oedema which is to be seen over a painful limb. It may in part be due to reflex impairment of tissue permeability but from time to time, in the absence of deep limb pain, there is clear evidence of lymphatic obstruction. The cutaneous areas distal to the site of obstruction have the typical 'peau d'orange' or 'pigskin' appearance of pitting oedema.

A case in which the diver presented $3\frac{1}{2}$ hours after surfacing with oedema over the left parotid region and later had tenderness and moderate enlargement of the parotid and anterior cervical glands (Fig. 25.1), responded well to recompression. A similar but bilateral parotid swelling associated with mild pyrexia followed a dive by another individual and, but for the response to recompression, would have been diagnosed as mumps. Another diver in this series reported an ache in the

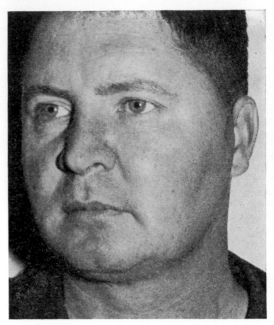

Fig. 25.1. Type I—Lymphatic manifestation before treatment

Unilateral pitting oedema anterior to left parotid area associated with soreness and enlarged tender submandibular glands which presented 230 min after surfacing from 244 ft (8·4 ATA) for 30 min. It was relieved at 33 ft (2 ATA) on 100% oxygen after 3 min

right axilla $1\frac{1}{2}$ hours after surfacing. On examination the central axillary glands were enlarged to walnut size and extremely tender. All signs and symptoms cleared during the first 8 min of treatment with pressure. Another case is illustrated in Fig. 25.2.

Malaise, anorexia and fatigue. As well as being an important causative factor in decompression sickness, a disproportionate degree of fatigue does appear to follow exposure to pressure *per se*. Prolonged and particularly deep repetitive diving followed by a decompression close to the theoretical limits may be totally asymptomatic except for an unusual fatigue. Fatigue, malaise and anorexia after a deep oxygen–helium dive have been considered as a warning that more serious symptoms might follow. These are difficult symptoms to assess and their presence may not always be appreciated as the following case history illustrates. Incidentally the following case history also illustrates that damaged tissues can have an increased susceptibility to decompression.

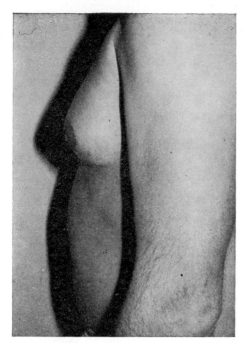

FIG. 25.2. Type I—Lymphatic manifestation before treatment

Marked unilateral oedema of left pectoral area extending to umbilicus and associated with mild ache over left nipple area which presented 120 min after surfacing from 72 ft (3·2 ATA) for 723 min. It was relieved at 66 ft (2·8 ATA) on 100% oxygen after 3 min

As part of an investigation into the cause of an epileptiform convulsion while diving, a 25-year-old diver had a lumbar puncture. The results were normal, though, during the procedure, his right leg had twitched for a second or two, indicating some nerve root irritation. Six days later, having been declared fully fit to resume diving, he dived on air to 50 ft (2·5 ATA) for 25 min. This is a very safe dive yet for 2 hours afterwards he noticed a strip of tingling down the length of the back of his right leg, though he did not report this. Some 20 days after the lumbar puncture he dived on air to 180 ft (6·5 ATA) for 15 min, another safe dive but requiring some decompression stoppages. After 45 min since surfacing he noticed the onset of analgesia in patches down the back of his right thigh and knee extending down to the outer aspect of his right foot. On examination there was an area of impaired sensation corresponding to the distribution of S1 and 2 from the gluteal region to the foot. There were no other physical signs. He was treated by recompression with complete relief and suffered no recurrence. After treatment the diver stated that during this incident he had felt

quite fit 'in himself' in contrast to the definite 'off colour' feeling which he had experienced during previous limb bends.

When sought, such malaise is a commonly admitted feature of decompression sickness. It was suggested by Dewey (1962) that the fatigue was a manifestation of adrenocortical exhaustion. An alternative explanation is based on the presence of intravascular gas in a number of divers after apparently safe dives as well as in cases of decompression sickness. If there is indeed some degree of sub-clinical pulmonary gas embolism in such persons then these symptoms may be considered analagous to similar symptoms reported in cases of mild pulmonary embolism due to other conditions (Hallenbeck, Elliott & Bove 1975).

Type II

This category includes all cases of more serious nature with central nervous system, peripheral neuropathy or respiratory involvement (Table 25.2). Since the site or sites of cavitation may be anywhere in the higher centres, the spinal cord or the cardiorespiratory system, the symptomatology is protean (Rivera 1964), may be multifocal and is always unpredictable. The magnitude of the

TABLE 25.2

Type II manifestations of decompression sickness. Presenting symptoms may occur in more than one category

Symptomatology	Number	Percentage
Dizziness	12	
Confusion	5	33
Disorientation	4	
Eye signs		
Nystagmus	2	
Diplopia	3	10
Tunnel vision	1	
Sensory impairment		
Hyperaesthesia	5	25
Paraesthesia	11	
Motor weakness or loss	8	16
Dysarthria	2	
Nausea and vomiting	3	5
Respiratory		
Dyspnoea	4	11
Coughing	3	
Total	63	—

lesion will determine the severity of the symptoms. One of these more serious conditions may be the only manifestation of decompression sickness but it is important to note that in about 30% of Type II cases joint pain is also present (Slark 1962).

Pulmonary decompression sickness. Respiratory decompression sickness, known to divers as the 'chokes', is probably the result of pulmonary bubble embolism. Inhalation may be limited by a sharp 'catch' which is pathognomonic. It is sometimes first noticed when the diver lights up a cigarette on surfacing. Perhaps the best description comes from the personal experience of Behnke (1945):

> About twenty years ago it was necessary to work for several hours at 4 atmospheres pressure about 3 days a week. Following decompression but often preceded by several hours of well-being I experienced substernal discomfort, at first only on deep inspiration, which frequently elicited the cough reflex... there were no respiratory signs or even symptoms (when deep inspirations were not attempted). . . . Either complete recovery occurred or, during the course of the next hour, depth of breathing became progressively less because of substernal distress, and rapid shallow breathing supervened. Deep inspiration at this stage induced paroxysmal coughing and to prevent asphyxia it was necessary to undergo recompression.

To this graphic description the present authors would only add that whereas a latency of several hours is described, the onset of respiratory decompression sickness is often relatively early and can occur within minutes of a severe decompression. It is also relevant to the earlier description of malaise and fatigue after decompression and its possible relationship to sub-clinical pulmonary embolism, that he adds, 'Concomitant with the onset of sub-sternal distress following a deep inspiration there occurred frequently a debilitating malaise. The contrast between the latent period of well-being and the abrupt onset of fatigue was unmistakable'.

Neurological decompression sickness. Schrotter (Heller, Mager & Schrotter 1900) describes a case in which paralysis and coma was preceded by respiratory difficulties and limb bends. Behnke and Shaw (1937) reported that neurological decompression sickness was often preceded by respiratory symptoms and, more recently, in another series of divers (Hallenbeck, Elliott & Bove 1975) there were six in whom there was a recorded difference between the times of onset of their pulmonary and of their respiratory symptoms. In five of these six, the respiratory symptoms preceded the symptoms of cord damage. Nevertheless, in a great many cases, the neurological symptoms and signs are the only manifestations of decompression sickness.

The commonest site for neurological lesions in divers is in the spinal cord, but cerebral manifestations are not uncommon. Disturbances of cerebral function may account for almost any bizarre symptoms or behaviour. Psychotic conditions have been simulated but visual blurring and headaches are more common. One specific decompression syndrome, which is referred to by divers as 'the staggers' is a disturbance of labyrinthine function with vertigo, nystagmus, nausea and vomiting. It may be associated with a tinnitus and partial deafness. Migraine-like symptoms have also been described, commonly in aviators (Engel et al. 1944; Fryer 1969) but also after decompression from depth (Anderson et al. 1965). The individuals concerned frequently gave a history of previous attacks of true migraine and said that the decompression manifestations were similar to the previous attacks but more serious. Scotomata and fortification spectra with unilateral headaches were related to electroencephalographic changes over the occipital cortex.

The most sinister development following a decompression is the insidious onset of peripheral sensory and motor symptoms. Paraesthesia may be noticed in a limb or possibly there may be a marginal degree of weakness. The feet may begin to feel 'woolly' or cold and what might be thought at first to be simple 'pins and needles' may spread rapidly until in less than half an hour the patient has become a paraplegic and has lost all sphincter control. The peripheral sensory and motor lesions are thought to be due to bubbles in the spinal cord but they do not always follow a typical segmental distribution and an isolated patch may occur in any limb. Experience has shown that girdle pains of the trunk indicate a cord lesion and should be treated as such.

Haemoconcentration and hypovolaemic shock. A possible mechanism for increased capillary permeability and for the loss of plasma into the extravascular shock as a consequence of intravascular bubbles was discussed in Chapter 23. Haemoconcentration is well documented as a phenomenon in some cases of acute decompression sickness but is not always present. In severe cases haematocrits of 58 to 68% have been reported (Brunner, Frick & Bühlmann 1964; Cockett & Nakamura 1964; Behnke 1967). Signs and symptoms of hypovolaemic shock from postural hypotension to oliguria can be anticipated, particularly in those who have required more than one recompression (Barnard et al. 1966).

Time of onset of symptoms

One might expect the greatest occurrence of symptoms to be during the time between leaving maximum pressure and reaching sea level. When atmospheric pressure is reached, elimination of inert gas continues until equilibrium is re-established, gas dynamic theory predicting that cavitation should be progressively less critical with time. In fact, the majority of cases present later than this and follow a latent period commencing at the time of reaching sea level. In Fig. 25.3 is shown a consecutive series of cases as related to their time of onset, time zero being the time of reaching sea level pressure. The distribution of cases with respect to time shows a marked similarity to those reported by Slark (1962). The longest latent period in the Canadian series was 15 hours and latent periods of up to 36 hours were reported by Welham and Waite (1951) and from the files of the US Navy by Rivera (1964). It remains possible that some at least of these long latent periods might be due in part to a failure to appreciate or to report some earlier manifestation. In saturation diving such latency is hidden since the decompressions are so lengthy that most symptoms are re-

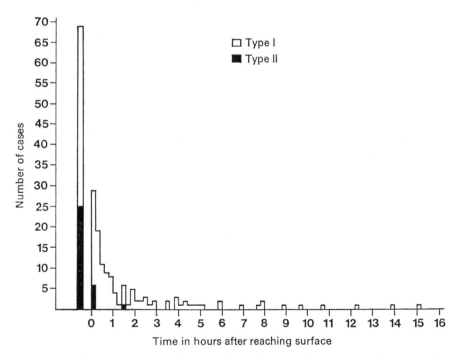

FIG. 25.3. Decompression sickness—time of onset of cases in relation to the time of reaching surface

196 cases from the Canadian Forces Institute of Aviation Medicine and Royal Canadian Navy Diving Establishments, July 1963 to October 1968. The cases which occurred during decompression are shown together before the time of surfacing

ported during the course of the prolonged decompression.

DIAGNOSIS

The diagnosis of acute decompression sickness is usually obvious. Doubt may occur in minor cases who have had a nominally safe decompression and then it may be tempting to ascribe the symptoms to some occupational, domestic, or athletic injury. This doubt could prompt a delay in the onset of treatment and hence allow time for the development of later complications. Little harm can come from recompression and the rapid response of a doubtful case to such treatment is not only diagnostic but is also wise management. A coincidental appendicitis (Behnke 1945) or ruptured spleen (Sonnenburg 1967) has been described and such conditions should be excluded as far as possible since most recompression chambers are totally unsuitable for surgery.

It needs to be emphasized that, in the absence of abnormal findings and particularly in consideration of the difficulties of making a totally satisfactory physical examination while at pressure, it is essential to treat the symptoms of a patient. Reduction of delay between the onset of symptoms and the application of recompression is most important to halt the progression of the illness and reduce the probability of residual damage.

Special investigations at this stage are contraindicated by the urgency of treatment. Radiography has demonstrated aeroarthrosis in aviators' decompression sickness but there was no significant correlation between the presence of air and the symptom of pain (Ferris & Engel 1951).

Differential diagnosis

Pulmonary barotrauma (see later) is responsible for an acute condition which may simulate decompression sickness and may account for a proportion of those cases of 'bends' which occur after nominally safe decompressions. Arterial air embolism is the most common manifestation of pulmonary barotrauma. The more serious cases lose consciousness within seconds of decompression and may die in spite of immediate and rigorous treatment. Less severe cases may mimic neurological lesions of decompression sickness

with the sudden onset of patches of numbness and of paralysis of one or more limbs within minutes of surfacing. Mediastinal emphysema and barotraumatic pneumothorax may occur. The patient usually complains of chest pain or dyspnoea on surfacing or has some haemoptysis. Surgical emphysema near the root of the neck is diagnostic of pulmonary barotrauma, but is not always present.

The treatment for both conditions is immediate recompression and thus a differential diagnosis is often made only retrospectively. However, if a firm diagnosis can be made at the start then the subsequent management will be simplified.

Mention must also be made of one case of Munchausen's syndrome (Kemp & Munro 1969) who some months later presented again elsewhere but this second time recompression was refused.

TREATMENT

The treatment of acute decompression sickness is by *immediate recompression*. In fact it was recognized as early as 1863 by Foley that the 'true specific' for caisson sickness was to return the patient to the raised environmental pressure but it was not till 1890 that Moir (1896) at the Hudson river tunnelling project provided the first 'medical lock'.

For many years it has been considered that the reduction of bubble size by the reapplication of raised environmental pressure should, if applied soon enough, be sufficient to restore the patient to full fitness. More recent studies have demonstrated that the bubble can very quickly trigger other events which may not be so responsive to reduction of bubble size. Nevertheless, whether due to compression of mechanically obstructive bubbles or to diminution of their surface area and reduction of bubble surface activity in the blood, there is no doubt that immediate recompression can be dramatically effective and that immediate recompression is the treatment of choice.

When the patient has been restored to fitness by the recompression, a relatively slow return to normal atmospheric pressure allows time for the adequate elimination of excess gas dissolved in the tissues of the body.

There are a number of recompression, or therapeutic, tables available. The selection of the one appropriate for the treatment of a particular case is determined by the nature of the manifestations, the type of dive which induced the illness and the availability of oxygen and other gases for the patient to breathe during his therapeutic recompression.

Particularly when treatment has been delayed, often because of the distance of the diving site from the nearest compression chamber, various supplementary treatments may be indicated but the use of such medications does not affect the principle that urgent recompression is the treatment of choice.

There are many alternative schedules available for the therapeutic recompression of divers and basically these can be considered as tables that return the patient to one of the following treatment depths.

1. *The depth of relief* of his symptoms or a few feet deeper than this. This has been especially used in the UK for divers whose symptoms arise during the course of a decompression from a deep oxy-helium dive. The depth of relief is usually found to be shallower than the depth of the original dive.

2. *The depth of the original exposure.* This has occasionally been used for divers when relief has not been obtained shallower and where there is, for some reason, reluctance to proceed deeper.

3. *An arbitrary depth.* The depth of 60 ft (2·8 ATA), when oxygen is available for treatment, and of 165 ft (6·0 ATA), using compressed air, are the treatment depths most commonly found in the Treatment Tables of Diving Manuals. These have

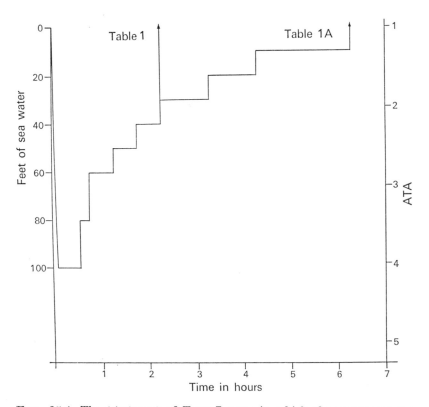

FIG. 25.4. The treatment of Type I cases in which the symptoms are relieved at depths less than 66 ft (3 ATA)

On USN Table 1 oxygen is breathed from 60 ft (2·8 ATA) to the surface. On USN Table 1A, from which the metric RN Table 51 was derived, compressed air is breathed throughout

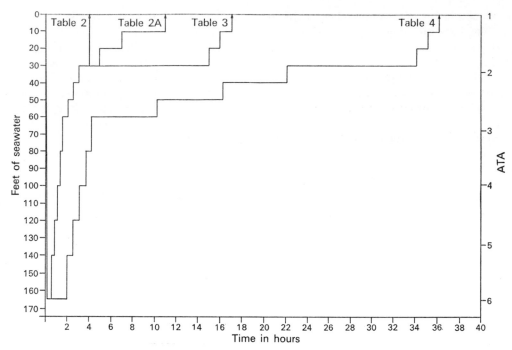

FIG. 25.5. The treatment of Type I cases in which the symptoms are relieved at depths greater than 66 ft (3 ATA) and the treatment of Type II cases

On USN Table 2 oxygen is breathed from 60 ft (2·8 ATA) to the surface. On USN Table 2A, from which the similar RN Table 53 was derived, compressed air is breathed throughout. USN Table 3 and the corresponding RN Table 54 are used for more serious cases. On this table oxygen may be breathed for the last hour at each of the last three stoppages. This is considered to reduce the incidence of recurrences and the incidence of decompression sickness in the attendant.

several practical advantages when treatment has to be carried out by divers remote from medical advice. They are also the most convenient to use since therapeutic recompression is a team effort requiring the special skills of hyperbaric or diving personnel and a standardized therapy is therefore the one most likely to succeed. Only when the management of the clinical condition or other aspects of a particular case proves difficult should these well-tried tables be abandoned in favour of some other regime and then only on the advice of a physician experienced in treating such cases.

Compressed air therapeutic tables

Generally speaking, physicians supervising the treatment of compressed air workers have advocated the use of the minimal pressure to ensure relief of symptoms. Physicians treating divers are faced with symptoms arising from a range of pressure and time exposures quite different from

those experienced by caisson workers and they have been forced to consider much higher recompression pressures in order to achieve relief. A decompression of a much longer time course is necessary and, for ease of supervision, the 'stop' system is adopted. The therapeutic tables, shown in Figs 25.4 and 25.5, were evolved by US Navy Medical Officers (Yarbrough & Behnke 1939; Van der Aue et al. 1945) and are in the *USN Diving Manual* (metric form, *RN Diving Manual*).

Once symptoms of decompression sickness occur, the mechanisms of inert gas exchange are impaired locally and also, probably, more generally. It is unfortunate that the use of these high recompression pressures (165 ft; 6 ATA) mean an additional exposure to raised inert gas partial pressures at a time when inert gas exchange is probably least efficient. The response of the patient to subsequent changes of ambient pressure can only be assessed by trial and error.

Any recurrence compounds the problem and the ultimate decompression of a serious or difficult case may be very prolonged if it is to be successful.

In the US Navy Therapeutic Table 4 (Fig. 25.5) there is an incidence of some 20% of cases of Type I decompression sickness in the attendant in addition to a high failure rate for the patient (Rivera 1964). It was shown during a series of 48-hour dives by the Canadian Armed Forces at Toronto that the maximum depth from which direct ascent appeared to be safe was an equivalent of 26·5 ft (1·8 ATA) of seawater. A number of modifications to that table exist, the simplest being to insist that both patient and attendant comply with the published option of breathing oxygen during the final hour at the 30, 20 and 10 ft (1·9, 1·6 and 1·3 ATA) stoppages. When oxygen is not available the Canadian modification of completing the final 10 hours of the prolonged stop at 26 ft (1·8 ATA) instead of at the published 30 ft (1·9 ATA) is also effective.

Treatment tables using oxygen

Ideally what is required is recompression to the point where effective circulation is restored and this pressure maintained for a sufficient time to ensure recovery. Yarbrough and Behnke (1939) introduced the long and short oxygen tables in which 100% oxygen was used between 60 ft (2·8 ATA) and the surface. These were the forerunners of the current Therapeutic Tables 1 and 2 (Figs 25.4 and 25.5).

Since then, a series of treatments using moderate pressures only and almost continuous breathing of 100% oxygen have been evolved by Goodman and Workman (1965). In 1964 the provisional regime (Fig. 25.6; Goodman 1967) was used for 2 years for all cases arising in the series in Toronto, and is still used in some centres. This regime had the advantage of assisting the relief of ischaemia in the most efficient way by avoiding further exposure to inert gas and also providing the maximum gradient for the elimination of the inert gas, thus shortening the treatment time dramatically. A linear ascent was considered to be of doubtful value since theory suggests that an exponential ascent profile is optimum; in practice when venting, unless frequent valve adjustments are made, the pressure in a chamber tends to follow such a profile. Oxygen is administered via well-fitting masks and low resistance demand regulators from a built-in breathing system (BIBS) manifold supplied by gas at 50 to 80 psi above ambient pressure.

At first this regime was cautiously reserved only for Type I cases of decompression sickness but the response was so consistently satisfactory that all but the most serious Type II cases were similarly treated. The regime was effective (5% failure to relieve symptoms) and had a low recurrence rate (7%).

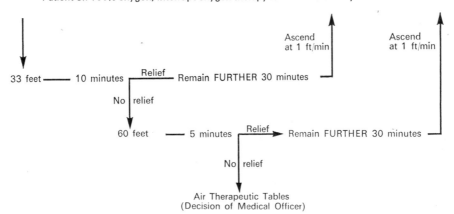

Patient on 100% oxygen; interrupt oxygen therapy for 5 minutes every 30 minutes.

Fɪɢ. 25.6. The original minimal-recompression oxygen-breathing treatment (Goodman 1967)

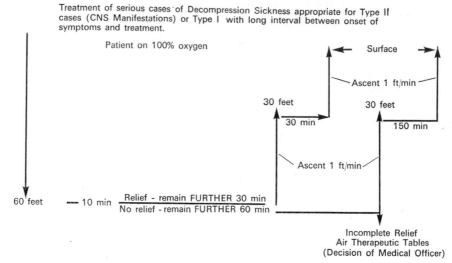

Treatment of serious cases of Decompression Sickness appropriate for Type II cases (CNS Manifestations) or Type I with long interval between onset of symptoms and treatment.

Interrupt 100% Oxygen for 5 minutes every 30 minutes. Substitute air or 20:80% Helium during break from 100% Oxygen.

FIG. 25.7. The revised minimal-recompression oxygen-breathing treatment (modified after Goodman & Workman 1965)

In 1966, following the work of Goodman and Workman (1965), the longer regime shown in Fig. 25.7 was adopted in Toronto for comparison. The breaks in the oxygen breathing cycle take advantage of rapid recovery time to prolong oxygen tolerance (Kaufman, Owen & Lambertsen 1956) as well as allowing time for drinks which are most welcome after very dry oxygen inhalation from the BIBS.

A summary of the results obtained in Canada using minimum pressure oxygen therapy (Figs 25.6 and 25.7) is given in Table 25.3. The effectiveness of these regimes has resulted in their adoption in principle by most recompression centres.

The mean ratio between depth of onset and depth of relief for those cases in the Canadian series arising during decompression was 1·5 for Type I and 1·9 for Type II cases (Table 25.4).

Treatments requiring oxygen–helium

The treatment tables using compressed air or oxygen are not sufficient for all cases of decompression sickness, in particular those that arise after a very deep dive when the depth of relief of symptoms may be deeper than the standard therapeutic depth 165 ft (6 ATA). In a number of cases the first symptom has occurred in the course of the

original decompression at a greater depth than this and thus recompression using oxygen–helium is again essential.

In such cases recompression is taken to the

TABLE 25.3

Summary of results using minimum pressure 100% oxygen therapy tables July 1964 to July 1972

	Type of case	
	I	II
Number of cases	205*	30†
Failure to relieve symptoms	4	4
Recurrences	17	1
Recurrences treated by repeated regimes	17	1
Mean interval from initiation of treatment to relief	10 min	13 min
Mean interval from onset of symptoms to initiation of treatment	90 min (longest 12 hours)	10 min
Evidence of oxygen toxicity	—	—
Treatment limited to 2 ATA (33 ft)	60	6

* 2 cases and † 3 cases followed oxygen–helium diving at less than 250 ft (8·6 ATA). All others followed compressed air diving.

TABLE 25.4

Relationship between depth of onset (when symptoms occurred during decompression) and depth of relief

Type I			Type II		
Depth (ATA)			Depth (ATA)		
Symptoms	Relief	Ratio	Symptoms	Relief	Ratio
1·06	1·36	1·3	1·51	2·82	1·9
1·18	1·36	1·2	1·06	1·91	1·8
1·18	2·0	1·7	1·3	2·82	2·2
1·15	2·0	1·7	1·3	2·0	1·5
1·15	1·91	1·7	1·58	2·82	1·8
1·32	1·91	1·4	1·46	2·82	1·9
1·15	1·91	1·7	1·18	2·82	2·4
1·10	1·85	1·7	1·16	2·0	1·7
1·15	1·3	1·1	1·37	2·82	2·1
1·61	2·82	1·7	1·3	1·91	1·5
1·3	1·91	1·5	1·97	2·82	1·4
1·3	1·91	1·5	1·27	2·0	1·6
1·21	2·0	1·7	1·06	2·0	1·9
1·28	2·0	1·6	1·64	2·82	1·7
1·28	1·46	1·1	1·82	2·82	1·6
1·46	2·07	1·4	1·82	2·82	1·6
1·15	2·03	1·8	1·18	2·82	2·4
1·18	1·85	1·6			
1·36	2·0	1·5			
1·3	2·0	1·5			
2·0	2·82	1·4			
1·2	2·0	1·7			
1·6	2·0	1·25			
1·84	2·5	1·4			
Mean ratio		1·5	Mean ratio		1·9

depth of the complete relief of symptoms. There is then a 20 to 30 min stay at that pressure before a slow decompression. Decompression sickness in one patient was not cured until he had been lowered in a submersible chamber to 450 ft (14·6 ATA) in the open sea (Fig. 25.8; Elliott 1967).

The subsequent decompression is at a rate determined by the condition of the patient and, after the experience of 30 such cases, it was found that most could return safely to the surface if an exponential decompression curve was followed. The exponential has a half-time of about 13 hours and corresponds to a drop of the absolute pressure in the ratio 1·3 to 1 over a period of 5 hours (Barnard 1967). Thus this curve entered at any depth after the relief of symptoms, provides a simple guide for the therapeutic decompression of all cases of decompression sickness occurring at great depth.

Not only does such therapy require a compression chamber able to withstand at least the maximum pressure of the original dive, but also it requires a chamber in which it is possible to monitor and maintain a comfortable temperature and humidity and a respirable oxygen–helium atmosphere.

The management of musculoskeletal decompression sickness

If oxygen is not available the patient must be treated on the conventional compressed air tables (see Figs 25.4 and 25.5). If pain is fully relieved at 66 ft (3 ATA), pressure is increased to 100 ft (4 ATA) and the subsequent decompression is in accordance with USN Therapeutic Table 1A or very similar tables in the diving manuals of other navies. If pain is not fully relieved, pressure is increased to 165 ft (6 ATA) and the patient is treated on USN Table 2A. These tables are usually effective.

If oxygen is available the patient breathes oxygen from the surface and is compressed to 60 ft (2·8 ATA). If the symptoms are fully relieved within 10 min of arrival at this depth the patient is treated in accordance with the therapy indicated in Fig. 25.7. If symptoms are not fully relieved in this time the physician has the choice of following North American practice and continuing with a more prolonged oxygen table or following the more conservative British practice by changing from oxygen breathing, compressing the patient to 165 ft (6 ATA) and treating with the appropriate compressed air table. While the longer minimal-recompression table of Goodman and Workman (1965) is certainly effective in the majority of cases, it is the experience of some medical officers that, following deep diving, the greater pressures of the air tables are more effective in achieving rapid and total relief.

It is usual for the pain to respond quickly with a rapid decrease of the pain to a dull ache, then complete relief shortly thereafter. Any guarding disappears, power and full range of painless movement are restored. If, however, the delays in onset of treatment have allowed the secondary effects of tissue hypoxia to be established, relief of pain may

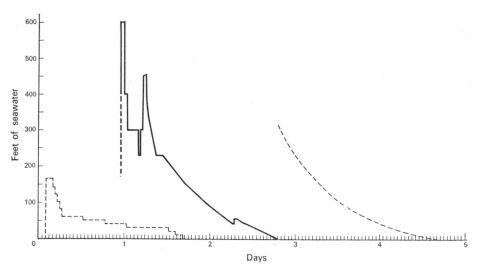

FIG. 25.8. The treatment of a case of decompression sickness which presented at 230 ft (8 ATA)

The stepped interrupted line indicates RN Table 54 to the same scale and the curved interrupted line represents the exponential guide to the decompression given. It can be seen that one small further recompression was needed at 42 ft (2·3 ATA) when the rate shown by the curve had been exceeded (after Elliott 1967)

not be complete and residual symptoms, often described as bruising, can be expected.

When recompression is first applied the symptoms may change in character and, on occasions, even become worse. Occasionally paraesthesia radiating to more distal parts of an affected limb may be reported before resolution is complete and may erroneously suggest a worsening or an additional complication. Careful neurological examination will reveal no additional peripheral signs and the symptoms soon disappear.

Rarely, usually following deep sea diving, the response to recompression is inadequate and the physician must decide whether to remain longer at 165 ft (6 ATA) or whether further recompression would be of benefit. If the effect of greater pressure is tried then there is possibly a need for oxygen–helium breathing and the subsequent decompression would follow the lengthy exponential already described. For bends pain alone, in the absence of serious symptoms, this decompression curve has been required only for those cases which began while still under pressure from the original deep oxygen–helium dive.

While the intensity or persistence of pain of many Type I lesions is usually a sufficient spur to

seek medical attention there are some relatively mild cases which will respond symptomatically to analgesics. This offers a temptation to conceal symptoms especially at the end of a long hard day. Nevertheless, it is important to treat all such symptoms with recompression as it is possible that the chronic sequelae of aseptic bone necrosis might thereby be avoided. Fortunately the motivation and training of divers generally encourages them to seek proper treatment rather than to avoid it.

It is also important to examine all cases carefully to establish the true nature and extent of the lesion. In the Toronto series, examination of four cases presenting with only the symptoms of a Type I manifestation revealed the additional signs of neurological involvement which requires more vigorous treatment.

The management of cutaneous and lymphatic decompression sickness

Recompression will always relieve an incidental focal irritation but when pruritus is the only symptom of decompression sickness continued observation is all that is required. The visible vascular changes may not always resolve during treatment, although this is usually the case in the mild forms. Recurrences have not been observed. Symptomatic relief of lymphatic obstruction is rapid, but complete resolution of the oedema may not occur by the time the short form of oxygen treatment is terminated. No recurrences of this type of lesion have been noted.

The management of respiratory decompression sickness

If there are respiratory symptoms, with or without evidence of Type I manifestations, the patient is to be treated by immediate recompression either using the prolonged oxygen table (Fig. 25.7) or by recompression to 165 ft (6 ATA) using USN Tables 3 or 4 (Fig. 25.5) or similar tables in other diving manuals. Most cases report complete relief within a few minutes.

The management of neurological decompression sickness

If there are neurological symptoms, with or without evidence of Type I manifestations, the patient is to be treated by immediate recompression using the tables recommended above for the respiratory cases.

The use of oxygen at 60 ft (2·8 ATA) for serious cases is still not fully accepted by all physicians with diving experience but is considered by many to be the treatment of choice. This is particularly so in those cases in which delay has occurred before recompression. After deep diving, however, the tendency is to treat on the shallow oxygen table only if response is rapid and complete and otherwise to continue the recompression to greater pressures.

If these therapies do not succeed then greater pressure may be successful, especially if the depth of the original dive was greater than the conventional therapeutic depth of 165 ft (6 ATA). In Fig. 25.9 is shown the treatment to the depth of the original dive, 270 ft (9·2 ATA), where full and immediate relief of symptoms was obtained. The subsequent decompression was at first too rapid and exceeded the 1·3 ratio but the slight recur-

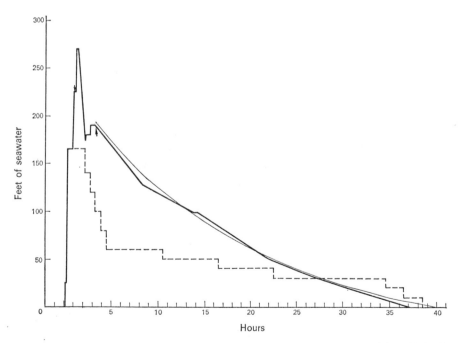

FIG. 25.9. The treatment of a case of decompression sickness with relief of symptoms at 270 ft (9·2 ATA)

The interrupted line indicates RN Table 54 to the same scale and the thin curved line is the same exponential shown in Fig. 25.8. Oxygen–helium was breathed by the patient during the period indicated between the two arrows

rence was relieved by a second recompression. The subsequent decompression was by a series of linear rates of ascent close to the exponential curve which had previously been successful for oxygen–helium therapeutic decompressions. On this occasion air was breathed for most of the ascent which was uneventful.

A case described by Barnard and Elliott (1966) illustrates some phenomena which cannot be entirely explained by current hypotheses of decompression sickness. It demonstrated quite effectively that recompression can be associated with a marked deterioration in the clinical condition of the patient. The diver had recently completed a decompression from a dive to 600 ft (19·2 ATA) during which he had developed some joint pain which was relieved by recompression. His recompression for neurological symptoms which developed after surfacing was associated during the compression with the onset of pain in joints not previously affected and of paralysis and numbness below the waist. At 165 ft (6 ATA) there was no further deterioration but neither was there any improvement. Recompression to 300 ft (10 ATA) achieved complete relief and the subsequent decompression using oxygen–helium was relatively uneventful.

During long treatments, fluids and food must be given and urinary output measured and maintained, bearing in mind not only the frequency of bladder involvement in spinal cord lesions for which catheterization may be required but also the rare danger of hypovolaemic renal failure. Rest is important and, when ambient pressure is held constant, sleep should be encouraged with periodic awakening to assess clinical progress or detect a possible relapse.

The management of relapse or recurrence during treatment

New symptoms or the recurrence of previous ones during or after a therapeutic recompression should be sought and are an indication for a further immediate recompression. Recompression must be applied as often as symptoms recur even to the extent of the heroic repetitions of treatment described by Rivera (1964) and Golding et al. (1960). These cases are the difficult ones and

specialist opinion should be sought. Repetition of the longer oxygen treatments may be preferred or, depending on the history, deeper recompression may be indicated.

The experience of Kidd directing the treatment of cases followed throughout by an on-line analogue computer (Stubbs & Kidd 1966) or of those in which the sequence of incident dive and subsequent therapeutic pressure-time course has been fed into an artificial time analogue computer, is that a reasonably accurate estimate of 'tissue inert gas pressure' can be made. When the subsequent decompression profile is adjusted so that ambient pressure equals the 'tissue inert gas pressure', theoretically no further cavitation can occur and in these circumstances the decompression has proved to be remarkably successful. Account is taken of variations induced by the gas inhaled (oxygen or oxygen–helium mixtures). While practical experience in guiding decompression from complicated and prolonged therapy in this manner has been limited to some 20 cases arising from diving to 350 ft (11·6 ATA) at the most, the close correlation between computer predictions and the protocols of others who deal with cases arising from deeper diving gives confidence for wider application.

The effect of delay upon prognosis

The importance of reducing the delay between onset of symptoms and the institution of recompression treatment was strikingly shown by Rivera (1964). A 90% probability of relief from initial treatment administered within ½ hour of onset fell to 50% when the delay exceeded 6 hours. Similarly, the probability of residual symptoms remaining even after repeated therapy rose from 1% if treated within ½ hour of onset to 13% if the delay exceeded 6 hours. The longer the delay in applying recompression treatment the greater the depth likely to be necessary for complete relief (Doll & Berghage 1967).

Nevertheless, considerable improvement can be achieved even after quite lengthy delays. The vertigo and nystagmus of one British civilian diver which began soon after a no-stop ascent from a 130 ft (5 ATA) untimed dive were completely relieved by recompression 5 days later.

Management when recompression is not available

While immediate recompression is the treatment of choice for all forms of acute decompression sickness, much diving takes place remote from recompression facilities. Since Type I manifestations may herald the onset of serious decompression sickness it is justifiable to consider any case of decompression sickness, especially one occurring remote from a recompression chamber, as a medical emergency.

The patient should be given 100% oxygen even though, perhaps due to its vasoconstrictive effect, it may be associated with some initial worsening of the condition. Through the local equivalent of a Rescue Coordination Centre, assistance with transport and specialist advice should be sought. Arrangements should be made for transfer to a definitive treatment centre, preferably using a portable recompression chamber. If no such chamber is available for the patient it is important that any air transport has a cabin pressure below 1000 ft (0·96 ATA) in order to avoid the dangers to the patient of a further decompression.

In the absence of any recompression the prognosis is not always poor. Before the introduction of recompression as an effective treatment Bauer (1870) stated that of 25 paraplegics 4 died but most recovered in 1 to 4 weeks. Similarly, Gal (1872) stated that those paralysed as a result of helmeted sponge diving would either recover over a period from 5 days to 3 months or die from bedsores or cystitis. With modern supportive therapy there is therefore some chance of recovery in a proportion of cases.

Supplementary forms of therapy

Difficulties in the treatment of acute decompression sickness usually arise only when the recompression has been delayed. Appropriate drug and fluid therapy is therefore indicated when recompression is not immediately available or when recompression has not been completely effective. Although the successful use of drugs in decompression sickness has been reported (Saumarex, Bolt & Gregory 1973), there is still no rational basis on which to plan such treatment and it is in this area of research that one can hope for significant progress during the next few years. It is entirely possible that a given drug may be useful at one stage of the illness, but harmful at another. In the meanwhile some guidelines to treatment can be offered, provided that it is understood that these are provisional and subject to future revision.

Intravenous plasma or low molecular weight dextran has been used successfully on many occasions (Brunner, Frick & Bühlmann 1964; Barnard et al. 1966; Cockett et al. 1970) particularly in cases in which there has been evidence of haemoconcentration. There is a tendency at present, perhaps in view of its additional beneficial effects on platelet stability and blood viscosity, to begin intravenous dextran at an early stage of the illness. Nevertheless, some caution is advisable especially when there is evidence of respiratory decompression sickness, because of a risk of precipitating pulmonary oedema.

Heparin can have some useful therapeutic effects in decompression sickness (Barthelemy 1963; Cockett, Pauley & Roberts 1972) but its mechanisms of action are complex and its efficacy in decompression sickness has not yet been proved. When given prophylactically in small animals its success in preventing decompression sickness has been related to its anti-lipaemic rather than to its anti-coagulative properties (Philp, Gowdey & Prasad 1967). Therefore it should be possible, by the use of a small dosage (2000 u), to avoid the possible dangers of haemorrhage in, for instance, a vestibular end-organ already damaged by decompression sickness.

Other drugs such as steroids have been advocated on the principle that they are useful in the treatment of shock and prevention of CNS oedema. Hypothermia has been advocated (Erde 1963) but, though of possible value in neurological cases where recompression is not available, has not been adopted for the use in recompression chambers. Theoretical reasons exist for a number of other drugs to be tried (Lambertsen 1968), a list to which can be added drugs based on their possible effects on the pathophysiological consequences of blood–bubble interface; but while drugs that, for instance, reduce platelet aggregation can be shown to be effective when given prophylactically (Ackles, Philp & Inwood 1973), there is no evidence yet that such drugs would be a useful therapeutic tool.

Drugs may also be indicated for symptomatic relief of labyrinthine dysfunction or, rarely, limb pain, provided that care is taken to avoid such treatment concealing the progress of the illness. For this reason they should be given only either when maximal recompression therapy has failed or when recompression cannot be used.

The management of residua

In spite of recompression, but occasionally because of inadequate treatment, a number of divers still have residual symptoms or signs on completion of therapeutic recompression. These may be circulatory and respond to continued intravenous therapy or, more commonly, neurological. The majority of such remaining weaknesses, patches of numbness and difficulties with bladder control resolve within a few weeks. The degree of restoration of function is considered to be excellent in comparison with that following other forms of transverse myelitis and trauma. However, any damage which persists beyond some 6 months after the incident must be considered as permanent.

Obviously such persons should not be allowed to dive again but, for one reason or another, some have not accepted the advice of their medical practitioners and have returned to professional diving apparently without further mishap. This is not to be encouraged since one would expect the neurological scars to increase the susceptibility of the patient to further decompression sickness. A compromise, when the patient is aware of this risk and accepts it, has been to reintroduce him to pressure with a graduated series of chamber dives under medical supervision before returning him to diving which is limited to within the accepted areas of safety of the compressed air tables.

DECOMPRESSION BAROTRAUMA

SINUS BAROTRAUMA

The gases which expand within the paranasal sinuses during a reduction of environmental pressure normally vent through their natural openings. Obstruction results in a rise of pressure within that space relative to the environmental pressure surrounding it. This results in acute pain

and, theoretically at least, the possibility of gas being forced from that sinus into the systemic veins. Gas pockets at the roots of the carious teeth can cause a similar problem but, like the gas within the middle ear, barotrauma at these sites are more commonly associated with the volume changes of compression.

PULMONARY BAROTRAUMA ('BURST LUNG')

Causes

It was shown by Malhotra and Wright (1960), using primates as experimental animals, that if during a decrease in ambient pressure by more than approximately 50 mm Hg (3·5 ft of seawater; 0·1 ATS), the gas expanding within the alveoli may rupture into the circulation, the interstitial tissues or the pleural space. Ascent to the surface following respiration of gas under pressure holds the same hazard for man. Should the rate at which gas is exhaled be exceeded, alveolar rupture will result.

The primary pulmonary damage is multifocal and the following secondary effects may present singly or in combination:

> Air embolism.
> Mediastinal and, later, subcutaneous emphysema.
> Pneumothorax.
> Pneumopericardium.

Factors which provoke the alveolar trauma include:

> Voluntary or involuntary breath-holding.
> Pre-existing pulmonary abnormality, such as cysts and broncholiths which should have been diagnosed radiologically before exposure to raised environmental pressure.
> The residua of recent upper respiratory infections.

Intrapulmonary trapping of air and, more significantly, the radiological presence of extra-alveolar air have been demonstrated in a proportion of symptom-free persons following simple immersion and apparently normal ascents (Liebow et al. 1959; James 1968; Dahlbach & Lundgren 1972).

Even after practice of the correct ascent techniques clinical cases of pulmonary barotrauma occur in fit persons during routine submarine escape training. It also occurs during the relatively slow decompression from a simulated dive in a compression chamber (Moses 1964). Occasionally a cough or sneeze during ascent may momentarily increase intrapulmonary pressure beyond its safe limit. A similar mechanism may be responsible for chest symptoms in a diver who, when recovering his breathing apparatus after a 'ditching drill', takes a breath from the mouthpiece while the demand regulator is supplying gas at the greater pressure of the full length of air hose below him.

The depth from which an ascent is initiated is not especially significant but since the rate of gas expansion increases as the surface is approached, many cases occur in shallow water and death has been recorded from as shallow as 7 ft (1·2 ATA).

TABLE 25.5
Manifestations of 'burst lung' accidents from submarine escape training

Substernal pain	40
Unconsciousness or dizziness	32
Focal paralyses	18
Convulsions and incontinence	17
Mediastinal emphysema	14
Focal anaesthesia, paraesthesia, pain	13
Dyspnoea	9
Pneumothorax	8
Visual disturbances	7
Focal pareses	4
'Syncope'	5

Data from Moses (1964).

Table 25.5 shows the order of frequency of presenting signs and symptoms found by Moses (1964) from submarine escape training. Table 25.6 tabulates the signs and symptoms from a series of divers (Kidd 1974).

Pulmonary manifestations

Chest pain and coughing of blood-stained froth or frank haemoptyses immediately upon surfacing are the usual symptoms. If mediastinal emphysema is gross or there is pneumothorax, dyspnoea from both cardiac or pulmonary causes may be

TABLE 25.6
Manifestations of 25 'burst lung' accidents from diving

Substernal pain	20
Blood-stained froth	19
Dyspnoea	16
Pulmonary oedema	10
Death	5
Haemoptysis	4
Focal paralyses	4
Mediastinal emphysema	4
Focal anaesthesia, paraesthesia, pain	3
Pneumothorax	3
Unconsciousness or dizziness	2
'Syncope'	2
Convulsions	2
Deafness	1

Data from Kidd (1974).

moderate or severe. The presence of subcutaneous emphysema at the root of the neck can be regarded as diagnostic of pulmonary barotrauma. If the patient is being examined at depth in a compression chamber the physical signs normally elicited by percussion and auscultation may be distorted. Radiological examination is possible at depth in a few compression chambers and is invaluable. In addition to demonstrating mediastinal emphysema or a pneumothorax, the X-ray is likely to reveal a diffuse miliary appearance of the lungs (Fig. 25.10) or, in others, a few large basal intrapulmonary cysts. Chest radiographs should be taken after treatment as a routine to confirm the diagnosis (Fig. 25.11) (Table 25.7). While the patient will be asymptomatic after treatment, his chest X-ray may show resolving pulmonary lesions for 24 to 48 hours thereafter. In a number of individuals the chest X-ray remains normal.

It is important to note that in an individual presenting with arterial air embolism there may be no immediate symptoms or signs indicating the preceding pulmonary barotrauma. In such cases treated by recompression, the pulmonary manifestations become clinically evident during the subsequent slow decompression, or retrospectively by radiograph.

Neurological manifestations

A common presentation, associated with rapid buoyant ascents, is loss of consciousness on arrival

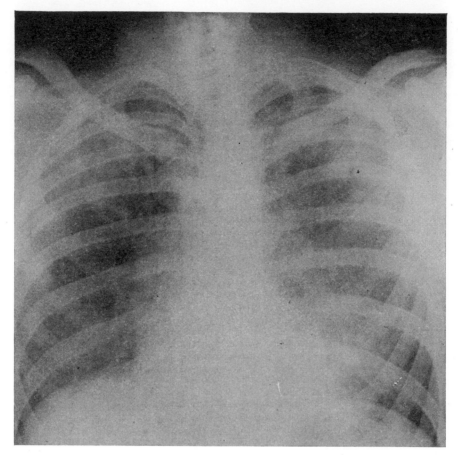

FIG. 25.10. Chest radiograph (Case No. 11, Table 25.7) immediately after successful treatment by recompression

at the surface. This may lead to epileptiform convulsions and apnoea. Cerebral air embolism can lead to various neurological manifestations depending upon the site of the emboli. Indeed, the symptoms and signs of air embolism reflect not only the severity of the accident but also to a certain extent the posture of the body in the water at the time of the pulmonary rupture. Disturbances of vision or speech are fairly common and neurological deficits from hemiparesis to ill-defined weaknesses occur.

Diagnosis

The diagnosis, due to unfamiliarity with the condition, may occasionally be overlooked. It is important to remind divers that pulmonary barotrauma and its complications can occur after any

exposure to pressure. Unlike decompression sickness it does not require some threshold exposure of depth and time but can and does occur in the course of diving which is within the safe 'no-stop' limits for decompression.

In differentiating between barotrauma and decompression sickness in an individual the following points may be useful. The consequences of barotrauma always present instantly or within a few minutes of surfacing and usually occur after a relatively rapid ascent through the water. Respiratory distress, retrosternal pain and haemoptysis are common. The presence of pneumothorax, subcutaneous emphysema in the neck, mediastinal shift or cardiac tamponade are diagnostic. Loss of consciousness is often the presenting sign. While the neurological manifestations

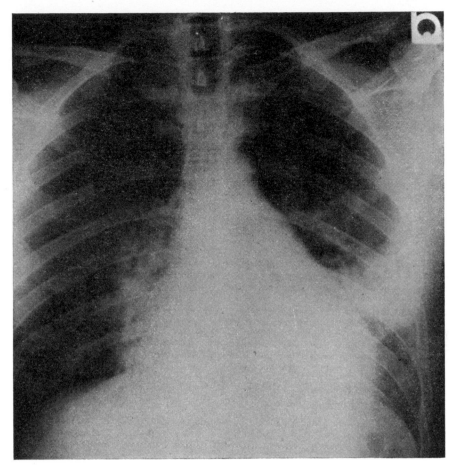

FIG. 25.11. Chest radiograph (Case No. 8, Table 25.7) immediately after successful treatment by recompression

from 'burst lung' are usually of cerebral origin (whereas those from decompression sickness are predominantly spinal), cord lesions identical to 'Brown–Sequard' type cord hemisection have been observed as primary or secondary effects.

Treatment

It is generally stated that the treatment of barotrauma is by immediate recompression and there can be no doubt of the importance of the high standards of preparedness at submarine escape training centres where a suspect casualty can be in the recompression chamber within 15 seconds of his arrival at the surface. This is because the greatest immediate danger from pulmonary damage is death due to cerebral air

embolism. An individual who loses consciousness on arrival at the surface may often recover during the recompression, while the rare fatalities have usually happened within a minute or two of surfacing. Nevertheless, although recompression of a case of pulmonary barotrauma is considered to be life-saving, recompression may not be indicated for the patient with only minor pulmonary manifestations which are not increasing in severity.

Some mild cases of pulmonary damage recover untreated. If dyspnoea occurs then recompression can bring immediate symptomatic relief by reduction of the intrathoracic volume of extrapulmonary air. Pleurocentesis may be necessary, particularly for those in whom the presence of a pneumothorax first becomes apparent during the pro-

TABLE 25.7

25 cases of burst lung

Case no.	Following diving exposure					Following chamber exposure				
	Incident depth (ft) Max. Min.		Chest X-ray	R_X	Outcome	Incident depth (ft) Max. Min.		Chest X-ray	R_X	Outcome
	Civilian									
1	15	0	None	2+5	Good	100	0	Pos.	5	Good
2	150	0	Pos.	5	Good	20	5	Pos.	5A	Good
3	130	0	Pos.	4+C	Good	40	0	None	None	Died
4	60	0	Pos.	5+5+C	Good					
5	10	0	Pos.	5	Residual					
6	20	0	Pos.	DOA	—					
7	30	5	None	None	Died					
8	50	0	Pos.	5A	Good					
9	20	0	Pos.	6+C	Good					
10	35	5	Pos.	None	Good					
11	10	0	Pos.	5	Good					
12	10	0	Pos.	None	Good					
13	30	0	Pos.	4	Good					
14	70	0	Pos.		Died					
15	40	0	Neg.		Died					
	Military									
1	15	0	Pos.	5	Good					
2	10	0	Pos.	5	Good					
3	25	15	Pos.	5	Good	20	10	Pos.	5	Good
4	30	10	Pos.	4+C	Good	20	15	Pos.	5	Residual cord lesion
5	11	0	Pos.	None	Died					

Average time of onset—all within 10 min of surfacing.
Average time from onset to institution of therapy—30 min (longest 8 hours).
R_X code: 2 to 5A—Canadian/USN Therapeutic Recompression Table Regimes; C—Therapeutic decompression guided by analogue decompression computer; DOA—dead on arrival.
Data from Kidd (1974).

longed decompression from a therapeutic recompression which had been administered for neurological reasons. It must be remembered that there is always pulmonary damage and the added mechanical respiratory difficulty of recompression can add to the patient's difficulties. Oxygen–helium mixtures are advocated to relieve this whenever possible.

In submarine escape training accidents unconsciousness and death have occurred within seconds of arrival at the surface from buoyant ascents made at some 9 ft/sec (3 m/sec) and therefore, at escape training centres, emergency arrangements enable recompression to begin immediately following the onset of any suspicious symptom or sign. The chamber is taken as fast as possible directly to 165 ft (6 ATA) for experience has shown that to delay or halt for any reason is to diminish the chances of recovery. The dramatic response of the majority of cases is an ample justification for the occasional recompression of one for whom this might have been unnecessary and for whom the subsequent decompression can then be shortened. However, following diving accidents, in which unconsciousness is a less frequent complication (compare Tables 25.5 & 25.6), Canadian experience has demonstrated that successful therapy is often achieved before that depth is reached (Table 25.7), particularly when circumstances have dictated some unavoidable delay before the recompression. The patient should be kept at 165 ft (6 ATA) until recovery is assured. This is usually certain in less than one minute. Subsequent decompression can be in accordance with one of the long therapeutic air tables but, at many centres, patients are rapidly decompressed to 60 ft (2·8 ATA), 100% oxygen given and subsequent management of the decompression follows a therapeutic oxygen table. There is no data for comparison available yet on the respective relapse rates on these alternative regimes but all recent Canadian experience favours the latter (Table 25.7). If recovery is not complete within minutes at 165 ft (6 ATA) consideration may be given to further recompression to the maximum depth of the chamber provided that the chamber has appropriate life-support systems and an experienced team of operators.

If there is no recompression chamber available at the site of the accident, the patient should be transferred without delay since persistent manifestations may respond to recompression hours after the original injury.

If apnoea occurs, respiratory assistance is necessary but positive pressure breathing, usually mouth-to-mouth, should not be started prematurely or too vigorously because of the real possibility of aggravating the respiratory embarrassment from the already damaged lung. If coma persists after 2 hours at maximum therapeutic pressure, improvement is unlikely and decompression should begin. This is considered valid even for cases having frequent epileptiform convulsions. Catheterization may be required. In one such case recovery of consciousness occurred during the decompression. The profile of decompression should be derived from the best advice available (computer centres) or modified USN Table 4. After each reduction of pressure on the selected table, the patient's condition should be reviewed for evidence of relapse and for the beginnings of respiratory effects due to expansion of extrapulmonary gas, for which recompression and possibly pleurocentesis may be indicated.

While there is no evidence that dextran, heparin or the other drugs mentioned for decompression sickness would have any specific beneficial effect in arterial air embolism, there are a few ancillary therapies that can be useful. Sedation of a patient subject to epileptiform convulsions may be required during a prolonged decompression. Anti-inflammatory steroid drugs with a specific pulmonary site of action, such as methyl prednisolone, in doses of 5 mg/kg/24 hours intravenously, divided in six equal doses, have been strongly advocated to reduce pulmonary oedema and secondary infection (Sladen & Zauder 1971), and may reduce cerebral oedema.

Residual effects

It should be noted that of the 25 cases of pulmonary barotrauma in Table 25.7, 16 are known to be currently diving without limitation. As a rule, no diving should be permitted for 2 months after the incident and successful passing of a stringent medical examination. Submarine escape training, however, should not be undertaken again following an incident of pulmonary barotrauma.

REFERENCES

ACKLES, K. N., PHILP, R. B. & INWOOD, M. J. (1973) Effects of orally-administered pyrimido-pyrimidine derivatives (RA 233 and VK 744) on platelet function in human subjects decompressed from a hyperbaric environment. In *Blood-Bubble Interaction in Decompression Sickness*. Proceedings of an International Symposium. Ed. K. N. Ackles. Toronto: Defence Research Board, Canada.

ALDRICH, C. J. (1900) Compressed air illness; caisson disease. *Int. Clin.* (ser. 10), **2**, 73–78.

ANDERSON, B., Jr, HEYMAN, A., WHALEN, R. E. & SALTZMAN, H. A. (1965) Migraine-like phenomena after decompression from hyperbaric environment. *Neurology, Minneap.* **15**, 1035–1040.

BARNARD, E. E. P. (1967) The treatment of decompression sickness developing at extreme pressures. In *Proc. 3rd Symp. Underwater Physiology*. Ed. C. J. Lambertsen. Baltimore: Williams & Wilkins.

BARNARD, E. E. P. & ELLIOTT, D. H. (1966) Decompression sickness: paradoxical response to recompression therapy. *Br. med. J.* **2**, 809–810.

BARNARD, E. E. P., HANSON, J. M., ROWTON-LEE, M. A., MORGAN, A. G., POLAK, A. & TIDY, D. R. (1966) Post decompression shock due to extravasation of plasma. *Br. med. J.* **2**, 154–155.

BARTHELEMY, L. (1963) Blood coagulation and chemistry during experimental dives and treatment of diving accidents with heparin. In *Proc. 2nd Symp. Underwater Physiology*. (Publ. 1181.) Ed. C. J. Lambertsen & L. J. Greenbaum. Washington: Natl Acad. Sci.-Natl Res. Council.

BAUER, L. (1870) Pathological effects upon the brain and spinal cord of men exposed to the action of largely increased atmospheric pressure. *St Louis med. surg. J.* **VII**, 234–245.

BEHNKE, A. R. (1945) Decompression sickness incident to deep sea diving and high altitude ascent. *Medicine, Baltimore* **24**, 381–402.

BEHNKE, A. R. (1947) *A Review of Physiology and Clinical Data Pertaining to Decompression Sickness.* Project X-443, Report No. 4. Bethesda: US Medical Research Institute.

BEHNKE, A. R. (1951) Decompression sickness following exposures to high pressures. In *Decompression Sickness*. Ed. J. F. Fulton. London and Philadelphia: Saunders.

BEHNKE, A. R. (1967) Work in compressed air: medical aspects. *J. occup. Med.* **9**, 630–631.

BEHNKE, A. R. & SHAW, L. A. (1937) The use of oxygen in the treatment of compressed air illness. *Nav. med. Bull.* **35**, 61–73.

BERGHAGE, T. E. (1966) *Summary Statistics: US Navy Diving Accidents.* US Navy Experimental Diving Unit. Report No. 1–66.

BERT, P. (1878) *Barometric Pressure—Researches in Experimental Physiology.* Translated by M. A. H. Hitchcock & F. A. Hitchcock (1943). Columbus, Ohio.

BRUNNER, F. P., FRICK, P. G. & BÜHLMANN, A. A. (1964) Post decompression shock due to extravasation of plasma. *Lancet* **1**, 1071–1073.

COCKETT, A. T. K. & NAKAMURA, R. M. (1964) A new concept in the treatment of decompression sickness (dysbarism). *Lancet* **1**, 1102.

COCKETT, A. T. K., PAULEY, S. M. & ROBERTS, A. P. (1972) Advances in treatment of decompression sickness. In *Third International Conference on Hyperbaric and Underwater Physiology*. Ed. X. Fructus. pp. 156–159. Paris: Doin.

COCKETT, A. T. K., SAUNDERS, J. C., DEPENBUSCH, F. L. & PAULEY, S. M. (1970) Combined treatment in decompression sickness. In *Proceedings of the Fourth International Congress on Hyperbaric Medicine*. Ed. J. Wada & T. Iwa. pp. 89–92. Baltimore: Williams & Wilkins.

DAHLBACH, G. O. & LUNDGREN, C. E. G. (1972) Pulmonary air trapping induced by water immersion. *Aerospace Med.* **43**, 768–771.

DEWEY, W. A. (1962) Decompression sickness—an emerging recreational hazard. *New Engl. J. Med.* **267**, 759–820.

DOLL, R. E. & BERGHAGE, T. E. (1967) *Interrelationships of Several Parameters of Decompression Sickness.* US Navy Experimental Diving Unit. Research Report 7–65.

ENGEL, G. L., WEBB, J. P., FERRIS, E. B., ROMANO, J., RYDER, H. & BLANKENHORN, M. A. (1944) A migraine-like syndrome complicating decompression sickness. Scintillating scotomas, focal neurologic signs and headache; clinical and electroencephalographic observations. *War Med., Chicago* **5**, 304–314.

ELLIOTT, D. H. (1967) The bends: current concepts in the treatment of decompression sickness. *J. Bone Jt Surg.* **49B**, 588–590.

ERDE, A. (1963) Experience with moderate hypothermia in the treatment of nervous system symptoms of decompression sickness. In *Proc. 2nd Symp. Underwater Physiology*. (Publ. 1181.) Ed. C. J. Lambertsen & L. J. Greenbaum. Washington: Natl Acad. Sci.-Natl Res. Council.

FERRIS, E. G. & ENGEL, G. L. (1951) Clinical nature of high altitude decompression sickness. In *Decompression Sickness*. Ed. J. F. Fulton. London and Philadelphia: Saunders.

FOLEY, A. E. (1863) *Du travail dans l'air comprimé. Étude médicale, hygienique et biologique faite au pont d'Argenteuil.* Bert: Paris.

FRYER, D. I. (1969) *Sub-atmospheric Decompression Sickness in Man.* NATO AGARDOgraph 125.

GAL, A. (1872) *Des dangers du travail dans l'air comprimé et des moyens de les prévenir.* Thesis by Montpellier. Quoted by Bert (1878).

GOLDING, F. C., GRIFFITHS, P., HEMPLEMAN, H. V., PATON, W. D. M. & WALDER, D. N. (1960) Decompression sickness during construction of the Dartford Tunnel. *Br. J. indust. Med.* **17**, 167–180.

GOODMAN, M. W. (1967) Minimal recompression, oxygen breathing method for the therapy of decompression sickness. In *Proc. 3rd Symp. Underwater Physiology*. Ed. C. J. Lambertsen. Baltimore: Williams & Wilkins.

GOODMAN, M. W. & WORKMAN, R. D. (1965) *Minimal Recompression, Oxygen Breathing Approach to Treatment of Decompression Sickness in Divers and Aviators.* US Navy Experimental Diving Unit, Research Report 5–65.

HALLENBECK, J. M., ELLIOTT, D. H. & BOVE, A. A. (1975). Decompression sickness studies in the dog. In *Underwater Physiology. Vth Symp. Underwater Physiology*. Ed. C. J. Lambertsen. Bethesda: Fedn Am. Socs exp. Biol.

HELLER, R., MAGER, W. & SCHROTTER, H. VON (1900) *Luftdruckerkrankungen mit besonderer Berucksichtigung der Sogenannten Caissonkrankheit.* Wein: A. Holder.

JAMES, J. E. (1968) *Extra-alveolar Air Resulting from Submarine Escape Training.* US Navy Submarine Medical Centre. Report No. 550.

KAUFMAN, B. D., OWEN, S. G. & LAMBERTSEN, C. J. (1956) The effects of brief interruptions of pure oxygen breathing upon central nervous system tolerance to oxygen. *Fedn Proc. Fedn Am. Socs exp. Biol.* **15**, 107.

KEMP, J. H. & MUNRO, J. G. (1969) Munchausen's Syndrome caisson disease. *Br. J. indust. Med.* **26**, 81–83.

KIDD, D. J. (1974) Pathology and management of burst lung. *Proceedings, Surgeon Generals Conference Canadian Forces Medical Service.*

KIDD, D. J., STUBBS, R. A. & WEAVER, R. S. (1971) Comparative approaches to prophylactic decompression in underwater physiology. In *Underwater Physiology. Proc. 4th Symp. Underwater Physiology*. Ed. C. J. Lambertsen. New York and London: Academic Press.

KLINTSEVICH, G. N. (1965) Some problems in the origin, diagnosis and treatment of decompression sickness in divers (In Russian.) *Voenno-med Sb.* **9**, 71–74.

LAMBERTSEN, C. J. (1968) Concepts for advances in the therapy of bends in undersea and aerospace activity. *Aerospace Med.* **39**, 1086–1093.

LANPHIER, E. H. (1966) Decompression sickness. In *Fundamentals of Hyperbaric Medicine*. (Publ. 1298.) Washington: Natl Acad. Sci.-Natl Res. Council.

LIEBOW, A. A., STARK, J. E., VOGEL, J. & SCHAEFER, K. E. (1959) Intrapulmonary trapping in submarine escape training casualties. *US arm. Forces med. J.* **10**, 265.

MALHOTRA, M. C. & WRIGHT, C. A. M. (1960) Arterial air embolism during decompression and its prevention. *Proc. R. Soc. B* **154**, 418–427.

MILES, S. (1966) *Underwater Medicine.* London: Staples Press.

MOIR, E. W. (1896) Tunnelling by compressed air. *Jl R. Soc. Arts* **45**, 15.

MOSES, H. (1964) *Casualties in Individual Submarine Escape.* US Naval Submarine Medical Centre. Report No. 438.

PHILP, R. B., GOWDEY, C. W. & PRASAD, M. (1967) Changes in blood lipid concentration and cell counts following decompression sickness in rats and the influence of dietary lipid. *Canad. J. Physiol. Pharmac.* **45**, 1047–1059.

RASHBASS, C. (1957) *Aetiology of Itching on Decompression.* Medical Research Council, RN Personnel Research Committee Report. UPS 167, London.

RIVERA, J. C. (1964) Decompression sickness among divers: an analysis of 935 cases. *Milit. Med.* **129**, 314–334.

ROSE, R. J. (1962) *Survey of Work in Compressed Air during the Construction of the Auckland Harbour Bridge.* Special Report No. 6. Medical Statistics Branch, Dept of Health, Wellington, New Zealand.

SAUMAREX, R. C., BOLT, J. F. & GREGORY, R. J. (1973) Neurological decompression sickness treated without recompression. *Br. med. J.* **1**, 151–152.

SLARK, A. G. (1962) *Treatment of 137 Cases of Decompression Sickness.* Medical Research Council, RN Personnel Research Committee Report 63/1030. London.

SLADEN, A. & ZAUDER, H. L. (1971) Methylprednisolone therapy for pulmonary edema following near drowning. *J. Am. med. Ass.* **215**, 1793–1795.

SONNENBURG, R. E. (1967) Splenic rupture as an incidental complication of decompression sickness: Report of a case. *Milit. Med.* **132**, 452–455.

STUBBS, R. A. & KIDD, D. J. (1966) Computer analogues of decompression. In *Proc. 3rd Symp. Underwater Physiology.* Ed. C. J. Lambertsen. Baltimore: Williams & Wilkins.

TRIGER, M. (1845) Influence de l'air comprimé sur la santé. *Anns Hyg. publ. Méd. lég.* **33**, 463.

VAN DER AUE, O. E., WHITE, W. A., HAYTER, R., BRINTON, F. S., KELLAR, R. J. & BEHNKE, A. R. (1945) *Physiologic Factors Underlying the Prevention and Treatment of Decompression Sickness.* Research Project Report X-443, No. 1. Washington: US Navy Experimental Diving Unit.

WELHAM, W. & WAITE, C. L. (1951) Decompression sickness, report of two unusual cases. *US arm. Forces med. J.* **2**, 1201–1204.

YARBROUGH, O. D. & BEHNKE, A. R. (1939) The treatment of compressed air illness utilizing oxygen. *J. ind. Hyg. Toxicol.* **21**, 213–218.

Decompression Sickness in Compressed Air Workers

P. D. GRIFFITHS

The term decompression sickness applies to the abnormal signs and symptoms that may appear in man within 24 hours following decompression to atmospheric pressure from a raised environmental pressure. Called in the past 'caisson disease' or 'compressed air illness' the commonest form of this condition is popularly known as 'the bends'.

The dangers to which men have been exposed by working at raised atmospheric pressure on civil engineering contracts may be fully realized by reading the reports on such contracts published during the last hundred years. Leonard Hill (1912) gave a resumé of many of these reports showing that in earlier days the risk to these workers of death or permanent paralysis was very high.

During recent years the use of various decompression procedures, which in some instances have been combined with a limitation of the length of shift worked in compressed air, have improved the situation to the extent that if the medical services are well organized the immediate dangers of decompression may be considered to be much reduced though not eliminated.

It is very unusual for decompression sickness to follow exposure to pressures below 2 ATA (14·5 psi gauge; 33 ft) and timed decompression is not usually required from such pressures. For men working at pressures above 2 ATA, particularly when working shifts of over 4 hours which is probably the minimum economic period, there is no known decompression procedure that will protect all men at all times. Thus, with our present knowledge, when men are working at these higher pressures cases of decompression sickness will always occur, particularly so when the standard working shift period is as long as 6 to 8 hours.

Reference to the early literature shows that as long ago as 1878 Bert wrote 'Immediate recompression is the only satisfactory treatment for the condition', and this is still true today. Duffner (1962) states that a medical recompression lock was first installed at a tunnel site in 1893. Although reports on subsequent civil engineering contracts confirm that men suffering from decompression sickness were treated by recompression, it would appear that both before and after the turn of the century the therapeutic procedures on these contracts were, to say the least, uncontrolled and unsatisfactory.

The most recent British Regulations (*Work in Compressed Air*, Special Regulations 1958) still do not recommend any therapeutic procedures because the authorities issuing these regulations are concerned only with the prevention, and not the treatment, of industrial disease. These regulations, however, do state that a medical recompression lock and medical attendants must be provided when the working pressure is above 2·2 ATA (18 psi gauge; 40 ft).

During the last 25 years the therapeutic procedures laid down in the US Naval Diving Regulations [1945] have been used in the USA on civil engineering contracts and later in the chapter these methods will be compared with the unofficial but generally accepted treatment procedures used in Great Britain during the last few years.

The overall decompression sickness rate reported from various large contracts in Great Britain on which working pressures between 2·2 ATA (18 psi gauge; 40 ft) and 4 ATA (43 psi gauge; 100 ft) have been used and on which the shift periods have been up to 8 hours, has usually been between 1·5% and 2% of man-decompressions. So, on a large contract of this kind some hundreds of cases of decompression sickness may require treatment.

As all authorities are not yet agreed concerning the basic pathological principles underlying decompression sickness, it is understandable that the regulations regarding length of exposure and man-lock decompression procedures should not be the same in all countries.

Following research during the last 15 years or so, the regulations concerning work in compressed air have been revised in most countries, the trend being towards longer decompression procedures, the inclusion of decompression procedures from the lower working pressures and the shortening of the shift periods as the working pressure increases. These amendments have not solved all the problems but it does appear that they have resulted in a decrease in the incidence of the more serious forms of decompression sickness and probably in the incidence of aseptic necrosis of bone.

In Great Britain the 1958 Regulations have not been altered, but revised and more prolonged decompression procedures, which have been approved by H.M. Factory Inspectorate, have been in use since 1966.

MEDICAL SERVICES

Whatever regulations are in force or procedures are approved they must be considered to be part of preventive medicine and so of interest to the medical officer. The carrying out of these regulations and procedures is the responsibility of the Contractor but it is to the advantage of all concerned if the medical officer and his staff can share some of this responsibility, in particular by checking man-lock registers and charts from the man-lock recording gauges.

The untoward signs and symptoms that may follow decompression should be explained tactfully to all men working in compressed air. They should be instructed to wear a disc with emergency treatment instructions, as required by the Regulations, in case they should be found unconscious, and to return immediately to the site medical centre should they develop pain or symptoms of any kind during the 24 hours following decompression. They should be advised not to go to hospital where recompression locks are very rarely available.

There is no doubt that the eventual health of the men will depend very largely upon the efficiency of the site medical service.

CLASSIFICATION OF DECOMPRESSION SICKNESS

Type I (the bends)

The man has pain in one or more of his limbs but he neither feels nor looks ill. The intensity of the pain can range from very severe to slight and in the latter case the men may refer to the attack as being one of 'the niggles'. The pain is more common in the legs than the arms and the actual site is usually described by the patient as being near a joint, but only rarely in the area of the hip joint. Occasionally the pain is described as being down the length of the arm or leg. There may be localized areas of tenderness.

The pain may commence during the final stages of the man-lock decompression or at any time during the 24 hours following decompression, the average time being about 2 hours after leaving the man-lock.

Type II

The man has symptoms other than pain in the limbs and usually he feels and appears to be ill. Characteristically the cardiovascular, neurological, respiratory or gastro-intestinal systems are affected. The first symptom may be fainting in the man-lock towards the end of the decompression. In the great majority of cases the symptoms commence within $\frac{3}{4}$ hour of the completion of decompression and only rarely are they delayed for a period of several hours.

The fact that these more serious cases usually develop symptoms early is an important diagnostic point, and is also a reason for encouraging men, even if not enforced by regulation, to remain on the site for at least 1 hour after the completion of decompression.

Although the initial treatment for all forms of decompression sickness is recompression, the subsequent treatment of a Type II case is more prolonged and more difficult than that of a Type I case and therefore it is important to decide which type of case is being considered. This is not usually difficult, but if there is any doubt the patient should be treated as though suffering from the more serious Type II condition.

A Type II case of decompression sickness may present in any one of a number of different ways. Loss of consciousness may occur during the later stages of man-lock decompression or soon after its completion. The patient may collapse with the signs and symptoms of shock. He may complain of giddiness which is known as 'the staggers'. Difficulty in breathing with substernal distress may be described as 'tightness of the chest' and is known as 'the chokes'. Visual symptoms are usually described as flashes of light or spots before the eyes. Headache is an important symptom that must not be ignored. Stomach pains with or without vomiting are another presentation. Tingling, numbness in the limbs, weakness or paralysis of the limbs are serious manifestations. The symptoms of coronary artery occlusion are also to be considered as Type II decompression sickness.

The signs and symptoms of Type II decompression sickness are so varied that there may be some difficulty in making the correct diagnosis but if the man has been exposed to compressed air in the previous 24 hours he should be assumed to have decompression sickness and be recompressed at once. Should adequate recompression not relieve his symptoms then the diagnosis may have to be reconsidered.

An example of the difficulties that may arise was provided by a man who, on decompression after working for an 8-hour shift at 2·8 ATA (26 psi gauge; 60 ft), collapsed and presented with the signs and symptoms of a perforated gastric ulcer but who recovered completely 5 min after being recompressed to working pressure.

Many compressed air workers tend to drink alcohol heavily and a man suffering from the 'staggers' may be wrongly arrested for drunkenness. The police must be informed concerning this possibility and instructed to return such a man immediately to the medical centre at the site and the medical staff should be instructed that any man recently exposed to compressed air who has symptoms of any kind should be recompressed whether he be drunk or sober.

The frequency of Type II cases appears to be 3 to 5 per 10 000 man decompressions from pressures above 2 ATA (14·5 psi gauge; 33 ft).

Minor signs and symptoms following decompression

In addition to the Type I and Type II decompression sickness mentioned above, certain minor complications may be encountered.

A bluish mottling of the skin of the trunk is commonly seen. Most marked in the upper abdominal area it may spread down the proximal parts of the limbs. It may be associated with any of the symptoms mentioned above or may occur alone and is known as 'bruising' or 'staining'.

An irritation of the skin over the chest, neck or face similar to that felt after a nettle sting may be reported. It usually occurs in men who are fat and may precede and accompany skin mottling.

A localized swelling may occur, usually in the neck and shoulder regions. Palpation will confirm that this is due to gas in the subcutaneous tissues and it may disappear on recompression.

A squelching noise heard on movement at the knee or shoulder joint is often clearly audible to other people and is due to gas in or around a joint. It appears to be of no consequence and disappears after a few hours.

These conditions are termed minor but they should be taken into serious consideration when assessing the fitness of a man to continue working in compressed air because they are evidence that for the man in question the decompression procedure, even though correct according to the tables, was inadequate.

TREATMENT OF DECOMPRESSION SICKNESS

Although differing in detail, the various methods of treatment have the same basic principles—recompression to remove all signs and symptoms, followed by a very carefully controlled decompression to prevent their recurrence.

High pressure treatment

This method is based upon that described in the *US Navy Diving Manual* (Table 26.1). It can be used for all types of decompression sickness following exposure to any working pressure. The method has been in satisfactory use for 20 years and though it has not cured all cases it must be realized that, particularly for some serious cases when treatment is long delayed, there may be no successful procedure. The reported rates of recurrence after this form of treatment vary considerably.

The argument in support of the high pressure treatment is that it provides the greatest reduction in the size of the causative bubble. The arguments against are that it causes yet more gas absorption by the tissues, that the treatment of simple cases is lengthy and that medical locks have to be designed to withstand a high pressure.

Minimum effective pressure treatment

In Great Britain there are no therapeutic procedures laid down in the Regulations but a method

TABLE 26.1

High pressure recompression treatment

	'Bends'—pain only		Serious symptoms	
Compress 10 psi g/min	Pain relieved at pressures less than 30 psi g	Pain relieved at pressures greater than 30 psi g	Serious symptoms include any one of the following: 1. Unconsciousness 2. Convulsions	
Decompress 1 min between stops	Use column 1A if O_2 is not available	Use column 2A if O_2 is not available. If pain does not improve within 30 min at 75 psi g the case is probably not bends. Decompress according column 2 or 2A	3. Weakness or inability to use arms or legs 4. Any visual disturbances 5. Dizziness 6. Loss of speech or hearing 7. Severe shortness of breath or 'chokes'	
			Symptoms relieved within 30 min at 75 psi g Use column 3	Symptoms not relieved within 30 min at 75 psi g Use column 4

Stops		1	1A	2	2A	3	4
psi g	ft			*Time in minutes unless otherwise indicated*			
75	168			30 (air)	30 (air)	30 (air)	30 to 120 (air)
65	146			12 (air)	12 (air)	12 (air)	30 (air)
55	123			12 (air)	12 (air)	12 (air)	30 (air)
45	101	30 (air)	30 (air)	12 (air)	12 (air)	12 (air)	30 (air)
35	78	12 (air)	12 (air)	12 (air)	12 (air)	12 (air)	30 (air)
25	56	30 (O_2)	30 (air)	30 (O_2)	30 (air)	30 (O_2 or air)	6 hours (air)
22	49	30 (O_2)	30 (air)	30 (O_2)	30 (air)	30 (O_2 or air)	6 hours (air)
18	41	30 (O_2)	30 (air)	30 (O_2)	30 (air)	30 (O_2 or air)	6 hours (air)
14	31	5 (O_2)	60 (air)	60 (O_2)	2 hours (air)	12 hours (air)	First 11 hours air Then 1 hour O_2 or air
8	18	5 (O_2)	60 (air)	5 (O_2)	2 hours (air)	2 hours (air)	First 1 hour air Then 1 hour O_2 or air
4	9	5 (O_2)	2 hours (air)	5 (O_2)	4 hours (air)	2 hours (air)	First 1 hour air Then 1 hour O_2 or air
0	0	5 (O_2)	1 min (air)	5 (O_2)	1 min (air)	1 min (air)	1 min (O_2)

involving the use of comparatively low pressures has been generally accepted and used on many contracts with good results during the last 15 years.

Treatment of Type I cases. The patient is recompressed to 0·07 ATS or 2 psi (4·5 ft) above the working pressure. If the pains are not completely relieved in 15 min the pressure is raised by 0·07 ATS or 2 psi; if the pain still persists the pressure is raised another 0·07 ATS or 2 psi and this is repeated if necessary at 15 min intervals. It is on only rare occasions that a pressure as high as 0·7 ATS (10 psi; 22 ft) above working pressure is required. The pressure at which the patient becomes completely free from pain is maintained for 10 min before decompression is started.

Therapeutic decompression of Type I cases. There are various methods of therapeutic decompression but recent experience suggests that the following is the most satisfactory in that it appears to result in the smallest number of recurrences.

The pressure is reduced at a rate of 0·07 ATS every 2 min (or 1 psi/min) to half the effective gauge pressure used and then reduced at the rate of 0·07 ATS every 25 min (or 1 psi/15 min). Should the symptoms return during the last stages of decompression or after it is completed, the patient must be recompressed again. This recompression can be to the previously effective pressure but it is preferable to recompress the patient slowly to a new effective pressure which is usually considerably lower than before. When the effective pressure has been maintained for 10 min, medical decompression is carried out as before. However, should the minimum effective pressure be below half the maximum pressure previously used, the phase of rapid decompression should be omitted and the decompression should be at the rate of 0·07 ATS every 25 min (or 1 psi/15 min).

Very rarely pain, usually in the region of a knee joint, may be intensified by recompression. Should this happen, the pressure must be reduced until the acute pain has subsided when very slow recompression should be tried again.

In spite of the apparently successful treatment of the acute effects of decompression sickness many compressed air workers are found to be suffering from chronic effects at a later date. The parts so affected are the bones (discussed in Chapter 27) and possibly the nervous system.

If limb bends are not treated by recompression the pain will disappear within a few days. Nevertheless it is generally accepted that all cases should be treated by recompression and that men should be encouraged to return for treatment, even when the pain is only slight, rather than to take alcohol and analgesics, for it may be that men with untreated bends are more liable to develop aseptic necrosis of bone at a later date.

Treatment of Type II cases. These cases are serious because permanent paralysis or death can result. The need for recompression is urgent and treatment must be prolonged and careful. Prompt treatment is rendered easier by the fact that the majority of men suffering from this type of illness develop symptoms before leaving the site.

A man who faints or becomes ill during decompression in the man-lock must be recompressed at once, and any men in the lock with him. No attempt should be made to get men being decompressed with him out of the lock as this may cause delay in treatment which could prove fatal. The affected man is then removed to the working chamber and his companions can be decompressed again in the usual way. The patient may be kept in the working chamber under medical supervision until symptom-free when he may be decompressed very slowly. The decompression procedure depends upon the condition of the patient but it must not be less in time than that recommended for Type I cases of decompression sickness. The man should be watched carefully during the decompression and recompressed if symptoms recur. When the decompression is completed successfully the patient must be transferred to the medical centre for observation and further recompression if necessary. Although this procedure has at times been used successfully, it has two disadvantages in that a pressure above the working chamber pressure is not available and a lock is occupied for a considerable time. Ideally a one-man portable compression chamber should be available for transporting the patient from the working chamber to the medical recompression lock.

Should a man collapse and appear to be dangerously ill on leaving the man-lock at the end of decompression, immediate recompression in the man-lock or even in the muck-lock (providing the latter has suitable controls) is preferable to wasting valuable minutes by transporting him to a distant medical lock. For this reason the medical lock should always be as near as possible to the man-lock.

The basic principles of treatment of Type II cases are immediate recompression to working pressure, or a higher pressure if required, the maintenance of the effective pressure for at least 30 min after all abnormal signs and symptoms have disappeared and then decompression carried out very slowly and very carefully.

The majority of cases, particularly if detected early and treated promptly, respond dramatically to recompression. If response is poor higher pressure must be used, even up to the safe working pressure of the lock. Recompression treatment should be continued, even for a period of days, so long as there continues to be improvement, however slight.

The patient should not be transferred to hospital, where treatment can be only symptomatic, until it is certain that any residual symptoms are either not due to decompression sickness or can no longer be improved by compression.

Therapeutic decompression of Type II cases. Decompression should not be commenced without authority from the doctor.

The following procedure is prolonged but has proved to be satisfactory and it is extremely rare for a patient who has received this treatment in full to require further recompression.

1. Reduce from the effective pressure to 2 ATA (or 15 psi gauge) at the rate of 0·07 ATS every 25 min (or 1 psi/15 min).
2. Retain at this pressure for 4 hours (called 'soaking').
3. Reduce to atmospheric pressure at the rate of 0·07 ATS every 45 min (or 1 psi/30 min), soaking for (a) 1½ hours at 0·54 ATS (or 8 psi), (b) 1 hour at 0·27 ATS (or 4 psi), (c) 1 hour at 0·13 ATS (or 2 psi).

During these procedures the patient must be observed constantly and should symptoms or signs return he must be recompressed at once. This recompression is not necessarily back to the original effective pressure but it must be sufficient to remove all signs and symptoms. Then, after half an hour at the effective pressure, decompression is started again.

After treatment is completed the patient should remain under observation for at least 2 hours before being taken home and he should be warned to return should any further symptoms develop.

It is advisable that any man, whatever his status, who has suffered from Type II decompression sickness should not be exposed to a pressure above 2 ATA (14·5 psi; 33 ft).

Results of minimum effective pressure treatment

Type I cases. Of over 3000 cases treated in this manner approximately 7% have required more than one therapeutic recompression because of recurrence of symptoms. Some men complained of a residual 'soreness' after treatment. This 'soreness' is quite different from the pain of 'bends' and is not relieved by further recompression.

Type II cases. Only one man has been reported to have required a second recompression after receiving the complete treatment recommended. All the men concerned were considered to be fit and symptom-free on the completion of treatment but in many cases a full neurological investigation was not carried out.

Minimal recompression oxygen-breathing method

In 1965 Goodman and Workman published a report in which they stated that recompression to the comparatively low pressure of 26·7 psi (2·8 ATA; 60 ft) combined with the breathing of oxygen should, when properly administered (Table 26.2), be effective in 98% of cases of decompression sickness.

Sealey (1967) reports that, over a period of 27 months on the Seattle Tunnel contract, 108 cases of bends were treated by this method and that of these only one required a pressure greater than the recommended 26·7 psi (2·8 ATA; 60 ft) to relieve symptoms. This is a satisfactory result, particularly as it involved a comparatively short period of time in the medical recompression lock.

On civil engineering contracts in Great Britain the administration of oxygen has never been part of the routine therapeutic procedure because of the risk of fire and the possibility of oxygen in-

TABLE 26.2

Minimal-pressure, oxygen recompression treatment of decompression sickness

Depth (ft)	Time (min)	Breathing media	Total elapsed time (min)
Method used when relief of symptoms is complete within 10 min at 60 ft			
60	20	O_2	20
60	5	air	25
60	20	O_2	45
60–30	20	O_2	75
30	5	air	80
30	20	O_2	100
30	5	air	105
30–0	30	O_2	135
Method used when relief of symptoms is not complete within 10 min at 60 ft			
60	20	O_2	20
60	5	air	25
60	20	O_2	45
60	5	air	60
60	20	O_2	70
60	5	air	75
60–30	30	O_2	105
30	15	air	120
30	60	O_2	180
30	15	air	195
30	60	O_2	255
30–0	30	O_2	285

Commence O_2 breathing prior to descent. Depth-time schedules should be followed with care.

Compression: rapid descent is desirable but do not exceed rate tolerated by patient. Descent time, usually 1 to 2 min, is not counted as time at 60 ft. Do not halt the descent to verify a report of symptom relief.

Decompression: ascents are continuous at uniform 1 ft/min. Do not compensate for slowing of the rate by subsequent acceleration. Do compensate if the rate is exceeded. If necessary, halt ascent and hold depth while ventilating the chamber.

Inside tender: tender routinely breathes chamber air. If treatment schedule is lengthened (see below), or if the treatment constitutes a repetitive dive for the tender, he must breathe O_2 for the final 30 min, from 30 ft to the surface.

Relief of symptoms: if completeness of relief is at all doubtful after 10 min O_2 breathing at 60 ft use the 285-min schedule.

If symptoms recur, fresh symptoms appear, or the patient's condition worsens, return to 60 ft and use the 285-min method.

If relief is not complete at 60 ft, proceed with the 285-min schedule, observing closely for any changes of the patient's condition, or lengthen the schedule (see below), or recompress to 135 ft and commit the patient to USN Treatment Table 2A, or Table 4 if symptoms are not relieved within 30 min.

A medical officer qualified in diving, or the diving supervisor (diving officer; master diver) can extend the 285-min schedule with a fourth O_2–air sequence (20 min O_2—5 min air) at 60 ft, or a third air–O_2 sequence (15 min air—60 min O_2) at 30 ft, or both.

tolerance. It would also entail full-time medical supervision which is not always available.

OTHER METHODS OF TREATMENT

Intravenous therapy

On occasions there have been reports of men suffering from very severe decompression sickness who have not responded to recompression but who have been cured by the administration of considerable quantities of intravenous blood plasma. Cockett and Nakamura (1964) reporting such a case suggested that all cases of decompression sickness are associated with some degree of haemoconcentration. Barnard et al. (1966) reported the successful treatment of a case of Type II decompression sickness by intravenous therapy after a recompression to 165 ft (6 ATA; 72 psi gauge) which had failed to cure his hypotension and oliguria.

Cases requiring this form of therapy are fortunately rare but facilities for giving intravenous plasma should be available at all medical centres concerned with decompression sickness. This treatment should always be additional and not an alternative to recompression.

The use of drugs

Few drugs are used in the treatment of decompression sickness. Simple analgesics may be given to assist in the relief of the pain of bends but not as an alternative to recompression.

In 1963 Barthelemy suggested that heparin in doses of 50 to 100 mg twice daily was useful in the recompression of very severe cases of decompression sickness or air embolism 'when the functional or vital prognosis is bad'.

Neurological lesions

In 1959 Rozsahegyi examined 100 men $2\frac{1}{2}$ to 5 years after they had suffered from a neurological form of Type II decompression sickness when working on the Budapest Metro contract. He reported that the majority of these men had symptoms and objective signs, that only 13 were 'reasonably well' and 14 were unable to work. The Budapest contract was a very large one but the number of neurological cases and the high proportion of men suffering permanent disability suggest that both the man-lock decompressions and immediate therapeutic procedures may have been inadequate. In Britain no attempt has been made to follow up the considerable number of men who have suffered from Type II decompression sickness and been considered fit after therapeutic recompression, but if the treatment procedures are to be fully justified then it is obviously important that this should be done.

REFERENCES

BARNARD, E. E. P., HANSON, J. M., ROWTON-LEE, M. A., MORGAN, A. G., POLAK, A. & TIDY, D. R. (1966) Post decompression shock due to extravasation of plasma. *Br. med. J.* **2**, 154–155.

BARTHELEMY, L. (1963) The use of heparin in the treatment of diving accidents. In *Proc. 2nd Symp. Underwater Physiology.* (Publ. 1181.) Ed. C. J. Lambertsen & L. J. Greenbaum. Washington: Natl Acad. Sci.-Natl Res. Council.

BERT, P. (1878) *La Pression Barometrique.* Paris: Masson.

COCKETT, A. T. K. & Nakumura, R. M. (1964) New concepts in the treatment of decompression sickness (dysbarism). *Lancet* **1**, 1102.

DUFFNER, G. J. (1962) *Decompression Sickness and its Prevention among Compressed Air Workers.* Seattle: Metropolitan Engineers Report.

GOODMAN, M. W. & WORKMAN, R. D. (1965) *Minimal Recompression, Oxygen Breathing Approach to the Treatment of Decompression Sickness in Divers and Aviators.* Research report. 5–65, US Navy Experimental Diving Unit, Washington, D.C.

HILL, L. (1912) *Caisson Disease*, Chapters 4 and 5. London: Arnold.

ROZSAHEGYI, I. (1959) Late consequences of neurological forms of decompression sickness. *Br. J. indust. Med.* **16**, 311–317.

SEALEY, J. L. (1967) Personal communication.

Regulations

Work in Compressed Air (1958) Amended Industrial Code Rule 22. New York State.

Work in Compressed Air, Special Regulations (1958) Ministry of Labour and National Service S.I. No. 61. London: H.M.S.O.

27

Dysbaric Osteonecrosis: Aseptic Necrosis of Bone

R. I. McCALLUM

Exposure to compressed air at pressures substantially greater than normal atmospheric pressure is known to be associated with death of portions of the long bones (aseptic necrosis or avascular necrosis of bone, caisson disease of bone, etc.[1]) in a proportion of those so exposed. So much is fact but much that has been confidently stated about bone necrosis, particularly its pathogenesis, is still conjectural or hypothetical and lacks objective evidence.

Although men have been exposed to compressed air in diving, tunnelling or caisson work since the end of the eighteenth century, recognition that bone disease might follow depended on the introduction of radiographic examination into clinical medicine. X-rays were discovered in 1895, and the first reports of bone necrosis from exposure to compressed air were published in 1911 by Bassoe in the United States of America and by Bornstein and Plate (1911–12) in Germany.

Bassoe (1911), in a paper to the Chicago Neurological Society, described chronic joint pain and stiffness in 11 out of 161 caisson workers whom he studied for the Illinois State Commission on Occupational Diseases. One of the 11 men had developed a disabling hip condition immediately after his second shift in compressed air 12 years previously. The radiological picture was described as typical of arthritis deformans.

Bornstein and Plate (1911–12) described 3 cases of joint disease in a group of 500 compressed air workers employed in the construction of the Elbe Tunnel in Hamburg. One man had bone necrosis in a hip, another man had a lesion in his right shoulder and the third man had bilateral hip lesions. Only the joints in which there were symptoms appear to have been radiographed. Two of the men were engineers aged 28 and 32 years respectively and one a fitter aged 28 years, and all had suffered from the bends at one time or another. The maximum pressure to which they had been exposed was 3·4 ATA (25 m). They had worked for various periods up to 8 hours a day but no details are given of the decompression procedure.

It is interesting now to note that Bornstein and Plate suggested that the main medical task at the next major compressed air project should be the systematic radiographic examination of the bones of all men with decompression sickness, a task which has only been attempted during the last decade.

NATURAL HISTORY

Bone necrosis in the compressed air worker or diver begins as a symptomless lesion detectable only by radiography. It occurs typically in the humerus, femur or tibia although lesions in other bones have been described, and as pointed out by

---

[1] For a full list of the 40 or more terms used to describe this condition see Werts and Shilling (1972).

Bell, Edson and Hornick (1942) it may be found in men who do not give a history of acute decompression sickness. Bone necrosis may follow a single exposure to compressed air and this was shown dramatically following the escape of five men from a submarine sunk in 120 ft (4·7 ATA; James 1945). The men spent $2\frac{1}{2}$ to 3 hours in gradually increasing air pressure before escaping, and all of them suffered from the bends. Twelve years later three men who could be traced were found to have bone lesions.

Lesions in the shafts or areas away from the joint surface of the humerus and femoral heads continue to be symptomless and practically never cause disability. One patient with pain in a very large medullary lesion has been reported by Golding (1966). Lesions near the joint surface (juxta-articular) of the humeral or femoral head are likely to give rise to symptoms of pain, stiffness and limitation of movement as a result of fracture and collapse of the weight-bearing area, or sequestration of part of the head of the bone. Osteoarthritis soon follows and is markedly disabling, especially if the femoral head is affected. Serious loss of function in the hip or shoulder joint necessitates surgical treatment. As the lesions are often bilateral and symmetrical, disability can be severe, especially if both femoral heads collapse. When the articular surface of a humerus is affected the joint may still function although movement is limited and painful. The whole process from the first radiographic appearance of the lesion to loss of continuity in the joint surface may take only 3 or 4 months to 2 or 3 years or perhaps longer. A more definite time range cannot be given until much more complete radiological studies with sufficiently frequent radiographs of the bones of men at risk are available. The notable exception to this picture is the total freedom of the knee joint from juxta-articular lesions and joint involvement, in spite of the frequent occurrence of large area of necrosis in the lower end of the femur and less often in the upper tibia.

Since the early descriptions of the natural history, radiology, pathology and pathogenesis of bone necrosis little new knowledge has been added. In recent years, however, the extent of the problem and its seriousness have been much better appreciated and the difficulties in providing a satisfactory explanation of the pathogenesis and of means of prevention have become apparent.

Bone necrosis in association with compressed air exposure has now an extensive literature (Werts & Shilling 1972). Many of the early accounts relate to single or small series of cases, usually describing men with symptoms and disability in the hip or shoulder who have consequently sought medical or surgical treatment. Later studies such as those of Cavigneaux et al. (1949) and Golding et al. (1960) have reported symptomless lesions detected by radiographic investigation of groups of workers while employed in compressed air. There has also been a rather slow recognition that naval and other divers are liable to bone necrosis (Slørdahl 1953; Alnor 1963).

Elliott and Harrison (1970) have reviewed reports on bone necrosis in divers, the earliest of which was in 1941. Reports have come mainly from Germany, Scandinavia and France, but lesions in divers have also been reported in China and Poland (Elliott 1971). The British Royal Navy has carried out radiological examinations of the joints of 383 of its professional divers. Definite bone lesions have been found in 16 men and there were also 7 doubtful lesions (Harrison 1971). It is interesting that none of the men had lesions in the femoral head. In a control series of divers no lesions were found. As in compressed air workers, bone necrosis occurs more frequently in divers who have had acute decompression sickness and it is also more prevalent in those who have taken part in experimental trials involving dives to 600 ft (182·9 m) using oxy-helium (Elliott 1971).

Ohta and Matsunaga (1974) have described bone lesions in Japanese shell fish divers. These men dive professionally from the age of 18 to 50 years throughout the whole year to depths of 60 or 70 m and may spend 4 hours on the sea bed in the morning and another 4 hours in the afternoon. In the past no decompression schedules have been used and bends have been very common, as have deaths from decompression sickness. The divers have treated bends symptomatically or by returning to depth, although cold has limited this considerably. Altogether 301 divers were examined and 152 (50·5%) were found to have definite bone necrosis whilst another 16 had doubtful changes.

The proportion of men with bone lesions increased with age particularly over 30 years, and with diving experience especially in excess of 10 years. The lesions were most frequent in the upper humerus. While there was a statistically significant association between bone lesions and the bends, there was no such relationship between bone lesions and paraplegia nor between the site of the bend and a bone lesion. No definite bone lesions was seen in men who did not go deeper than 20 m (3 ATA) while those who usually dived to over 30 m (4 ATA) had significantly more bone lesions. Thus the exposure to compressed air of these divers and the prevalence of bone necrosis is comparable with that of compressed air workers in tunnels and caissons. The authors quote Japanese reports of bone lesions in divers affecting between 38% and 76·6% of the men and they emphasize the importance of the length of compressed air experience and working depth. In their series the proportion of men with juxta-articular lesions was higher than that in compressed air workers.

The authors point out that the position of the bone in a radiograph may determine whether it is seen to be juxta-articular or not and thus how it is classified.

Bone lesions have been reported from exposure to lowered atmospheric pressure (Hodgson et al. 1968) but are rare. Realization of the size of the problem in tunnel workers in the United Kingdom came during the construction of the Dartford road tunnel under the river Thames between 1957 and 1959 (Golding et al., 1960), and in the USA in connection with the building of the third tube of the Lincoln Tunnel which began in 1955 (Behnke 1967).

The building of two road tunnels under the river Clyde at Glasgow in Scotland between 1958 and 1963 gave an opportunity of taking radiographs of the major joints of a group of 223 compressed air workers employed at a single contract who had no previous exposure to work in raised atmospheric pressure (Decompression Sickness Panel Report, MRC 1966). Of these men 38 (17%) were found to have bone lesions and 12 men are known to be seriously disabled by them. The risk of bone necrosis appears to be non-existent or negligible in men exposed only to pressures below about 17 psi gauge (2·16 ATA).

At the Clyde Tunnels, for example, only 4 men had bone necrosis whose maximum working pressure did not exceed 25 psi gauge (2·5 ATA) at any time, whereas with maximum pressures greater than this level 34 men had bone lesions. In addition to maximum pressure experienced, bone lesions were associated with the number of decompressions and the number of treated attacks of bends, but it was impossible to separate these three factors.

The effect of length of shift in compressed air is difficult to evaluate because so few of the men involved have not at one time or another worked a full shift of 8 hours in compressed air.

Bone necrosis has been reported from all the major compressed air contracts in the United Kingdom carried out since 1948 and has been found in men who were employed in other contracts carried out prior to these. Radiological examination of men who have worked regularly in compressed air in tunnels or caissons over a period of years shows that at least 50% of them have bone lesions. The Decompression Sickness Central Registry at the University of Newcastle upon Tyne, England, has radiographs of the major joints of 1700 compressed air workers and bone lesions of aseptic necrosis are present in 334 men (20%). About 17% of the men so affected have disabling lesions but the proportion of juxta-articular and thus potentially disabling lesions given by different authors varies from 10% (Decompression Sickness Panel Report, MRC 1966) to 49% (Davidson & Griffiths 1970) and even 71% (Nellen & Kindwall 1972). It seems likely that an element of selection is responsible for such divergent figures.

RADIOLOGY

The radiographic picture of well-established aseptic necrosis of bone in divers and compressed air workers is characterized by multiple well-defined areas of density with rather ill-defined margins. These areas are often bilateral and symmetrical. Dead bone is indistinguishable radiographically from live bone, and it is regenerating new bone on dead trabeculae which produces the opacities typical of bone necrosis. Good descriptions of the radiology of this condition in its relatively advanced stages have been given by Taylor (1943) and Poppel and Robinson (1956) and are well illustrated in the Decompression Sickness Panel Report, MRC (1966) and by Davidson and Griffiths (1970). Very early bone lesions appear as faint densities and are difficult or impossible to reproduce convincingly in half-tone plates. For this reason no early lesions are reproduced here. Indeed they are difficult to demonstrate to the inexperienced even in good radiographs which are the only means of studying them.

For practical reasons radiography has been confined mainly to the large joints of the arms and legs. These are the joints that are important clinically. Radiation dosage must be kept within safe limits, and the time involved in carrying out the examination is important, particularly in construction site conditions. Little is known therefore of changes in bone areas other than those usually examined, but lesions have been described in the os calcis (Poppel & Robinson 1956) and around the elbow joint (El Ghawabi et al. 1971) but do not appear to have clinical significance.

Problems arise in the recognition of the earliest radiographic abnormality of bone necrosis because of poor technique. There may be a lack of clear bone detail, and poor positioning in the shoulders may lead to unnecessary superimposition of the glenoid or acromion shadow on the articular surface of the humerus. In the Decompression Sickness Central Registry (Griffiths 1971) bone radiographs are seen from all over the United Kingdom and from overseas. They vary so much in quality of detail and in care of positioning that the Registry has issued suggestions for guidance of radiographers to improve the quality of the films it receives (see appendix). These suggestions are concerned mainly with the projections of the shoulders, hips and knees which are the most likely to show the bone lesions clearly. The frog-leg position for films of the head of the femur is helpful. Here the limb is rotated externally to show clearly the upper and inner segment of the femoral head which is so frequently affected in aseptic necrosis. Early juxta-articular lesions in the femoral head are inevitably difficult to detect and tomography may help to show them more clearly (Nellen & Kindwall 1972). Radio-

graphy of the bones of compressed air workers employed on isolated construction sites distant from hospital X-ray facilities is probably best carried out by an adequately equipped mobile X-ray unit.

Radiological classification of bone necrosis

Surveys by the British Medical Research Council Decompression Sickness Panel on tunnel workers employed in compressed air have produced a mass of radiographic data on bone necrosis. From these a working classification of bone lesions (Decompression Sickness Panel Report, MRC 1966) has been constructed, and has been found to be of practical value in the study of bone lesions in tunnel workers and in deep sea divers both in the United Kingdom and in the United States of America. An album of illustrative radiographs by Griffiths (1968) gives examples of the main types of bone lesions found in compressed air workers.

Periodic radiographic examinations of the joints in relatively young men, particularly when the hips are included, raises the question of radiation dose. It appears acceptable in terms of dosage to skin, gonads and bone marrow to carry out not more than three routine examinations of the major joints per year provided that gonad protection is used. At present there is no other diagnostic method to equal conventional radiography in the detection and follow-up study of bone necrosis but there is a need for some means of detecting bone damage at a much earlier stage than is now possible. An 0·8 mm focal spot may confirm radiographic bone detail and enable small deviations from normal structure to be seen more easily. Other techniques may have to be used such as bone scans using radioactive isotopes, e.g. ^{85}Sr or ^{18}Fl, both of which are being tried experimentally for the detection of bone necrosis.

Radiological lesions have been divided into two main descriptive groups (Decompression Sickness Panel Report, MRC 1966) based on their position and radiographic appearance: (A) juxta-articular, and (B) head, neck and shaft lesions.

This division is on clinical grounds and does not imply any difference in their pathogenesis. Groups A and B have been further subdivided as described below.

Juxta-articular lesions

A1. *Dense areas with an intact articular cortex.* These occur in the head of the humerus or femur close to or involving the articular cortex. In their earliest stage lesions may be difficult to detect in the femoral head because of the acetabular shadows but tomography or a magnification film may demonstrate them more clearly.

A2. *Spherical segmental opacity.* This is seen typically in the humeral head and is shaped like the segment of a sphere.

A3. *Linear opacity.* This is found typically in the humeral head as a curved or serpiginous shadow of varied thickness and density and there may be other small dense areas distal to it.

A4. *Structural failure.* This may follow A1, A2 or A3 and is accompanied by pain and stiffness in the joint. There are three main appearances:

(a) A fine transradiant subcortical line under the articular cortex of the humeral or femoral head. The cortex and underlying bone have not collapsed.

(b) Collapse of the articular cortex which may involve up to half of its extent, sometimes with a stepped depression in the head of the bone. A large triangular opacity is usually present in the adjacent bone.

(c) Sequestration of part of the cortex may occur by fracture through the necrotic area in the subchrondral zone.

A5. *Osteo-arthritis.* Osteophyte formation occurs at the lower part of the articular cortex of the humerous and in the hip at the margin of the femoral head. It is typical of bone necrosis with osteo-arthritis that the width of the joint space remains normal in the earlier stages. At an advanced stage the picture is similar to that of osteoarthritis from a variety of causes.

Head, neck and shaft lesions

B1. *Dense areas.* The common sites for these lesions are the neck and proximal shaft of the femur and humerus, but they also occur elsewhere in the long bones.

B2. *Irregular calcified areas.* They are often large, bilateral and prominent because of extensive irregular calcification but in their early stages they present as vague shadows seen best in the distal femur in lateral views. They also occur in the proximal part of the humerus and tibia.

B3. *Transradiant areas and cysts.* These are seen occasionally in the head and neck of the femur and humerus and may best be shown by tomography.

B4. *Endosteal or cortical thickening.* This appearance was described by Fournier, Jullien and Leandri (1965). It is seen in the distal part of the femur usually associated with a shaft lesion (B2).

Recognition of the earliest radiological change requires not only well-positioned films of good quality to show fine bone detail but also familiarity with the fine deviations from normal which may be learnt from the study of sets of serial films of the same individuals extending over a period of years. Fig. 27.1 (a–e) is a series of radiographs from the Decompression Sickness Central Registry showing the left humeral head of a tunnel fitter aged 32 years. Between November 1964 and September 1965, he worked 344 shifts of 6 to 9 hours each in compressed air. The maximum pressure he experienced was 35 psi gauge (3·39 ATA) for $7\frac{3}{4}$ hours, and 100 of his shifts were at pressures above 27 psi gauge (2·84 ATA). He was decompressed according to a modified British Statutory Table (Decompression Sickness Panel Report, MRC 1971). These early changes may be more easily visible when the films are viewed on an illuminated screen from a distance of 6 or 7 ft, and tend to disappear on approaching closer. In the radiography of pneumoconiosis an elaborate system of scrutiny of the same films by two or more experienced observers has been developed to reduce over or under diagnosis of early lesions. A similar but at present simpler approach is desirable for the diagnosis of early bone lesions, particularly where groups of compressed air workers or divers are being screened. Each observer works alone but where opinions differ on a particular film a combined opinion is sought by the observers viewing the film together.

Other changes which have been described as characteristic are some types of bone cyst, and local or general rarefaction of bone (demineralization) (Alnor, Herget & Seusing 1964; Fournier, Jullien & Leandri 1965). However, other observers consider that these changes occur also in people having had no compressed air exposure and that

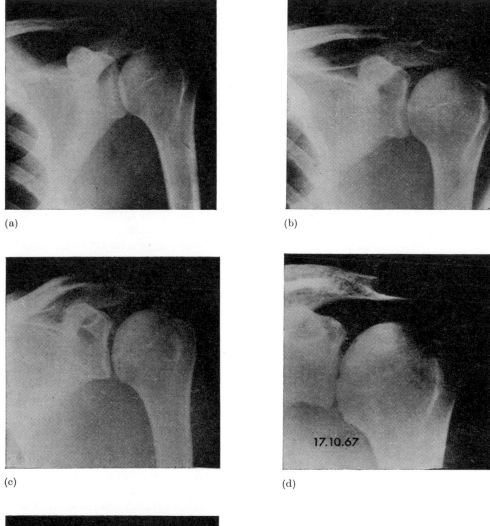

(a)   (b)   (c)   (d)

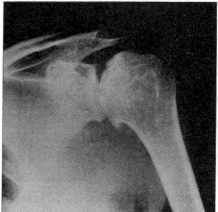

(e)

FIG. 27.1. Progression of bone necrosis

(a) Radiograph of left humeral head in November 1964, 3 months after the individual began work in compressed air. The bone appears normal but in retrospect faint mottling is present which was probably the beginning of the radiographically visible lesions.

(b) August 1965. There is an early juxta-articular opacity (A1).

(c) November 1966. The opacity is now more marked and there is a slight break in the articular surface (A4).

(d) October 1967. Damage to the articular surface is now more evident and there is a trans-radiant band below the cortex.

(e) November 1973. Gross bone damage and osteoarthritis are now present.

they are due to a variety of other causes. In the humerus, for example, cysts may occur on the anatomical neck from traumatic tears to the rotator cuff (Golding 1962).

The relative distribution of 600 lesions in compressed air workers has been studied by Davidson and Golding (1969). Lesions were commonest in the head of the humerus (34·5%), next in the lower end of the femur (29·6%), head of femur (11%) and shaft of humerus (11·4%), upper end of tibia (10·5%) and upper end of femur (3%). Lesions were bilateral in about a third of patients. Records of the Decompression Sickness Registry give a slightly different picture (Table 27.1) with the lower end of the femoral shaft as much the most frequent site.

TABLE 27.1

Relative frequency of sites of radiographic bone lesions in 334 compressed air workers. Decompression Sickness Central Registry, University of Newcastle upon Tyne.

Site	Percentage
Femur, distal shaft	39
Humerus, head	26
Femur, head	15
Tibia	14
Humerus, neck/shaft	4
Femur, neck/shaft	2

Alnor, Herget and Seusing (1964) described bone lesions in 72 divers out of a group of 131. Single lesions occurred in 15 men and multiple lesions in 57 men. The upper end of the humerus was the commonest site (right 59; left 58). Next common was the lower end of the femur (right 20, left 18), the upper end of the femur (right 10, left 8), and then the upper tibia (right 2, left 2).

DIFFERENTIAL DIAGNOSIS

Aseptic necrosis of bone from work in compressed air is indistinguishable by itself from necrosis due to other causes. However, in men with a history of work in compressed air or diving the probability of bone necrosis being due to compressed air is obviously very high. Most other causes of bone necrosis are likely to be rare and unusual in men who are relatively young and fit,

and who have passed the usual medical checks. Nevertheless, in individual cases it may be necessary to carry out appropriate investigations into other possible causes. These include alcoholism, steroid treatment, sickle cell anaemia, rheumatoid arthritis, Gaucher's disease (lipoid storage splenohepatomegaly), and phenylbutazone treatment. Alcoholism is difficult to define and steroid treatment is widely used so that the role played by these factors can be difficult to assess. It is likely that some cases diagnosed in the past as 'idiopathic' bone necrosis have been unrecognized aseptic necrosis from exposure to compressed air. Other illnesses which may also be relevant are diabetes mellitus, cirrhosis of the liver, hepatitis, pancreatitis, gout, syphilis, alkaptanuria, arteriosclerosis and treatment with ionizing radiation for an unrelated disease. Even in the presence of one of the above conditions an occupational cause of bone necrosis in a compressed air worker may be difficult to disprove.

There can be confusion between opacities due to bone necrosis and bone islands which are developmental in origin and of obscure cause. They are well-defined round or oval areas of cortical bone and lie in the medulla, partly connected with the cortex. Bone islands are quite common, certainly more frequent than the 42 examples in 5000 consecutive patients reported by Kim and Barry (1964). Fournier, Jullien and Leandri (1965) considered bone islands to be more common in compressed air workers than in the general population but Nellen and Kindwall (1972) found that bone islands were equally prevalent in men with and without previous compressed air experience. The prevalence of bone islands clearly requires further epidemiological investigation in compressed air workers and divers and more data from a large series of bone radiographs of a normal population matched for age.

A review of Decompression Sickness Central Registry radiographs of the shoulders, hips and knee joints of 100 experienced commercial divers and 100 control subjects not previously exposed to compressed air shows about 30% of both groups to have bone islands (Griffiths, personal communication). Unlike those in the ilium reported by Blank and Lieber (1965), which increased in size over a period of years, the 100 examples of bone islands in the films of 1700 men in the Decompression Sickness Central Registry have not so far altered in size over 2 to 5 years.

PATHOLOGY

The first description of the pathology of aseptic necrosis in a compressed air worker was given by Kahlstrom, Burton and Phemister (1939). They described in detail its histology in a 61-year-old man who died of a bronchogenic carcinoma and whose exposure to compressed air had occurred in 1901, 35 years before. While employed in the construction of a water tunnel he suffered severe pains in his limbs which left him with a limp. Both hip joints were extensively damaged, and there were lesions in the lower part of both femora. The head and upper shaft of the left humerus and the upper left tibia were also affected.

Macroscopically the affected articular surfaces showed flattening, the cartilage thin or absent and there was osteophyte formation. Sections of the damaged areas of bone showed cystic areas containing necrotic and gelatinous material. Encapsulated areas of necrotic bone were bounded by dense fibrous calcified walls and surrounded by sclerosed cancellous bone. These changes were interpreted as resulting from massive necrosis of a large area of bone with later invasion, absorption, and replacement of dead bone by cancellous bone and cysts, and with calcification of tissue at the periphery. Dead articular cartilage had been replaced by a thin layer of fibrocartilage, and secondary villous synovitis and loose bodies were present.

Kahlstrom, Burton and Phemister (1939) also described the histology of the excised left femoral head of a man who had worked in a caisson 4 years previously and had been rapidly decompressed in an emergency. Pain in his hips and legs, resulting from the bends caused by this decompression, had persisted in spite of treatment in a pressure chamber. The heads of both femora and humeri had radiological evidence of bone damage. Histological examination showed aseptic necrosis of bone with invasion and partial absorption by connective tissue.

More recently a detailed study of symptomless bone lesions in the heads of the left humerus and right femur of an active compressed air worker was made by Catto (Decompression Sickness Panel Report MRC 1966). An important new finding was that the whole of the humeral head had at one time been dead but that revascularization had occurred in all but a shallow layer. A band of dense fibrous tissue separated the necrotic from the revascularized area, and unresorbed dead trabeculae adjacent to the fibrous tissue on the revascularized side were covered with a thick layer of living bone. Similar changes were seen in the femoral head. It is noteworthy that there was no evidence of thrombosis or recanalization in any blood vessel, nor have other bone specimens from divers and compressed air workers which have been studied histologically provided any such evidence so far.

Little of importance has been added to the pathological picture since 1939 because of a dearth of histological material from lesions which are known with certainty to be of very recent origin. It is therefore important to obtain bone specimens from divers or compressed air workers whenever possible. Such material is most likely to be available from men actively engaged in diving or compressed air work who die accidentally (Bennison, Catton & Fryer 1965; Decompression Sickness Panel Report, MRC 1966). Examination of bone specimens is included in the suggested procedure for post-mortem examination of divers and compressed air workers drawn up by the Decompression Sickness Panel and circulated by the Association of Clinical Pathologists to pathologists and forensic experts in the United Kingdom. Amongst other recommendations it is suggested that where there is radiographic evidence of lesions a number of specimens should be taken from both affected and apparently unaffected areas, and that where possible at least a whole femur and humerus should be removed and fixed for histological study.

PATHOGENESIS

The actual way in which bone necrosis of compressed air workers and divers is caused is not clearly indicated by its pathology and has proved extraordinarily elusive, in spite of much speculation and numerous animal experiments. Bornstein and Plate (1911–1912) were the first to put forward the hypothesis that bone necrosis resulted from the formation of gas bubbles in the ends of limb bones in which there was a poor blood supply. They envisaged a marked nutritional disturbance from the presence of bubbles in bone tissue and vessels but thought that actual infarction was unlikely because of the absence of end arteries. They also pointed out that the areas of damaged bone were too extensive to be the result of obstruction of a single vessel. In spite of Bornstein and Plate's reservations about infarction, however, some authors still assume that it occurs in bone necrosis.

Kahlstrom, Burton and Phemister (1939), from their histological study, concluded that aseptic necrosis was due to an accumulation of either intra or extravascular nitrogen gas in the bones although they gave no direct evidence of this. They considered that the changes in the femoral head were similar to those resulting from slipped epiphyses, some cases of traumatic dislocation of the hip, fracture of the femoral neck, or idiopathic bone necrosis in adults. They commented particularly on the number and extent of the shaft lesions. In favour of the nitrogen embolism theory they pointed out the frequency of lesions in the femoral heads 'where end arteries are known to be frequently found', and the lesions in the lower end of the femur and in the tibia and fibula, sparing the epiphysis, which suggested blockage of parts of their nutrient arteries. Against the simple embolic theory was the very large size of the necrotic areas (as noted by Bornstein & Plate), their symmetry, and the absence of evidence of infarction in spleen and kidneys. Kahlstrom and his colleagues also remarked that with such extensive embolism in bones, death might have been expected from brain, lung, kidney or intestinal embolism. Finally, there was no involvement of the trunk bones. On the other hand extravascular gas in limb bones rich in fatty marrow might press on blood vessels and cause obstruction. They quoted Bornstein's observation that the bone marrow circulation is sluggish so that gas would not be removed very quickly.

Rózsahegyi (1965) considered that bends and bone necrosis resulted from two different disease processes and he associated the sites of bone lesions with a high fat content in the marrow of the humerus and femur.

Evidence that true end arteries occur in bone is equivocal and there appears to be free anastomosis between the vessels of the diaphysis, metaphysis and epiphysis and the marrow. Although bone is a vascular tissue, the femoral and humeral heads are relatively poorly supplied with arteries and this may play a part in the occurrence of structural failure in juxta-articular bone necrosis. However, any theory of causation must also explain the occurrence of lesions in other areas, such as the femoral and humeral shafts or the tibia, which are comparatively well vascularized, unless it can be shown that there are two different mechanisms in operation. The possibility that there might be a predisposition to bone necrosis in either the femoral head or the lower end of the femoral shaft, depending on whether the individual's legs were short or long, has been investigated (Decompression Sickness Panel Report, MRC 1971). The theory was that during decompression men with short legs sat with the level of the knees below that of the hips while men with long legs sat with the knees above hip level. If gas bubbles caused bone necrosis then leg length might determine the site. No significant association was found between the site of a lesion in the femur and leg length.

Decompression sickness and bone lesions

The occurrence of bends pains and bone lesions in the same regions of the limbs suggests that they are closely related (Fryer 1969), but it is unexpectedly difficult to establish a connection between them. It is generally accepted that acute decompression sickness (Types I and II) is caused by gas bubbles (Gersh & Catchpole 1951) but the adequacy of this mechanism by itself to explain the whole range of signs and symptoms associated with decompression is considered in another chapter (23). The site of the bubble in bends has been placed variously in peripheral vessels, sensory nerves, nutrient arteries to nerves, dorsal nerve roots, joint spaces or extravascularly in tendinous tissues or ligaments. It has been suggested that pain might result from obstruction of venous outflow from the medulla of a long bone causing severe distortion and stagnation (Fryer 1969), or by a gas bubble under the periosteum of a bone distorting and stimulating nerve endings (Walder 1969). Alnor, Herget and Seusing (1964) saw no relationship between an attack of the bends and the site of a bone lesion. They pointed out that severe decompression sickness (DCS) often occur without a subsequent bone lesion while men with no history of bends or of only mild bends can have bone lesions. On the other hands the depths to which the divers have been and the time spent at depth are important. Disabling bone necrosis has been described as immediately following bends at the same site (Bornstein & Plate 1911–1912; Thomson & Young 1958), but it is possible in these cases that there was confusion between the bends pain and that from a juxta-articular lesion with structural failure. In a group of 290 men with bone necrosis, 36% had never been treated for DCS (Walder 1969). This, however, is usually only recorded when the pain is severe enough for men to report for treatment. On the other hand, it may be mild enough to be ignored ('niggles') or made tolerable with the help of analgesics. Although most men have the bends at one time or another a few individuals do not admit to having had them at all. The pain of bends is felt most commonly in the region of the knees (Fryer 1969), and rather less often in the shoulders. Bone necrosis is perhaps most common in the shoulders (Davidson & Griffiths 1970), although data from the Decompression Sickness Central Registry show more lesions in the distal femur than in the humerus. Attempts to relate particular attacks of bends to bone lesions are frustrated because of the time-lag of at least several months between the inception of the lesion and the earliest radiographic sign. In the men who were first exposed to compressed air at the Clyde Tunnels there was no statistically significant relationship between the site of a bone lesion and the site of bends (Decompression Sickness Panel Report, MRC 1966), and the probability of a man having a bone lesion did not increase with the number of attacks of bends that he had. Similarly, there was no tendency for Type II decompression sickness to be associated with bone lesions in this group of men.

The natural history of bone necrosis as understood so far suggests a widespread or generalized phenomenon which can affect nearly the whole of the femoral and humeral heads and large areas of the lower femur and upper tibia, in addition to other bone sites. The generalized nature of the cause is reinforced by the symmetrical tendency of the lesions. There is evidence also that if a fuller radiological examination of the skeleton was regularly carried out in compressed air workers and divers, lesions would be found more frequently in the distal ends of the radius, ulna and tibia. There is also some evidence that healing of bone damage can occur before radiographically visible lesions can develop. (Decompression Sickness Panel Report, MRC 1966). Questions which still require an answer are:

What is the nature of the insult to bone, how does it occur and in what circumstances?

What determines the sites of the lesions and their tendency to symmetry?

What factors cause a lesion to progress to involve an articular surface and cause disability?

Why is the knee joint never involved?

Experimental bone necrosis

There have been many attempts to produce embolic bone lesions in experimental animals either by injecting gas into the circulation (Kahlstrom, Burton & Phemister 1939), or by rapid decompression from a high pressure to induce intravascular gas bubbles (Gersh 1945; Colonna & Jones 1948; Antopol et al. 1964), or with solid carbon particles introduced into the circulation (Kistler 1934). Much of this work has been carried out in small animals over short periods of time and the results have been difficult to interpret in human terms. More recently Antopol and Chryssanthou (1972) produced bone necrosis in mice by exposing them repeatedly to compressed air over a period of 5 months. They found that the bone necrosis was independent of decompression sickness and suggested that altered immunity was the basis of the bone changes. Necrotic bone changes could also occur in control obese mice not subjected to pressure. Wünsche and Scheele (1973a) produced cystic changes in the limb bones of albino rats following repeated exposures to 12 kp/cm² (13 ATA) for an hour. Cox (1973) used radiopaque glass microspheres of less than 120 μm in diameter to simulate embolic arterial obstruction in the lower limbs of rabbits. Necrotic lesions were produced in the femoral heads and shafts but not in the lower end of the femora. Cortical thickening and occasional sub-periosteal new bone formation was seen but no evidence of thrombosis was reported.

A more convincing model for the study of bone necrosis would be larger animals exposed to compressed air repeatedly over weeks or months. Goats have been used experimentally for many years and subjected to bend-producing compression/decompression experiments (Boycott, Damant & Haldane 1908) but damage to their bones has not been reported. Phemister (Kahlstrom, Burton & Phemister 1939) failed to produce bone necrosis in dogs by inducing arterial air embolism, and this was regarded as evidence that bone lesions in compressed air workers were due to extravascular gas liberation rather than intravascular embolism. Reeves et al. (1972) tried to produce bone necrosis in long-term experiments on mongrel dogs given repeated compressed air exposure over a 5-year period. Decompression sickness occurred after 50% of these exposures. Erosions and necrosis occurred in articular cartilage with alteration in the shape of the femoral head and dense bone sclerosis but there was no necrosis of cortical or cancellous bone. This was thought to be because there had been an insufficient mean pressure ratio and because bends had been adequately treated. Aseptic bone necrosis has been shown to occur as a specific disease in young dogs, but no control animals were used.

Bone changes have recently been described in miniature pigs subjected to repeated compression/decompression over many weeks. Seven pigs repeatedly decompressed at varying rates from several hours exposure at 60 ft (2·8 ATA) developed sclerotic and radiolucent areas in radiographs of the metaphyses of femora and humeri after 2 or 3 months (Stegall & Smith 1975). Aseptic necrosis was diagnosed at biopsy in one pig. Blood fibrinogen concentration, thrombin time and platelet counts decreased while the creatine phosphokinase (CPK) level increased markedly. There was also evidence that disseminated intravascular coagulation could occur

without decompression sickness. Wünsche and Scheele (1973) subjected 37 miniature pigs to compressed air at 5 kp/cm^2 (6 ATA) for 125 minutes daily for between 68 and 360 days. Cystic and fibrotic changes were found in the long bones of 29% of the animals but none in 6 controls. The histological changes which they described include bone necrosis, pseudocyst formation, sclerosis of bone, periosteal thickening and new bone formation in connective tissue. These experiments are the most encouraging yet and their further extension and evaluation in relation to bone necrosis in humans is of the utmost importance. Although there appear to be many similarities with human bone necrosis, the periosteal changes which have been described in miniature pigs are not typical of the bone lesions in compressed air workers or divers.

Other theories

Alternatives to the theory of vascular obstruction by gas bubbles which have been put forward include: fat embolism, haemoconcentration and increased coagulability of the blood, changes in blood enzymes, and the osmotic effect of gases dissolved in the tissues.

Fat embolism. Fat and bone marrow embolism in decompression sickness is well documented. Clay (1963), for example, described bone marrow emboli in pulmonary arteries or arterioles in dogs subjected to high atmospheric pressure and rapid decompression. Disruption of the femoral marrow by bubbles was thought to be the source of embolic fat.

Fat embolism in humans in association with severe decompression sickness has been demonstrated in the lungs, kidney and brain (Bennison, Catton & Fryer 1965; Fryer 1969), but Fryer regards fat emboli, at least in altitude cases, as not being clinically significant. Striking similarities in the clinical picture of fat embolism and decompression sickness are seen by Pauley and Cockett (1970) who suggest that nitrogen bubbles provoke damage to fatty tissue especially in liver. Disruption of liver cells may lead to formation of fat emboli in the portal circulation. This mechanism could provide a common explanation for bone lesions, not only in compressed air workers but in a number of different conditions associated with bone necrosis, such as alcoholism or sickle cell diseases, in all of which there is hepatic damage.

Although fat and marrow emboli certainly occur in decompression sickness, areas of bone necrosis have not been shown to occur as a direct result. Fat emboli appear to be frequent from a variety of causes and one would therefore expect bone necrosis to be much commoner than it is. It has been suggested by Jones (1971) that an important factor in bone necrosis is not a single episode of fat embolism but repeated showers of fat emboli over a period of months or years. However, while in many cases of bone necrosis there is repeated exposure to compressed air over quite long periods, in a number of well-attested cases bone necrosis has occurred after only one exposure (James 1945; Rose 1962). Furthermore, trauma to bone or chronic alcoholism are common conditions, but bone necrosis comparable to that seen in compressed air workers or divers is unusual.

Blood changes in decompression. Decompression can be accompanied by complex changes in the blood and circulation and it is possible that some of these play a part in the pathogenesis of bone necrosis.

Intravascular erthyrocyte agglutination, made worse by increased CO_2, was reported in experimental animals (kangaroos and tadpoles) decompressed from high pressures by Swindle in 1937. Human red cell agglutination has been considered as the primary abnormality in decompression sickness but this was not confirmed experimentally (Gersh & Catchpole 1951). Platelet thrombi may occur in air embolism and Philp, Schacham and Gowdey (1971) have shown that severe decompression sickness in rats is accompanied by microthrombi of platelet and red cell aggregates in the smaller lung vessels. Serotonin plus adenosine diphosphate (ADP), which are known to aggregate platelets, significantly shortened the survival time of air-injected rabbits and increased thrombocytopenia. They postulated that intravascular bubble formation could cause a syndrome similar to disseminated intravascular coagulation. Martin (1973) described a drop in the level of blood platelets and a rise in the enzyme creatine phosphokinase (CPK) 3 days after a safe dive, but there was no change in blood

coagulability. While all these observations are of the greatest interest they do not yet give any clear lead in determining the pathogenesis of bone necrosis.

Intramedullary pressure and gas osmosis. During alterations in ambient pressure the body tissues in general behave like a fluid in transmitting pressure evenly and instantaneously. Bone is the only rigid structure and it is possible therefore that transient pressure differentials could occur which might damage the bone. Harrelson and Hills (1970) measured femoral marrow pressures during compression and decompression of dogs. On compression to 35 psi gauge for 1·3 to 5·3 min there was a marked fall in marrow pressure (average 43·8%). Taking intramedullary pressure as an index of blood flow these findings suggest a relative bone ischaemia during compression. Arterial pressure was recorded at the same time and although it also fell during compression and rose during decompression, there was no statistically significant correlation between arterial and marrow pressures.

Harrelson and Hills (1970) considered these findings consistent with a hypothesis of gas induced osmosis. They suggest that the cause of bone necrosis may lie in compression rather than decompression, but the significance of these interesting observations in relation to bone necrosis is not clear at present. Compression normally takes only a few minutes, but bone deprived of its blood supply may survive at least 6 hours so that some factor other than a transient pressure change would have to be involved. The osmotic effect of gas in the tissues at pressures above atmospheric in altering the distribution of body water have been studied experimentally by Hills (1971a). Using excised tissues (bladder and peritoneum) water was shown to move towards increased gas concentrations. Nitrogen can also induce osmotic pressure in tissues (Hills 1971b) and might be of importance in the mechanism for production of bone necrosis.

Nitrogen may act directly on bone as a poison by abolishing the biosynthesis of collagen from proline (Deiss, Holmes & Johnston 1962), but one would expect a general effect on bone tissue rather than the localized lesions which occur. Hills and Straley (1972) studied blood flow in the tibia at various conditions of atmospheric pressures. They found an increase in blood flow 4 to 7 min after compression to 4 ATA in air and a reversal of this situation upon return to normal atmospheric pressure or exposure to pure oxygen. However, they concluded that the amount of interference with blood supply was not sufficient to produce aseptic necrosis of bone. The pathology of bone necrosis as it occurs in persons never exposed to compressed air might be expected to throw some light on the pathogenesis of the condition in divers and compressed air workers. Chronic hip disease from bone necrosis of unknown cause (idiopathic) has aroused very considerable interest (*Proceedings of the Conference on Aseptic Necrosis of the Femoral Head.* St Louis, Missouri 1964; Zinn 1971) but the mechanism by which it occurs appears to be as mysterious as that in compressed air workers.

TREATMENT

The treatment of bone necrosis and the management of patients with this condition is at present very unsatisfactory. Bone necrosis not involving an articular surface or affecting the shafts of bone requires no treatment, as it does not cause symptoms or disability. Some juxta-articular lesions do not progress to cause symptoms and disability, but it is not at present possible to forecast which lesions will fall into that category.

In early juxta-articular lesions the question arises whether a period of immobilization of the joint to achieve complete avoidance of weight bearing and other mechanical stresses can prevent a break in the articular surface or deformation of the joint. This is difficult to put to the test in symptomless and otherwise fit men because the duration of immobilization would have to be above 6 months, and there is no guarantee of the effectiveness of such a regimen were it possible to carry it out in practice. The pathology of juxta-articular bone necrosis suggests that in many cases the repair process has halted, leaving an avascular area which will never revascularize even with prolonged immobilization.

Removing a core of bone from the dead area of the femoral head and packing the cavity with cancellous bone from the ilium has been tried

(Barnes 1967) but the results have not been successful. Osteotomy of the femur may also give relief of pain for a time but some limitation of movement remains.

It is likely that most men with severe juxta-articular lesions of the femoral head will eventually require a prosthetic replacement. In the head of the humerus pinning the loose fragment (Fig. 27.2) may be successful, but in the long term osteo-arthritis and some permanent disability from limitation of movement can be expected.

A difficult question is whether a man with a symptomless lesion or lesions should be allowed to continue work as a diver or compressed air worker. Such men are often young, physically fit and at the peak of their earning capacity so that the decision to abandon a well-paid job is a serious step. At present there is no evidence to judge whether or not a man who already has bone necrosis is any more or less likely to acquire other bone lesions if he continues exposure to compressed air than a man with normal bone radiographs. However, it

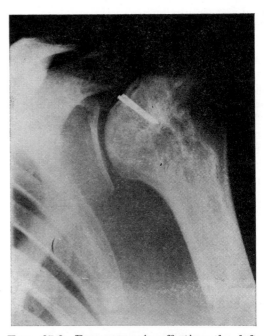

FIG. 27.2. Bone necrosis affecting the left shoulder of a compressed air worker aged 31 years. A loose fragment of articular surface has been pinned to the underlying bone. Joint movement is almost full but some discomfort remains.

can be argued that if bone lesions are discovered, particularly a juxta-articular one in the head of a femur, continued exposure could substantially increase the risk of disability were fresh lesions to occur, as they may do (Decompression Sickness Panel Report, MRC 1974). A man with a definite lesion of bone necrosis should at least have an opportunity to discuss the situation with a medical specialist familiar with the condition so that a personal decision to continue in his job or not can be made.

There is also the viewpoint of an employer to be considered: if he knows that a man has bone necrosis he may not be willing to employ him at all because of possible medico-legal complications should a further bone lesion appear, or at least not without a legally binding disclaimer of the employer's responsibility in such an event.

PREVENTION

Until recently most decompression tables were designed to reduce or eliminate decompression sickness (Types I and II) only.

Bone necrosis has occurred during the use of a variety of different decompression schedules, many of which employ decompression times much in excess of those required by the British Regulations (*Work in Compressed Air*, Special Regulations 1958) which appear to give no protection at all against bone necrosis. There is some confusion in making a distinction between an essentially faulty table and faulty, inexpert, or careless use of a table which may or may not be adequate. If the table is inherently inadequate there can be no adequate decompressions and it is difficult to ascribe bone necrosis to deviations from its strict use, particularly if it is not known in what precise respects the table is deficient. It has been confirmed that bubbles occur during most decompressions (Evans, Barnard & Walder 1972), including those in which no complications follow. This seems to imply that there may be no truly safe decompressions.

A solution to the bone necrosis problem in tunnel and caisson workers has been sought in freshly designed decompression tables based on re-examination of the basic principles which have been adopted in the past and in the light of new concepts of the behaviour of gas at pressure in body tissue. The trend is towards much longer decompression times than before and to decompressions in a step pattern rather than a smooth curve. In seeking to prevent bone necrosis by better decompression procedure the assumption has been made that it is the decompression phase only of the compression/decompression cycle that is crucial and that a reduction in gas bubble formation would reduce the risk of bone necrosis.

Two new sets of decompression tables for tunnelling or caisson work in compressed air have attracted widespread attention during the last 5 years, one of them American, the Washington State Tables, and the other British, the Blackpool Trial Tables of the Medical Research Council Decompression Sickness Panel. It appears that some bone changes have occured in men decompressed by the Washington State Tables (State of Washington 1963). These lesions were in the shafts of the humerus and femur and in one man a juxta-articular lesion in a hip joint (Sealey 1969; Behnke 1969). More detailed information about follow-up examinations of men decompressed according to this table is still required to form a sound opinion on its adequacy in respect of bone necrosis. It is known that 5 cases of bone necrosis have occurred in men whose only compressed air exposure was at a contract where the Blackpool Trial Tables were used (Decompression Sickness Panel Report, MRC 1974).

Information on the prevalence of bone necrosis in divers decompressed on a particular table is extremely difficult to obtain because of the variety of methods in use and the lack of adequate radiographic data.

There is, therefore, little sound evidence that decompression procedures in present use can be relied upon to prevent bone necrosis, however strictly they are followed.

EPIDEMIOLOGY

In the past little or no attention has been paid to the evaluation of compression/decompression procedures in tunnelling or caisson work by epidemiological techniques. This is perhaps because the essentially empirical nature of these procedures and the sporadic occurrence of compressed air work in Europe, North America and elsewhere has made such an approach difficult. Until comparatively recently commercial diving has been carried out on too small a scale and at too many widely scattered points for dependable data to be collected. Naval diving has also suffered from similar limitations. In order to find a procedure which will prevent bone necrosis, one type of decompression table must be compared with another. This can only be achieved by comparing bone radiographs of suitably matched groups, each using a decompression table under study, in conditions where there are as few other variables as possible.

The more closely the bones of compressed air workers or divers are studied radiologically or pathologically, the more evidence of bone damage is found. From the epidemiological point of view however, the studies of compressed air workers which have been carried out hitherto are most unsatisfactory. The proportion of compressed air workers who have had radiographs taken of their joints is often less than 30% at best, and essential follow-up radiographs can be obtained in only a small minority. In the bone radiographs of compressed air workers and divers in the Decompression Sickness Central Registry, 72% are of men who have had only one radiographic examination (Table 27.2).

The earliest radiological signs of bone necrosis occur about 4 or 5 months after the first exposure

to compressed air but lesions may appear up to about $2\frac{1}{2}$ years after leaving the work (Golding 1966) so that it is essential for 6-monthly radiographic examinations to continue for about 3 years. This again has not been achieved for a large enough proportion of the men to give reasonably good data. Comparisons of the prevalence of bone necrosis in one contract with another are perhaps best made at the same interval of time after the compressed air work has finished. However, former compressed air workers living in an area in which there is awareness of the hazard are much more likely to have bone necrosis correctly diagnosed than if they live in an area in which there is little experience of or interest in the condition.

Labour at a tunnel or bridge site is often largely casual and consists of men recruited locally plus a number of groups of men who move from one part of the country to another, wherever the work is. Commercial divers may also move from one centre to another or overseas to follow the demand for their services. Follow-up of these men can be difficult if they have no fixed address in the area in which they are employed and a home address may be difficult to ascertain. If men remain in the same type of work it is likely that a follow-up radiographic examination can be carried out sooner or later. Apart from the almost insuperable difficulties in obtaining extensive bone radiography of sufficient men to give a good epidemiological base-line, environmental, clinical and social variables can make sound comparisons of one decompression procedure with another very uncertain. Thus differences between civil engineering projects in working pressures, shift length and use of decanting must be considered, and the effects of physique, obesity, alcohol intake and acclimatization may also have to be taken into account. The identification of casual mobile workers, particularly when compressed air work or diving is being carried out at more than one centre at the same time, can be difficult.

APPENDIX

Radiographic technique

The Decompression Sickness Panel recommendations emphasize the importance of good definition

TABLE 27.2

Frequency of radiographic examination of shoulder, hip and knee joints of compressed air workers

No. of radiographic examinations	No. of men examined
1	1223
2	281
3	119
4	50
5	16
6	5
7	1
8	4
9	1
	1700

of the trabecular structure of bone as this is essential for detection of early changes.

Their suggestions for the projections required are as follows:

1. *Anteroposterior projection of each shoulder joint*. The patient is placed in a supine position with the trunk rotated at an angle of approximately 45 degrees, to bring the shoulder to be radiographed in contact with the table. The arm is partially abducted and the elbow is flexed. Centre 1 inch below the coracoid process of the scapula, and cone to show as much humerus as possible, bringing in the lateral diaphragms to show only the head and shaft of the humerus. This view should show a clear joint space, and the acromion should not overlap the head of the humerus.

2. *Anteroposterior projection of each hip joint*. The gonads must be protected from ionizing radiation by the use of a lead shield.

The patient is placed in a supine position with the feet at 90° to the table top. Use 12 inch × 10 inch (30 × 24 cm) film coned. The edge of the gonad protector should be as near the femoral head as possible, but not in any way obscuring it. Centre the cone over the head of the femur, that is 1 inch below the mid-point of a line joining the anterior superior iliac spine and the upper border of the pubic symphysis.

3. *Anteroposterior and lateral projections of each knee*. Centre at the level of the upper border of the patella. The field should include the distal femur from a point proximal to the mid point and the proximal tibia and fibula to the mid point or just beyond.

Nellen and Kindwall (1972), in describing their radiographic technique, advocate a 0·3 or 0·6 mm focus tube and Bucky grid for good bone detail. They recommend an anteroposterior view of the shoulder as described by Grashey (1912) taken with the trunk rotated 45° from the table so that the rays are tangential to the glenoid to show the articular surface of the humeral head.

REFERENCES

ALNOR, P. C. (1963) Die chronischen Skelettveranderungen bei tauchern. *Beitr. klin. Chir.* **207**, 475–485.

ALNOR, P. C., HERGET, R. & SEUSING, J. (1964) *Druckluft Erkrankungen*. München: Barth.

ANTOPOL, W. & CHRYSSANTHOU, P. (1972) Experimental production of aseptic bone necrosis in mice. Preprint of 1972 Annual Scientific Meeting, Aerospace Medical Association.

ANTOPOL, W., KALBERER, J., KOOPERSTEIN, S., SUGAAR, S. & CHRYSSANTHOU, C. (1964) Studies on dysbarism 1. Development of decompression syndrome in genetically obese mice. *Am. J. Path.* **45**, 11–127.

BARNES, R. (1967) Surgical treatment of bone lesions in compressed air workers. In *Decompression of Compressed Air Workers in Civil Engineering*. Ed. R. I. McCallum. Newcastle upon Tyne: Oriel Press.

BASSOE, P. (1911) Compressed air disease. *J. nerv. ment. Dis.* **38**, 368–369.

BEHNKE, A. R. (1967) Split shift and short shift decompression: New York State experience. In *Decompression of Compressed Air Workers in Civil Engineering*. Ed. R. I. McCallum. Newcastle upon Tyne: Oriel Press.

BEHNKE, A. R. (1969) In Discussion (p. 87) *Proc. 4th int. Congr. on Hyperbaric Med.*, Sapporo, Japan, Ed. J. Wada & T. Iwa, Baltimore: Williams & Wilkins.

BELL, A. L. L., EDSON, G. N. & HORNICK, N. (1942) Characteristic bone and joint changes in compressed air workers: a survey of symptomless cases. *Radiology* **38**, 698–707.

BENNISON, W. H., CATTON, M. J. & FRYER, D. I. (1965) Fatal decompression sickness in a compressed air worker. *J. Path. Bact.* **89**, 319–329.

BLANK, N. & LIEBER, A. (1965) The significance of growing bone islands. *Radiology* **85**, 508–511.

BORNSTEIN, A. & PLATE, E. (1911–12) Über chronische Gelenkveränderungen, entstanden durch Presslufterkrankung. *Fortschr. Geb. RöntgStrahl.* **18**, 197–206.

BOYCOTT, A. E., DAMANT, G. C. C. & HALDANE, J. S. (1908) The prevention of compressed air illness. *J. Hyg., Camb.* **8**, 342–443.

CAVIGNEAUX, A., CHARLES, A., FUCHS, S. & TARA, S. (1949) Les lésions osseuses ignorées des tubistes. *Archs Mal. prof. Méd. trav.* **10**, 359–361.

CLAY, J. R. (1963) Histopathology of experimental decompression sickness. *Aerospace Med.* **34**, 1107–1110.

COLONNA, P. C. & JONES, E. D. (1948) Aeroembolism of bone marrow: experimental study. *Archs Surg., Chicago* **56**, 161–171.

COX, P. T. (1973) Simulated caisson disease of bone. *Förvarsmedicin* **9**, 520–524.

DAVIDSON, J. K. & GRIFFITHS, P. D. (1970) Caisson disease of bone. *X-ray Focus* **10**, 2–11.

DAVIDSON, J. K. & GOLDING, F. C. (1969) Aseptic necrosis of bone in compressed air workers: caisson disease of bone. In *Symposium Ossium*. Ed. A. M. Jellife & B. Strickland. Edinburgh: Livingstone.

Decompression Sickness Panel Report, MRC (1966) Bone lesions in compressed air workers with special reference to men who worked on the Clyde Tunnels 1958 to 1963. *J. Bone and Jt Surg.* **48B**, 207–235.

Decompression Sickness Panel Report, MRC (1971) Decompression sickness and aseptic necrosis of bone. Investigations carried out during and after the construction of the Tyne Road Tunnel (1962–66). *Br. J. ind. Med.* **28**, 1–21.

Decompression Sickness Panel Report, MRC (1974) Construction Industry Research and Information Association, London.

DEISS, W. P., HOLMES, L. B. & JOHNSTON, C. C. jun. (1962) Bone matrix biosynthesis in vitro. 1. Labeling of hexosamine and collagen of normal bone. *J. biol. Chem.* **237**, 3555–3559.

EL GHAWABI, S. H., MANSOUR, M. B., YOUSSEF, F. L., EL GHAWABI, M. H. & ABD EL LATIF, M. M. (1971) Decompression sickness in caisson workers. *Br. J. ind. Med.* **28**, 323–329.

ELLIOTT, D. H. (1971) The role of decompression inadequacy in aseptic bone necrosis of naval divers. *Proc. R. Soc. Med.* **64**, 26–28.

ELLIOTT, D. H. & HARRISON, J. A. B. (1970) Bone necrosis—an occupational hazard of diving. *Jl. r. nav. med. Serv.* **56**, 140–161.

EVANS, A., BARNARD, E. E. P. & WALDER, D. N. (1972) Detection of gas bubbles in man at decompression. *Aerospace Med.* **43**, 1095–1096.

FRYER, D. I. (1969) *Subatmospheric decompression sickness in man.* Advisory Group for Aerospace Research and Development, NATO. Slough: Technivision Services.

FOURNIER, A. M., JULLIEN, G. & LEANDRI, M. (1965) *La maladie ostéo-articulaire des caissons.* Paris: Masson.

GERSH, I. (1945) Gas bubbles in bone and associated structures, lung and spleen of guinea pigs decompressed rapidly from high pressure atmospheres. *J. Cell comp. physiol.* **26**, 101–117.

GERSH, I. & CATCHPOLE, H. R. (1951) Decompression sickness: physical factors and pathologic consequences. In *Decompression Sickness.* Ed. F. J. Fulton. Philadelphia & London: Saunders.

GOLDING, F. C. (1962) The shoulder—the forgotten joint. *Br. J. Radiol.* **35**, 149–158.

GOLDING, F. C. (1966) Radiology and orthopaedic surgery. *J. Bone Jt Surg.* **48B**, 320–332.

GOLDING, F. C., GRIFFITHS, P. D., HEMPLEMAN, H. V., PATON. W. D. M. & WALDER, D. N. (1960) Decompression sickness during the construction of the Dartford Tunnel. *Br. J. ind. Med.* **17**, 167–180.

GRASHEY, R. (1912) Atlas typischer Röntgenbilder von normalen Menschen ausgewählt und erklärt nach chirurgisch-praktischen Gesichtspuncten. In Lehmann's *Medizinische Helanen.* Vol. 5, 2nd Edition. München: Lehmann.

GRIFFITHS, P. D. (1968) *Radiographic Appearance of Bone Lesions in Compressed Air Workers.* Limited publication by Dr C. T. Fagan, Dept. of Radiology, University of Texas Medical Branch, Galveston, Texas 77550, USA.

GRIFFITHS, P. D. (1971) An exposure to risk registry for compressed air workers. *Trans. Soc. occup. Med.* **21**, 123–125.

HARRELSON, J. M. & HILLS, B. A. (1970) Changes in bone marrow pressure in response to hyperbaric exposure. *Aerospace Med.* **41**, 1018–1021.

HARRISON, J. A. B. (1971) Aseptic bone necrosis in naval divers: radiographic findings. *Proc. R. Soc. Med.* **64**, 24–26.

HILLS, B. A. (1971a) Gas-induced osmosis as a factor influencing the distribution of body water. *Clin. Sci.* **40**, 175–191.

HILLS, B. A. (1971b) Osmosis induced by nitrogen. *Aerospace Med.* **42**, 664–666.

HILLS, B. A. & STRALEY, R. (1972) Aseptic osteonecrosis: a study of tibial blood flow under various environmental conditions. *Aerospace Med.* **43**, 724–728.

HODGSON, C. J., DAVIS, J. C., RANDOLPH, C. L. & CHAMBERS, G. H. (1968) Seven year follow-up X-ray survey for bone changes in low pressure chamber operators. *Aerospace Med.* **39**, 417–421.

JAMES, C. C. M. (1945) Late bone lesions in caisson disease. Three cases in submarine personnel. *Lancet*, **2**, 6–8.

JONES, J. P. (1971) Alcoholism, hypercortisonism, fat embolism and osseous avascular necrosis. In *Idiopathic Ischaemic Necrosis of the Femoral Head in Adults.* Ed. W. M. Zinn. Stuttgart: Thieme.

KAHLSTROM, S. C., BURTON, C. C. & PHEMISTER, D. B. (1939) Aseptic necrosis of bone. I. Infarction of bones in caisson disease resulting in encapsulated and calcified areas in diaphyses and in arthritis deformans. *Surg. Gynec. Obstet.* **68**, 129–146.

KIM, S. K. & BARRY, W. F. (1964) Bone islands. *Am. J. Roentg.* **92**, 1301–1306.

KISTLER, G. H. (1934) Sequences of experimental infarction of the femur in rabbits. *Proc. Inst. Med. Chicago* **10**, 110–113.

MARTIN, K. J. (1973) Decompression sickness. Observations on haematological and biochemical parameters. *J. clin. Path.* **25**, 1004–1005.

NELLEN, J. R. & KINDWALL, E. P. (1972) Aseptic necrosis of bone secondary to occupational exposure to compressed air. Roentgenologic findings in 59 cases. *Am. J. Roentg. radium Ther. nucl. Med.* **115**, 512–524.

OHTA, Y. & MATSUNAGA, H. (1974) Bone lesions in divers. *J. Bone Jt Surg.* **56B**, 3–16.

PAULEY, S. M. & COCKETT, A. T. K. (1970) Role of lipids in decompression sickness. *Aerospace Med.* **41**, 55–60.

PHILP, R. B. & SCHACHAM, P. & GOWDEY, C. W. (1971) Involvement of platelets and microthrombi in experimental decompression sickness—similarities with disseminated intravascular coagulation. *Aerospace Med.* **42**, 494–502.

POPPEL, M. H. & ROBINSON, W. T. (1956) The roentgen manifestations of caisson disease. *Am. J. Roentg.* **76**, 74–80.

Proceedings of the Conference on Aseptic Necrosis of the Femoral Head, St. Louis, Missouri (1964), National Institutes of Health, United States Public Health Service.

REEVES, E., MCKEE, A. E., STUNKARD, J. A. & SCHILLING, P. W. (1972) Radiographic and pathologic studies for aseptic bone necrosis in dogs incurring decompression sickness. *Aerospace Med.* **43**, 61–66.

ROSE, R. J. (1962) *Survey of Work in Compressed Air During the Construction of the Auckland Harbour Bridge.* Special Report No. 6, Department of Health, Wellington, New Zealand.

RÓZSAHEGYI, I. (1956) Die chronische Osteoarthropathie der Caissonarbeiter. *Arch. Gewerbepath. Gewerbehyg.* **14**, 483–510.

SEALEY, J. L. (1969) In Discussion (p. 87), *Proc. 4th int. Congr. Hyperbaric Med.*, Sapporo, Japan. Ed. J. Wada & T. Iwa. Baltimore: Williams & Wilkins.

SLØRDAHL, J. (1953) Aseptic necrosis of bone in caisson disease. *Tidsskr norske Laegeforen* **73**, 300–304.

STATE OF WASHINGTON (1963) *Safety Standards for Compressed Air Work*, Chapter 20, part 2. Department of Labor and Industries, Division of Safety.

STEGALL, P. J. & SMITH, K. H. (1975) In *Proc. 5th Symp. Underwater Physiology.* Freeport, Bahamas (In press.)

SWINDLE, P. F. (1937) Occlusion of blood vessels by agglutinated red cells, mainly as seen in tadpoles and very young kangaroos. *Am. J. Physiol.* **120**, 59–74.

TAYLOR, H. K. (1943) Aseptic necrosis and bone infarcts in caisson and noncaisson workers. *N.Y. St. J. Med.* **43**, 2390–2398.

THOMSON, I. D. & YOUNG, A. B. (1958) Aseptic necrosis of bone in caisson disease. *Br. J. ind. Med.* **15**, 270–272.

WALDER, D. N. (1969) *Work in Compressed Air, Including Diving. Safety on Construction Sites*, pp. 49–55. London: Inst. Civil Engineers.

WERTS, M. F. & SHILLING, C. W. (1972) *Dysbaric Osteonecrosis. An Annotated Bibliography*. George Washington University, Dept. Medicine & Public Affairs. Biological Sciences Communication Project, 2001 S. Street, N.W. Washington, D.C. 20009.

Work in Compressed Air, Special Regulations (1958) London: H.M.S.O.

WÜNSCHE, O. & SCHEELE, G. (1973a) *Kritische Dekompression aus Überdruck Skelettuntersuchungen an Albinoratten*. Forschungsbericht Nr. 107. Ärztliche Forschungsstelle für Druckluftarbeiten im Institut für Flugmedizin. Bonn, Bad Godesberg.

WÜNSCHE, O. & SCHEELE, G. (1973b) *Skelettveränderungen nach kritischer Decompression aus überdruck bei Zwergschweinen*. Forschungsberichte des Landes Nordrhein-Westfalen Nr. 2384. Westdeutscher. Verlag: Opladen.

ZINN, W. M. (Ed.) (1971) *Idiopathic ischemic necrosis of the femoral head in adults*. Stuttgart: Thieme.

28

Auditory and Vestibular Function in Diving

J. C. FARMER AND W. G. THOMAS

Vestibular and auditory problems seen in diving and high pressure work are in many respects paradoxical. Man is primarily a terrestrial being, and the evolution of the external and middle ear has given man a mechanism which overcomes to a remarkable degree the impedance mismatch of sound transmission between air and water. The human ear is essentially a pressure transducer, capable of responding to minute changes in atmospheric pressure (in the order of 2×10^{-4} dynes/cm^2). The amplitude of vibration of the ear drum at the threshold of hearing is approximately 10^{-9} cm, or about one-half the diameter of a hydrogen molecule (Bekesy & Rosenblith 1951). Yet, as man returns to the sea in increasing numbers, he is subjected to enormous pressure changes. The existence of the external and middle ear as a pressure transducer for the transmission of sound, therefore, becomes a liability.

In terrestrial environments, the perception of position and motion is dependent upon the central nervous system integration of information from the visual, proprioceptive, and vestibular systems. During underwater conditions, visual and proprioceptive input to the central integration mechanism frequently becomes distorted; thus, proper spacial orientation under such conditions becomes more dependent upon the information received from the vestibular system. When dysfunction of this system occurs, the subsequent vertigo with nausea and possible vomiting can present significant and potentially life-threatening dangers to the diver.

The relationship between changes in atmospheric pressure and dysfunction of the peripheral auditory system has been generally known for hundreds of years (Lester & Gomez 1898; Boot 1913; Vail 1929; Almour 1942; Shilling & Everley 1942; Behnke 1945; Haines & Harris 1946; Fields 1958; Taylor 1959; Heller 1960; Palmgren 1960; MacFie 1964; Bayliss 1968; Simmons 1968; Soss 1971; Stucker & Echols 1971; Freeman & Edmonds 1972). Most of the literature has referred to otologic injury during diving in terms of aural barotrauma or aerotitis media, thought to be a reversible middle ear problem. Some reports of permanent inner ear injury with neurosensory deafness have appeared. However, much of the literature has discounted the possibility of permanent inner ear injury during diving or has ignored the problem entirely.

Labyrinthine disturbances during diving have also been frequently mentioned in diving literature. Kennedy (1972) has edited a most detailed and comprehensive bibliography on this subject. A more recent writing by this author suggests that the vestibular system is becoming more implicated in human compressed gas exposures (Kennedy 1973). These works should be consulted to appreciate the full scope of the previous literature. Most of the reports are not well documented or they describe symptoms which would suggest possible dysfunction or injury to the vestibular system only as incidental observations. The main symptom of vestibular dysfunction, true vertigo, has often not been differentiated from other vague symptoms of balance disturbances such as dizziness, light-headedness, unsteadiness, faintness and swaying. Even when vertigo has been specifically described adequate evaluations have frequently not been done to either differentiate endorgan from central vestibular system dysfunction or to properly determine whether such affected individuals are suitable for further diving after apparent recovery. These deficiencies and most of the previous literature are very understandable, for dizzy patients often represent complex and perplexing diagnostic problems even to otologic physicians.

ANATOMY AND PHYSIOLOGY OF THE AUDITORY AND VESTIBULAR SYSTEMS

A complete and thorough description of the physics and physiology of the auditory and vestibular systems is impossible within the context of this chapter. Therefore, only a selection of the highlights that may have a direct relationship to diving or high pressure work will be discussed.

Middle ear

The medial wall of the middle ear contains the oval window, an oval-shaped opening into the inner ear. This window is covered and occupied by the footplates of the stapes. Inferior to the oval window is a rounded prominence called the promontory, formed by the lateral projection of the basal turn of the chochlea. Below the promontory is the round window, a circular opening covered by a thin membrane into the basal turn of the scala tympani of the cochlea. The contents of the middle ear space include the ossicles (malleus, incus, and stapes), two muscles (tensor tympani and stapedius) and several ligaments (Fig. 28.1). The middle ear mechanism is extremely important in man since it acts as an impedance-matching device between sound pressures in air and the extremely high input impedance of the inner ear fluids. This impedance matching is accomplished primarily in three ways: (1) the area difference between the tympanic membrane and the footplate of the stapes (17:1), which serves to increase the force acting on the oval window; (2) the lever effect of the ossicular change (1·3:1) resulting from the difference in the lengths of the long processes of the malleus and incus relative to the axis of rotation of the ossicular chain; and (3) the difference in the phase relationships of sound impinging upon the oval and round windows, resulting from the direct connection to the oval window through the ossicles.

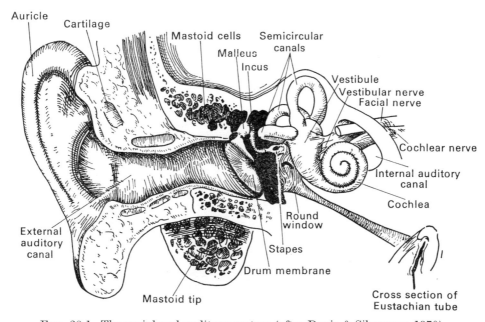

FIG. 28.1. The peripheral auditory system (after Davis & Silverman 1970)

The combined external and middle ear mechanisms, because of their collective volumes, masses, compliances, shapes, etc., have a broad resonance in the mid-frequency range, which enhances the auditory threshold in this area. Alterations in gas pressure or density, changes in the velocity characteristics of the gas medium, volume changes, middle ear effusions, or disruption of the tympanic membrane–ossicular chain complex, cause changes in these mechanisms with resulting changes in auditory thresholds.

Eustachian tube

Pressure equalization between the middle ear air space and the ambient pressure is accomplished through the Eustachian tube. The main function of this tube is to ventilate the middle ear cleft. The pharyngeal ostium is normally closed except when opened by positive middle ear pressure. The tube is also opened by the muscular actions of the pharyngeal and palatine muscles during swallowing. The tube is lined with a respiratory ciliated epithelium, which beats downward toward the nasopharynx. In high pressure work, the proper function of this tube is extremely important in maintaining pressure equalization between the middle ear space and the rapidly changing ambient pressure. Failure to maintain adequate ventilation through the Eustachian tube can result in middle ear or even inner ear barotrauma.

Inner ear

The inner ear consists of a system of interconnected membranous labyrinths which are located within the bony labyrinth, a system of spaces within the petrous portion of the temporal bone (Fig. 28.2). The membranous labyrinth (Fig. 28.3) is divided into two parts: the pars superior containing the vestibular system, which consists of the semicircular canals and utricle; and the pars inferior containing the saccule and the auditory system, or the cochlea. Although these

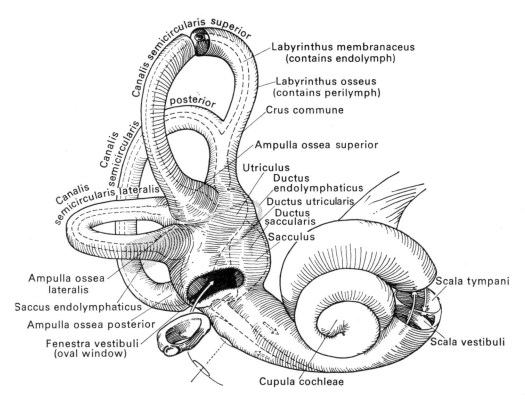

FIG. 28.2. The bony and membranous labyrinth (after *Internal Ear*. Chicago: Abbott Laboratories)

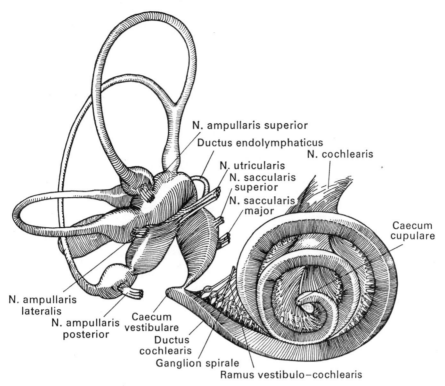

N. ampullaris superior

Ductus endolymphaticus

N. cochlearis

N. utricularis
N. saccularis
superior
N. saccularis
major

Caecum
cupulare

N. ampullaris
lateralis

N. ampullaris
posterior

Caecum
vestibulare

Ductus
cochlearis

Ganglion spirale

Ramus vestibulo–cochlearis

FIG. 28.3. The membranous labyrinth (after *Internal Ear*. Chicago: Abbott Laboratories)

two systems are different functionally, they are similar anatomically and share common fluid compartments and blood supplies.

The cochlea is a snail-like coil, composed of approximately $2\frac{1}{2}$ turns in a flat spiral. The canal within the bony cochlea is approximately 35 mm in length and ends blindly at the apex. This canal (Fig. 28.4) is partially divided into two cavities or scalae, the upper or scala vestibuli and the lower or scala tympani. Between these two scalae is located the scala media which contains the sensory cells of hearing and their supporting structures, the organ of Corti. The scala media or space within the cochlear duct terminates just short of the apex of the cochlear coil where the scalae vestibuli and tympani are joined in an area known as the helicotrema. At the basal end of the cochlear, the scala vestibuli communicates with the bone vestibule within which lies the saccule. The oval window is located in the lateral bony vestibular wall and is covered by the bony stapes footplate, thus separating the vestibule from the

middle ear space. The scala tympani terminates at its basal end at the round window, covered by the round window membrane which separates this scala from the middle ear space. The scalae vestibuli and tympani are filled with perilymphatic fluid, which is similar in chemical composition to cerebrospinal fluid with a relatively high sodium and low potassium content. The scala media is filled with endolymph, which is similar in chemical composition to intracellular fluid with a relative high potassium and low sodium content. The scala media is divided from the scala vestibuli by a thin membrane (Reisner's membrane), and from the scala tympani by a bony shelf protruding from the inner wall (the spiral lamina) and by a fibrous membrane (the basilar membrane) which supports the organ of Corti and attaches by the spiral ligament to the outer bony cochlear wall. The outer wall of the scala media contains a very vascular strip called the stria vascularis which is thought to be involved in the secretion and possibly the reabsorption of endolymph.

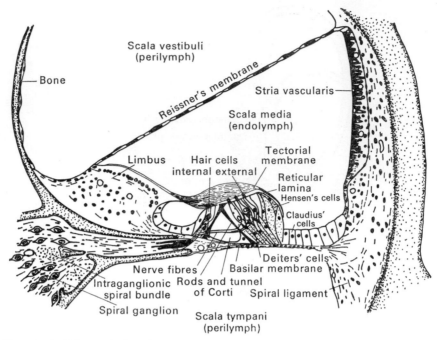

FIG. 28.4. Schematic drawing of a cross section of a cochlear turn (after Davis & Silverman 1970)

The organ of Corti is a rather complicated structure containing the sensory cells of hearing, the hair cells, and the supporting cells of the hair cells, Claudius' cells, Hensen's cells, Deiters' cells, etc. The hair cells can be divided into two anatomical and possibly functional groups, the outer hair cells and the inner hair cells. The outer hair cells are arranged in three to four rows and are cylindrical in shape. The inner hair cells are arranged in one to two rows and are flask shaped. Dendrites of the primary auditory neurons travel from the hair cells via the basilar membrane to the cell bodies of these neurons composing the spiral ganglion located in the modiolus or the centre of the cochlear spiral. The axons travel via the auditory division of the eighth cranial nerve through the internal auditory canal to the dorsal and ventral cochlear nuclei located in the brain stem and containing the secondary auditory neurons which innervate higher centres.

Cochlear function

Thus the membranous cochlea is encased in bone and filled with a practically incompressible fluid. Therefore, any increase in pressure caused by stapedial movement must find a release mechanism. This pressure release is accomplished through the round window membrane, which acts in phase opposition to the oval window. Slow changes in ambient pressure find release through the helicotrema and round window. However, more rapid changes in ambient pressure (i.e. frequencies within the audio range) accomplish release of pressure by displacing the scala media or cochlear duct toward the scala tympani. This process distorts the contents of the cochlear duct and bends the hair-bearing ends of the hair cells with a shearing force between the basilar membrane and the tectorial membrane lying on top of the hair cells. This shearing motion is accomplished by slightly different anchor points of the basilar membrane and the tectorial membrane. The shearing of the hairs is thought by many to be the final stimulus in depolarizing the hair cells.

The basilar membrane is very narrow at the base of the cochlea and becomes progressively wider toward the apex. This combination of progressive changes in elasticity and width of the basilar membrane tends to give certain analytical properties. A disturbance in the fluid of the inner ear produces a travelling wave of pressure which progresses from the base toward the apex and reaches a maximum at some point along the cochlear partition (Bekesy 1960). The maximum displacement of the travelling wave is determined by the stimulus frequency and the analytical properties of the basilar membrane, governed by the progressive changes in elasticity and mass from base to apex. The maximum displacement of the travelling wave is associated with frequency of stimulation, maximum displacement for high frequencies occurring near the base and that for the low frequencies occurring near the apex. The travelling wave is thought to change the resistance of the basilar membrane, allowing current to flow between the endolymph with its positive potential and the negative intercellular potential of the hair cell. Movement within the fluids of the cochlea is highly, though not critically, damped. This allows rapid transmission of information which is necessary for the ear to analyse complex acoustic signals like speech. Direct observation of the travelling wave indicates a rather broad maximum, somewhat inconsistent with the fine frequency discrimination exhibited by the ear. This has led many researchers to suggest neural sharpening and/or lateral inhibition to produce this precise frequency discrimination.

Innervation of the organ of Corti is very complex. It is extremely difficult to trace in detail the precise course of nerve fibres from the main auditory nerve trunk to the region of the hair cells. Several distinct fibre groups have been identified; some innervate inner hair cells and others innervate outer hair cells (Engstrom, Ades & Anderson 1966). It is not yet possible to describe all the nerve fibres of the organ of Corti in terms of their functional properties, nor even according to the direction they propagate impulses. Different types of nerve endings have been described at the base of the hair cells. An afferent function is assumed for Type 1 nerve endings, while Type 2 endings are thought to be efferent.

The presence of centrifugal pathways and nerve endings at the hair cell level greatly increases the potential for analysis by the ear. Each inner hair cell is innervated by one or two radial fibres and each radial fibre is connected to one or two hair cells. The outer hair cells have numerous innervations, with multiple connections of a single fibre extending over half a turn of the cochlea in some regions. The complex innervation of hair cells and the presence of efferent pathways at this level may help to explain some of the phenomena exhibited by the ear, such as attention, fine frequency discrimination, and loudness discrimination. Most of the phenomena related to localization of sound in space, loudness summation, and time and phase differences are assumed to occur at higher centres in the auditory system, especially at the brain stem level.

Blood supply

The blood supply to the inner ear (Axelsson 1968) comes through the labyrinthine or internal auditory artery, a branch of either the basilar or inferior cerebellar arteries. This is an end-artery system supplying only the inner ear and has no collaterals with other vessels. The blood supply of the membranous labyrinth is separate from that of the bony labyrinth, which is supplied from the arteries of the tympanic plexus located in the mucous membrane covering the medial wall of the middle ear cavity. The internal auditory artery branches into the vestibular artery, the cochlear artery, and the vestibulocochlear artery. The vestibular branch goes to parts of the utricle and semicircular canals, plus the saccule. The cochlear branch supplies the upper two turns of the cochlea. The vestibulocochlear branch supplies part of the basal cochlear turn, plus parts of the saccule, utricle and semicircular canals (Donaldson & Miller 1973).

The major blood supply to the organ of Corti (Axelsson 1968) is derived from vessels within the stria vascularis and the spiral vessels underneath the basilar membrane. Arterioles, branches from the arteries of the modiolus, branch into two groups at the osseous spiral lamina. One group of vessels goes underneath the basilar membrane, and the second group runs within the periosteal lining of the bony cochlear wall across the scala vestibuli to the regions of the spiral ligament where arterioles divide into four capillary networks along the lateral bony wall of the cochlea. The first group of capillaries supplies the region of the spiral ligament adjacent to the insertion of Reisner's membrane. A second group forms a capillary bed in the stria vascularis. The third group supplies the vessels of the spiral prominence, and the fourth group supplies the lower portion of the spiral ligament. There is a remarkable linear continuity of capillary beds in the cochlea from the basal to the apical end. However, some capillary beds, especially those in stria vascularis and spiral prominence, seem to be isolated from the others.

Interestingly, the individual structures of the organ of Corti do not have blood vessels. It is generally felt that the neuroepithelium of this organ receives oxygen and nutrients indirectly by diffusion from out of the spiral vessels underlying the basilar membrane or from the capillary networks in the lateral wall of the bony cochlea.

The arteries and veins have separate channels and do not accompany each other within the cochlea. The venous drainage (Axelsson 1968) appears to be more complicated and is thought to be by venules which course through the bone of the scala tympani and terminate in a posterior spiral vein. Venous blood is collected by this vein and emptied into a larger cochlear vein which runs in a bony channel parallel to the cochlea aqueduct. There is some evidence to show that collaterals do exist between the cochlear veins and the dural veins.

Saccule, utricle, semicircular canals, endolymphatic duct and sac

The remainder of the membranous labyrinth consists of the endolymphatic duct and sac, the utricle, the semicircular canals, and the cochlear duct. These structures are joined (Fig. 28.3): the saccule communicates inferiorly with the cochlear duct by the ductus reuniens and superiorly with the endolymphatic duct via the saccular duct; the utricle communicates anteriorly with the endolymphatic duct by means of the utricular duct and posteriorly with the semicircular canals by direct connection. The endolymphatic duct thus arises at the junction of the utricular and saccular ducts. Communication between the utricle and the utricular duct is thought to be limited by an intraductal fold called the endolymphatic valve of Bast. The endolymphatic duct connects with the endolymphatic sac which lies on the posterior surface of the temporal bone in the posterior cranial fossa where it is located between the layers of the dura. It is variable in size and shape and has a rugose lumen. The exact function of the endolymphatic duct is disputed; most observers feel that it is concerned with the reabsorption of endolymph.

The utricle and the saccule each contain a structure known as the macular which consists of flat sensory areas containing sensory receptors and hair cells. The hairs of these cells project into an otolithic membrane which lies over each macular and is made up of crystals of calcium carbonate, the otoconia. The macular of the saccule lies in a vertical plane and is perpendicular to the macular of the utricle which lies in a horizontal plane. The utricle and saccule seem to be best equipped to serve as sensory receptors of linear acceleration, including gravity.

There are three semicircular canals, each of which is a tubular structure having an enlargement at one end, the ampula. Each canal opens into the utricle directly at the ampulary end; however, at the opposite end, the posterior and superior ducts open into the utricle through a common crus. The ampula of each canal consists of a transverse ridge of tissue, the crista, containing sensory epithelium and supportive structures. In the crista are hair cells similar to those found in the macular of the saccule and utricle. These hairs insert into a gelatinous cupula which lies on top of the ridge of sensory cells. The cupula extends from the surface of the ridge to the roof of the ampula so that any movement of the endolymph which fills the canal moves the cupula relative to the surface of the sensory ridge of epithelium. This causes bending of the hairs and a change in the constant resting discharge rate of the neuroepithelium. The canals respond to head movements in which there is angular acceleration. Since the density of the cupulae and endolymph are equal, gravity does not affect the cupulae.

Vestibular function

Each semicircular canal is paired with the same canal on the opposite side so that any movement of the head in which there is angular acceleration causes a displacement of endolymph on both sides in such a way that the discharge rate on one side is increased while the rate on the other side is decreased. The degree of increase and decrease is the same; thus equal, but opposite, information is transmitted to various centres in the central nervous system. This change in the discharge rate of each side is interpreted in the cerebral cortex as a movement of specific direction and speed. The eye muscle nuclei also receive this information and move the eyes compensatorily to retain the field of last gaze. The anterior horn cells in the spinal cord acting upon signals over the vestibulospinal tracts adjust the trunk and limb muscles. The cerebellum adjusts the muscle tone to compensate for the change in position.

Thus, the vestibular end organs are dynamic structures in three ways: (1) they respond to linear and radial acceleration; (2) they are constantly discharging a resting pattern of signals to the brain with movement causing a change in this pattern of signals which is distributed to the brain and interpreted; and (3) there are two vestibular end organs, each of which is constantly signalling the brain with a difference in the signal pattern between the right and left side being produced by acceleration (McCabe 1973).

Vestibular dysfunction

When a sudden pathological decrease in the function of one vestibular end organ occurs, the involved structure ceases to deliver its equal but opposite signals to the brain. Thus, the two sides begin to discharge at rest with unequal intensities and the brain perceives this as hyperfunction of the non-injured side. This state is interpreted in the cerebral cortex as a condition of constant motion or vertigo (McCabe 1973).

Generally, vestibular end organ diseases involve the entire end organ. The resulting sensation of motion may be a pitching, yawing, or rolling sensation. However, a rotational component is always present because of the predominance of the central nervous system innervation from the six semicircular canals over the four otolithic organs, the two saccules and two utricles. This imbalance of information from each side is transmitted to the eye muscle nuclei and reticular formation, and the eyes are deviated in a direction of last gaze to retain orientation. This is the slow component of vestibular nystagmus. However, the rotary sensation continues and the eyes cannot continue to rotate indefinitely because of anatomical limitations. Therefore, at the limit of gaze in any one direction, inhibitor neurons in the reticular formation inhibit the incoming flow from the vestibular nuclei, with simultaneous activation from reticular activating neurons directing the ocular muscle nuclei to quickly return the eye balls to the point of gaze from which the slow component originally began. This fast second phase of eye deviation is the quick component of vestibular nystagmus. The same imbalance of information causes staggering and ataxia due to the transmission of these impulses from the vestibular nuclei to the spinal cord anterior horn cells. In addition, impulses from the vestibular nuclei play on the dorsal efferent nucleus of the tenth cranial nerve causing initial inhibition with cessation of motor activity in the gut. If the imbalance is large and continuous, this nucleus becomes heavily stimulated and nausea and vomiting occurs. The cerebellum responds to this imbalance of information by inhibition of some of the vestibular nuclei thus partially decreasing the magnitude of these symptoms (McCabe 1973).

Fortunately, compensation will occur over a period of time, usually 2 to 4 weeks, after an acute vestibular injury. This restoration of equilibrium can be accomplished in three basic ways: (1) a return of the affected end organ to its previous healthy state; (2) continued central suppression of the healthy, uninjured side by central nervous system inhibitory centres; (3) the initiation of a new resting electrical activity in the hypofunctioning system, either in the end organ or the centrally located vestibular nuclei, which balances the unaffected and relatively hyperactive side.

When compensation is completed after permanent injury, the symptoms disappear except for varying degrees of motion intolerance. The speed at which compensation occurs is dependent upon the severity of the original injury causing the imbalance and the ability of the central nervous system to respond (McCabe 1973).

When dizziness occurs in divers, a systematic approach to the evaluation and management must be undertaken, keeping in mind the above described anatomical and physiological relation-

ships of the vestibular system. To develop such
an approach, several points should be noted:

1. Dysfunction in many body systems such as
cardiovascular system, the extravestibular neurological tracts, the pulmonary system and the
hormonal system, can produce dizziness. Thus,
the first distinction that should be made in the
evaluation of a dizzy individual is whether the
individual is experiencing non-vestibular dizziness (i.e. altered spacial awareness) or true vestibular vertigo with the sensation of rotary motion
of the subject or his environment.

2. With vestibular dysfunction of any severity
there will always be present simultaneous, classical, labyrinthine nystagmus with a well-defined
quick and slow component. If such nystagmus is
not demonstrated, either by visual observation or
electronystagmography of a patient during a dizzy
spell, the dizziness is not due to vestibular system
dysfunction.

3. Vestibular system pathology does not produce continuous and non-episodic dizziness for
longer than 2 to 3 weeks. If dizziness is continuous
and lasts for a longer period of time, the cause is
not due to vestibular system dysfunction for, as
noted above, compensation usually occurs after
acute injury.

4. Vestibular system dysfunction is frequently
accompanied by nausea, vomiting, visual disturbances, presyncope, difficulty with standing or
walking, etc. The simultaneous presence of these
symptoms does not necessarily mean a more
widespread central nervous system injury.

5. Once it has been established that dizziness
is due to vestibular dysfunction, the next distinction which should be made is whether the pathology is located in the end organ or the central
vestibular pathways. In a few cases this determination is not difficult, for there are other
accompanying neurological signs which point to a
centrally located lesion. However, in many cases
such accompanying signs are lacking and this
determination is more difficult. The presence of
accompanying auditory symptoms or signs of
damage to the tympanic membrane or the middle
ear as seen by otoscopic examination is more frequently, but not always, associated with end
organ injury. The presence of vertical nystagmus
almost always indicates central pathology. In

addition, the presence of a nystagmus during
position testing which has no latency, is non-
fatigable and is direction changing, is suggestive
of a central pathology.

6. Further evaluation, such as electronystagmography, pure tone and speech audiometry,
temporal bone and skull radiography and complete neurological examination, should be done as
soon as feasible.

7. The subsidence of symptoms of vertigo after
an acute injury to the vestibular system over a
period of days or weeks is the result of the normal
compensatory mechanism of the central nervous
system in responding to such injury. Thus, this
disappearance of symptoms does not necessarily
mean that the injured part of the vestibular system has been restored to its previous healthy state.
Certain motions or positions can and frequently
do cause vertigo and loss of spacial orientation in
individuals who have fully compensated from
permanent injury. Therefore, all divers (and
flyers) who experience vestibular injury should be
evaluated by specialists in vestibular problems
after their symptoms have apparently disappeared. Only in this way can rational judgments
be made regarding an individual's suitability for
exposure to future situations in diving or flying in
which spacial disorientation might endanger his
life or the lives of others.

AUDITORY FUNCTION IN DIVING

Several studies have reported reversible depth-
related conductive hearing loss as a function of
pressure and/or depth in hyperbaric chambers.
Fluur and Adolfson (1966) reported threshold
elevations of 30 to 40 dB in the middle frequency
range on 26 experienced divers at simulated sea
depths of 330 ft (11 ATA) under hyperbaric air.
No change was noted in bone conduction and
Fluur and Adolfson postulated that the increased
ambient pressure caused a decrease in the conduction of sound through the middle ear. Farmer,
Thomas and Preslar (1971) reported reversible
and depth-related conductive hearing losses in
six experienced divers at depths up to 600 ft
(19·2 ATA) in helium–air. This study reported
maximum elevation in thresholds of 26 dB in the
lower frequencies with less threshold shift in the

higher frequencies. There was a greater variability in thresholds during compression with less variation after 6 days on the bottom. Cochlear function as measured by sensory acuity levels and frequency difference limens was not altered at pressure.

Thomas, Summitt and Farmer (1974) studied 33 different divers under eight different saturation dives in helium–air-filled chambers. The dives included one dive to 300 ft (10 ATA), four separate dives to 600 ft (19·2 ATA), two dives to 805 ft (25·4 ATA), and one dive to 1000 ft (31·3 ATA). A total of 400 air conduction and 300 bone conduction studies were done at 26 different depths: 11 depths during compression and 15 depths during decompression. Each earphone was calibrated separately to an equivalent depth of 1000 ft (31·3 ATA) in helium–air, using the microphone corrections reported by Thomas, Preslar and Farmer (1972). Bone conduction was again done using the sensory acuity level technique of Jerger and Tillman (1960). Fig. 28.5 shows the results at four different depths during compression. Only four depths are shown for clarity, with the value for the remaining seven depths falling in between the values shown. The results at 500 and 1000 Hz show a progressive hearing loss which is related to depth, while 2000 Hz shows little or no change as a function of depth. The hearing loss at 3000 Hz is present at 100 ft (4 ATA) and shows little additional loss with increasing depth. The hearing level at 4000 Hz shows approximately 10 dB of loss at 100 ft, with additional loss at greater depths. The results at 6000 Hz show a significant

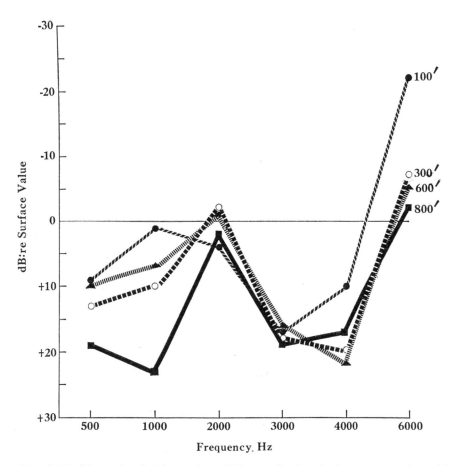

FIG. 28.5. Mean thresholds at four different depths during compression. All thresholds are measured relative to surface threshold (Thomas et al. 1974)

improvement in hearing in the first 100 ft (4 ATA) with this improvement decreasing toward the initial surface value with increasing depth. Although the data tend to indicate a decrease in auditory thresholds as a function of depth, there was no significant difference between the values for any depth below 100 ft (4 ATA). It appears that the greatest amount of hearing loss occurs during the first 1 or 2 ATS. This is similar to the phenomena reported by Brandt and Hollien (1967, 1969) regarding underwater hearing thresholds under wet conditions at depths from 12 ft to 105 ft (1·3 to 4·2 ATA).

Fig. 28.6 shows the threshold shift of each of the frequencies tested. This figure shows a general trend of depth related threshold shifts for 500, 1000, 3000 and 4000 Hz which is fairly symmetrical during compression and decompression. The results at 2000 Hz show little or no change in threshold while 6000 Hz shows an initial improvement in threshold during the first 100 ft (4 ATA) with a decrease toward the initial surface value with greater depth. This frequency also showed an improvement in threshold as surface is approached during decompression, reaching a maximum at 72 ft (3·2 ATA). Waterman and Smith (1970) noted an improvement at

8000 Hz when divers were tested at surface inside a sound treated room while breathing an 80% helium 20% oxygen mixture. Although 8000 Hz was not tested in the Thomas, Summitt and Farmer study, this phenomenon is noted at 6000 Hz.

The mean auditory thresholds on the bottom during four different saturation dives are shown in Fig. 28.7. Although this figure tends to show depth related changes in thresholds, there are no significant differences between 300 and 1000 ft (10 and 31 ATA). Fig. 28.8 shows the mean bone conduction thresholds (sensory acuity levels) and range for each of the frequencies tested. There was no significant difference in the bone conduction thresholds at depth from surface values at any frequency tested. These results would tend to agree with the previous research, indicating that the threshold shifts represent a conductive hearing loss which is reversible and, to some extent, depth related.

None of the hearing losses seen in the helium–oxygen dives (Thomas et al. 1974) even at 1000 ft (31 ATA) were as great as the 30 to 40 dB hearing losses noted by Fluur and Adolphson at 330 ft (11 ATA) of hyperbaric air. This difference is thought to be due, in part, to the difference in density between helium and air; i.e. the less dense

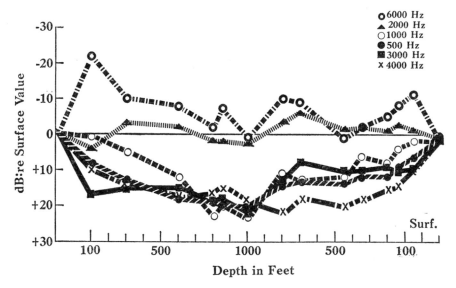

FIG. 28.6. Mean thresholds for six different frequencies as a function of depth. All thresholds are measured relative to surface threshold (Thomas, Summitt & Farmer 1974)

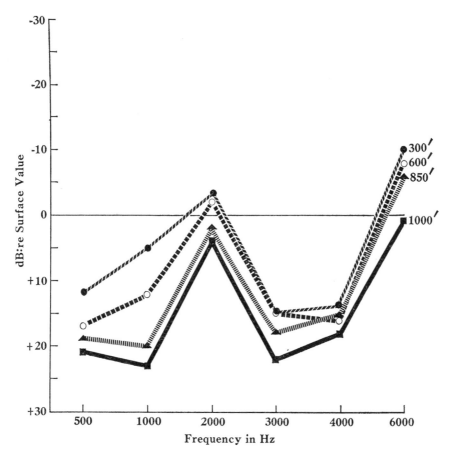

FIG. 28.7. Mean auditory thresholds on the bottom during four different saturation dives (Thomas, Summitt & Farmer 1974)

helium mixtures do not impede the motion of the tympanic membrane and ossicular chain as much as air at the same pressures. Also, calibration studies on standard audiometric earphones under conditions of increased atmospheric pressures in both air and helium (Thomas, Preslar & Farmer 1975) indicate a great variability (± 5 dB) between earphones as a function of pressure and within the same earphone during different pressurizations and between compression and decompression. This variability would indicate that audiometric thresholds taken with standard earphones should be evaluated with caution. The great variability in earphone performance may account for some of the differences in threshold measurement.

Auditory thresholds measured under wet, underwater conditions rather than in dry pressure chambers present more technical problems. First, the stimulus is presented in the 'field' rather than with earphones. The acoustic radiation patterns in water, scatter and the distance from the sound source to the listener become quite critical. Thus, there is somewhat less control of the stimulus. In addition, questions have been raised regarding the mechanism of underwater hearing. Several authors have suggested that this mechanism is by bone conduction (Hamilton 1957; Wainwright 1958; Sivian 1943; Montague & Strickland 1961; Brandt & Hollien 1967, 1969). When the ear is submerged in water rather than in air, several factors might possibly be operating which would change the sensitivity, resonance and the impedance of the ear. The middle ear mechanism is primarily an

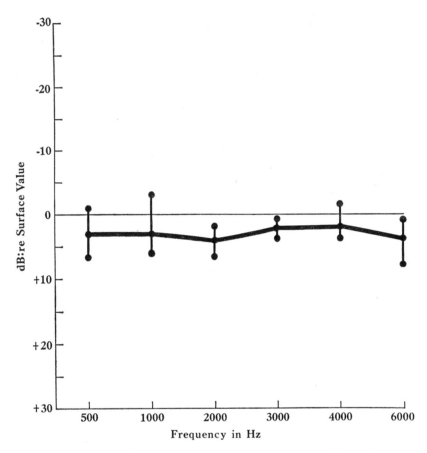

F IG. 28.8. Bone conduction thresholds (sensory acuity levels) as a function of frequency. Because of the similarity of the data for all depths, the mean threshold averaged over all depths and the range from the highest to lowest scores are plotted. All measures are relative to sensory acuity level measures at surface (Thomas, Summitt & Farmer 1974)

impedance-matching device which restores most of the energy lost when air-borne sound is transmitted into the inner ear fluids where there is an extremely high input impedance. This impedance matching is primarily accomplished by an increase in force resulting from the area differences between the tympanic membrane and the footplate of the stapes and from the architure and suspension of the ossicles. However, when the ear is submerged under water, an additional water–air interface is created. Water filling the external auditory canal may create an additional impedance mismatch, resulting in decreased sensitivity. The presence of water in the external canal may also produce mass loading on the tympanic membrane which would

result in a further decrease in sensitivity as a function of frequency. The resonance characteristics of the ear would also be changed with a downward shift in the resonance frequency and a flattening of the response characteristics.

Underwater thresholds have been measured at various depths from 10 to 105 ft (1·3 to 4·2 ATA). The mean underwater thresholds found have been variable. Sivian (1943) indicated a 45 to 55 dB shift in underwater thresholds compared to separate thresholds in air. Hamilton (1957) showed a hearing loss ranging from 44 dB to 60 dB for frequencies from 250 Hz to 4000 Hz. A study by Wainwright (1958) showed underwater thresholds ranging from 69 dB to 88 dB sound pressure level (SPL) in two divers, with minimal threshold changes occurring at 1000 Hz. Montague and Strickland (1961) in a study of underwater hearing of seven experienced divers at 25 ft (1·7 ATA), found threshold changes ranging from 60 dB to 80 dB SPL with the greatest changes occurring in the mid-frequencies. A more complete set of data has resulted from the studies of Brandt and Hollien (1967, 1969). Auditory thresholds were measured at depths from 12 to 105 ft (1·3 to 4·2 ATA) on 14 different divers for frequencies from 125 to 8000 Hz. Data indicated threshold changes from 69 dB to 80 dB SPL with the mean threshold as 70 dB. The threshold difference increased with frequency, and no significant difference was found between threshold levels at 12 ft (1·3 ATA) and threshold levels at 105 ft (4·2 ATA). This lack of significant difference between threshold changes at shallow depths and deep depths is similar to the results of Thomas, Summitt and Farmer (1974) in dry helium–oxygen atmospheres in hyperbaric chambers. The smallest threshold changes would appear to occur in pressure chambers pressurized with helium–air. Greater changes occur under hyperbaric air (Fluur & Adolfson 1966) and the greatest changes occur when the ear is actually submerged in water. These changes are not unexpected when the differences in density and mass between these three media of helium–oxygen, air and water are considered in relation to their effects on the resonance and impedance of the ear.

Bennett (1962) has postulated that the ear submerged in water becomes a velocity sensitive mechanism rather than a pressure sensitive device. A shift from sound pressure phenomenon to particle velocity mechanisms would suggest an upward shift in acoustic pressure to 1 dyne/cm², resulting in a threshold difference of 72 dB. This is in close agreement with the previous findings quoted by Montague and Strickland (1961), Wainwright (1958) and Brandt and Hollien (1967, 1969). Bennett's hypothesis would seem to implicate a velocity-sensitive system. The problem was studied directly by Hollien and Brandt (1969) who measured underwater thresholds with and without air bubbles present in the external auditory canals. Their results indicated no significant difference between these two conditions which would

suggest a bone conduction-like mechanism responsible for underwater hearing since changes in the impedance characteristics of the middle ear did not seem to affect the auditory thresholds.

Change in the auditory evoked responses (AER) is a function of depth and gas mixture and has been reported by several authors in laboratory animals and man (Bennett & Glass 1961; Bennett 1964; Bennett, Ackles & Cripps 1969; Roger, Cabarrou & Gastaut 1955; Bevan 1971). Using cats, Bennett (1964) found that increased pressures using nitrogen–argon induced a reversible reduction of electroencephalographic spontaneous activity and auditory evoked potential. However, helium had no effect on either evoked potentials or spontaneous activity. Bennett hypothesized that the observed changes in the evoked responses resulted from increased partial pressure of the inert gas and not from the oxygen content. In addition, it was further hypothesized that the inert gases acted primarily on polysynaptic regions of the brain, such as the reticular system in dendritic connections of the cerebral cortex. Similar data have also been reported in human subjects. Bennett, Ackles and Cripps (1969) noted decreases in the AER of experienced divers while breathing compressed air, oxygen–helium, and oxygen–helium–nitrogen at 300 ft (10 ATA). The changes noted for the compressed air and oxygen–helium–nitrogen mixtures were very similar, while the decrease in the AER for the oxygen–helium was considerably less. Decreases in the AER were also noted while breathing oxygen at 1, 2 and 3 ATA. These decreases in the measured AER were explained by narcosis in compressed air and oxygen–helium–nitrogen mixtures and conduction deficiencies in the brain when breathing pure oxygen. Bevan (1971) also noted reductions in the amplitude of the AER during dives in hyperbaric air, while the contingent negative variation was not affected. It is, of course, interesting to speculate on changes in the AER in relation to changes in the synaptic and dendritic regions of the brain or in relation to changes in nerve conduction. Indeed, by other methods, such as visual evoked responses (Bennett & Towse 1971), these CNS changes have been confirmed. However, audiometric studies in hyperbaric air (Fluur & Adolfson 1966) and in helium–air (Farmer, Thomas &

Preslar 1971; Thomas, Summitt & Farmer 1974) have shown a reversible depth-related conductive hearing loss with no demonstrable changes in cochlear function. This loss is greater in air than in helium atmospheres. These changes in the conduction mechanism of the middle ear could cause a decrease in the amplitude of the AER, since this amplitude is related to the intensity of the input signal. Thus, AER techniques should not be used to investigate the effects of hyperbaric inert gases upon central nervous system function without knowledge of the magnitude of the conductive hearing losses and appropriate correction of the stimulus strengths.

STUDIES OF OTOLOGIC FUNCTION IN ANIMALS DURING DIVING CONDITIONS

Miller (1971), McCormick et al. (1972a, b) and Thomas, Prazma and Farmer (1973) have studied the effects of increased pressure and different gas mixtures on cochlear potentials in laboratory animals. Miller reported losses in sensitivity after pressurization to 11 ATA in air and helium–air. Generally, this loss in cochlear microphonics did not recover after return to surface except in two animals. McCormick attempted to produce decompression sickness in guinea pigs experimentally by shortening decompression tables. The animals in these experiments did not recover. Thomas, Prazma and Farmer (1973) have found mixed results from recordings of cochlear microphonics and eighth nerve action potentials on guinea pigs under hyperbaric air. Responses to air conduction and bone conduction sounds at pressures to 3 ATA were recorded with the middle ear intact and with the middle ear removed. The bulla was opened in all cases for placement of the round window electrode. With the middle ear intact, cochlear microphonics showed a progressive loss to 3 ATA with additional losses as the animal was returned to the surface. With the middle ear removed, the cochlear microphonics for air conduction showed a progressive loss at 3 ATA with recovery as the animal was returned to the surface. Cochlear microphonics from bone conduction stimuli showed no changes as a function of pressure. Eighth nerve action potentials, particularly

with N_2, showed a decrease with exposures to 3 ATA with recovery as the animal was brought to the surface. The recovery was less complete when the middle ear was intact.

Extensive otologic studies in animals under diving conditions are only just beginning. During the next 5 years, many studies of animal auditory and vestibular function as related to changes in depth, changes in gas mixtures, alterations in rates of compression, etc. will be completed and will add much to our knowledge in these fields.

AURAL BAROTRAUMA OR BAROTITIS MEDIA

The most common otologic problem associated with diving is related to aural barotrauma resulting from a pressure differential between the middle ear and the external environment. This problem is generally noted during compression and reflects the inability to clear the ears. With an intact tympanic membrane, the Eustachian tube provides the only means of equalizing air pressure between the middle ear and the changing ambient pressure. During compression or descent, the ambient pressure increases rapidly and the pressure in the middle ear may become negative relative to this increasing ambient pressure. The nasopharyngeal ostium of the Eustachian tube acts as a valve which is normally closed. A positive pressure in the middle ear usually opens the Eustachian tube without difficulty. However, with a negative pressure in the middle ear, opening of the Eustachian tube is more difficult because of the valve action in the nasopharynx. With a pressure differential of approximately 90 mm of mercury, it is impossible to open the tube voluntarily (Armstrong & Heim 1937; Keller 1958). Pain usually occurs at a pressure differential of approximately 60 mm Hg of mercury and the tympanic membrane has been found to rupture at pressure differentials ranging from 100 to 500 mm Hg (Keller 1958). Varying degrees of pathological changes in the middle ear are seen. These include edema of the middle ear mucosa, submucosal hemorrhage, inflammation, and/or transudation of serous fluid into the middle ear. In addition to pain and fullness other symptoms include tinnitus, vertigo, and hearing loss. As noted in the introduction, the majority of the previous literature dealing with otologic problems in diving has indicated that these pathological changes are reversible and that the associated hearing loss is a conductive loss which is also reversible. However, recent work, as will be discussed below, has indicated that inner ear damage can occur during these conditions which is frequently permanent.

TRANSIENT VERTIGO DURING DIVING

Vertigo has been described in practically all phases of diving (Kennedy 1972). However, most of the reports are not well documented or have discussed vertigo only as an incidental observation. Also, true vertigo has not been specifically differentiated from other vague symptoms of balance disturbance, nor has adequate evaluation been done to differentiate end organ from central vestibular dysfunction. Possible causes which have been suggested for vertigo in divers include decompression sickness, hypoxia, hypercarbia, nitrogen narcosis, seasickness, alcoholic hangover, sensory deprivation, hyperventilation, impure breathing gas, unequal caloric stimulation, and difficulties with middle ear pressure equilibration. One can readily appreciate that these causes can encompass a wide range of varying pathological mechanisms. In order to better understand the mechanisms which can cause vertiginous problems in divers, this problem will be reviewed by separating those causes of transient vertigo from those situations in which permanent otologic damage has been seen. Similar pathophysiologic mechanisms are probably occurring in some of the transient and permanent cases, with the permanent forms of injury representing more severe changes than occur in the transient cases.

Edmonds (1973) has undertaken a detailed review of the various causes of vertigo in diving. His classification of this problem is basically broken down into those causes due to unequal vestibular stimulation, including caloric stimulations; barotrauma causes; decompression sickness; and those causes due to unequal vestibular responses to equal stimuli. This last classification covers subjects who, when exposed to conditions in which multiple vestibular stimuli were encountered, would develop vertigo as a result of one vestibular apparatus being relatively more sensitive than the other. Such individuals might have vertigo with caloric stimulation resulting from equal amounts of cold water entering the external ear canal. This would be particularly noted when the diver is swimming in a position in which the lateral semicircular canal is vertical in orientation. Edmonds further includes in this classification vertigo resulting from a unilateral hypofunctioning vestibular end organ in situations in which equal and symmetrical pressure changes occur in the middle ear cavities during ascent and descent. Also included are cases of vertigo or dizziness seen in nitrogen narcosis, although there is some doubt as to whether this dizziness includes vertigo and vestibular dysfunction. The vertigo, nausea, and tremor which is seen in the high pressure nervous syndrome, the vertigo seen during oxygen toxicity in association with other neurological dysfunctions, the disorientation seen during carbon dioxide toxicity which has not been verified as true vertigo by electronystagmography (Blackwood & Edmonds 1971), and sensory deprivation—all are included in the possible causes of vestibular dysfunction secondary to unequal vestibular responses.

A modification of Edmonds' classification is offered which separates the diving situations causing vertigo into those which have been described as causing true vestibular dysfunction of a transient nature and those which have been noted as causing permanent otologic injury. As noted above, it is quite possible and likely in some instances that the pathophysiological mechanisms involved are similar in both cases, with the mechanisms causing the permanent injury being more severe forms of those involved in transient changes.

Transient vertigo due to caloric stimulation

During most diving conditions, vestibular end organs are stimulated equally and vertigo does not occur except in those few individuals who, due to previous disease or injury, congenital defects or anatomical variations, have asymmetrical end organ sensitivities and will develop vertigo even though the stimuli are equal bilaterally. In certain situations, unequal stimulation with subsequent vertigo occurs, especially when there are preexisting pathological changes. Unequal entry of cold water in the external auditory canals, secondary to obstruction of one canal by cerumen, otitis externa, ear plugs etc., can produce a caloric response, particularly when the diver is oriented in a position in which the lateral semicircular canal is in a vertical plane. Tympanic membrane perforation, such as seen with trauma during descent or pre-existing middle ear disease, can result in unequal stimulation of one semicircular canal by the entry of cold water into the middle ear.

Transient vertigo resulting from unequal middle ear pressure equilibration

Transient vestibular dysfunction secondary to asymmetrical middle ear pressure equilibration has been described during descent and ascent by Lundgren (1965) who coined the term 'alternobaric vertigo', by Vorosmarti and Bradley (1970) and by Terry and Dennison (1966). Lundgren (1965) has attributed such vertigo to increased middle ear pressure on one side with resulting unequal vestibular end organ stimulation because such occurrences more frequently occur during ascent. Indeed, it has been noted that some individuals who have experienced 'alternobaric vertigo' can produce vertigo and vestibular nystagmus by performing the Valsalva manoeuver and unequally inflating the middle ears at 1 ATA. Many of these individuals have encountered difficulty with pressure equalization of the middle ear, usually unilaterally. Disappearance of the vertigo has been associated with stopping the ascent or descending again, or has followed a sudden hissing of air into one ear. Further work by Lundgren and by Tjernström (1973), using a special technique for measuring middle ear pressures during conditions of changing ambient pressure with simultaneous electronystagmographic recordings, has shown true vestibular nystagmus during conditions of asymmetrical equilibration of middle ear pressures during ascents from shallow depths.

Transient vertigo associated with the high pressure nervous syndrome

Transient symptoms of vestibular dysfunction, vertigo, tinnitus and nausea have been mentioned in association with the high pressure nervous syndrome (Bühlmann et al. 1970; Bennett & Towse 1971). Whether these symptoms represent disorders in the vestibular end organ or the primary vestibular neuron or locations central to these structures requires further investigation. A preliminary report on divers who exhibited the classical manifestations of the high pressure nervous syndrome during a 1600 ft (49·5 ATA) helium–oxygen dive in the spring of 1973 indicated that these symptoms were not accompanied by any demonstrable electronystagmographic abnormalities during positional testing, cold caloric testing and pendulum tracking. Further investigations of possible vestibular dysfunction during the high pressure nervous syndrome are needed.

PERMANENT OTOLOGIC INJURY IN DIVING

In recent years, reports of permanent cochlea and/or vestibular injury in multiple phases of diving have occurred with increased frequency. Analysis of these reports indicates that these permanent otological injuries should be classified as follows:

1. Injuries occurring during descent or compression.

2. Injuries occurring at stable deep depths.

3. Injuries occurring during ascent or decompression.

4. Injuries related to high background noise during diving conditions.

Injuries occurring during descent or compression

Freeman and Edmonds (1972) have described a series of five cases of cochlear damage occurring after shallow air dives. In each case there was associated difficulty with ear clearing during descent. Two cases also had vertigo. The depth and duration of these dives makes decompression sickness very unlikely. Each case is well documented with timely pre- and post-dive audiograms which demonstrate significant neurosensory hearing losses. The authors postulate that the sudden outward movement of the stapes, which occurs when the middle ear is suddenly cleared, damages the cochlea. They strongly advised that dives be abandoned whenever divers cannot easily clear their ears at shallow depths shortly after beginning of descent. Goodhill (1972) has suggested that, with a forcible Valsalva manoeuver, intracochlear pressure arises significantly either by the transmission of the accompanying increased cerebrospinal fluid pressures through a patent cochlear aqueduct or by the transmission by the round or oval windows of the sudden increase in middle ear pressure seen with sudden ear clearing. These two mechanisms singly or in combination could lead to cochlear membrane dysfunction or rupture of the annular ligament or round window membrane. Goodhill advised managing such cases with bed rest and head elevation and, if there was no hearing improvement in 48 hours, he advised an exploratory tympanotomy for closure of a possible perilymph fistula.

Later investigations by Edmonds, Freeman and Tonkin (1974) have actually demonstrated ruptured round windows in divers who developed cochlear and/or vestibular symptoms during a shallow no-decompression dive in which there were difficulties with middle ear clearing during compression. Subsequent surgery to repair these round window fistulae has resulted in improvement of hearing and/or disappearance of the vestibular dysfunction. It is possible that alternobaric vertigo during ascent represents a similar but less intense type of physiological mechanism as that postulated to explain the permanent damage associated with inner ear barotrauma. The fact that a high percentage of divers who have experienced alternobaric vertigo during ascent can reproduce these transient symptoms and vestibular nystagmus during a Valsalva manoeuver performed at 1 ATA supports this hypothesis.

Otologic problems occurring at stable deep depths

Inner ear problems occurring during deep diving which begin while at a stable and unchanging depth have been described by Sundmaker (1974) and Lambertsen (1975). These investigators describe three divers, each of whom sustained a unilateral loss of labyrinthine function while at a stable deep depth. These divers experienced the sudden onset of vertigo, nausea, and nystagmus in association with the breathing by mask of a mixture which included nitrogen or neon, while they remained in a helium atmosphere. The respired partial pressure of helium was therefore decreased and replaced by the second inert gas while the total pressure remained the same. Oxygen partial pressure was not changed and remained at a safe level. No auditory symptoms were noted and there were no problems with ear clearing during compression. Extensive follow-up evaluation after the dive revealed a total unilateral loss of labyrinthine function in one subject, a partial unilateral loss in another subject, and a recovery of function after an initial partial unilateral loss in the third subject. No losses of auditory function were noted and no evidence of central nervous system lesions were found.

As to the etiology of these injuries, two theories are postulated, both of which take into account the onset of symptoms shortly after the initiation of breathing a mixture in which helium is partially replaced by another inert gas. The first theory postulates that with the sudden addition of a second inert gas at a deep depth, the rate of increase in the concentration of the dissolved second gas in the perilymph and endolymph is significantly different because of the difference in blood supply to these areas. In this case, endolymph concentration would rise at a faster rate than the concentration in the perilymph. This would lead to a significant difference in osmotic pressure between these two spaces with the subsequent flux of water into the endolymphatic space resulting in disturbed function and injury. The second theory involves the counter-diffusion principle. When divers change from one breathing mixture to another, the diffusion of the new inert gas into those body tissues or spaces with the reverse diffusion of the previous inert gas which saturated the body tissues and fluids results in bubbles at various body interfaces such as the interfaces in the inner ear between the perilymph and endolymph. This bubble formation produces displacement and/or disruption of inner ear structures with subsequent disturbed function and injury. Such bubble formation resulting from the counter-diffusion of two inert gases would occur without changes in total ambient pressure. An analogous clinical situation, felt to involve this counter-diffusion principle, has been described by Blenkarn et al. (1971) who noted skin eruptions following the sequential breathing of various inert gases at constant ambient pressure of 7 ATA. This bullous eruption was considered to be the result of the formation of gas bubbles in the deeper layers of the skin.

The understanding of the mechanisms of inner ear injuries occurring during stable deep depths in association with changes in inert gas content will obviously require further investigation, If either of these two theories is correct, such injuries should be alleviated by avoiding changes in the inert gas content at deep depths.

Otologic injuries occurring during ascent or decompression

Classical descriptions of decompression sickness have mentioned otologic manifestations only in association with massive central nervous system decompression sickness where the inner ear symptoms were of secondary importance and, in many cases, were probably related to centrally located lesions. Otologic symptoms have not been felt to occur during decompression without other manifestations of decompression sickness. Such symptoms have usually been ignored. With more frequent exposures to deeper depths, reports of vertigo and hearing loss during and following decompression without other signs of decompression sickness have become more frequent. Bühlmann and Waldvogel (1967), reporting on 82 decompression accidents in a series of 211 dives, noted that the only neurological symptoms in the entire series consisted of vertigo, nausea, vomiting, and tinnitus in 11 cases. Hearing losses were noted in two of these cases. These symptoms appeared only with decompressions from the deepest dives, depths of 485 and 726 ft (15·7 and 23 ATA). Gehring and Bühlmann (1975) more recently have described 12 cases of inner ear symptoms consisting of vertigo, nausea and vomiting after 24 decompressions from depths ranging from 5·2 to 31 ATA. In four cases there were associated hearing loss and tinnitus. With dives using longer decompression schedules, such inner ear symptoms have not been noted.

Farmer and Thomas (1973) reported on 20 cases of vertigo and/or hearing loss during decompression. Ten of these cases had been previously reported by Rubenstein and Summitt (1971). In none of the cases did a diver have difficulty clearing his ears during compression and no cases were included in which there were ear symptoms while at the maximum depth or in which there were uncontrolled or rapid emergency ascents suggesting air emboli. Further, in none of these cases were there other neurological symptoms which might suggest a more extensive central nervous system involvement. The other associated symptoms included mild headache, skin rash, back pain, and knee pain in four of the 20 cases.

Eight of the cases presented with only vestibular symptoms occurring during or shortly after decompression. Six cases presented with hearing loss without vestibular symptoms either during or shortly after decompression. Six cases were noted in which there were both hearing loss and vestibular symptoms during decompression. Two of the six cases showing only hearing symptoms underwent prompt recompression treatment and demonstrated good recovery. The other four cases, which either were not recompressed or in which there was a significant delay in recompression treatment, demonstrated residual sensorineural hearing losses. In one case there was bilateral loss; all the other losses were unilateral. The six cases showing both hearing and vestibular symptoms were all recompressed without significant delay and all showed good recovery. In the eight cases showing only vestibular symptoms, relief was seen promptly in those three cases which were recompressed within 1 hour after the onset of symptoms. Thus in these 20 cases, there is a significant correlation between prompt recompression treatment, relief of symptoms, and lack of residual deficit. This, plus the fact that in each case symptoms began either during or shortly after decompression, suggests that these injuries are a form of decompression sickness and are related to bubble formation either in the perilymph or endolymph or in the internal auditory system. Otic barotrauma is an unlikely contributing factor in that no divers noted difficulties with ear clearing during compression. In trying to implicate other possible mechanisms of injury such as hemorrhage into the inner ear or vascular spasm or thrombosis, one would not expect to obtain relief with recompression.

Further investigations are needed to develop a

better understanding of these decompression events. Until new knowledge is obtained, isolated cochlear and/or vestibular symptoms appearing during or shortly after decompression should be considered forms of decompression sickness and should be recompressed promptly.

Otologic injuries related to high background noise during diving conditions

Numerous authors have reported sensorineural hearing losses in diving population (Coles & Knight 1961; Shilling & Everly 1942; Taylor 1959; Soss 1971; Haines & Harris 1946). Coles and Knight (1961), in a survey of Royal Navy divers, concluded that the high frequency neurosensory deafness in the usual diving population could be explained on the basis of previous non-diving exposures to loud noise, particularly that of gunfire. A selected subgroup of divers with no history of previous excessive noise exposure had thresholds which were similar to the normal British population when allowance was made for age. Italian investigators (Zannini, Odaglia & Giorgio 1975) recently reported that professional divers demonstrated much higher instances of high frequency hearing losses than the population as a whole. They did not attribute this to excessive noise exposure, but postulated instead that these losses were secondary to 'reflex vasomotor problems'. However, studies by Summitt and Reimers (1971) and Murray (1970) have demonstrated excessive noise levels in various diving conditions including pressure chambers and diving helmets. Noise levels inside diving helmets occasionally reach 113 DBA and in pressure chambers may reach 120 DBA during ventilation. When these levels are considered in relation to the acceptable damage risk criteria curves (Eldrige & Miller 1969), the allowable exposure times may be as short as 15 or 20 min before running the risk of permanent noise-induced hearing loss. Whether the previously noted reversible conductive hearing losses (Fluur & Adolfson 1966; Farmer, Thomas & Preslar 1971; Thomas, Preslar & Farmer 1974) from compressed gas environments is of sufficient magnitude to provide protective attenuation from excessive noise conditions encountered in diving is not known. In the study by Summitt and Reimers (1971), significant temporary threshold shifts were seen following a 190-ft (6·7 ATA) 64-min air dive and a 60-ft (2·8 ATA) 53-min air dive. These threshold shifts reverted back to pre-dive levels within 24 to 48 hours post-dive. In this situation, the temporary conduction hearing losses previously described apparently did not provide sufficient attenuation to protect the divers from the ambient noise of these dives. Whether or not the different degrees of conductive losses seen at deeper depths and under other diving conditions may serve to protect the diver from excessive noise, in a manner similar to ear plugs or ear muffs, requires further investigation.

In summary, permanent cochlear and/or vestibular damage can occur during all phases of diving, during compression, at stable deep depths, and during decompression. The exact pathophysiology of permanent inner ear injury during diving is not definitely established. The following mechanisms are suspected:

1. Permanent inner ear injury during compression seems to be related to difficulties with middle ear pressure equalization.

2. Permanent inner ear damage at stable deep depths seems to be related to changes in inspired inert gas composition.

3. Permanent cochlear and vestibular damage occurring during decompression seems to be a form of decompression sickness and can be the only manifestation of this problem.

4. Excessive background noise seems to be not uncommon during various diving conditions and can possibly contribute to cochlear damage and subsequent permanent neurosensory hearing losses.

SUMMARY OF OTOLOGIC FUNCTIONS IN DIVING

Since the peripheral auditory system is primarily a pressure transducer and has evolved as an impedance-matching mechanism between air and water, it is not surprising that serious problems are encountered in diving. The most frequent problem is associated with difficulties with middle ear pressure equalization. The subsequent creation of a pressure differential between the middle ear and the ambient environment can lead to transient cochlear and/or vestibular dysfunction or to more serious permanent problems related to the inner ear damage. During diving in which there is no apparent difficulty with middle ear pressure equalization, divers develop a reversible conductive hearing loss which is related to depth and gas mixture. This loss is apparently secondary to changes in gas density, resonance shift, and subsequent impedance mismatches between the surrounding environment and the inner ear.

The unique anatomical relationships of the inner ear, with delicate tissue spaces surrounded by bone, filled with fluid and supplied by an end artery system, makes this organ susceptible to various alterations during multiple phases of diving. Such alterations can lead to transient cochlear and/or vestibular dysfunction or permanent injury. It can include such pathological changes as rupture of the round window membrane, as seen during compression; the formation of gas bubbles in the intracochlear spaces as postulated to explain those injuries occurring at stable deep depths but associated with changes in inert gas composition; the formation of intravascular gas or platelet emboli in the arteriole supply or venous drainage or gas bubbles in the intracochlear fluid spaces during decompression; or possible hair cell damage secondary to excessive noise exposure. Possible direct alterations in the inner ear resulting from high inert gas concentrations might inhibit active or passive ion transport or result in fluid electrolyte changes. More detailed answers to these questions require further investigations of otologic functions under various diving conditions.

REFERENCES

ALMOUR, R. (1942) Industrial otology in caisson workers. *N.Y. St. J. Med.* **42**, 779–785.

ARMSTRONG, H. G. & HEIM, J. W. (1937) The effect of flight on the middle ear. *J. Am. med. Ass.* **109**, 417–421.

AXELSSON, A. (1968) The vascular anatomy of the cochlear in the guinea pig and in man. *Acta Oto-lar.* Suppl., 243.

BAYLISS, G. J. A. (1968) Aural barotrauma in naval divers. *Archs Otolar.* **88**, 49–55.

BEHNKE, A. R. (1945) Physiologic effect of pressure changes with reference to otolaryngology. *Archs Otolar.* **42**, 110–116.

BEKESY, G. V. (1960) *Experiments In Hearing.* New York: McGraw-Hill.

BEKESY, G. V. & ROSENBLITH, W. A. (1951) The mechanical properties of the ear. In *Handbook of Experimental Psychology.* Ed. S. S. Stevens. New York: John Wiley.

BENNETT, G. S. (1962) Remarks on the paper by Montague and Strickland. *J. acoust. Soc. Am.* **34**, 347.

BENNETT, P. B. (1964) The effects of high pressures of inert gases on auditory evoked potentials in cat cortex and reticular formation. *Electroenceph. clin. Neurophysiol.* **17**, 388–397.

BENNETT, P. B. (1975) Pharmacological effects of inert gases. In *Proc. 5th Symp. Underwater Physiology.* Ed. C. J. Lambertsen. Washington: (In press.)

BENNETT, P. B. & GLASS, A. (1961) Electroencephalographic and other changes induced by high partial pressures of nitrogen. *Electroenceph. clin. Neurophysiol.* **13**, 91–98.

BENNETT, P. B. & TOWSE, E. J. (1971) Performance efficiency of men breathing oxygen–helium at depths between 100 feet and 1500 feet. *Aerospace Med.* **42**, 147–156.

BENNETT, P. B., ACKLES, K. N. & CRIPPS, V. J. (1969) Effects of hyperbaric nitrogen and oxygen on auditory evoked responses in man. *Aerospace Med.* **40**, 521–525.

BEVAN, J. (1971) The human auditory evoked response and contigent negative variation in hyperbaric air. *Electroenceph. clin. Neurophysiol.* **30**, 198–204.

BLACKWOOD, F. & EDMONDS, C. (1971) *Otological Investigations in Diving.* Royal Australian Navy School of Underwater Medicine Project Report 2/71.

BLENKARN, G. D., AQUADRO, C., HILLS, B. A. & SALTZMAN, H. A. (1971) Urticaria following the sequential breathing of various inert gases at a constant pressure of 7 ATA; A possible manifestation of gas-induced osmosis. *Aerospace Med.* **42**, 141–146.

BOOT, G. W. (1913) Caisson workers' deafness. *Ann. Otol. Rhinol. Lar.* **22**, 1121–1132.

BRANDT, J. F. & HOLLIEN, H. (1967) Underwater hearing thresholds in man. *J. acoust. Soc. Am.* **42**, 966–971.

BRANDT, J. F. & HOLLIEN, H. (1969) Underwater hearing thresholds in man as a function of water depth. *J. acoust. Soc. Am.* **46**, 893–897.

BÜHLMANN, A. A. & WALDVOGEL, W. (1967) The treatment of decompression sickness. *Helv. med. Acta* **33**, 487–491.

BÜHLMANN, A. A., MATTHYS, H., OVERRATH, H. G., BENNETT, P. B., ELLIOTT, D. H. & GRAY, S. P. (1970) Saturation exposures at 31 ATA in a helium–oxygen atmosphere with excursions to 36 ATA. *Aerospace Med.* **41**, 394–402.

COLES, R. A. A. & KNIGHT, J. J. (1961) *Aural and Audiometric Survey of Qualified Divers and Submarine Escape Training Instructors.* Med. Res. Council (UK) Report RNPL 61/1011.

DAVIS, H. & SILVERMAN, S. R. (Eds) (1970) *Hearing and Deafness.* New York: Rhinehart & Winston.

DONALDSON, J. A. & MILLER, J. M. (1973) Anatomy of the ear. In *Otolaryngology, Vol. I, Basic Sciences and Related Disciplines.* Ed. M. M. Paparella & D. A. Shumrick. pp. 75–109. Philadelphia: Saunders.

EDMONDS, C. (1973) Vertigo in diving. In *The Use of Nystagmography in Aviation Medicine; AGARD Conference Proceedings* No. 128. Ed. F. E. Guedry. Naval Aerospace Medical Research Institute, Pensacola.

EDMONDS, C., FREEMAN, P., THOMAS, R., TONKIN, J. & BLACKWOOD, F. A. (1973) *Otological Aspects of Diving*. Sidney: Australian Medical Publishing Co.

EDMONDS, C., FREEMAN, P. & TONKIN, J. (1974) Fistula of the round window in diving. *Trans. Am. Acad. Ophth. Otol.*, 78, 444–447.

ELDRIDGE, D. H. & MILLER, J. D. (1969) Acceptable noise exposures—damage risk criteria. In *Noise As a Public Health Hazard*. Ed. W. D. Ward & J. E. Fricke. pp. 110–120 ASHA Rep. 4.

ENGSTROM, H., ADES, H. W. & ANDERSON, A. (1966) *Structural Pattern of the Organ of Corti*. Stockholm: Almqvist & Wiksells.

FARMER, J. C. & THOMAS, W. G. (1973) Vestibular injury during diving. *Försvarsmedecin* 9, 396–403.

FARMER, J. C., THOMAS, W. G. & PRESLAR, M. J. (1971) Human auditory responses during hyperbaric helium–oxygen exposures. *Surg. Forum* 22, 456–458.

FIELDS, F. A. (1958) Skin diving: its physiological and otolaryngological aspects. *Archs Otolar.* 68, 531–541.

FLUUR, E. & ADOLFSON, J. (1966) Hearing in hyperbaric air. *Aerospace Med.* 37, 783–785.

FREEMAN, P. & EDMONDS, C. (1972) Inner Ear Barotrauma. *Archs Otolar.* 95, 556–563.

GEHRING, H. & BÜHLMANN, A. A. (1975) So-called vertigo bends after oxygen–helium dives. In *Proc. 5th Symp. Underwater Physiology*. Ed. C. J. Lambertsen. Washington. (In press.)

GOODHILL, V. (1972) Letter to the editor: Inner ear barotrauma. *Archs Otolar.* 95, 588.

HAINES, H. L. & HARRIS, J. D. (1946) Aerotitis media in submariners. *Ann. Otol. Rhinol. Lar.* 55, 347–371.

HAMILTON, P. M. (1957) Underwater hearing thresholds. *J. acoust. Soc. Am.* 29, 792–794.

HELLER, M. F. (1960) Skin diving injury. *Archs Otolar.* 72, 358–360.

HOLLIEN, H. & BRANDT, J. F. (1969) Effects of air bubbles in the external auditory meatus on underwater hearing thresholds. *J. acoust. Soc. Am.* 46, 384–387.

JERGER, J. & TILLMAN, T. (1960). *A New Method for the Clinical Determination of Sensorineural Acuity Level*. Technical Documentary Report 60–31, USAF Aerospace Medical Center, Brooks Air Force Base, Texas.

KELLER, A. P. (1958) A study of the relationship of air pressures to myringo-rupture. *Laryngoscope, St Louis* 68, 2015–2029.

KENNEDY, R. S. (1972) *A Bibliography of the Role of the Vestibular Apparatus under Water and Pressure: Content-oriented and Annotated*. US Naval Med. Res. Inst. M4306.03. 5000 BAK9. Report No. 1.

KENNEDY, R. S. (1973) *The Role of the Vestibular Apparatus under Water and High Pressure*. US Naval Med. Res. Inst. M4306.03.5000BAK9. Report No. 3.

LAMBERTSEN, C. J. (1975) Collaborative investigation of limits of human tolerance to pressurization with helium, neon and nitrogen. Simulation of density equivalent to helium–oxygen respiration at depths to 2000, 3000, 4000 and 5000 feet of sea water. In *Proc. 5th Symp. Underwater Physiology*. Ed. C. J. Lambertsen. Washington. (In press.)

LESTER, J. C. & GOMEZ, V. (1898) Observations made in the caisson of the new East River bridge as to the effects of compressed air upon the human ear. *Archs Otolar.* 27, 1–19.

LUNDGREN, C. E. G. (1965) Alternobaric vertigo—a diving hazard. *Br. med. J.* 2, 511–513.

MACFIE, W. C. D. D. (1964) E.N.T. problems of diving. *Med. Servs J. Can.* 20, 845–861.

MCCABE, B. F. (1973) Vestibular physiology: its clinical application in understanding the dizzy patient. In *Otolaryngology Vol. 1, Basic Sciences and Related Disciplines*. Ed. M. M. Paparella & D. A. Schumrick. pp. 318–328. Philadelphia: Saunders.

MCCORMICK, J. G., HIGGINS, T. L., CLAYTON, R. M. & BRAUER, R. W. (1972a) Auditory and vestibular effects of helium–oxygen hyperbaric chamber dives to convulsion depths. *J. acoust. Soc. Am.* 51, 103.

MCCORMICK, J. G., HIGGINS, T. L. DAUGHERTY, H. S. & JOHNSON, P. E. (1972b) Cochlear dysfunction associated with decompression from 300 feet hyperbaric chamber dives. *J. acoust. Soc. Am.* 51, 103.

MILLER, H. E. (1971) Cochlear potentials at 11 atmospheres. *Laryngoscope* 81, 979–988.

MONTAGUE, W. E. & STRICKLAND, J. F. (1961) Sensitivity of the water-immersed ear to high and low level tones. *J. acoust. Soc. Am.* 33, 1376–1381.

MURRAY, T. (1970) *Noise Levels inside Navy Diving Chambers during Compression and Decompression*. US Navy Submarine Med. Center Report No. 643.

PALMGREN, R. (1960) Work under compression and in noisy environments. An otorhinolaryngologic investigation of construction workers building the Stockholm underground railway from 1953 to 1957. *Acta Oto-lar.* 51, 165–174.

ROGER, A., CABARROU, P. & GASTAUT, H. (1955) EEG changes in humans due to changes of surrounding atmospheric pressure. *Electroenceph. clin. Neurophysiol.* 7, 152.

RUBENSTEIN, C. J. & SUMMITT, J. K. (1971) Vestibular derangement in decompression. In *Proc. 4th Symp. Underwater Physiology*. Ed. C. J. Lambertsen. pp. 287–292. New York and London: Academic Press.

SHILLING, C. W. & EVERLEY, I. A. (1942) Auditory acuity in submarine personnel. *Nav. med. Bull.* 40, 664–686.

SIMMONS, F. BLAIR (1968) Theory of membrane breaks in sudden hearing loss. *Archs Otolar.* 88, 41–48.

SIVIAN, L. J. (1943) *On Hearing in Water vs. Hearing in Air, with some Experimental Evidence*. Report No. 6.1-NDRC-838. Office of Scientific Research and Development, National Defense Research Committee, Division 6, Section 6.1.

SOSS, S. L. (1971) Sensorineural hearing loss with diving. *Archs Otolar.* 93, 501–504.

STUCKER, F. J. & ECHOLS, W. B. (1971) Otolarygic problems of underwater exploration. *Milit. Med.* 136, 896–899.

SUMMITT, J. K. & REIMERS, J. D. (1971) Noise: a hazard to divers and hyperbaric chamber personnel. *Aerospace Med.* 42, 1173–1177.

SUNDMAKER, W. K. H. (1974) Vestibular function. *Special Summary Program—Predictive Studies III*. Univ. Pennsylvania. (In press.)

TAYLOR, G. D. (1959) The otolaryngologic aspects of skin and scuba diving. *Laryngoscope* 69, 809–859.

TERRY, L. & DENNISON, W. L. (1966) *Vertigo amongst Divers*. US Navy Submarine Med. Center Special Report, No. 66–2.

THOMAS, W. G., PRAZMA, T. & FARMER, J. C. (1973) Unpublished data.

THOMAS, W. G., PRESLAR, M. J. & FARMER, J. C. (1972) Calibration of condensor microphones under increased atmospheric pressures. *J. acoust Soc. Am.* **51**, 6–14.

THOMAS, W. G., PRESLAR, M. J. & FARMER, J. C. (1975) Calibration of earphones under increased atmospheric pressures. *J. acoust. Soc. Am.* (In press.)

THOMAS, W. G., SUMMITT, J. & FARMER, J. C. (1974) Human auditory thresholds during deep, saturation helium–oxygen dives. *J. acoust. Soc. Am.* **55**, 810–813.

TJERNSTRÖM, O. (1973) On alternobaric vertigo-experimental studies. *Försvarsmedecin* **9**, 410–415.

VAIL, H. H. (1929) Traumatic conditions of the ear in workers in an atmosphere of compressed air. *Archs Otolar.* **10**, 113–126.

VOROSMARTI, J. & BRADLEY, J. J. (1970) Alternobaric vertigo in military divers. *Milit. Med.* **135**, 182–185.

WAINWRIGHT, W. N. (1958) Comparison of hearing thresholds in air and in water. *J. acoust. Soc. Am.* **30**, 1025–1029.

WATERMAN, D. & SMITH, P. F. (1970) *An Investigation of the Effects of a Helium–oxygen Breathing Mixture on Hearing in Naval Personnel.* US Navy Submarine Med. Center, Mem. Rep. 70–7.

ZANNINI, D., ODAGLIA, G. & GIORGIO, S. (1975) Audiographic changes in professional divers. In *Proc. 5th Symp. Underwater Physiology.* Ed. C. J. Lambertsen. Washington. (In press.)

29

Diving Accidents

R. DE G. HANSON AND J. M. YOUNG

An accident may be regarded as an event which occurs by chance or which arises from an unknown cause but it is unfortunately true that more often it occurs through carelessness or ignorance. Some of the factors which commonly contribute to accidents underwater have been described previously (Miles 1962; Berghage 1966; Elliott 1966; Bayliss 1968) and it is the purpose of this review to summarize these various factors and their interactions. An increased awareness on the part of medical practitioners and divers to these dangers will, it is hoped, lead to better prevention of diving accidents. The principles of accident investigation are also included since it is important that the lessons which can be learned should be discovered and then adequately reported, leading, if possible, to improved diving safety. Though the various decompression disorders may be regarded as diving accidents they usually do not begin until after leaving the water and, since they are dealt with in detail elsewhere, they have not been further discussed in this chapter.

PRE-DIVE SAFETY PRECAUTIONS

Dive planning

The planning of a dive does not usually concern a doctor or physiologist directly. As discussed earlier, careful training and planning will remove many of the possible causes of accidents. Items which need to be considered in dive planning include: the experience and self-reliance of each diver; the equipment of the divers relative to their task; the diving area and its known hazards such as currents and underwater obstructions; the state of the weather; water temperature; visibility both above and below the surface; the boat or diving platform and the need for competent seamanship; the adequate provision of stand-by divers; the whereabouts of the nearest emergency treatment centre together with the mode of transport for casualties; the need to inform other authorities of the intention to dive; the necessity of keeping a diving log with a record of the exact time of entering and leaving the water and the depth–time profile of each dive.

Fitness to dive

The diver should be within 12 months of a medical examination undertaken specifically for fitness to dive. A candidate for professional diving training should be accepted only if he is fully fit for arduous physical work and fulfils certain behavioural standards. These are not easy to define and are best summarized by analogy: if you were to be in a life-threatening situation, is he a person to whom you would entrust your life?

The medical examination will *exclude* any candidate for initial diving training who is over 40 years of age or who has one of the following conditions:

A history of pneumothorax, a recent history of exposure to tuberculosis, emphysema, asthma or, indeed, any past or present chronic lung condition that might lead to alveolar air trapping.

Any chronic catarrh or recurrent sinus infection, perforated or immobile ear drums, chronic otitis media or recurrent otitis externa which does not respond to treatment.

Dental neglect.

Any chronic infective skin condition.

A history of epilepsy, cranial surgery, any neurological residua from head injury or any disease of the central nervous system.

Any psychiatric condition.

A systolic blood pressure greater than 140 mm Hg, a diastolic blood pressure greater than 90 mm Hg or any heart disease.

Excessive obesity.

Any renal, gastro-intestinal or endocrine disorder or any other detectable disease that, in a diving situation, might render him a potential danger to himself and thus to others.

The successful candidate will have a normal chest X-ray and will pass an exercise tolerance test such as stepping up on to a chair 5 times in 15 seconds after which the pulse should return to normal within 45 seconds. There are a number of supplementary investigations that may be requested. With the arm hanging in a relaxed position, the skin-fold thickness in the mid-triceps area should be less than 15 mm. An ECG may be required and may be combined with the stress of an exercise tolerance test. An audiogram and an EEG are required of some categories of divers not only to exclude current illness but also to be used as a base-line against which any future injury may be compared. Bone radiology should follow the recommendations laid down in Chapter 27. Any juxta-articular lesion of dysbaric osteonecrosis should contraindicate further diving. A successful test exposure to oxygen at some 3 bar is not regarded as evidence of tolerance to the toxic effects of oxygen because an individual's threshold for oxygen toxicity can vary considerably from one day to the next (Donald 1947).

Each year the trained diver should be re-examined to these standards and any deviation, especially if he continues to be employed over the age of 40 years, should disqualify him from further work underwater.

Fitness to dive on a particular day is usually decided by the diver himself on the basis of subjective feelings. A severe hangover can predispose to vomiting underwater or to subsequent decompression sickness. An upper respiratory tract in-fection can lead to aural barotrauma, vertigo and disorientation. A lower respiratory tract infection can lead to mucus causing alveolar air trapping. Any injury, including that to a nerve root by a prolapsed intervertebral disc, can lead to the localized formation of bubbles.

Any condition which keeps the diver off diving for a couple of days or longer should lead to a review of diving fitness by a doctor. The diver should also be re-examined after any diving accident or any manifestation of a decompression disorder before he may, after a suitable interval, resume diving.

USE OF PARTICULAR APPARATUS

Breath-hold diving

Breath-hold diving is the commonest form of diving among untrained persons and can lead to a number of the many accidents which can result from going underwater. The change of pressure with depth is greatest when near the surface so the breath-hold diver may suffer otitic and sinus barotrauma. The risk of hypothermia is greatest when no protective garments are worn and this is frequently so with snorkel divers. It has been shown that it is even possible for the body to absorb sufficient nitrogen during multiple breath-hold dives to develop decompression sickness (Paulev 1969). Because breath-hold diving appears to be so simple, the lack of dive planning is common and the 'thrill of the chase', especially in spear fishing, is a common cause of overexertion. Careless divers may then find themselves far from their original point of entry into the water and faced with a long return swim when already tired.

Equipment. The basic equipment for breath-hold diving, namely fins, mask and snorkel, can themselves be contributing factors in an accident. Fins should be carefully chosen as overlarge fins will hamper swimming and they should be firmly attached, as the loss of one will also hamper effective swimming.

The air space within the face mask will initially be at atmospheric pressure and will be subjected to increased hydrostatic pressure during the dive. The mask will tend to collapse on to the face to decrease contained volume and equalize the hydrostatic and air pressures. Some masks are fitted with collapsible bags of compensating air but most are not. A mask which has reached the limit of its compressibility will have a lower pressure within it than that of the surrounding water. This may be prevented by breathing out sufficient air through the nose into the mask to equalize the pressure, but this procedure requires some training. The consequence of a 'squeeze' of the face into the mask is usually subconjunctival oedema and possibly haemorrhage. Fortunately this normally requires no treatment except reassurance that the swelling will decrease within hours and that the haemorrhages will be reabsorbed in due course.

The design of the snorkel tube is critical in the prevention of accidents and a simple, single-bend or 'J'-tube is strongly recommended. The length of the tube should be sufficient for it to just clear the water when the diver is in a normal swimming position on the surface. It should be gently curving and the bore of the tube should be about $\frac{3}{4}$ inch (18 mm) internal diameter. This design is a compromise between the need to minimize both the external resistance to respiration and the respiratory dead space. Too narrow a tube will cause respiratory embarrassment through increased resistance but too wide a tube will increase respiratory dead space to an unacceptable degree. Any snorkel tube must cause some increase in expired ventilation to maintain adequate alveolar ventilation and it is common for an increase in alveolar P_{CO_2} to be present. Thus there is some limitation of exercise capability of which the diver should be aware.

Some snorkel tubes have an additional device to prevent the entry of water while diving, but any such device must increase the respiratory resistance and has the added risk of failure with an unexpected flooding of the mouth with water. Such flooding could cause glottal spasm and it is much safer if the diver is trained to expect the 'J'-tube to fill with water on each dive. To blow out that water on surfacing is both simple and safe. Unfortunately, the snorkel tube with a valve device usually costs more than the simple 'J'-tube and hence may be bought by the uninitiated on the assumption that the more expensive snorkel must be better.

Buoyancy. The density of the average unclothed human body is very little different from that of water and most people are just positively buoyant at the surface when their lungs are in the normal end-respiratory position. There are a few, however, who are negatively buoyant even at maximum inspiration in seawater.

Not everybody realizes that their net specific gravity will vary with the volume of air contained in their lungs and thus their buoyancy will decrease by about 2 kg between maximum inspiration and maximum expiration. It is important that a breath-hold diver appreciates that descent will compress his thoracic cavity in accordance with Boyle's Law and he will become increasingly negatively buoyant. Thus to return to the surface from below some 5 m (1·5 ATA) may require a positive upwards swimming action.

The first action on returning to surface after a breath-hold dive, either with or without a snorkel, is to exhale. This immediately reduces buoyancy and, if the diver is not careful, it could result in the inhalation of water. Shouting for help can have the same effect.

Hyperventilation. The breath-hold breaking point was defined by Mithoefer (1965) as the termination of breath-holding in response to the development of a net ventilatory stimulus too strong to be further resisted by voluntary effort, and this has been extensively studied by Lanphier and Rahn (1963a, b), Mithoefer (1965) and Craig and Harley (1968). Physiologically, it is correct to state that hyperventilation before a breath-hold dive will reduce alveolar P_{CO_2}, slightly increase alveolar P_{O_2}, and prolong the time before the breaking point is reached. In practical diving, however, this practice can be dangerous because, although P_{O_2} at the breaking point may be sufficient to maintain consciousness at that particular depth, the decrease in hydrostatic pressure on return to the surface will further reduce P_{O_2}. A typical accident is that in which the breath-hold diver arrives at the surface, loses consciousness and sinks down again.

Open circuit air diving ('scuba')

Self-contained open circuit compressed air apparatus with a simple demand valve is that used most commonly by amateur divers. Accidents which occur when using this type of apparatus may be more commonly associated with inexperience, but can result from particular predisposing factors.

Buoyancy. Buoyancy is again of importance in open circuit air (scuba) diving as a possible contributory cause of an accident. Not only must divers be aware that their relative buoyancy will vary with their lung volume, but also that their net weight will decrease as they use up the compressed air in their cylinders and thus that their buoyancy will increase slowly throughout the dive. This might be a source of difficulty at the end of a dive when they wish to ascend slowly or to remain at a shallow decompression.

For warmth many divers wear a 'wet suit' which contains air trapped in a neoprene layer and also provides some buoyancy. If the diver adjusts his weight to be neutrally buoyant at the surface, he will become negatively buoyant on descent because the air in the suit will be compressed by hydrostatic pressure. The sum of these effects could cause a total difference of as much as 10 kg buoyancy when comparing the diver at 20 m with full cylinders at maximum expiration with the same diver at the surface with nearly empty cylinders at full inspiration. The extra energy required to maintain a given depth, or some unnoticed alteration in depth, could contribute to an accident. Other divers wear a 'dry suit' and, while 'squeeze' and 'blow-up' are described with 'standard' diving with which they are more commonly associated, it should be remembered that a minor form of 'squeeze', involving the skin, and a 'blow-up' can occur if the suit inflation of a dry suit is not used correctly.

Nitrogen narcosis. The effects of nitrogen have been fully covered earlier in this volume, but must always be considered as a possible contributing factor to a scuba accident, especially in inexperienced divers. Irresponsibility should be avoided if amateur divers remain shallower than 40 m (5·0 ATA) and professional divers shallower than 60 m (7 ATA) when breathing compressed air.

Hyperventilation. Hyperventilation during a dive may play a part in causing an accident and be a result of simple anxiety. The usual symptoms of acute hypocapnia caused by hyperventilation are paraesthesia, muscle twitching, tetany, light-headedness, possible clouding of consciousness, and the onset or exacerbation of anxiety. Scintillating scotomata have also been reported, especially in bad visibility underwater.

It is also possible that a small amount of hyperventilation for some time could produce a slowly developing hypocapnia with symptoms. In one case (Fryer 1969) the patient was in a laboratory and 'surrounded by experienced respiratory physiologists' for an hour before symptoms occurred. The initial symptoms of hyperventilation are similar to those of incipient acute oxygen toxicity and could also be compatible with cerebral decompression sickness. The diagnosis may, therefore, be difficult. Often, hyperventilation can be suggested only retrospectively when the other possible causes of the symptoms have been eliminated and may sometimes be considered only after the dive supervisor has commented on the excessive consumption of gas by the diver. A degree of anxiety and concomitant hyperventilation is usually present in naïve and inexperienced divers and is best controlled by the reassurance of a companion and instructions to relax and breath slowly. The dangers of gross hyperventilation during a dive include loss of the mouthpiece during clouding of consciousness, the risk of pulmonary barotrauma caused by change of hydrostatic pressure with a closed glottis if in a tetanic phase, and a general diminution of self control and effectiveness. An inability to control anxiety and breathing, associated with a tendency to hyperventilate is sufficient to advise the discontinuance of diving.

Purity of breathing gas. A possible cause of diving accidents is the contamination of the air supply. Standards which are sufficiently stringent for long-term safety are laid down for the maximum amount of oil and other contaminants permissible in air for breathing (British Standard 4001). The diver's air should preferably be obtained from an oil-free compressor and should be filtered. Care must be taken to ensure that the exhaust gases from the compressor engine do not enter the air intake resulting in carbon monoxide contamination of the compressed air.

Standard diving

This refers to the traditional type of diving in which the diver wears a rigid helmet, weighted boots and is supplied with breathing gas by means of a hose. In this type of equipment it is important that the pressure of the air supply balances that at the depth of the diver. Failure to maintain this equilibrium may result in either a 'squeeze' or a 'blow-up'.

'Squeeze'. This condition arises if the hydrostatic pressure exceeds that of the air supply. A common cause is a fall from an underwater staging. A fall in shallow water is more serious than a fall of the same distance in deep water due to the greater volume change. The result of this increase in hydrostatic pressure tends to crush the rib cage, may force the diver's body into the rigid helmet and has led to death and severe injury.

'Blow-up'. A 'blow-up' will occur if the diver allows the pressure inside his diving suit to build up. A typical time for this accident to occur is during the ascent phase of the dive when the diver should be venting the air from his suit but may attempt to make himself lighter in order to make the ascent easier. The result of a blow-up is that the diver arrives on the surface precipitously, spread-eagled and incapable of helping himself. As a result of too rapid an ascent, the victim of a blow-up may also be suffering from a decompression disorder.

Carbon dioxide. If ventilation to the standard diver's helmet is not increased in proportion to the depth there can be a build up of carbon dioxide. This can give rise to the symptoms of hypercapnia which are described elsewhere in this volume.

Closed circuit breathing apparatus

Closed circuit breathing apparatus utilizes pure oxygen as the breathing medium, the diver breathing the oxygen to and from a 'counterlung' via a CO_2 absorber. As described in Chapter 4, the apparatus can be used either with a constant mass flow of oxygen into the counterlung or 'on demand', with oxygen being added to the counterlung when the volume of the counterlung is becoming insufficient. This apparatus has its usefulness but should be used by only highly trained and disciplined personnel.

Oxygen toxicity. The development of acute oxygen toxicity is an obvious risk when using this apparatus and, since an underwater convulsion could be fatal, a strict depth limitation of 8 m (1·8 ATA) should be imposed on its use. Nevertheless, convulsions can occur both under the water and on reaching the surface (Gillen 1966; Young 1970).

Hypoxia. The first effect of hypoxia is frequently a decrease in the powers of judgement so that warning symptoms (hyperpnoea, loss of muscular control, loss of concentration, possible visual defects) will either go unnoticed or will be considered trivial by the diver. For practical purposes it may be said that there are no reliable warnings. Unconsciousness follows, with possibly fatal results, unless the diver's companion or the surface attendant recognizes the problem and takes immediate life-saving action.

The development of hypoxia when breathing pure oxygen may seem to be a paradox, but it is not unknown for the cylinders of the diving apparatus to have been filled with the wrong gas.

Dilution hypoxia also can result from improper procedures. The volume of the counterlung is usually about 7 litres in order to ensure that the diver does not have a restriction of respiration through having insufficient gas for inspiration ('bottoming the lung'). This volume, together with the lungs of the diver, whose tissues are equilibrated with air, requires to be fully purged with oxygen before a dive because during the time that the diver is rebreathing from the set there will be a trend towards equilibrium between the gas in the counterlung and the gas dissolved in the tissues of the diver. However, after 2 min of oxygen breathing on the surface and a second purge before entering the water, the total amount of nitrogen given off during the dive is unlikely to be more than some 250 ml. This is relatively negligible and is within the safe limits. However, if purging with oxygen has not been carried out prior to diving, the set is still full of air. On commencing hard work the diver would rapidly consume not only his constant mass flow of oxygen but also the residual oxygen in the counterlung. He would still be able to breathe fully without 'bottoming the lung' and hence he would have no warning of the likelihood of hypoxia. If, however, the set had been correctly purged before diving, an oxygen consumption by the diver greater than the inlet flow would result in a noticeable reduction of the counterlung volume whereupon the diver would reinflate his counterlung with oxygen by using a by-pass valve.

It is even more important to ensure that the set and lungs are fully purged with oxygen before the dive if the closed circuit apparatus is being used 'on demand'. For then, when there is no constant inflow of oxygen to the counterlung, it is refilled with oxygen only when it is considered by the diver to contain insufficient gas for the required tidal volume.

Hypoxia should always remain as a possible explanation of any oxygen diving incident until it has been excluded.

Carbon dioxide effects. Closed circuit breathing sets vary in design but often have a single inspiration and expiration hose between the mouthpiece and the carbon dioxide absorption chamber which is in close relation to the counterlung. The volume of the common pathway may be 300 ml or more and represents an appreciable proportion of the resting tidal volume of the diver. This increased dead space will normally tend to increase alveolar Pco_2 and will result in an increased tidal ventilation. However, it is possible for the diver to breathe with a small tidal volume which barely clears gas out of the common respiratory hose and the CO_2 absorber, and hence there is a rapid build-up of CO_2.

A typical incident occurs a few minutes after the diver has entered the water. He may appear normal in routine tasks and movement but then suddenly becomes incoordinated or is found to be unresponsive to commands. On return to the surface he appears conscious and responsive, he is not cyanotic and has no noticeable hyperpnoea. On removing the mouthpiece from his lips and returning him to breathing air, the diver does not react for some 5 to 10 sec and then suddenly clutches his head and may lose consciousness. The unconscious state lasts for only a matter of seconds and may be accompanied by jactitations of a varying degree. On regaining consciousness the diver complains of violent frontal headache and has a retrograde amnesia for the events since the beginning of the dive. The diver may be slightly confused and shaky for up to an hour and the headache slowly regresses. Ophthalmological examination may reveal papilloedema during this time and an EEG may show slight abnormalities without focal lesions.

The jactitations on losing consciousness may be so extreme as to simulate an epileptiform attack and, because the dive was on pure oxygen, may give rise to suspicions of oxygen toxicity. However, the early onset of symptoms after entering the water, particularly if the diver has remained at a shallow depth, will make oxygen toxicity an unlikely explanation while the frontal headache is more typical of CO_2 poisoning.

A possible explanation of these events is that the high arterial Pco_2 causes dilation of cerebral circulation (Lambertsen et al. 1953) which tends to be counteracted by the constrictive effects of high Po_2. On return to air breathing there is a rapid decrease in arterial Pco_2, a reduction of cerebral circulation both because of the reduced Pco_2 and the longer lasting effects of high Po_2, and a simultaneous decrease in Po_2 which can result in cerebral hypoxia and hypoxic convulsions.

CO_2 absorbent. The commonly used absorbents for carbon dioxide are 'soda lime' and 'baralime', as granules of different sizes. They can absorb CO_2 only by chemical combination and the absorbent charge in a diving set will have a finite life, depending mainly upon the weight of the absorbent used. Diving with an absorbent which has either been partly used already or is not sufficient for the duration of the dive will be a further cause of CO_2 poisoning. The absorbent can also cause trouble if it has not been properly sieved, so that a fine dust of absorbent may be inhaled.

It is also important to ensure that the CO_2 absorbent does not come into contact with the water. The result is a hydroxide which the divers call a 'cocktail' and is dangerously disconcerting when it reaches the mouth. This is a possible contributory cause to any incident in closed circuit breathing apparatus and can be recognized by the burns which it leaves or by the symptoms which it causes.

Semi-closed circuit breathing apparatus

Semi-closed circuit breathing apparatus uses a similar principle to that of the closed circuit set. As described in Chapter 4, the breathing gas is a mixture of oxygen and inert gas which flows at a predetermined rate into the circuit. Pendulum breathing with a single hose and counterlung may be used or, more commonly for oxy-helium diving, there may be inspiratory and expiratory counterlungs each with uni-directional hoses. A carbon dioxide absorbent cannister is in the circuit and excess gas is vented into the water. One advantage of this apparatus is that it uses less gas than the conventional air or oxy-helium set. The gas may be oxygen-rich oxy-nitrogen for depths down to 55 m (6·5 ATA), the oxygen percentage being chosen to avoid toxic levels. For commercial divers using oxy-helium semi-closed apparatus at greater depths the oxygen percentage is related to depth and is less than 20%.

In addition to the specific problems of nitrogen or helium, the accidents which may occur to a diver breathing from semi-closed apparatus arise from similar causes to those already described for divers using closed circuit oxygen apparatus.

GENERAL CAUSES

The combination of factors

Very few accidents result from a single adverse factor, most are a result of a succession of contributory causes, each one of which might have been corrected individually but which, in combination, become insuperable and may lead, perhaps through panic, to a fatal outcome.

Disorientation

The reported frequency of vertigo in divers differs widely from survey to survey: 0·4% (Bayliss 1968); 11·9% (Vorosmarti & Bradley 1970); 22·9% (Coles & Knight 1961); 26% (Lundgren 1965); and 40% (Terry & Dennison 1966).

Either pressure or cold acting on the ear can give rise to vertigo. As described in Chapter 28, a common cause is overinflation of the middle ear while performing a Valsalva manoeuvre.

The occurrence of vertigo when visibility may be negligible, combined with the lack of proprioceptive input due to the relative weightlessness of the diver, may give rise to severe disorientation. If this happens, the diver may need to follow his bubbles to the surface or ask his attendant to assist him from the water.

Hypothermia

As discussed in Chapter 16, cold is well recognized as a major problem in deep diving (Rawlins & Tauber 1971) but it may also be a source of danger in relatively shallow situations. In addition to loss of manual dexterity owing to chilling of the extremities the diver may suffer from hypothermia and, as his core temperature drops, he may become confused, disorientated and withdrawn. However, the diver is not only at risk in the water but also after leaving it, when he may become hypothermic from 'wind-chill' by standing around in wet clothing or from the 'after-drop' due to blood beginning to recirculate through the chilled subcutaneous tissues. The diver who becomes cold and disorientated or withdrawn after leaving the water must be regarded as hypothermic and treated accordingly.

Exhaustion

In diving there may be many factors which increase the work-load on the diver and can lead to exhaustion. Among these are strong tidal streams, since a diver cannot cope with flows in excess of 1·5 to 2 knots, and increased breathing resistance. Regardless of the primary cause, exhaustion will potentiate many accidents: for instance, excess CO_2 may build up and cause CO_2 poisoning; extreme oxygen consumption in semi-closed apparatus may cause dilution hypoxia; the uptake of inert gas tends to be increased and thus there will be an increased risk of subsequent decompression sickness. The concentration of the diver upon his exhaustion will cause a narrowing of his perception and thus make him more susceptible to other perils.

Panic

In the underwater environment panic can lead to a fatality from a simple problem which should have been overcome. It may also lead to problems from hyperventilation or breath holding during ascent. Although panic is most common in the inexperienced diver, it can occur in anyone, no matter what his experience. It must be remembered that panic can occur not only in the diver but also in the attendant or supervisor. The best protection against panic is correct training to give those involved in diving operations confidence in themselves and in the other members of the team (Egstrom & Bachrach 1971).

Venomous marine animals

The term venomous is used in preference to poisonous since the latter term should be reserved for animals whose tissues are toxic when ingested. Venomous animals may be divided into two main groups, depending on whether the venoms are used for defence or for capture.

Venom for defence. This is the type of poison which is found in the spines of fish such as the sting-ray, weever fish and the stone-fish. It is also found in invertebrates such as sea-eggs and some marine worms. The venomous apparatus is usually found in spines on the back of the fish and the poison causes severe pain and discomfort. However, deaths do occur following stings from these fishes and treatment should be given as outlined later.

Venom for capture. As with the defensive type, this type of venom occurs in both invertebrates and vertebrates. These toxins are found in the jaws of animals such as octopus and sea-snakes. The bites are generally not painful apart from the initial wound, but cause numbness and eventual paralysis. The treatment in the case of sea-snakes is the use of the appropriate antivenin. Unfortunately, the structures of such poisons are very complex and no antivenin has yet been developed for some, including the blue-ringed octopus and cone shells.

In the case of the sea-snake there may be a latent period of from 20 min to several hours before the onset of symptoms. This has led to some victims failing to associate the initial bite with the subsequent illness. Early signs include a sensation of thickening of the tongue, ptosis and a general 'aching stiffness' of the muscles.

Jelly-fish and corals, which have nematocysts for the capture of their prey, have toxins which give rise to severe pain. They can be divided into three groups: *Hydrozoa*, e.g. Portuguese man-of-war; *Scyphozoa* (box jelly-fish), e.g. sea-wasp; *Anthozoa*, e.g. sea-anemones and corals.

A large specimen of the box jelly-fish may weigh as much as 6 or 7 lb (3 kg) and the tentacles can extend as far as 30 ft (9 m). Since there can be some 50 to 60 of these long invisible strands, a swimmer can be injured without knowing the cause.

The outcome of the stinging is governed by the size and species of jelly-fish, the amount of venom, and the state of the victim.

In severe cases there is little that can be done and death from shock and respiratory arrest may occur in minutes.

TREATMENT

Oxygen toxicity

Generally no treatment is needed at the surface apart from removing the diver's equipment and allowing him to breathe air. He must be prevented from injuring himself during the epileptiform convulsions. Recovery is generally rapid though there may be some degree of amnesia.

Carbon dioxide toxicity

As with oxygen poisoning all that is required is the return of the diver to the fresh air, though, as pointed out earlier, there may be a transient exacerbation of symptoms and it is likely that the diver will complain of a headache for some hours after the event.

Soda lime cocktail

The treatment of this condition consists of removal of the breathing apparatus as quickly as possible. After this has been done the diver's mouth should be washed with a dilute solution of vinegar or other weak acid. Exposed skin should be washed liberally with water and a drop of sterile liquid paraffin put into the victim's eyes. In all but the minor cases the diver should be kept under observation for any lung damage due to inhalation of the toxic fluid.

Hypothermia

A low-reading rectal thermometer should be readily available at medical centres associated with diving for the diagnosis and treatment of cases of acute hypothermia. Mild cases will recover if wet clothes are removed and the diver is wrapped in blankets or a sleeping bag and is allowed to regain warmth from his own metabolic heat. However, those with a rectal temperature of 30°C or less require active rewarming or they will die. The method of choice for active rewarming is to immerse the patient's trunk in a bath of hot water with a temperature of 40 to 42°C. The limbs should be kept out of the water and when the core temperature has risen above 33°C he should be removed from the bath, wrapped in blankets and allowed to rewarm naturally (Keatinge 1969). The indication for cardiac massage in the treatment of immersion hypothermia has been challenged by Golden (1973) who states that resuscitative efforts should not include external cardiac massage until such time as the deep body temperature exceeds 30°C.

Decompression disorders

Recompression and other treatment of pulmonary barotrauma, cerebral air embolism and decompression sickness have been dealt with in other chapters.

Venomous marine animals

Fishes. The toxins found in the stings of stone-fish, sting-rays and weever fish are heat labile. The relief given by applying heat to weever fish stings has been known for many years (Russell 1758), and Evans (1921) has reported that fishermen have relieved the symptoms by holding the affected limb over the funnel of the donkey engine. The treatment for sting-ray injuries is well established (Russell 1965) and consists of:

Washing the wound, since much of the venom can be removed this way.

Attempting to remove the sheath of the sting, if it is visible in the wound.

Immersing the limb in hot water for 30 to 90 min. If possible, tie a constraining band directly above the wound site.

Analgesics.

Debridement and suture of the wound.

This treatment could be used for the stings of other fish mentioned above and, in the case of stone-fish, it is also possible to obtain an antivenin.

Jelly-fish stings. The severe pain and shock that can occur in a serious case may put the swimmer or skin-diver at great risk. Sea wasp venom has been studied (Baxter & Lane 1970; Keen 1970) but no jelly-fish antivenins are readily available. Treatment should be carried out as outlined:

The prevention of drowning.

The treatment of shock with artificial respiration if needed.

Tourniquets may delay venom absorption.

Removal of tentacles (wearing gloves).

Wash with seawater or, preferably, fix with alcohol or vinegar. Fresh water, or rubbing with sand, may trigger off more nematocysts. Meat tenderizer has a reputation for being effective in first aid.

General supportive and analgesic treatment.

Corals. Injuries from coral can produce infected ulcers which may take a long time to heal. Wounds should be thoroughly cleaned and antibiotics used if secondary infection occurs.

Sea-urchins (sea eggs). The treatment of the painful injuries from spines is to remove the spines if possible and administer analgesics and anti-inflammatory agents.

Cone shells. No antivenin has been produced. Bites can lead to paralysis and death though usually the patients recover in about 6 hours (Thambirajah 1968).

Octopus. The most dangerous is the tiny blue-ringed octopus whose small bite is usually unnoticed by the victim. No antivenin has been developed and death occurs from respiratory paralysis. The only treatment is to ligature above the wound and give artificial respiration until the effect of the toxin wears off after many hours.

Drowning

This is very often the final stage in a diving accident. The problem of drowning or near drowning has been the subject of much discussion (Fuller 1962; Griffin 1966; Keatinge 1969; Rivers, Orr & Lea 1970; Martin & Barrett 1971). There are several important facts to be kept in mind. Immediate resuscitation is essential and 16% O_2 given at once by mouth-to-mouth expired air resuscitation is of greater value than any waiting for 100% O_2 to arrive. Secondly, admission to hospital is necessary, both for more definitive treatment such as intravenous plasma and bicarbonate, and for observation in anticipation of the possible onset of pulmonary or cerebral oedema. Figures given by Martin and Barrett (1971) demonstrate the importance of recognizing the dangers of secondary drowning.

INVESTIGATION OF
DIVING ACCIDENTS

The principle of accident investigation should be to evaluate the cause or causes of the accident on the basis of three possibilities: human biological failure, equipment failure, and faulty procedures.

THE DIVER

It is important to find out as much as possible from the man himself and other people. It unfortunately happens that the diver who is the focal point of the investigation is no longer able to act as a witness. Some of the facts which are important to discover are set out below:

Experience. This implies not only the man's experience as a diver but also his experience in doing that particular job under those particular conditions and diving with that particular equipment.

Recent medical history. This is obviously important as the diver may have had an illness or have been on a course of treatment which is incompatible with diving. For instance, he may be a diabetic, in which case the course of decompression sickness and other disorders would be complicated by disturbances of blood sugar levels.

Personal history. The diver's motivation should be considered as well as the possible effect of some emotional problem which he might have had.

Pre-dive activities. Consideration should be given to the diver's food and drink in relation to the dive. Miles (1962) tells the story of a diver who is alleged to have poisoned himself by exhaling the metabolic products of several pints of rough cider into his breathing bag. However, the real risk of a hangover is that it can lead to underwater vomiting and it is also associated with an increased risk of decompression sickness. Another consideration is whether the diver's pre-dive activities may have tired him excessively. One diver who failed to surface was eventually recovered from the warm shallow water where he had gone to sleep.

Medical examination

The diver should be examined as soon as possible after the incident. Both the examination and the record of it should be meticulous.

Post-mortem

If the diver is dead it is most important to get photographic evidence of any lesions at the earliest opportunity. A post-mortem examination and inquest must be carried out in accordance with the laws of the appropriate country. In general, the official pathologist welcomes any help or advice given on esoteric diving matters and the instructions of the Medical Research Council to Coroner's pathologists in the United Kingdom are given as an example. However, it needs to be emphasized that the discovery and location of gas bubbles at post-mortem are of doubtful significance at best, and are of *no* significance at all if the diver had died while under pressure.

External examination. Particular note should be taken of the presence of subcutaneous emphysema and also the appearance and distribution of abnormal blotching or marbling of the skin. (A colour photograph of any such markings would be extremely useful.)

Radiological examination. Whenever possible, radiography of the chest and major joints should be carried out before any internal examination. Chest radiography may show lung pathology, such as a cyst, and the presence of gas in the heart and blood vessels. Joint radiographs could indicate the choice of bones to be examined.

Internal examination.

1. *Central nervous system.* The calvarium should be opened before any other incision is made in order to prevent the accidental introduction of air into the body. Even then the unavoidable opening of the dural sinuses and the reflection of the dura usually leads to the presence of air bubbles in superficial cortical veins. The presence or absence of bubbles in cortical arteries should be noted. The post-mortem artefact of bubbles in cerebral veins can be averted only if the calvarium is opened under water.

The brain should be removed intact and placed in a bucket of 10% formalin. It should be suspended by the basilar artery using a paper clip or simply by passing a piece of string under this vessel and attaching the ends to the bucket handle. The formalin should be changed twice during the first 7 days. After 10 to 14 days the brain ($\pm$ spinal cord) can, if necessary, be sent by post to a reference laboratory, wrapped in formalin-soaked gauze or wool and enclosed in a biscuit tin or other rigid container. If possible the whole of the spinal cord should be removed and placed in the same container as the brain.

2. *Chest and abdomen.* It is advised that the trachea should be tied and occluded through a neck incision before the chest is opened.

(a) *Heart.* It is particularly important to note the quantity and distribution of gas in the heart and thoracic blood vessels. The heart should be examined under water in the conventional manner for the presence of gas in the chambers and coronary vessels and it must also be carefully examined for evidence of valvular or non-valvular communication between the left and right compartments.

(b) *Lungs.* Particular interest centres around the presence or absence of localized or generalized air trapping in the lungs and also the role of fat embolism in decompression sickness. The heart and lungs should be removed with care and any local distension or collapse or any evidence of sub-pleural spread of air noted. The heart–lung preparation should, if possible, be preserved in its entirety for subsequent dissection. In any event, the whole of both lungs should be retained for later examination. This can be achieved by irrigating the lungs using 10% formol saline down the bronchial tree with a pressure head of 25 to 30 cm and leaving for up to three days. Should even this be impossible, adequate blocks from all lobes should be withheld from paraffin processing and be processed in formalin for later fat studies.

(c) *Blood vessels.* Arteries and veins should be examined for the presence of gas in such sites as the alimentary canal, the brain and the kidneys. The consistency of the blood should be noted for haemoconcentration, and a sample kept for carbon monoxide estimation.

3. *Skeletal system.* There is a particular interest in caisson disease of bone. Therefore, where possible, at least the head of a humerus and if possible the head of a femur should be removed and fixed for subsequent examination. Where there is radiological evidence of bone disease, as many specimens as possible should be obtained from both affected and unaffected regions.

4. *Other systems.* Where possible, other organs should be preserved in their entirety, or portions retained for examination. This particularly applies to the kidneys and the endocrine system. Unprocessed blocks of kidney, pituitary gland and areas of skin which show blotchy changes should be preserved in formalin for studies of systemic fat embolism in decompression sickness. Specimens of voluntary muscles should also be obtained.

THE DIVE

This part of the investigation should cover the conduct of the dive itself and the climatic conditions at the time.

The following headings are suggested:

    Diver's narrative.
    Witness narrative.
    Object of dive.
    Depth and duration of dive.
    Frequency of dives.
    Tides and sea state.
    Water temperature.

THE EQUIPMENT

The general conditions of the apparatus should be noted. The gas valves must be shut off and the number of turns needed must be noted. Any relief valve must be sealed. Once the set has been sealed it should be sent, if possible, to have the breathing gases analysed. If appropriate, it is important to warn the analyst that the gas may be pure oxygen because analysis by chemical absorption (Scholander or Lloyd–Haldane Apparatus) would be harmful to the apparatus.

RECORDS

It is important that diving accidents are reported to a central authority so that the causes may be analysed. For this reason the reporting system should be simple and capable of analysis. If the system is too complex there is a likelihood that the reporting forms will not be completed correctly. If the facts are analysed carefully, the reporting and recording system has considerable potential value in the prevention of further similar incidents.

REFERENCES

BAYLISS, G. J. A. (1968) Aural barotrauma in naval divers. *Archs Otolar.* **88,** 141–147.

BERGHAGE, T. E. (1966) *Summary statistics: U.S. Navy Diving Accidents.* US Navy Experimental Diving Unit Research Report 1–66.

CRAIG, A. B. & HARLEY, A. D. (1968) Alveolar gas exchanges during breath-hold dives. *J. appl. Physiol.* **24,** 182–189.

COLES, R. R. A. & KNIGHT, J. J. (1961) *Aural and Audiometric Survey of Qualified Divers and Submarine Escape Training Tank Instructors.* Royal Naval Personnel Research Report, RNP 61/1011.

DANZIGER, R. E., SALLEE, T. L., UDDIN, D. E., FLYNN, E. T., & ALEXANDER, J. M. (1971) Case of mumps during hyperbaric exposure. *Aerospace Med.* **42,** 1335–1337.

DONALD, K. W. (1947) Oxygen poisoning in man. *Br. med. J.* **1,** 667–672.

EGSTROM, G. H. & BACHRACH, A. J. (1971) Diver panic. *Skin Diver* **20,** 36–39.

ELLIOTT, D. H. (1966) *Diving accidents.* In *Diving Manual,* 5th edition. pp. 111–117. Ed. B. Eaton. London: BSAC.

EVANS, H. M. (1921) The poison organs and venoms of venomous fish. *Br. med. J.* No. 3174, 690–2.

FRYER, D. I. (1969) *Subatmospheric Decompression Sickness in Man.* NATO Agardograph 125. pp. 235–238. Slough: Technivision Services.

FULLER, R. H. (1962) The clinical pathology of human near-drowning. *Proc. R. Soc. Med.* **56,** 34–38.

GILLEN, H. W. (1966) Oxygen convulsions in man. In *Proceedings of 3rd International Conference on Hyperbaric Medicine.* Ed. I. W. Brown, Jr. & B. G. Cox. (Publ. 1404.) pp. 217–222. Washington, D.C.: Natl Acad. Sci.-Natl Res. Council.

GOLDEN, F. St.G. (1973) Recognition and treatment of immersion hypothermia. *Proc. R. Soc. Med.* **66,** 1058–1061.

GRIFFIN, C. E. (1966) Near-drowning: its pathophysiology and treatment in man. *Milit. Med.* **131,** 12–21.

KEATINGE, W. R. (1969) *Survival in Cold Water,* pp. 87–99. Oxford & Edinburgh: Blackwell.

KIDD, D. J. & ELLIOTT, D. H. (1969) Clinical manifestations and treatment of decompression sickness in divers. In *The Physiology and Medicine of Diving,* pp. 464–490. London: Baillière Tindall & Cassell.

LAMBERTSEN, C. J., KOUGH, R. H., COOPER, D. Y., EMMEL, G. L., LOESCHCKE, H. H. & SCHMIDT, C. F. (1953) Oxygen toxicity. Effects in man of oxygen inhalation at 1 and 3·5 atmospheres upon blood gas transport, cerebral circulation and cerebral metabolism. *J. appl. Physiol.* **5,** 471–486.

LANPHIER, E. H. & RAHN, H. (1969a) Alveolar gas exchange during breath-hold diving. *J. appl. Physiol.* **18,** 471–477.

LANPHIER, E. H. & RAHN, H. (1969b) Alveolar gas exchange during breath-holding in air. *J. appl. Physiol.* **18,** 478–482.

LUNDGREN, C. E. G. (1965) Alternabaric vertigo—a diving hazard. *Br. med. J.* **2,** 511–513.

MARTIN, C. M. & BARRETT, O. (1971) Drowning and near-drowning: a review of ten years' experience in a large army hospital. *Milit. Med.* **136,** 439–442.

MILES, S. (1962) *Underwater Medicine,* pp. 186–199. London: Staples Press.

MITHOEFER, J. C. (1965) Breath holding. In *Handbook of Physiology, Section 3; Respiration.* Ed. W. O. Fenn & H. Rahn. pp. 1011–1025. American Physiological Society.

PAULEV, P. E. (1969) Respiratory and cardiovascular effects of breath-holding. *Acta physiol. scand. Suppl.* 324, 1–116.

RAWLINS, J. S. P. & TAUBER, J. F. (1971) Thermal balance at depth. In *Underwater Physiology. Proc. 4th Symp. Underwater Physiology.* Ed. C. J. Lambertsen. pp. 435–442. New York: Academic Press.

RIVERA, J. C. (1963) *Decompression Sickness among Divers: an Analysis of 935 Cases.* US Navy Experimental Diving Unit Research Report, 1–63.

RUSSELL, F. E. (1965) Marine toxins and venomous and poisonous animals. In *Advances in Marine Biology.* Ed. F. S. Russell. pp. 255–384. New York and London: Academic Press.

RUSSELL, P. (1758) Cited by RUSSELL, F. E. (1965).

SLARK, A. G. (1962) *Treatment of 137 Cases of Decompression Sickness.* Royal Naval Physiological Laboratory Research Report. 8/62.

TERRY, L. & DENNISON, W. L. (1966) *Vertigo Among Divers.* USN Submarine Medical Centre Special Report No. 66/2.

THAMBIRAJAH, A. (1968) *Dangerous Marine Animals.* Report H.23. R.A.N. School of Underwater Medicine, H.M.A.S. Penguin.

RIVERS, J. F., ORR, G. & LEE, H. A. (1970) Drowning: its clinical sequelae and management. *Br. med. J.* **2,** 157–161.

VOROSMARTI, J. & BRADLEY, M. E. (1970) Alternobaric vertigo in military divers. *Milit. Med.* **135,** 182–185.

YOUNG, J. M. (1970) Oxygen poisoning in a hyperbaric environment. *Jl. nav. med. Serv.* **56,** 39–47.

Index

125-A-3

1996 EDITION

ARMS CONTROL AND DISARMAMENT AGREEMENTS

TEXTS AND HISTORIES OF THE NEGOTIATIONS

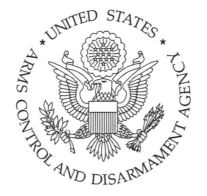

UNITED STATES ARMS CONTROL AND DISARMAMENT AGENCY

FOREWORD

This is the revised sixth edition of a publication originally issued in 1972. It contains the texts of the Geneva Protocol of 1925 and, in chronological order, all major arms control agreements concluded after World War II in which the United States has been a participant up to May 1988. The text of each agreement is preceded by a brief narrative discussion prepared by the United States Arms Control and Disarmament Agency and is followed by a list of signatories and parties.

CONTENTS

INCIDENTS AT SEA AGREEMENT, May 25, 1972*
Agreement Between the Government of the United States of America and the Government of the Union of Soviet Socialist Republics on the Prevention of Incidents On and Over the High Seas

STRATEGIC ARMS LIMITATION TALKS (SALT I)

ABM TREATY, May 26, 1972*
Treaty Between the United States of America and the Union of Soviet Socialist Republics on the Limitation of Anti-Ballistic Missile Systems

INTERIM AGREEMENT, May 26, 1972*
Interim Agreement Between the United States of America and the Union of Soviet Socialist Republics on Certain Measures With Respect to the Limitation of Strategic Offensive Arms

PREVENTION OF NUCLEAR WAR AGREEMENT, June 22, 1973*
Agreement Between the United States of America and the Union of Soviet Socialist Republics on the Prevention of Nuclear War

ABM PROTOCOL, July 3, 1974*
Protocol to the Treaty Between the United States of America and the Union of Soviet Socialist Republics on the Limitation of Anti-Ballistic Missile Systems

THRESHOLD TEST BAN TREATY, July 3, 1974*
Treaty Between the United States of America and the Union of Soviet Socialist Republics on the Limitation of Underground Nuclear Weapon Tests (and Protocol Thereto)

"HOT LINE" EXPANSION AGREEMENT, July 17, 1984*
Agreement Between the United States of America and the Union of Soviet Socialist
Republics To Expand the U.S.-USSR Direct Communications Link

CONFIDENCE- AND SECURITY-BUILDING MEASURES DOCUMENT, September 19, 1986*
Document of the Stockholm Conference on Confidence- and Security-Building Measures
and Disarmament in Europe Convened in Accordance With the Relevant Provisions of the
Concluding Document of the Madrid Meeting of the Conference on Security and
Cooperation in Europe

NUCLEAR RISK REDUCTION CENTERS, September 15, 1987*
Agreement Between the United States of America and the Union of Soviet Socialist
Republics on the Establishment of Nuclear Risk Reduction Centers (and Protocols Thereto)

INTERMEDIATE-RANGE NUCLEAR FORCES, December 8, 1987*
Treaty Between the United States of America and the Union of Soviet Socialist Republics
on the Elimination of Their Intermediate-Range and Shorter-Range Missiles

BALLISTIC MISSILE LAUNCH NOTIFICATION AGREEMENT, May 31, 1988*
Agreement Between the United States of America and the Union of Soviet Socialist
Republics on Notifications of Launches of Intercontinental Ballistic Missiles and
Submarine-Launched Ballistic Missiles

* Date signed

Efforts to prevent or limit war have a long history and have taken many forms. Men have tried to erect religious and ethical barriers against war, to outlaw it, to create codes and tribunals for peaceful arbitration and settlement of disputes. Nations have tried to avert war by withdrawing into isolation or neutrality, or by joining with others in leagues and alliances for the collective defense of peace and security.

In past eras efforts to control weapons of war were seldom successful or lasting. The coming of the nuclear era, however, brought such vast new dimensions of potential destructiveness that concepts of waging war and keeping the peace were transformed.

Until comparatively recent times, disarmament and arms control were chiefly measures imposed by the victors on the vanquished. Only rarely was arms limitation the result of freely negotiated agreement.

A notable example of freely negotiated and successful arms control in "modern" times was the Rush-Bagot agreement of 1817 between the United States and Great Britain, limiting naval forces on the Great Lakes and Lake Champlain to a few vessels on each side.

In the late 19th century the control of armaments took on new importance. The techniques of industrialization applied to the manufacture of weapons, mounting imperialist rivalries, nationalism, competing alliance systems -- all contributed to an increasingly dangerous and costly arms race.

At the invitation of Tsar Nicholas II, International Peace Conferences met at The Hague in 1899 and 1907. The Hague Conferences brought advances in codifying the rules of war and in establishing institutions and procedures for settling international disputes -- notably the Permanent Court of Arbitration at The Hague, antecedent of the Permanent Court of International Justice and of the present International Court of Justice.

Declarations signed at the 1899 conference prohibited the use of dum-dum bullets, asphyxiating gases, and the launching of projectiles and explosives from balloons or by other new methods of similar nature. The use of poison or poisoned weapons was forbidden by regulations annexed to both the 1899 and the 1907 conventions and a convention prohibiting or restricting the use of specific automatic contact mines and torpedoes was adopted in 1907.

The Hague Conferences were the first attempts at a worldwide approach to the problems of war and peace. They were the outgrowth of recognition that the control of modern weapons and the effects of modern warfare concerned the interests of all nations and required their collective action. Plans for a third conference, however, fell victim to the antagonisms and military competition that preceded World War I, as did many of the arms control declarations.

World War I was fought on a scale previously unknown, and new weapons -- tanks, submarines, aircraft, poison gas -- increased its deadliness. The war gave fresh momentum to the creation of international peacekeeping institutions and to negotiations for disarmament. Following the cessation of hostilities, the Covenant of the League of Nations declared that "the maintenance of peace requires the reduction of national armaments to the lowest point consistent with national safety and the enforcement by common action of international obligations." The Treaty of Versailles imposed drastic limitations on Germany's armament and demilitarized the Rhineland. In a series of postwar negotiations the Allied powers sought to impose agreed restrictions on certain weapons.

In 1921, at the initiative of the United States, a conference was convened at Washington to discuss arms limitations, one of its purposes being to curb an emerging naval race among the victorious allies. The resulting agreement established fixed ratios and tonnage limits for the capital ships of the leading naval powers, and a freeze on naval fortifications and bases in the western Pacific. In 1930 a subsequent treaty signed in London limited other classes of warships and provided for a third naval conference in 1935. That conference was unable to reach any effective agreement, and the naval treaties expired in 1936, following Japanese refusal to continue the arrangements.

The use of poison gas in the battles of World War I had evoked especially strong condemnation. In 1925, as the result of a U.S.

initiative, a protocol was signed at Geneva prohibiting the use in war of poison gas and bacteriological weapons. By World War II most countries had ratified it, including all the great powers except the United States and Japan. The protocol was generally observed during that war, although Italy used poison gas in the Ethiopian war. Japan ratified the protocol in 1970; U.S. ratification took place in 1975. When the protocol was originally submitted to the U.S. Senate in 1926, there was strong lobbying against it, and Senate action was not completed. It was resubmitted by President Nixon in 1970, but disagreement about the protocol's application to riot-control agents and herbicides delayed Senate consent to ratification. (The administration took the position the protocol did not apply to these.)

In 1928 the Kellogg-Briand Pact, initiated by the United States and France and signed by 63 nations, renounced war as an instrument of national policy. The pact included no provisions for ensuring compliance with its obligations, and many signatories attached sweeping qualifications or unilateral interpretations, which made the agreement meaningless.

In 1932, after 7 years of preparation, a general disarmament conference was held under the auspices of the League of Nations. A wide variety of measures to limit armed forces, weapons, and expenditures was proposed, including a French proposal for an international police force under the League, a Soviet proposal for general and complete disarmament, and the U.S. plan to reduce forces and to abolish chemical warfare, tanks, bombers, and heavy artillery. No agreement was achieved. Germany demanded the right to rearm unless other nations disarmed to her level, and after Hitler came to power, Germany left the conference and the League. Sporadic sessions of the conference continued until 1937, when it dissolved in deadlock.

New levels of violence and devastation were reached in World War II. Even before its close, the nations fighting the Axis powers began a new effort to prevent war through a system of collective security. The U.N. Charter envisaged international forces under the Security Council to keep the peace. "Armed forces, assistance and facilities" were to be contributed by all U.N. members. Unlike the Covenant of the League,

the Charter gave disarmament no immediate priority; the five great powers would maintain their armaments, policing the disarmament of Germany and Japan and maintaining the peace until the United Nations had developed its own effective military forces. Under Article II the General Assembly was "to consider the general principles of cooperation in the maintenance of international peace and security, including the principles governing disarmament and the regulation of armaments," and make recommendations to the Security Council. Article 47 provided that the Military Staff Committee would advise the Security Council on "the regulation of armaments and possible disarmament." Only in these two articles does the word "disarmament" occur.

The Charter of the United Nations was signed at San Francisco on June 26, 1945; on August 6, a new weapon exploded over Hiroshima. Its stupendous power, shattering old concepts of war and weaponry, imposed new urgencies and demanded new perspectives on international efforts to control armaments.

The first U.S. proposal for the control of nuclear weapons recognized that this new force involved the interests of the entire world community. In 1946 the U.S. representative to the U.N. Atomic Energy Commission, Bernard Baruch, presented a U.S. plan that called for placing all the atomic resources of the world under the ownership or control of an independent international authority. It would have exclusive authority over all the stages of nuclear production, from mining to manufacture, and over the eventual destruction of all nuclear weapons. If the plan were adopted, the United States, the only nuclear power, would give up its atomic arsenal. All nations would submit to inspection by the international authority. If violations called for action by the Security Council, the veto could not be exercised. The plan was to be carried out in stages; the control system was to be in effective operation before the nuclear weapons were removed from the U.S. arsenal.

Although the plan was endorsed by a large majority of U.N. members, the Soviet Union objected to the ownership, staging, and enforcement provisions. Soviet counterproposals left nuclear activities under the control of national governments. The international authority would be empowered only to conduct periodic inspection of declared nuclear facilities. The United States and most other nations considered the Soviet plan's verification provisions altogether inadequate, and negotiations became deadlocked.

Meanwhile, the development of technology brought new dangers and complexities. In September 1949 President Truman announced that the Soviet Union had detonated a nuclear device. In 1952 the United States exploded the first hydrogen device. The first atomic bomb had the power of 15,000 tons of TNT-15 kilotons. The destructive power of the new weapons was measured in megatons, the equivalent of millions of tons of TNT. In 1953 the Soviet Union announced that they too had exploded a hydrogen bomb. Rivalry in nuclear weapons was paralleled by rivalry in the development of delivery systems.

Among earlier efforts of the nuclear era to control armaments were broad, inclusive proposals, including (by 1959) proposals for "General and Complete Disarmament," with carefully interlocked stages for reducing or eliminating weapons and armed forces, and with precisely stipulated timing to ensure that the process of disarming would not leave any nation's security weakened. This exacting requirement for establishing the pace and order of reductions and ensuring their equitable impact put great difficulties in the way of agreements. Each nation defined its security needs differently; each possessed differing arrays of weapons and armed forces designed to defend its particular interests. Disparities and differences were accompanied by strong ideological conflicts that intensified wariness and suspicion. And the obstacle of verification stubbornly persisted.

The General Assembly's sessions devoted increasing attention to disarmament issues, and the non-nuclear powers demonstrated heightened concern as the spread of nuclear technology and the continued testing of weapons sharpened world awareness of the implications of nuclear warfare. Successive subsidiary bodies were created as forums for arms control negotiations. The U.N. Disarmament Commission, created in 1952, operated at first chiefly through a subcommittee of five -- the United States, Great Britain, France, Canada and the Soviet Union. As debates continued without agreement, membership in disarmament bodies were

broadened and efforts were made to blunt the sharpness of East-West division by the participation of nonaligned, non-nuclear nations. The Eighteen Nation Disarmament Committee (ENDC), which began meeting in 1962, became the Conference of the Committee on Disarmament (CCD) in 1969, when its membership was enlarged. The ENDC and the CCD played important roles in achieving the multinational agreements that finally emerged. The Committee on Disarmament (CD), a still larger forum comprising 40 member states was established in 1978 and began negotiations in 1979. France was a member of both the ENDC and the CCD but had never taken its seat in either. It is today an active participant in CD meetings. China has also been an active participant since January 1980. The Committee on Disarmament became the Conference on Disarmament in 1984.

The creation of such active organizations for multilateral negotiations marked a step forward; so did the convening of special meetings with the participation of experts to deal with particular issues, such as the Geneva Conference on the Discontinuance of Nuclear Tests. The broad continuing effort was supported by active diplomatic exchanges and high-level meetings among the nuclear powers. The special responsibility of the major nuclear powers was subsequently manifested in bilateral talks between the United States and the Soviet Union: Strategic Arms Limitations Talks (SALT, 1969-1979); Intermediate Range Nuclear Force Talks (INF, 1980-1987); Strategic Arms Reduction Talks (START, 1982-1991); the Nuclear and Space Talks (NST, 1985-1991); and the Nuclear Testing Talks (NTT, 1987-1990).

By the middle of the 1950s, past production of nuclear materials could no longer be reliably accounted for, and control systems could not ensure that none had been diverted to clandestine weapons manufacture or illegal stockpiles. A point of no return seemed to have been passed. As negotiations and debate continued, emphasis thus shifted gradually from programs of comprehensive disarmament to more limited measures. This brought a new flexibility and pragmatism into negotiations and, while general and complete disarmament remained a goal, willingness to consider partial solutions of limited scope helped to make solid step-by-step progress possible.

Moreover, advanced technology brought qualitative and quantitative changes in weaponry that radically altered concepts of national security and supplied a compelling incentive for pursuing arms control agreements. In the past it was the generally accepted assumption that more armed strength equaled more security. But this equation is no longer valid. More armaments do not guarantee more security. They may in fact have an opposite effect, creating new dangers by causing a potential adversary to overreact in his own weapons program -- in response to what he perceives as a threat to his own security. The continuing arms race also increases the possibility of an accident.

Arms control is no longer an intermittent enterprise. It has become a central and continuing concern of governments and an integral aspect of foreign policy and national security. Thus the United States -- the first government to do so -- established a separate agency in 1961 to deal with disarmament issues. The U.S. Arms Control and Disarmament Agency (ACDA) is charged with formulating, coordinating and carrying out arms control policies, with conducting and coordinating research, with preparation and management of U.S. participation in negotiations; and with public dissemination of information about arms control.

Some of the agreements printed here have been signed by almost all the world's nations. Others have been negotiated among the chief nuclear powers, who bear the greatest responsibility for averting conflict that would tragically affect nations and peoples everywhere. Some of the treaties are essentially "nonarmament" agreements, designed to keep free of conflict and nuclear weaponry the environments that science has made newly accessible and significant, and whose resources must be preserved for all -- for example, outer space or the seabed -- or geographic regions where nuclear weapons have not been introduced -- Antarctica and Latin America. Some agreements reflect a growing concern with the need to prevent a war that might occur through accident, unauthorized or lawless action, human error, or mechanical failure. And some reflect a conscious decision by the major nuclear powers to limit their own strategic offensive and defensive weapons.

PROTOCOL FOR THE PROHIBITION OF THE USE IN WAR OF ASPHYXIATING, POISONOUS OR OTHER GASES, AND OF BACTERIOLOGICAL METHODS OF WARFARE

At the end of World War I, the victorious Allies decided to reaffirm in the Versailles Treaty (1919) the prewar prohibition of the use of poisonous gases (see Introduction) and to forbid Germany to manufacture or import them. Similar provisions were included in the peace treaties with Austria, Bulgaria, and Hungary.

Drawing upon the language of these peace treaties, the United States -- at the Washington Disarmament Conference of 1922 -- took the initiative of introducing a similar provision into a treaty on submarines and noxious gases. The U.S. Senate gave its advice and consent to ratification of this treaty without a dissenting vote. It never entered into force, however, since French ratification was necessary, and France objected to the submarine provisions.

At the 1925 Geneva Conference for the Supervision of the International Traffic in Arms, the United States similarly took the initiative of seeking to prohibit the export of gases for use in war. At French suggestion it was decided to draw up a protocol on non-use of poisonous gases and at the suggestion of Poland the prohibition was extended to bacteriological weapons. Signed on June 17, 1925, the Geneva Protocol thus restated the prohibition previously laid down by the Versailles and Washington treaties and added a ban on bacteriological warfare.

Before World War II the protocol was ratified by many countries, including all the great powers except the United States and Japan. When they ratified or acceded to the protocol, some nations -- including the United Kingdom, France, and the USSR -- declared that it would cease to be binding on them if their enemies, or the allies of their enemies, failed to respect the prohibitions of the protocol. Although Italy was a party to the protocol, it used poison gas in the Ethiopian war. Nevertheless, the protocol was generally observed in World War II. Referring to reports that the Axis powers were considering the use of gas, President Roosevelt said on June 8, 1943:

Use of such weapons has been outlawed by the general opinion of civilized mankind.

This country has not used them, and I hope that we never will be compelled to use them. I state categorically that we shall under no circumstances resort to the use of such weapons unless they are first used by our enemies.

Although the Senate Foreign Relations Committee favorably reported the protocol in 1926, there was strong lobbying against it, and the Senate never voted on it. After the war, President Truman withdrew it from the Senate, together with other inactive older treaties. Little attention was paid to the protocol for several years thereafter. During the Korean war the Communist side accused the United States of using bacteriological weapons in Korea, but at the same time they rejected American proposals for international investigation of their charges. In the Security Council, the Soviet Union introduced a draft resolution calling on all U.N. members to ratify the protocol. At that time the United States was not willing to agree to prohibit the use of any weapons of mass destruction unless they could be eliminated through a disarmament agreement with effective safeguards. On June 26, 1952, the Soviet resolution was rejected by a vote of 1 to 0, with 10 abstentions (including the United States, the United Kingdom, and France).

In 1966 the Communist countries strongly criticized the United States for using tear gas and chemical herbicides in Vietnam. In the General Assembly, Hungary charged that the use in war of these agents was prohibited by the Geneva Protocol and other provisions of international law. The United States denied that the protocol applied to nontoxic gases or chemical herbicides. Joined by Canada, Italy, and the United Kingdom, the United States introduced amendments to a Hungarian resolution that would have made the use of any chemical and bacteriological weapons an international crime. In its final form the resolution called for "strict observance by all states of the principles and objectives" of the protocol, condemned "all actions contrary to those objectives," and invited all states to accede to the protocol. During the debate the U.S. Representative stated that it would be up to each country to decide whether or how to adhere to the protocol, "in the light of constitutional and other considerations."

Interpretation of the protocol remained a thorny problem. In his foreword to a U.N. report on chemical and biological weapons (July 1, 1969),

Secretary General Thant recommended a renewed appeal for accession to the protocol and a "clear affirmation" that it covered the use in war of all chemical and biological weapons, including tear gas and other harassing agents. Discussion in the Conference of the Committee on Disarmament (CCD) showed that most members agreed with the Thant recommendations. Swedish Ambassador Myrdal, a strong advocate of the broad interpretation, stressed the danger of escalation if nonlethal chemical agents were permitted. She also pointed out that the military use of tear gases should be distinguished from their use for riot control and that there was a similar difference between using herbicides in war and employing them for peaceful purposes. On the other hand, U.K. Disarmament Minister Mulley held that only the parties to the protocol were entitled to say what it meant.

In the General Assembly, the 12 nonaligned members of the CCD, joined by 9 other nations, introduced a resolution condemning as contrary to international law the use in international armed conflict of all chemical and biological agents. Opposing the resolution, the U.S. Representative reaffirmed the American interpretation of the protocol and took the position that it was inappropriate for the General Assembly to interpret treaties by means of a resolution. The 21-nation resolution was adopted on December 16, 1969, by a vote of 80 to 3 (Australia, Portugal, the United States), and 36 abstentions (including France and the United Kingdom). France and many other abstainers accepted the broad interpretation of the protocol but considered the resolution undesirable on other grounds.

While the General Assembly debate was still underway, President Nixon announced on November 25, 1969, that he would resubmit the protocol to the Senate. He reaffirmed U.S. renunciation of the first use of lethal chemical weapons and extended this renunciation to incapacitating chemicals. It was on this occasion that he also announced the unilateral U.S. renunciation of bacteriological (biological) methods of warfare.

Some support for the American interpretation of the protocol now came from the United Kingdom and Japan. During the 1930 discussion at Geneva in the Preparatory Commission for the Disarmament Conference, the United Kingdom had taken the position that the protocol covered

tear gas. In February 1970 the British Foreign Secretary told Parliament that this was still the British position, but that the riot-control agent CS, unlike older tear gases, was not harmful to man and was therefore not covered by the protocol. During the Diet debate on Japanese ratification of the protocol, Foreign Minister Aichi took the position that it did not prohibit riot-control agents and herbicides. Japan ratified the protocol in May 1970.

In a report of August 11, 1970, to the President, Secretary of State Rogers recommended that the protocol be ratified with a reservation of the right to retaliate with gas if an enemy state or its allies violated the protocol. He also reaffirmed the position that the protocol did not apply to the use in war of riot-control agents and herbicides. President Nixon resubmitted the protocol to the Senate on August 19.

The Foreign Relations Committee did not accept the Administration's interpretation regarding riot-control agents and herbicides. In a letter of April 15, 1971, to the President, Chairman Fulbright said many members thought that it would be in the interest of the United States either to ratify the protocol without "restrictive understandings" or to postpone action until this became possible. The Committee thus deferred action. It also held in abeyance the Biological Weapons Convention, which was submitted to it on August 10,1972, pending resolution of this issue.

In the latter part of 1974, the Ford Administration launched a new initiative to obtain Senate consent to ratification of the protocol (and simultaneously of the Biological Weapons Convention). The new approach was set forth to the Committee by ACDA Director Fred Ikle on December 10, when he announced that the President, while reaffirming the Administration's view as to the scope of the protocol, was prepared "to renounce as a matter of national policy: (1) first use of herbicides in war except use, under regulations applicable to their domestic use, for control of vegetation within U.S. bases and installations or around their immediate defensive perimeters; (2) first use of riot-control agents in war except in defensive military modes to save lives such as:

(a) Use of riot-control agents in riot-control circumstances to include controlling rioting prisoners of war. This exception would permit use of riot-control agents in riot situations in areas under direct and distinct U.S. military control;

(b) Use of riot-control agents in situations where civilian casualties can be reduced or avoided. This use would be restricted to situations in which civilians are used to mask or screen attacks;

(c) Use of riot-control agents in rescue missions. The use of riot-control agents would be permissible in the recovery of remotely isolated personnel such as downed aircrews (and passengers);

(d) Use of riot-control agents in rear echelon areas outside the combat zone to protect convoys from civil disturbances, terrorists and paramilitary organizations."

In addition, Dr. Ikle testified that "the President, under an earlier directive still in force, must approve in advance any use of riot-control agents and chemical herbicides in war."

Two days later, on December 12, the Committee voted unanimously to send the protocol and the convention to the Senate floor and on December 16 the Senate voted its approval, also unanimously. The Committee, in recommending advice and consent to ratification of the protocol, indicated that it attached particular importance to Dr. Ikle's response to the following question posed in connection with his December 10 testimony:

Question: "Assuming the Senate were to give its advice and consent to ratification on the grounds proposed by the Administration, what legal impediment would there be to subsequent Presidential decisions broadening the permissible uses of herbicides and riot-control agents?

Answer: "There would be no formal legal impediment to such a decision. However, the policy which was presented to the Committee will be inextricably linked with the history of Senate consent to ratification of the Protocol with its consent dependent upon its observance. If a future administration should change this policy without Senate consent whether in practice or by a formal policy change, it would be inconsistent with the history of the ratification, and could have extremely grave political repercussions and as a result is extremely unlikely to happen."

The protocol and the convention were ratified by President Ford on January 22, 1975. The U.S. instrument of ratification of the convention was deposited on March 26, 1975, and of the protocol on April 10, 1975.

Responding to the extensive use of chemical weapons between belligerents in the Iran-Iraq war and the increasing number of chemical weapon-capable states, President Reagan, in an address to the U.N. General Assembly on September 26, 1988, urged the Parties to the Protocol and all other concerned states to convene a conference to review the rapid deterioration of respect for international norms against chemical weapon use. Hosted by France, 149 states met in Paris, January 7-11, 1989, for a Conference on Chemical Weapons Use. In the Final Declaration, the states "solemnly affirm their commitments not to use chemical weapons and condemn such use." Among other things, they also recognized the importance of the Geneva Protocol, reaffirmed the prohibitions as established in it, and called upon all states which have not yet done so to accede to the Protocol.

PROTOCOL FOR THE PROHIBITION OF THE USE IN WAR OF ASPHYXIATING, POISONOUS OR OTHER GASES, AND OF BACTERIOLOGICAL METHODS OF WARFARE

Signed at Geneva June 17, 1925
Entered into force February 8, 1928
Ratification advised by the U.S. Senate December 16, 1974
Ratified by U.S. President January 22, 1975
U.S. ratification deposited with the
  Government of France April 10, 1975
Proclaimed by U.S. President April 29, 1975

The Undersigned Plenipotentiaries, in the name of their respective Governments:

Whereas the use in war of asphyxiating, poisonous or other gases, and of all analogous liquids, materials or devices, has been justly condemned by the general opinion of the civilized world; and

Whereas the prohibition of such use has been declared in Treaties to which the majority of Powers of the World are Parties; and

To the end that this prohibition shall be universally accepted as a part of International Law, binding alike the conscience and the practice of nations;

Declare:

That the High Contracting Parties, so far as they are not already Parties to Treaties prohibiting such use, accept this prohibition, agree to extend this prohibition to the use of bacteriological methods of warfare and agree to be bound as between themselves according to the terms of this declaration.

The High Contracting Parties will exert every effort to induce other States to accede to the present Protocol. Such accession will be notified to the Government of the French Republic, and by the latter to all signatory and acceding Powers, and will take effect on the date of the notification by the Government of the French Republic.

The present Protocol, of which the French and English texts are both authentic, shall be ratified as soon as possible. It shall bear today's date.

The ratifications of the present Protocol shall be addressed to the Government of the French Republic, which will at once notify the deposit of such ratification to each of the signatory and acceding Powers.

The instruments of ratification of and accession to the present Protocol will remain deposited in the archives of the Government of the French Republic.

The present Protocol will come into force for each signatory Power as from the date of deposit of its ratification, and, from that moment, each Power will be bound as regards other powers which have already deposited their ratifications.

IN WITNESS WHEREOF the Plenipotentiaries have signed the present Protocol.

DONE at Geneva in a single copy, this seventeenth day of June, One Thousand Nine Hundred and Twenty-Five.

STATES PARTIES TO THE PROTOCOL FOR THE PROHIBITION OF THE USE IN WAR OF ASPHYXIATING, POISONOUS OR OTHER GASES, AND OF BACTERIOLOGICAL METHODS OF WARFARE, DONE AT GENEVA JUNE 17, 1925

States which have deposited instruments of ratification or accession, or continue to be bound as the result of succession agreements concluded by them or by reason of notification given by them to the Secretary-General of the United Nations:

Afghanistan-Dec. 9, 1986
Angola-Oct. 23, 1990
Antigua and Barbuda-Nov. 1, 1981
Argentina-May 12, 1969
1 [a] [b] Australia-Jan. 22, 1930
Austria-May 9, 1928

1 [a] [b] [2] Bahamas, The-July 10, 1973
Bahrain-Dec. 9, 1988
Bangladesh-May 20, 1989
2 Barbados-June 22, 1976
1 [a] [b] Belgium-Dec. 4, 1928
Belize-Sept. 21, 1981
Benin-Dec. 9, 1986
6 Bhutan-June 12, 1978
Bolivia-Aug. 13, 1985
1 [a] [b] [2] Botswana-Sept. 30, 1966
Brazil-Aug. 28, 1970
1 [a] [b] Bulgaria-Mar. 7, 1934
Burkina Faso (Upper Volta)-Mar. 3, 1971
1 [a] [b] [2] Burma-Jan. 4, 1948

Cambodia-Mar. 15, 1983
Cameroon-July 20, 1989
1 [a] [b] Canada-May 6, 1930
Cape Verde-May 20, 1991
Central African Republic-July 31, 1970
1 [a] [b] Chile-July 2, 1935
1 [a] [b] China, People's Republic of-Aug. 9, 1952
8 China (Taiwan)-Aug. 7, 1929
7 Comoros
Cuba-June 24, 1966
Cyprus-Dec. 12, 1966
1 [b] Czechoslovakia-Aug. 16, 1938

Denmark-May 5, 1930
7 Djibouti
Dominica-Nov. 8, 1978
Dominican Republic-Dec. 8, 1970

Ecuador-Sept. 16, 1970
Egypt-Dec. 6, 1928
1 [a] [b] Estonia-Aug. 28, 1931
Ethiopia-Sept. 18, 1935
Equatorial Guinea-May 20, 1989

1 [a] [b] Fiji-Mar. 21, 1973
Finland-June 26, 1929
1 [a] [b] [3] France-May 9, 1926

Gambia, The-Nov. 16, 1966
Germany (GDR/FRG)-Apr. 25, 1929
Ghana-May 3, 1967
Greece-May 30, 1931
1 [a] [b] Grenada-May 20, 1989
Guatemala
Guinea-Bissau-May 20, 1989
1 [a] [b] [2] Guyana

Holy See-Oct. 18, 1966
Hungary-Oct. 11, 1952

Iceland-Nov. 2, 1967
1 [a] [b] India-Apr. 9, 1930
Indonesia-Jan. 26, 1971
Iran-July 4, 1929
1 [a] [b] Iraq-Sept. 8, 1931
Ireland-Aug. 18, 1930
1 [a] [b] Israel-Feb. 20, 1969
Italy-Apr. 3, 1928
Ivory Coast-July 27, 1970

Jamaica-July 31, 1970
Japan-May 21, 1970
1 [a] [b] [d] Jordan-Jan. 20, 1977

Kenya-July 6, 1970
Kiribati-July 12, 1979
Korea, North-Jan.4, 1989
1 [a] [b] Korea, South-Jan. 4, 1989
1 [a] [b] [d] Kuwait-Dec. 15, 1971

Laos-May 20, 1989
Latvia-June 3, 1931
Lebanon-Apr. 17, 1969
Lesotho-Mar. 15, 1972
Liberia-Apr. 2, 1927
1 [b] [d] Libya-Dec. 29, 1971
Liechenstein-Nov. 6, 1991
Lithuania-June 15, 1933
Luxembourg-Sept. 1, 1936

Madagascar-Aug. 12, 1967
Malawi-Sept. 14, 1970
Malaysia-Dec. 10, 1970
Maldives (Islands)-Jan. 6, 1967
Mali-Nov. 19, 1966
Malta-Oct. 15, 1970
Mauritius-Jan. 8, 1971
Mexico-Mar. 15, 1932
Monaco-Jan. 6, 1967
1 [b] Mongolia-Dec. 6, 1968
Morocco-Oct. 13, 1970

Nepal-May 9, 1969
1 [c] [4] Netherlands, The-Oct. 31, 1930

1 [a b]   New Zealand-Jan. 22, 1930
          Nicaragua-Oct. 5, 1990
          Niger-Apr. 19, 1967
1 [a b]   Nigeria-Oct. 15, 1968
          Norway-July 27, 1932

          Pakistan-June 9, 1960
          Panama-Dec. 4, 1970
1 [a b]   Papua New Guinea-Sept. 16, 1975
          Paraguay-Jan. 14, 1969
          Peru-Aug. 13, 1985
          Philippines-May 29, 1973
          Poland-Feb. 4, 1929
1 [a b]   Portugal-July 1, 1930

          Qatar-Sept. 16, 1976

1 [a b]   Romania-Aug. 23, 1929
          Russia (See USSR)
          Rwanda-June 25, 1964

          St. Kitts & Nevis-Sept. 19, 1983
          St. Lucia-Dec. 21, 1988
          St. Vincent & The Grenadines-Oct. 27,
          1979
          Saudi Arabia-Jan. 27, 1971
1 [a b 2] Seychelles-June 29, 1976
          Sierra Leone-Mar. 20, 1967
1 [a b 2] Singapore-Aug. 9, 1965
          Solomon Islands-July 7, 1978
1 [a b]   South Africa-Jan. 22, 1930
1 [a b]   Spain-Aug. 22, 1929
          Sri Lanka-Jan. 20, 1954
          Sudan-Dec. 17, 1980
1 [c 4]   Suriname-Sept. 25, 1975
1 [a b 2] Swaziland-Sept. 6, 1968
          Sweden-Apr. 25, 1930
          Switzerland-July 12, 1932
1 [d]   Syrian Arab Republic-Dec. 17, 1968

          Tanzania-Apr. 22, 1963
          Thailand-June 6, 1931
          Togo-Apr. 5, 1971
          Tonga-July 28, 1971
          Trinidad and Tobago-Nov. 30, 1970
          Tunisia-July 12, 1967
          Turkey-Oct. 5, 1929
          Tuvalu-Oct. 1, 1978

          Uganda-May 24, 1965
1 [a b]   Union of Soviet Socialist Republics-Apr. 5, 1928
1 [a b 5] United Kingdom-Apr. 9, 1930
1 [c]   United States-Apr. 10, 1975
          Uruguay-Apr. 12, 1977

          Venezuela-Feb. 8, 1928
1 [a b]   Vietnam-Sept. 23, 1980

1 [b]   Yemen Arab Republic (Sana)-Mar. 17, 1971
          Yugoslavia-Apr. 12, 1929

1 [a b 2] Zambia-Oct. 24, 1964
          Zimbabwe-Apr. 18, 1980

---

[1] a,b,c,d   With reservations to Protocol as follows:
   a- binding only as regards relations with other parties.
   b- to cease to be binding in regard to any enemy States
       whose armed forces or allies do not observe provisions.
   c- to cease to be binding as regards use of chemical
       agents with respect to any enemy State whose armed
       forces or allies do not observe provisions.
   d- does not constitute recognition of or involve treaty
       relations with Israel.
[2] By virtue of agreement with former parent State or
notification to the Secretary General of the United Nations of
succession to treaty rights and obligations upon
independence.
[3] Applicable to all French territories.
[4] Applicable to Suriname and Curacao.
[5] It does not bind India or any British Dominion which is a
separate member of the League of Nations and does not
separately sign or adhere the Protocol. It is applicable to all
colonies.
[6] Deposited accession on June 12, 1978, but the French
Government asked that accession take effect on date of
notification by them Feb. 19, 1979.
[7] Included in declaration by France. Continued application
has apparently not been determined.
[8] Effective Jan. 1, 1979, the United States recognized the
Government of the People's Republic of China as the sole
legal government of China.

THE ANTARCTIC TREATY

The Antarctic Treaty, the earliest of the post-World War II arms limitation agreements, has significance both in itself and as a precedent. It internationalized and demilitarized the Antarctic Continent and provided for its cooperative exploration and future use. It has been cited as an example of nations exercising foresight and working in concert to prevent conflict before it develops. Based on the premise that to exclude armaments is easier than to eliminate or control them once they have been introduced, the treaty served as a model, in its approach and even provisions, for later "nonarmament" treaties -- the treaties that excluded nuclear weapons from outer space, from Latin America, and from the seabed.

By the 1950s seven nations -- Argentina, Australia, Chile, France, New Zealand, Norway, and the United Kingdom -- claimed sovereignty over areas of Antarctica, on the basis of discovery, exploration, or geographic propinquity. Claims of Argentina, Chile, and the United Kingdom overlapped. Eight other nations -- the United States, the Soviet Union, Belgium, Germany, Poland, Sweden, Japan, and South Africa -- had engaged in exploration but had put forward no specific claims. The United States did not recognize the claims of other governments and reserved the right to assert claims based on exploration by its citizens. The Soviet Union took a similar position.

Activities in the Antarctic had generally been conducted peacefully and cooperatively. Yet the possibility that exploitable economic resources might be found meant the possibility of future rivalry for their control. Moreover, isolated and uninhabited, the continent might at some time become a potential site for emplacing nuclear weapons.

Fortunately, scientific interests rather than political, economic, or military concerns dominated the expeditions sent to Antarctica after World War II. Fortunately, too, international scientific associations were able to work out arrangements for effective cooperation. In 1956 and 1957, for example, American meteorologists "wintered over" at the Soviet post Mirnyy, while Soviet meteorologists "wintered over" at Little America. These cooperative activities culminated in the International Geophysical Year of 1957-1958 (IGY), a joint scientific effort by 12

nations -- Argentina, Australia, Belgium, Chile, France, Japan, New Zealand, Norway, South Africa, the Soviet Union, the United Kingdom, and the United States -- to conduct studies of the Earth and its cosmic environment.

In these years the desire to keep the continent demilitarized was general and some diplomatic discussion of the possibility had taken place. On May 3, 1958, the United States proposed to the other 11 nations participating in the IGY that a conference be held, based on the points of agreement that had been reached in informal discussions:

(1) that the legal *status quo* of the Antarctic Continent remain unchanged;

(2) that scientific cooperation continue;

(3) that the continent be used for peaceful purposes only.

All accepted the U.S. invitation. The Washington Conference on Antarctica met from October 15 to December 1, 1959. No insurmountable conflicts or issues divided the conference, and negotiations culminated in a treaty signed by all 12 nations on December 1, 1959. Approved by the U.S. Senate, U.S. ratification was deposited August 18, 1960, and the treaty entered into force on June 23, 1961, when the formal ratifications of all the participating nations had been received.

The treaty provides that Antarctica shall be used for peaceful purposes only. It specifically prohibits "any measures of a military nature, such as the establishment of military bases and fortifications, the carrying out of military maneuvers, as well as the testing of any type of weapons." Military personnel or equipment, however, may be used for scientific research or for any other peaceful purpose. Nuclear explosions and the disposal of radioactive waste material in Antarctica are prohibited, subject to certain future international agreements on these subjects. All Contracting Parties entitled to participate in the meetings referred to in Article IX of the treaty have the right to designate observers to carry out inspections in all areas of Antarctica, including all stations, installations and equipment, and ships and aircraft at discharge or embarkation points. Each observer has complete freedom of access at any time to any or all areas of Antarctica. Contracting Parties may also carry out aerial inspections. There are provisions for amending the treaty; for referring disputes that cannot be handled by direct talks, mediation, arbitration, or other peaceful means to the International Court of Justice; and for calling a conference in 30 years to review the operation of the treaty if any parties request it.

Argentina, Australia, New Zealand, the Soviet Union, the United Kingdom, and the United States have all exercised the right of inspection. The United States conducted inspections in 1971, 1975, 1977, 1980, 1983, 1985, and 1989. All American inspections included Soviet facilities. The 1985 inspection concentrated on the Antarctic Peninsula area where the U.S. team inspected stations belonging to the United Kingdom, the Soviet Union, the People's Republic of China, Argentina, Chile, and Poland. The 1989 inspection was conducted in the Ross Sea area, visiting six (only five are named) stations of France, Italy, New Zealand, the Federal Republic of Germany, and the Soviet Union, as well as 12 sites of historic and scientific interest. In February 1995, the 10th inspection since inspections began in 1963 was conducted. In a circumnavigation of the South Pole, eight sites were visited to allow teams to observe environmental conditions at research stations. No military activities, armaments, or prohibited nuclear activities were observed, and all scientific programs were in accord with previously published plans. The observed activities at each station were in compliance with the provisions and spirit of the Antarctic Treaty.

Fifteen consultative meetings have been held in accordance with Article IX of the treaty. Numerous recommendations on measures in furtherance of the principles and objectives of the treaty have been adopted, many of which have now entered into force. There are now 24 Contracting Parties entitled to participate in these meetings: the original 12 signatory states plus Brazil, China, Germany, Finland, India, Italy, Republic of Korea, Peru, Poland, Spain, Sweden, and Uruguay.

ANTARCTIC TREATY

Signed at Washington December 1, 1959
Ratification advised by U.S. Senate August 10, 1960
Ratified by U.S. President August 18, 1960
U.S. ratification deposited at Washington August 18, 1960
Proclaimed by U.S. President June 23, 1961
Entered into force June 23, 1961

The Governments of Argentina, Australia, Belgium, Chile, the French Republic, Japan, New Zealand, Norway, the Union of South Africa, the Union of Soviet Socialist Republics, the United Kingdom of Great Britain and Northern Ireland, and the United States of America,

Recognizing that it is in the interest of all mankind that Antarctica shall continue forever to be used exclusively for peaceful purposes and shall not become the scene or object of international discord;

Acknowledging the substantial contributions to scientific knowledge resulting from international cooperation in scientific investigation in Antarctica;

Convinced that the establishment of a firm foundation for the continuation and development of such cooperation on the basis of freedom of scientific investigation in Antarctica as applied during the International Geophysical Year accords with the interests of science and the progress of all mankind;

Convinced also that a treaty ensuring the use of Antarctica for peaceful purposes only and the continuance of international harmony in Antarctica will further the purposes and principles embodied in the Charter of the United Nations;

Have agreed as follows:

Article I

1. Antarctica shall be used for peaceful purposes only. There shall be prohibited, *inter alia*, any measures of a military nature, such as the establishment of military bases and fortifications, the carrying out of military maneuvers, as well as the testing of any type of weapons.

2. The present treaty shall not prevent the use of military personnel or equipment for scientific research or for any other peaceful purposes.

Article II

Freedom of scientific investigation in Antarctica and cooperation toward that end, as applied during the International Geophysical Year, shall continue, subject to the provisions of the present treaty.

Article III

1. In order to promote international cooperation in scientific investigation in Antarctica, as provided for in Article II of the present treaty, the Contracting Parties agree that, to the greatest extent feasible and practicable:

(a) information regarding plans for scientific programs in Antarctica shall be exchanged to permit maximum economy and efficiency of operations;

(b) scientific personnel shall be exchanged in Antarctica between expeditions and stations;

(c) scientific observations and results from Antarctica shall be exchanged and made freely available.

2. In implementing this Article, every encouragement shall be given to the establishment of cooperative working relations with those Specialized Agencies of the United Nations and other international organizations having a scientific or technical interest in Antarctica.

Article IV

1. Nothing contained in the present treaty shall be interpreted as:

(a) a renunciation by any Contracting Party of previously asserted rights of or claims to territorial sovereignty in Antarctica;

(b) a renunciation or diminution by any Contracting Party of any basis of claim to territorial sovereignty in Antarctica which it may have whether as a result of its activities or those of its nationals in Antarctica, or otherwise;

(c) prejudicing the position of any Contracting Party as regards its recognition or non-recognition of any other State's right of or claim or basis of claim to territorial sovereignty in Antarctica.

2. No acts or activities taking place while the present treaty is in force shall constitute a basis for asserting, supporting or denying a claim to territorial sovereignty in Antarctica or create any rights of sovereignty in Antarctica. No new claim, or enlargement of an existing claim, to territorial sovereignty in Antarctica shall be asserted while the present treaty is in force.

Article V

1. Any nuclear explosions in Antarctica and the disposal there of radioactive waste material shall be prohibited.

2. In the event of the conclusion of international agreements concerning the use of nuclear energy, including nuclear explosions and the disposal of radioactive waste material, to which all of the Contracting Parties whose representatives are entitled to participate in the meetings provided for under Article IX are parties, the rules established under such agreements shall apply in Antarctica.

Article VI

The provisions of the present treaty shall apply to the area south of 60° South Latitude, including all ice shelves, but nothing in the present treaty shall prejudice or in any way affect the rights, or the exercise of the rights, of any State under international law with regard to the high seas within that area.

Article VII

1. In order to promote the objectives and ensure the observance of the provisions of the present treaty, each Contracting Party whose representatives are entitled to participate in the meetings referred to in Article IX of the treaty shall have the right to designate observers to carry out any inspection provided for by the present Article. Observers shall be nationals of the Contracting Parties which designate them. The names of observers shall be communicated to every other Contracting Party having the right to designate observers, and like notice shall be given of the termination of their appointment.

2. Each observer designated in accordance with the provisions of paragraph 1 of this Article shall have complete freedom of access at any time to any or all areas of Antarctica.

3. All areas of Antarctica, including all stations, installations and equipment within those areas, and all ships and aircraft at points of discharging or embarking cargoes or personnel in Antarctica, shall be open at all times to inspection by any observers designated in accordance with paragraph 1 of this Article.

4. Aerial observation may be carried out at any time over any or all areas of Antarctica by any of the Contracting Parties having the right to designate observers.

5. Each Contracting Party shall, at the time when the present treaty enters into force for it, inform the other Contracting Parties, and thereafter shall give them notice in advance, of

(a) all expeditions to and within Antarctica, on the part of its ships or nationals, and all expeditions to Antarctica organized in or proceeding from its territory;

(b) all stations in Antarctica occupied by its nationals; and

(c) any military personnel or equipment intended to be introduced by it into Antarctica subject to the conditions prescribed in paragraph 2 of Article I of the present treaty.

Article VIII

1. In order to facilitate the exercise of their functions under the present treaty, and without prejudice to the respective positions of the Contracting Parties relating to jurisdiction over all other persons in Antarctica, observers designated under paragraph 1 of Article VII and scientific personnel exchanged under subparagraph 1(b) of Article III of the treaty, and members of the staffs accompanying any such persons, shall be subject only to the jurisdiction of the Contracting Party of which they are nationals in respect of all acts or omissions occurring while they are in Antarctica for the purpose of exercising their functions.

Without prejudice to the provisions of paragraph 1 of this Article, and pending the adoption of measures in pursuance of subparagraph 1(e) of Article IX, the Contracting Parties concerned in any case of dispute with regard to the exercise of jurisdiction in Antarctica shall immediately consult together with a view to reaching a mutually acceptable solution.

Article IX

1. Representatives of the Contracting Parties named in the preamble to the present treaty shall meet at the City of Canberra within two months after the date of entry into force of the treaty, and thereafter at suitable intervals and places, for the purpose of exchanging information, consulting together on matters of common interest pertaining to Antarctica, and formulating and considering, and recommending to their Governments, measures in furtherance of the principles and objectives of the treaty, including measures regarding:

(a) use of Antarctica for peaceful purposes only;

(b) facilitation of scientific research in Antarctica;

(c) facilitation of international scientific cooperation in Antarctica;

(d) facilitation of the exercise of the rights of inspection provided for in Article VII of the treaty;

(e) questions relating to the exercise of jurisdiction in Antarctica;

(f) preservation and conservation of living resources in Antarctica.

2. Each Contracting Party which has become a party to the present treaty by accession under Article XIII shall be entitled to appoint representatives to participate in the meetings referred to in paragraph 1 of the present Article, during such time as that Contracting Party demonstrates its interest in Antarctica by conducting substantial scientific research activity there, such as the establishment of a scientific station or the despatch of a scientific expedition.

3. Reports from the observers referred to in Article VII of the present treaty shall be transmitted to the representatives of the Contracting Parties participating in the meetings referred to in paragraph 1 of the present Article.

4. The measures referred to in paragraph 1 of this Article shall become effective when approved by all the Contracting Parties whose representatives were entitled to participate in the meetings held to consider those measures.

5. Any or all of the rights established in the present treaty may be exercised from the date of entry into force of the treaty whether or not any measures facilitating the exercise of such rights have been proposed, considered or approved as provided in this Article.

Article X

Each of the Contracting Parties undertakes to exert appropriate efforts, consistent with the Charter of the United Nations, to the end that no one engages in any activity in Antarctica contrary to the principles or purposes of the present treaty.

Article XI

1. If any dispute arises between two or more of the Contracting Parties concerning the interpretation or application of the present treaty, those Contracting Parties shall consult among themselves with a view to having the dispute resolved by negotiation, inquiry, mediation, conciliation, arbitration, judicial settlement or other peaceful means of their own choice.

2. Any dispute of this character not so resolved shall, with the consent, in each case, of all parties to the dispute, be referred to the International Court of Justice for settlement; but failure to reach agreement on reference to the International Court shall not absolve parties to the dispute from the responsibility of continuing to seek to resolve it by any of the various peaceful means referred to in paragraph 1 of this Article.

Article XII

1. (a) The present treaty may be modified or amended at any time by unanimous agreement of the Contracting Parties whose representatives are entitled to participate in the meetings provided for under Article IX. Any such modification or amendment shall enter into force when the depositary Government has received notice from all such Contracting Parties that they have ratified it.

(b) Such modification or amendment shall thereafter enter into force as to any other Contracting Party when notice of ratification by it has been received by the depositary Government. Any such Contracting Party from which no notice of ratification is received within a period of two years from the date of entry into force of the modification or amendment in accordance with the provisions of subparagraph 1(a) of this Article shall be deemed to have withdrawn from the present treaty on the date of the expiration of such period.

2. (a) If after the expiration of thirty years from the date of entry into force of the present treaty, any of the Contracting Parties whose representatives are entitled to participate in the meetings provided for under Article IX so requests by a communication addressed to the depositary Government, a Conference of all the Contracting Parties shall be held as soon as practicable to review the operation of the treaty.

(b) Any modification or amendment to the present treaty which is approved at such a Conference by a majority of the Contracting Parties there represented, including a majority of those whose representatives are entitled to participate in the meetings provided for under Article IX, shall be communicated by the depositary Government to all the Contracting Parties immediately after the termination of the Conference and shall enter into force in accordance with the provisions of paragraph 1 of the present Article.

(c) If any such modification or amendment has not entered into force in accordance with the provisions of subparagraph 1(a) of this Article within a period of two years after the date of its communication to all the Contracting Parties, any Contracting Party may at any time after the expiration of that period give notice to the depositary Government of its withdrawal from the present treaty; and such withdrawal shall take effect two years after the receipt of the notice of the depositary Government.

Article XIII

1. The present treaty shall be subject to ratification by the signatory States. It shall be open for accession by any State which is a Member of the United Nations, or by any other State which may be invited to accede to the treaty with the consent of all the Contracting Parties whose representatives are entitled to participate in the meetings provided for under Article IX of the treaty.

2. Ratification of or accession to the present treaty shall be effected by each State in accordance with its constitutional processes.

3. Instruments of ratification and instruments of accession shall be deposited with the Government of the United States of America, hereby designated as the depositary Government.

4. The depositary Government shall inform all signatory and acceding States of the date of each deposit of an instrument of ratification or accession, and the date of entry into force of the treaty and of any modification or amendment thereto.

5. Upon the deposit of instruments of ratification by all the signatory States, the present treaty shall enter into force for those States and for States which have deposited instruments of accession. Thereafter the treaty shall enter into force for any acceding State upon the deposit of its instrument of accession.

6. The present treaty shall be registered by the depositary Government pursuant to Article 102 of the Charter of the United Nations.

Article XIV

The present treaty, done in the English, French, Russian and Spanish languages, each version being equally authentic, shall be deposited in the archives of the Government of the United States of America, which shall transmit duly certified copies thereof to the Governments of the signatory and acceding States.

IN WITNESS WHEREOF the undersigned Plenipotentiaries, duly authorized, have signed the present treaty.

DONE at Washington this first day of December, one thousand nine hundred and fifty-nine.

ANTARCTIC TREATY

Country	Date of Signature	Date of Deposit of Ratification	Date of Deposit of Accession
Argentina	12/01/59	06/23/61	
Australia	12/01/59	06/23/61	
Austria			08/25/87
Belgium	12/01/59	07/26/60	
Brazil			05/16/75
Bulgaria			09/11/78
Chile	12/01/59	06/23/61	
China			06/08/83
Cuba			08/16/84
Czechoslovakia			06/14/62
Denmark			05/20/65
Ecuador			09/15/87
Finland			05/15/84
France	12/01/59	09/16/60	
German Democratic Republic			11/19/74
Germany, Federal Republic of			02/05/79
Greece			01/08/87
Hungary			01/27/84
India			08/19/83
Italy			03/18/81
Japan	12/01/59	08/04/60	
Korea, Democratic People's Republic of			01/21/87
Korea, Republic of			11/28/86
Netherlands			03/30/67
New Zealand	12/01/59	11/01/60	
Norway	12/01/59	08/24/60	
Papua New Guinea			03/16/81
Peru			04/10/81
Poland			06/08/61
Romania			09/15/71

ANTARCTIC TREATY -- Continued

Country	Date of Signature	Date of Deposit of Ratification	Date of Deposit of Accession
South Africa	12/01/59	06/21/60	
Spain			03/31/82
Sweden			04/24/84
Union of Soviet Socialist Republics	12/01/59	11/02/60	
United Kingdom	12/01/59	05/31/60	
United States	12/01/59	08/18/60	
Uruguay			01/11/80
Total	12	12	25

**MEMORANDUM OF UNDERSTANDING
BETWEEN THE UNITED STATES OF AMERICA
AND THE UNION OF SOVIET SOCIALIST
REPUBLICS REGARDING THE
ESTABLISHMENT OF A DIRECT
COMMUNICATIONS LINK
(WITH ANNEX)**

The need for ensuring quick and reliable communication directly between the heads of government of nuclear-weapons states first emerged in the context of efforts to reduce the danger that accident, miscalculation, or surprise attack might trigger a nuclear war. These risks, arising out of conditions which are novel in history and peculiar to the nuclear-armed missile age, can of course threaten all countries, directly or indirectly.

The Soviet Union had been the first nation to propose, in 1954, specific safeguards against surprise attack; it also expressed concern about the danger of accidental war. At Western initiative, a Conference of Experts on Surprise Attack was held in Geneva in 1958, but recessed without achieving conclusive results, although it stimulated technical research on the issues involved.

In its "Program for General and Complete Disarmament in a Peaceful World," presented to the General Assembly by President Kennedy on September 25, 1961, the United States proposed a group of measures to reduce the risks of war. These included advance notification of military movements and maneuvers, observation posts at major transportation centers and air bases, and additional inspection arrangements. An international commission would be established to study possible further measures to reduce risks, including "failure of communication."

The United States draft Treaty outline submitted to the ENDC[1] on April 18, 1962, added a proposal for the exchange of military missions to improve communications and understanding. It also proposed "establishment of rapid and reliable communications" among the heads of government and with the Secretary General of the United Nations.

The Soviet draft Treaty on general and complete disarmament (March 15, 1962) offered no provisions covering the risk of war by surprise attack, miscalculation, or accident. On July 16, however, the Soviet Union introduced amendments to its draft that called for (1) a ban on joint maneuvers involving the forces of two or more states and advance notification of substantial military movements, (2) exchange of military missions, and (3) improved communications between heads of government and with the U.N. Secretary General. These measures were not separable from the rest of the Soviet program.

The Cuban missile crisis of October 1962 compellingly underscored the importance of prompt, direct communication between heads of state. On December 12 of that year, a U.S. working paper submitted to the ENDC urged consideration of a number of measures to reduce the risk of war. These measures, the United States argued, offered opportunities for early agreement and could be undertaken either as a group or separately. Included was establishment of communications links between major capitals to ensure rapid and reliable communications in times of crisis. The working paper suggested that it did not appear either necessary or desirable to specify in advance all the situations in which a special communications link might be used:

> . . . In the view of the United States, such a link should, as a general matter, be reserved for emergency use; that is to say, for example, that it might be reserved for communications concerning a military crisis which might appear directly to threaten the security of either of the states involved and where such developments were taking place at a rate which appeared to preclude the use of normal consultative procedures. Effectiveness of the link would not be degraded through use for other matters.

On June 20, 1963, at Geneva the U.S. and Soviet representatives to the ENDC completed negotiations and signed the "Memorandum of Understanding Between the United States of America and the Union of Soviet Socialist Republics Regarding the Establishment of a Direct Communications Link." The memorandum

---

[1] Eighteen-Nation Disarmament Committee, which met at Geneva from 1962 on. In 1969, with the addition of new members, the name was changed to Conference of the Committee on Disarmament (CCD). A yet larger group, the Committee on Disarmament, was established in 1978-79. In 1984 the Committee on Disarmament changed its name to the Conference on Disarmament.

provided that each government should be responsible for arrangements for the link on its own territory, including continuous functioning of the link and prompt delivery of communications to its head of government. An annex set forth the routing and components of the link and provided for allocation of costs, exchange of equipment, and other technical matters. The direct communications link would comprise:

(1) two terminal points with teletype equipment;

(2) a full-time duplex wire telegraph circuit (Washington-London-Copenhagen-Stockholm-Helsinki-Moscow); and

(3) a full-time duplex radiotelegraph circuit (Washington-Tangier-Moscow).

If the wire circuit should be interrupted, messages would be transmitted by the radio circuit. If experience showed the need for an additional wire circuit, it might be established by mutual agreement.

The "Hot Line" agreement, the first bilateral agreement between the United States and the Soviet Union that gave concrete recognition to the perils implicit in modern nuclear-weapons systems, was a limited but practical step to bring those perils under rational control.

The communications link has proved its worth since its installation. During the Arab-Israeli war in 1967, for example, the United States used it to prevent possible misunderstanding of U.S. fleet movements in the Mediterranean. It was used again during the 1973 Arab-Israeli war. The significance of the hot line is further attested by the 1971, 1984 and 1988 agreements to modernize it. These agreements are discussed in following sections.

MEMORANDUM OF UNDERSTANDING BETWEEN THE UNITED STATES OF AMERICA AND THE UNION OF SOVIET SOCIALIST REPUBLICS REGARDING THE ESTABLISHMENT OF A DIRECT COMMUNICATIONS LINK

Signed at Geneva June 20, 1963
Entered into force June 20, 1963

For use in time of emergency the Government of the United States of America and the Government of the Union of Soviet Socialist Republics have agreed to establish as soon as technically feasible a direct communications link between the two Governments.

Each Government shall be responsible for the arrangements for the link on its own territory. Each Government shall take the necessary steps to ensure continuous functioning of the link and prompt delivery to its head of government of any communications received by means of the link from the head of government of the other party.

Arrangements for establishing and operating the link are set forth in the Annex which is attached hereto and forms an integral part hereof.

DONE in duplicate in the English and Russian languages at Geneva, Switzerland, this 20th day of June, 1963.

FOR THE GOVERNMENT OF THE UNITED STATES OF AMERICA:

CHARLES C. STELLE
Acting Representative of the United States of America to the Eighteen-Nation Committee on Disarmament

FOR THE GOVERNMENT OF THE SOVIET SOCIALIST REPUBLICS:

SEMYON K. TSARAPKIN
Acting Representative of the Union of Soviet Socialist Republics to the Eighteen-Nation Committee on Disarmament

(SEAL)

ANNEX

TO THE MEMORANDUM OF UNDERSTANDING BETWEEN THE UNITED STATES OF AMERICA AND THE UNION OF SOVIET SOCIALIST REPUBLICS REGARDING THE ESTABLISHMENT OF A DIRECT COMMUNICATIONS LINK

The direct communications link between Washington and Moscow established in accordance with the Memorandum, and the operation of such link, shall be governed by the following provisions:

1. The direct communications link shall consist of:

a. Two terminal points with telegraph-teleprinter equipment between which communications shall be directly exchanged;

b. One full-time duplex wire telegraph circuit, routed Washington-London-Copenhagen-Stockholm-Helsinki-Moscow, which shall be used for the transmission of messages;

c. One full-time duplex radiotelegraph circuit, routed Washington-Tangier-Moscow, which shall be used for service communications and for coordination of operations between the two terminal points.

If experience in operating the direct communications link should demonstrate that the establishment of an additional wire telegraph circuit is advisable, such circuit may be established by mutual agreement between authorized representatives of both Governments.

2. In case of interruption of the wire circuit, transmission of messages shall be effected via the radio circuit, and for this purpose provision shall be made at the terminal points for the capability of prompt switching of all necessary equipment from one circuit to another.

3. The terminal points of the link shall be so equipped as to provide for the transmission and reception of messages from Moscow to Washington in the Russian language and from Washington to Moscow in the English language. In this connection, the USSR shall furnish the United States four sets of telegraph terminal equipment, including page printers, transmitters, and reperforators, with one year's supply of spare parts and all necessary special tools, test equipment, operating instructions, and other technical literature, to provide for transmission and reception of messages in the Russian language.

The United States shall furnish the Soviet Union four sets of telegraph terminal equipment, including page printers, transmitters, and reperforators, with one year's supply of spare parts and all necessary special tools, test equipment, operating instructions and other technical literature, to provide for transmission and reception of messages in the English language.

The equipment described in this paragraph shall be exchanged directly between the parties without any payment being required therefor.

4. The terminal points of the direct communications link shall be provided with encoding equipment. For the terminal point in the USSR, four sets of such equipment (each capable of simplex operation), with one year's supply of spare parts, with all necessary special tools, test equipment, operating instructions and other technical literature, and with all necessary blank tape, shall be furnished by the United States to the USSR against payment of the cost thereof by the USSR.

The USSR shall provide for preparation and delivery of keying tapes to the terminal point of the link in the United States for reception of messages from the USSR. The United States shall provide for the preparation and delivery of keying tapes to the terminal point of the link in the USSR for reception of messages from the United States. Delivery of prepared keying tapes to the terminal points of the link shall be effected through the Embassy of the USSR in Washington (for the terminal of the link in the USSR) and through the Embassy of the United States in Moscow (for the terminal of the link in the United States).

5. The United States and the USSR shall designate the agencies responsible for the arrangements regarding the direct communications link, for its technical maintenance, continuity and reliability, and for the timely transmission of messages.

Such agencies may, by mutual agreement, decide matters and develop instructions relating to the technical maintenance and operation of the direct communications link and effect arrangements to improve the operation of the link.

6. The technical parameters of the telegraph circuits of the link and of the terminal equipment, as well as the maintenance of such circuits and equipment, shall be in accordance with CCITT and CCIR recommendations.

Transmission and reception of messages over the direct communications link shall be effected in accordance with applicable recommendations of international telegraph and radio communications regulations, as well as with mutually agreed instructions.

7. The costs of the direct communications link shall be borne as follows:

a. The USSR shall pay the full cost of leasing the portion of the telegraph circuit from Moscow to Helsinki and 50 percent of the cost of leasing the portion of the telegraph circuit from Helsinki to London. The United States shall pay the full cost of leasing the portion of the telegraph circuit from Washington to London and 50 percent of the cost of leasing the portion of the telegraph circuit from London to Helsinki.

b. Payment of the cost of leasing the radio telegraph circuit between Washington and Moscow shall be effected without any transfer of payments between the parties. The USSR shall bear the expenses relating to the transmission of messages from Moscow to Washington. The United States shall bear the expenses relating to the transmission of messages from Washington to Moscow.

TREATY BANNING NUCLEAR WEAPON TESTS IN THE ATMOSPHERE, IN OUTER SPACE AND UNDER WATER

The Test Ban Treaty of 1963 prohibits nuclear weapons tests "or any other nuclear explosion" in the atmosphere, in outer space, and under water. While not banning tests underground, the Treaty does prohibit nuclear explosions in this environment if they cause "radioactive debris to be present outside the territorial limits of the State under whose jurisdiction or control" the explosions were conducted. In accepting limitations on testing, the nuclear powers accepted as a common goal "an end to the contamination of man's environment by radioactive substances."

Efforts to achieve a test ban agreement had extended over eight years. They involved complex technical problems of verification and the difficulties of reconciling deep-seated differences in approach to arms control and security. The uneven progress of the negotiations reflected, moreover, contemporaneous fluctuations in East-West political relationships.

Prior to SALT, no arms control measure since World War II had enlisted so intensely the sustained interest of the international community. The United States in November 1952, and the Soviet Union in August of the following year, exploded their first hydrogen devices, and rising concern about radioactive fallout and the prospect of even more powerful explosions spurred efforts to halt testing. Succeeding events gave the dangers of fallout concrete and human meaning. In March 1954 the United States exploded an experimental thermonuclear device at Bikini atoll, expected to have the power of eight million tons of TNT. The actual yield was almost double that predicted, about 15 megatons, and the area of dangerous fallout greatly exceeded original estimates. A Japanese fishing vessel, the *Lucky Dragon*, was accidentally contaminated, and its crew suffered from radiation sickness, as did the inhabitants of an atoll in the area. In another such accident, radioactive rain containing debris from a Soviet hydrogen bomb test fell on Japan.

As knowledge of the nature and effects of fallout increased, and as it became apparent that no region was untouched by radioactive debris, the issue of continued nuclear tests drew widened and intensified public attention. Apprehension was expressed about the possibility of a cumulative contamination of the environment and of resultant genetic damage.

Efforts to negotiate an international agreement to end nuclear tests began in the Subcommittee of Five (the United States, the United Kingdom, Canada, France, and the Soviet Union) of the U.N. Disarmament Commission in May 1955, when the Soviet Union included discontinuance of weapons tests in its proposals.

Public interest in the course of the negotiations was active and sustained. In individual statements and proposals, and in international meetings, governments pressed for discontinuance of nuclear tests. A dozen resolutions of the General Assembly addressed the issue, repeatedly urging conclusion of an agreement to ban tests under a system of international controls.

Test Ban and General Disarmament

The relation of a test ban to other aspects of disarmament was for a time a troubling issue. The initial Soviet proposal of a test ban on May 10, 1955, was part of a comprehensive plan to reduce conventional forces and armaments and to eliminate nuclear weapons. Later that year, in the General Assembly, the Soviet Union advocated a separate test ban. The three Western powers, over the next three years, made discontinuance of tests contingent on progress in other measures of arms control, particularly a cut-off in the production of fissionable materials for weapons and safeguards against surprise attack. They insisted that a test ban could not be enforced "in the absence of more general control agreements."

In January 1959 the United States and the United Kingdom dropped the linkage between a test ban and other arms control agreements; France, however, did not. The French continued to maintain that until there was agreement on nuclear disarmament -- including an end to weapons production, reconversion of stocks, and a ban on possession and use -- French plans to conduct tests would go forward. The Soviet Union abruptly reversed its position in June 1961, when Premier Khrushchev declared during his meeting with President Kennedy in Vienna that the test-ban question must be linked with general and complete disarmament. The Soviet Union refused to modify this position until November, when it proposed a separate test ban with no controls whatever, pending agreement on general and complete disarmament.

Verification

The central and most persistent barrier to a Treaty on cessation of tests, however, was the issue of verifying compliance, of agreeing to establish a system of controls and inspection -- particularly with regard to underground explosions -- that could guarantee against testing in secret. The Western powers were determined to ensure that no agreement would be vulnerable to clandestine violation. In test-ban negotiations, as well as in other arms control efforts, they considered that it would be dangerous to their security to accept simple pledges without the means of knowing that they would be observed.

It was further believed that such pledges would mislead concerned world opinion with illusions of secure progress toward disarmament.

Writing to President Eisenhower on October 17, 1956, Premier Bulganin had stated the fundamental Soviet position. "Since any explosion of an atomic or hydrogen bomb cannot, in the present state of scientific knowledge, be produced without being recorded in other countries," there could be an immediate agreement to prohibit tests without any provision for international control. He said:

> Would not the best guarantee against the violation of such an agreement be the mere fact that secret testing of nuclear weapons is impossible and that consequently a government undertaking the solemn obligation to stop making tests could not violate it without exposing itself to the entire world as the violator of an international agreement?

The Western countries were not convinced that existing technology for detecting nuclear explosions was adequate to monitor compliance, or that the mere force of world opinion would provide insurance against violations. In his response, President Eisenhower stated that "to be effective, and not simply a mirage," disarmament plans required systems of inspection and control. And in a public statement a few days later, he said:

> A simple agreement to stop H-bomb tests cannot be regarded as automatically self-enforcing on the unverified assumption that such tests can instantly and surely be detected. It is true that tests of very

large weapons would probably be detected when they occur . . . It is, however, impossible -- in my view of the vast Soviet landmass that can screen future tests -- to have positive assurance of such detection, except in the case of the largest weapons.

On June 14, 1957, the Soviet Union for the first time offered test ban proposals that included international control. The proposals were very general: establishment of an international supervisory commission and control posts, on the basis of reciprocity, on the territories of the three nuclear powers and in the Pacific Ocean area. The Western powers suggested that a group of experts work out the details of a control system, while the delegates considered a temporary test ban in relation to other disarmament measures.

The Soviet Union continued to press for an immediate suspension of tests, and the United States for agreement on a control system as a necessary accompanying measure. In March 1958 the Soviet Union announced that it was discontinuing all tests and appealed to the parliaments of other nuclear powers to take similar action. It added, however, that the Soviet Union would "naturally be free" to resume testing if other nuclear powers did not stop their tests. Succeeding Bulganin as Premier, Nikita Khrushchev called on President Eisenhower to end tests. President Eisenhower rejected the proposal, stating that some tests could be conducted "under conditions of secrecy," and renewed the proposal for an experts' group to study control problems. After further summit correspondence and diplomatic exchange, Khrushchev agreed to a conference of experts. Meanwhile U.S. and British tests continued.

The Geneva Conference of Experts met in July and August 1958, attended by representatives from the United States, the United Kingdom, Canada, France, the Soviet Union, Poland, Czechoslovakia, and Romania. They agreed on the technical characteristics of a control system to monitor a ban on tests in the atmosphere, under water, and underground. Their report proposed an elaborate network of 170-180 land control posts and 10 shipborne posts, as well as regular and special aircraft flights. It recognized that on-site inspections would be needed to determine whether some seismic events were caused by earthquakes or explosions.

The United States and Britain welcomed the experts' report and declared their willingness to negotiate an agreement for suspension of tests and the establishment of an international control system on the basis of the report. They were prepared to suspend tests for a year from the beginning of negotiations unless the Soviet Union resumed testing. The suspension could continue on a year-to-year basis, provided that the inspection system was installed and functioning, and "satisfactory progress" was being made on major arms-control measures. Premier Khrushchev's response was to attack the United States and U.K. for continuing their tests, and for linking the test ban to other matters. He announced that the Soviet Union was released from its self-imposed pledge. The USSR resumed tests, and the series continued until November 3.

The negotiating powers refrained from testing for the next three years. The "moratorium" was marked by several public statements of intent, by the United States, the United Kingdom, and the Soviet Union, in varying degrees of specificity and with various caveats. At the end of December 1959 President Eisenhower announced that the United States would no longer consider itself bound by the "voluntary moratorium" but would give advance notice if it decided to resume testing. The Soviet Government stated on August 28 and Premier Khrushchev repeated on December 30, 1959, that the Soviet Union would not resume testing if the Western powers did not. France conducted its first test on February 13, 1960, two more later in the year, and a fourth on April 25, 1961. On May 15, 1961, the Soviet Government stated that if France continued testing, the Soviet Union might be compelled to test. On August 30, 1961, although neither the United States nor the United Kingdom had resumed testing and France had not continued to test, the Soviet Union announced that it would resume testing. It did so on September 1, thus ending the moratorium. The United States resumed testing two weeks later.

Throughout the various conferences and exchanges on a test ban, the complexity of the central problem brought successive deadlocks, break-offs, and renewals of discussion, shifts in position, searches for compromise and new approaches, and for new techniques of verifications, and successive suspensions and resumptions of tests. The United States continued to be unwilling to accept the Soviet basic

proposition that a test ban could be agreed to and controls instituted subsequently, or to accept indefinite test suspensions that were tantamount to endorsing an uncontrolled prohibition. New data from U.S. underground tests, moreover, had shown that techniques recommended earlier for distinguishing between explosions and earthquakes were less effective than had been believed and that a reliable control system to monitor seismic events that registered under 4.75 on the Richter scale required further research and confirmed the need for on-site inspections.

Among the salient points of disagreement on a control system were:

The Veto. The Soviet Union initially sought to have all substantive operations of the system subject to veto; the United States insisted that the fact-finding process of inspection, to be effective, must be as automatic as possible.

On-Site Inspections. The Soviet Union placed a limit on permitted inspections in its territory, refusing to allow more than three per year. The United States and the United Kingdom held that the number must be determined by scientific fact and detection capability. As new information became available, the United States eventually indicated that it could accept a minimum of seven, but the Soviet Union rejected this quota. There was disagreement, as well, over the size of the area to be inspected, the nationality and composition of inspection teams, and the criteria for identifying events that required inspection.

Control Posts. Although the United States and the United Kingdom had originally proposed that the control posts should be internationally owned and operated, they later agreed to national ownership and operation of the posts, as the Soviet Union insisted, with international monitoring and supervision.

There were unresolved differences about the number and location of posts and about the number and location of the automatic seismic observation stations ("black boxes") with which it was proposed to supplement them. The Soviet Union also claimed that national control posts and automatic observation devices made any international inspection unnecessary, a position that the United States and the United Kingdom were not willing to accept.

The Organization of the Control Commission. In March 1961 the Soviet Union recommended replacing the single administrator of the proposed Control Commission with a "troika," a tripartite administrative council, consisting of one neutral, one Western, and one Communist member (a proposal paralleling the Soviet effort the previous year to replace the U.N. Secretary-General with a tripartite commission). This three-headed administration would be able to function even in routine matters only by unanimous agreement, an arrangement that the Western powers argued was unworkable and would make the Control Commission helpless. The Soviet Union eventually abandoned this demand.

The effort to achieve a test ban, and to resolve the stubborn issues involved, had been pursued in a wide variety of channels. Successive General Assembly sessions had debated the issue. It had been a major item on the agenda of the U.N. Disarmament Commission and its Subcommittee of Five (later ten). The United States, the United Kingdom, and the Soviet Union had engaged in a long tripartite effort --The Conference on the Discontinuance of Nuclear Weapon Tests -- in almost continuous session in Geneva from October 31, 1958, to January 29, 1962. Under its auspices three technical working groups of experts had investigated and reported on various aspects of control: one on high altitude tests, another on underground tests, the third on seismic research programs to improve detection capabilities.

After the three-power conference adjourned in January 1962, unable to complete the drafting of a Treaty because of the Soviet Union's claim that national means of detection were adequate for all environments, the principal forum for negotiations became the newly formed Eighteen-Nation Disarmament Committee (ENDC), which began its meetings at Geneva under the aegis of the General Assembly in March 1962. On the U.S. side, overall direction of the negotiations was assumed by William C. Foster, first Director of the newly created U.S. Arms Control and Disarmament Agency. Soviet insistence that the West accept Premier Khrushchev's quota of three annual inspections, however, brought these talks to an impasse. The United States and the United Kingdom, in high-level correspondence with the Soviet Union, then sought to arrange three-power talks. Finally, on June 10, 1963, President Kennedy announced

that agreement had been reached to hold three-power meetings on the test ban in Moscow. He also pledged that the United States would not be the first to resume tests in the atmosphere.

At this time a shift of Soviet interest to a ban that did not deal with underground tests emerged, although the Soviet Union had rejected an Anglo-American proposal for an agreement of this kind the year before. Premier Khrushchev disclosed this in a speech on July 2, 1963, when he called for an agreement outlawing tests in the atmosphere, in outer space, and under water -- environments where both sides agreed their existing verification systems could adequately police a ban.

The three-power meetings began on July 15. The long years of discussion had clarified views and greatly reduced areas of disagreement, and a Treaty was negotiated within 10 days. It was initialed on July 25 and formally signed at Moscow on August 5, 1963, by U.S. Secretary of State Dean Rusk, the Foreign Minister of the USSR, Andrei Gromyko, and the Foreign Minister of the U.K., Lord Home. On September 24, after extensive hearings and almost three weeks of floor debate, the Senate consented to ratification of the Treaty by a vote of 80 to 19. It was ratified by President Kennedy on October 7, 1963, and entered into force on October 10 when the three original signatories deposited their instruments of ratification.

The parties to the Treaty undertake "not to carry out any nuclear weapon test explosion, or any other nuclear explosion," in the atmosphere, under water, or in outer space, or in any other environment if the explosion would cause radioactive debris to be present outside the borders of the state conducting the explosion. As explained by Acting Secretary of State Ball in a subsequent report to President Kennedy, "The phrase 'any other nuclear explosion' includes explosions for peaceful purposes. Such explosions are prohibited by the Treaty because of the difficulty of differentiating between weapon test explosions and peaceful explosions without additional controls."

The Treaty is of unlimited duration. Article II notes that any party may propose amendments, and that, if so requested by one-third or more of the states Party, the Depositary Governments are to convene a conference to consider the

amendment. This article stipulates that any
amendment must be approved by a majority of
Parties, including the three Original Parties.
Article III opens the Treaty to all states, and most
of the countries of the world are parties to it. The
Treaty has not been signed by France or by the
People's Republic of China.

In August 1988, six countries (Mexico,
Indonesia, Peru, Sri Lanka, Yugoslavia, and
Venezuela) presented a proposal to the three
Depositary Governments to amend the LTBT and
to have a special amendment conference to
consider this proposal. Their proposal was to
extend the LTBT's prohibitions to all
environments, transforming the LTBT into a
comprehensive test ban. By late March 1989 the
Depositary Governments had received the
requisite number of requests, in accordance with
Article II of the Treaty, to convene such a
conference for consideration of the proposed
amendment. The Conference was held in
January 1991. The United States, strongly
opposed to using the LTBT as a vehicle for
negotiating a comprehensive test ban, made it
clear to all participants that it would block any
attempt to amend the LTBT by consensus.

TREATY BANNING NUCLEAR WEAPON TESTS IN THE ATMOSPHERE, IN OUTER SPACE AND UNDER WATER

Signed at Moscow August 5, 1963
Ratification advised by U.S. Senate September 24, 1963
Ratified by U.S. President October 7, 1963
U.S. ratification deposited at Washington, London, and Moscow October 10, 1963
Proclaimed by U.S. President October 10, 1963
Entered into force October 10, 1963

The Governments of the United States of America, the United Kingdom of Great Britain and Northern Ireland, and the Union of Soviet Socialist Republics, hereinafter referred to as the "Original Parties,"

Proclaiming as their principal aim the speediest possible achievement of an agreement on general and complete disarmament under strict international control in accordance with the objectives of the United Nations which would put an end to the armaments race and eliminate the incentive to the production and testing of all kinds of weapons, including nuclear weapons,

Seeking to achieve the discontinuance of all test explosions of nuclear weapons for all time, determined to continue negotiations to this end, and desiring to put an end to the contamination of man's environment by radioactive substances,

Have agreed as follows:

Article I

1. Each of the Parties to this Treaty undertakes to prohibit, to prevent, and not to carry out any nuclear weapon test explosion, or any other nuclear explosion, at any place under its jurisdiction or control:

(a) in the atmosphere; beyond its limits, including outer space; or under water, including territorial waters or high seas; or

(b) in any other environment if such explosion causes radioactive debris to be present outside the territorial limits of the State under whose jurisdiction or control such explosion is conducted. It is understood in this connection that the provisions of this subparagraph are without prejudice to the conclusion of a Treaty resulting in the permanent banning of all nuclear test explosions, including all such explosions underground, the conclusion of which, as the Parties have stated in the Preamble to this Treaty, they seek to achieve.

2. Each of the Parties to this Treaty undertakes furthermore to refrain from causing, encouraging, or in any way participating in, the carrying out of any nuclear weapon test explosion, or any other nuclear explosion, anywhere which would take place in any of the environments described, or have the effect referred to, in paragraph 1 of this Article.

Article II

1. Any Party may propose amendments to this Treaty. The text of any proposed amendment shall be submitted to the Depositary Governments which shall circulate it to all Parties to this Treaty. Thereafter, if requested to do so by one-third or more of the Parties, the Depositary Governments shall convene a conference, to which they shall invite all the Parties, to consider such amendment.

2. Any amendment to this Treaty must be approved by a majority of the votes of all the Parties to this Treaty, including the votes of all of the Original Parties. The amendment shall enter into force for all Parties upon the deposit of instruments of ratification by a majority of all the Parties, including the instruments of ratification of all of the Original Parties.

Article III

1. This Treaty shall be open to all States for signature. Any State which does not sign this Treaty before its entry into force in accordance with paragraph 3 of this Article may accede to it at any time.

2. This Treaty shall be subject to ratification by signatory States. Instruments of ratification and instruments of accession shall be deposited with the Governments of the Original Parties -- the United States of America, the United Kingdom of Great Britain and Northern Ireland, and the Union of Soviet Socialist Republics -- which are hereby designated the Depositary Governments.

3. This Treaty shall enter into force after its ratification by all the Original Parties and the deposit of their instruments of ratification.

4. For States whose instruments of ratification or accession are deposited subsequent to the entry into force of this Treaty, it shall enter into force on the date of the deposit of their instruments of ratification or accession.

5. The Depositary Governments shall promptly inform all signatory and acceding States of the date of each signature, the date of deposit of each instrument of ratification of and accession to this Treaty, the date of its entry into force, and the date of receipt of any requests for conferences or other notices.

6. This Treaty shall be registered by the Depositary Governments pursuant to Article 102 of the Charter of the United Nations.

Article IV

This Treaty shall be of unlimited duration.

Each Party shall in exercising its national sovereignty have the right to withdraw from the Treaty if it decides that extraordinary events, related to the subject matter of this Treaty, have jeopardized the supreme interests of its country. It shall give notice of such withdrawal to all other Parties to the Treaty three months in advance.

Article V

This Treaty, of which the English and Russian texts are equally authentic, shall be deposited in the archives of the Depositary Governments. Duly certified copies of this Treaty shall be transmitted by the Depositary Governments to the Governments of the signatory and acceding States.

IN WITNESS WHEREOF the undersigned, duly authorized, have signed this Treaty.

DONE in triplicate at the city of Moscow the fifth day of August, one thousand nine hundred and sixty-three.

For the Government of the United States of America

DEAN RUSK

For the Government of the United Kingdom of Great Britain and Northern Ireland

HOME

For the Government of the Union of Soviet Socialist Republics

A. GROMYKO

Limited Test Ban Treaty

Country	Date[1] of Signature	Date of Deposit[1] of Ratification	Date of Deposit[1] of Accession
Afghanistan	08/08/63	03/12/64	
Algeria	08/14/63		
Argentina	08/08/63		11/21/86
Australia	08/08/63	11/12/63	
Austria	09/11/63	07/17/64	
Bahamas, The			07/16/76
Bangladesh			03/11/85
Belgium	08/08/63	03/01/66	
Benin	08/27/63	12/15/64	
Bhutan			06/08/78
Bolivia	08/08/63	08/04/65	
Botswana			01/05/68
Brazil	08/08/63	12/15/64	
Bulgaria	08/08/63	11/13/63	
Burkina Faso	08/30/63		
Burma	08/14/63	11/15/63	
Burundi	10/04/63		
Byelorussian S.S.R.[2]	10/08/63	12/16/63	
Cameroon	08/27/63		
Canada	08/08/63	01/28/64	
Cape Verde			10/24/79
Central African Republic			12/22/64
Chad	08/26/63	03/01/65	
Chile	08/08/63	10/06/65	
China (Taiwan)[4]	08/23/63	05/18/64	
Colombia	08/16/63	10/17/85	
Costa Rica	08/09/63	07/10/67	
Cote d'Ivoire	09/05/63	07/05/65	
Cyprus	08/08/63	04/15/65	
Czechoslovakia	08/08/63	10/14/63	
Denmark	08/09/63	01/15/64	
Dominican Republic	09/16/63	06/03/64	
Ecuador	09/27/63	05/06/64	
Egypt	08/08/63	01/10/64	
El Salvador	08/21/63	12/03/64	
Ethiopia	08/09/63		
Fiji			07/18/72
Finland	08/08/63	01/09/64	
Gabon	09/10/63	02/20/64	
Gambia, The			04/27/65
German Democratic Republic	08/08/63	12/30/63	
Germany, Federal Republic of	08/19/63	12/01/64	
Ghana	08/08/63	11/27/63	

Limited Test Ban Treaty -- Continued

Country	Date[1] of Signature	Date of Deposit[1] of Ratification	Date of Deposit[1] of Accession
Greece	08/08/63	12/18/63	
Guatemala	09/23/63	01/06/64	
Haiti	10/09/63		
Honduras	08/08/63	10/02/64	
Hungary	08/08/63	10/21/63	
Iceland	08/12/63	04/29/64	
India	08/08/63	10/10/63	
Indonesia	08/23/63	01/20/64	
Iran	08/08/63	05/05/64	
Iraq	08/13/63	11/30/64	
Ireland	08/08/63	12/18/63	
Israel	08/08/63	01/15/64	
Italy	08/08/63	12/10/64	
Jamaica	08/13/63		11/22/91
Japan	08/14/63	06/15/64	
Jordan	08/12/63	05/29/64	
Kenya			06/10/65
Korea, Republic of	08/30/63	07/24/64	
Kuwait	08/20/63	05/20/65	
Laos	08/12/63	02/10/65	
Lebanon	08/12/63	05/14/65	
Liberia	08/08/63	05/19/64	
Libya	08/09/63	07/15/68	
Luxembourg	08/13/63	02/10/65	
Madagascar	09/23/63	03/15/65	
Malawi			11/26/64
Malaysia	08/08/63	07/15/64	
Mali	08/23/63		
Malta			11/25/64
Mauritania	09/13/63	04/06/64	
Mauritius			04/30/69
Mexico	08/08/63	12/27/63	
Mongolia	08/08/63	11/01/63	
Morocco	08/27/63	02/01/66	
Nepal	08/26/63	10/07/64	
Netherlands	08/09/63	09/14/64	
New Zealand	08/08/63	10/10/63	
Nicaragua	08/13/63	01/26/65	
Niger	09/24/63	07/03/64	
Nigeria	08/30/63	02/17/67	
Norway	08/09/63	11/21/63	
Pakistan	08/14/63		03/03/88
Panama	09/20/63	02/24/66	
Papua New Guinea			03/16/81
Paraguay	08/15/63		

Limited Test Ban Treaty -- Continued

Country	Date[1] of Signature	Date of Deposit[1] of Ratification	Date of Deposit[1] of Accession
Peru	08/23/63	07/20/64	
Philippines	08/08/63	11/10/65	
Poland	08/08/63	10/14/63	
Portugal	10/09/63		
Romania	08/08/63	12/12/63	
Rwanda	09/19/63	12/27/63	
San Marino	09/17/63	07/03/64	
Senegal	09/20/63	05/06/64	
Seychelles			03/12/85
Sierra Leone	09/04/63	02/21/64	
Singapore			07/12/68
Somalia	08/19/63		
South Africa			10/10/63
Spain	08/13/63	12/17/64	
Sri Lanka	08/22/63	02/05/64	
Sudan	08/09/63	03/04/66	
Swaziland			05/29/69
Sweden	08/12/63	12/09/63	
Switzerland	08/26/63	01/16/64	
Syria	08/13/63	06/01/64	
Tanzania	09/16/63	02/06/64	
Thailand	08/08/63	11/15/63	
Togo	09/18/63	12/07/64	
Tonga			07/07/71
Trinidad & Tobago	08/12/63	07/14/64	
Tunisia	08/08/63	05/26/65	
Turkey	08/09/63	07/08/65	
Uganda	08/29/63	03/24/64	
Ukrainian S.S.R.[2]	10/08/63	12/30/63	
Union of Soviet Socialist Republics	08/05/63	10/10/63	
United Kingdom	08/05/63	10/10/63	
United States	08/05/63	10/10/63	
Uruguay	08/12/63	02/25/63	
Venezuela	08/16/63	02/22/65	
Western Samoa	09/05/63	01/15/65	
Yemen Arab Republic (Sanaa)	08/13/63		
Yemen, People's Democratic Republic of (Aden)			06/01/79
Yugoslavia	08/08/63	01/15/64	

Limited Test Ban Treaty -- Continued

Country	Date[1] of Signature	Date of Deposit[1] of Ratification	Date of Deposit[1] of Accession
Zaire	08/08/63	10/28/63	
Zambia			1/11/65
Total[3]	108	94	23

See footnotes on page 350.

TREATY ON PRINCIPLES GOVERNING THE ACTIVITIES OF STATES IN THE EXPLORATION AND USE OF OUTER SPACE, INCLUDING THE MOON AND OTHER CELESTIAL BODIES

The Outer Space Treaty, as it is known, was the second of the so-called "nonarmament" treaties; its concepts and some of its provisions were modeled on its predecessor, the Antarctic Treaty. Like that Treaty it sought to prevent "a new form of colonial competition" and the possible damage that self-seeking exploitation might cause.

In early 1957, even before the launching of Sputnik in October, developments in rocketry led the United States to propose international verification of the testing of space objects. The development of an inspection system for outer space was part of a Western proposal for partial disarmament put forward in August 1957. The Soviet Union, however, which was in the midst of testing its first ICBM and was about to orbit its first Earth satellite, did not accept these proposals.

Between 1959 and 1962 the Western powers made a series of proposals to bar the use of outer space for military purposes. Their successive plans for general and complete disarmament included provisions to ban the orbiting and stationing in outer space of weapons of mass destruction. Addressing the General Assembly on September 22, 1960, President Eisenhower proposed that the principles of the Antarctic Treaty be applied to outer space and celestial bodies.

Soviet plans for general and complete disarmament between 1960 and 1962 included provisions for ensuring the peaceful use of outer space. The Soviet Union, however, would not separate outer space from other disarmament issues, nor would it agree to restrict outer space to peaceful uses unless U.S. foreign bases at which short-range and medium-range missiles were stationed were eliminated also.

The Western powers declined to accept the Soviet approach; the linkage, they held, would upset the military balance and weaken the security of the West.

After the signing of the Limited Test Ban Treaty, the Soviet Union's position changed. It ceased to link an agreement on outer space with the question of foreign bases. On September 19, 1963, Foreign Minister Gromyko told the General Assembly that the Soviet Union wished to conclude an agreement banning the orbiting of objects carrying nuclear weapons. Ambassador Stevenson stated that the United States had no intention of orbiting weapons of mass destruction, installing them on celestial bodies or stationing them in outer space. The General Assembly unanimously adopted a resolution on October 17, 1963, welcoming the Soviet and U.S. statements and calling upon all states to refrain from introducing weapons of mass destruction into outer space.

The United States supported the resolution, despite the absence of any provisions for verification; the capabilities of its space-tracking systems, it was estimated, were adequate for detecting launchings and devices in orbit.

Seeking to sustain the momentum for arms control agreements, the United States in 1965 and 1966 pressed for a Treaty that would give further substance to the U.N. resolution.

On June 16, 1966, both the United States and the Soviet Union submitted draft treaties. The U.S. draft dealt only with celestial bodies; the Soviet draft covered the whole outer space environment. The United States accepted the Soviet position on the scope of the Treaty, and by September agreement had been reached in discussions at Geneva on most Treaty provisions. Differences on the few remaining issues -- chiefly involving access to facilities on celestial bodies, reporting on space activities, and the use of military equipment and personnel in space exploration -- were satisfactorily resolved in private consultations during the General Assembly session by December.

On the 19th of that month the General Assembly approved by acclamation a resolution commending the Treaty. It was opened for signature at Washington, London, and Moscow on January 27, 1967. On April 25 the Senate gave unanimous consent to its ratification, and the Treaty entered into force on October 10, 1967.

The substance of the arms control provisions is in Article IV. This article restricts activities in two ways:

First, it contains an undertaking not to place in orbit around the Earth, install on the moon or any other celestial body, or otherwise station in outer space, nuclear or any other weapons of mass destruction.

Second, it limits the use of the moon and other celestial bodies exclusively to peaceful purposes and expressly prohibits their use for establishing military bases, installation, or fortifications; testing weapons of any kind; or conducting military maneuvers.

After the Treaty entered into force, the United States and the Soviet Union collaborated in jointly planned and manned space enterprises.

TREATY ON PRINCIPLES GOVERNING THE ACTIVITIES OF STATES IN THE EXPLORATION AND USE OF OUTER SPACE, INCLUDING THE MOON AND OTHER CELESTIAL BODIES

Signed at Washington, London, Moscow, January 27, 1967
Ratification advised by U.S. Senate April 25, 1967
Ratified by U.S. President May 24, 1967
U.S. ratification deposited at Washington, London, and Moscow October 10, 1967
Proclaimed by U.S. President October 10, 1967
Entered into force October 10, 1967

The States Parties to this Treaty,

Inspired by the great prospects opening up before mankind as a result of man's entry into outer space,

Recognizing the common interest of all mankind in the progress of the exploration and use of outer space for peaceful purposes,

Believing that the exploration and use of outer space should be carried on for the benefit of all peoples irrespective of the degree of their economic or scientific development,

Desiring to contribute to broad international co-operation in the scientific as well as the legal aspects of the exploration and use of outer space for peaceful purposes,

Believing that such co-operation will contribute to the development of mutual understanding and to the strengthening of friendly relations between States and peoples,

Recalling resolution 1962 (XVIII), entitled "Declaration of Legal Principles Governing the Activities of States in the Exploration and Use of Outer Space," which was adopted unanimously by the United Nations General Assembly on 13 December 1963,

Recalling resolution 1884 (XVIII), calling upon States to refrain from placing in orbit around the Earth any objects carrying nuclear weapons or any other kinds of weapons of mass destruction or from installing such weapons on celestial bodies, which was adopted unanimously by the United Nations General Assembly on 17 October 1963,

Taking account of United Nations General Assembly resolution 110 (II) of 3 November 1947, which condemned propaganda designed or likely to provoke or encourage any threat to the peace, breach of the peace or act of aggression, and considering that the aforementioned resolution is applicable to outer space,

Convinced that a Treaty on Principles Governing the Activities of States in the Exploration and Use of Outer Space, including the Moon and Other Celestial Bodies, will further the Purposes and Principles of the Charter of the United Nations,

Have agreed on the following:

Article I

The exploration and use of outer space, including the moon and other celestial bodies, shall be carried out for the benefit and in the interests of all countries, irrespective of their degree of economic or scientific development, and shall be the province of all mankind.

Outer space, including the moon and other celestial bodies, shall be free for exploration and use by all States without discrimination of any kind, on a basis of equality and in accordance with international law, and there shall be free access to all areas of celestial bodies.

There shall be freedom of scientific investigation in outer space, including the moon and other celestial bodies, and States shall facilitate and encourage international co-operation in such investigation.

Article II

Outer space, including the moon and other celestial bodies, is not subject to national appropriation by claim of sovereignty, by means of use or occupation, or by any other means.

Article III

States Parties to the Treaty shall carry on activities in the exploration and use of outer space, including the moon and other celestial bodies, in accordance with international law, including the Charter of the United Nations, in the interest of maintaining international peace and security and promoting international co-operation and understanding.

Article IV

States Parties to the Treaty undertake not to place in orbit around the Earth any objects carrying nuclear weapons or any other kinds of weapons of mass destruction, install such weapons on celestial bodies, or station such weapons in outer space in any other manner.

The Moon and other celestial bodies shall be used by all States Parties to the Treaty exclusively for peaceful purposes. The establishment of military bases, installations and fortifications, the testing of any type of weapons and the conduct of military maneuvers on celestial bodies shall be forbidden. The use of military personnel for scientific research or for any other peaceful purposes shall not be prohibited. The use of any equipment or facility necessary for peaceful exploration of the Moon and other celestial bodies shall also not be prohibited.

Article V

States Parties to the Treaty shall regard astronauts as envoys of mankind in outer space and shall render to them all possible assistance in the event of accident, distress, or emergency landing on the territory of another State Party or on the high seas. When astronauts make such a landing, they shall be safely and promptly returned to the State of registry of their space vehicle.

In carrying on activities in outer space and on celestial bodies, the astronauts of one State Party shall render all possible assistance to the astronauts of other States Parties.

States Parties to the Treaty shall immediately inform the other States Parties to the Treaty or the Secretary-General of the United Nations of any phenomena they discover in outer space, including the Moon and other celestial bodies, which could constitute a danger to the life or health of astronauts.

Article VI

States Parties to the Treaty shall bear international responsibility for national activities in outer space, including the Moon and other celestial bodies, whether such activities are carried on by governmental agencies or by non-governmental entities, and for assuring that

national activities are carried out in conformity with the provisions set forth in the present Treaty. The activities of non-governmental entities in outer space, including the Moon and other celestial bodies, shall require authorization and continuing supervision by the appropriate State Party to the Treaty. When activities are carried on in outer space, including the Moon and other celestial bodies, by an international organization, responsibility for compliance with this Treaty shall be borne both by the international organization and by the States Parties to the Treaty participating in such organization.

Article VII

Each State Party to the Treaty that launches or procures the launching of an object into outer space, including the Moon and other celestial bodies, and each State Party from whose territory or facility an object is launched, is internationally liable for damage to another State Party to the Treaty or to its natural or juridical persons by such object or its component parts on the Earth, in air space or in outer space, including the Moon and other celestial bodies.

Article VIII

A State Party to the Treaty on whose registry an object launched into outer space is carried shall retain jurisdiction and control over such object, and over any personnel thereof, while in outer space or on a celestial body. Ownership of objects launched into outer space, including objects landed or constructed on a celestial body, and of their component parts, is not affected by their presence in outer space or on a celestial body or by their return to the Earth. Such objects or component parts found beyond the limits of the State Party to the Treaty on whose registry they are carried shall be returned to that State Party, which shall, upon request, furnish identifying data prior to their return.

Article IX

In the exploration and use of outer space, including the Moon and other celestial bodies, States Parties to the Treaty shall be guided by the principle of co-operation and mutual assistance and shall conduct all their activities in outer space, including the Moon and other celestial bodies, with due regard to the corresponding interests of all other States Parties to the Treaty. States Parties to the Treaty shall pursue studies of outer space, including the Moon and other celestial bodies, and conduct exploration of them so as to avoid their harmful contamination and also adverse changes in the environment of the Earth resulting from the introduction of extraterrestrial matter and, where necessary, shall adopt appropriate measures for this purpose. If a State Party to the Treaty has reason to believe that an activity or experiment planned by it or its nationals in outer space, including the Moon and other celestial bodies, would cause potentially harmful interference with activities of other States Parties in the peaceful exploration and use of outer space, including the Moon and other celestial bodies, it shall undertake appropriate international consultations before proceeding with any such activity or experiment. A State Party to the Treaty which has reason to believe that an activity or experiment planned by another State Party in outer space, including the Moon and other celestial bodies, would cause potentially harmful interference with activities in the peaceful exploration and use of outer space, including the Moon and other celestial bodies, may request consultation concerning the activity or experiment.

Article X

In order to promote international co-operation in the exploration and use of outer space, including the Moon and other celestial bodies, in conformity with the purposes of this Treaty, the States Parties to the Treaty shall consider on a basis of equality any requests by other States Parties to the Treaty to be afforded an opportunity to observe the flight of space objects launched by those States.

The nature of such an opportunity for observation and the conditions under which it could be afforded shall be determined by agreement between the States concerned.

Article XI

In order to promote international co-operation in the peaceful exploration and use of outer space, States Parties to the Treaty conducting activities in outer space, including the Moon and other celestial bodies, agree to inform the Secretary-General of the United Nations as well as the public and the international scientific community,

to the greatest extent feasible and practicable, of the nature, conduct, locations and results of such activities. On receiving the said information, the Secretary-General of the United Nations should be prepared to disseminate it immediately and effectively.

Article XII

All stations, installations, equipment and space vehicles on the Moon and other celestial bodies shall be open to representatives of other States Parties to the Treaty on a basis of reciprocity. Such representatives shall give reasonable advance notice of a projected visit, in order that appropriate consultations may be held and that maximum precautions may be taken to assure safety and to avoid interference with normal operations in the facility to be visited.

Article XIII

The provisions of this Treaty shall apply to the activities of States Parties to the Treaty in the exploration and use of outer space, including the Moon and other celestial bodies, whether such activities are carried on by a single State Party to the Treaty or jointly with other States, including cases where they are carried on within the framework of international intergovernmental organizations.

Any practical questions arising in connection with activities carried on by international inter-governmental organizations in the exploration and use of outer space, including the Moon and other celestial bodies, shall be resolved by the States Parties to the Treaty either with the appropriate international organization or with one or more States members of that international organization, which are Parties to this Treaty.

Article XIV

1. This Treaty shall be open to all States for signature. Any State which does not sign this Treaty before its entry into force in accordance with paragraph 3 of this article may accede to it at any time.

2. This Treaty shall be subject to ratification by signatory States. Instruments of ratification and instruments of accession shall be deposited with the Governments of the United States of America,

the United Kingdom of Great Britain and Northern Ireland and the Union of Soviet Socialist Republics, which are hereby designated the Depositary Governments.

3. This Treaty shall enter into force upon the deposit of instruments of ratification by five Governments including the Governments designated as Depositary Governments under this Treaty.

4. For States whose instruments of ratification or accession are deposited subsequent to the entry into force of this Treaty, it shall enter into force on the date of the deposit of their instruments of ratification or accession.

5. The Depositary Governments shall promptly inform all signatory and acceding States of the date of each signature, the date of deposit of each instrument of ratification of and accession to this Treaty, the date of its entry into force and other notices.

6. This Treaty shall be registered by the Depositary Governments pursuant to Article 102 of the Charter of the United Nations.

Article XV

Any State Party to the Treaty may propose amendments to this Treaty. Amendments shall enter into force for each State Party to the Treaty accepting the amendments upon their acceptance by a majority of the States Parties to the Treaty and thereafter for each remaining State Party to the Treaty on the date of acceptance by it.

Article XVI

Any State Party to the Treaty may give notice of its withdrawal from the Treaty one year after its entry into force by written notification to the Depositary Governments. Such withdrawal shall take effect one year from the date of receipt of this notification.

Article XVII

This Treaty, of which the English, Russian, French, Spanish and Chinese texts are equally authentic, shall be deposited in the archives of the Depositary Governments. Duly certified copies of this Treaty shall be transmitted by the Depositary Governments to the Governments of the signatory and acceding States.

IN WITNESS WHEREOF the undersigned, duly authorized, have signed this Treaty.

DONE in triplicate, at the cities of Washington, London and Moscow, this twenty-seventh day of January one thousand nine hundred sixty-seven.

OUTER SPACE TREATY

Country	Date[1] of Signature	Date of Deposit[1] of Ratification	Date of Deposit[1] of Accession
Afghanistan	01/27/67	03/21/88	
Antigua and Barbuda			01/01/81
Argentina	01/27/67	03/26/69	
Australia	01/27/67	10/10/67	
Austria	02/20/67	02/26/68	
Bahamas, The			08/11/76
Bangladesh			01/17/86
Barbados			09/12/68
Belgium	01/27/67	03/30/73	
Benin			06/19/86
Bolivia	01/27/67		
Botswana	01/27/67		
Brazil	01/30/67	03/05/69	
Brunei			01/18/84
Bulgaria	01/27/67		03/28/67
Burkina Faso	03/03/67	06/18/68	
Burma	05/22/67	03/18/70	
Burundi	01/27/67		
Byelorussian S.S.R.[2]	02/10/67	10/31/67	
Cameroon	01/27/67		
Canada	01/27/67	10/10/67	
Central African Republic	01/27/67		
Chile	01/27/67	10/08/81	
China, People's Republic of			12/30/83
China (Taiwan)[4]	01/27/67	07/24/70	
Colombia	01/27/67		
Cuba			06/03/77
Cyprus	01/27/67	07/05/72	
Czechoslovakia	01/27/67	05/11/67	
Denmark	01/27/67	10/10/67	
Dominica			11/8/78
Dominican Republic	01/27/67	11/21/68	
Ecuador	01/27/67	03/07/69	
Egypt	01/27/67	10/10/67	
El Salvador	01/27/67	01/15/69	
Ethiopia	01/27/67		
Fiji			07/14/72
Finland	01/27/67	07/12/67	
France	09/25/67	08/05/70	
Gambia, The	06/02/67		
German Democratic Republic	01/27/67	02/02/67	
Germany, Federal Republic of	01/27/67	02/10/71	

OUTER SPACE TREATY -- Continued

Country	Date[1] of Signature	Date of Deposit[1] of Ratification	Date of Deposit[1] of Accession
Ghana	01/27/67		
Greece	01/27/67	01/19/71	
Grenada			02/07/74
Guinea-Bissau			08/20/76
Guyana	02/03/67		
Haiti	01/27/67		
Holy See	04/05/67		
Honduras	01/27/67		
Hungary	01/27/67	06/26/67	
Iceland	01/27/67	02/05/68	
India	03/03/67	01/18/82	
Indonesia	01/27/67		
Iran	01/27/67		
Iraq	02/27/67	12/04/68	
Ireland	01/27/67	07/17/68	
Israel	01/27/67	02/18/77	
Italy	01/27/67	05/04/72	
Jamaica	06/29/67	08/06/70	
Japan	01/27/67	10/10/67	
Jordan	02/02/67		
Kenya			01/19/84
Korea, Republic of	01/27/67	10/13/67	
Kuwait			06/07/72
Laos	01/27/67	11/27/72	
Lebanon	02/23/67	03/31/69	
Lesotho	01/27/67		
Libya			07/03/68
Luxembourg	01/27/67		
Madagascar			08/22/68
Malaysia	02/20/67		
Mali			06/11/68
Mauritius			04/07/69
Mexico	01/27/67	01/31/68	
Mongolia	01/27/67	10/10/67	
Morocco			12/21/67
Nepal	02/03/67	10/10/67	
Netherlands	02/10/67	10/10/69	
New Zealand	01/27/67	05/31/68	
Nicaragua	01/27/67		
Niger	02/01/67	04/17/67	
Nigeria			11/14/67
Norway	02/03/67	07/01/69	

OUTER SPACE TREATY -- Continued

Country	Date[1] of Signature	Date of Deposit[1] of Ratification	Date of Deposit[1] of Accession
Pakistan	09/12/67	04/08/68	
Panama	01/27/67		
Papua New Guinea			10/27/80
Peru	06/30/67	02/28/79	
Philippines	01/27/67		
Poland	01/27/67	01/30/68	
Romania	01/27/67	04/09/68	
Rwanda	01/27/67		
Saint Christopher-Nevis			09/19/83
Saint Lucia			02/22/79
San Marino	04/21/67	10/29/68	
Saudi Arabia			12/17/76
Seychelles			01/05/78
Sierra Leone	01/27/67	07/13/67	
Singapore			09/10/76
Solomon Islands			07/07/78
Somalia	02/02/67		
South Africa	03/01/67	09/30/68	
Spain			11/27/68
Sri Lanka	03/10/69	11/18/86	
Swaziland			10/22/68
Sweden	01/27/67	10/11/67	
Switzerland	01/27/67	12/18/69	
Syria			11/19/68
Thailand	01/27/67	09/05/68	
Togo	01/27/67		
Tonga			06/22/71
Trinidad and Tobago	07/24/67		
Tunisia	01/27/67	03/28/68	
Turkey	01/27/67	03/27/68	
Uganda			04/24/68
Ukrainian S.S.R.[2]	02/10/67	10/31/67	
Union of Soviet Socialist Republics	01/27/67	10/10/67	
United Kingdom	01/27/67	10/10/67	
United States	01/27/67	10/10/67	
Uruguay	01/27/67	08/31/70	
Venezuela	01/27/67	03/03/70	
Vietnam			06/20/80
Yemen, People's Democratic Republic of (Aden)			06/01/79
Yugoslavia	01/27/67		

OUTER SPACE TREATY -- Continued

Country	Date[1] of Signature	Date of Deposit[1] of Ratification	Date of Deposit[1] of Accession
Zaire	01/27/67		
Zambia			08/20/73
Total[3]	91	62	36

See footnotes on page 350.

TREATY FOR THE PROHIBITION OF NUCLEAR WEAPONS IN LATIN AMERICA

The Treaty for the Prohibition of Nuclear Weapons in Latin America (also known as the Treaty of Tlatelolco) obligates Latin American parties not to acquire or possess nuclear weapons, nor to permit the storage or deployment of nuclear weapons on their territories by other countries. Besides the agreement among the Latin American countries themselves, there are two Additional Protocols dealing with matters that concern non-Latin American countries. Protocol I involves an undertaking by non-Latin American countries that have territories in the nuclear-free zone. Protocol II involves an undertaking by those powers which possess nuclear weapons. The United States is a party to both protocols.

The United States has favored the establishment of nuclear-weapon-free zones where, inter alia, they would limit the spread of nuclear weapons; they would not disturb existing security arrangements; provisions exist for adequate verification; the initiative for such zones originates in the geographical area concerned; and all states important to the denuclearization of the area participate. Considering that Soviet proposals for the denuclearization of Central Europe and other areas have not met these criteria, the United States has opposed them. From the start, however, the United States supported and encouraged Latin American countries in this undertaking.

In mid-1962, the Brazilian representative to the UN General Assembly proposed making Latin America a nuclear-weapon-free zone. At the seventeenth regular session of the General Assembly, during the October Cuban missile crisis, a draft resolution calling for such a zone was submitted by Brazil and supported by Bolivia, Chile, and Ecuador. While asserting support for the principle, Cuba stipulated certain conditions, including the requirement that Puerto Rico and the Panama Canal Zone be included in the zone, and that foreign military bases, especially Guantanamo Naval Base, be eliminated. The draft resolution was not put to a vote at the General Assembly that year.

On April 29, 1963, at the initiative of the President of Mexico, the Presidents of five Latin American countries -- Bolivia, Brazil, Chile, Ecuador, and Mexico -- announced that they were prepared to sign a multilateral agreement that would make Latin America a nuclear-weapon-free zone. On November 27, 1963, this declaration received the support of the UN General Assembly, with the United States voting in the affirmative.

The Latin American nations followed this initiative by extensive and detailed negotiations among themselves. At the Mexico City Conference (November 23-27, 1964) a Preparatory Commission for the Denuclearization of Latin America was created, with instructions to prepare a draft Treaty. Important differences among the Latin American countries emerged over questions of defining the boundaries of the nuclear-weapon-free zone, transit guarantees, and safeguards on peaceful nuclear activities.

On February 14, 1967, the Treaty was signed at a regional meeting of Latin American countries at Tlatelolco, a section of Mexico City. On December 5, 1967, the UN General Assembly endorsed it by a vote of 82-0 with 28 abstentions, the United States voting in support of the Treaty. As of January 1, 1989, the Treaty had entered into force for 23 Latin American states. Belize and Guyana were not invited to accede to the Treaty because a special regime is foreseen for those political entities whose territories are wholly or partially the subject of disputes or claims by an extracontinental state and one or more Latin American states. When all eligible states ratify the Treaty, it will enter into force for all of them, as specified in Article 28. Alternatively, under that article, any Latin American state may bring the Treaty into force for itself at any time by waiving that provision.

The basic obligations of the Treaty are contained in Article I:

1. The contracting parties undertake to use exclusively for peaceful purposes the nuclear material and facilities which are under their jurisdiction, and to prohibit and prevent in their respective territories;

(a) The testing, use, manufacture, production, or acquisition by any means whatsoever of any nuclear weapons, by the parties themselves, directly or indirectly, on behalf of anyone else or in any other way; and

(b)   The receipt, storage, installation, deployment, and any form of possession of any nuclear weapons, directly or indirectly, by the parties themselves, by anyone on their behalf or in any other way.

2. The contracting parties also undertake to refrain from engaging in, encouraging or authorizing, directly or indirectly, or in any way participating in the testing, use, manufacture, production, possession, or control of any nuclear weapon.

Important provisions in the Treaty deal with verification. Treaty parties undertake to negotiate agreements with the International Atomic Energy Agency for application of its safeguards to their nuclear activities. The Treaty also establishes an organization to help ensure compliance with Treaty provisions -- the Agency for the Prohibition of Nuclear Weapons in Latin America (OPANAL) -- with a General Conference, a Council, and a Secretariat as its permanent organs. The five-member elected Council is empowered to perform "special inspections."

Of the accompanying protocols, Protocol I calls on nations outside the Treaty zone to apply the denuclearization provisions of the Treaty to the territories in the zone "for which de jure or de facto they are internationally responsible." All four powers having such territories have signed -- the United Kingdom, the Netherlands, France, and the United States. All except France have ratified. The U.S. Protocol I territories include Puerto Rico, the U.S. Virgin Islands, and the naval base at Guantanamo Bay. Since the entry into force of the Panama Canal Treaties on October 1, 1979, U.S. obligations to the former Canal Zone have been governed by those treaties and by Protocol II to the Treaty of Tlatelolco.

President Carter signed Protocol I for the United States in 1977. In November 1981, the Senate completed its review of the Protocol and gave its advice and consent to ratification subject to certain understandings which were supported by the executive branch and are outlined below. President Reagan ratified Protocol I in November 1981, and the U.S. instrument of ratification was deposited in Mexico City on November 23, 1981.

Senate advice and consent to ratification of Protocol I was made subject to three understandings:

— That the provisions of the Treaty made applicable by the protocol do not affect the rights of the contracting parties to grant or deny transport and transit privileges to their own or other vessels or aircraft regardless of cargo or armaments;

— That the provisions of the Treaty made applicable by the protocol do not affect the rights of the contracting parties regarding the exercise of freedom of the seas or passage through or over waters subject to the sovereignty of a State;

— That the understandings and declarations the United States attached to ratification of Protocol II apply also to its ratification of Protocol I.

In Protocol II, nuclear-weapon states undertake (1) to respect the denuclearized status of the zone; (2) not to contribute to acts involving violation of obligations of the parties; and (3) not to use or threaten to use nuclear weapons against the contracting parties. France, the United Kingdom, the United States, China, and the Soviet Union are parties to Protocol II.

The United States signed Protocol II on April 1, 1968. When President Nixon transmitted it to the Senate on August 13, 1970, he recommended that the Senate give its advice and consent subject to certain understandings and declarations. The Senate Foreign Relations Committee revised the statement slightly during its hearings on the Protocol in September 1970 and February 1971, and the full Senate made its consent to ratification, on April 19, 1971, subject to the revised statement. The President ratified the Protocol on May 8, 1971, and the United States deposited the instrument of ratification on May 12, 1971, subject to the following understandings and declarations:

— The Treaty and its protocols have no effect upon the international status of territorial claims.

— The Treaty does not affect the rights of the contracting parties to grant or deny transport and transit privileges to non-contracting parties.

— With respect to the undertaking in Article 3 of Protocol II not to use or threaten to use nuclear weapons against the Treaty parties, the United States would "have to consider that an armed attack by a Contracting Party, which it was assisted by a nuclear-weapon state, would be incompatible with the Contracting Party's corresponding obligations under Article I of the Treaty."

— Considering the technology for producing nuclear explosive devices for peaceful purposes to be indistinguishable from that for making nuclear weapons, the United States regards the Treaty's prohibitions as applying to all nuclear explosive devices. However, the Treaty would not prevent the United States, as a nuclear-weapon state, from making nuclear explosion services for peaceful purposes available "in a manner consistent with our policy of not contributing to the proliferation of nuclear weapons capabilities."

— Although not required to do so, the United States will act, with respect to the territories of Protocol I adherents that are within the Treaty zone, in the same way as Protocol II requires it to act toward the territories of the Latin American Treaty parties.

The Treaty of Tlatelolco was first amended at a special general conference in July 1990 to attach the phrase "and the Caribbean" to the title. The Treaty was amended again in May 1991 to replace paragraph 2 of Article 25. The original Treaty paragraph had excluded political entities "part or all of which whose territory" is in dispute with "an extra-continental country and one or more Latin American States" prior to the opening of signature of the Treaty. This clause effectively excluded Belize and Guyana from membership. Belize (formerly British Honduras) attained its independence from the UK in 1981; Guyana gained independence from Britain in 1966, but has ongoing territorial disputes with Venezuela and Suriname.

This amendment replaced the original text with the following: "The condition of State Party to the Treaty of Tlatelolco shall be restricted to independent states which are situated within the zone of application of the Treaty in accordance with Article 4 of same, and with Paragraph 1 of the present Article, and which were members of the United Nations as of December 10, 1985, as well as the nonautonomous territories mentioned in Document OAS/CER.P, AG/DOC. 1939/85 of November 5, 1985, once they attain their independence."

— The referenced OAS document lists the Bermuda, Cayman, Turks and Caicos and British Virgin Islands, Montserrat, Guadeloupe, Martinique, French Guiana, St. Pierre, Miquelon, Netherlands Antilles (Aruba, Bonaire, Curaçao, Saba, St. Eustatius, St. Martin), Greenland, and U.S. Virgin Islands as "nonautonomous territories" in one sense or another; Anguilla, with ties to the UK, is considered something of special case, more than "nonautonomous" but less than independent. Greenland is not within the zone of application, and as such would not be eligible for membership should it one day achieve independence from Denmark.

This amendment, adopted by consensus at the 1991 General Conference, has not yet been ratified by all of the current contracting parties to the Treaty.

The third amending of the Treaty occurred at a special general conference in August 1992, when amendments to Articles 14-16 and 19 were adopted. The most significant of these was a change in Article 16 designating the IAEA as having the sole authority to conduct special inspections of Tlatelolco parties; the original text gave this authority both to the IAEA and to OPANAL, the Treaty's executive agency.

The complete text of this third set of the amendments is reproduced below:

Article 14

2. The Contracting Parties shall simultaneously transmit to the Agency a copy of the reports sent to the International Atomic Energy Agency in relation to matters subject to the present Treaty which are relevant to the Agency's work.

3. The information provided by the Contracting Parties cannot be divulged or communicated to third parties, totally or partially, by the recipients of the reports except with the express consent of the former.

Article 15

1. At the request of any of the Parties, and with the authorization of the Council, the Secretary General may request any of the Contracting Parties to provide the Agency with complementary or supplementary information regarding any extraordinary fact or circumstance

which affects compliance with the present Treaty, explaining the reasons he/they had for such action. The Contracting Parties commit themselves to cooperate quickly and fully with the Secretary General.

2. The Secretary General will immediately inform the Council and the Contracting Parties about such requests and their respective replies.

Article 16

1. The International Atomic Energy Agency has the power of carrying out special inspections in conformity with Article 12 and with the agreements referred to in Article 13 of this Treaty.

2. At the request of any of the Contracting Parties, and following the procedures established under Article 15 of the present Treaty, the Council may submit to the consideration of the International Atomic Energy Agency a requisition that the latter initiate the arrangements required for the carrying out of a special inspection.

3. The Secretary General shall request the General Director of the International Atomic Energy Agency to transmit to him in a timely manner the information sent by the former to the IAEA Board of Governors regarding the conclusion of the said special inspection. The Secretary General shall promptly impart such information to the Council.

4. By the Agency or the Secretary General, the Council shall transmit such information to all of the Contracting Parties.

Article 19

The Agency may conclude agreements with the International Atomic Energy Agency as are authorized by the General Conference and as it considers appropriate to facilitate the efficient operation of the Control System established by this Treaty.

Article 20

1. The Agency may also enter into relations with any international organization or body, especially any which may be established in the future to supervise disarmament or measures for the control of armaments in any party of the world.

2. The Contracting Parties may, when they see fit, request the advice of the Inter-American Nuclear Energy Commission on all technical matters connected with the application of this Treaty with which the Commission is competent to deal under its Statute.

TREATY FOR THE PROHIBITION OF NUCLEAR WEAPONS IN LATIN AMERICA

Signed at Mexico City February 14, 1967
Entered into force April 22, 1968

Preamble

In the name of their peoples and faithfully interpreting their desires and aspirations, the Governments of the States which sign the Treaty for the Prohibition of Nuclear Weapons in Latin America,

Desiring to contribute, so far as lies in their power, towards ending the armaments race, especially in the field of nuclear weapons, and towards strengthening a world at peace, based on the sovereign equality of States, mutual respect and good neighbourliness,

Recalling that the United Nations General Assembly, in its Resolution 808 (IX), adopted unanimously as one of the three points of a coordinated programme of disarmament "the total prohibition of the use and manufacture of nuclear weapons and weapons of mass destruction of every type,"

Recalling that military denuclearized zones are not an end in themselves but rather a means for achieving general and complete disarmament at a later stage,

Recalling United Nations General Assembly Resolution 1911 (XVIII), which established that the measures that should be agreed upon for the denuclearization of Latin America should be taken "in the light of the principles of the Charter of the United Nations and of regional agreements,"

Recalling United Nations General Assembly Resolution 2028 (XX), which established the principle of an acceptable balance of mutual responsibilities and duties for the nuclear and non-nuclear powers, and

Recalling that the Charter of the Organization of American States proclaims that it is an essential purpose of the Organization to strengthen the peace and security of the hemisphere,

Convinced:

That the incalculable destructive power of nuclear weapons has made it imperative that the legal prohibition of war should be strictly observed in practice if the survival of civilization and of mankind itself is to be assured,

That nuclear weapons, whose terrible effects are suffered, indiscriminately and inexorably, by military forces and civilian population alike, constitute, through the persistence of the radioactivity they release, an attack on the integrity of the human species and ultimately may even render the whole earth uninhabitable,

That general and complete disarmament under effective international control is a vital matter which all the peoples of the world equally demand,

That the proliferation of nuclear weapons, which seems inevitable unless States, in the exercise of their sovereign rights, impose restrictions on themselves in order to prevent it, would make any agreement on disarmament enormously difficult and would increase the danger of the outbreak of a nuclear conflagration,

That the establishment of militarily denuclearized zones is closely linked with the maintenance of peace and security in the respective regions,

That the military denuclearization of vast geographical zones, adopted by the sovereign decision of the States comprised therein, will exercise a beneficial influence on other regions where similar conditions exist,

That the privileged situation of the signatory States, whose territories are wholly free from nuclear weapons, imposes upon them the inescapable duty of preserving that situation both in their own interest and for the good of mankind,

That the existence of nuclear weapons in any country of Latin America would make it a target for possible nuclear attacks and would inevitably set off, throughout the region, a ruinous race in nuclear weapons which would involve the unjustifiable diversion, for warlike purposes, of the limited resources required for economic and social development,

That the foregoing reasons, together with the traditional peace-loving outlook of Latin America, give rise to an inescapable necessity that nuclear energy should be used in that region exclusively for peaceful purposes, and that the Latin American countries should use their right to the greatest and most equitable possible access to this new source of energy in order to expedite the economic and social development of their peoples,

Convinced finally:

That the military denuclearization of Latin America -- being understood to mean the undertaking entered into internationally in this Treaty to keep their territories forever free from nuclear weapons -- will constitute a measure which will spare their peoples from the squandering of their limited resources on nuclear armaments and will protect them against possible nuclear attacks on their territories, and will also constitute a significant contribution towards preventing the proliferation of nuclear weapons and a powerful factor for general and complete disarmament, and

That Latin America, faithful to its tradition of universality, must not only endeavour to banish from its homelands the scourge of a nuclear war, but must also strive to promote the well-being and advancement of its peoples, at the same time co-operating in the fulfillment of the ideals of mankind, that is to say, in the consolidation of a permanent peace based on equal rights, economic fairness and social justice for all, in accordance with the principles and purposes set forth in the Charter of the United Nations and in the Charter of the Organization of American States.

Have agreed as follows:

Obligations

Article 1

1. The Contracting Parties hereby undertake to use exclusively for peaceful purposes the nuclear material and facilities which are under their jurisdiction, and to prohibit and prevent in their respective territories:

   (a) The testing, use, manufacture, production or acquisition by any means whatsoever of any

nuclear weapons, by the Parties themselves, directly or indirectly, on behalf of anyone else or in any other way, and

   (b) The receipt, storage, installation, deployment and any form of possession of any nuclear weapons, directly or indirectly, by the Parties themselves, by anyone on their behalf or in any other way.

2. The Contracting Parties also undertake to refrain from engaging in, encouraging or authorizing, directly or indirectly, or in any way participating in the testing, use, manufacture, production, possession or control of any nuclear weapon.

Definition of the Contracting Parties

Article 2

For the purposes of this Treaty, the Contracting Parties are those for whom the Treaty is in force.

Definition of territory

Article 3

For the purposes of this Treaty, the term "territory" shall include the territorial sea, air space and any other space over which the State exercises sovereignty in accordance with its own legislation.

Zone of application

Article 4

1. The zone of application of this Treaty is the whole of the territories for which the Treaty is in force.

2. Upon fulfillment of the requirements of article 28, paragraph 1, the zone of application of this Treaty shall also be that which is situated in the western hemisphere within the following limits (except the continental part of the territory of the United States of America and its territorial waters): starting at a point located at 35° north latitude, 75° west longitude; from this point directly southward to a point at 30° north latitude, 75° west longitude; from there, directly eastward to a point at 30° north latitude, 50° west longitude; from there, along a loxodromic line to a point at 5° north latitude, 20° west longitude;

from there directly southward to a point 60°
south latitude, 20° west longitude; from there,
directly westward to a point at 60° south latitude,
115° west longitude; from there, directly
northward to a point at 0° latitude, 115° west
longitude; from there, along a loxodromic line to a
point at 35° north latitude, 150° west longitude;
from there, directly eastward to a point at 35°
north latitude, 75° west longitude.

Definition of nuclear weapons

Article 5

For the purposes of this Treaty, a nuclear
weapon is any device which is capable of
releasing nuclear energy in an uncontrolled
manner and which has a group of characteristics
that are appropriate for use for warlike purposes.
An instrument that may be used for the transport
or propulsion of the device is not included in this
definition if it is separable from the device and not
an indivisible part thereof.

Meeting of signatories

Article 6

At the request of any of the signatory States or
if the Agency established by article 7 should so
decide, a meeting of all the signatories may be
convoked to consider in common questions which
may affect the very essence of this instrument,
including possible amendments to it. In either
case, the meeting will be convoked by the
General Secretary.

Organization

Article 7

1. In order to ensure compliance with the
obligations of this Treaty, the Contracting Parties
hereby establish an international organization to
be known as the "Agency for the Prohibition of
Nuclear Weapons in Latin America," hereinafter
referred to as "the Agency." Only the Contracting
Parties shall be affected by its decisions.

2. The Agency shall be responsible for the
holding of periodic or extraordinary consultations
among Member States on matters relating to the
purposes, measures and procedures set forth in
this Treaty and to the supervision of compliance
with the obligations arising therefrom.

3. The Contracting Parties agree to extend to
the Agency full and prompt cooperation in
accordance with the provisions of this Treaty, of
any agreements they may conclude with the
Agency and of any agreements the Agency may
conclude with any other international organization
or body.

4. The headquarters of the Agency shall be in
Mexico City.

Organs

Article 8

1. There are hereby established as principal
organs of the Agency a General Conference, a
Council and a Secretariat.

2. Such subsidiary organs as are considered
necessary by the General Conference may be
established within the purview of this Treaty.

The General Conference

Article 9

1. The General Conference, the supreme organ
of the Agency, shall be composed of all the
Contracting Parties; it shall hold regular sessions
every two years, and may also hold special
sessions whenever this Treaty so provides or, in
the opinion of the Council, the circumstances so
require.

2. The General Conference:

(a) May consider and decide on any matters or
questions covered by this Treaty, within the limits
thereof, including those referring to powers and
functions of any organ provided for in this Treaty.

(b) Shall establish procedures for the control
system to ensure observance of this Treaty in
accordance with its provisions.

(c) Shall elect the Members of the Council and
the General Secretary.

(d) May remove the General Secretary from
office if the proper functioning of the Agency so
requires.

(e) Shall receive and consider the biennial and

special reports submitted by the Council and the General Secretary.

(f) Shall initiate and consider studies designed to facilitate the optimum fulfillment of the aims of this Treaty, without prejudice to the power of the General Secretary independently to carry out similar studies for submission to and consideration by the Conference.

(g) Shall be the organ competent to authorize the conclusion of agreements with Governments and other international organizations and bodies.

3. The General Conference shall adopt the Agency's budget and fix the scale of financial contributions to be paid by Member States, taking into account the systems and criteria used for the same purpose by the United Nations.

4. The General Conference shall elect its officers for each session and may establish such subsidiary organs as it deems necessary for the performance of its functions.

5. Each Member of the Agency shall have one vote. The decisions of the General Conference shall be taken by a two-thirds majority of the Members present and voting in the case of matters relating to the control system and measures referred to in article 20, the admission of new Members, the election or removal of the General Secretary, adoption of the budget and matters related thereto. Decisions on other matters, as well as procedural questions and also determination of which questions must be decided by a two-thirds majority, shall be taken by a simple majority of the Members present and voting.

6. The General Conference shall adopt its own rules of procedure.

The Council

Article 10

1. The Council shall be composed of five Members of the Agency elected by the General Conference from among the Contracting Parties, due account being taken of equitable geographic distribution.

2. The Members of the Council shall be elected for a term of four years. However, in the first election three will be elected for two years. Outgoing Members may not be reelected for the following period unless the limited number of States for which the Treaty is in force so requires.

3. Each Member of the Council shall have one representative.

4. The Council shall be so organized as to be able to function continuously.

5. In addition to the functions conferred upon it by this Treaty and to those which may be assigned to it by the General Conference, the Council shall, through the General Secretary, ensure the proper operation of the control system in accordance with the provisions of this Treaty and with the decisions adopted by the General Conference.

6. The Council shall submit an annual report on its work to the General Conference as well as such special reports as it deems necessary or which the General Conference requests of it.

7. The Council shall elect its officers for each session.

8. The decisions of the Council shall be taken by a simple majority of its Members present and voting.

9. The Council shall adopt its own rules of procedure.

The Secretariat

Article 11

1. The Secretariat shall consist of a General Secretary, who shall be the chief administrative officer of the Agency, and of such staff as the Agency may require. The term of office of the General Secretary shall be four years and he may be re-elected for a single additional term. The General Secretary may not be a national of the country in which the Agency has its headquarters. In case the office of General Secretary becomes vacant, a new election shall be held to fill the office for the remainder of the term.

2. The staff of the Secretariat shall be appointed by the General Secretary, in accordance with rules laid down by the General Conference.

3. In addition to the functions conferred upon him by this Treaty and to those which may be assigned to him by the General Conference, the General Secretary shall ensure, as provided by article 10, paragraph 5, the proper operation of the control system established by this Treaty, in accordance with the provisions of the Treaty and the decisions taken by the General Conference.

4. The General Secretary shall act in that capacity in all meetings of the General Conference and of the Council and shall make an annual report to both bodies on the work of the Agency and any special reports requested by the General Conference or the Council or which the General Secretary may deem desirable.

5. The General Secretary shall establish the procedures for distributing to all Contracting Parties information received by the Agency from governmental sources and such information from non-governmental sources as may be of interest to the Agency.

6. In the performance of their duties the General Secretary and the staff shall not seek or receive instructions from any Government or from any other authority external to the Agency and shall refrain from any action which might reflect on their position as international officials responsible only to the Agency; subject to their responsibility to the Agency, they shall not disclose any industrial secrets or other confidential information coming to their knowledge by reason of their official duties in the Agency.

7. Each of the Contracting Parties undertakes to respect the exclusively international character of the responsibilities of the General Secretary and the staff and not to seek to influence them in the discharge of their responsibilities.

Control system

Article 12

1. For the purpose of verifying compliance with the obligations entered into by the Contracting Parties in accordance with article 1, a control system shall be established which shall be put into effect in accordance with the provisions of articles 13-18 of this Treaty.

2. The control system shall be used in particular for the purpose of verifying:

(a) That devices, services and facilities intended for peaceful uses of nuclear energy are not used in the testing or manufacture of nuclear weapons,

(b) That none of the activities prohibited in article 1 of this Treaty are carried out in the territory of the Contracting Parties with nuclear materials or weapons introduced from abroad, and

(c) That explosions for peaceful purposes are compatible with article 18 of this Treaty.

IAEA safeguards

Article 13

Each Contracting Party shall negotiate multilateral or bilateral agreements with the International Atomic Energy Agency for the application of its safeguards to its nuclear activities. Each Contracting Party shall initiate negotiations within a period of 180 days after the date of the deposit of its instrument of ratification of this Treaty. These agreements shall enter into force, for each Party, not later than eighteen months after the date of the initiation of such negotiations except in case of unforeseen circumstances or *force majeure*.

Reports of the Parties

Article 14

1. The Contracting Parties shall submit to the Agency and to the International Atomic Energy Agency, for their information, semi-annual reports stating that no activity prohibited under this Treaty has occurred in their respective territories.

2. The Contracting Parties shall simultaneously transmit to the Agency a copy of any report they may submit to the International Atomic Energy Agency which relates to matters that are the subject of this Treaty and to the application of safeguards.

3. The Contracting Parties shall also transmit to the Organization of American States, for its information, any reports that may be of interest to it, in accordance with the obligations established by the Inter-American System.

Special reports requested by the General Secretary

Article 15

1. With the authorization of the Council, the General Secretary may request any of the Contracting Parties to provide the Agency with complementary or supplementary information regarding any event or circumstance connected with compliance with this Treaty, explaining his reasons. The Contracting Parties undertake to co-operate promptly and fully with the General Secretary.

2. The General Secretary shall inform the Council and the Contracting Parties forthwith of such requests and of the respective replies.

Special inspections

Article 16

1. The International Atomic Energy Agency and the Council established by this Treaty have the power of carrying out special inspections in the following cases:

(a) In the case of the International Atomic Energy Agency, in accordance with the agreements referred to in article 13 of this Treaty;

(b) In the case of the Council:

(i) When so requested, the reasons for the request being stated, by any Party which suspects that some activity prohibited by this Treaty has been carried out or is about to be carried out, either in the territory of any other Party or in any other place on such latter Party's behalf, the Council shall immediately arrange for such an inspection in accordance with article 10, paragraph 5.

(ii) When requested by any Party which has been suspected of or charged with having violated this Treaty, the Council shall immediately arrange for the special inspection requested in accordance with article 10, paragraph 5.

The above requests will be made to the Council through the General Secretary.

2. The costs and expenses of any special inspection carried out under paragraph 1, sub-paragraph (b), sections (i) and (ii) of this article shall be borne by the requesting Party or Parties, except where the Council concludes on the basis of the report on the special inspection that, in view of the circumstances existing in the case, such costs and expenses should be borne by the agency.

3. The General Conference shall formulate the procedures for the organization and execution of the special inspections carried out in accordance with paragraph 1, sub-paragraph (b), sections (i) and (ii) of this article.

4. The Contracting Parties undertake to grant the inspectors carrying out such special inspections full and free access to all places and all information which may be necessary for the performance of their duties and which are directly and intimately connected with the suspicion of violation of this Treaty. If so requested by the authorities of the Contracting Party in whose territory the inspection is carried out, the inspectors designated by the General Conference shall be accompanied by representatives of said authorities, provided that this does not in any way delay or hinder the work of the inspectors.

5. The Council shall immediately transmit to all the Parties, through the General Secretary, a copy of any report resulting from special inspections.

6. Similarly, the Council shall send through the General Secretary to the Secretary-General of the United Nations, for transmission to the United Nations Security Council and General Assembly, and to the Council of the Organization of American States, for its information, a copy of any report resulting from any special inspection carried out in accordance with paragraph 1, sub-paragraph (b), sections (i) and (ii) of this article.

7. The Council may decide, or any Contracting Party may request, the convening of a special session of the General Conference for the purpose of considering the reports resulting from any special inspection. In such a case, the General Secretary shall take immediate steps to convene the special session requested.

8. The General Conference, convened in special session under this article, may make recommendations to the Contracting Parties and submit reports to the Secretary-General of the United Nations to be transmitted to the United Nations Security Council and the General Assembly.

Use of nuclear energy for peaceful purposes

Article 17

Nothing in the provisions of this Treaty shall prejudice the rights of the Contracting Parties, in conformity with this Treaty, to use nuclear energy for peaceful purposes, in particular for their economic development and social progress.

Explosions for peaceful purposes

Article 18

1. The Contracting Parties may carry out explosions of nuclear devices for peaceful purposes -- including explosions which involve devices similar to those used in nuclear weapons -- or collaborate with third parties for the same purpose, provided that they do so in accordance with the provisions of this article and the other articles of the Treaty, particularly articles 1 and 5.

2. Contracting Parties intending to carry out, or to cooperate in carrying out, such an explosion shall notify the Agency and the International Atomic Energy Agency, as far in advance as the circumstances require, of the date of the explosion and shall at the same time provide the following information:

(a) The nature of the nuclear device and the source from which it was obtained,

(b) The place and purpose of the planned explosion,

(c) The procedures which will be followed in order to comply with paragraph 3 of this article,

(d) The expected force of the device, and

(e) The fullest possible information on any possible radioactive fall-out that may result from the explosion or explosions, and measures which will be taken to avoid danger to the population, flora, fauna and territories of any other Party or

Parties.

3. The General Secretary and the technical personnel designated by the Council and the International Atomic Energy Agency may observe all the preparations, including the explosion of the device, and shall have unrestricted access to any area in the vicinity of the site of the explosion in order to ascertain whether the device and the procedures followed during the explosion are in conformity with the information supplied under paragraph 2 of this article and the other provisions of this Treaty.

4. The Contracting Parties may accept the collaboration of third parties for the purpose set forth in paragraph 1 of the present article, in accordance with paragraphs 2 and 3 thereof.

Relations with other international organizations

Article 19

1. The Agency may conclude such agreements with the International Atomic Energy Agency as are authorized by the General Conference and as it considers likely to facilitate the efficient operation of the control system established by this Treaty.

2. The Agency may also enter into relations with any international organization or body, especially any which may be established in the future to supervise disarmament or measures for the control of armaments in any part of the world.

3. The Contracting Parties may, if they see fit, request the advice of the International American Nuclear Energy Commission on all technical matters connected with the application of this Treaty with which the Commission is competent to deal under its Statute.

Measures in the event of violation of the Treaty

Article 20

1. The General Conference shall take note of all cases in which, in its opinion, any Contracting Party is not complying fully with its obligations under this Treaty and shall draw the matter to the attention of the Party concerned, making such recommendations as it deems appropriate.

2. If, in its opinion, such non-compliance

constitutes a violation of this Treaty which might endanger peace and security, the General Conference shall report thereon simultaneously to the United Nations Security Council and the General Assembly through the Secretary-General of the United Nations, and to the Council of the Organization of American States. The General Conference shall likewise report to the International Atomic Energy Agency for such purposes as are relevant in accordance with its Statute.

United Nations and Organization of American States

Article 21

None of the provisions of this Treaty shall be construed as impairing the rights and obligations of the Parties under the Charter of the United Nations or, in the case of States Members of the Organization of American States, under existing regional treaties.

Privileges and immunities

Article 22

1. The Agency shall enjoy in the territory of each of the Contracting Parties such legal capacity and such privileges and immunities as may be necessary for the exercise of its functions and the fulfillment of its purposes.

2. Representatives of the Contracting Parties accredited to the Agency and officials of the Agency shall similarly enjoy such privileges and immunities as are necessary for the performance of their functions.

3. The Agency may conclude agreements with the Contracting Parties with a view to determining the details of the application of paragraphs 1 and 2 of this article.

Notification of other agreements

Article 23

Once this Treaty has entered into force, the Secretariat shall be notified immediately of any international agreement concluded by any of the Contracting Parties on matters with which this Treaty is concerned; the Secretariat shall register it and notify the other Contracting Parties.

Settlement of disputes

Article 24

Unless the Parties concerned agree on another mode of peaceful settlement, any question or dispute concerning the interpretation or application of this Treaty which is not settled shall be referred to the International Court of Justice with the prior consent of the Parties to the controversy.

Signature

Article 25

1. This Treaty shall be open indefinitely for signature by:

(a) All the Latin American Republics, and

(b) All other sovereign States situated in their entirety south of latitude 35° north in the western hemisphere; and, except as provided in paragraph 2 of this article, all such States which become sovereign, when they have been admitted by the General Conference.

2. The General Conference shall not take any decision regarding the admission of a political entity part or all of whose territory is the subject, prior to the date when this Treaty is opened for signature, of a dispute or claim between an extra-continental country and one or more Latin American States, so long as the dispute has not been settled by peaceful means.

Ratification and deposit

Article 26

1. This Treaty shall be subject to ratification by signatory States in accordance with their respective constitutional procedures.

2. This Treaty and the instruments of ratification shall be deposited with the Government of the Mexican United States, which is hereby designated the Depositary Government.

3. The Depositary Government shall send certified copies of this Treaty to the Governments of signatory States and shall notify them of the deposit of each instrument of ratification.

Reservations

Article 27

This Treaty shall not be subject to reservations.

Entry into force

Article 28

1. Subject to the provisions of paragraph 2 of this article, this Treaty shall enter into force among the States that have ratified it as soon as the following requirements have been met:

(a) Deposit of the instruments of ratification of this Treaty with the Depositary Government by the Governments of the States mentioned in article 25 which are in existence on the date when this Treaty is opened for signature and which are not affected by the provisions of article 25, paragraph 2;

(b) Signature and ratification of Additional Protocol I annexed to this Treaty by all extra-continental or continental States having *de jure* or *de facto* international responsibility for territories situated in the zone of application of the Treaty;

(c) Signature and ratification of the Additional Protocol II annexed to this Treaty by all powers possessing nuclear weapons;

(d) Conclusion of bilateral or multilateral agreements on the application of Safeguards System of the International Atomic Energy Agency in accordance with article 13 of this Treaty.

2. All signatory States shall have the imprescriptible right to waive, wholly or in part, the requirements laid down in the preceding paragraph. They may do so by means of a declaration which shall be annexed to their respective instrument of ratification and which may be formulated at the time of deposit of the instrument or subsequently. For those States which exercise this right, this Treaty shall enter into force upon deposit of the declaration, or as soon as those requirements have been met which have not been expressly waived.

3. As soon as this Treaty has entered into force in accordance with this provisions of paragraph 2 for eleven States, the Depositary Government shall convene a preliminary meeting of those States in order that the Agency may be set up and commence its work.

4. After the entry into force of this Treaty for all the countries of the zone, the rise of a new power possessing nuclear weapons shall have the effect of suspending the execution of this Treaty for those countries which have ratified it without waiving requirements of paragraph 1, sub-paragraph (c) of this article, and which request such suspension; the Treaty shall remain suspended until the new power, on its own initiative or upon request by the General Conference, ratifies the annexed Additional Protocol II.

Amendments

Article 29

1. Any Contracting Party may propose amendments to this Treaty and shall submit its proposals to the Council through the General Secretary, who shall transmit them to all the other Contracting Parties and, in addition, to all other signatories in accordance with article 6. The Council, through the General Secretary, shall immediately following the meeting of signatories convene a special session of the General Conference to examine the proposals made, for the adoption of which a two-thirds majority of the Contracting Parties present and voting shall be required.

2. Amendments adopted shall enter into force as soon as the requirements set forth in article 28 of this Treaty have been complied with.

Duration and denunciation

Article 30

1. This Treaty shall be of a permanent nature and shall remain in force indefinitely, but any Party may denounce it by notifying the General Secretary of the Agency if, in the opinion of the denouncing State, there have arisen or may arise circumstances connected with the content of this Treaty or of the annexed Additional Protocols I and II which affect its supreme interests or the peace and security of one or more Contracting Parties.

2. The denunciation shall take effect three months after the delivery to the General Secretary of the Agency of the notification by the Government of the signatory State concerned. The General Secretary shall immediately communicate such notification to the other Contracting Parties and to the Secretary-General of the United Nations for the information of the United Nations Security Council and the General Assembly. He shall also communicate it to the Secretary-General of the Organization of American States.

Authentic texts and registration

Article 31

This Treaty, of which the Spanish, Chinese, English, French, Portuguese and Russian texts are equally authentic, shall be registered by the Depositary Government in accordance with article 102 of the United Nations Charter. The Depositary Government shall notify the Secretary-General of the United Nations of the signatures, ratification and amendments relating to this Treaty and shall communicate them to the Secretary-General of the Organization of American States for its information.

Transitional Article

Denunciation of the declaration referred to article 28, paragraph 2, shall be subject to the same procedures as the denunciation of this Treaty, except that it will take effect on the date of delivery of the respective notification.

IN WITNESS WHEREOF the undersigned Plenipotentiaries, having deposited their full powers, found in good and due form, sign this Treaty on behalf of their respective Governments.

DONE at Mexico, Distrito Federal, on the Fourteenth day of February, one thousand nine hundred and sixty-seven.

ADDITIONAL PROTOCOL I TO THE TREATY FOR THE PROHIBITION OF NUCLEAR WEAPONS IN LATIN AMERICA

Signed by the United States at Washington May 26, 1977
Ratification advised by U.S. Senate November 13, 1981
Ratified by U.S. President November 19, 1981
U.S. ratification deposited at Mexico City November 23, 1981
Proclaimed by U.S. President December 4, 1981

The undersigned Plenipotentiaries, furnished with full powers by their respective Governments,

Convinced that the Treaty for the Prohibition of Nuclear Weapons in Latin America, negotiated and signed in accordance with the recommendations of the General Assembly of the United Nations in Resolution 1911 (XVIII) of 27 November 1963, represents an important step towards ensuring the non-proliferation of nuclear weapons,

Aware that the non-proliferation of nuclear weapons is not an end in itself but, rather, a means of achieving general and complete disarmament at a later stage, and

Desiring to contribute, so far as lies in their power, towards ending the armaments race, especially in the field of nuclear weapons, and towards strengthening a world at peace, based on mutual respect and sovereign equality of States,

Have agreed as follows:

Article 1. To undertake to apply the statute of denuclearization in respect of warlike purposes as defined in articles 1, 3, 5 and 13 of the Treaty for the Prohibition of Nuclear Weapons in Latin America in territories for which, de jure or de facto, they are internationally responsible and which lie within the limits of the geographical zone established in that Treaty.

Article 2. The duration of this Protocol shall be the same as that of the Treaty for the Prohibition of Nuclear Weapons in Latin America of which this Protocol is an annex, and the provisions regarding ratification and denunciation contained in the Treaty shall be applicable to it.

Article 3. This Protocol shall enter into force, for the States which have ratified it, on the date of the deposit of their respective instruments of ratification.

IN WITNESS WHEREOF the undersigned Plenipotentiaries, having deposited their full powers, found in good and due form, sign this Protocol on behalf of their respective Governments.

ADDITIONAL PROTOCOL II TO THE TREATY FOR THE PROHIBITION OF NUCLEAR WEAPONS IN LATIN AMERICA

Signed by the United States at Mexico City April 1, 1968
Ratification advised by U.S. Senate April 19, 1971
Ratified by U.S. President May 8, 1971
U.S. ratification deposited at Mexico City May 12, 1971
Proclaimed by U.S. President June 11, 1971

The undersigned Plenipotentiaries, furnished with full powers by their respective Governments,

Convinced that the Treaty for the Prohibition of Nuclear Weapons in Latin America, negotiated and signed in accordance with the recommendations of the General Assembly of the United Nations in Resolution 1911 (XVIII) of 27 November 1963, represents an important step towards ensuring the non-proliferation of nuclear weapons,

Aware that the non-proliferation of nuclear weapons is not an end in itself but, rather, a means of achieving general and complete disarmament at a later stage, and

Desiring to contribute, so far as lies in their power, towards ending the armaments race, especially in the field of nuclear weapons, and towards promoting and strengthening a world at peace, based on mutual respect and sovereign equality of States,

Have agreed as follows:

Article 1. The statute of denuclearization of Latin America in respect or warlike purposes, as defined, delimited and set forth in the Treaty for the Prohibition of Nuclear Weapons in Latin America of which this instrument is an annex, shall be fully respected by the Parties to this Protocol in all its express aims and provisions.

Article 2. The Governments represented by the undersigned Plenipotentiaries undertake, therefore, not to contribute in any way to the performance of acts involving a violation of the obligations of article 1 of the Treaty in the territories to which the Treaty applies in accordance with article 4 thereof.

Article 3. The Governments represented by the undersigned Plenipotentiaries also undertake not to use or threaten to use nuclear weapons against the Contracting Parties of the Treaty for the Prohibition of Nuclear Weapons in Latin America.

Article 4. The duration of this Protocol shall be the same as that of the Treaty for the Prohibition of Nuclear Weapons in Latin America of which this protocol is an annex, and the definitions of territory and nuclear weapons set forth in articles 3 and 5 of the Treaty shall be applicable to this Protocol, as well as the provisions regarding ratification, reservations, denunciation, authentic texts and registration contained in articles 26, 27, 30 and 31 of the Treaty.

Article 5. This Protocol shall enter into force, for the States which have ratified it, on the date of the deposit of their respective instruments of ratification.

IN WITNESS WHEREOF the undersigned Plenipotentiaries, having deposited their full powers, found in good and due form, sign this Additional Protocol on behalf of their respective Governments.

PROCLAMATION BY PRESIDENT NIXON ON RATIFICATION OF ADDITIONAL PROTOCOL II TO THE TREATY FOR THE PROHIBITION OF NUCLEAR WEAPONS IN LATIN AMERICA

BY THE PRESIDENT OF THE UNITED STATES OF AMERICA

A PROCLAMATION

Considering that:

Additional Protocol II to the Treaty for the Prohibition of Nuclear Weapons in Latin America, done at the City of Mexico on February 14, 1967, was signed on behalf of the United States of America on April 1, 1968, the text of which Protocol is word for word as follows:

[The text of the Protocol appears here.]

The Senate of the United States of America by its resolution of April 19, 1971, two-thirds of the Senators present concurring, gave its advice and consent to the ratification of Additional Protocol II, with the following understandings and declarations:

I

That the United States Government understands the reference in Article 3 of the Treaty to "its own legislation" to relate only to such legislation as is compatible with the rules of international law and as involves an exercise of sovereignty consistent with those rules, and accordingly that ratification of Additional Protocol II by the United States Government could not be regarded as implying recognition, for the purposes of this Treaty and its protocols or for any other purpose, of any legislation which did not, in the view of the United States, comply with the relevant rules of international law.

That the United States Government takes note of the Preparatory Commission's interpretation of the Treaty, as set forth in the Final Act, that, governed by the principles and rules of international law, each of the Contracting Parties retains exclusive power and legal competence, unaffected by the terms of the Treaty, to grant or deny non-Contracting Parties transit and transport privileges.

That as regards the undertaking in Article 3 of

Protocol II not to use or threaten to use nuclear weapons against the Contracting Parties, the United States Government would have to consider that an armed attack by a Contracting Party, in which it was assisted by a nuclear-weapon state, would be incompatible with the Contracting Party's corresponding obligations under Article I of the Treaty.

II

That the United States Government considers that the technology of making nuclear explosive devices for peaceful purposes is indistinguishable from the technology of making nuclear weapons, and that nuclear weapons and nuclear explosive devices for peaceful purposes are both capable of releasing nuclear energy in an uncontrolled manner and have the common group of characteristics of large amounts of energy generated instantaneously from a compact source. Therefore, the United States Government understands the definition contained in Article 5 of the Treaty as necessarily encompassing all nuclear explosive devices. It is also understood that Articles 1 and 5 restrict accordingly the activities of the Contracting Parties under paragraph 1 of Article 18.

That the United States Government understands that paragraph 4 of Article 18 of the Treaty permits, and that United States adherence to Protocol II will not prevent, collaboration by the United States with Contracting Parties for the purpose of carrying out explosions of nuclear devices for peaceful purposes in a manner consistent with a policy of not contributing to the proliferation of nuclear weapons capabilities. In this connection, the United States Government notes Article V of the Treaty on the Non-Proliferation of Nuclear Weapons, under which it joined in an undertaking to take appropriate measures to ensure that potential benefits of peaceful applications of nuclear explosions would be made available to non-nuclear-weapon states party to that Treaty, and reaffirms its willingness to extend such undertaking, on the same basis, to states precluded by the present Treaty from manufacturing or acquiring any nuclear explosive device.

III

That the United States Government also declares that, although not required by Protocol II, it will act with respect to such territories of Protocol I adherents as are within the geographical area defined in paragraph 2 of Article 4 of the Treaty in the same manner as Protocol II requires it to act with respect to the territories of Contracting Parties.

The President ratified Additional Protocol II on May 8, 1971, with the above recited understandings and declarations, in pursuance of the advice and consent of the Senate.

It is provided in Article 5 of Additional Protocol II that the Protocol shall enter into force, for the States which have ratified it, on the date of the deposit of their respective instruments of ratification.

The instrument of ratification of the United Kingdom of Great Britain and Northern Ireland was deposited on December 11, 1969 with understandings and a declaration, and the instrument of ratification of the United States of America was deposited on May 12, 1971 with the above recited understandings and declarations.

In accordance with Article 5 of Additional Protocol II, the Protocol entered into force for the United States of America on May 12, 1971, subject to the above recited understandings and declarations.

NOW, THEREFORE, I, Richard Nixon, President of the United States of America, proclaim and make public Additional Protocol II to the Treaty for the Prohibition of Nuclear Weapons in Latin America to the end that it shall be observed and fulfilled with good faith, subject to the above recited understandings and declarations, on and after May 12, 1971 by the United States of America and by the citizens of the United States of America and all other persons subject to the jurisdiction thereof.

IN TESTIMONY WHEREOF, I have signed this proclamation and caused the Seal of the United States of America to be affixed.

DONE at the city of Washington this eleventh day of June in the year of our Lord one thousand nine hundred seventy-one and of the Independence of the United States of America the one hundred ninety-fifth.

(Seal)

TREATY FOR THE PROHIBITION OF NUCLEAR WEAPONS IN LATIN AMERICA

Country	Date of Signature	Date of Deposit of Ratification
Antigua & Barbuda	10/11/83	10/11/83 [1]
Argentina	09/27/67	
Bahamas, The		07/16/76 [a]
Barbados	10/18/68	04/25/69
Belize	02/14/92	
Bolivia	02/14/67	02/18/69
Brazil	05/09/67	01/29/68 [b]
Chile	02/14/67	10/09/74 [b]
Colombia	02/14/67	08/04/72
Costa Rica	02/14/67	08/25/69
Dominica	05/02/89	
Dominican Republic	07/29/67	06/14/68
Ecuador	02/14/67	02/11/69
El Salvador	02/14/67	04/22/68
Grenada	04/29/75	06/20/75
Guatemala	02/14/67	02/06/70
Haiti	02/14/67	05/23/69
Honduras	02/14/67	09/23/68
Jamaica	10/26/67	06/26/69
Mexico	02/14/67	09/20/67
Nicaragua	02/15/67	10/24/68
Panama	02/14/67	06/11/71
Paraguay	04/26/67	03/19/69
Peru	02/14/67	03/04/69
St. Lucia	08/25/92	
St. Vincent/Grenadines	02/14/92	02/14/92
Suriname	02/13/76	06/10/77
Trinidad & Tobago	06/27/67	12/03/70 [c]
Uruguay	02/14/67	08/20/68
Venezuela	02/14/67	03/23/70
TOTAL	29	26 (24 in force)

[1] See footnotes on page 350.
[a] This is date of notification of succession. The declaration of waiver was deposited 4/26/77, which is date of entry into force for the Bahamas.
[b] Not in force. No declaration of waiver under Art. 28, para 2.
[c] The declaration of waiver was deposited 6/27/75, which is date of entry into force for Trinidad and Tobago.

Additional Protocol I to the Treaty for the Prohibition of Nuclear Weapons in Latin America

Country	Date of Signature	Date of Deposit of Ratification
France	03/02/79	08/24/92
Netherlands	04/01/68	07/26/71
United Kingdom	12/20/67	12/11/69
United States	05/26/77	11/23/81

Additional Protocol II to the Treaty for the Prohibition of Nuclear Weapons in Latin America

Country	Date of Signature	Date of Deposit of Ratification
China, People's Republic of	08/21/73	06/12/74
France	07/18/73	03/22/74
Union of Soviet Socialist Republics	05/18/78	01/08/79
United Kingdom	12/20/67	12/11/69
United States	04/01/68	05/12/71

TREATY ON THE NON-PROLIFERATION OF NUCLEAR WEAPONS

The need to prevent the spread of nuclear weapons was evident from the first days of the nuclear era. On November 15, 1945, the United States, the United Kingdom, and Canada proposed the establishment of a U.N. Atomic Energy Commission for the purpose of "entirely eliminating the use of atomic energy for destructive purposes." The Baruch plan of 1946, offered by the United States, sought to forestall nuclear arms proliferation by placing all nuclear resources under international ownership and control.

But the early postwar efforts to achieve agreement on nuclear disarmament failed. The Soviet Union in 1949, the United Kingdom in 1952, France in 1960, and the People's Republic of China in 1964, became nuclear-weapon states. And increasingly it was becoming apparent that earlier assumptions about the scarcity of nuclear materials and the difficulty of mastering nuclear technology were inaccurate.

Other developments and prospects further underscored the threat of nuclear proliferation. In the early 1960s the search for peaceful applications of nuclear energy had brought advances in the technology of nuclear reactors for the generation of electric power. By 1966 such nuclear reactors were operating or under construction in five countries. It was estimated that by 1985 more than 300 nuclear power reactors would be operating, under construction, or on order. Nuclear reactors produce not only power, but plutonium -- a fissionable material which can be chemically separated and used in the manufacture of nuclear weapons. By 1985 it was estimated that the quantity of plutonium being produced worldwide would make possible the construction of 15 to 20 nuclear bombs daily, depending upon the level of the technology employed.

If the diversion of nuclear materials from peaceful purposes was not prevented by an international nuclear nonproliferation regime, and if a growing number of nations came to possess nuclear weapon arsenals, it was believed that the risks of nuclear war as a result of accident, unauthorized use, or escalation of regional conflicts would greatly increase. The possession of nuclear weapons by many countries would add a grave new dimension of threat to world security.

A succession of initiatives beginning in the 1950s by both nuclear and non-nuclear powers sought to check proliferation. Indeed the effort to achieve a nuclear test ban -- culminating in the Treaty of 1963 -- had as one of its main purposes inhibiting the spread of nuclear weapons. But much before that, in August 1957, the Western powers (Canada, France, the United Kingdom, and the United States) submitted a "package" of measures in the Subcommittee of the United Nations Disarmament Commission, which included a commitment "not to transfer out of its control any nuclear weapons, or to accept transfer to it of such weapons," except for self-defense.

Although the Soviet Union opposed proliferation, it claimed that this Western formula would allow an aggressor to judge his own actions, and to use nuclear weapons "under cover of the alleged right of self-defense." It therefore sought to couple a ban on transfer of nuclear weapons to other states with a prohibition on stationing nuclear weapons in foreign countries.

In 1961 the UN General Assembly unanimously approved an Irish resolution calling on all states, particularly the nuclear powers, to conclude an international agreement to refrain from transfer or acquisition of nuclear weapons. In addition, the general disarmament plans which had been submitted by the United States and the Soviet Union during the period 1960 -1962 included provisions banning the transfer and acquisition of nuclear weapons.

The United States, on January 21, 1964, outlined a program to halt the nuclear arms race in a message from President Johnson to the Eighteen-Nation Disarmament Committee (ENDC). This program, unlike the 1957 proposal, was not a "package." It included a nondissemina-tion and nonacquisition proposal -- based on the Irish resolution -- and safeguards on international transfers of nuclear materials for peaceful purposes, combined with acceptance by the major nuclear powers that their peaceful nuclear activities undergo increasingly "the same inspection they recommend for other states."

An issue that was to be the principal stumbling block for the next three years was the proposed multilateral nuclear force (MLF) then under discussion by the United States and its NATO allies. The Soviet Union strongly objected to this plan and maintained that no agreement could be reached on nonproliferation so long as the United States held open the possibility of such nuclear-sharing arrangements in NATO. These arrangements would constitute proliferation, the Soviet Union contended, and were devices for giving the Federal Republic of Germany access to or control of nuclear weapons.

On August 17, 1965, the United States submitted a draft nonproliferation Treaty to the ENDC. This draft obliged the nuclear-weapon powers not to transfer nuclear weapons to the national control of any non-nuclear country not having them. Non-nuclear nations would undertake to facilitate the application of International Atomic Energy Agency (IAEA) or equivalent safeguards to their peaceful nuclear activities.

A Soviet draft Treaty was submitted to the General Assembly on September 24. In an accompanying memorandum, the Soviet Union declared that the greatest danger of proliferation was posed by the MLF and the alternative British proposal for an Atlantic nuclear force (ANF). The Soviet draft prohibited the transfer of nuclear weapons "directly or indirectly, through third States or groups of States not possessing nuclear weapons." It also barred nuclear powers from transferring "nuclear weapons, or control over them or their emplacement or use" to military units of non-nuclear allies, even if these were placed under joint command. The draft included no safeguards provisions.

In March 1966, the United States tabled amendments to its draft Treaty in the ENDC, seeking to clarify and emphasize the Western view that collective defense arrangements would not violate the principle of nonproliferation. The U.S. representative stressed that the United States would not relinquish its veto over the use of U.S. weapons. The Soviet Union objected that the amendments did not prevent the transfer of nuclear weapons through such alliance arrangements as the MLF, the ANF, or units placed under joint command. The U.S. retention of a veto, the Soviet representative argued, did not provide security against dissemination.

Despite strong disagreement on the issue of collective defense arrangements, it was apparent that both sides recognized the desirability of an agreement on nuclear nonproliferation. Moreover, the interest of non-nuclear powers in such a Treaty was increasingly manifest. It was shown in 1964 at the African summit conference and at the Cairo conference of nonaligned states and expressed in a series of resolutions in the General Assembly urging that nuclear non-proliferation receive priority attention. In May 1966, the U.S. Senate unanimously passed a resolution sponsored by Senator Pastore of Rhode Island and 55 other Senators commending efforts to reach a nuclear nonproliferation agreement and supporting continued efforts.

In the fall of 1966 the U.S. and Soviet co-chairmen of the ENDC began private talks, and by the end of the year they had reached tentative agreement on the basic nontransfer and nonacquisition provisions of a Treaty, as well as on a number of other aspects.

There followed a long and arduous series of consultations between the United States and its allies. The allies raised a number of questions regarding the effect of the Treaty on NATO nuclear defense arrangements, and the United States gave its interpretations. The United States considered that the Treaty covered nuclear weapons and/or nuclear explosive devices, but not delivery systems. It would not prohibit NATO consultation and planning on nuclear defense, nor ban deployment of U.S.-owned and -controlled nuclear weapons on the territory of non-nuclear NATO members. It would not "bar succession by a new federated European state to the nuclear status of one of its members." The allies' questions and the United States answers were provided to the Soviet Union, which did not challenge the U.S. interpretations.

On August 24, 1967, the United States and the Soviet Union were able to submit separate but identical texts of a draft Treaty to the ENDC. Other ENDC members proposed numerous amendments, largely reflecting the concerns of the non-nuclear states. In response to these, the drafts underwent several revisions, and the co-chairmen tabled a joint draft on March 11, 1968. With additional revisions, the joint draft was submitted to the U.N. General Assembly, where it was extensively debated. Further suggestions for strengthening the Treaty were made, and in the light of these, the United States and the Soviet Union submitted a new revised version, the seventh, to the First Committee of the General Assembly on May 31. The General Assembly on June 12 approved a resolution commending the text and requesting the depositary governments (the U.S., U.K., and Soviet Union) to open it for signature. France abstained in the General Assembly vote, stating that while France would not sign the Treaty, it "would behave in the future in this field exactly as the States adhering to the Treaty."

In the course of these extended negotiations, the concerns of the non-nuclear powers centered particularly on three main issues:

Safeguards. There was general agreement that the Treaty should include provisions designed to detect and deter the diversion of nuclear materials from peaceful to weapons use. Two problems were involved. One was to reconcile the Soviet insistence that all non-nuclear parties accept IAEA[1] safeguards with the desire of the non-nuclear members of EURATOM[2] (Belgium, the Federal Republic of Germany, Italy, Luxembourg, and the Netherlands) to preserve their regional system. To meet this concern, the final draft provided that non-nuclear parties could negotiate safeguards agreements with IAEA either individually or together with other states.[3]

The other problem was to satisfy the widespread concern among non-nuclear states that IAEA safeguards might place them at a commercial and industrial disadvantage in developing nuclear energy for peaceful use, since the nuclear powers would not be required to accept safeguards. To help allay these misgivings, the United States offered, on December 2, 1967, to permit the IAEA to apply its safeguards, when such safeguards were applied under the NPT, in all nuclear facilities in the United States, excluding only those with "direct national security significance." The United Kingdom announced that it would take similar action. Its safeguards agreement with the IAEA was concluded in 1976 and is now in force. The U.S.-IAEA agreement, signed on November 18, 1977, was submitted by the President to the Senate for its advice and consent to ratification on February 9, 1978, and entered into force on December 9, 1980. In 1977, France opened negotiations with the IAEA, and a safeguards

agreement entered into force on September 12, 1981. In June 1982, the Soviet Union announced its readiness to put some of its nuclear installations under IAEA safeguards, and on June 10, 1985, its safeguards agreement with the IAEA entered into force. In September 1985 China declared at the IAEA that it would place some of its civil nuclear facilities under international safeguards, and a safeguards agreement was approved by the IAEA Board of Governors in September 1988.

Balanced Obligations. Throughout the negotiations most non-nuclear states held that their renunciation of nuclear weapons should be accompanied by a commitment on the part of the nuclear powers to reduce their nuclear arsenals and to make progress on measures toward comprehensive disarmament. General provisions were included in the Treaty affirming the intentions of the parties to negotiate in good faith to achieve a cessation of the nuclear arms race, nuclear disarmament, and general and complete disarmament.

Further, to meet objections about possible discriminatory effects, the Treaty stipulated that parties were to participate in, and have fullest access to materials and information for, peaceful uses of nuclear energy. The Treaty also provided that any potential benefits of nuclear explosions for peaceful purposes would be made available to non-nuclear weapon parties on a nondiscriminatory basis.

Security Assurances. Non-nuclear-weapon states sought guarantees that renunciation of nuclear arms would not place them at a permanent military disadvantage and make them vulnerable to nuclear intimidation. But, it was argued, the security interests of the various states, and groups of states, were not identical; an effort to frame provisions within the Treaty that would meet this diversity of requirements for

---

[1] International Atomic Energy Agency, a U.N.-sponsored agency headquartered at Vienna.
[2] European Atomic Energy Community, an organization established by the original European Common Market partners for cooperation in nuclear energy matters.
[3] EURATOM and the IAEA began negotiations in 1971. An IAEA-EURATOM safeguards agreement was signed in April 1973 and entered into force on February 21, 1977.

unforeseeable future contingencies would create inordinate complexities. To resolve the issue, the United States, the Soviet Union, and the United Kingdom submitted in the ENDC, on March 7, 1968, a tripartite proposal that security assurances take the form of a U.N. Security Council resolution, supported by declarations of the three powers. The resolution, noting the security concerns of states wishing to subscribe to the Non-Proliferation Treaty, would recognize that nuclear aggression, or the threat of nuclear aggression, would create a situation requiring immediate action by the Security Council, especially by its permanent members.

Following submission of the Treaty itself to the U.N. General Assembly, the tripartite resolution was submitted to the Security Council. In a formal declaration, the United States asserted its intention to seek immediate Security Council actions to provide assistance to any non-nuclear-weapon state party to the Treaty that was the object of nuclear aggression or threats. The Soviet Union and the United Kingdom made similar declarations. France abstained from voting on the Security Council resolution; the French representative said that France did not intend its abstention to be an obstacle to adoption of the tripartite proposal, but that France did not believe the nations would receive adequate security guarantees without nuclear disarmament.

In addition to this "positive" security assurance, the United States in 1978 issued a policy statement on "negative" security assurances in connection with the U.N. Special Session on Disarmament. Secretary of State Vance made the following statement on June 12, 1978:

After reviewing the current status of the discussions in the United Nations Special Session on Disarmament, after consultations with our principal allies, and on the basis of studies made in preparation for the Special Session, the President has decided to elaborate the U.S. position on the question of security assurances. His objective is to encourage support for halting the spread of nuclear weapons, to increase international security and stability, and to create a more positive environment for success of the Special Session. To this end, the President declares:

"The United States will not use nuclear weapons against any non-nuclear weapon state party to the NPT or any comparable internationally binding commitment not to acquire nuclear explosive

devices, except in the case of an attack on the United States, its territories or armed forces, or its allies, by such a state allied to a nuclear weapon state, or associated with a nuclear weapon state in carrying out or sustaining the attack."

In 1982, then-ACDA Director Eugene Rostow reaffirmed the assurance in the Geneva-based Committee on Disarmament. It is the U.S. view that this formulation preserves U.S. security commitments and advances U.S. collective security, as well as enhances the prospect for more effective arms control and disarmament.

This declaration has been reaffirmed by every successive Administration, most recently at the 1990 NPT Review Conference.

The Treaty was opened for signature on July 1, 1968, and signed on that date by the United States, the United Kingdom, the Soviet Union, and 59 other countries. On July 9, President Johnson transmitted it to the Senate, but prospects for early U.S. ratification dimmed after the Soviet invasion of Czechoslovakia in August. The Senate adjourned without voting on the Treaty. In February, 1969, President Nixon requested Senate approval of the Treaty, and in March the Senate gave its advice and consent to ratification. The Treaty entered into force with the deposit of U.S. ratification on March 5, 1970. In broadest outline, the basic provisions of the Treaty are designed to:

— prevent the spread of nuclear weapons (Articles I and II);

— provide assurance, through international safeguards, that the peaceful nuclear activities of states which have not already developed nuclear weapons will not be diverted to making such weapons (Article III);

— promote, to the maximum extent consistent with the other purposes of the Treaty, the peaceful uses of nuclear energy, to include the potential benefits of any peaceful application of nuclear explosion technology being made available to non-nuclear parties under appropriate international observation (Articles IV and V);

— express the determination of the parties that the Treaty should lead to further progress in comprehensive arms control and nuclear disarmament measures (Article VI).

Article VIII provides for a conference to be held five years after entry into force of the Treaty to review the operation of the Treaty with a view to assuring that the purposes of the Preamble and the provisions of the Treaty are being realized. Four such review conferences have been held since the Treaty entered into force. The first review conference, held in Geneva in May 1975, produced a strong reaffirmation of support for the Treaty by the parties thereto. It also expressed solid support for IAEA safeguards and recommended that greater efforts be made to make them universal and more effective. The 1975 conference urged common export requirements designed to extend safeguards to all peaceful nuclear activities, so-called "comprehensive safeguards" in importing non-nuclear-weapon states not party to the Treaty, and urged all suppliers and recipients to accept these requirements. It also concluded that NPT adherence should facilitate access to peaceful nuclear assistance and credit arrangements.

At the second review conference, which was held in Geneva August 11 - September 7, 1980, a thorough exchange of views on progress toward fulfillment of the Treaty's objectives was heard. Although the participants failed to agree on a final document, the national statements of the parties present and the ensuing debate revealed continued strong support for the NPT and its objectives.

The third review conference was held August 27 - September 21, 1985, in Geneva. The conference adopted by consensus a Final Declaration which reaffirmed the parties' support for the NPT and their appreciation of its essential contribution to international peace and security.

The 1985 conference reaffirmed the importance of preventing the further spread of nuclear weapons and concluded that the Treaty continued to meet this basic objective. It also affirmed that the nonproliferation and safeguards commitments of the NPT provide an essential framework for peaceful nuclear cooperation and acknowledged that there has been appreciable bilateral cooperation and multilateral technical assistance in the area of peaceful nuclear uses. Ways to strengthen peaceful nuclear cooperation were identified. The conference also strongly endorsed the IAEA and its safeguards system, as well as efforts to enhance further their effectiveness. Although it was unable to agree that

comprehensive safeguards should be a precondition for significant nuclear exports to non-NPT, non-nuclear-weapon states, the conference agreed not only on the desirability of such safeguards in non-nuclear-weapon states, but also that effective steps should be taken to achieve them.

As expected, evaluation of the progress made since 1970 in achieving the arms control and disarmament goals of Article VI evoked great disappointment and produced the most criticism. In particular, virtually all parties present supported immediate negotiations on and urgent conclusion of, a comprehensive nuclear test ban (CTB). The United States, while stating its commitment to the long-term goal of a CTB, stressed its conviction that deep reductions in existing nuclear arsenals should have the highest priority, and that it would continue to negotiate seriously and flexibly to this end in the Geneva negotiations. Both views were set out in the Final Declaration.

The NPT emerged from the 1985 review conference widely recognized as an arms control success, and the results of the conference reinforced the international norm of nonproliferation.

The fourth NPT review conference was held August 1990, in Geneva. A comprehensive and thorough review of the operation of the NPT over the previous five years was conducted during the conference, which once again affirmed that the NPT was a vital instrument for preserving global stability and security. The conference made progress on some important issues on which there was consensus, including the need for full-scope IAEA safeguards as a condition of significant nuclear supply, tighter export controls on nuclear technology transfers, and the need for scrupulous adherence to the obligations of the Treaty. Consensus was also achieved on such issues as negative security assurances and positive security assurances, prohibition of attacks on nuclear facilities, cooperation in the peaceful uses of nuclear energy, the importance of IAEA safeguards and effective export controls, and on nuclear safety. A very important result of the conference was the strong commitment by a clear majority of participating states to the importance of extending the life of the NPT in 1995. Unfortunately, this conference also demonstrated that a small number of states might be willing to risk damage to the Treaty by linking its extension to negotiations of other arms control measures, such as a Comprehensive Test Ban Treaty (CTB).

Article X (2). In accordance with the terms of the NPT, a conference was held in 1995 to decide whether the NPT should continue in force indefinitely or be extended for an additional fixed period or periods. On May 11, more than 170 countries attending the 1995 NPT Review and Extension Conference in New York decided to extend the Treaty indefinitely and without conditions.

The NPT remains the cornerstone of international efforts to prevent the further spread of nuclear weapons. With over 180 parties, it is the most widely adhered to arms control agreement in history. This impressive membership, which continues to grow, is a concrete reflection of the growing international support for nuclear nonproliferation.

TREATY ON THE NON-PROLIFERATION OF NUCLEAR WEAPONS

Signed at Washington, London, and Moscow July 1, 1968
Ratification advised by U.S. Senate March 13, 1969
Ratified by U.S. President November 24, 1969
U.S. ratification deposited at Washington, London, and Moscow March 5, 1970
Proclaimed by U.S. President March 5, 1970
Entered into force March 5, 1970

The States concluding this Treaty, hereinafter referred to as the "Parties to the Treaty",

Considering the devastation that would be visited upon all mankind by a nuclear war and the consequent need to make every effort to avert the danger of such a war and to take measures to safeguard the security of peoples,

Believing that the proliferation of nuclear weapons would seriously enhance the danger of nuclear war,

In conformity with resolutions of the United Nations General Assembly calling for the conclusion of an agreement on the prevention of wider dissemination of nuclear weapons,

Undertaking to cooperate in facilitating the application of International Atomic Energy Agency safeguards on peaceful nuclear activities,

Expressing their support for research, development and other efforts to further the application, within the framework of the International Atomic Energy Agency safeguards system, of the principle of safeguarding effectively the flow of source and special fissionable materials by use of instruments and other techniques at certain strategic points,

Affirming the principle that the benefits of peaceful applications of nuclear technology, including any technological by-products which may be derived by nuclear-weapon States from the development of nuclear explosive devices, should be available for peaceful purposes to all Parties of the Treaty, whether nuclear-weapon or non-nuclear weapon States,

Convinced that, in furtherance of this principle, all Parties to the Treaty are entitled to participate in the fullest possible exchange of scientific information for, and to contribute alone or in cooperation with other States to, the further development of the applications of atomic energy for peaceful purposes,

Declaring their intention to achieve at the earliest possible date the cessation of the nuclear arms race and to undertake effective measures in the direction of nuclear disarmament,

Urging the cooperation of all States in the attainment of this objective,

Recalling the determination expressed by the Parties to the 1963 Treaty banning nuclear weapon tests in the atmosphere, in outer space and under water in its Preamble to seek to achieve the discontinuance of all test explosions of nuclear weapons for all time and to continue negotiations to this end,

Desiring to further the easing of international tension and the strengthening of trust between States in order to facilitate the cessation of the manufacture of nuclear weapons, the liquidation of all their existing stockpiles, and the elimination from national arsenals of nuclear weapons and the means of their delivery pursuant to a Treaty on general and complete disarmament under strict and effective international control,

Recalling that, in accordance with the Charter of the United Nations, States must refrain in their international relations from the threat or use of force against the territorial integrity or political independence of any State, or in any other manner inconsistent with the Purposes of the United Nations, and that the establishment and maintenance of international peace and security are to be promoted with the least diversion for armaments of the world's human and economic resources,

Have agreed as follows:

Article I

Each nuclear-weapon State Party to the Treaty undertakes not to transfer to any recipient whatsoever nuclear weapons or other nuclear explosive devices or control over such weapons or explosive devices directly, or indirectly; and not in any way to assist, encourage, or induce any non-nuclear weapon State to manufacture or otherwise acquire nuclear weapons or other nuclear explosive devices, or control over such weapons or explosive devices.

Article II

Each non-nuclear-weapon State Party to the Treaty undertakes not to receive the transfer from any transferor whatsoever of nuclear weapons or other nuclear explosive devices or of control over such weapons or explosive devices directly, or indirectly; not to manufacture or otherwise acquire nuclear weapons or other nuclear explosive devices; and not to seek or receive any assistance in the manufacture of nuclear weapons or other nuclear explosive devices.

Article III

1. Each non-nuclear-weapon State Party to the Treaty undertakes to accept safeguards, as set forth in an agreement to be negotiated and concluded with the International Atomic Energy Agency in accordance with the Statute of the International Atomic Energy Agency and the Agency's safeguards system, for the exclusive purpose of verification of the fulfillment of its obligations assumed under this Treaty with a view to preventing diversion of nuclear energy from peaceful uses to nuclear weapons or other nuclear explosive devices. Procedures for the safeguards required by this article shall be followed with respect to source or special fissionable material whether it is being produced, processed or used in any principal nuclear facility or is outside any such facility. The safeguards required by this article shall be applied to all source or special fissionable material in all peaceful nuclear activities within the territory of such State, under its jurisdiction, or carried out under its control anywhere.

2. Each State Party to the Treaty undertakes not to provide: (a) source or special fissionable material, or (b) equipment or material especially designed or prepared for the processing, use or production of special fissionable material, to any non-nuclear-weapon State for peaceful purposes, unless the source or special fissionable material shall be subject to the safeguards required by this article.

3. The safeguards required by this article shall be implemented in a manner designed to comply with article IV of this Treaty, and to avoid hampering the economic or technological development of the Parties or international cooperation in the field of peaceful nuclear activities, including the international exchange of nuclear material and equipment for the processing, use or production of nuclear material for peaceful purposes in accordance with the provisions of this article and the principle of safeguarding set forth in the Preamble of the Treaty.

4. Non-nuclear-weapon States Party to the Treaty shall conclude agreements with the International Atomic Energy Agency to meet the requirements of this article either individually or together with other States in accordance with the Statute of the International Atomic Energy Agency. Negotiation of such agreements shall commence within 180 days from the original entry into force of this Treaty. For States depositing their instruments of ratification or accession after the 180-day period, negotiation of such agreements shall commence not later than the date of such deposit. Such agreements shall enter into force not later than eighteen months after the date of initiation of negotiations.

Article IV

1. Nothing in this Treaty shall be interpreted as affecting the inalienable right of all the Parties to the Treaty to develop research, production and use of nuclear energy for peaceful purposes without discrimination and in conformity with articles I and II of this Treaty.

2. All the Parties to the Treaty undertake to facilitate, and have the right to participate in, the fullest possible exchange of equipment, materials and scientific and technological information for the peaceful uses of nuclear energy. Parties to the Treaty in a position to do so shall also cooperate in contributing alone or together with other States or international organizations to the further development of the applications of nuclear energy for peaceful purposes, especially in the territories of non-nuclear-weapon States Party to the Treaty, with due consideration for the needs of the developing areas of the world.

Article V

Each party to the Treaty undertakes to take appropriate measures to ensure that, in accordance with this Treaty, under appropriate international observation and through appropriate international procedures, potential benefits from any peaceful applications of nuclear explosions will be made available to non-nuclear-weapon

States Party to the Treaty on a nondiscriminatory basis and that the charge to such Parties for the explosive devices used will be as low as possible and exclude any charge for research and development. Non-nuclear-weapon States Party to the Treaty shall be able to obtain such benefits, pursuant to a special international agreement or agreements, through an appropriate international body with adequate representation of non-nuclear-weapon States. Negotiations on this subject shall commence as soon as possible after the Treaty enters into force. Non-nuclear-weapon States Party to the Treaty so desiring may also obtain such benefits pursuant to bilateral agreements.

Article VI

Each of the Parties to the Treaty undertakes to pursue negotiations in good faith on effective measures relating to cessation of the nuclear arms race at an early date and to nuclear disarmament, and on a Treaty on general and complete disarmament under strict and effective international control.

Article VII

Nothing in this Treaty affects the right of any group of States to conclude regional treaties in order to assure the total absence of nuclear weapons in their respective territories.

Article VIII

1. Any Party to the Treaty may propose amendments to this Treaty. The text of any proposed amendment shall be submitted to the Depositary Governments which shall circulate it to all Parties to the Treaty. Thereupon, if requested to do so by one-third or more of the Parties to the Treaty, the Depositary Governments shall convene a conference, to which they shall invite all the Parties to the Treaty, to consider such an amendment.

2. Any amendment to this Treaty must be approved by a majority of the votes of all the Parties to the Treaty, including the votes of all nuclear-weapon States Party to the Treaty and all other Parties which, on the date the amendment is circulated, are members of the Board of Governors of the International Atomic Energy Agency. The amendment shall enter into force for each Party that deposits its instrument of

ratification of the amendment upon the deposit of such instruments of ratification by a majority of all the Parties, including the instruments of ratification of all nuclear-weapon States Party to the Treaty and all other Parties which, on the date the amendment is circulated, are members of the Board of Governors of the International Atomic Energy Agency. Thereafter, it shall enter into force for any other Party upon the deposit of its instrument of ratification of the amendment.

3. Five years after the entry into force of this Treaty, a conference of Parties to the Treaty shall be held in Geneva, Switzerland, in order to review the operation of this Treaty with a view to assuring that the purposes of the Preamble and the provisions of the Treaty are being realized. At intervals of five years thereafter, a majority of the Parties to the Treaty may obtain, by submitting a proposal to this effect to the Depositary Governments, the convening of further conferences with the same objective of reviewing the operation of the Treaty.

Article IX

1. This Treaty shall be open to all States for signature. Any State which does not sign the Treaty before its entry into force in accordance with paragraph 3 of this article may accede to it at any time.

2. This Treaty shall be subject to ratification by signatory States. Instruments of ratification and instruments of accession shall be deposited with the Governments of the United States of America, the United Kingdom of Great Britain and Northern Ireland and the Union of Soviet Socialist Republics, which are hereby designated the Depositary Governments.

3. This Treaty shall enter into force after its ratification by the States, the Governments of which are designated Depositaries of the Treaty, and forty other States signatory to this Treaty and the deposit of their instruments of ratification. For the purposes of this Treaty, a nuclear-weapon State is one which has manufactured and exploded a nuclear weapon or other nuclear explosive device prior to January 1, 1967.

4. For States whose instruments of ratification or accession are deposited subsequent to the entry into force of this Treaty, it shall enter into

force on the date of the deposit of their instruments of ratification or accession.

5. The Depositary Governments shall promptly inform all signatory and acceding States of the date of each signature, the date of deposit of each instrument of ratification or of accession, the date of the entry into force of this Treaty, and the date of receipt of any requests for convening a conference or other notices.

6. This Treaty shall be registered by the Depositary Governments pursuant to article 102 of the Charter of the United Nations.

Article X

1. Each Party shall in exercising its national sovereignty have the right to withdraw from the Treaty if it decides that extraordinary events, related to the subject matter of this Treaty, have jeopardized the supreme interests of its country. It shall give notice of such withdrawal to all other Parties to the Treaty and to the United Nations Security Council three months in advance. Such notice shall include a statement of the extraordinary events it regards as having jeopardized its supreme interests.

2. Twenty-five years after the entry into force of the Treaty, a conference shall be convened to decide whether the Treaty shall continue in force indefinitely, or shall be extended for an additional fixed period or periods. This decision shall be taken by a majority of the Parties to the Treaty.

Article XI

This Treaty, the English, Russian, French, Spanish and Chinese texts of which are equally authentic, shall be deposited in the archives of the Depositary Governments. Duly certified copies of this Treaty shall be transmitted by the Depositary Governments to the Governments of the signatory and acceding States.

IN WITNESS WHEREOF the undersigned, duly authorized, have signed this Treaty.

DONE in triplicate, at the cities of Washington, London and Moscow, this first day of July one thousand nine hundred sixty-eight.

TREATY ON THE NON-PROLIFERATION OF NUCLEAR WEAPONS

Country	Date of[a] Signature	Date of Deposit[a] of Ratification	Date of Deposit[a] of Accession (A) or Succession(S)
Afghanistan*	07/01/68	02/04/70	
Albania**			09/12/90(A)
Algeria			01/12/95(A)
Antigua and Barbuda			06/17/85(S)
Argentina			02/10/95(A)
Armenia			07/15/93(A)
Australia*	02/27/70	01/23/73	
Austria*	07/01/68	06/27/69	
Azerbaijan			09/22/92(A)
Bahamas, The			08/11/76(S)
Bahrain			11/03/88(A)
Bangladesh*			08/31/79(A)
Barbados	07/01/68	02/21/80	
Belarus			07/22/93(A)
Belgium*	08/20/68	05/02/75	
Belize			08/09/85(S)
Benin	07/01/68	10/31/72	
Bhutan*			05/23/85(A)
Bolivia	07/01/68	05/26/70	
Bosnia & Herzegovina			08/15/94(S)
Botswana	07/01/68	04/28/69	
Brunei*			03/26/85(A)
Bulgaria*	07/01/68	09/05/69	
Burkina Faso	11/25/68	03/03/70	
Burundi			03/19/71(A)
Cameroon	07/17/68	01/08/69	
Canada*	07/23/68	01/08/69	
Cape Verde			10/24/79(A)
Central African Republic			10/25/70(A)
Chad	07/01/68	03/10/71	
Chile			05/25/95(A)
China			03/09/92(A)
Colombia**	07/01/68	04/08/86	
Comoros			10/04/95(A)
Congo, People's Republic of (Brazzaville)			10/23/78(A)
Costa Rica*	07/01/68	03/03/70	
Croatia			06/29/92(S)
Cyprus*	07/01/68	02/10/70	
Czech Republic*			01/01/93(S)
Denmark*	07/01/68	01/03/69	
Dominica			08/10/84(S)
Dominican Republic*	07/01/68	07/24/71	
Ecuador*	07/09/68	03/07/69	
Egypt*	07/01/68	02/26/81[1]	
El Salvador*	07/01/68	07/11/72	
Equatorial Guinea			11/01/84(A)
Eritrea			03/03/95(A)
Estonia			01/07/92(A)
Ethiopia*	09/05/68	02/05/70	

TREATY ON THE NON-PROLIFERATION OF NUCLEAR WEAPONS -- Continued

Country	Date of[a] Signature	Date of Deposit[a] of Ratification	Date of Deposit[a] of Accession (A) or Succession(S)
Fiji*			07/14/72(S)
Finland*	07/01/68	02/05/69	
Former Yugoslav Republic of Macedonia			04/12/95(A)
France			08/03/92(A)
Gabon			02/19/74(A)
Gambia*, The	09/04/68	05/12/75	
Georgia			03/07/94(A)
Germany*, Federal Republic of	11/28/69	05/02/75[1,2]	
Ghana*	07/01/68	05/04/70	
Greece*	07/01/68	03/11/70	
Grenada			09/02/75(S)
Guatemala*	07/26/68	09/22/70	
Guinea			04/29/85(A)
Guinea-Bissau			08/20/76(S)
Guyana			10/19/93(A)
Haiti	07/01/68	06/02/70	
Holy See*			02/25/71(A)[1]
Honduras*	07/01/68	05/16/73	
Hungary*, Republic of	07/01/68	05/27/69	
Iceland*	07/01/68	07/18/69	
Indonesia*	03/02/70	07/12/79[1]	
Iran*	07/01/68	02/02/70	
Iraq*	07/01/68	10/29/69	
Ireland*	07/01/68	07/01/68	
Italy*	01/28/69	05/02/75[1]	
Ivory Coast*	07/01/68	03/06/73	
Jamaica*	04/14/69	03/05/70	
Japan*	02/03/70	06/08/76[1]	
Jordan*	07/10/68	02/11/70	
Kampuchea			06/02/72(A)
Kazakstan			02/14/94(A)
Kenya	07/01/68	06/11/70	
Kiribati*			04/18/85(S)
Korea, Democratic People's Republic of			12/12/85(A)
Korea*, Republic of	07/01/68	04/23/75	
Kuwait	08/15/68	11/17/89	
Kyrgyzstan			07/05/94(A)
Laos	07/01/68	02/20/70	
Latvia			01/31/92(A)
Lebanon*	07/01/68	07/15/70	
Lesotho*	07/09/68	05/20/70	
Liberia	07/01/68	03/05/70	
Libya*	07/18/68	05/26/75	
Liechtenstein*			04/20/78(A)[1]

TREATY ON THE NON-PROLIFERATION OF NUCLEAR WEAPONS -- Continued

Country	Date of[a] Signature	Date of Deposit[a] of Ratification	Date of Deposit[a] of Accession (A) or Succession(S)
Lithuania			09/23/91(A)
Luxembourg*	08/14/68	05/02/75	
Madagascar*	08/22/68	10/08/70	
Malawi*			02/18/86(S)
Malaysia*	07/01/68	03/05/70	
Maldive Islands*	09/11/68	04/07/70	
Mali	07/14/69	02/10/70	
Malta*	04/17/69	02/06/70	
Marshall Islands			01/30/95(A)
Mauritania			10/26/93(A)
Mauritius*	07/01/68	04/08/69	
Mexico*	07/26/68	01/21/69[1]	
Micronesia			04/14/95(A)
Moldova			10/11/94(A)
Monaco			03/13/95(A)
Mongolia*	07/01/68	05/14/69	
Morocco*	07/01/68	11/27/70	
Mozambique			09/04/90(A)
Myanmar (Burma)			12/02/92(A)
Namibia			10/02/92(A)
Nauru*			06/07/82(A)
Nepal*	07/01/68	01/05/70	
Netherlands*	08/20/68	05/02/75[3]	
New Zealand*	07/01/68	09/10/69	
Nicaragua*	07/01/68	03/06/73	
Niger			10/09/92(A)
Nigeria*	07/01/68	09/27/68	
Norway*	07/01/68	02/05/69	
Palau			04/12/95(A)
Panama	07/01/68	01/13/77	
Papua New Guinea*			01/25/82(A)
Paraguay*	07/01/68	02/04/70	
Peru*	07/01/68	03/03/70	
Philippines*	07/01/68	10/05/72	
Poland*	07/01/68	06/12/69	
Portugal*			12/15/77(A)
Qatar			04/03/89(A)
Romania*	07/01/68	02/04/70	
Russia[5]	07/01/68	03/05/70	
Rwanda			05/20/75(A)

TREATY ON THE NON-PROLIFERATION OF NUCLEAR WEAPONS -- Continued

Country	Date of[a] Signature	Date of Deposit[a] of Ratification	Date of Deposit[a] of Accession (A) or Succession(S)
St. Kitts and Nevis			03/22/93(A)
St. Lucia*			12/28/79(S)
St. Vincent and the Grenadines			11/06/84(S)
San Marino	07/01/68	08/10/70	
Sao Tome and Principe			07/20/83(A)
Saudi Arabia			10/03/88(A)
Senegal*	07/01/68	12/17/70	
Seychelles			03/12/85(A)
Sierra Leone			02/26/75(A)
Singapore*	02/05/70	03/10/76	
Slovakia			01/01/93(S)
Slovenia			04/07/92(A)
Solomon Islands			06/17/81(S)
Somalia	07/01/68	03/05/70	
South Africa*			07/10/91(A)
Spain*			11/05/87(A)
Sri Lanka*	07/01/68	03/05/79	
Sudan*	12/24/68	10/31/73	
Suriname*			06/30/76(S)[b]
Swaziland*	06/24/69	12/11/69	
Sweden*	08/19/68	01/09/70	
Switzerland*	11/27/69	03/09/77[1]	
Syrian Arab Republic	07/01/68	09/24/69	
Taiwan[7]	07/01/68	01/27/70[5]	
Tajikistan			01/17/95(A)
Tanzania			05/31/91(A)
Thailand*			12/02/72(A)
Togo	07/01/68	02/26/70	
Tonga			07/07/71(S)
Trinidad and Tobago	08/20/68	10/30/86	
Tunisia*	07/01/68	02/26/70	
Turkey*	01/28/69	04/17/80[1]	
Tuvalu*			01/19/79(S)
Turkmenistan			09/29/94(A)
Uganda			10/20/82(A)
Ukraine			12/05/94(A)
United Kingdom	07/01/68	11/27/68[4]	
United States	07/01/68	03/05/70	
Uruguay*	07/01/68	08/31/70	
Uzbekistan*			05/02/92
Vanuatu			08/26/95(A)
Venezuela*	07/01/68	09/25/75	
Vietnam*, Socialist Republic of			06/14/82(A)
Western Samoa*			03/17/75(A)

TREATY ON THE NON-PROLIFERATION OF NUCLEAR WEAPONS -- Continued

Country	Date of[a] Signature	Date of Deposit[a] of Ratification	Date of Deposit[a] of Accession (A) or Succession(S)
Yemen[6]	11/14/68	06/01/79	
Yugoslavia, Socialist Federal Republic of	07/10/68	03/04/70	
Zaire*	07/22/68	08/04/70	
Zambia			05/15/91(A)
Zimbabwe			09/26/91(A)

TOTAL: 181 (Total does not include Taiwan or SFR Yugoslavia, which has dissolved.)

NOTES:

[a] - Dates given are the earliest dates on which a country signed the Treaty or deposited its instrument of ratification or accession -- whether in Washington, London, or Moscow. In the case of a country that was a dependent territory which became a party through succession, the date given is the date on which the country gave notice that it would continue to be bound by the terms of the Treaty.

[b] - Effective 11/25/75.

[1] With Statement.

[2] The former German Democratic Republic, which united with the Federal Republic of Germany on 10/3/90, had signed the NPT on 7/1/68 and deposited its instrument of ratification on 10/31/69.

[3] Extended to Netherlands Antilles and Aruba.

[4] Extended to Aguilla and territories under the territorial sovereignty of the United Kingdom.

[5] Russia has given notice that it would continue to exercise the rights and fulfill the obligations of the former Soviet Union arising from the NPT.

[6] The Republic of Yemen resulted from the union of the Yemen Arab Republic and the People's Democratic Republic of Yemen. The table indicates the date of signature and ratification by the People's Democratic Republic of Yemen; the first of these two states to become a party to the NPT. The Yemen Arab Republic signed the NPT on 9/23/68 and deposited its instrument of ratification on 5/14/86.

[7] On 1/27/70, an instrument of ratification was deposited in the name of the Republic of China. Effective 1/1/79, the United States recognized the People's Republic of China as the sole legal government of China. The authorities on Taiwan state that they will continue to abide by the provisions of the Treaty and the United States regards them as bound by the obligations imposed by the Treaty.

* Entries with asterisk have NPT safeguards agreements that have entered into force as of 10/31/92.

** Non-NPT, full-scope safeguards agreement in force.

TREATY ON THE PROHIBITION OF THE EMPLACEMENT OF NUCLEAR WEAPONS AND OTHER WEAPONS OF MASS DESTRUCTION ON THE SEABED AND THE OCEAN FLOOR AND IN THE SUBSOIL THEREOF

Like the Antarctic Treaty, the Outer Space Treaty, and the Latin American Nuclear-Free Zone, the Seabed Treaty sought to prevent the introduction of international conflict and nuclear weapons into an area hitherto free of them. Reaching agreement on the seabed, however, involved problems not met in framing the other two agreements.

In the 1960s, advances in the technology of oceanography and greatly increased interest in the vast and virtually untapped resources of the ocean floor led to concern that the absence of clearly established rules of law might lead to strife. And there were concurrent fears that nations might use the seabed as a new environment for military installations, including those capable of launching nuclear weapons.

In keeping with a proposal submitted to the U.N. Secretary General by Ambassador Pardo of Malta in August 1967, the U.N. General Assembly, on December 18, 1967, established an ad hoc committee to study ways of reserving the seabed for peaceful purposes, with the objective of ensuring "that the exploration and use of the seabed and the ocean floor should be conducted in accordance with the principles and purposes of the Charter of the United Nations, in the interests of maintaining international peace and security and for the benefit of all mankind." The Committee was given permanent status the following year. At the same time, seabed-related military and arms control issues were referred to the ENDC and its successor, the CCD.[1] In a message of March 18, 1969, President Nixon said the American delegation to the ENDC should seek discussion of the factors necessary for an international agreement prohibiting the emplacement of weapons of mass destruction on the seabed and ocean floor and pointed out that an agreement of this kind would, like the Antarctic and Outer Space treaties, "prevent an arms race before it has a chance to start."

---

[1] As noted elsewhere, the Geneva-based ENDC (Eighteen-Nation Disarmament Committee) became known as the CCD (Conference of the Committee on Disarmament) after its enlargement in 1969.

On March 18, 1969, the Soviet Union presented a draft Treaty that provided for the complete demilitarization of the seabed beyond a 12-mile limit and making all seabed installations open to Treaty parties on the basis of reciprocity. The U.S. draft Treaty, submitted on May 22, prohibited the emplacement of nuclear weapons and other weapons of mass destruction on the seabed and ocean floor beyond a three-mile band. This, the United States held, was the urgent problem, and complete demilitarization would not be verifiable.

As can be seen, the two drafts differed importantly on what was to be prohibited. The Soviet draft would have banned all military uses of the seabed. It would have precluded, for example, submarine surveillance systems that were fixed to the ocean floor. The United States regarded these as essential to its defense.

The two drafts also differed on the issue of verification. Using as a model the provisions for verification in the Outer Space Treaty, the Soviets proposed that all installations and structures be open to inspection, provided that reciprocal rights to inspect were granted. The United States contended that on the Moon no claims of national jurisdiction existed and that provisions suitable for the Moon would not be adequate for the seabed, where many claims of national jurisdiction already existed and many kinds of activities were in progress or possible. Moreover, the United States felt that to attempt to inspect for the emplacement of all kinds of weapons would make the problems connected with verification virtually insuperable.

On the other hand, the United States stated the case that any structures capable of handling nuclear devices would necessarily be large and elaborate; their installation would require extensive activity, difficult to conceal; and there would probably be a number of devices involved, as it would not be worth violating the Treaty simply to install one or two weapons. Violations, therefore, would be readily observed and evoke the appropriate steps -- first an effort to deal directly with the problem through consultations with the country violating the Treaty; if that failed, recourse to cooperative action; and, as a last resort, appeal to the Security Council.

Comments on the two drafts in the ENDC, U.S. consultations with its NATO allies, and private U.S.-Soviet talks at the ENDC eventually led to the framing of a joint draft by the United States and the Soviet Union, submitted on October 7, 1969, to the CCD. This joint draft underwent intensive discussion and was three times revised in response to suggestions made in the CCD and at the United Nations.

Discussion centered on a few difficult issues. In international law there was much confusion about how territorial waters were to be defined. Some countries claimed up to 200 miles, and international conventions on the subject contained ambiguities. In its final form the Treaty adopted a 12-mile limit to define the seabed area.

The verification provisions also were a subject of intensive discussion. Coastal states were concerned about whether their rights would be protected. Smaller states had doubts as to their ability to check on violations. Some felt that the United Nations should play a larger role. Some wondered whether the verification procedures would really be effective. Reassurances were given to the coastal states. Smaller states could apply for assistance to another state to help it in case of a suspected violation.

The verification procedures are set forth in Article III. Parties may undertake verification using their own means, with the assistance of other parties, or through appropriate international procedures within the framework of the United Nations and in accordance with its Charter. These provisions permit parties to assure themselves the Treaty obligations are being fulfilled without interfering with legitimate seabed activities.

After more than two years of negotiation, the final draft was approved by the U.N. General Assembly on December 7, 1970, by a vote of 104 to 2 (El Salvador, Peru), with two abstentions (Ecuador and France).

Article I sets forth the principal obligation of the Treaty. It prohibits parties from emplacing nuclear weapons or weapons of mass destruction on the seabed and the ocean floor beyond a 12-mile coastal zone. Article II provides that the "seabed zone" is to be measured in accordance with the provisions of the 1958 Convention on the Territorial Sea and the Contiguous Zone. To make clear that none of the Treaty's provisions

should be interpreted as supporting or prejudicing the positions of any party regarding law-of-the-sea issues, a broad disclaimer provision to this effect was included as Article IV.

In recognition of the feeling that efforts to achieve a more comprehensive agreement should continue, Article V of the Treaty bound parties to work for further measures to prevent an arms race on the seabed.

The Seabed Arms Control Treaty was opened for signature in Washington, London, and Moscow on February 11, 1971. It entered into force May 18, 1972, when the United States, the United Kingdom, the Soviet Union, and more than 22 nations had deposited instruments of ratification.

Article VII included a provision for a review conference to be held in five years. The Seabed Arms Control Treaty Review Conference was held in Geneva June 20 - July 1, 1977. The Conference concluded that the first five years in the life of the Treaty had demonstrated its effectiveness. The Second Review Conference, held in Geneva in September 1983, concluded that the Treaty continued to be an important and effective arms control measure. The Third Review Conference was held in Geneva in September 1989 and confirmed results of previous meetings. It was agreed that the next review conference would be convened in Geneva not earlier than 1996.

TREATY ON THE PROHIBITION OF THE EMPLACEMENT OF NUCLEAR WEAPONS AND OTHER WEAPONS OF MASS DESTRUCTION ON THE SEABED AND THE OCEAN FLOOR AND IN THE SUBSOIL THEREOF

Signed at Washington, London, and Moscow February 11, 1971
Ratification advised by U.S. Senate February 15, 1972
Ratified by U.S. President April 26, 1972
U.S. ratification deposited at Washington, London, and Moscow May 18, 1972
Proclaimed by U.S. President May 18, 1972
Entered into force May 18, 1972

The States Parties to this Treaty,

Recognizing the common interest of mankind in the progress of the exploration and use of the seabed and the ocean floor for peaceful purposes,

Considering that the prevention of a nuclear arms race on the seabed and the ocean floor serves the interests of maintaining world peace, reduces international tensions and strengthens friendly relations among States,

Convinced that this Treaty constitutes a step towards the exclusion of the seabed, the ocean floor and the subsoil thereof from the arms race,

Convinced that this Treaty constitutes a step towards a Treaty on general and complete disarmament under strict and effective international control, and determined to continue negotiations to this end,

Convinced that this Treaty will further the purposes and principles of the Charter of the United Nations, in a manner consistent with the principles of international law and without infringing the freedoms of the high seas,

Have agreed as follows:

Article I

1. The States Parties to this Treaty undertake not to emplant or emplace on the seabed and the ocean floor and in the subsoil thereof beyond the outer limit of a seabed zone, as defined in article II, any nuclear weapons or any other types of weapons of mass destruction as well as structures, launching installations or any other facilities specifically designed for storing, testing or using such weapons.

2. The undertakings of paragraph 1 of this article shall also apply to the seabed zone referred to in the same paragraph, except that within such seabed zone, they shall not apply either to the coastal State or to the seabed beneath its territorial waters.

3. The States Parties to this Treaty undertake not to assist, encourage or induce any State to carry out activities referred to in paragraph 1 of this article and not to participate in any other way in such actions.

Article II

For the purpose of this Treaty, the outer limit of the seabed zone referred to in article I shall be coterminous with the twelve-mile outer limit of the zone referred to in part II of the Convention on the Territorial Sea and the Contiguous Zone, signed at Geneva on April 29, 1958, and shall be measured in accordance with the provisions of part I, section II, of that Convention and in accordance with international law.

Article III

1. In order to promote the objectives of and insure compliance with the provisions of this Treaty, each State Party to the Treaty shall have the right to verify through observations the activities of other States Parties to the Treaty on the seabed and the ocean floor and in the subsoil thereof beyond the zone referred to in article I, provided that observation does not interfere with such activities.

2. If after such observation reasonable doubts remain concerning the fulfillment of the obligations assumed under the Treaty, the State Party having such doubts and the State Party that is responsible for the activities giving rise to the doubts shall consult with a view to removing the doubts. If the doubts persist, the State Party having such doubts shall notify the other States Parties, and the Parties concerned shall cooperate on such further procedures for verification as may be agreed, including appropriate inspection of objects, structures, installations or other facilities that reasonably may be expected to be of a kind described in article I. The Parties in the region of the activities, including any coastal State, and any other Party so requesting, shall be entitled to participate in

such consultation and cooperation. After completion of the further procedures for verification, an appropriate report shall be circulated to other Parties by the Party that initiated such procedures.

3. If the State responsible for the activities giving rise to the reasonable doubts is not identifiable by observation of the object, structure, installation or other facility, the State Party having such doubts shall notify and make appropriate inquiries of States Parties in the region of the activities and of any other State Party. If it is ascertained through these inquiries that a particular State Party is responsible for the activities, that State Party shall consult and cooperate with other Parties as provided in paragraph 2 of this article. If the identity of the State responsible for the activities cannot be ascertained through these inquiries, then further verification procedures, including inspection, may be undertaken by the inquiring State Party, which shall invite the participation of the Parties in the region of the activities, including any coastal State, and of any other Party desiring to cooperate.

4. If consultation and cooperation pursuant to paragraphs 2 and 3 of this article have not removed the doubts concerning the activities and there remains a serious question concerning fulfillment of the obligations assumed under this Treaty, a State Party may, in accordance with the provisions of the Charter of the United Nations, refer the matter to the Security Council, which may take action in accordance with the Charter.

5. Verification pursuant to this article may be undertaken by any State Party using its own means, or with the full or partial assistance of any other State Party, or through appropriate international procedures within the framework of the United Nations and in accordance with its Charter.

6. Verification activities pursuant to this Treaty shall not interfere with activities of other States Parties and shall be conducted with due regard for rights recognized under international law, including the freedoms of the high seas and the rights of coastal States with respect to the exploration and exploitation of their continental shelves.

Article IV

Nothing in this Treaty shall be interpreted as supporting or prejudicing the position of any State Party with respect to existing international conventions, including the 1958 Convention on the Territorial Sea and the Contiguous Zone, or with respect to rights or claims which such State Party may assert, or with respect to recognition or non-recognition of rights or claims asserted by any other State, related to waters off its coasts, including, *inter alia*, territorial seas and contiguous zones, or to the seabed and the ocean floor, including continental shelves.

Article V

The Parties to this Treaty undertake to continue negotiations in good faith concerning further measures in the field of disarmament for the prevention of an arms race on the seabed, the ocean floor and the subsoil thereof.

Article VI

Any State Party may propose amendments to this Treaty. Amendments shall enter into force for each State Party accepting the amendments upon their acceptance by a majority of the States Parties to the Treaty and, thereafter, for each remaining State Party on the date of acceptance by it.

Article VII

Five years after the entry into force of this Treaty, a conference of Parties to the Treaty shall be held at Geneva, Switzerland, in order to review the operation of this Treaty with a view to assuring that the purposes of the preamble and the provisions of the Treaty are being realized. Such review shall take into account any relevant technological developments. The review conference shall determine, in accordance with the views of a majority of those Parties attending, whether and when an additional review conference shall be convened.

Article VIII

Each State Party to this Treaty shall in exercising its national sovereignty have the right to withdraw from this Treaty if it decides that extraordinary events related to the subject matter of this Treaty have jeopardized the supreme interests of its country. It shall give notice of such withdrawal to all other States Parties to the Treaty and to the United Nations Security Council three months in advance. Such notice shall include a statement of the extraordinary events it considers to have jeopardized its supreme interests.

Article IX

The provisions of this Treaty shall in no way affect the obligations assumed by States Parties to the Treaty under international instruments establishing zones free from nuclear weapons.

Article X

1. This Treaty shall be open for signature to all States. Any State which does not sign the Treaty before its entry into force in accordance with paragraph 3 of this article may accede to it at any time.

2. This Treaty shall be subject to ratification by signatory States. Instruments of ratification and of accession shall be deposited with the Governments of the United States of America, the United Kingdom of Great Britain and Northern Ireland, and the Union of Soviet Socialist Republics, which are hereby designated the Depositary Governments.

3. This Treaty shall enter into force after the deposit of instruments of ratification by twenty-two Governments, including the Governments designated as Depositary Governments of this Treaty.

4. For states whose instruments of ratification or accession are deposited after the entry into force of this Treaty, it shall enter into force on the date of the deposit of their instruments of ratification or accession.

5. The Depositary Governments shall promptly inform the Governments of all signatory and acceding States of the date of each signature, of the date of deposit of each instrument of ratification or of accession, of the date of the entry into force of this Treaty, and of the receipt of other notices.

6. This Treaty shall be registered by the Depositary Governments pursuant to Article 102 of the Charter of the United Nations.

Article XI

This Treaty, the English, Russian, French, Spanish and Chinese texts of which are equally authentic, shall be deposited in the archives of the Depositary Governments. Duly certified copies of this Treaty shall be transmitted by the Depositary Governments to the Governments of the States signatory and acceding thereto.

IN WITNESS WHEREOF the undersigned, being duly authorized thereto, have signed this Treaty.

DONE in triplicate, at the cities of Washington, London and Moscow, this eleventh day of February, one thousand nine hundred seventy-one.

SEABED ARMS CONTROL TREATY

Country	Date[1] of Signature	Date of Deposit[1] of Ratification	Date of Deposit[1] of Accession
Afghanistan	02/11/71	04/22/71	
Algeria			01/27/92
Antigua & Barbuda		03/21/83	11/16/88
Argentina	09/03/71		
Australia	02/11/71	01/23/73	
Austria	02/11/71	08/10/72	
Bahamas, The			06/07/89
Belgium	02/11/71	11/20/72	
Benin	03/18/71	07/02/86	
Bolivia	02/11/71		
Botswana	02/11/71	11/10/72	
Brazil	09/03/71	05/10/88	
Bulgaria	02/11/71	04/16/71	
Burma	02/11/71		
Burundi	02/11/71		
Byelorussian S.S.R.[2]	03/03/71	09/14/71	
Cameroon	11/11/71		
Canada	02/11/71	05/17/72	
Cape Verde			10/24/79
Central African Republic	02/11/71	07/09/81	
China, People's Republic of			02/28/91
China (Taiwan)[4]	02/11/71	02/22/72	
Colombia	02/11/71		
Congo, People's Republic of (Brazzaville)			10/23/78
Costa Rica	02/11/71		
Côte d'Ivoire			01/14/72
Croatia*			10/08/91
Cyprus	02/11/71	11/17/71	
Cuba			06/03/77
Czechoslovakia	02/11/71	01/11/72	
Denmark	02/11/71	06/15/71	
Dominican Republic	02/11/71	02/11/72	
Equatorial Guinea	06/04/71		
Ethiopia	02/11/71	07/14/77	
Finland	02/11/71	06/08/71	
Gambia, The	05/18/71		
German Democratic Republic	02/11/71	07/27/71	
Germany, Federal Republic of	06/08/71	11/18/75	
Ghana	02/11/71	08/09/72	
Greece	02/11/71	05/28/85	
Guatemala	02/11/71		
Guinea	02/11/71		
Guinea-Bissau			08/20/76

SEABED ARMS CONTROL TREATY -- Continued

Country	Date[1] of Signature	Date of Deposit[1] of Ratification	Date of Deposit[1] of Accession
Honduras	02/11/71		
Hungary	02/11/71	08/13/71	
Iceland	02/11/71	05/30/72	
India			07/20/73
Iran	02/11/71	08/26/71	
Iraq	02/22/71	09/13/72	
Ireland	02/11/71	08/19/71	
Italy	02/11/71	09/03/74	
Jamaica	10/11/71	07/30/86	
Japan	02/11/71	06/21/71	
Jordan	02/11/71	08/17/71	
Kampuchea	02/11/71		
Korea, Republic of	02/11/71	06/25/86	
Laos	02/11/71	10/19/71	
Latvia			08/18/92
Lebanon	02/11/71		
Lesotho	09/08/71	04/03/73	
Liberia	02/11/71		
Liechtenstein			05/30/91
Luxembourg	02/11/71	11/11/82	
Madagascar	09/14/71		
Malaysia	05/20/71	06/21/72	
Mali	02/11/71		
Malta	02/11/71	05/04/71	
Mauritius	02/11/71	04/23/71	
Mexico			3/23/84
Mongolia	02/11/71	10/08/71	
Morocco	02/11/71	07/26/71	
Nepal	02/11/71	07/06/71	
Netherlands	02/11/71	01/14/76	
New Zealand	02/11/71	02/24/72	
Nicaragua	02/11/71	02/07/73	
Niger	02/11/71	08/09/71	
Norway	02/11/71	06/28/71	
Panama	02/11/71	03/20/74	
Paraguay	02/23/71		
Philippines			11/05/92
Poland	02/11/71	11/15/71	
Portugal			06/24/75
Qatar			11/12/74
Romania	02/11/71	07/10/72	
Rwanda	02/11/71	05/20/75	

SEABED ARMS CONTROL TREATY -- Continued

Country	Date[1] of Signature	Date of Deposit[1] of Ratification	Date of Deposit[1] of Accession
St. Christopher-Nevis			09/19/83[1]
St. Lucia			02/22/79[1]
St. Vincent and the Grenadines			10/27/79[1]
São Tomé and Principe			08/24/79
Saudi Arabia	01/07/72	06/23/72	
Senegal	03/17/71		
Seychelles			03/12/85[1]
Sierra Leone	02/11/71		
Singapore	05/05/71	09/10/76	
Slovenia*			04/13/92
Slovak Republic*			10/08/91
Solomon Islands			07/07/78[1]
South Africa	02/11/71	11/14/73	
Spain			07/15/87
Sudan	02/11/71		
Swaziland	02/11/71	08/09/71	
Sweden	02/11/71	04/28/72	
Switzerland	02/11/71	05/04/76	
Tanzania	02/11/71		
Togo	04/02/71	06/28/71	
Tunisia	02/11/71	10/22/71	
Turkey	02/25/71	10/19/72	
Ukrainian S.S.R.[2]	03/03/71	09/03/71	
Union of Soviet Socialist Republics	02/11/71	05/18/72	
United Kingdom	02/11/71	05/18/72	
United States	02/11/71	05/18/72	
Uruguay	02/11/71		
Vietnam			06/20/80
Yemen Arab Republic (Sanaa)	02/23/71		
Yemen, People's Democratic Republic of (Aden)	02/23/71	06/01/79	
Yugoslavia	03/02/71	10/25/73	
Zambia			10/09/72
Total [3]	89	66	28

* notification of succession
  See footnotes on page 350.

AGREEMENT ON MEASURES TO REDUCE THE RISK OF OUTBREAK OF NUCLEAR WAR BETWEEN THE UNITED STATES OF AMERICA AND THE UNION OF SOVIET SOCIALIST REPUBLICS

The very existence of nuclear-weapon systems, even under the most sophisticated command-and-control procedures, obviously is a source of constant concern. Despite the most elaborate precautions, it is conceivable that technical malfunction or human failure, a misinterpreted incident or unauthorized action, could trigger a nuclear disaster or nuclear war. In the course of the Strategic Arms Limitation Talks (SALT), the United States and the Soviet Union reached two agreements that manifest increasing recognition of the need to reduce such risks, and that complement the central goal of the negotiations.

In early sessions, discussions parallel to the main SALT negotiations showed a degree of mutual concern regarding the problem of accidental war that indicated encouraging prospects of accord. These preliminary explorations resulted in the establishment of two special working groups under the direction of the two SALT delegations. One group focused on arrangements for exchanging information to reduce uncertainties and prevent misunderstandings in the event of a nuclear incident. The other addressed a related topic -- ways to improve the direct communications link between Washington and Moscow. By the summer of 1971, major substantive issues had been resolved, and draft international agreements were referred by the SALT delegations to their governments. Both agreements were signed in Washington on September 30, 1971, and came into force on that date.

The Agreement on Measures To Reduce the Risk of Outbreak of Nuclear War between the United States of America and the Union of Soviet Socialist Republics covers three main areas:

— A pledge by each party to take measures each considers necessary to maintain and improve its organizational and technical safeguards against accidental or unauthorized use of nuclear weapons;

— Arrangements for immediate notification should a risk of nuclear war arise from such incidents, from detection of unidentified objects on early warning systems, or from any accidental, unauthorized, or other unexplained incident involving a possible detonation of a nuclear weapon; and

— Advance notification of any planned missile launches beyond the territory of the launching party and in the direction of the other party.

The agreement provides that for urgent communication "in situations requiring prompt clarification" the "Hot Line" will be used. The duration of the agreement is not limited, and the parties undertake to consult on questions that may arise and to discuss possible amendments aimed at further reduction of risks.

AGREEMENT ON MEASURES TO REDUCE THE RISK OF OUTBREAK OF NUCLEAR WAR BETWEEN THE UNITED STATES OF AMERICA AND THE UNION OF SOVIET SOCIALIST REPUBLICS

Signed at Washington September 30, 1971
Entered into force September 30, 1971

The United States of America and the Union of Soviet Socialist Republics, hereinafter referred to as the Parties:

Taking into account the devastating consequences that nuclear war would have for all mankind, and recognizing the need to exert every effort to avert the risk of outbreak of such a war, including measures to guard against accidental or unauthorized use of nuclear weapons,

Believing that agreement on measures for reducing the risk of outbreak of nuclear war serves the interests of strengthening international peace and security, and is in no way contrary to the interests of any other country,

Bearing in mind that continued efforts are also needed in the future to seek ways of reducing the risk of outbreak of nuclear war,

Have agreed as follows:

Article 1

Each Party undertakes to maintain and to improve, as it deems necessary, its existing organizational and technical arrangements to guard against the accidental or unauthorized use of nuclear weapons under its control.

Article 2

The Parties undertake to notify each other immediately in the event of an accidental, unauthorized or any other unexplained incident involving a possible detonation of a nuclear weapon which could create a risk of outbreak of nuclear war. In the event of such an incident, the Party whose nuclear weapon is involved will immediately make every effort to take necessary measures to render harmless or destroy such weapon without its causing damage.

Article 3

The Parties undertake to notify each other immediately in the event of detection by missile warning systems of unidentified objects, or in the event of signs of interference with these systems or with related communications facilities, if such occurrences could create a risk of outbreak of nuclear war between the two countries.

Article 4

Each Party undertakes to notify the other Party in advance of any planned missile launches if such launches will extend beyond its national territory in the direction of the other Party.

Article 5

Each Party, in other situations involving unexplained nuclear incidents, undertakes to act in such a manner as to reduce the possibility of its actions being misinterpreted by the other Party. In any such situation, each Party may inform the other Party or request information when in its view, this is warranted by the interests of averting the risk of outbreak of nuclear war.

Article 6

For transmission of urgent information, notifications and requests for information in situations requiring prompt clarification, the Parties shall make primary use of the Direct Communications Link between the Governments of the United States of America and the Union of Soviet Socialist Republics.

For transmission of other information, notification and requests for information, the Parties, at their own discretion, may use any communications facilities, including diplomatic channels, depending on the degree of urgency.

Article 7

The Parties undertake to hold consultations, as mutually agreed, to consider questions relating to implementation of the provisions of this Agreement, as well as to discuss possible amendments thereto aimed at further implementation of the purposes of this Agreement.

Article 8

This Agreement shall be of unlimited duration.

Article 9

This Agreement shall enter into force upon signature.

DONE at Washington on September 30, 1971, in two copies, each in the English and Russian languages, both texts being equally authentic.

FOR THE UNITED STATES OF AMERICA:
WILLIAM P. ROGERS

FOR THE UNION OF SOVIET SOCIALIST REPUBLICS:
A. GROMYKO

AGREEMENT BETWEEN THE UNITED STATES OF AMERICA AND THE UNION OF SOVIET SOCIALIST REPUBLICS ON MEASURES TO IMPROVE THE U.S.A.-USSR DIRECT COMMUNICATIONS LINK (WITH ANNEX, SUPPLEMENTING AND MODIFYING THE MEMORANDUM OF UNDERSTANDING WITH ANNEX, OF JUNE 20,1963)

The United States and the Soviet Union had agreed in 1963 to establish, for use in time of emergency, a direct communications link between the two governments. The original "Hot Line" agreement provided for a wire telegraph circuit, routed Washington-London-Copenhagen-Stockholm-Helsinki-Moscow, and as a backup system a radio telegraph circuit routed Washington-Tangier-Moscow. These circuits had one terminal in the United States and one in the Soviet Union.

Concern about the risk that nuclear accidents, ambiguous incidents, or unauthorized actions might lead to the outbreak of nuclear war contributed to concern about the reliability and survivability of the "Hot Line," which had shown its value in emergency situations. The advances in satellite communications technology that had occurred since 1963, moreover, offered the possibility of greater reliability than the arrangements originally agreed upon. Hence, when the SALT delegations established a special working group under their direction to work on "accidents measures," a similar group was established to consider ways to improve the Washington-Moscow direct communications link.

The understandings reached by this group were reported to the SALT delegations in the summer of 1971 and became a formal agreement to improve the "Hot Line" at the same time that the related agreement on steps to reduce the risks of accidental war was concluded.

The terms of the agreement, with its annex detailing the specifics of operation, equipment, and allocation of costs, provided for establishment of two satellite communications circuits between the United States and the Soviet Union, with a system of multiple terminals in each country. The United States was to provide one circuit via the Intelsat system, and the Soviet Union a circuit via its Molniya II system. The agreement of 1963 was to remain in force "except to the extent that its provisions are modified by this Agreement and Annex thereto." The original circuits were to be maintained until it was agreed that the operation of the satellite circuits made them no longer necessary.

On September 30, 1971, the agreement was signed in Washington. The two satellite communications circuits became operational in January 1978. The radio circuit provided for in the 1963 agreement was then terminated, but the wire telegraph circuit has been retained as a backup.

AGREEMENT BETWEEN THE UNITED STATES OF AMERICA AND THE UNION OF SOVIET SOCIALIST REPUBLICS ON MEASURES TO IMPROVE THE U.S.A.-USSR DIRECT COMMUNICATIONS LINK

Signed at Washington September 30, 1971
Entered into force September 30, 1971

The United States of America and the Union of Soviet Socialist Republics, hereinafter referred to as the Parties,

Noting the positive experience gained in the process of operating the existing Direct Communications Link between the United States of America and the Union of Soviet Socialist Republics, which was established for use in time of emergency pursuant to the Memorandum of Understanding Regarding the Establishment of a Direct Communications Link, signed on June 20, 1963,

Having examined, in a spirit of mutual understanding, matters relating to the improvement and modernization of the Direct Communications Link,

Having agreed as follows:

Article 1

1. For the purpose of increasing the reliability of the Direct Communications Link, there shall be established and put into operation the following:

(a) two additional circuits between the United States of America and the Union of Soviet Socialist Republics each using a satellite communications system, with each Party selecting a satellite communications system of its own choice,

(b) a system of terminals (more than one) in the territory of each Party for the Direct Communications Link, with the locations and number of terminals in the United States of America to be determined by the United States side, and the locations and number of terminals in the Union of Soviet Socialist Republics to be determined by the Soviet side.

2. Matters relating to the implementation of the aforementioned improvements of the Direct Communications Link are set forth in the Annex which is attached hereto and forms an integral part hereof.

Article 2

Each Party confirms its intention to take all possible measures to assure the continuous and reliable operation of the communications circuits and the system of terminals of the Direct Communications Link for which it is responsible in accordance with this Agreement and the Annex hereto, as well as to communicate to the head of its Government any messages received via the Direct Communications Link from the head of Government of the other Party.

Article 3

The Memorandum of Understanding Between the United States of America and the Union of Soviet Socialist Republics Regarding the Establishment of a Direct Communications Link, signed on June 20, 1963, with the Annex thereto, shall remain in force, except to the extent that its provisions are modified by this Agreement and Annex hereto.

Article 4

The undertakings of the Parties hereunder shall be carried out in accordance with their respective Constitutional processes.

Article 5

This Agreement, including the Annex hereto, shall enter into force upon signature.

DONE at Washington on September 30, 1971, in two copies, each in the English and Russian languages, both texts being equally authentic.

FOR THE UNITED STATES OF AMERICA:
WILLIAM P. ROGERS

FOR THE UNION OF SOVIET SOCIALIST REPUBLICS:
A. GROMYKO

ANNEX TO THE AGREEMENT BETWEEN THE UNITED STATES OF AMERICA AND THE UNION OF SOVIET SOCIALIST REPUBLICS ON MEASURES TO IMPROVE THE U.S.A.-USSR DIRECT COMMUNICATIONS LINK

Improvements to the U.S.A.-USSR Direct Communications Link shall be implemented in accordance with the provisions set forth in this Annex.

I. CIRCUITS

(a) Each of the original circuits established pursuant to paragraph 1 of the Annex to the Memorandum of Understanding, dated June 20, 1963, shall continue to be maintained and operated as part of the Direct Communications Link until such time, after the satellite communications circuits provided for herein become operational, as the agencies designated pursuant to paragraph III (hereinafter referred to as the "designated agencies") mutually agree that such original circuit is no longer necessary. The provisions of paragraph 7 of the Annex to the Memorandum of Understanding, dated June 20, 1963, shall continue to govern the allocation of the costs of maintaining and operating such original circuits.

(b) Two additional circuits shall be established using two satellite communications systems. Taking into account paragraph I (e) below, the United States side shall provide one circuit via the Intelsat system and the Soviet side shall provide one circuit via the Molniya II system. The two circuits shall be duplex telephone band-width circuits conforming to CCITT standards, equipped for secondary telegraphic multiplexing. Transmission and reception of messages over the Direct Communications Link shall be effected in accordance with applicable recommendations of international communications regulations, as well as with mutually agreed instructions.

(c) When the reliability of both additional circuits has been established to the mutual satisfaction of the designated agencies, they shall be used as the primary circuits of the Direct Communications Link for transmission and reception of teleprinter messages between the United States and the Soviet Union.

(d) Each satellite communications circuit shall utilize an earth station in the territory of the

United States, a communications satellite transponder, and an earth station in the territory of the Soviet Union. Each Party shall be responsible for linking the earth stations in its territory to its own terminals of the Direct Communications Link.

(e) For the circuits specified in paragraph I (b):

— The Soviet side will provide and operate at least one earth station in its territory for the satellite communications circuit in the Intelsat system, and will also arrange for the use of suitable earth station facilities in its territory for the satellite communications circuit in the Molniya II system. The United States side, through a governmental agency or other United States legal entity, will make appropriate arrangements with Intelsat with regard to access for the Soviet Intelsat earth station to the Intelsat space segment, as well as for the use of the applicable portion of the Intelsat space segment.

— The United States side will provide and operate at least one earth station in its territory for the satellite communications circuit in the Molniya II system, and will also arrange for the use of suitable earth station facilities in its territory for the satellite communications circuit in the Intelsat system.

(f) Each earth station shall conform to the performance specifications and operating procedures at the corresponding satellite communications system and the ratio of antenna gain to the equivalent noise temperature should be no less than 31 decibels. Any deviation from these specifications and procedures which may be required in any unusual situation shall be worked out and mutually agreed upon by the designated agencies of both Parties after consultation.

(g) The operational commissioning dates for the satellite communications circuits based on the Intelsat and Molniya II systems shall be as agreed upon by the designated agencies of the Parties through consultations.

(h) The United States side shall bear the costs of: (1) providing and operating the Molniya II earth station in its territory; (2) the use of the Intelsat earth station in its territory; and (3) the transmission of messages via the Intelsat system. The Soviet side shall bear the costs of:

(1) providing and operating the Intelsat earth station in its territory; (2) the use of the Molniya II earth station in its territory; and (3) the transmission of messages via the Molniya II system. Payment of the costs of the satellite communications circuits shall be effected without any transfer of payments between the Parties.

(i) Each Party shall be responsible for providing to the other Party notification of any proposed modification or replacement of the communications satellite system containing the circuit provided by it that might require accommodation by earth stations using that system or otherwise affect the maintenance or operation of the Direct Communications Link. Such notification should be given sufficiently in advance to enable the designated agencies to consult and to make, before the modification or replacement is effected, such preparation as may be agreed upon for accommodation by the affected earth stations.

II. TERMINALS

(a) Each Party shall establish a system of terminals in its territory for the exchange of messages with the other Party, and shall determine the locations and number of terminals in such a system. Terminals of the Direct Communications Link shall be designated "U.S.A." and "USSR."

(b) Each Party shall take necessary measures to provide for rapidly switching circuits among terminal points in such a manner that only one terminal location is connected to the circuits at any one time.

(c) Each Party shall use teleprinter equipment from its own sources to equip the additional terminals for the transmission and reception of messages from the United States to the Soviet Union in the English language and from the Soviet Union to the United States in the Russian language.

(d) The terminals of the Direct Communications Link shall be provided with encoding equipment. One-time tape encoding equipment shall be used for transmissions via the Direct Communications Link. A mutually agreed quantity of encoding equipment of a modern and reliable type selected by the United States side, with spares, test equipment, technical literature and operating

supplies, shall be furnished by the United States side to the Soviet side against payment of the cost thereof by the Soviet side; additional spares for the encoding equipment supplied will be furnished as necessary.

(e) Keying tapes shall be supplied in accordance with the provisions set forth in paragraph 4 of the Annex to the Memorandum of Understanding, dated June 20, 1963. Each Party shall be responsible for reproducing and distributing additional keying tapes for its system of terminals and for implementing procedures which ensure that the required synchronization of encoding equipment can be effected from any one terminal at any time.

III. OTHER MATTERS

Each Party shall designate the agencies responsible for arrangements regarding the establishment of the additional circuits and the systems of terminals provided for in this Agreement and Annex, for their operation and for their continuity and reliability. These agencies shall, on the basis of direct contacts:

(a) arrange for the exchange of required performance specifications and operating procedures for the earth stations of the communications systems using Intelsat and Molniya II satellites;

(b) arrange for testing, acceptance and commissioning of the satellite circuits and for operation of these circuits after commissioning; and,

(c) decide matters and develop instructions relating to the operation of the secondary teleprinter multiplex system used on the satellite circuits.

CONVENTION ON THE PROHIBITION OF THE DEVELOPMENT, PRODUCTION AND STOCKPILING OF BACTERIOLOGICAL (BIOLOGICAL) AND TOXIN WEAPONS AND ON THEIR DESTRUCTION

Biological and chemical weapons have generally been associated with each other in the public mind, and the extensive use of poison gas in World War I (resulting in over a million casualties and over 100,000 deaths) led to the Geneva Protocol of 1925 prohibiting the use of both poison gas and bacteriological methods in warfare. At the 1932 - 1937 Disarmament Conference, unsuccessful attempts were made to work out an agreement that would prohibit the production and stockpiling of biological and chemical weapons. During World War II, new and more toxic nerve gases were developed, and research and development was begun on biological weapons. Neither side used such weapons. President Roosevelt, in a statement warning the Axis powers against the use of chemical weapons, declared:

> Use of such weapons has been outlawed by the general opinion of civilized mankind. This country has not used them, and I hope we never will be compelled to use them. I state categorically that we shall under no circumstances resort to the use of such weapons unless they are first used by our enemies.

In the postwar negotiations on general disarmament, biological and chemical weapons were usually considered together with nuclear and conventional weapons. Both the United States and Soviet Union, in the 1962 sessions of the Eighteen-Nation Disarmament Committee (ENDC), offered plans for general and complete disarmament that included provisions for eliminating chemical and biological weapons.

An issue that long hindered progress was whether chemical and biological weapons should continue to be linked. A British draft convention submitted to the ENDC on July 10, 1969, concentrated on the elimination of biological weapons only. A draft convention proposed in the General Assembly by the Soviet Union and its allies on September 19 dealt with both chemical and biological weapons. The Soviet representative argued that they had been treated together in the Geneva Protocol and in the General Assembly resolutions and report, and should continue to be dealt with in the same

instrument. A separate biological weapons convention, he warned, might serve to intensify the chemical arms race.

The United States supported the British position and stressed the difference between the two kinds of weapons. Unlike biological weapons, chemical weapons had actually been used in modern warfare. Many states maintained chemical weapons in their arsenals to deter the use of this type of weapon against them, and to provide a retaliatory capability if deterrence failed. Many of these nations, the United States pointed out, would be reluctant to give up this capability without reliable assurance that other nations were not developing, producing, and stockpiling chemical weapons.

While the United States did not consider prohibition of one of these classes of weapons less urgent or important than the other, it held that biological weapons presented less intractable problems, and an agreement on banning them should not be delayed until agreement on a reliable prohibition of chemical weapons could be reached.

Shortly after President Nixon took office, he ordered a review of U.S. policy and programs regarding biological and chemical warfare. On November 25, 1969, the President declared that the United States unilaterally renounced first use of lethal or incapacitating chemical agents and weapons and unconditionally renounced all methods of biological warfare. Henceforth the U.S. biological program would be confined to research on strictly defined measures of defense, such as immunization. The Department of Defense was ordered to draw up a plan for the disposal of existing stocks of biological agents and weapons. On February 14, 1970, the White House announced extension of the ban to cover toxins (substances falling between biologicals and chemicals in that they act like chemicals but are ordinarily produced by biological or microbic processes).

The U.S. action was widely welcomed internationally, and the example was followed by others. Canada, Sweden, and the United Kingdom stated that they had no biological weapons and did not intend to produce any. It was generally recognized, however, that unilateral actions could not take the place of a binding international commitment. A number of nations, including the Soviet Union and its allies, continued to favor a comprehensive agreement covering both chemical and biological weapons.

Discussion throughout 1970 in the General Assembly and the Conference of the Committee on Disarmament (CCD) -- as the ENDC was named after its enlargement to 26 members in August 1969 -- produced no agreement. A breakthrough came on March 30, 1971, however, when the Soviet Union and its allies changed their position and introduced a revised draft convention limited to biological weapons and toxins. It then became possible for the co-chairmen of the CCD -- the U.S. and Soviet representatives -- to work out an agreed draft, as they had done with the Non-Proliferation and the Seabed Treaties. On August 5, the United States and the Soviet Union submitted separate but identical texts.

On December 16, the General Assembly approved a resolution, adopted by a vote of 110 to 0, commending the convention and expressing hope for the widest possible adherence.

The French representative abstained, explaining that the convention, though a step forward, might weaken the Geneva Protocol ban on the use of chemical weapons, and he did not consider that adequate international controls were provided. He announced, however, that France would enact domestic legislation prohibiting biological weapons, and this was done in June of the next year.

The People's Republic of China did not participate in the negotiations on the convention and did not sign it. At the 1972 General Assembly its representative attacked the convention as a "sham," and criticized it for not prohibiting chemical weapons.

The convention was opened for signature at Washington, London, and Moscow on April 10, 1972. President Nixon submitted it to the Senate on August 10, calling it "the first international agreement since World War II to provide for the actual elimination of an entire class of weapons from the arsenals of nations." The Senate Foreign Relations Committee delayed action on the convention, however, holding it for consideration after resolution of the herbicide and riot-control issues involved in the Geneva Protocol (see section on the Geneva Protocol).

In the latter part of 1974 the Ford Administration undertook a new initiative to obtain Senate consent to ratification of both the Geneva Protocol and the Biological Weapons Convention, and ACDA Director Fred Ikle testified with respect to both instruments before the Senate Foreign Relations Committee on December 10. Soon thereafter the Committee voted unanimously to send the two measures to the Senate floor, and on December 16 the Senate voted its approval, also unanimously.

President Ford signed instruments of ratification for the two measures on January 22, 1975.

Under the terms of the convention, the parties undertake not to develop, produce, stockpile, or acquire biological agents or toxins "of types and in quantities that have no justification for prophylactic, protective, and other peaceful purposes," as well as weapons and means of delivery. All such material is to be destroyed within nine months of the convention's entry into force. In January 1976, all heads of Federal departments and agencies certified to the President that as of December 26, 1975, their respective departments and agencies were in full compliance with the convention.

The parties are to consult and cooperate in solving any problems that arise. Complaints of a breach of obligations may be lodged with the Security Council, and parties undertake to cooperate with any investigation the Council initiates. If the Security Council finds that a state has been endangered by a violation, the parties are to provide any assistance requested.

Nothing in the convention is to be interpreted as lessening the obligations imposed by the Geneva Protocol, and the parties undertake to pursue negotiations for a ban on chemical weapons.

In addition, articles provide for exchange of information on peaceful uses, amendment and review, and accession and withdrawal. The convention is of unlimited duration.

At the second Review Conference in September 1986, the parties agreed to implement data exchange measures to enhance confidence and to promote cooperation in areas of permitted biological activities. In accordance with the Final Declaration of that Review Conference, an ad hoc meeting of scientific and technical experts was held March 31 - April 15, 1987, to develop procedures for implementing annual data exchanges.

At the third Review Conference in September 1991 it was agreed to reaffirm and extend confidence building measures agreed at the second Review Conference and to create an Ad Hoc Group of Governmental Experts open to all parties to identify, examine, and evaluate from a scientific and technical standpoint potential verification measures with respect to the prohibitions of the convention. The Ad Hoc Group met four times in 1992 and 1993, completing its work and submitting a consensus report circulated to all States Parties. As provided in the mandate, a majority of States Parties called for a Special Conference to discuss the final report and consider further actions. The Special Conference, held in September 1994, agreed to establish an Ad Hoc Group, open to all States Parties, to consider appropriate measures, and draft proposals to strengthen the Convention in a legally binding instrument. The Ad Hoc Group convened two substantive sessions in 1995, with additional meetings scheduled for 1996. The Ad Hoc Group will prepare a report, to be considered at the Fourth Review Conference of the BWC in the Fall of 1996.

CONVENTION ON THE PROHIBITION OF THE DEVELOPMENT, PRODUCTION AND STOCKPILING OF BACTERIOLOGICAL (BIOLOGICAL) AND TOXIN WEAPONS AND ON THEIR DESTRUCTION

Signed at Washington, London, and Moscow April 10, 1972
Ratification advised by U.S. Senate December 16, 1974
Ratified by U.S. President January 22, 1975
U.S. ratification deposited at Washington, London, and Moscow March 26, 1975
Proclaimed by U.S. President March 26, 1975
Entered into force March 26, 1975

The States Parties to this Convention,

Determined to act with a view to achieving effective progress towards general and complete disarmament, including the prohibition and elimination of all types of weapons of mass destruction, and convinced that the prohibition of the development, production and stockpiling of chemical and bacteriological (biological) weapons and their elimination, through effective measures, will facilitate the achievement of general and complete disarmament under strict and effective international control,

Recognizing the important significance of the Protocol for the Prohibition of the Use in War of Asphyxiating, Poisonous or Other Gases, and of Bacteriological Methods of Warfare, signed at Geneva on June 17, 1925, and conscious also of the contribution which the said Protocol has already made, and continues to make, to mitigating the horrors of war,

Reaffirming their adherence to the principles and objectives of that Protocol and calling upon all States to comply strictly with them,

Recalling that the General Assembly of the United Nations has repeatedly condemned all actions contrary to the principles and objectives of the Geneva Protocol of June 17, 1925,

Desiring to contribute to the strengthening of confidence between peoples and the general improvement of the international atmosphere,

Desiring also to contribute to the realization of the purposes and principles of the Charter of the United Nations,

Convinced of the importance and urgency of eliminating from the arsenals of States, through effective measures, such dangerous weapons of mass destruction as those using chemical or bacteriological (biological) agents,

Recognizing that an agreement on the prohibition of bacteriological (biological) and toxin weapons represents a first possible step towards the achievement of agreement on effective measures also for the prohibition of the development, production and stockpiling of chemical weapons, and determined to continue negotiations to that end,

Determined, for the sake of all mankind, to exclude completely the possibility of bacteriological (biological) agents and toxins being used as weapons,

Convinced that such use would be repugnant to the conscience of mankind and that no effort should be spared to minimize this risk,

Have agreed as follows:

Article I

Each State Party to this Convention undertakes never in any circumstances to develop, produce, stockpile or otherwise acquire or retain:

(1) Microbial or other biological agents, or toxins whatever their origin or method of production, of types and in quantities that have no justification for prophylactic, protective or other peaceful purposes;

(2) Weapons, equipment or means of delivery designed to use such agents or toxins for hostile purposes or in armed conflict.

Article II

Each State Party to this Convention undertakes to destroy, or to divert to peaceful purposes, as soon as possible but not later than nine months after the entry into force of the Convention, all agents, toxins, weapons, equipment and means of delivery specified in article I of the Convention, which are in its possession or under its jurisdiction or control. In implementing the provisions of this article all necessary safety precautions shall be observed to protect populations and the environment.

Article III

Each State Party to this Convention undertakes not to transfer to any recipient whatsoever, directly or indirectly, and not in any way to assist, encourage, or induce any State, group of States or international organizations to manufacture or otherwise acquire any of the agents, toxins, weapons, equipment or means of delivery specified in article I of the Convention.

Article IV

Each State Party to this Convention shall, in accordance with its constitutional processes, take any necessary measures to prohibit and prevent the development, production, stockpiling, acquisition, or retention of the agents, toxins, weapons, equipment and means of delivery specified in article I of the Convention, within the territory of such State, under its jurisdiction or under its control anywhere.

Article V

The States Parties to this Convention undertake to consult one another and to cooperate in solving any problems which may arise in relation to the objective of, or in the application of the provisions of, the Convention. Consultation and cooperation pursuant to this article may also be undertaken through appropriate international procedures within the framework of the United Nations and in accordance with its Charter.

Article VI

(1) Any State Party to this Convention which finds that any other State Party is acting in breach of obligations deriving from the provisions of the Convention may lodge a complaint with the Security Council of the United Nations. Such a complaint should include all possible evidence confirming its validity, as well as a request for its consideration by the Security Council.

(2) Each State Party to this Convention undertakes to cooperate in carrying out any investigation which the Security Council may initiate, in accordance with the provisions of the Charter of the United Nations, on the basis of the complaint received by the Council. The Security Council shall inform the States Parties to the Convention of the results of the investigation.

Article VII

Each State Party to this Convention undertakes to provide or support assistance, in accordance with the United Nations Charter, to any Party to the Convention which so requests, if the Security Council decides that such Party has been exposed to danger as a result of violation of the Convention.

Article VIII

Nothing in this Convention shall be interpreted as in any way limiting or detracting from the obligations assumed by any State under the Protocol for the Prohibition of the Use in War of Asphyxiating, Poisonous or Other Gases, and of Bacteriological Methods of Warfare, signed at Geneva on June 17, 1925.

Article IX

Each State Party to this Convention affirms the recognized objective of effective prohibition of chemical weapons and, to this end, undertakes to continue negotiations in good faith with a view to reaching early agreement on effective measures for the prohibition of their development, production and stockpiling and for their destruction, and on appropriate measures concerning equipment and means of delivery specifically designed for the production or use of chemical agents for weapons purposes.

Article X

(1) The States Parties to this Convention undertake to facilitate, and have the right to participate in, the fullest possible exchange of equipment, materials and scientific and technological information for the use of bacteriological (biological) agents and toxins for peaceful purposes. Parties to the Convention in a position to do so shall also cooperate in contributing individually or together with other States or international organizations to the further development and application of scientific discoveries in the field of bacteriology (biology) for prevention of disease, or for other peaceful purposes.

(2) This Convention shall be implemented in a manner designed to avoid hampering the economic or technological development of States Parties to the Convention or international

cooperation in the field of peaceful bacteriological (biological) activities, including the international exchange of bacteriological (biological) agents and toxins and equipment for the processing, use or production of bacteriological (biological) agents and toxins for peaceful purposes in accordance with the provisions of the Convention.

Article XI

Any State Party may propose amendments to this Convention. Amendments shall enter into force for each State Party accepting the amendments upon their acceptance by a majority of the States Parties to the Convention and thereafter for each remaining State Party on the date of acceptance by it.

Article XII

Five years after the entry into force of this Convention, or earlier if it is requested by a majority of Parties to the Convention by submitting a proposal to this effect to the Depositary Governments, a conference of States Parties to the Convention shall be held at Geneva, Switzerland, to review the operation of the Convention, with a view to assuring that the purposes of the preamble and the provisions of the Convention, including the provisions concerning negotiations on chemical weapons, are being realized. Such review shall take into account any new scientific and technological developments relevant to the Convention.

Article XIII

(1) This Convention shall be of unlimited duration.

(2) Each State Party to this Convention shall in exercising its national sovereignty have the right to withdraw from the Convention if it decides that extraordinary events, related to the subject matter of the Convention, have jeopardized the supreme interests of its country. It shall give notice of such withdrawal to all other States Parties to the Convention and to the United Nations Security Council three months in advance. Such notice shall include a statement of the extraordinary events it regards as having jeopardized its supreme interests.

Article XIV

(1) This Convention shall be open to all States for signature. Any State which does not sign the Convention before its entry into force in accordance with paragraph (3) of this Article may accede to it at any time.

(2) This Convention shall be subject to ratification by signatory States. Instruments of ratification and instruments of accession shall be deposited with the Governments of the United States of America, the United Kingdom of Great Britain and Northern Ireland and the Union of Soviet Socialist Republics, which are hereby designated the Depositary Governments.

(3) This Convention shall enter into force after the deposit of instruments of ratification by twenty-two Governments, including the Governments designated as Depositaries of the Convention.

(4) For States whose instruments of ratification or accession are deposited subsequent to the entry into force of this Convention, it shall enter into force on the date of the deposit of their instruments of ratification or accession.

(5) The Depositary Governments shall promptly inform all signatory and acceding States of the date of each signature, the date of deposit of each instrument of ratification or of accession and the date of the entry into force of this Convention, and of the receipt of other notices.

(6) This Convention shall be registered by the Depositary Governments pursuant to Article 102 of the Charter of the United Nations.

Article XV

This Convention, the English, Russian, French, Spanish and Chinese texts of which are equally authentic, shall be deposited in the archives of the Depositary Governments. Duly certified copies of the Convention shall be transmitted by the Depositary Governments to the Governments of the signatory and acceding states.

IN WITNESS WHEREOF the undersigned, duly authorized, have signed this Convention.

DONE in triplicate, at the cities of Washington, London and Moscow, this tenth day of April, one thousand nine hundred and seventy-two.

Biological Weapons Convention

Country	Date[1] of Signature	Date of Deposit[1] of Ratification	Date of Deposit[1] of Accession
Afghanistan	04/10/72	03/26/75	
Albania			06/03/92
Argentina	08/01/72	11/27/79	
Armenia			06/07/94
Australia	04/10/72	10/05/77	
Austria	04/10/72	08/10/73	
Bahamas			11/26/86
Bahrain			10/28/88
Bangladesh			03/12/85
Barbados	02/16/73	02/16/73	
Belarus	04/10/72	03/26/75	
Belgium	04/10/72	03/15/79	
Belize			10/20/86
Benin	04/10/72	04/25/75	
Bhutan			06/08/78
Bolivia	04/10/72	10/30/75	
Bosnia Herzegovina			08/15/94
Botswana	04/10/72	02/05/92	
Brazil	04/10/72	02/27/73	
Brunei			01/31/91
Bulgaria	04/10/72	08/02/72	
Burkina Faso			04/17/91
Burundi	04/10/72		
Cambodia (Kampuchea)	04/10/72	03/09/83	
Canada	04/10/72	09/18/72	
Cape Verde			10/20/77
Central African Republic	04/10/72		
Chile	04/10/72	04/22/80	
China, People's Republic of			11/15/84
Colombia	04/10/72	12/19/83	
Congo			10/23/78
Costa Rica	04/10/72	12/17/73	
Cote d'Ivoire	05/23/72		
Croatia			10/08/91
Cuba	04/12/72	04/21/76	
Cyprus	04/10/72	11/06/73	
Czech Republic			01/01/93
Denmark	04/10/72	03/01/73	
Dominica			11/08/78
Dominican Republic	04/10/72	02/23/73	
Ecuador	06/14/72	03/12/75	
Egypt	04/10/72		
El Salvador	04/10/72	12/31/91	
Equatorial Guinea			01/16/89
Estonia			06/21/93
Ethiopia	04/10/72	06/26/75	
Fiji	02/22/73	09/04/73	
Finland	04/10/72	02/04/74	
France			09/27/84

Biological Weapons Convention -- Continued

Country	Date[1] of Signature	Date of Deposit[1] of Ratification	Date of Deposit[1] of Accession
Gabon	04/10/72		
Gambia, The	06/02/72	11/21/91	
Germany	04/10/72	11/28/72	
Ghana	04/10/72	06/06/75	
Greece	04/10/72	12/10/75	
Grenada			10/22/86
Guatemala	05/09/72	09/19/73	
Guinea-Bissau			08/20/76
Guyana	01/03/73		
Haiti	04/10/72		
Honduras	04/10/72	03/14/79	
Hungary	04/10/72	12/27/72	
Iceland	04/10/72	02/15/73	
India	01/15/73	07/15/74	
Indonesia	06/20/72	04/01/92	
Iran	04/10/72	08/22/73	
Iraq	05/11/72	04/18/91	
Ireland	04/10/72	10/27/72	
Italy	04/10/72	05/30/75	
Jamaica			08/13/75
Japan	04/10/72	06/08/82	
Jordan	04/10/72	06/02/75	
Kenya			09/30/81
Korea, Democratic People's Republic of			03/13/87
Korea, Republic of	04/10/72	06/25/87	
Kuwait	04/14/72	07/18/72	
Laos	04/10/72	03/20/73	
Lebanon	04/10/72	06/13/75	
Lesotho	04/10/72	09/06/77	
Liberia	04/10/72		
Libya			01/19/82
Liechtenstein			05/30/91
Luxembourg	04/10/72	03/23/76	
Madagascar	10/13/72		
Malawi	04/10/72		
Malaysia	04/10/72	09/26/91	
Maldives			07/01/93
Mali	04/10/72		
Malta	09/11/72	04/07/75	
Mauritius	04/10/72	08/07/72	
Mexico	04/10/72	04/08/74	
Mongolia	04/10/72	09/05/72	
Morocco	05/02/72		
Myanmar (Burma)	04/10/72		

Biological Weapons Convention -- Continued

Country	Date[1] of Signature	Date of Deposit[1] of Ratification	Date of Deposit[1] of Accession
Nepal	04/10/72		
Netherlands	04/10/72	06/22/81	
New Zealand	04/10/72	12/13/72	
Nicaragua	04/10/72	08/07/75	
Niger	04/21/72	06/23/72	
Nigeria	07/03/72	07/03/73	
Norway	04/10/72	08/01/73	
Oman			03/31/92
Pakistan	04/10/72	09/25/74	
Panama	05/02/72	03/20/74	
Papua New Guinea			10/27/80
Paraguay			06/09/76
Peru	04/10/72	06/05/85	
Philippines	04/10/72	05/21/73	
Poland	04/10/72	01/25/73	
Portugal	06/29/72	05/15/75	
Qatar	11/14/72	04/17/75	
Romania	04/10/72	07/25/79	
Russia	04/10/72	03/26/75	
Rwanda	04/10/72	05/20/75	
St. Kitts and Nevis			04/02/91
St. Lucia			11/26/86
San Marino	09/12/72	03/11/75	
São Tomé & Principe			08/24/79
Saudi Arabia	04/12/72	05/24/72	
Senegal	04/10/72	03/26/75	
Serbia-Montenergo (formerly Yugoslavia)	04/10/72	10/25/73	
Seychelles			10/24/79
Sierra Leone	11/07/72	06/29/76	
Singapore	06/19/72	12/02/75	
Slovak Republic			01/01/93
Slovenia			04/07/92*
Solomon Islands			09/04/81
Somalia	07/03/72		
South Africa	04/10/72	11/03/75	
Spain	04/10/72	06/20/79	
Sri Lanka	04/10/72	11/18/76	
Suriname			02/06/93
Swaziland			06/18/91
Sweden	02/27/75	02/05/76	
Switzerland	04/10/72	05/04/76	
Syria	04/14/72		

* with effect from 06/25/91

Biological Weapons Convention -- Continued

Country	Date[1] of Signature	Date of Deposit[1] of Ratification	Date of Deposit[1] of Accession
Taiwan	04/10/72	02/09/73	
Tanzania	08/16/72		
Thailand	01/17/73	05/28/75	
Togo	04/10/72	11/10/76	
Tonga			09/30/81
Tunisia	04/10/72	05/18/73	
Turkey	04/10/72	11/05/74	
Uganda			05/12/92
Ukraine	04/10/72	03/26/75	
United Arab Emirates	09/28/72		
United Kingdom	04/10/72	03/26/75	
United States	04/10/72	03/26/75	
Uruguay			04/06/81
Vanuatu			10/12/90
Venezuela	04/10/72	10/18/78	
Vietnam			06/20/80
Yemen	04/26/72	06/01/79	
Zaire	04/10/72	09/16/75	
Zimbabwe			11/05/90
Total	109	91	45

See footnotes on page 350.

AGREEMENT BETWEEN THE GOVERNMENT OF THE UNITED STATES OF AMERICA AND THE GOVERNMENT OF THE UNION OF SOVIET SOCIALIST REPUBLICS ON THE PREVENTION OF INCIDENTS ON AND OVER THE HIGH SEAS

In the late 1960s, there were several incidents between forces of the U.S. Navy and the Soviet Navy. These included planes of the two nations passing near one another, ships bumping one another, and both ships and aircraft making threatening movements against those of the other side. In March 1968 the United States proposed talks on preventing such incidents from becoming more serious. The Soviet Union accepted the invitation in November 1970, and the talks were conducted in two rounds -- October 1, 1971, in Moscow and May 17, 1972, in Washington, D.C. The Agreement was signed by Secretary of the Navy John Warner and Soviet Admiral Sergei Gorshkov during the Moscow summit meeting in 1972.

Specifically, the agreement provides for:

• steps to avoid collision;

• not interfering in the "formations" of the other party;

• avoiding maneuvers in areas of heavy sea traffic;

• requiring surveillance ships to maintain a safe distance from the object of investigation so as to avoid "embarrassing or endangering the ships under surveillance";

• using accepted international signals when ships maneuver near one another;

• not simulating attacks at, launching objects toward, or illuminating the bridges of the other party's ships;

• informing vessels when submarines are exercising near them; and

• requiring aircraft commanders to use the greatest caution and prudence in approaching aircraft and ships of the other party and not permitting simulated attacks against aircraft or ships, performing aerobatics over ships, or dropping hazardous objects near them.

The agreement also provides for: (1) notice three to five days in advance, as a rule, of any projected actions that might "represent a danger to navigation or to aircraft in flight"; (2) information on incidents to be channeled through naval attaches assigned to the respective capitals; and (3) annual meetings to review the implementation of the Agreement.

The protocol to this agreement grew out of the first meeting of the Consultative Committee established by the agreement. Each side recognized that its effectiveness could be enhanced by additional understandings relating to nonmilitary vessels. In the protocol signed in Washington, D.C., on May 22, 1973, each party pledged not to make simulated attacks against the nonmilitary ships of the other.

Like other confidence-building measures, the Incidents at Sea Agreement does not directly affect the size, weaponry, or force structure of the parties. Rather, it serves to enhance mutual knowledge and understanding of military activities; to reduce the possibility of conflict by accident, miscalculation, or the failure of communication; and to increase stability in times of both calm and crisis. In 1983, Secretary of the Navy John Lehman cited the accord as "a good example of functional navy-to-navy process" and credited this area of Soviet-American relations with "getting better rather than worse." In 1985, he observed that the frequency of incidents was "way down from what it was in the 1960s and early 1970s."

AGREEMENT BETWEEN THE GOVERNMENT
OF THE UNITED STATES OF AMERICA AND
THE GOVERNMENT OF THE UNION OF
SOVIET SOCIALIST REPUBLICS ON THE
PREVENTION OF INCIDENTS ON AND OVER
THE HIGH SEAS

Signed at Moscow May 25, 1972
Entered into force May 25, 1972

The Government of the United States of
America and the Government of the Union of
Soviet Socialist Republics,

Desiring to assure the safety of navigation of
the ships of their respective armed forces on the
high seas and flight of their military aircraft over
the high seas, and

Guided by the principles and rules of
international law,

Have decided to conclude this Agreement and
have agreed as follows:

Article I

For the purpose of this Agreement, the
following definitions shall apply:

1. "Ship" means:

(a) A warship belonging to the naval forces of
the Parties bearing the external marks
distinguishing warships of its nationality, under
the command of an officer duly commissioned by
the government and whose name appears in the
Navy list, and manned by a crew who are under
regular naval discipline;

(b) Naval auxiliaries of the Parties, which
include all naval ships authorized to fly the naval
auxiliary flag where such a flag has been
established by either Party.

2. "Aircraft" means all military manned
heavier-than-air and lighter-than-air craft,
excluding space craft.

3. "Formation" means an ordered arrangement
of two or more ships proceeding together and
normally maneuvered together.

Article II

The Parties shall take measures to instruct the
commanding officers of their respective ships to
observe strictly the letter and spirit of the
International Regulations for Preventing Collisions
at Sea, hereinafter referred to as the Rules of the
Road. The Parties recognize that their freedom to
conduct operations on the high seas is based on
the principles established under recognized
international law and codified in the 1958 Geneva
Convention on the High Seas.

Article III

1. In all cases ships operating in proximity to
each other, except when required to maintain
course and speed under the Rules of the Road,
shall remain well clear to avoid risk of collision.

2. Ships meeting or operating in the vicinity of a
formation of the other Party shall, while
conforming to the Rules of the Road, avoid
maneuvering in a manner which would hinder the
evolutions of the formation.

3. Formations shall not conduct maneuvers
through areas of heavy traffic where
internationally recognized traffic separation
schemes are in effect.

4. Ships engaged in surveillance of other ships
shall stay at a distance which avoids the risk of
collision and also shall avoid executing
maneuvers embarrassing or endangering the
ships under surveillance. Except when required to
maintain course and speed under the Rules of
the Road, a surveillant shall take positive early
action so as, in the exercise of good seamanship,
not to embarrass or endanger ships under
surveillance.

5. When ships of both Parties maneuver in
sight of one another, such signals (flag, sound,
and light) as are prescribed by the Rules of the
Road, the International Code of Signals, or other
mutually agreed signals, shall be adhered to for
signalling operations and intentions.

6. Ships of the Parties shall not simulate
attacks by aiming guns, missile launchers,
torpedo tubes, and other weapons in the direction
of a passing ship of the other Party, not launch

any object in the direction of passing ships of the other Party, and not use searchlights or other powerful illumination devices to illuminate the navigation bridges of passing ships of the other Party.

7. When conducting exercises with submerged submarines, exercising ships shall show the appropriate signals prescribed by the International Code of Signals to warn ships of the presence of submarines in the area.

8. Ships of one Party when approaching ships of the other Party conducting operations as set forth in Rule 4 (c) of the Rules of the Road, and particularly ships engaged in launching or landing aircraft as well as ships engaged in replenishment underway, shall take appropriate measures not to hinder maneuvers of such ships and shall remain well clear.

Article IV

Commanders of aircraft of the Parties shall use the greatest caution and prudence in approaching aircraft and ships of the other Party operating on and over the high seas, in particular, ships engaged in launching or landing aircraft, and in the interest of mutual safety shall not permit: simulated attacks by the simulated use of weapons against aircraft and ships, or performance of various aerobatics over ships, or dropping various objects near them in such a manner as to be hazardous to ships or to constitute a hazard to navigation.

Article V

1. Ships of the Parties operating in sight of one another shall raise proper signals concerning their intent to begin launching or landing aircraft.

2. Aircraft of the Parties flying over the high seas in darkness or under instrument conditions shall, whenever feasible, display navigation lights.

Article VI

Both Parties shall:

1. Provide through the established system of radio broadcasts of information and warning to mariners, not less than 3 to 5 days in advance as a rule, notification of actions on the high seas which represent a danger to navigation or to aircraft in flight.

2. Make increased use of the informative signals contained in the International Code of Signals to signify the intentions of their respective ships when maneuvering in proximity to one another. At night, or in conditions of reduced visibility, or under conditions of lighting and such distances when signal flags are not distinct, flashing light should be used to inform ships of maneuvers which may hinder the movements of others or involve a risk of collision.

3. Utilize on a trial basis signals additional to those in the International Code of Signals, submitting such signals to the Intergovernmental Maritime Consultative Organization for its consideration and for the information of other States.

Article VII

The Parties shall exchange appropriate information concerning instances of collision, incidents which result in damage, or other incidents at sea between ships and aircraft of the Parties. The United States Navy shall provide such information through the Soviet Naval Attache in Washington and the Soviet Navy shall provide such information through the United States Naval Attache in Moscow.

Article VIII

This Agreement shall enter into force on the date of its signature and shall remain in force for a period of three years. It will thereafter be renewed without further action by the Parties for successive periods of three years each.

This Agreement may be terminated by either Party upon six months written notice to the other Party.

Article IX

The Parties shall meet within one year after the date of the signing of this Agreement to review the implementation of its terms. Similar consultations shall be held thereafter annually, or more frequently as the Parties may decide.

Article X

The Parties shall designate members to form a Committee which will consider specific measures in conformity with this Agreement. The Committee will, as a particular part of its work, consider the practical workability of concrete fixed distances to be observed in encounters between ships, aircraft, and ships and aircraft. The Committee will meet within six months of the date of signature of this Agreement and submit its recommendations for decision by the Parties during the consultations prescribed in Article IX.

DONE in duplicate on the 25th day of May 1972 in Moscow in the English and Russian languages each being equally authentic.

FOR THE GOVERNMENT OF THE UNITED STATES OF AMERICA:
John W. Warner
Secretary of the Navy

FOR THE GOVERNMENT OF THE UNION OF SOVIET SOCIALIST REPUBLICS:
Sergei G. Gorshkov
Commander-in-Chief of the Navy

PROTOCOL TO THE AGREEMENT BETWEEN THE GOVERNMENT OF THE UNITED STATES OF AMERICA AND THE GOVERNMENT OF THE UNION OF SOVIET SOCIALIST REPUBLICS ON THE PREVENTION OF INCIDENTS ON AND OVER THE HIGH SEAS SIGNED MAY 25, 1972

Signed at Washington May 22, 1973
Entered into force May 22, 1973

The Government of the United States of America and the Government of the Union of Soviet Socialist Republics, herein referred to as the Parties,

Having agreed on measures directed to improve the safety of navigation of the ships of their respective armed forces on the high seas and flight of their military aircraft over the high seas,

Recognizing that the objectives of the Agreement may be furthered by additional understandings, in particular concerning actions of naval ships and military aircraft with respect to the non-military ships of each Party,

Further agree as follows:

Article I

The Parties shall take measures to notify the non-military ships of each Party on the provisions of the Agreement directed at securing mutual safety.

Article II

Ships and aircraft of the Parties shall not make simulated attacks by aiming guns, missile launchers, torpedo tubes and other weapons at non-military ships of the other Party, nor launch nor drop any objects near non-military ships of the other Party in such a manner as to be hazardous to these ships or to constitute a hazard to Navigation.

Article III

This Protocol will enter into force on the day of its signing and will be considered as an integral part of the Argument between the Government of the United States of America and the Government of the Union of Soviet Socialist Republics on the Prevention of Incidents On and Over the High Seas which was signed in Moscow on May 25, 1972.

DONE on the 22nd of May, 1973 in Washington, in two copies, each in the English and the Russian language, both texts having the same force.

FOR THE GOVERNMENT OF THE UNITED STATES OF AMERICA:
J.P. Weinel
Vice Admiral, U.S. Navy

FOR THE GOVERNMENT OF THE UNION OF SOVIET SOCIALIST REPUBLICS:
Alekseyev, Admiral

STRATEGIC ARMS LIMITATION TALKS (SALT I)

SALT I, the first series of Strategic Arms Limitation Talks, extended from November 1969 to May 1972. During that period the United States and the Soviet Union negotiated the first agreements to place limits and restraints on some of their central and most important armaments. In a Treaty on the Limitation of Anti-Ballistic Missile Systems, they moved to end an emerging competition in defensive systems that threatened to spur offensive competition to still greater heights. In an Interim Agreement on Certain Measures With Respect to the Limitation of Strategic Offensive Arms, the two nations took the first steps to check the rivalry in their most powerful land- and submarine-based offensive nuclear weapons.

The earliest efforts to halt the growth in strategic arms met with no success. Strategic weapons had been included in the U.S. and Soviet proposals for general and complete disarmament. But the failure of these comprehensive schemes left strategic arms unrestrained. The United States was the first to suggest dissociating them from comprehensive disarmament plans -- proposing, at the Geneva-based Eighteen-Nation Disarmament Committee in January 1964, that the two sides should "explore a verified freeze of the number and characteristics of their strategic nuclear offensive and defensive vehicles."

The competition in offensive and defensive armaments continued. By 1966 the Soviet Union had begun to deploy an antiballistic missile defense around Moscow; and that year the People's Republic of China successfully tested a nuclear missile. In the United States, research and development were leading to U.S. deployment of its own ABM system.

In March 1967, after an exchange of communication with Soviet leaders, President Johnson announced that Premier Kosygin had indicated a willingness to begin discussions. Attempts to get talks underway, however, were not successful.

On September 18, 1967, the United States announced that it would begin deployment of a "thin" antiballistic missile (ABM) system. The Administration emphasized that the deployment was intended to meet a possible limited Chinese ICBM threat, to underscore U.S. security assurances to its allies by reinforcing the U.S. deterrent capability, and to add protection against "the improbable but possible accidental launch of an intercontinental missile by one of the nuclear powers." This program for limited ABM defense brought sharply divided views in public and congressional debate regarding the efficacy and desirability of an ABM system and its possible effects on the arms race.

In announcing the U.S. decision, Secretary of Defense McNamara said,

Let me emphasize -- and I cannot do so too strongly -- that our decision to go ahead with a limited ABM deployment in no way indicates that we feel an agreement with the Soviet Union on the limitation of strategic nuclear offensive and defensive forces is in any way less urgent or desirable.

Through diplomatic channels in Washington and Moscow, discussions with Soviet representatives in the ENDC, and exchanges at the highest levels of the two governments, the United States continued to press for a Soviet commitment to discuss strategic arms limitation. But it was not until the following year that evidence of a Soviet reassessment of its position emerged. On July 1, 1968, President Johnson announced, at the signing of the Non-Proliferation Treaty, that agreement had been reached with the Soviet Union to begin discussions on limiting and reducing both strategic nuclear weapons delivery systems and defense against ballistic missiles. The date and place for the talks had not yet been announced, when, on August 20, the Soviet Union began its invasion of Czechoslovakia, an event that postponed the talks indefinitely.

On January 20, 1969, the day that President Nixon assumed office, a statement by the Soviet Foreign Ministry expressed willingness to discuss strategic arms limitations. The new President promptly voiced his support for talks, and initiated, under the aegis of the National Security Council, an extensive and detailed review of the strategic, political, and verification aspects of the problem.

In October, the White House and the Kremlin announced that the Strategic Arms Limitation Talks would begin in Helsinki on November 17,

1969, "for preliminary discussion of the questions involved." The Director of ACDA, Gerard Smith, was named to head the U.S. delegation and led it throughout the two and a half-year series of SALT I negotiations.

In the first session of the talks, from November 17 to December 22, each side gained a better understanding of the other's views and of the range of questions to be considered. It was agreed that the talks would be private, to encourage a free and frank exchange, and the stage was set for the main negotiations, which opened in Vienna in April 1970. Sessions thereafter alternated between Helsinki and Vienna until the first accords were reached in May 1972. (When SALT II began, in November 1972, to reduce the administrative burdens involved in shifting sites it was agreed to hold them henceforth in one place -- Geneva.)

Soviet and American weapons systems were far from symmetrical. The Soviet Union had continued its development and deployment of heavy ballistic missiles and had overtaken the U.S. lead in land-based ICBMs. During the SALT I years alone Soviet ICBMs rose from around 1,000 to around 1,500, and they were being deployed at the rate of some 200 annually. Soviet submarine-based launchers had quadrupled. The huge payload capacity of some Soviet missiles ("throw-weight") was seen as a possible threat to U.S. land-based strategic missiles even in heavily protected ("hardened") launch-sites.

The United States had not increased its deployment of strategic missiles since 1967 (when its ICBMs numbered 1,054 and its SLBMs 656), but it was conducting a vigorous program of equipping missiles with "Multiple Independently-targeted Re-entry Vehicles" (MIRV). "MIRVs" permit an individual missile to carry a number of warheads directed at separate targets. MIRVs thus gave the United States a lead in numbers of warheads. The United States also retained a lead in long-range bombers. The Soviet Union had a limited ABM system around Moscow; the United States had shifted from its earlier plan for a "thin" ABM defense of certain American cities and instead began to deploy ABMs at two land-based ICBM missile sites to protect its retaliatory forces. (The full program envisaged 12 ABM complexes.)

Besides these asymmetries in their strategic

forces, the defense needs and commitments of the two parties differed materially. The United States had obligations for the defense of allies overseas, such as Western Europe and Japan, while the Soviet Union's allies were its near neighbors. All these circumstances made for difficulties in equating specific weapons, or categories of weapons, and in defining overall strategic equivalence.

Two initial disagreements presented obstacles. The Soviet representatives sought to define as "strategic" -- i.e., negotiable in SALT-- any U.S. or Soviet weapons system capable of reaching the territory of the other side. This would have included U.S. "forward-based systems," chiefly short-range or medium-range bombers on aircraft carriers or based in Europe, but it would have excluded, for example, Soviet intermediate-range missiles aimed at Western Europe. The United States held that weapons to be negotiated in SALT comprised intercontinental systems. Its forward-based forces served to counter Soviet medium-range missiles and aircraft aimed at U.S. allies. To accept the Soviet approach would have prejudiced alliance commitments.

After initial attempts to reach a comprehensive agreement failed, the Soviets sought to restrict negotiations to antiballistic missile systems, maintaining that limitations on offensive systems should be deferred. The U.S. position was that to limit ABM systems but allow the unrestricted growth of offensive weapons would be incompatible with the basic objectives of SALT and that it was essential to make at least a beginning at limiting offensive systems as well. A long deadlock on the question was finally broken by exchanges at the highest levels of both governments. On May 20, 1971, Washington and Moscow announced that an understanding had been reached to concentrate on a permanent Treaty to limit ABM systems, but at the same time to work out certain limitations on offensive systems, and to continue negotiations for a more comprehensive and long-term agreement on the latter.

In a summit meeting in Moscow, after two and a half years of negotiation, the first round of SALT was brought to a conclusion on May 26, 1972, when President Nixon and General Secretary Brezhnev signed the ABM Treaty and the Interim Agreement on strategic offensive arms.

Intensive research had gone into finding ways of verifying possible agreements without requiring access to the territory of the other side. Both the ABM Treaty and the Interim Agreement stipulate that compliance is to be assured by "national technical means of verification." Moreover, the agreements include provisions that are important steps to strengthen assurance against violations: both sides undertake not to interfere with national technical means of verification. In addition, both countries agree not to use deliberate concealment measures to impede verification.

The basic provisions of each SALT I agreement are briefly reviewed in sections that follow. The two accords differ in their duration and inclusiveness. The ABM Treaty "shall be of unlimited duration," but each Party has the right to withdraw on six months' notice if it decides that its supreme interests are jeopardized by "extraordinary events related to the subject matter of this Treaty." The Interim Agreement was for a five-year span, and covered only certain major aspects of strategic weaponry. The agreements are linked not only in their strategic effects, but in their relationship to future negotiations for limitations on strategic offensive arms. A formal statement by the United States stressed the critical importance it attached to achieving more complete limitations on strategic offensive arms.

The two agreements were accompanied by a number of "Agreed Statements" that were agreed upon and initialed by the Heads of the Delegations. When the two agreements were submitted to the U.S. Congress, they were also accompanied by common understandings reached and unilateral statements made during the negotiations. These were intended to clarify specific provisions of the agreements or parts of the negotiating record. The three groups of items are reproduced here with the texts of the agreements.

TREATY BETWEEN THE UNITED STATES OF AMERICA AND THE UNION OF SOVIET SOCIALIST REPUBLICS ON THE LIMITATION OF ANTI-BALLISTIC MISSILE SYSTEMS

In the Treaty on the Limitation of Anti-Ballistic Missile Systems the United States and the Soviet Union agree that each may have only two ABM deployment areas,[1] so restricted and so located that they cannot provide a nationwide ABM defense or become the basis for developing one. Each country thus leaves unchallenged the penetration capability of the other's retaliatory missile forces.

The Treaty permits each side to have one limited ABM system to protect its capital and another to protect an ICBM launch area. The two sites defended must be at least 1,300 kilometers apart, to prevent the creation of any effective regional defense zone or the beginnings of a nationwide system.

Precise quantitative and qualitative limits are imposed on the ABM systems that may be deployed. At each site there may be no more than 100 interceptor missiles and 100 launchers. Agreement on the number and characteristics of radars to be permitted had required extensive and complex technical negotiations, and the provisions governing these important components of ABM systems are spelled out in very specific detail in the Treaty and further clarified in the "Agreed Statements" accompanying it.

Both Parties agreed to limit qualitative improvement of their ABM technology, e.g., not to develop, test, or deploy ABM launchers capable of launching more than one interceptor missile at a time or modify existing launchers to give them this capability, and systems for rapid reload of launchers are similarly barred. These provisions, the Agreed Statements clarify, also ban interceptor missiles with more than one independently guided warhead.

There had been some concern over the possibility that surface-to-air missiles (SAMs) intended for defense against aircraft might be improved, along with their supporting radars, to the point where they could effectively be used against ICBMs and SLBMs, and the Treaty prohibits this. While further deployment of radars intended to give early warning of strategic ballistic missile attack is not prohibited, such radars must be located along the territorial boundaries of each country and oriented outward, so that they do not contribute to an effective ABM defense of points in the interior.

Further, to decrease the pressures of technological change and its unsettling impact on the strategic balance, both sides agree to prohibit development, testing, or deployment of sea-based, air-based, or space-based ABM systems and their components, along with mobile land-based ABM systems. Should future technology bring forth new ABM systems "based on other physical principles" than those employed in current systems, it was agreed that limiting such systems would be discussed, in accordance with the Treaty's provisions for consultation and amendment.

The Treaty also provides for a U.S.-Soviet Standing Consultative Commission to promote its objectives and implementation. The commission was established during the first negotiating session of SALT II, by a Memorandum of Understanding dated December 21, 1972. Since then both the United States and the Soviet Union have raised a number of questions in the Commission relating to each side's compliance with the SALT I agreements. In each case raised by the United States, the Soviet activity in question has either ceased or additional information has allayed U.S. concern.

Article XIV of the Treaty calls for review of the Treaty five years after its entry into force, and at five-year intervals thereafter. The first such review was conducted by the Standing Consultative Commission at its special session in the fall of 1977. At this session, the United States and the Soviet Union agreed that the Treaty had operated effectively during its first five years, that it had continued to serve national security interests, and that it did not need to be amended at that time.

The most recent Treaty review was completed in October 1993. Following that review, numerous sessions of the Standing Consultative Commission have been held to work out Treaty succession -- to "multilateralize" the Treaty -- as a result of the break-up of the Soviet Union and to negotiate a demarcation between ABM and non-ABM systems.

---

[1] Subsequently reduced to one area (See section on ABM Protocol)

TREATY BETWEEN THE UNITED STATES OF AMERICA AND THE UNION OF SOVIET SOCIALIST REPUBLICS ON THE LIMITATION OF ANTI-BALLISTIC MISSILE SYSTEMS

Signed at Moscow May 26, 1972
Ratification advised by U.S. Senate August 3, 1972
Ratified by U.S. President September 30, 1972
Proclaimed by U.S. President October 3, 1972
Instruments of ratification exchanged October 3, 1972
Entered into force October 3, 1972

The United States of America and the Union of Soviet Socialist Republics, hereinafter referred to as the Parties,

Proceeding from the premise that nuclear war would have devastating consequences for all mankind,

Considering that effective measures to limit anti-ballistic missile systems would be a substantial factor in curbing the race in strategic offensive arms and would lead to a decrease in the risk of outbreak of war involving nuclear weapons,

Proceeding from the premise that the limitation of anti-ballistic missile systems, as well as certain agreed measures with respect to the limitation of strategic offensive arms, would contribute to the creation of more favorable conditions for further negotiations on limiting strategic arms,

Mindful of their obligations under Article VI of the Treaty on the Non-Proliferation of Nuclear Weapons,

Declaring their intention to achieve at the earliest possible date the cessation of the nuclear arms race and to take effective measures toward reductions in strategic arms, nuclear disarmament, and general and complete disarmament,

Desiring to contribute to the relaxation of international tension and the strengthening of trust between States,

Have agreed as follows:

Article I

1. Each Party undertakes to limit anti-ballistic missile (ABM) systems and to adopt other measures in accordance with the provisions of this Treaty.

2. Each Party undertakes not to deploy ABM systems for a defense of the territory of its country and not to provide a base for such a defense, and not to deploy ABM systems for defense of an individual region except as provided for in Article III of this Treaty.

Article II

1. For the purpose of this Treaty an ABM system is a system to counter strategic ballistic missiles or their elements in flight trajectory, currently consisting of:

(a) ABM interceptor missiles, which are interceptor missiles constructed and deployed for an ABM role, or of a type tested in an ABM mode;

(b) ABM launchers, which are launchers constructed and deployed for launching ABM interceptor missiles; and

(c) ABM radars, which are radars constructed and deployed for an ABM role, or of a type tested in an ABM mode.

2. The ABM system components listed in paragraph 1 of this Article include those which are:

(a) operational;

(b) under construction;

(c) undergoing testing;

(d) undergoing overhaul, repair or conversion; or

(e) mothballed.

Article III

Each Party undertakes not to deploy ABM systems or their components except that:

(a) within one ABM system deployment area having a radius of one hundred and fifty kilometers and centered on the Party's national capital, a Party may deploy: (1) no more than one hundred ABM launchers and no more than one hundred ABM interceptor missiles at launch sites, and (2) ABM radars within no more than six ABM radar complexes, the area of each complex being circular and having a diameter of no more than three kilometers; and

(b) within one ABM system deployment area having a radius of one hundred and fifty kilometers and containing ICBM silo launchers, a Party may deploy: (1) no more than one hundred ABM launchers and no more than one hundred ABM interceptor missiles at launch sites, (2) two large phased-array ABM radars comparable in potential to corresponding ABM radars operational or under construction on the date of signature of the Treaty in an ABM system deployment area containing ICBM silo launchers, and (3) no more than eighteen ABM radars each having a potential less than the potential of the smaller of the above-mentioned two large phased-array ABM radars.

Article IV

The limitations provided for in Article III shall not apply to ABM systems or their components used for development or testing, and located within current or additionally agreed test ranges. Each Party may have no more than a total of fifteen ABM launchers at test ranges.

Article V

1. Each Party undertakes not to develop, test, or deploy ABM systems or components which are sea-based, air-based, space-based, or mobile land-based.

2. Each Party undertakes not to develop, test or deploy ABM launchers for launching more than one ABM interceptor missile at a time from each launcher, not to modify deployed launchers to provide them with such a capacity, not to develop, test, or deploy automatic or semi-automatic or other similar systems for rapid reload of ABM launchers.

Article VI

To enhance assurance of the effectiveness of the limitations on ABM systems and their components provided by the Treaty, each Party undertakes:

(a) not to give missiles, launchers, or radars, other than ABM interceptor missiles, ABM launchers, or ABM radars, capabilities to counter strategic ballistic missiles or their elements in

flight trajectory, and not to test them in an ABM mode; and

(b) not to deploy in the future radars for early warning of strategic ballistic missile attack except at locations along the periphery of its national territory and oriented outward.

Article VII

Subject to the provisions of this Treaty, modernization and replacement of ABM systems or their components may be carried out.

Article VIII

ABM systems or their components in excess of the numbers or outside the areas specified in this Treaty, as well as ABM systems or their components prohibited by this Treaty, shall be destroyed or dismantled under agreed procedures within the shortest possible agreed period of time.

Article IX

To assure the viability and effectiveness of this Treaty, each Party undertakes not to transfer to other States, and not to deploy outside its national territory, ABM systems or their components limited by this Treaty.

Article X

Each Party undertakes not to assume any international obligations which would conflict with this Treaty.

Article XI

The Parties undertake to continue active negotiations for limitations on strategic offensive arms.

Article XII

1. For the purpose of providing assurance or compliance with the provisions of this Treaty, each Party shall use national technical means of verification at its disposal in a manner consistent with generally recognized principles of international law.

2. Each Party undertakes not to interfere with the national technical means of verification of the

other Party operating in accordance with paragraph 1 of this Article.

3. Each Party undertakes not to use deliberate concealment measures which impede verification by national technical means of compliance with the provisions of this Treaty. This obligation shall not require changes in current construction, assembly, conversion, or overhaul practices.

Article XIII

1. To promote the objectives and implementation of the provisions of this Treaty, the Parties shall establish promptly a Standing Consultative Commission, within the framework of which they will:

(a) consider questions concerning compliance with the obligations assumed and related situations which may be considered ambiguous;

(b) provide on a voluntary basis such information as either Party considers necessary to assure confidence in compliance with the obligations assumed;

(c) consider questions involving unintended interference with national technical means of verification;

(d) consider possible changes in the strategic situation which have a bearing on the provisions of this Treaty;

(e) agree upon procedures and dates for destruction or dismantling of ABM systems or their components in cases provided for by the provisions of this Treaty;

(f) consider, as appropriate, possible proposals for further increasing the viability of this Treaty; including proposals for amendments in accordance with the provisions of this Treaty;

(g) consider, as appropriate, proposals for further measures aimed at limiting strategic arms.

2. The Parties through consultation shall establish, and may amend as appropriate, Regulations for the Standing Consultative Commission governing procedures, composition and other relevant matters.

Article XIV

1. Each Party may propose amendments to this Treaty. Agreed amendments shall enter into force in accordance with the procedures governing the entry into force of this Treaty.

2. Five years after entry into force of this Treaty, and at five-year intervals thereafter, the Parties shall together conduct a review of this Treaty.

Article XV

1. This Treaty shall be of unlimited duration.

2. Each Party shall, in exercising its national sovereignty, have the right to withdraw from this Treaty if it decides that extraordinary events related to the subject matter of this Treaty have jeopardized its supreme interests. It shall give notice of its decision to the other Party six months prior to withdrawal from the Treaty. Such notice shall include a statement of the extraordinary events the notifying Party regards as having jeopardized its supreme interests.

Article XVI

1. This Treaty shall be subject to ratification in accordance with the constitutional procedures of each Party. The Treaty shall enter into force on the day of the exchange of instruments of ratification.

2. This Treaty shall be registered pursuant to Article 102 of the Charter of the United Nations.

DONE at Moscow on May 26, 1972, in two copies, each in the English and Russian languages, both texts being equally authentic.

FOR THE UNITED STATES OF AMERICA:
RICHARD NIXON
President of the United States of America

FOR THE UNION OF SOVIET SOCIALIST REPUBLICS:
L. I. BREZHNEV
General Secretary of the Central Committee of the CPSU

AGREED STATEMENTS, COMMON UNDERSTANDINGS, AND UNILATERAL STATEMENTS REGARDING THE TREATY BETWEEN THE UNITED STATES OF AMERICA AND THE UNION OF SOVIET SOCIALIST REPUBLICS ON THE LIMITATION OF ANTI-BALLISTIC MISSILES

1. AGREED STATEMENTS

The document set forth below was agreed upon and initialed by the Heads of the Delegations on May 26, 1972 (letter designations added):

Agreed Statements Regarding the Treaty Between the United States of America and the Union of Soviet Socialist Republics on the Limitation of Anti-Ballistic Missile Systems

[A]

The Parties understand that, in addition to the ABM radars which may be deployed in accordance with subparagraph (a) of Article III of the Treaty, those non-phased-array ABM radars operational on the date of signature of the Treaty within the ABM system deployment area for defense of the national capital may be retained.

[B]

The Parties understand that the potential (the product of mean emitted power in watts and antenna area in square meters) of the smaller of the two large phased-array ABM radars referred to in subparagraph (b) of Article III of the Treaty is considered for purposes of the Treaty to be three million.

[C]

The Parties understand that the center of the ABM system deployment area centered on the national capital and the center of the ABM system deployment area containing ICBM silo launchers for each Party shall be separated by no less than thirteen hundred kilometers.

[D]

In order to insure fulfillment of the obligation not to deploy ABM systems and their components except as provided in Article III of the Treaty, the Parties agree that in the event ABM systems based on other physical principles and including components capable of substituting for ABM interceptor missiles, ABM launchers, or ABM radars are created in the future, specific limitations on such systems and their components would be subject to discussion in accordance with Article XIII and agreement in accordance with Article XIV of the Treaty.

[E]

The Parties understand that Article V of the Treaty includes obligations not to develop, test or deploy ABM interceptor missiles for the delivery by each ABM interceptor missile of more than one independently guided warhead.

[F]

The Parties agree not to deploy phased-array radars having a potential (the product of mean emitted power in watts and antenna area in square meters) exceeding three million, except as provided for in Articles III, IV, and VI of the Treaty, or except for the purposes of tracking objects in outer space or for use as national technical means of verification.

[G]

The Parties understand that Article IX of the Treaty includes the obligation of the United States and the USSR not to provide to other States technical descriptions or blueprints specially worked out for the construction of ABM systems and their components limited by the Treaty.

2. COMMON UNDERSTANDINGS

Common understanding of the Parties on the following matters was reached during the negotiations:

A. Location of ICBM Defenses

The U.S. Delegation made the following statement on May 26, 1972:

Article III of the ABM Treaty provides for each side one ABM system deployment area centered on its national capital and one ABM system deployment area containing ICBM silo launchers. The two sides have registered agreement on the following statement: "The Parties understand that the center of the ABM system deployment area centered on the national capital and the center of the ABM system deployment area containing ICBM silo launchers for each Party shall be

separated by no less than thirteen hundred kilometers."
In this connection, the U.S. side notes that its ABM
system deployment area for defense of ICBM silo
launchers, located west of the Mississippi River, will be
centered in the Grand Forks ICBM silo launcher
deployment area. (See Agreed Statement [C].)

B. ABM Test Ranges

The U.S. Delegation made the following
statement on April 26, 1972:

Article IV of the ABM Treaty provides that "the
limitations provided for in Article III shall not apply to
ABM systems or their components used for
development or testing, and located within current or
additionally agreed test ranges." We believe it would be
useful to assure that there is no misunderstanding as
to current ABM test ranges. It is our understanding that
ABM test ranges encompass the area within which
ABM components are located for test purposes. The
current U.S. ABM test ranges are at White Sands, New
Mexico, and at Kwajalein Atoll, and the current Soviet
ABM test range is near Sary Shagan in Kazakhstan.
We consider that non-phased array radars of types
used for range safety or instrumentation purposes may
be located outside of ABM test ranges. We interpret
the reference in Article IV to "additionally agreed test
ranges" to mean that ABM components will not be
located at any other test ranges without prior
agreement between our Governments that there will
be such additional ABM test ranges.

On May 5, 1972, the Soviet Delegation stated
that there was a common understanding on what
ABM test ranges were, that the use of the types
of non-ABM radars for range safety or
instrumentation was not limited under the Treaty,
that the reference in Article IV to "additionally
agreed" test ranges was sufficiently clear, and
that national means permitted identifying current
test ranges.

C. Mobile ABM Systems

On January 29, 1972, the U.S. Delegation
made the following statement:

Article V(1) of the Joint Draft Text of the ABM Treaty
includes an undertaking not to develop, test, or deploy
mobile land-based ABM systems and their
components. On May 5, 1971, the U.S. side indicated
that, in its view, a prohibition on development of mobile
ABM systems and components would rule out the
deployment of ABM launchers and radars which were
not permanent fixed types. At that time, we asked for
the Soviet view of this interpretation. Does the Soviet

side agree with the U.S. side's interpretation put
forward on May 5, 1971?

On April 13, 1972, the Soviet Delegation said
there is a general common understanding on this
matter.

D. Standing Consultative Commission

Ambassador Smith made the following
statement on May 22, 1972:

The United States proposes that the sides agree
that, with regard to initial implementation of the ABM
Treaty's Article XIII on the Standing Consultative
Commission (SCC) and of the consultation Articles to
the Interim Agreement on offensive arms and the
Accidents Agreement,[1] agreement establishing the SCC
will be worked out early in the follow-on SALT
negotiations; until that is completed, the following
arrangements will prevail: when SALT is in session,
any consultation desired by either side under these
Articles can be carried out by the two SALT
Delegations; when SALT is not in session, *ad hoc*
arrangements for any desired consultations under these
Articles may be made through diplomatic channels.

Minister Semenov replied that, on an *ad
referendum* basis, he could agree that the U.S.
statement corresponded to the Soviet
understanding.

E. Standstill

On May 6, 1972, Minister Semenov made the
following statement:

In an effort to accommodate the wishes of the U.S.
side, the Soviet Delegation is prepared to proceed on
the basis that the two sides will in fact observe the
obligations of both the Interim Agreement and the ABM
Treaty beginning from the date of signature of these
two documents.

In reply, the U.S. Delegation made the following
statement on May 20, 1972:

---

[1] See Article 7 of Agreement to Reduce the Risk of Outbreak
of Nuclear War Between the United States of America and the
Union of Soviet Socialist Republics, signed September 30,
1971.

The United States agrees in principle with the Soviet statement made on May 6 concerning observance of obligations beginning from date of signature but we would like to make clear our understanding that this means that, pending ratification and acceptance, neither side would take any action prohibited by the agreements after they had entered into force. This understanding would continue to apply in the absence of notification by either signatory of its intention not to proceed with ratification or approval.

The Soviet Delegation indicated agreement with the U.S. statement.

3. UNILATERAL STATEMENTS

The following noteworthy unilateral statements were made during the negotiations by the United States Delegation:

A. Withdrawal from the ABM Treaty

On May 9, 1972, Ambassador Smith made the following statement:

The U.S. Delegation has stressed the importance the U.S. Government attaches to achieving agreement on more complete limitations on strategic offensive arms, following agreement on an ABM Treaty and on an Interim Agreement on certain measures with respect to the limitation of strategic offensive arms. The U.S. Delegation believes that an objective of the follow-on negotiations should be to constrain and reduce on a long-term basis threats to the survivability of our respective strategic retaliatory forces. The USSR Delegation has also indicated that the objectives of SALT would remain unfulfilled without the achievement of an agreement providing for more complete limitations on strategic offensive arms. Both sides recognize that the initial agreements would be steps toward the achievement of complete limitations on strategic arms. If an agreement providing for more complete strategic offensive arms limitations were not achieved within five years, U.S. supreme interests could be jeopardized. Should that occur, it would constitute a basis for withdrawal from the ABM Treaty. The United States does not wish to see such a situation occur, nor do we believe that the USSR does. It is because we wish to prevent such a situation that we emphasize the importance the U.S. Government attaches to achievement of more complete limitations on strategic offensive arms. The U.S. Executive will inform the Congress, in connection with Congressional consideration of the ABM Treaty and the Interim Agreement, of this statement of the U.S. position.

B. Tested in an ABM Mode

On April 7, 1972, the U.S. Delegation made the following statement:

Article II of the Joint Text Draft uses the term "tested in an ABM mode," in defining ABM components, and Article VI includes certain obligations concerning such testing. We believe that the sides should have a common understanding of this phrase. First, we would note that the testing provisions of the ABM Treaty are intended to apply to testing which occurs after the date of signature of the Treaty, and not to any testing which may have occurred in the past. Next, we would amplify the remarks we have made on this subject during the previous Helsinki phase by setting forth the objectives which govern the U.S. view on the subject, namely, while prohibiting testing of non-ABM components for ABM purposes: not to prevent testing of ABM components, and not to prevent testing of non-ABM components for non-ABM purposes. To clarify our interpretation of "tested in an ABM mode," we note that we would consider a launcher, missile or radar to be "tested in an ABM mode" if, for example, any of the following events occur: (1) a launcher is used to launch an ABM interceptor missile, (2) an interceptor missile is flight tested against a target vehicle which has a flight trajectory with characteristics of a strategic ballistic missile flight trajectory, or is flight tested in conjunction with the test of an ABM interceptor missile or an ABM radar at the same test range, or is flight tested to an altitude inconsistent with interception of targets against which air defenses are deployed, (3) a radar makes measurements on a cooperative target vehicle of the kind referred to in item (2) above during the reentry portion of its trajectory or makes measurements in conjunction with the test of an ABM interceptor missile or an ABM radar at the same test range. Radars used for purposes such as range safety or instrumentation would be exempt from application of these criteria.

C. No-Transfer Article of ABM Treaty

On April 18, 1972, the U.S. Delegation made the following statement:

In regard to this Article [IX], I have a brief and I believe self-explanatory statement to make. The U.S. side wishes to make clear that the provisions of this Article do not set a precedent for whatever provision may be considered for a Treaty on Limiting Strategic Offensive Arms. The question of transfer of strategic offensive arms is a far more complex issue, which may require a different solution.

D. No Increase in Defense of Early Warning Radars

On July 28, 1970, the U.S. Delegation made the following statement:

Since Hen House radars [Soviet ballistic missile early warning radars] can detect and track ballistic missile warheads at great distances, they have a significant ABM potential. Accordingly, the United States would regard any increase in the defenses of such radars by surface-to-air missiles as inconsistent with an agreement.

INTERIM AGREEMENT BETWEEN THE UNITED STATES OF AMERICA AND THE UNION OF SOVIET SOCIALIST REPUBLICS ON CERTAIN MEASURES WITH RESPECT TO THE LIMITATION OF STRATEGIC OFFENSIVE ARMS

As its title suggests, the "Interim Agreement Between the United States and the Union of Soviet Socialist Republics on Certain Measures With Respect to the Limitation of Offensive Arms" was limited in duration and scope. It was intended to remain in force for five years. (See preceding section on SALT.) Both countries undertook to continue negotiations for a more comprehensive agreement as soon as possible, and the scope and terms of any new agreement were not to be prejudiced by the provisions of the 1972 accord.

Thus the Interim Agreement was seen essentially as a holding action, designed to complement the ABM Treaty by limiting competition in offensive strategic arms and to provide time for further negotiations. The agreement essentially freezes at existing levels the number of strategic ballistic missile launchers, operational or under construction, on each side, and permits an increase in SLBM launchers up to an agreed level for each party only with the dismantling or destruction of a corresponding number of older ICBM or SLBM launchers.

In view of the many asymmetries in the two countries' forces, imposing equivalent limitations required rather complex and precise provisions. At the date of signing, the United States had 1,054 operational land-based ICBMs, and none under construction; the Soviet Union had an estimated 1,618 operational and under construction. Launchers under construction could be completed. Neither side would start construction of additional fixed land-based ICBM launchers during the period of the agreement -- this, in effect, also bars relocation of existing launchers. Launchers for light or older ICBMs cannot be converted into launchers for modern heavy ICBMs. This prevents the Soviet Union from replacing older missiles with missiles such as the SS-9, which in 1972 was the largest and most powerful missile in the Soviet inventory and a source of particular concern to the United States.

Within these limitations, modernization and replacement are permitted, but in the process of modernizing, the dimensions of silo launchers cannot be significantly increased.

Mobile ICBMs are not covered. The Soviet Union held that since neither side had such systems, a freeze should not apply to them; it also opposed banning them in a future comprehensive agreement. The United States held they should be banned because of the verification difficulties they presented. In a formal statement, the U.S. delegation declared that the United States would consider deployment of land-mobile ICBMs during the period of the agreement as inconsistent with its objectives.

Article III and the protocol limit launchers for submarine-launched ballistic missiles (SLBMs) and modern ballistic missile submarines. The United States is permitted to reach a ceiling of 710 SLBM launchers on 44 submarines, from its base level of 656 SLBM launchers on 41 ballistic missile submarines, by replacing 54 older ICBM launchers. The Soviet Union, beyond the level of 740 SLBM launchers on modern nuclear-powered submarines, may increase to 950. But these additional launchers are permitted only as replacements for older ICBM or SLBM launchers, which must be dismantled or destroyed under agreed procedures.

In a unilateral statement, the Soviet Union asserted that if the U.S. NATO allies increased the number of their modern submarines, the Soviet Union would have a right to increase the number of its submarines correspondingly. The United States declared that it did not accept this claim.

INTERIM AGREEMENT BETWEEN THE UNITED STATES OF AMERICA AND THE UNION OF SOVIET SOCIALIST REPUBLICS ON CERTAIN MEASURES WITH RESPECT TO THE LIMITATION OF STRATEGIC OFFENSIVE ARMS

Signed at Moscow May 26, 1972
Approval authorized by U.S. Congress September 30, 1972
Approved by U.S. President September 30, 1972
Notices of acceptance exchanged October 3, 1972
Entered into force October 3, 1972

The United States of America and the Union of Soviet Socialist Republics, hereinafter referred to as the Parties,

Convinced that the Treaty on the Limitation of Anti-Ballistic Missile Systems and this Interim Agreement on Certain Measures with Respect to the Limitation of Strategic Offensive Arms will contribute to the creation of more favorable conditions for active negotiations on limiting strategic arms as well as to the relaxation of international tension and the strengthening of trust between States,

Taking into account the relationship between strategic offensive and defensive arms,

Mindful of their obligations under Article VI of the Treaty on the Non-Proliferation of Nuclear Weapons,

Have agreed as follows:

Article I

The Parties undertake not to start construction of additional fixed land-based intercontinental ballistic missile (ICBM) launchers after July 1, 1972.

Article II

The Parties undertake not to convert land-based launchers for light ICBMs, or for ICBMs of older types deployed prior to 1964, into land-based launchers for heavy ICBMs of types deployed after that time.

Article III

The Parties undertake to limit submarine-launched ballistic missile (SLBM) launchers and modern ballistic missile submarines to the numbers operational and under construction on the date of signature of this Interim Agreement, and in addition to launchers and submarines constructed under procedures established by the Parties as replacements for an equal number of ICBM launchers of older types deployed prior to 1964 or for launchers on older submarines.

Article IV

Subject to the provisions of this Interim Agreement, modernization and replacement of strategic offensive ballistic missiles and launchers covered by this Interim Agreement may be undertaken.

Article V

1. For the purpose of providing assurance of compliance with the provisions of this Interim Agreement, each Party shall use national technical means of verification at its disposal in a manner consistent with generally recognized principles of international law.

2. Each Party undertakes not to interfere with the national technical means of verification of the other Party operating in accordance with paragraph 1 of this Article.

3. Each Party undertakes not to use deliberate concealment measures which impede verification by national technical means of compliance with the provisions of this Interim Agreement. This obligation shall not require changes in current construction, assembly, conversion, or overhaul practices.

Article VI

To promote the objectives and implementation of the provisions of this Interim Agreement, the Parties shall use the Standing Consultative Commission established under Article XIII of the Treaty on the Limitation of Anti-Ballistic Missile Systems in accordance with the provisions of that Article.

Article VII

The Parties undertake to continue active negotiations for limitations on strategic offensive arms. The obligations provided for in this Interim Agreement shall not prejudice the scope or terms of the limitations on strategic offensive arms which may be worked out in the course of further negotiations.

Article VIII

1. This Interim Agreement shall enter into force upon exchange of written notices of acceptance by each Party, which exchange shall take place simultaneously with the exchange of instruments of ratification of the Treaty on the Limitation of Anti-Ballistic Missile Systems.

2. This Interim Agreement shall remain in force for a period of five years unless replaced earlier by an agreement on more complete measures limiting strategic offensive arms. It is the objective of the Parties to conduct active follow-on negotiations with the aim of concluding such an agreement as soon as possible.

3. Each Party shall, in exercising its national sovereignty, have the right to withdraw from this Interim Agreement if it decides that extraordinary events related to the subject matter of this Interim Agreement have jeopardized its supreme interests. It shall give notice of its decision to the other Party six months prior to withdrawal from this Interim Agreement. Such notice shall include a statement of the extraordinary events the notifying Party regards as having jeopardized its supreme interests.

DONE at Moscow on May 26, 1972, in two copies, each in the English and Russian languages, both texts being equally authentic.

FOR THE UNITED STATES OF AMERICA:
RICHARD NIXON
President of the United States of America

FOR THE UNION OF SOVIET SOCIALIST REPUBLICS:
L.I. BREZHNEV
General Secretary of the
Central Committee of the CPSU

PROTOCOL TO THE INTERIM AGREEMENT BETWEEN THE UNITED STATES OF AMERICA AND THE UNION OF SOVIET SOCIALIST REPUBLICS ON CERTAIN MEASURES WITH RESPECT TO THE LIMITATION OF STRATEGIC OFFENSIVE ARMS

The United States of America and the Union of Soviet Socialist Republics, hereinafter referred to as the Parties,

Having agreed on certain limitations relating to submarine-launched ballistic missile launchers and modern ballistic missile submarines, and to replacement procedures, in the Interim Agreement,

Have agreed as follows:

The Parties understand that, under Article III of the Interim Agreement, for the period during which that Agreement remains in force:

The United States may have no more than 710 ballistic missile launchers on submarines (SLBMs) and no more than 44 modern ballistic missile submarines. The Soviet Union may have no more than 950 ballistic missile launchers on submarines and no more than 62 modern ballistic missile submarines.

Additional ballistic missile launchers on submarines up to the above-mentioned levels, in the United States -- over 656 ballistic missile launchers on nuclear-powered submarines, and in the USSR -- over 740 ballistic missile launchers on nuclear-powered submarines, operational and under construction, may become operational as replacements for equal numbers of ballistic missile launchers of older types deployed prior to 1964 or of ballistic missile launchers on older submarines.

The deployment of modern SLBMs on any submarine, regardless of type, will be counted against the total level of SLBMs permitted for the United States and the USSR.

This Protocol shall be considered an integral part of the Interim Agreement.

DONE at Moscow this 26th day of May, 1972

FOR THE UNITED STATES OF AMERICA:
RICHARD NIXON
President of the United States of America

FOR THE UNION OF SOVIET SOCIALIST REPUBLICS:
L.I. BREZHNEV
General Secretary of the
Central Committee of the CPSU

AGREED STATEMENTS, COMMON UNDERSTANDINGS, AND UNILATERAL STATEMENTS REGARDING THE INTERIM AGREEMENT BETWEEN THE UNITED STATES OF AMERICA AND THE UNION OF SOVIET SOCIALIST REPUBLICS ON CERTAIN MEASURES WITH RESPECT TO THE LIMITATION OF STRATEGIC OFFENSIVE ARMS

1. Agreed Statements

The document set forth below was agreed upon and initialed by the Heads of the Delegations on May 26, 1972 (letter designations added):

AGREED STATEMENTS REGARDING THE INTERIM AGREEMENT BETWEEN THE UNITED STATES OF AMERICA AND THE UNION OF SOVIET SOCIALIST REPUBLICS ON CERTAIN MEASURES WITH RESPECT TO THE LIMITATION OF STRATEGIC OFFENSIVE ARMS

[A]

The Parties understand that land-based ICBM launchers referred to in the Interim Agreement are understood to be launchers for strategic ballistic missiles capable of ranges in excess of the shortest distance between the northeastern border of the continental United States and the north-western border of the continental USSR.

[B]

The Parties understand that fixed land-based ICBM launchers under active construction as of the date of signature of the Interim Agreement may be completed.

[C]

The Parties understand that in the process of modernization and replacement the dimensions of land-based ICBM silo launchers will not be significantly increased.

[D]

The Parties understand that during the period of the Interim Agreement there shall be no significant increase in the number of ICBM or SLBM test and training launchers, or in the number of such launchers for modern land-based heavy ICBMs. The Parties further understand that construction or conversion of ICBM launchers at test ranges shall be undertaken only for purposes of testing and training.

[E]

The Parties understand that dismantling or destruction of ICBM launchers of older types deployed prior to 1964 and ballistic missile launchers on older submarines being replaced by new SLBM launchers on modern submarines will be initiated at the time of the beginning of sea trials of a replacement submarine, and will be completed in the shortest possible agreed period of time. Such dismantling or destruction, and timely notification thereof, will be accomplished under procedures to be agreed in the Standing Consultative Commission.

2. Common Understandings

Common understanding of the Parties on the following matters was reached during the negotiations:

A. Increase in ICBM Silo Dimensions

Ambassador Smith made the following statement on May 26, 1972:

The Parties agree that the term "significantly increased" means that an increase will not be greater than 10-15 percent of the present dimensions of land-based ICBM silo launchers.

Minister Semenov replied that this statement corresponded to the Soviet understanding.

B. Standing Consultative Commission

Ambassador Smith made the following statement on May 22, 1972:

The United States proposes that the sides agree that, with regard to initial implementation of the ABM Treaty's Article XIII on the Standing Consultative Commission (SCC) and of the consultation Articles to the Interim Agreement on offensive arms and the Accidents Agreement,[1] agreement establishing the SCC will be worked out early in the follow-on SALT negotiations; until that is completed, the following arrangements will prevail: when SALT is in session, any consultation desired by either side under these Articles can be carried out by the two SALT Delegations; when SALT is not in session, ad hoc arrangements for any desired consultations under these Articles may be made through diplomatic channels.

Minister Semenov replied that, on an *ad referendum* basis, he could agree that the U.S. statement corresponded to the Soviet understanding.

C. Standstill

On May 6, 1972, Minister Semenov made the following statement:

In an effort to accommodate the wishes of the U.S. side, the Soviet Delegation is prepared to proceed on the basis that the two sides will in fact observe the obligations of both the Interim Agreement and the ABM Treaty beginning from the date of signature of these two documents.

In reply, the U.S. Delegation made the following statement on May 20, 1972:

The United States agrees in principle with the Soviet statement made on May 6 concerning observance of obligations beginning from date of signature but we would like to make clear our understanding that this means that, pending ratification and acceptance, neither side would take any action prohibited by the agreements after they had entered into force. This understanding would continue to apply in the absence of notification by either signatory of its intention not to proceed with ratification or approval.

The Soviet Delegation indicated agreement with the U.S. statement.

3. Unilateral Statements

(a) The following noteworthy unilateral statements were made during the negotiations by the United States Delegation:

A. Withdrawal from the ABM Treaty

On May 9, 1972, Ambassador Smith made the following statement:

The U.S. Delegation has stressed the importance the U.S. Government attaches to achieving agreement on more complete limitations on strategic offensive arms, following agreement on an ABM Treaty and on an Interim Agreement on certain measures with respect to the limitation of strategic offensive arms. The U.S. Delegation believes that an objective of the follow-on negotiations should be to constrain and reduce on a long-term basis threats to the survivability of our respective strategic retaliatory forces. The USSR Delegation has also indicated that the objectives of SALT would remain unfulfilled without the achievement of an agreement providing for more complete limitations on strategic offensive arms. Both sides recognize that the initial agreements would be steps toward the achievement of more complete limitations on strategic arms. If an agreement providing for more complete strategic offensive arms limitations were not achieved within five years, U.S. supreme interests could be jeopardized. Should that occur, it would constitute a basis for withdrawal from the ABM Treaty. The United States does not wish to see such a situation occur, nor do we believe that the USSR does. It is because we wish to prevent such a situation that we emphasize the importance the U.S. Government attaches to achievement of more complete limitations on strategic offensive arms. The U.S. Executive will inform the Congress, in connection with Congressional consideration of the ABM Treaty and the Interim Agreement, of this statement of the U.S. position.

B. Land-Mobile ICBM Launchers

The U.S. Delegation made the following statement on May 20, 1972:

In connection with the important subject of land-mobile ICBM launchers, in the interest of concluding the Interim Agreement the U.S. Delegation now withdraws its proposal that Article I or an agreed statement explicitly prohibit the deployment of mobile land-based ICBM launchers. I have been instructed to inform you that, while agreeing to defer the question of limitation of operational land-mobile ICBM launchers to the subsequent negotiations on more complete limitations on strategic offensive arms, the United States would consider the deployment of operational land-mobile ICBM launchers during the period of the Interim Agreement as inconsistent with the objectives of that Agreement.

C. Covered Facilities

The U.S. Delegation made the following statement on May 20, 1972:

I wish to emphasize the importance that the United States attaches to the provisions of Article V, including in particular their application to fitting out or berthing submarines.

D. "Heavy" ICBM's

The U.S. Delegation made the following statement on May 26, 1972:

The U.S. Delegation regrets that the Soviet Delegation has not been willing to agree on a common definition of a heavy missile. Under these circumstances, the U.S. Delegation believes it necessary to state the following: The United States would consider any ICBM having a volume significantly greater than that of the largest light ICBM now operational on either side to be a heavy ICBM. The United States proceeds on the premise that the Soviet side will give due account to this consideration.

On May 17, 1972, Minister Semenov made the following unilateral "Statement of the Soviet Side":

Taking into account that modern ballistic missile submarines are presently in the possession of not only the United States, but also of its NATO allies, the Soviet Union agrees that for the period of effectiveness of the Interim 'Freeze' Agreement the United States and its NATO allies have up to 50 such submarines with a total of up to 800 ballistic missile launchers thereon (including 41 U.S. submarines with 656 ballistic missile launchers). However, if during the period of effectiveness of the Agreement U.S. allies in NATO should increase the number of their modern submarines to exceed the numbers of submarines they would have operational or under construction on the date of signature of the Agreement, the Soviet Union will have the right to a corresponding increase in the number of its submarines. In the opinion of the Soviet side, the solution of the question of modern ballistic missile submarines provided for in the Interim Agreement only partially compensates for the strategic imbalance in the deployment of the nuclear-powered missile submarines of the USSR and the United States. Therefore, the Soviet side believes that this whole question, and above all the question of liquidating the American missile submarine bases outside the United States, will be appropriately resolved in the course of follow-on negotiations.

On May 24, Ambassador Smith made the following reply to Minister Semenov:

The United States side has studied the "statement made by the Soviet side" of May 17 concerning compensation for submarine basing and SLBM submarines belonging to third countries. The United States does not accept the validity of the considerations in that statement.

On May 26 Minister Semenov repeated the unilateral statement made on May 17. Ambassador Smith also repeated the U.S. rejection on May 26.

AGREEMENT BETWEEN THE UNITED STATES OF AMERICA AND THE UNION OF SOVIET SOCIALIST REPUBLICS ON THE PREVENTION OF NUCLEAR WAR

From the onset of the SALT negotiations between the United States and the Soviet Union, the two countries began the process of reshaping their relations on the basis of peaceful cooperation. One of the primary goals in this relationship was the prevention of war, especially nuclear war. During the last session of the Moscow summit meeting in May 1972, the countries exchanged some general ideas on how to accomplish this objective. These discussions were continued throughout the next year and were concluded in a formal agreement during General Secretary Brezhnev's visit to the United States June 18-25, 1973.

In the Agreement on the Prevention of Nuclear War, signed in Washington on June 22, 1973, the United States and the Soviet Union agreed to make the removal of the danger of nuclear war and the use of nuclear weapons an "objective of their policies," to practice restraint in their relations toward each other and toward all countries, and to pursue a policy dedicated toward stability and peace. It was viewed as a preliminary step toward preventing the outbreak of nuclear war or military conflict by adopting an attitude of international cooperation.

The agreement basically covers two main areas:

1. It outlines the general conduct of both countries toward each other and toward third countries regarding the avoidance of nuclear war. In this respect it is a bilateral agreement with multilateral implications.

2. The Parties agreed that in a situation in which the two great nuclear countries find themselves in a nuclear confrontation or in which, either as a result of their policies toward each other or as the result of developments elsewhere in the world, there is a danger of a nuclear confrontation between them or any other country, they are committed to consult with each other in order to avoid this risk.

The agreement further provides that these consultations may be communicated to the United Nations and to other countries, a clause the United States, of course, applies to its allies. Article VI stipulates that nothing in the agreement shall affect formal alliance obligations or the inherent right of countries to defend themselves.

AGREEMENT BETWEEN THE UNITED STATES OF AMERICA AND THE UNION OF SOVIET SOCIALIST REPUBLICS ON THE PREVENTION OF NUCLEAR WAR

Signed at Washington June 22, 1973
Entered into force June 22, 1973

The United States of America and the Union of Soviet Socialist Republics, hereinafter referred to as the Parties,

Guided by the objectives of strengthening world peace and international security,

Conscious that nuclear war would have devastating consequences for mankind,

Proceeding from the desire to bring about conditions in which the danger of an outbreak of nuclear war anywhere in the world would be reduced and ultimately eliminated,

Proceeding from their obligations under the Charter of the United Nations regarding the maintenance of peace, refraining from the threat or use of force, and the avoidance of war, and in conformity with the agreements to which either Party has subscribed,

Proceeding from the Basic Principles of Relations between the United States of America and the Union of Soviet Socialist Republics signed in Moscow on May 29, 1972,

Reaffirming that the development of relations between the United States of America and the Union of Soviet Socialist Republics is not directed against other countries and their interests,

Have agreed as follows:

Article I

The United States and the Soviet Union agree that an objective of their policies is to remove the danger of nuclear war and of the use of nuclear weapons.

Accordingly, the Parties agree that they will act in such a manner as to prevent the development of situations capable of causing a dangerous exacerbation of their relations, as to avoid military confrontations, and as to exclude the outbreak of nuclear war between them and between either of the Parties and other countries.

Article II

The Parties agree, in accordance with Article I and to realize the objective stated in that Article, to proceed from the premise that each Party will refrain from the threat or use of force against the other Party, against the allies of the other Party and against other countries, in circumstances which may endanger international peace and security. The Parties agree that they will be guided by these considerations in the formulation of their foreign policies and in their actions in the field of international relations.

Article III

The Parties undertake to develop their relations with each other and with other countries in a way consistent with the purposes of this Agreement.

Article IV

If at any time relations between the Parties or between either Party and other countries appear to involve the risk of a nuclear conflict, or if relations between countries not parties to this Agreement appear to involve the risk of nuclear war between the United States of America and the Union of Soviet Socialist Republics or between either Party and other countries, the United States and the Soviet Union, acting in accordance with the provisions of this Agreement, shall immediately enter into urgent consultations with each other and make every effort to avert this risk.

Article V

Each Party shall be free to inform the Security Council of the United Nations, the Secretary General of the United Nations and the Governments of allied or other countries of the progress and outcome of consultations initiated in accordance with Article IV of this Agreement.

Article VI

Nothing in this Agreement shall affect or impair:

(a) the inherent right of individual or collective self-defense as envisaged by Article 51 of the Charter of the United Nations,*

(b) the provisions of the Charter of the United Nations, including those relating to the maintenance or restoration of international peace and security, and

(c) the obligations undertaken by either Party towards its allies or other countries in treaties, agreements, and other appropriate documents.

Article VII

This Agreement shall be of unlimited duration.

Article VIII

This Agreement shall enter into force upon signature.

DONE at Washington on June 22, 1973, in two copies, each in the English and Russian languages, both texts being equally authentic.

FOR THE UNITED STATES OF AMERICA:
RICHARD NIXON
President of the United States of America

FOR THE UNION OF SOVIET SOCIALIST REPUBLICS:
L.I. BREZHNEV
General Secretary of the Central Committee, CPSU

---

* TS 993; 59 Stat. 1044.

PROTOCOL TO THE TREATY BETWEEN THE UNITED STATES OF AMERICA AND THE UNION OF SOVIET SOCIALIST REPUBLICS ON THE LIMITATION OF ANTI-BALLISTIC MISSILE SYSTEMS

At the 1974 Summit meeting, the United States and the Soviet Union signed a protocol that further restrained deployment of strategic defensive armaments. The 1972 ABM Treaty had permitted each side two ABM deployment areas, one to defend its national capital and another to defend an ICBM field. The 1974 ABM Protocol limits each side to one site only.

The Soviet Union had chosen to maintain its ABM defense of Moscow, and the United States chose to maintain defense of its ICBM emplacements near Grand Forks, North Dakota. To allow some flexibility, the protocol allows each side to reverse its original choice of an ABM site. That is, the United States may dismantle or destroy its ABM system at Grand Forks and deploy an ABM defense of Washington. The Soviet Union, similarly, can decide to shift to an ABM defense of a missile field rather than of Moscow. Each side can make such a change only once. Advance notice must be given, and this may be done only during a year in which a review of the ABM Treaty is scheduled. The Treaty prescribes reviews every five years; the first year for such a review began October 3, 1977.

Upon entry into force, the protocol became an integral part of the 1972 ABM Treaty, of which the verification and other provisions continue to apply. Thus the deployments permitted are governed by the Treaty limitations on numbers and characteristics of interceptor missiles, launchers, and supporting radars. The system the United States chose to deploy (Grand Forks) has actually been on an inactive status since 1976.

PROTOCOL TO THE TREATY BETWEEN THE UNITED STATES OF AMERICA AND THE UNION OF SOVIET SOCIALIST REPUBLICS ON THE LIMITATION OF ANTI-BALLISTIC MISSILE SYSTEMS

Signed at Moscow July 3, 1974
Ratification advised by U.S. Senate November 10, 1975
Ratified by U.S. President March 19, 1976
Instruments of ratification exchanged May 24, 1976
Proclaimed by U.S. President July 6, 1976
Entered into force May 24, 1976

The United States of America and the Union of Soviet Socialist Republics, hereinafter referred to as the Parties,

Proceeding from the Basic Principles of Relations between the United States of America and the Union of Soviet Socialist Republics signed on May 29, 1972,

Desiring to further the objectives of the Treaty between the United States of America and the Union of Soviet Socialist Republics on the Limitation of Anti-Ballistic Missile Systems signed on May 26, 1972, hereinafter referred to as the Treaty,

Reaffirming their conviction that the adoption of further measures for the limitation of strategic arms would contribute to strengthening international peace and security,

Proceeding from the premise that further limitation of anti-ballistic missile systems will create more favorable conditions for the completion of work on a permanent agreement on more complete measures for the limitation of strategic offensive arms,

Have agreed as follows:

Article I

1. Each Party shall be limited at any one time to a single area of the two provided in Article III of the Treaty for deployment of anti-ballistic missile (ABM) systems or their components and accordingly shall not exercise its right to deploy an ABM system or its components in the second of the two ABM system deployment areas permitted by Article III of the Treaty, except as an exchange of one permitted area for the other in accordance with Article II of this Protocol.

2. Accordingly, except as permitted by Article II of this Protocol: the United States of America shall not deploy an ABM system or its components in the area centered on its capital, as permitted by Article III(a) of the Treaty, and the Soviet Union shall not deploy an ABM system or its components in the deployment area of intercontinental ballistic missile (ICBM) silo launchers as permitted by Article III(b) of the Treaty.

Article II

1. Each Party shall have the right to dismantle or destroy its ABM system and the components thereof in the area where they are presently deployed and to deploy an ABM system or its components in the alternative area permitted by Article III of the Treaty, provided that prior to initiation of construction, notification is given in accord with the procedure agreed to in the Standing Consultative Commission, during the year beginning October 3, 1977, and ending October 2, 1978, or during any year which commences at five year intervals thereafter, those being the years of periodic review of the Treaty, as provided in Article XIV of the Treaty. This right may be exercised only once.

2. Accordingly, in the event of such notice, the United States would have the right to dismantle or destroy the ABM system and its components in the deployment area of ICBM silo launchers and to deploy an ABM system or its components in an area centered on its capital, as permitted by Article III(a) of the Treaty, and the Soviet Union would have the right to dismantle or destroy the ABM system and its components in the area centered on its capital and to deploy an ABM system or its components in an area containing ICBM silo launchers, as permitted by Article III(b) of the Treaty.

3. Dismantling or destruction and deployment of ABM systems or their components and the notification thereof shall be carried out in accordance with Article VIII of the ABM Treaty and procedures agreed to in the Standing Consultative Commission.

Article III

The rights and obligations established by the Treaty remain in force and shall be complied with by the Parties except to the extent modified by this Protocol. In particular, the deployment of an ABM system or its components within the area selected shall remain limited by the levels and other requirements established by the Treaty.

Article IV

This Protocol shall be subject to ratification in accordance with the constitutional procedures of each Party. It shall enter into force on the day of the exchange of instruments of ratification and shall thereafter be considered an integral part of the Treaty.

DONE at Moscow on July 3, 1974, in duplicate, in the English and Russian languages, both texts being equally authentic.

FOR THE UNITED STATES OF AMERICA:
RICHARD NIXON
President of the United States of America

FOR THE UNION OF SOVIET SOCIALIST REPUBLICS:
L.I. BREZHNEV
General Secretary of the Central Committee of the CPSU

TREATY BETWEEN THE UNITED STATES OF AMERICA AND THE UNION OF SOVIET SOCIALIST REPUBLICS ON THE LIMITATION OF UNDERGROUND NUCLEAR WEAPON TESTS (AND PROTOCOL THERETO)

The Treaty on the Limitation of Underground Nuclear Weapon Tests, also known as the Threshold Test Ban Treaty (TTBT), was signed in July 1974. It establishes a nuclear "threshold," by prohibiting tests having a yield exceeding 150 kilotons (equivalent to 150,000 tons of TNT).

The threshold is militarily important since it removes the possibility of testing new or existing nuclear weapons going beyond the fractional-megaton range. In the 1960s, many tests above 150 kilotons were conducted by both countries. The mutual restraint imposed by the Treaty reduced the explosive force of new nuclear warheads and bombs which could otherwise be tested for weapons systems. Of particular significance was the relationship between explosive power of reliable, tested warheads and first-strike capability.

The task of negotiating a comprehensive test ban remained on the agenda of the U.S. Government, and, in Article I, the parties to the Threshold Test Ban Treaty undertook an obligation to continue negotiations toward that goal.

The first proposal for stopping nuclear weapon tests was made in 1955, and the first major negotiations with the Soviet Union for an effectively controlled test ban began in Geneva in 1958, with the United Kingdom also participating. The Conference on the Discontinuance of Nuclear Weapon Tests produced no agreement. The problem of working out verification procedures to ensure compliance with a complete ban on nuclear weapon tests in all environments proved to be intractable at that time. The procedures deemed necessary by the United States and the United Kingdom were not acceptable to the Soviet Union.

In 1963 the Limited Test Ban Treaty (LTBT) was signed by the Soviet Union, the United States, and the United Kingdom. This Treaty prohibits nuclear weapon testing in the atmosphere, in outer space and under water. The parties also agreed not to carry out any nuclear weapon test, or any other nuclear explosion, in any other environment -- i.e., underground -- that would cause radioactive debris to be present beyond the borders of the country in which the explosion took place.

Underground nuclear explosions were not prohibited by the 1963 Treaty, although both in the Treaty preamble and Article I, the LTBT parties pledged to seek "the discontinuance of all test explosions of nuclear weapons for all time...."

The United States and Soviet Union agreed in the spring of 1974 to pursue the possibilities of further restrictions on nuclear testing. Accordingly, a team of U.S. experts was sent to Moscow for technical talks.

Agreement on the Threshold Test Ban Treaty was reached during the summit meeting in Moscow in July 1974. The Treaty included a protocol which detailed technical data to be exchanged and which limited weapon testing to specific designated test sites to assist verification. The data to be exchanged included information on the geographical boundaries and geology of the testing areas. Geological data -- including such factors as density of rock formation, water saturation, and depth of the water table -- are useful in verifying test yields because the seismic signal produced by a given underground nuclear explosion varies with these factors at the test location. After an actual test has taken place, the geographic coordinates of the test location are to be furnished to the other party, to help in placing the test in the proper geological setting and thus in assessing the yield.

The Treaty also stipulates that data will be exchanged on a certain number of tests for calibration purposes. By establishing the correlation between stated yields of explosions at the specified sites and the seismic signals produced, this exchange improved assessments by both parties of the yields of explosions based primarily on the measurements derived from their seismic instruments. The tests used for calibration purposes may be tests conducted in the past or new tests.

Agreement to exchange the detailed data described above represented a significant degree of direct cooperation by the two major nuclear powers in the effort to control nuclear weapons. For the first time, each party agreed to make available to the other data relating to its nuclear weapons test program.

The technical problems associated with a yield threshold were recognized by the sides in the spring of 1974. In this context the Soviet Union mentioned the idea of some kind of a "mistakes" understanding concerning occasional, minor, unintended breaches. Discussions on the subject of such an understanding took place in the autumn of 1974 and in the spring of 1976. The Soviet Union was informed by the United States that the understanding reached would be included as part of the public record associated with submitting the Treaty to the Senate for advice and consent to ratification. The entire understanding is as follows:

Both Parties will make every effort to comply fully with all the provisions of the TTB Treaty. However, there are technical uncertainties associated with predicting the precise yields of nuclear weapons tests. These uncertainties may result in slight, unintended breaches of the 150 kiloton threshold. Therefore, the two sides have discussed this problem and agreed that: (1) one or two slight, unintended breaches per year would not be considered a violation of the Treaty; (2) such breaches would be a cause for concern, however, and, at the request of either Party, would be the subject for consultations.

The Soviet Union was also informed that while the United States would not consider such a slight, unintentional breach a violation, the United States would carefully review each such breach to ensure that it is not part of a general attempt to exceed the confines of the Treaty.

The understanding in its entirety was included in the transmittal documents which accompanied the TTB Treaty and the PNE Treaty when they were submitted to the Senate for advice and consent to ratification on July 29, 1976.

Although the TTBT was signed in 1974, it was not sent to the U.S. Senate for advice and consent to ratification until July 1976. Submission was held in abeyance until the companion Treaty on underground nuclear explosions for peaceful purposes (PNET) had been successfully negotiated in accordance with Article III of the TTBT.

For many years, neither the United States nor the Soviet Union ratified the TTBT or the PNE Treaty. However, in 1976 each party separately announced its intention to observe the Treaty limit of 150 kilotons, pending ratification.

The United States and the Soviet Union began negotiations in November 1987 to reach agreement on additional verification provisions that would make it possible for the United States to ratify the treaties. Agreement on additional verification provisions, contained in new protocols, substituting for the original protocols, was reached in June 1990. The TTBT and PNET entered into force on December 11, 1990.* The TTBT verification protocol provides for the use of the hydrodynamic yield measurement method with respect to all tests having a planned yield exceeding 50 kilotons, as well as seismic monitoring and, with respect to all tests having a planned yield exceeding 35 kilotons, on-site inspection.

---

* The full text of the 1990 Protocols will appear in the next edition of this series.

TREATY BETWEEN THE UNITED STATES OF AMERICA AND THE UNION OF SOVIET SOCIALIST REPUBLICS ON THE LIMITATION OF UNDERGROUND NUCLEAR WEAPON TESTS

Signed at Moscow July 3, 1974
Ratified December 8, 1990
Entered into force December 11, 1990

The United States of America and the Union of Soviet Socialist Republics, hereinafter referred to as the Parties,

Declaring their intention to achieve at the earliest possible date the cessation of the nuclear arms race and to take effective measures toward reductions in strategic arms, nuclear disarmament, and general and complete disarmament under strict and effective international control,

Recalling the determination expressed by the Parties to the 1963 Treaty Banning Nuclear Weapon Tests in the Atmosphere, in Outer Space and Under Water in its Preamble to seek to achieve the discontinuance of all test explosions of nuclear weapons for all time, and to continue negotiations to this end,

Noting that the adoption of measures for the further limitation of underground nuclear weapon tests would contribute to the achievement of these objectives and would meet the interests of strengthening peace and the further relaxation of international tension,

Reaffirming their adherence to the objectives and principles of the Treaty Banning Nuclear Weapon Tests in the Atmosphere, in Outer Space and Under Water and of the Treaty on the Non-Proliferation of Nuclear Weapons,

Have agreed as follows:

Article I

1. Each Party undertakes to prohibit, to prevent, and not to carry out any underground nuclear weapon test having a yield exceeding 150 kilotons at any place under its jurisdiction or control, beginning March 31, 1976.

2. Each Party shall limit the number of its underground nuclear weapon tests to a minimum.

3. The Parties shall continue their negotiations with a view toward achieving a solution to the problem of the cessation of all underground nuclear weapon tests.

Article II

1. For the purpose of providing assurance of compliance with the provisions of this Treaty, each Party shall use national technical means of verification at its disposal in a manner consistent with the generally recognized principles of international law.

2. Each Party undertakes not to interfere with the national technical means of verification of the other Party operating in accordance with paragraph 1 of this Article.

3. To promote the objectives and implementation of the provisions of this Treaty the Parties shall, as necessary, consult with each other, make inquiries and furnish information in response to such inquiries.

Article III

The provisions of this Treaty do not extend to underground nuclear explosions carried out by the Parties for peaceful purposes. Underground nuclear explosions for peaceful purposes shall be governed by an agreement which is to be negotiated and concluded by the Parties at the earliest possible time.

Article IV

This Treaty shall be subject to ratification in accordance with the constitutional procedures of each Party. This Treaty shall enter into force on the day of the exchange of instruments of ratification.

Article V

1. This Treaty shall remain in force for a period of five years. Unless replaced earlier by an agreement in implementation of the objectives specified in paragraph 3 of Article I of this Treaty, it shall be extended for successive five-year periods unless either Party notifies the other of its termination no later than six months prior to the expiration of the Treaty. Before the expiration of this period the Parties may, as necessary, hold consultations to consider the situation relevant to

the substance of this Treaty and to introduce possible amendments to the text of the Treaty.

2. Each Party shall, in exercising its national sovereignty, have the right to withdraw from this Treaty if it decides that extraordinary events related to the subject matter of this Treaty have jeopardized its supreme interests. It shall give notice of its decision to the other Party six months prior to withdrawal from this Treaty. Such notice shall include a statement of the extraordinary events the notifying Party regards as having jeopardized its supreme interests.

3. This Treaty shall be registered pursuant to Article 102 of the Charter of the United Nations.

DONE at Moscow on July 3, 1974, in duplicate, in the English and Russian languages, both texts being equally authentic.

FOR THE UNITED STATES OF AMERICA:
RICHARD NIXON
The President of the United States of America

FOR THE UNION OF SOVIET SOCIALIST REPUBLICS:
L. BREZHNEV
General Secretary of the Central Committee of the CPSU

PROTOCOL TO THE TREATY BETWEEN THE UNITED STATES OF AMERICA AND THE UNION OF SOVIET SOCIALIST REPUBLICS ON THE LIMITATION OF UNDERGROUND NUCLEAR WEAPON TESTS

The United States of America and the Union of Soviet Socialist Republics, hereinafter referred to as the Parties,

Having agreed to limit underground nuclear weapon tests,

Have agreed as follows:

1. For the Purpose of ensuring verification of compliance with the obligations of the Parties under the Treaty by national technical means, the Parties shall, on the basis of reciprocity, exchange the following data:

a. The geographic coordinates of the boundaries of each test site and of the boundaries of the geophysically distinct testing areas therein.

b. Information on the geology of the testing areas of the sites (the rock characteristics of geological formations and the basic physical properties of the rock, i.e., density, seismic velocity, water saturation, porosity and the depth of water table).

c. The geographic coordinates of underground nuclear weapon tests, after they have been conducted.

d. Yield, date, time, depth and coordinates for two nuclear weapon tests for calibration purposes from each geophysically distinct testing area where underground nuclear weapon tests have been and are to be conducted. In this connection the yield of such explosions for calibration purposes should be as near as possible to the limit defined in Article I of the Treaty and not less than one-tenth of that limit. In the case of testing areas where data are not available on two tests for calibration purposes, the data pertaining to one such test shall be exchanged, if available, and the data pertaining to the second test shall be exchanged as soon as possible after the second test having a yield in the above-mentioned range. The provisions of this Protocol shall not require the Parties to conduct tests solely for calibration purposes.

2. The Parties agree that the exchange of data pursuant to subparagraphs a, b, and d of paragraph 1 shall be carried out simultaneously with the exchange of instruments of ratification of the Treaty, as provided in Article IV of the Treaty, having in mind that the Parties shall, on the basis of reciprocity, afford each other the opportunity to familiarize themselves with these data before the exchange of instruments of ratification.

3. Should a Party specify a new test site or testing area after the entry into force of the Treaty, the data called for by subparagraphs a and b of paragraph 1 shall be transmitted to the other Party in advance of use of that site or area. The data called for by subparagraph d of paragraph 1 shall also be transmitted in advance of use of that site or area if they are available; if they are not available, they shall be transmitted as soon as possible after they have been obtained by the transmitting Party.

4. The Parties agree that the test sites of each Party shall be located at places under its jurisdiction or control and that all nuclear weapon tests shall be conducted solely within the testing areas specified in accordance with paragraph 1.

5. For the purposes of the Treaty, all underground nuclear explosions at the specified test sites shall be considered nuclear weapon tests and shall be subject to all the provisions of the Treaty relating to nuclear weapon tests. The provisions of Article III of the Treaty apply to all underground nuclear explosions conducted outside of the specified test sites, and only to such explosions.

This Protocol shall be considered an integral part of the Treaty.

DONE at Moscow on July 3, 1974.

FOR THE UNITED STATES OF AMERICA: RICHARD M. NIXON
The President of the United States of America

FOR THE UNION OF SOVIET SOCIALIST REPUBLICS: L. BREZHNEV
General Secretary of the Central Committee of the CPSU

TREATY BETWEEN THE UNITED STATES OF AMERICA AND THE UNION OF SOVIET SOCIALIST REPUBLICS ON UNDERGROUND NUCLEAR EXPLOSIONS FOR PEACEFUL PURPOSES (AND PROTOCOL THERETO)

In preparing the Threshold Test Ban Treaty (TTBT) in July 1974, the United States and the Soviet Union recognized the need to establish an appropriate agreement to govern underground nuclear explosions for peaceful purposes (PNEs). There is no essential distinction between the technology of a nuclear explosive device which would be used as a weapon and the technology of a nuclear explosive device used for a peaceful purpose.

Negotiations on the PNE agreement contemplated in Article III of the TTBT began in Moscow on October 7, 1974, and after six negotiating sessions over a period of 18 months, resulted in the Treaty on Underground Nuclear Explosions for Peaceful Purposes in April 1976. The agreement consists of a Treaty, a detailed protocol to the Treaty, and an agreed statement delineating certain important activities which do not constitute a peaceful application as that term is used in the Treaty.

The PNE Treaty governs all nuclear explosions carried out at locations outside the weapons test sites specified under the Threshold Test Ban Treaty.

In the PNE Treaty the United States and the Soviet Union agreed: not to carry out any individual nuclear explosions having a yield exceeding 150 kilotons; not to carry out any group explosion (consisting of a number of individual explosions) having an aggregate yield exceeding 1,500 kilotons; and not to carry out any group explosion having an aggregate yield exceeding 150 kilotons unless the individual explosions in the group could be identified and measured by agreed verification procedures. The parties also reaffirmed their obligations to comply fully with the Limited Test Ban Treaty of 1963.

The parties reserve the right to carry out nuclear explosions for peaceful purposes in the territory of another country if requested to do so, but only in full compliance with the yield limitations and other provisions of the PNE Treaty and in accord with the Non-Proliferation Treaty.

Articles IV and V of the PNE Treaty set forth the agreed verification arrangements. In addition to the use of national technical means, the Treaty states that information and access to sites of explosions will be provided by each side, and includes a commitment not to interfere with verification means and procedures.

The protocol to the PNE Treaty sets forth the specific agreed arrangements for ensuring that no weapon-related benefits precluded by the Threshold Test Ban Treaty are derived by carrying out a nuclear explosion used for peaceful purposes, including provisions for use of the hydrodynamic yield measurement method, seismic monitoring and on-site inspection.

The agreed statement that accompanies the Treaty specifies that a "peaceful application" of an underground nuclear explosion would not include the developmental testing of any nuclear explosive. Such testing must be carried out at the nuclear weapon test sites specified by the terms of the TTBT, and therefore, is treated as the testing of a nuclear weapon.

The provisions of the PNE Treaty, together with those of the TTBT, establish a comprehensive system of regulations to govern all underground nuclear explosions of the United States and the Soviet Union. The interrelationship of the TTBT and the PNE Treaty is further recognized by their identical five-year durations, and by the provision that neither party may withdraw from the PNE Treaty while the TTBT remains in force. Conversely, either party may withdraw from the PNE Treaty upon termination of the TTBT.

The PNET and the TTBT were both submitted to the Senate for its advice and consent on June 28, 1990. Following the Senate's approval of the treaties, the United States and the Soviet Union exchanged instruments of ratification and the treaties entered into force on December 11, 1990.

A Joint Consultative Commission was established to discuss any questions of compliance, to develop further details of the on-site inspection process as needed, and to facilitate cooperation in various areas related to which might be mutually beneficial.

TREATY BETWEEN THE UNITED STATES OF AMERICA AND THE UNION OF SOVIET SOCIALIST REPUBLICS ON UNDERGROUND NUCLEAR EXPLOSIONS FOR PEACEFUL PURPOSES

Signed at Washington and Moscow May 28, 1976
Entered into force December 11, 1990

The United States of America and the Union of Soviet Socialist Republics, hereinafter referred to as the Parties,

Proceeding from a desire to implement Article III of the Treaty Between the United States of America and the Union of Soviet Socialist Republics on the Limitation of Underground Nuclear Weapon Tests, which calls for the earliest possible conclusion of an agreement on underground nuclear explosions for peaceful purposes,

Reaffirming their adherence to the objectives and principles of the Treaty Banning Nuclear Weapon Tests in the Atmosphere, in Outer Space and Under Water, the Treaty on Non-Proliferation of Nuclear Weapons, and the Treaty on the Limitation of Underground Nuclear Weapon Tests, and their determination to observe strictly the provisions of these international agreements,

Desiring to assure that underground nuclear explosions for peaceful purposes shall not be used for purposes related to nuclear weapons,

Desiring that utilization of nuclear energy be directed only toward peaceful purposes,

Desiring to develop appropriately cooperation in the field of underground nuclear explosions for peaceful purposes,

Have agreed as follows:

Article I

1. The Parties enter into this Treaty to satisfy the obligations in Article III of the Treaty on the Limitation of Underground Nuclear Weapon Tests, and assume additional obligations in accordance with the provisions of this Treaty.

2. This Treaty shall govern all underground nuclear explosions for peaceful purposes conducted by the Parties after March 31, 1976.

Article II

For the purposes of this Treaty:

(a) "explosion" means any individual or group underground nuclear explosion for peaceful purposes;

(b) "explosive" means any device, mechanism or system for producing an individual explosion;

(c) "group explosion" means two or more individual explosions for which the time interval between successive individual explosions does not exceed five seconds and for which the emplacement points of all explosives can be interconnected by straight line segments, each of which joins two emplacement points and each of which does not exceed 40 kilometers.

Article III

1. Each Party, subject to the obligations assumed under this Treaty and other international agreements, reserves the right to:

(a) carry out explosions at any place under its jurisdiction or control outside the geographical boundaries of test sites specified under the provisions of the Treaty on the Limitation of Underground Nuclear Weapon Tests; and

(b) carry out, participate or assist in carrying out explosions in the territory of another State at the request of such other State.

2. Each Party undertakes to prohibit, to prevent and not to carry out at any place under its jurisdiction or control, and further undertakes not to carry out, participate or assist in carrying out anywhere:

(a) any individual explosion having a yield exceeding 150 kilotons;

(b) any group explosion:

(1) having an aggregate yield exceeding 150 kilotons except in ways that will permit identification of each individual explosion and determination of the yield of each individual explosion in the group in accordance with the provisions of Article IV of and the Protocol to this Treaty;

(2) having an aggregate yield exceeding one and one-half megatons;

(c) any explosion which does not carry out a peaceful application;

(d) any explosion except in compliance with the provisions of the Treaty Banning Nuclear Weapon Tests in the Atmosphere, in Outer Space and Under Water, the Treaty on the Non-Proliferation of Nuclear Weapons, and other international agreements entered into by that Party.

3. The question of carrying out any individual explosion having a yield exceeding the yield specified in paragraph 2(a) of this article will be considered by the Parties at an appropriate time to be agreed.

Article IV

1. For the purpose of providing assurance of compliance with the provisions of this Treaty, each Party shall:

(a) use national technical means of verification at its disposal in a manner consistent with generally recognized principles of international law; and

(b) provide to the other Party information and access to sites of explosions and furnish assistance in accordance with the provisions set forth in the Protocol to this Treaty.

2. Each Party undertakes not to interfere with the national technical means of verification of the other Party operating in accordance with paragraph 1(a) of this article, or with the implementation of the provisions of paragraph 1(b) of this article.

Article V

1. To promote the objectives and implementation of the provisions of this Treaty, the Parties shall establish promptly a Joint Consultative Commission within the framework of which they will:

(a) consult with each other, make inquiries and furnish information in response to such inquiries, to assure confidence in compliance with the obligations assumed;

(b) consider questions concerning compliance with the obligations assumed and related situations which may be considered ambiguous;

(c) consider questions involving unintended interference with the means for assuring compliance with the provisions of this Treaty;

(d) consider changes in technology or other new circumstances which have a bearing on the provisions of this Treaty; and

(e) consider possible amendments to provisions governing underground nuclear explosions for peaceful purposes.

2. The Parties through consultation shall establish, and may amend as appropriate, Regulations for the Joint Consultative Commission governing procedures, composition and other relevant matters.

Article VI

1. The Parties will develop cooperation on the basis of mutual benefit, equality, and reciprocity in various areas related to carrying out underground nuclear explosions for peaceful purposes.

2. The Joint Consultative Commission will facilitate this cooperation by considering specific areas and forms of cooperation which shall be determined by agreement between the Parties in accordance with their constitutional procedures.

3. The Parties will appropriately inform the International Atomic Energy Agency of results of their cooperation in the field of underground nuclear explosions for peaceful purposes.

Article VII

1. Each Party shall continue to promote the development of the international agreement or agreements and procedures provided for in Article V of the Treaty on the Non-Proliferation of Nuclear Weapons, and shall provide appropriate assistance to the International Atomic Energy Agency in this regard.

2. Each Party undertakes not to carry out, participate or assist in the carrying out of any explosion in the territory of another State unless that State agrees to the implementation in its territory of the international observation and

procedures contemplated by Article V of the Treaty on the Non-Proliferation of Nuclear Weapons and the provisions of Article IV of and the Protocol to this Treaty, including the provision by that State of the assistance necessary for such implementation and of the privileges and immunities specified in the Protocol.

Article VIII

1. This Treaty shall remain in force for a period of five years, and it shall be extended for successive five-year periods unless either Party notifies the other of its termination no later than six months prior to its expiration. Before the expiration of this period the Parties may, as necessary, hold consultations to consider the situation relevant to the substance of this Treaty. However, under no circumstances shall either Party be entitled to terminate this Treaty while the Treaty on the Limitation of Underground Nuclear Weapon Tests remains in force.

2. Termination of the Treaty on the Limitation of Underground Nuclear Weapon Tests shall entitle either Party to withdraw from this Treaty at any time.

3. Each Party may propose amendments to this Treaty. Amendments shall enter into force on the day of the exchange of instruments of ratification of such amendments.

Article IX

1. This Treaty, including the Protocol which forms an integral part hereof, shall be subject to ratification in accordance with the constitutional procedures of each Party. This Treaty shall enter into force on the day of the exchange of instruments of ratification which exchange shall take place simultaneously with the exchange of instruments of ratification of the Treaty on the Limitation of Underground Nuclear Weapon Tests.

2. This Treaty shall be registered pursuant to Article 102 of the Charter of the United Nations.

DONE at Washington and Moscow, on May 28, 1976, in duplicate, in the English and Russian languages, both texts being equally authentic.

FOR THE UNITED STATES OF AMERICA:
GERALD R. FORD
The President of the United States of America

FOR THE UNION OF SOVIET SOCIALIST REPUBLICS:
L. BREZHNEV
General Secretary of the Central Committee of the CPSU

PROTOCOL TO THE TREATY BETWEEN THE UNITED STATES OF AMERICA AND THE UNION OF SOVIET SOCIALIST REPUBLICS ON UNDERGROUND NUCLEAR EXPLOSIONS FOR PEACEFUL PURPOSES

The United States of America and the Union of Soviet Socialist Republics, hereinafter referred to as the Parties,

Having agreed to the provisions in the Treaty on Underground Nuclear Explosions for Peaceful Purposes, hereinafter referred to as the Treaty,

Have agreed as follows:

Article I

1. No individual explosion shall take place at a distance, in meters, from the ground surface which is less than 30 times the 3.4 root of its planned yield in kilotons.

2. Any group explosion with a planned aggregate yield exceeding 500 kilotons shall not include more than five individual explosions, each of which has a planned yield not exceeding 50 kilotons.

Article II

1. For each explosion, the Party carrying out the explosion shall provide the other Party:

(a) not later than 90 days before the beginning of emplacement of the explosives when the planned aggregate yield of the explosion does not exceed 100 kilotons, or not later than 180 days before the beginning of emplacement of the explosives when the planned aggregate yield of the explosion exceeds 100 kilotons, with the following information to the extent and degree of precision available when it is conveyed:

(1) the purpose of the planned explosion;

(2) the location of the explosion expressed in geographical coordinates with a precision of four or less kilometers, planned date and aggregate yield of the explosion;

(3) the type or types of rock in which the explosion will be carried out, including the degree of liquid saturation of the rock at the point of emplacement of each explosive; and

(4) a description of specific technological features of the project, of which the explosion is a part, that could influence the determination of its yield and confirmation of purpose; and

(b) not later than 60 days before the beginning of emplacement of the explosives the information specified in subparagraph 1(a) of this article to the full extent and with the precision indicated in that subparagraph.

2. For each explosion with a planned aggregate yield exceeding 50 kilotons, the Party carrying out the explosion shall provide the other Party, not later than 60 days before the beginning of emplacement of the explosives, with the following information:

(a) the number of explosives, the planned yield of each explosive, the location of each explosive to be used in a group explosion relative to all other explosives in the group with a precision of 100 or less meters, the depth of emplacement of each explosive with a precision of one meter and the time intervals between individual explosions in any group explosion with a precision of one-tenth second; and

(b) a description of specific features of geological structure or other local conditions that could influence the determination of the yield.

3. For each explosion with a planned aggregate yield exceeding 75 kilotons, the Party carrying out the explosion shall provide the other Party, not later than 60 days before the beginning of emplacement of the explosives, with a description of the geological and geophysical characteristics of the site of each explosion which could influence determination of the yield, which shall include: the depth of the water table; a stratigraphic column above each emplacement point; the position of each emplacement point relative to nearby geological and other features which influenced the design of the project of which the explosion is a part; and the physical parameters of the rock, including density, seismic velocity, porosity, degree of liquid saturation, and rock strength, within the sphere centered on each emplacement point and having a radius, in meters, equal to 30 times the cube root of the planned yield in kilotons of the explosive emplaced at that point.

4. For each explosion with a planned aggregate yield exceeding 100 kilotons, the Party carrying out the explosion shall provide the other Party, not later than 60 days before the beginning of emplacement of the explosives, with:

(a) information on locations and purposes of facilities and installations which are associated with the conduct of the explosion;

(b) information regarding the planned date of the beginning of emplacement of each explosive; and

(c) a topographic plan in local coordinates of the areas specified in paragraph 7 of Article IV, at a scale of 1:24,000 or 1:25,000 with a contour interval of 10 meters or less.

5. For application of an explosion to alleviate the consequences of an emergency situation involving an unforeseen combination of circumstances which calls for immediate action for which it would not be practicable to observe the timing requirements of paragraphs 1, 2 and 3 of this article, the following conditions shall be met:

(a) the Party deciding to carry out an explosion for such purposes shall inform the other Party of that decision immediately after it has been made and describe such circumstances;

(b) the planned aggregate yield of an explosion for such purpose shall not exceed 100 kilotons; and

(c) the Party carrying out an explosion for such purpose shall provide to the other Party the information specified in paragraph 1 of this article, and the information specified in paragraphs 2 and 3 of this article if applicable, after the decision to conduct the explosion is taken, but not later than 30 days before the beginning of emplacement of the explosives.

6. For each explosion, the Party carrying out the explosion shall inform the other Party, not later than two days before the explosion, of the planned time of detonation of each explosive with a precision of one second.

7. Prior to the explosion, the Party carrying out the explosion shall provide the other Party with timely notification of changes in the information provided in accordance with this article.

8. The explosion shall not be carried out earlier than 90 days after notification of any change in the information provided in accordance with this article which requires more extensive verification procedures than those required on the basis of the original information, unless an earlier time for carrying out the explosion is agreed between the Parties.

9. Not later than 90 days after each explosion the Party carrying out the explosion shall provide the other Party with the following information:

(a) the actual time of the explosion with a precision of one-tenth second and its aggregate yield;

(b) when the planned aggregate yield of a group explosion exceeds 50 kilotons, the actual time of the first individual explosion with a precision of one-tenth second, the time interval between individual explosions with a precision of one milli-second and the yield of each individual explosion; and

(c) confirmation of other information provided in accordance with paragraphs 1, 2, 3 and 4 of this article and explanation of any changes or corrections based on the results of the explosion.

10. At any time, but not later than one year after the explosion, the other Party may request the Party carrying out the explosion to clarify any item of the information provided in accordance with this article. Such clarification shall be provided as soon as practicable, but not later than 30 days after the request is made.

Article III

1. For the purposes of this Protocol:

(a) "designated personnel" means those nationals of the other Party identified to the Party carrying out an explosion as the persons who will exercise the rights and functions provided for in the Treaty and this Protocol; and

(b) "emplacement hole" means the entire interior of any drill-hole, shaft, adit or tunnel in which an explosive and associated cables and other equipment are to be installed.

2. For any explosion with a planned aggregate yield exceeding 100 kilotons but not exceeding 150 kilotons if the Parties, in consultation based on information provided in accordance with Article II and other information that may be introduced by either Party, deem it appropriate for the confirmation of the yield of the explosion, and for any explosion with a planned aggregate yield exceeding 150 kilotons, the Party carrying out the explosion shall allow designated personnel within the areas and at the locations described in Article V to exercise the following rights and functions:

(a) confirmation that the local circumstances, including facilities and installations associated with the project, are consistent with the stated peaceful purposes;

(b) confirmation of the validity of the geological and geophysical information provided in accordance with Article II through the following procedures:

(1) examination by designated personnel of research and measurement data of the Party carrying out the explosion and of rock core or rock fragments removed from each emplacement hole, and of any logs and drill core from existing exploratory holes which shall be provided to designated personnel upon their arrival at the site of the explosion;

(2) examination by designated personnel of rock core or rock fragments as they become available in accordance with the procedures specified in subparagraph 2(b)(3) of this article; and

(3) observation by designated personnel of implementation by the Party carrying out the explosion of one of the following four procedures, unless this right is waived by the other Party:

(i) construction of that portion of each emplacement hole starting from a point nearest the entrance of the emplacement hole which is at a distance, in meters, from the nearest emplacement point equal to 30 times the cube root of the planned yield in kilotons of the explosive to be emplaced at that point and continuing to the completion of the emplacement hole; or

(ii) construction of that portion of each emplacement hole starting from a point nearest the entrance of the emplacement hole which is at a distance, in meters, from the nearest emplacement point equal to six times the cube root of the planned yield in kilotons of the explosive to be emplaced at that point and continuing to the completion of the emplacement hole as well as the removal of rock core or rock fragments from the wall of an existing exploratory hole, which is substantially parallel with and at no point more than 100 meters from the emplacement hole, at locations specified by designated personnel which lie within a distance, in meters, from the same horizon as each emplacement point of 30 times the cube root of the planned yield in kilotons of the explosive to be emplaced at that point; or

(iii) removal of rock core or rock fragments from the wall of each emplacement hole at locations specified by designated personnel which lie within a distance, in meters, from each emplacement point of 30 times the cube root of the planned yield in kilotons of the explosive to be emplaced at each such point; or

(iv) construction of one or more new exploratory holes so that for each emplacement hole there will be a new exploratory hole to the same depth as that of the emplacement of the explosive, substantially parallel with and at no point more than 100 meters from each emplacement hole, from which rock cores would be removed at locations specified by designated personnel which lie within a distance, in meters, from the same horizon as each emplacement point of 30 times the cube root of the planned yield in kilotons of the explosive to be emplaced at each such point:

(c) observation of the emplacement of each explosive, confirmation of the depth of its emplacement and observation of the stemming of each emplacement hole;

(d) unobstructed visual observation of the area of the entrance to each emplacement hole at any time from the time of emplacement of each explosive until all personnel have been withdrawn from the site for the detonation of the explosion; and

(e) observation of each explosion.

3. Designated personnel, using equipment provided in accordance with paragraph 1 of Article IV, shall have the right, for any explosion with a planned aggregate yield exceeding 150 kilotons, to determine the yield of each individual explosion in a group explosion in accordance with the provisions of Article VI.

4. Designated personnel, when using their equipment in accordance with paragraph 1 of Article IV, shall have the right, for any explosion with planned aggregate yield exceeding 500 kilotons, to emplace, install and operate under the observation and with the assistance of personnel of the Party carrying out the explosion, if such assistance is requested by designated personnel, a local seismic network in accordance with the provisions of paragraph 7 of Article IV. Radio links may be used for the transmission of data and control signals between the seismic stations and the control center. Frequencies, maximum power output of radio transmitters, directivity of antennas and times of operation of the local seismic network radio transmitters before the explosion shall be agreed between the Parties in accordance with Article X and time of operation after the explosion shall conform to the time specified in paragraph 7 of Article IV.

5. Designated personnel shall have the right to:

(a) acquire photographs under the following conditions:

(1) the Party carrying out the explosion shall identify to the other Party those personnel of the Party carrying out the explosion who shall take photographs as requested by designated personnel;

(2) photographs shall be taken by personnel of the Party carrying out the explosion in the presence of designated personnel and at the time requested by designated personnel for taking such photographs. Designated personnel shall determine whether these photographs are in conformity with their requests and, if not, additional photographs shall be taken immediately;

(3) photographs shall be taken with cameras provided by the other Party having built-in, rapid developing capability and a copy of each photograph shall be provided at the completion of the development process to both Parties;

(4) cameras provided by designated personnel shall be kept in agreed secure storage when not in use; and

(5) the request for photographs can be made, at any time, of the following:

(i) exterior views of facilities and installations associated with the conduct of the explosion as described in subparagraph 4(a) of Article II;

(ii) geological samples used for confirmation of geological and geophysical information, as provided for in subparagraph 2(b) of this article and the equipment utilized in the acquisition of such samples;

(iii) emplacement and installation of equipment and associated cables used by designated personnel for yield determination;

(iv) emplacement and installation of the local seismic network used by designated personnel;

(v) emplacement of the explosives and the stemming of the emplacement hole; and

(vi) containers, facilities and installations for storage and operation of equipment used by designated personnel;

(b) photographs of visual displays and records produced by the equipment used by designated personnel and photographs within the control centers taken by cameras which are component parts of such equipment; and

(c) receive at the request of designated personnel and with the agreement of the Party carrying out the explosion supplementary photographs taken by the Party carrying out the explosion.

Article IV

1. Designated personnel in exercising their rights and functions may choose to use the following equipment of either Party, of which choice the Party carrying out the explosion shall be informed not later than 150 days before the beginning of emplacement of the explosives:

(a) electrical equipment for yield determination and equipment for a local seismic network as described in paragraphs 3, 4 and 7 of this article; and

(b) geologist's field tools and kits and equipment for recording of field notes.

2. Designated personnel shall have the right in exercising their rights and functions to utilize the following additional equipment which shall be provided by the Party carrying out the explosion, under procedures to be established in accordance with Article X to ensure that the equipment meets the specifications of the other Party: portable short-range communication equipment, field glasses, optical equipment for surveying and other items which may be specified by the other Party. A description of such equipment and operating instructions shall be provided to the other Party not later than 90 days before the beginning of emplacement of the explosives in connection with which such equipment is to be used.

3. A complete set of electrical equipment for yield determination shall consist of:

(a) sensing elements and associated cables for transmission of electrical power, control signals and data;

(b) equipment of the control center, electrical power supplies and cables for transmission of electrical power, control signals and data; and

(c) measuring and calibration instruments, maintenance equipment and spare parts necessary for ensuring the functioning of sensing elements, cables and equipment of the control center.

4. A complete set of equipment for the local seismic network shall consist of:

(a) seismic stations each of which contains a seismic instrument, electrical power supply and associated cables and radio equipment for receiving and transmission of control signals and data or equipment for recording control signals and data;

(b) equipment of the control center and electrical power supplies; and

(c) measuring and calibration instruments, maintenance equipment and spare parts necessary for ensuring the functioning of the complete network.

5. In case designated personnel, in accordance with paragraph 1 of this article, choose to use equipment of the Party carrying out the explosion for yield determination or for a local seismic network, a description of such equipment and installation and operating instructions shall be provided to the other Party not later than 90 days before the beginning of emplacement of the explosives in connection with which such equipment is to be used. Personnel of the Party carrying out the explosion shall emplace, install and operate the equipment in the presence of designated personnel. After the explosion, designated personnel shall receive duplicate copies of the recorded data. Equipment for yield determination shall be emplaced in accordance with Article VI. Equipment for a local seismic network shall be emplaced in accordance with paragraph 7 of this article.

6. In case designated personnel, in accordance with paragraph 1 of this article, choose to use their own equipment for yield determination and their own equipment for a local seismic network, the following procedures shall apply:

(a) the Party carrying out the explosion shall be provided by the other Party with the equipment and information specified in subparagraphs (a)(1) and (a)(2) of this paragraph not later than 150 days prior to the beginning of emplacement of the explosives in connection with which such equipment is to be used in order to permit the Party carrying out the explosion to familiarize itself with such equipment, if such equipment and information has not been previously provided, which equipment shall be returned to the other Party not later than 90 days before the beginning of emplacement of the explosives. The equipment and information to be provided are:

(1) one complete set of electrical equipment for yield determination as described in paragraph 3 of this article, electrical and mechanical design information, specifications and installation and operating instructions concerning this equipment; and

(2) one complete set of equipment for the local seismic network described in paragraph 4 of this article, including one seismic station, electrical and mechanical design information, specifications and installation and operating instructions concerning this equipment;

(b) not later than 35 days prior to the beginning of emplacement of the explosives in connection with which the following equipment is to be used, two complete sets of electrical equipment for yield determination as described in paragraph 3 of this article and specific installation instructions for the emplacement of the sensing elements based on information provided in accordance with subparagraph 2(a) of Article VI and two complete sets of equipment for the local seismic network as described in paragraph 4 of this article, which sets of equipment shall have the same components and technical characteristics as the corresponding equipment specified in subparagraph 6(a) of this article, shall be delivered in sealed containers to the port of entry;

(c) The Party carrying out the explosion shall choose one of each of the two sets of equipment described above which shall be used by designated personnel in connection with the explosions;

(d) the set or sets of equipment not chosen for use in connection with the explosion shall be at the disposal of the Party carrying out the explosion for a period that may be as long as 30 days after the explosion at which time such equipment shall be returned to the other Party;

(e) the set or sets of equipment chosen for use shall be transported by the Party carrying out the explosion in the sealed containers in which this equipment arrived, after seals of the Party carrying out the explosion have been affixed to them, to the site of the explosion, so that this equipment is delivered to designated personnel for emplacement, installation and operation not later than 20 days before the beginning of emplacement of the explosives. This equipment shall remain in the custody of designated personnel in accordance with paragraph 7 of Article V or in agreed secure storage. Personnel of the Party carrying out the explosion shall have the right to observe the use of this equipment by designated personnel during the time the equipment is at the site of the explosion. Before the beginning of emplacement of the explosives, designated personnel shall demonstrate to personnel of the Party carrying out the explosion that this equipment is in working order;

(f) each set of equipment shall include two sets of components for recording data and associated calibration equipment. Both of these sets of components in the equipment chosen for use shall simultaneously record data. After the explosion, and after duplicate copies of all data have been obtained by designated personnel and the Party carrying out the explosion, one of each of the two sets of components for recording data and associated calibration equipment shall be selected, by an agreed process of chance, to be retained by designated personnel. Designated personnel shall pack and seal such components for recording data and associated calibration equipment which shall accompany them from the site of the explosion to the port of exit; and

(g) all remaining equipment may be retained by the Party carrying out the explosion for a period that may be as long as 30 days, after which time this equipment shall be returned to the other Party.

7. For any explosion with a planned aggregate yield exceeding 500 kilotons, a local seismic network, the number of stations of which shall be determined by designated personnel but shall not exceed the number of explosives in the group plus five, shall be emplaced, installed and operated at agreed sites of emplacement within an area circumscribed by circles of 15 kilometers in radius centered on points on the surface of the earth above the points of emplacement of the explosives during a period beginning not later than 20 days before the beginning of emplacement of the explosives and continuing after the explosion not later than three days unless otherwise agreed between the Parties.

8. The Party carrying out the explosion shall have the right to examine in the presence of designated personnel all equipment, instruments

and tools of designated personnel specified in subparagraph 1(b) of this article.

9. The Joint Consultative Commission will consider proposals that either Party may put forward for the joint development of standardized equipment for verification purposes.

Article V

1. Except as limited by the provisions of paragraph 5 of this article, designated personnel in the exercise of their rights and functions shall have access along agreed routes:

(a) for an explosion with a planned aggregate yield exceeding 100 kilotons in accordance with paragraph 2 of Article III:

(1) to the locations of facilities and installations associated with the conduct of the explosion provided in accordance with subparagraph 4(a) of Article II; and

(2) to the locations of activities described in paragraph 2 of Article III; and

(b) for any explosion with a planned aggregate yield exceeding 150 kilotons, in addition to the access described in subparagraph 1(a) of this article:

(1) to other locations within the area circumscribed by circles of 10 kilometers in radius centered on points on the surface of the earth above the points of emplacement of the explosives in order to confirm that the local circumstances are consistent with the stated peaceful purposes;

(2) to the locations of the components of the electrical equipment for yield determination to be used for recording data when, by agreement between the Parties, such equipment is located outside the area described in subparagraph 1(b)(1) of this article; and

(3) to the sites of emplacement of the equipment of the local seismic network provided for in paragraph 7 of Article IV.

2. The Party carrying out the explosion shall notify the other Party of the procedure it has chosen from among those specified in subparagraph 2(b)(3) of Article III not later than

30 days before beginning the implementation of such procedure. Designated personnel shall have the right to be present at the site of the explosion to exercise their rights and functions in the areas and at the locations described in paragraph 1 of this article for a period of time beginning two days before the beginning of the implementation of the procedure and continuing for a period of three days after the completion of this procedure.

3. Except as specified in paragraph 5 of this article, designated personnel shall have the right to be present in the areas and at the locations described in paragraph 1 of this article:

(a) for an explosion with a planned aggregate yield exceeding 100 kilotons but not exceeding 150 kilotons, in accordance with paragraph 2 of Article III, at any time beginning five days before the beginning of emplacement of the explosives and continuing after the explosion and after safe access to evacuated areas has been established according to standards determined by the Party carrying out the explosion for a period of two days; and

(b) for any explosion with a planned aggregate yield exceeding 150 kilotons, at any time beginning 20 days before the beginning of emplacement of the explosives and continuing after the explosion and after safe access to evacuated areas has been established according to standards determined by the Party carrying out the explosion for a period of:

(1) five days in the case of an explosion with a planned aggregate yield exceeding 150 kilotons but not exceeding 500 kilotons; or

(2) eight days in the case of an explosion with a planned aggregate yield exceeding 500 kilotons.

4. Designated personnel shall not have the right to be present in those areas from which all personnel have been evacuated in connection with carrying out an explosion, but shall have the right to re-enter those areas at the same time as personnel of the Party carrying out the explosion.

5. Designated personnel shall not have or seek access by physical, visual or technical means to the interior of the canister containing an explosive, to documentary or other information descriptive of the design of an explosive nor to

equipment for control and firing of explosives. The Party carrying out the explosion shall not locate documentary or other information descriptive of the design of an explosive in such ways as to impede the designated personnel in the exercise of their rights and functions.

6. The number of designated personnel present at the site of an explosion shall not exceed:

(a) for the exercise of their rights and functions in connection with the confirmation of the geological and geophysical information in accordance with the provisions of subparagraph 2(b) and applicable provisions of paragraph 5 of Article III -- the number of emplacement holes plus three;

(b) for the exercise of their rights and functions in connection with confirming that the local circumstances are consistent with the information provided and with the stated peaceful purposes in accordance with the provisions in subparagraphs 2(a), 2(c), 2(d) and 2(e) and applicable provisions of paragraph 5 of Article III -- the number of explosives plus two;

(c) for the exercise of their rights and functions in connection with confirming that the local circumstances are consistent with the information provided and with the stated peaceful purposes in accordance with the provisions in subparagraphs 2(a), 2(c), 2(d) and 2(e) and applicable provisions of paragraph 5 of Article III and in connection with the use of electrical equipment for determination of the yield in accordance with paragraph 3 of Article III -- the number of explosives plus seven; and

(d) for the exercise of their rights and functions in connection with confirming that the local circumstances are consistent with the information provided and with the stated peaceful purposes in accordance with the provisions in subparagraphs 2(a), 2(c), 2(d) and 2(e) and applicable provisions of paragraph 5 of Article III and in connection with the use of electrical equipment for determination of the yield in accordance with paragraph 3 of Article III and with the use of the local seismic network in accordance with paragraph 4 of Article III -- the number of explosives plus 10.

7. The Party carrying out the explosion shall have the right to assign its personnel to accompany designated personnel while the latter exercise their rights and functions.

8. The Party carrying out an explosion shall assure for designated personnel telecommunications with their authorities, transportation and other services appropriate to their presence and to the exercise of their rights and functions at the site of the explosion.

9. The expenses incurred for the transportation of designated personnel and their equipment to and from the site of the explosion, telecommunications provided for in paragraph 8 of this article, their living and working quarters, subsistence and all other personal expenses shall be the responsibility of the Party other than the Party carrying out the explosion.

10. Designated personnel shall consult with the Party carrying out the explosion in order to coordinate the planned program and schedule of activities of designated personnel with the program of the Party carrying out the explosion for the conduct of the project so as to ensure that designated personnel are able to conduct their activities in an orderly and timely way that is compatible with the implementation of the project. Procedures for such consultations shall be established in accordance with Article X.

Article VI

For any explosion with a planned aggregate yield exceeding 150 kilotons, determination of the yield of each explosive used shall be carried out in accordance with the following provisions:

1. Determination of the yield of each individual explosion in the group shall be based on measurements of the velocity of propagation, as a function of time, of the hydrodynamic shock wave generated by the explosion, taken by means of electrical equipment described in paragraph 3 of Article IV.

2. The Party carrying out the explosion shall provide the other Party with the following information:

(a) not later than 60 days before the beginning of emplacement of the explosives, the length of each canister in which the explosive will be contained in the corresponding emplacement hole, the dimensions of the tube or other device used to emplace the canister and the cross-sectional dimensions of the emplacement hole to a distance, in meters, from the emplacement point 10 times the cube root of its yield in kilotons;

(b) not later than 60 days before the beginning of emplacement of the explosives, a description of materials, including their densities, to be used to stem each emplacement hole; and

(c) not later than 30 days before the beginning of emplacement of the explosives, for each emplacement hole of a group explosion, the local coordinates of the point of emplacement of the explosive, the entrance of the emplacement hole, the point of the emplacement hole most distant from the entrance, the location of the emplacement hole at each 200 meters distance from the entrance and the configuration of any known voids larger than one cubic meter located within the distance, in meters, of 10 times the cube root of the planned yield in kilotons measured from the bottom of the canister containing the explosive. The error in these coordinates shall not exceed one percent of the distance between the emplacement hole and the nearest other emplacement hole or one percent of the distance between the point of measurement and the entrance of the emplacement hole, whichever is smaller, but in no case shall the error be required to be less than one meter.

3. The Party carrying out the explosion shall emplace for each explosive that portion of the electrical equipment for yield determination described in subparagraph 3(a) of Article IV, supplied in accordance with paragraph 1 of Article IV, in the same emplacement hole as the explosive in accordance with the installation instructions supplied under the provisions of paragraph 5 or 6 of Article IV. Such emplacement shall be carried out under the observation of designated personnel. Other equipment specified in subparagraph 3(b) of Article IV shall be emplaced and installed:

(a) by designated personnel under the observation and with the assistance of personnel of the Party carrying out the explosion, if such assistance is requested by designated personnel; or

(b) in accordance with paragraph 5 of Article IV.

4. That portion of the electrical equipment for yield determination described in subparagraph 3(a) of Article IV that is to be emplaced in each emplacement hole shall be located so that the end of the electrical equipment which is farthest from the entrance to the emplacement hole is at a distance, in meters, from the bottom of the canister containing the explosive equal to 3.5 times the cube root of the planned yield in kilotons of the explosive when the planned yield is less than 20 kilotons and three times the cube root of the planned yield in kilotons of the explosive when the planned yield is 20 kilotons or more. Canisters longer than 10 meters containing the explosive shall only be utilized if there is prior agreement between the Parties establishing provisions for their use. The Party carrying out the explosion shall provide the other Party with data on the distribution of density inside any other canister in the emplacement hole with a transverse cross-sectional area exceeding 10 square centimeters located within a distance, in meters, of 10 times the cube root of the planned yield in kilotons of the explosion from the bottom of the canister containing the explosive. The Party carrying out the explosion shall provide the other Party with access to confirm such data on density distribution within any such canister.

5. The Party carrying out an explosion shall fill each emplacement hole, including all pipes and tubes contained therein which have at any transverse section an aggregate cross-sectional area exceeding 10 square centimeters in the region containing the electrical equipment for yield determination and to a distance, in meters, of six times the cube root of the planned yield in kilotons of the explosive from the explosive emplacement point, with material having a density not less than seven-tenths of the average density of the surrounding rock, and from that point to a distance of not less than 60 meters from the explosive emplacement point with material having a density greater than one gram per cubic centimeter.

6. Designated personnel shall have the right to:

(a) confirm information provided in accordance with subparagraph 2(a) of this article;

(b) confirm information provided in accordance with subparagraph 2(b) of this article and be provided, upon request, with a sample of each batch of stemming material as that material is put into the emplacement hole; and

(c) confirm the information provided in accordance with subparagraph 2(c) of this article by having access to the data acquired and by observing, upon their request, the making of measurements.

7. For those explosives which are emplaced in separate holes, the emplacement shall be such that the distance D, in meters, between any explosive and any portion of the electrical equipment for determination of the yield of any other explosive in the group shall be not less than 10 times the cube root of the planned yield in kilotons of the larger explosive of such a pair of explosives. Individual explosions shall be separated by time intervals, in milliseconds, not greater than one-sixth the amount by which the distance D, in meters, exceeds 10 times the cube root of the planned yield in kilotons of the larger explosive of such a pair of explosives.

8. For those explosives in a group which are emplaced in a common emplacement hole, the distance, in meters, between each explosive and any other explosive in that emplacement hole shall be not less than 10 times the cube root of the planned yield in kilotons of the larger explosive of such a pair of explosives, and the explosives shall be detonated in sequential order, beginning with the explosive farthest from the entrance to the emplacement hole, with the individual detonations separated by time intervals, in milliseconds, of not less than one times the cube root of the planned yield in kilotons of the largest explosive in this emplacement hole.

Article VII

1. Designated personnel with their personal baggage and their equipment as provided in Article IV shall be permitted to enter the territory of the Party carrying out the explosion at an entry port to be agreed upon by the Parties, to remain in the territory of the Party carrying out the explosion for the purpose of fulfilling their rights and functions provided for in the Treaty and this Protocol, and to depart from an exit port to be agreed upon by the Parties.

2. At all times while designated personnel are in the territory of the Party carrying out the explosion, their persons, property, personal baggage, archives and documents as well as their temporary official and living quarters shall be accorded the same privileges and immunities as provided in Articles 22, 23, 24, 29, 30, 31, 34 and 36 of the Vienna Convention on Diplomatic Relations of 1961 to the persons, property, personal baggage, archives and documents of diplomatic agents as well as to the premises of diplomatic missions and private residences of diplomatic agents.

3. Without prejudice to their privileges and immunities it shall be the duty of designated personnel to respect the laws and regulations of the State in whose territory the explosion is to be carried out insofar as they do not impede in any way whatsoever the proper exercising of their rights and functions provided for by the Treaty and this Protocol.

Article VIII

The Party carrying out an explosion shall have sole and exclusive control over and full responsibility for the conduct of the explosion.

Article IX

1. Nothing in the Treaty and this Protocol shall affect proprietary rights in information made available under the Treaty and this Protocol and in information which may be disclosed in preparation for and carrying out of explosions; however, claims to such proprietary rights shall not impede implementation of the provisions of the Treaty and this Protocol.

2. Public release of the information provided in accordance with Article II or publication of material using such information, as well as public release of the results of observation and measurements obtained by designated personnel, may take place only by agreement with the Party carrying out an explosion; however, the other Party shall have the right to issue statements after the explosion that do not divulge information in which the Party carrying out the explosion has rights which are referred to in paragraph 1 of this article.

Article X

The Joint Consultative Commission shall establish procedures through which the Parties will, as appropriate, consult with each other for the purpose of ensuring efficient implementation of this Protocol.

DONE at Washington and Moscow, on May 28, 1976.

FOR THE UNITED STATES OF AMERICA:
GERALD R. FORD
The President of the United States of America.

FOR THE UNION OF SOVIET SOCIALIST REPUBLICS:
L. BREZHNEV
General Secretary of the Central Committee of the CPSU.

AGREED STATEMENT

May 13, 1976

The Parties to the Treaty Between the United States of America and the Union of Soviet Socialist Republics on Underground Nuclear Explosions for Peaceful Purposes, hereinafter referred to as the Treaty, agree that under subparagraph 2(c) of Article III of the Treaty:

(a) Development testing of nuclear explosives does not constitute a "peaceful application" and any such development tests shall be carried out only within the boundaries of nuclear weapon test sites specified in accordance with the Treaty Between the United States of America and the Union of Soviet Socialist Republics on the Limitation of Underground Nuclear Weapon Tests;

(b) Associating test facilities, instrumentation or procedures related only to testing of nuclear weapons or their effects with any explosion carried out in accordance with the Treaty does not constitute a "peaceful application."

CONVENTION ON THE PROHIBITION OF MILITARY OR ANY OTHER HOSTILE USE OF ENVIRONMENTAL MODIFICATION TECHNIQUES

Use of environmental modification techniques for hostile purposes does not play a major role in military planning at the present time. Such techniques might be developed in the future, however, and would pose a threat of serious damage unless action was taken to prohibit their use. In July 1972 the U.S. Government renounced the use of climate modification techniques for hostile purposes, even if their development were proved to be feasible in the future.

Both the U.S. Senate and the House of Representatives held hearings, beginning in 1972, and the Senate adopted a resolution in 1973 calling for an international agreement "prohibiting the use of any environmental or geophysical modification activity as a weapon of war...." In response to this resolution, the President ordered the Department of Defense to undertake an in-depth review of the military aspects of weather and other environmental modification techniques. The results of this study and a subsequent interagency study led to the U.S. Government's decision to seek agreement with the Soviet Union to explore the possibilities of an international agreement.

During the summit meeting in Moscow in July 1974, President Nixon and General Secretary Brezhnev formally agreed to hold bilateral discussions on how to bring about "the most effective measures possible to overcome the dangers of the use of environmental modification techniques for military purposes." Three sets of discussions were held in 1974 and 1975, resulting in agreement on a common approach and common language.

In August 1975, the chief representatives of the U.S. and the Soviet delegations to the Conference of the Committee on Disarmament (CCD) tabled, in parallel, identical draft texts of a "Convention on the Prohibition of Military or any Other Hostile Use of Environmental Modification Techniques."

The Convention defines environmental modification techniques as changing -- through the deliberate manipulation of natural processes

-- the dynamics, composition or structure of the earth, including its biota, lithosphere, hydro-sphere, and atmosphere, or of outer space. Changes in weather or climate patterns, in ocean currents, or in the state of the ozone layer or ionosphere, or an upset in the ecological balance of a region are some of the effects which might result from the use of environmental modification techniques.

Intensive negotiations held in the CCD during the spring and summer of 1976 resulted in a modified text and, in addition, to understandings regarding four of the Treaty articles. These were transmitted to the U.N. General Assembly for consideration during the fall session.

Article I sets forth the basic commitment: "Each State Party to this Convention undertakes not to engage in military or any other hostile use of environmental modification techniques having widespread, long-lasting or severe effects as the means of destruction, damage or injury to any other State Party." An understanding defines the terms "widespread, long-lasting or severe." "Widespread" is defined as "encompassing an area on the scale of several hundred square kilometers"; "long-lasting" is defined as "lasting for a period of months, or approximately a season"; and "severe" is defined as "involving serious or significant disruption or harm to human life, natural and economic resources or other assets."

With regard to peaceful uses of environmental modification techniques, the convention provides that the parties shall have the right to participate in the fullest possible exchange of scientific and technological information.

In addition to the provision for mutual consultation regarding complaints and for resource to the Security Council, the revised draft establishes the framework for a Consultative Committee of Experts, which would meet on an *ad hoc* basis when so requested by a party, in order to clarify the nature of activities suspected to be in violation of the convention. Responding to the suggestion of many delegations, the revised text incorporates a provision for periodic conferences to review the Convention's operation.

During the 1976 fall session, the U.N. General Assembly held extensive debate on the draft

Convention, including several resolutions relating thereto. On December 10, the General Assembly adopted a resolution by a vote of 96 to 8, with 30 abstentions, which referred the Convention to all member nations for their consideration, signature, and ratification, and requested the U.N. Secretary-General to open the Convention for signature.

The U.N. Secretary-General officiated at the signing ceremony in Geneva on May 18. The United States joined 33 other nations in signing the Convention. The Convention entered into force on October 5, 1978, when the 20th state to sign the Convention deposited its instrument of ratification. President Carter transmitted the Convention to the Senate on September 22, 1978.

The Senate gave its advice and consent to ratification on November 28, 1979, by a vote of 98-0. The President ratified the Convention December 13, 1979. The Convention entered into force for the United States on January 17, 1980, when the U.S. instrument of ratification was deposited in New York.

CONVENTION ON THE PROHIBITION OF MILITARY OR ANY OTHER HOSTILE USE OF ENVIRONMENTAL MODIFICATION TECHNIQUES

Signed in Geneva May 18, 1977
Entered into force October 5, 1978
Ratification by U.S. President December 13, 1979
U.S. ratification deposited at New York January 17, 1980

The States Parties to this Convention,

Guided by the interest of consolidating peace, and wishing to contribute to the cause of halting the arms race, and of bringing about general and complete disarmament under strict and effective international control, and of saving mankind from the danger of using new means of warfare,

Determined to continue negotiations with a view to achieving effective progress towards further measures in the field of disarmament,

Recognizing that scientific and technical advances may open new possibilities with respect to modification of the environment,

Recalling the Declaration of the United Nations Conference on the Human Environment adopted at Stockholm on 16 June 1972,

Realizing that the use of environmental modification techniques for peaceful purposes could improve the interrelationship of man and nature and contribute to the preservation and improvement of the environment for the benefit of present and future generations,

Recognizing, however, that military or any other hostile use of such techniques could have effects extremely harmful to human welfare,

Desiring to prohibit effectively military or any other hostile use of environmental modification techniques in order to eliminate the dangers to mankind from such use, and affirming their willingness to work towards the achievement of this objective,

Desiring also to contribute to the strengthening of trust among nations and to the further improvement of the international situation in accordance with the purposes and principles of the Charter of the United Nations,

Have agreed as follows:

Article I

1. Each State Party to this Convention undertakes not to engage in military or any other hostile use of environmental modification techniques having widespread, long-lasting or severe effects as the means of destruction, damage or injury to any other State Party.

2. Each State Party to this Convention undertakes not to assist, encourage or induce any State, group of States or international organization to engage in activities contrary to the provisions of paragraph 1 of this article.

Article II

As used in Article I, the term "environmental modification techniques" refers to any technique for changing -- through the deliberate manipulation of natural processes -- the dynamics, composition or structure of the Earth, including its biota, lithosphere, hydrosphere and atmosphere, or of outer space.

Article III

1. The provisions of this Convention shall not hinder the use of environmental modification techniques for peaceful purposes and shall be without prejudice to the generally recognized principles and applicable rules of international law concerning such use.

2. The States Parties to this Convention undertake to facilitate, and have the right to participate in, the fullest possible exchange of scientific and technological information on the use of environmental modification techniques for peaceful purposes. States Parties in a position to do so shall contribute, alone or together with other States or international organizations, to international economic and scientific co-operation in the preservation, improvement, and peaceful utilization of the environment, with due consideration for the needs of the developing areas of the world.

Article IV

Each State Party to this Convention undertakes to take any measures it considers necessary in accordance with its constitutional processes to prohibit and prevent any activity in violation of the provisions of the Convention anywhere under its jurisdiction or control.

Article V

1. The States Parties to this Convention undertake to consult one another and to cooperate in solving any problems which may arise in relation to the objectives of, or in the application of the provisions of, the Convention. Consultation and cooperation pursuant to this article may also be undertaken through appropriate international procedures within the framework of the United Nations and in accordance with its Charter. These international procedures may include the services of appropriate international organizations, as well as of a Consultative Committee of Experts as provided for in paragraph 2 of this article.

2. For the purposes set forth in paragraph 1 of this article, the Depositary shall, within one month of the receipt of a request from any State Party to this Convention, convene a Consultative Committee of Experts. Any State Party may appoint an expert to the Committee whose functions and rules of procedure are set out in the annex, which constitutes an integral part of this Convention. The Committee shall transmit to the Depositary a summary of its findings of fact, incorporating all views and information presented to the Committee during its proceedings. The Depositary shall distribute the summary to all States Parties.

3. Any State Party to this Convention which has reason to believe that any other State Party is acting in breach of obligations deriving from the provisions of the Convention may lodge a complaint with the Security Council of the United Nations. Such a complaint should include all relevant information as well as all possible evidence supporting its validity.

4. Each State Party to this Convention undertakes to cooperate in carrying out any investigation which the Security Council may initiate, in accordance with the provisions of the Charter of the United Nations, on the basis of the complaint received by the Council. The Security Council shall inform the States Parties of the results of the investigation.

5. Each State Party to this Convention undertakes to provide or support assistance, in accordance with the provisions of the Charter of the United Nations, to any State Party which so requests, if the Security Council decides that such Party has been harmed or is likely to be harmed as a result of violation of the Convention.

Article VI

1. Any State Party to this Convention may propose amendments to the Convention. The text of any proposed amendment shall be submitted to the Depositary who shall promptly circulate it to all States Parties.

2. An amendment shall enter into force for all States Parties to this Convention which have accepted it, upon the deposit with the Depositary of instruments of acceptance by a majority of States Parties. Thereafter it shall enter into force for any remaining State Party on the date of deposit of its instrument of acceptance.

Article VII

This Convention shall be of unlimited duration.

Article VIII

1. Five years after the entry into force of this Convention, a conference of the States Parties to the Convention shall be convened by the Depositary at Geneva, Switzerland. The conference shall review the operation of the Convention with a view to ensuring that its purposes and provisions are being realized, and shall in particular examine the effectiveness of the provisions of paragraph 1 of Article I in eliminating the dangers of military or any other hostile use of environmental modification techniques.

2. At intervals of not less than five years thereafter, a majority of the States Parties to the Convention may obtain, by submitting a proposal to this effect to the Depositary, the convening of a conference with the same objectives.

3. If no conference has been convened pursuant to paragraph 2 of this article within ten years following the conclusion of a previous conference, the Depositary shall solicit the views

of all States Parties to the Convention, concerning the convening of such a conference. If one third or ten of the States Parties, whichever number is less, respond affirmatively, the Depositary shall take immediate steps to convene the conference.

Article IX

1. This Convention shall be open to all States for signature. Any State which does not sign the Convention before its entry into force in accordance with paragraph 3 of this article may accede to it at any time.

2. This Convention shall be subject to ratification by signatory States. Instruments of ratification or accession shall be deposited with the Secretary-General of the United Nations.

3. This Convention shall enter into force upon the deposit of instruments of ratification by twenty Governments in accordance with paragraph 2 of this article.

4. For those States whose instruments of ratification or accession are deposited after the entry into force of this Convention, it shall enter into force on the date of the deposit of their instruments of ratification or accession.

5. The Depositary shall promptly inform all signatory and acceding States of the date of each signature, the date of deposit of each instrument of ratification or accession and the date of the entry into force of this Convention and of any amendments thereto, as well as of the receipt of other notices.

6. This Convention shall be registered by the Depositary in accordance with Article 102 of the Charter of the United Nations.

Article X

This Convention, of which the English, Arabic, Chinese, French, Russian, and Spanish texts are equally authentic, shall be deposited with the Secretary-General of the United Nations, who shall send certified copies thereof to the Governments of the signatory and acceding States.

IN WITNESS WHEREOF, the undersigned, being duly authorized thereto by their respective governments, have signed this Convention, opened for signature at Geneva on the eighteenth day of May, one thousand nine hundred and seventy-seven.

DONE at Geneva on May 18, 1977.

ANNEX TO THE CONVENTION CONSULTATIVE COMMITTEE OF EXPERTS

1. The Consultative Committee of Experts shall undertake to make appropriate findings of fact and provide expert views relevant to any problem raised pursuant to paragraph 1 of Article V of this Convention by the State Party requesting the convening of the Committee.

2. The work of the Consultative Committee of Experts shall be organized in such a way as to permit it to perform the functions set forth in paragraph 1 of this annex. The Committee shall decide procedural questions relative to the organization of its work, where possible by consensus, but otherwise by a majority of those present and voting. There shall be no voting on matters of substance.

3. The Depositary or his representative shall serve as the Chairman of the Committee.

4. Each expert may be assisted at meetings by one or more advisers.

5. Each expert shall have the right, through the Chairman, to request from States, and from international organizations, such information and assistance as the expert considers desirable for the accomplishment of the Committee's work.

UNDERSTANDINGS REGARDING THE CONVENTION[1]

Understanding Relating to Article I

It is the understanding of the Committee that, for the purposes of this Convention, the terms, "widespread", "long-lasting" and "severe" shall be interpreted as follows:

(a) "widespread": encompassing an area on the scale of several hundred square kilometres;

(b) "long-lasting": lasting for a period of months, or approximately a season;

(c) "severe": involving serious or significant disruption or harm to human life, natural and economic resources or other assets.

It is further understood that the interpretation set forth above is intended exclusively for this Convention and is not intended to prejudice the interpretation of the same or similar terms if used in connexion with any other international agreement.

Understanding Relating to Article II

It is the understanding of the Committee that the following examples are illustrative of phenomena that could be caused by the use of environmental modification techniques as defined in Article II of the Convention: earthquakes, tsunamis; an upset in the ecological balance of a region; changes in weather patterns (clouds, precipitation, cyclones of various types and tornadic storms); changes in climate patterns; changes in ocean currents; changes in the state of the ozone layer; and changes in the state of the ionosphere.

It is further understood that all the phenomena listed above, when produced by military or any other hostile use of environmental modification techniques, would result, or could reasonably be expected to result, in widespread, long-lasting or severe destruction, damage or injury. Thus, military or any other hostile use of environmental modification techniques as defined in Article II, so as to cause those phenomena as a means of destruction, damage or injury to another State Party, would be prohibited.

It is recognized, moreover, that the list of examples set out above is not exhaustive. Other phenomena which could result from the use of environmental modification techniques as defined in Article II could also be appropriately included. The absence of such phenomena from the list does not in any way imply that the undertaking contained in Article I would not be applicable to those phenomena, provided the criteria set out in that article were met.

Understanding Relating to Article III

It is the understanding of the Committee that this Convention does not deal with the question whether or not a given use of environmental modification techniques for peaceful purposes is in accordance with generally recognized principles and applicable rules of international law.

Understanding Relating to Article VIII

It is the understanding of the Committee that a proposal to amend the Convention may also be considered at any conference of Parties held pursuant to Article VIII. It is further understood that any proposed amendment that is intended for such consideration should, if possible, be submitted to the Depositary no less than 90 days before the commencement of the conference.

---

[1] These are not incorporated into the Convention but are part of the negotiating record and were included in the report transmitted by the CCD to the U.N. General Assembly in September 1976.

Environmental Modification Convention

Country	Date[1] of Signature	Date of Deposit[1] of Ratification	Date of Deposit[1] of Accession
Afghanistan			10/22/85
Algeria			12/19/91
Antigua and Barbuda			10/25/88
Argentina			03/20/87
Australia	05/31/78	09/07/84	
Austria			01/17/90
Bangladesh			10/03/79
Belgium	05/18/77	07/12/82	
Benin	06/10/77	06/30/86	
Bolivia	05/18/77		
Brazil	11/09/77	10/12/84	
Brunei			01/01/84[1]
Bulgaria	05/18/77	05/31/78	
Byelorussian S.S.R.[2]	05/18/77	06/07/78	
Canada	05/18/77	06/11/81	
Cape Verde			10/03/79
Chile			04/26/94
Cuba	09/23/77	04/10/78	
Cyprus	10/07/77	04/12/78	
Czechoslovakia	05/18/77	05/12/78	
Czech Republic			02/22/93
Denmark	05/18/77	04/19/78	
Dominica		11/09/92	11/08/78[1]
Egypt			04/01/82
Ethiopia	05/18/77		
Finland	05/18/77	05/12/78	
German Democratic Republic	05/18/77	05/25/78	
Germany, Federal Republic of	05/18/77	05/24/83	
Ghana	03/21/78	06/22/78	
Greece			08/23/83
Guatemala			03/21/88
Holy See	05/27/77		
Hungary	05/18/77	04/19/78	
Iceland	05/18/77		
India	12/10/77	12/15/78	
Iran	05/18/77		
Iraq	08/15/77		
Ireland	05/18/77	12/16/82	
Italy	05/18/77	11/27/81	

Environmental Modification Convention -- Continued

Country	Date[1] of Signature	Date of Deposit[1] of Ratification	Date of Deposit[1] of Accession
Japan			06/09/82
Korea, Democratic People's Republic of			11/08/84
Korea, Republic of			12/02/86
Kuwait			01/02/80
Laos	04/13/78	10/05/78	
Lebanon	05/18/77		
Liberia	05/18/77		
Luxembourg	05/18/77		
Malawi			10/05/78
Mauritius			12/09/92
Mongolia	05/18/77	05/19/78	
Morocco	05/18/77		
Netherlands	05/18/77	04/15/83	
New Zealand			09/07/84
Nicaragua	08/11/77		
Niger			02/17/93
Norway	05/18/77	02/15/79	
Pakistan			02/27/86
Papua New Guinea			10/28/80
Poland	05/18/77	06/08/78	
Portugal	05/18/77		
Romania	05/18/77	05/06/83	
St. Christopher-Nevis			09/19/83[1]
St. Lucia		05/27/93	02/22/79[1]
St. Vincent and the Grenadines			10/27/79[1]
São Tomé and Principe			10/05/79
Sierra Leone	04/12/78		
Solomon Islands		06/18/81	06/18/81
Spain	05/18/77	07/19/78	
Sri Lanka	06/08/77	04/25/78	
Sweden			04/27/84
Switzerland			08/05/88
Syria	08/04/77		
Tunisia	05/11/78	05/11/78	
Turkey	05/18/77		

Environmental Modification Convention -- Continued

Country	Date[1] of Signature	Date of Deposit[1] of Ratification	Date of Deposit[1] of Accession
Uganda	05/18/77		
Ukrainian S.S.R.[2]	05/18/77	06/13/78	
Union of Soviet Socialist Republics	05/18/77	05/30/78	
United Kingdom	05/18/77	05/16/78	
United States	05/18/77	01/17/80	
Uruguay			09/16/93
Uzbekistan	05/26/93		
Vietnam			08/26/80
Yemen Arab Republic (Sanaa)	05/18/77	07/20/77	
Yemen, People's Democratic of (Aden)			06/12/79
Zaire	02/28/78		
Total[3]	51	36	34

See footnotes on page 350.

AGREEMENT BETWEEN THE UNITED STATES
OF AMERICA AND THE INTERNATIONAL
ATOMIC ENERGY AGENCY FOR THE
APPLICATION OF SAFEGUARDS IN THE
UNITED STATES (AND PROTOCOL THERETO)

The Agreement between the United States and
the International Atomic Energy Agency (IAEA)
for the Application of Safeguards in the United
States and its accompanying protocol stemmed
from the Eighteen-Nation Disarmament
Committee's (ENDC's) negotiation of the Treaty
on the Non-
Proliferation of Nuclear Weapons (NPT). In 1967,
during preliminary NPT negotiations, Japan and
the non-nuclear weapons states of the European
Community opposed the NPT provision that
requires only non-nuclear weapons states party to
the Treaty to accept IAEA safeguards in all of
their peaceful nuclear activities.

The widespread concern was that the absence
of any requirement for IAEA safeguards in
nuclear-weapons states would place the non-
nuclear weapons states at a commercial and
industrial disadvantage in developing nuclear
energy for peaceful uses, due to interference of
these safeguards with efficient operation of their
commercial activities and by compromise of their
industrial and trade secrets through IAEA
personnel's access to their facilities and records.
Efforts to devise acceptable Treaty provisions for
IAEA safeguards in nuclear-weapons states were
unsuccessful, and by late 1967, the safeguards
issue had become a serious obstacle to
acceptance of the NPT by major industrialized
non-nuclear weapon states.

In an effort to break that impasse and allay the
concerns embodied in the impasse, President
Johnson on December 2, 1967, stated that the
United States was not asking any country to
accept safeguards that the United States was
unwilling to accept and that . . ." when such
safeguards are applied under the Treaty, the
United States will permit the International Atomic
Energy Agency to apply its safeguards to all
nuclear activities in the United States -- excluding
only those with direct national security
significance." The United Kingdom announced a
similar offer on December 4, 1967. These two
offers were instrumental in gaining acceptance of
the NPT by key industrialized countries, and their
importance was emphasized in public statements
by the Federal Republic of Germany, Japan, and

others. The U.S. offer would be delineated in a
separate, formal agreement to be concluded with
the IAEA.

Soon after the NPT entered into force in March
1970, a Safeguards Committee established by the
IAEA Board of Governors undertook to advise the
Board concerning the form and content of the
safeguards agreements to be concluded with the
non-nuclear weapon states party to the NPT.
Nearly 50 governments participated in the
Committee's work, which continued until 1971.
One of the most difficult matters that the
Committee addressed was that of financing the
increase in the IAEA's safeguards activities
resulting from the entry into force of the NPT. It
was recognized that the number of facilities in the
United States and the United Kingdom that would
be eligible for IAEA safeguards within the terms
of these two countries' offers would equal the
total number of facilities in all non-nuclear
weapon states. Thus, if the IAEA were to apply
its safeguards in all of the facilities under the
offers, it would require a doubling of its budget for
its safeguards activities. Subsequently, a number
of non-nuclear weapon states, led by Australia,
proposed that the objective of the two offers could
be achieved at reasonable cost to the IAEA if the
IAEA carried out full inspections of only those
facilities in the United States and the United
Kingdom that were of advanced design or were
sensitive in terms of international competition.
Under the proposal endorsed by Italy, Japan, and
the Federal Republic of Germany, the IAEA could
apply something less than the full regime of
inspections to all other eligible facilities not of
advanced design or sensitive in terms of
international competition in the two offering
countries. Australia's proposal to the Committee
achieved a balance between the costs of
implementing the offers and attainment of the
offers' objectives.

By March 1971, the Safeguards Committee
completed its formulation of detailed provisions
for the individual safeguards agreements. The
Board approved the document, and shortly
thereafter Austria and Finland negotiated
safeguards agreements with the IAEA which
became the models for future such agreements.
They were also used in the development of the
voluntary offer agreements with the United States
and the United Kingdom.

In order for the U.S. offer to achieve its

purpose, it was essential that the IAEA, in applying its safeguards in a particular type of U.S. facility, use the same procedures it follows in similar facilities in non-nuclear weapon states. Many of the model provisions could therefore be incorporated into the U.S.-IAEA safeguards agreement without change.

However, other provisions required adaptation in light of fundamental differences between the terms of the U.S. offer and the obligations of non-nuclear weapon states party to the NPT. These differences reflect several facts: 1) The U.S. offer excludes activities of direct national security significance and does not contain any limitations on use of nuclear material by the United States. (Therefore, the agreement provides that at any time the United States can remove a facility from the list of those eligible for safeguards should the facility become associated with activities of direct national security significance, and the United States can transfer nuclear material from eligible facilities to any location including non-eligible facilities.) 2) The United States has sole authority to decide which U.S. facilities are eligible for safeguards, and the IAEA has sole authority to decide which eligible facilities will be selected for safeguards (although the IAEA is obliged to take into account the requirement that the U.S. Government avoid discriminatory treatment between U.S. commercial firms similarly situated). 3) The United States had made separate commitments to provide to the IAEA, for safeguards purposes, information on imports and exports of nuclear material.

The U.S.-IAEA agreement itself addresses only the selection of facilities for the application of the full regime of safeguards procedures, including routine inspections. Australia and several other key non-nuclear weapon states had also proposed in the Safeguards Committee that all of the eligible facilities should bear some burden of safeguards. In further consultations it appeared that a satisfactory arrangement would be for the facilities not selected for the application of safeguards to submit design information, permit IAEA inspectors to verify such information in the facility, maintain accounting records, and provide accounting reports to the IAEA. The IAEA, however, was concerned that this would overwhelm its staff. Consequently, the concept of a secondary selection was introduced, whereby complete flexibility was provided to the IAEA, so that any or all of the eligible facilities could be

required to submit the specified information, maintain records, etc. For ease of drafting, and to maintain the distinction between "safeguards," which includes routine inspections by the IAEA, and only the submission of information and maintenance of records, the provision dealing with the secondary category of selected facilities are grouped into a protocol to the agreement. The technical provisions in the protocol follow closely the comparable provisions in the agreement itself.

In September 1976, the U.S.-IAEA agreement was submitted to the IAEA Board of Governors for the Board's approval. The Director General informed the Board that in selecting facilities in which the IAEA would apply the full regime of safeguards (including inspections) the IAEA would take into account the need to avoid discrimination among commercial firms in the United States. The IAEA, he stated, would also observe the criteria for selection that had been proposed by Australia and others -- facilities of advanced design and those sensitive in terms of international competition. The Board, acting by consensus, authorized the Director General to conclude the agreement with the United States.

The agreement was submitted to the U.S. Senate on February 9, 1978. Its advice and consent to ratification was given unanimously, with understandings, on July 2, 1980. One of the understandings was that the President establish an appropriate interagency mechanism for dealing with the implementation of the agreement in the United States. The result was the creation of the "Interagency Steering Group for International Safeguards" to deal with policy matters and two subgroups. The first, the "Safeguards Agreement Working Group" was to monitor implementation and take necessary actions relating to implementation, the second, a "Negotiating Team" to negotiate the necessary subsidiary arrangements for implementing the agreement. Each of these three groups was chaired by the Department of State. In 1994 these groups were reformulated as a structure of interagency subcommittees and subgroups organized under the "International Atomic Energy Agency Steering Committee," chaired by the U.S. Ambassador to the IAEA.

The safeguards agreement entered into force on December 9, 1980. At that time the United States submitted to the IAEA a list of the more than 200 eligible facilities, including facilities licensed by the Nuclear Regulatory Commission and eligible license-exempt facilities of the Department of Energy. The IAEA is notified whenever an addition or removal is made to the list.

In early 1981, the IAEA made its initial selection of facilities in which the full regime of safeguards, including inspections, was applied, pursuant to the agreement proper. Two operating commercial reactors and one commercial fuel fabrication facility were selected. The facilities submitted design information, and negotiations were begun regarding each of the detailed "facility attachments," the detailed description of safeguards implementation at that particular facility. While those negotiations proceeded, the IAEA carried out ad hoc inspections in the facilities as permitted by the agreement. These first facility attachments entered into force in early 1982. Also at that time, the IAEA made its first selections under the protocol of two commercial fuel fabrication plants.

From then until 1988 the IAEA followed a practice of selecting for safeguards at approximately two-year intervals a different commercial fuel fabrication plant and two power reactors. Each time new facilities were selected, the current one was removed from selection under the agreement, and the fabrication was removed from selection under the protocol. In August 1981, the IAEA also selected for safeguards a decommissioned government-owned research reactor in which a quantity of plutonium was stored, satisfying an existing obligation of the United States and the IAEA for safeguards on two kilograms of plutonium.

In July 1983, the United States added the Portsmouth Gas Centrifuge Enrichment Plant (GCEP) to the eligible list, and the following August it was selected by the IAEA for safeguards. IAEA safeguards activities were performed at GCEP between August 1983 and July 1985. These activities included limited frequency, unannounced access by IAEA inspectors to the cascade halls. The Department of Energy terminated the gas centrifuge project in June 1985 and following the removal of nuclear material from the facility in July 1985, the facility was removed from the eligible list.

By the end of 1984 all commercial plants fabricating fuel for power reactors had been selected under either the agreement or the protocol.

In September 1993, President Clinton announced that the United States would place material deemed excess to its defense needs under IAEA safeguards. This historic initiative was designed to demonstrate the transparency and irreversibility of the dismantlement process and underscore the U.S. commitment to fulfill its obligations under the Non-Proliferation Treaty. Since that announcement, high-enriched uranium at the Y-12 Plant in Oak Ridge, Tennessee and plutonium at Hanford Site, Washington have been placed under IAEA safeguards. Additional plutonium at Rocky Flats, Colorado will also be placed under IAEA safeguards. The IAEA is also scheduled to conduct verification activities on high-enriched uranium transferred from Kazakstan to the United States in 1994 under "Project Sapphire." Finally, the United States is working to place its gaseous diffusion plants under IAEA safeguards as well. Each of these activities is, in whole or in part, conducted under the authority of the U.S.-IAEA Safeguards Agreement. This agreement, in its flexibility, will continue to be a crucial agreement for shaping U.S. nonproliferation and arms control policy throughout the next century.

AGREEMENT BETWEEN THE UNITED STATES OF AMERICA AND THE INTERNATIONAL ATOMIC ENERGY AGENCY FOR THE APPLICATION OF SAFEGUARDS IN THE UNITED STATES

Signed at Vienna November 18, 1977
Ratification advised by U.S. Senate July 2, 1980
Ratified by U.S. President July 31, 1980
Entered into force December 9, 1980
Proclaimed by U.S. President December 31, 1980

Whereas the United States of America (hereinafter referred to as the "United States") is a Party to the Treaty on the Non-Proliferation of Nuclear Weapons (hereinafter referred to as the "Treaty") which was opened for signature at London, Moscow and Washington on 1 July 1968 and which entered into force on 5 March 1970[1];

Whereas States Parties to the Treaty undertake to co-operate in facilitating the application of International Atomic Energy Agency (hereinafter referred to as the "Agency") safeguards on peaceful nuclear activities;

Whereas non-nuclear-weapon States Parties to the Treaty undertake to accept safeguards, as set forth in an agreement to be negotiated and concluded with the Agency, on all source or special fissionable material in all their peaceful nuclear activities for the exclusive purpose of verification of the fulfillment of their obligations under the Treaty with a view to preventing diversion of nuclear energy from peaceful uses to nuclear weapons or other nuclear explosive devices;

Whereas the United States, a nuclear-weapon State as defined by the Treaty, has indicated that at such time as safeguards are being generally applied in accordance with paragraph 1 of Article III of the Treaty, the United States will permit the Agency to apply its safeguards to all nuclear activities in the United States -- excluding only those with direct national security significance -- by concluding a safeguards agreement with the Agency for that purpose;

Whereas the United States has made this offer and has entered into this agreement for the purpose of encouraging widespread adherence to the Treaty by demonstrating to non-nuclear-weapon States that they would not be placed at a commercial disadvantage by reason of the application of safeguards pursuant to the Treaty;

Whereas the purpose of a safeguards agreement giving effect to this offer by the United States would thus differ necessarily from the purposes of safeguards agreements concluded between the Agency and non-nuclear-weapon States Party to the Treaty;

Whereas it is in the interest of Members of the Agency, that, without prejudice to the principles and integrity of the Agency's safeguards system, the expenditure of the Agency's financial and other resources for implementation of such an agreement not exceed that necessary to accomplish the purpose of the Agreement;

Whereas the Agency is authorized, pursuant to Article III of the Statute of the International Atomic Energy Agency[2] (hereinafter referred to as the "Statute"), to conclude such a safeguards agreement;

Now, therefore, the United States and the Agency have agreed as follows:

PART I

Article 1

(a) The United States undertakes to permit the Agency to apply safeguards, in accordance with the terms of this Agreement, on all source or special fissionable material in all facilities within the United States, excluding only those facilities associated with activities with direct national security significance to the United States, with a view to enabling the Agency to verify that such material is not withdrawn, except as provided for in this Agreement, from activities in facilities while such material is being safeguarded under this Agreement.

(b) The United States shall, upon entry in force of this Agreement, provide the Agency with a list of facilities within the United States not associated with activities with direct national security significance to the United States and may, in accordance with the procedures set forth in Part II of this Agreement, add facilities to or remove facilities from that list as it deems appropriate.

---

[1] TIAS 6839; 21 UST 483.

[2] Done October 26, 1956. TIAS 3873, 5284, 7668; 8 UST 1095; 14 UST 135; 24 UST 1637

(c) The United States may, in accordance with the procedures set forth in this Agreement, withdraw nuclear material from activities in facilities included in the list referred to in Article 1(b).

Article 2

(a) The Agency shall have the right to apply safeguards, in accordance with the terms of this Agreement, on all source or special fissionable material in all facilities within the United States, excluding only those facilities associated with activities with direct national security significance to the United States, with a view to enabling the Agency to verify that such material is not withdrawn, except as provided for in this Agreement, from activities in facilities while such material is being safeguarded under this Agreement.

(b) The Agency shall, from time to time, identify to the United States those facilities, selected from the then current list provided by the United States in accordance with Article 1(b), in which the Agency wishes to apply safeguards, in accordance with the terms of this Agreement.

(c) In identifying facilities and in applying safeguards thereafter on source or special fissionable material in such facilities, the Agency shall proceed in a manner which the Agency and the United States mutually agree takes into account the requirement on the United States to avoid discriminatory treatment as between United States commercial firms similarly situated.

Article 3

(a) The United States and the Agency shall co-operate to facilitate the implementation of the safeguards provided for in this Agreement.

(b) The source or special fissionable material subject to safeguards under this Agreement shall be that material in those facilities which shall have been identified by the Agency at any given time pursuant to Article 2(b).

(c) The safeguards to be applied by the Agency under this Agreement on source or special fissionable material in facilities in the United States shall be implemented by the same procedures followed by the Agency in applying its safeguards on similar material in similar facilities

in non-nuclear-weapon States under agreements pursuant to paragraph 1 of Article III of the Treaty.

Article 4

The safeguards provided for in this Agreement shall be implemented in a manner designed:

(a) To avoid hampering the economic and technological development of the United States or international co-operation in the field of peaceful nuclear activities, including international exchange of nuclear material;

(b) To avoid undue interference in peaceful nuclear activities of the United States and in particular in the operation of facilities; and

(c) To be consistent with prudent management practices required for the economic and safe conduct of nuclear activities.

Article 5

(a) The agency shall take every precaution to protect commercial and industrial secrets and other confidential information coming to its knowledge in the implementation of this Agreement.

(b) (i) The Agency shall not publish or communicate to any State, organization or person any information obtained by it in connection with the implementation of this Agreement, except that specific information relating to the implementation thereof may be given to the Board of Governors of the Agency (hereinafter referred to as "the Board") and to such Agency staff members as require such knowledge by reason of their official duties in connection with safeguards, but only to the extent necessary for the Agency to fulfill its responsibilities in implementing this Agreement.

(ii) Summarized information on nuclear material subject to safeguards under this Agreement may be published upon the decision of the Board if the United States agrees thereto.

Article 6

(a) The Agency shall, in implementing safeguards pursuant to this Agreement, take full account of technological developments in the field of safeguards, and shall make every effort to ensure optimum cost-effectiveness and the application of the principle of safeguarding effectively the flow of nuclear material subject to safeguards under this Agreement by use of instruments and other techniques at certain strategic points to the extent that present or future technology permits.

(b) In order to ensure optimum cost-effectiveness, use shall be made, for example, of such means as:

(i) Containment as a means of defining material balance areas for accounting purposes;

(ii) Statistical techniques and random sampling in evaluating the flow of nuclear material; and

(iii) Concentration of verification procedures on those stages in the nuclear fuel cycle involving the production, processing, use or storage of nuclear material from which nuclear weapons or other nuclear explosive devices could readily be made, and minimization of verification procedures in respect of other nuclear material, on condition that this does not hamper the Agency in applying safeguards under this Agreement.

Article 7

(a) The United States shall establish and maintain a system of accounting for and control of all nuclear material subject to safeguards under this Agreement.

(b) The Agency shall apply safeguards in accordance with Article 3(c) in such a manner as to enable the Agency to verify, in ascertaining that there has been no withdrawal of nuclear material, except as provided for in this Agreement, from activities in facilities while such material is being safeguarded under this Agreement, findings of the accounting and control system of the United States. The Agency's verification shall include, inter alia, independent measurements and observations conducted by the Agency in accordance with the procedures specified in Part II. The Agency, in its verification, shall take due account of the technical effectiveness of the system of the United States.

Article 8

(a) In order to ensure the effective

implementation of safeguards under this Agreement, the United States shall, in accordance with the provisions set out in Part II, provide the Agency with information concerning nuclear material subject to safeguards under this Agreement and the features of facilities relevant to safeguarding such material.

(b) (i) The Agency shall require only the minimum amount of information and data consistent with carrying out its responsibilities under this Agreement.

(ii) Information pertaining to facilities shall be the minimum necessary for safeguarding nuclear material subject to safeguards under this Agreement.

(c) If the United States so requests, the Agency shall be prepared to examine on premises of the United States design information which the United States regards as being of particular sensitivity. Such information need not be physically transmitted to the Agency provided that it remains readily available for further examination by the Agency on premises of the United States.

Article 9

(a) (i) The Agency shall secure the consent of the United States to the designation of Agency inspectors to the United States.

(ii) If the United States, either upon proposal of a designation or at any other time after designation has been made, objects to the designation, the Agency shall propose to the United States an alternative designation or designations.

(iii) If, as a result of the repeated refusal of the United States to accept the designation of Agency inspectors, inspections to be conducted under this Agreement would be impeded, such refusal shall be considered by the Board, upon referral by the Director General of the Agency (hereinafter referred to as "the Director General") with a view to its taking appropriate action.

(b) The United States shall take the necessary steps to ensure that Agency inspectors can effectively discharge their functions under this Agreement.

(c) The visits and activities of Agency inspectors shall be so arranged as:

(i) To reduce to a minimum the possible inconvenience and disturbance to the United States and to the peaceful nuclear activities inspected; and

(ii) To ensure protection of industrial secrets or any other confidential information coming to the inspectors' knowledge.

Article 10

The provisions of the International Organizations Immunities Act of the United States of America[3] shall apply to Agency inspectors performing functions in the United States under this Agreement and to any property of the Agency used by them.

Article 11

Safeguards shall terminate on nuclear material upon determination by the Agency that the material has been consumed, or has been diluted in such a way that it is no longer usable for any nuclear activity relevant from the point of view of safeguards, or has become practically irrecoverable.

Article 12

(a) If the United States intends to exercise its right to withdraw nuclear material from activities in facilities identified by the Agency pursuant to Articles 2(b) and 39(b) other than those facilities removed, pursuant to Article 34(b)(i) from the list provided for by Article 1(b) and to transfer such material to a destination in the United States other than to a facility included in the list established and maintained pursuant to Articles 1(b) and 34, the United States shall notify the Agency in advance of such withdrawal. Nuclear material in respect of which such notification has been given shall cease to be subject to safeguards under this Agreement as from the time of its withdrawal.

(b) Nothing in this Agreement shall affect the right of the United States to transfer material subject to safeguards under this Agreement to destinations not within or under the jurisdiction of the United States. The United States shall provide the Agency with information with respect to such transfers in accordance with Article 89. The Agency shall keep records of each such transfer and, where applicable, of the reapplication of safeguards to the transferred nuclear material.

Article 13

Where nuclear material subject to safeguards under this Agreement is to be used in non-nuclear activities, such as the production of alloys or ceramics, the United States shall agree with the Agency, before the material is so used, on the circumstances under which the safeguards on such material may be terminated.

Article 14

The United States and the Agency will bear the expenses incurred by them in implementing their respective responsibilities under this Agreement. However, if the United States or persons under its jurisdiction incur extraordinary expenses as a result of a specific request by the Agency, the Agency shall reimburse such expenses provided that it has agreed in advance to do so. In any case the Agency shall bear the cost of any additional measuring or sampling which inspectors may request.

Article 15

In carrying out its functions under this Agreement within the United States, the Agency and its personnel shall be covered to the same extent as nationals of the United States by any protection against third-party liability provided under the Price-Anderson Act,[4] including insurance or other indemnity coverage that may be required by the Price-Anderson Act with respect to nuclear incidents.

Article 16

Any claim by the United States against the Agency or by the Agency against the United States in respect to any damage resulting from the implementation of safeguards under this Agreement, other than damage arising out of a nuclear incident, shall be settled in accordance with international law.

---

[3] 59 Stat. 669; U.S.C. § 288 note.
[4] 71 Stat. 576; 42 U.S.C. 2210.

Article 17

If the Board, upon report of the Director General, decides that an action by the United States is essential and urgent in order to ensure compliance with this Agreement, the Board may call upon the United States to take the required action without delay, irrespective of whether procedures have been invoked pursuant to Article 21 for the settlement of a dispute.

Article 18

If the Board, upon examination of relevant information reported to it by the Director General, determines there has been any non-compliance with this Agreement, the Board may call upon the United States to remedy forthwith such non-compliance. In the event there is a failure to take fully corrective action within a reasonable time, the Board may make the reports provided for in paragraph C of Article XII of the Statute and may also take, where applicable, the other measures provided for in that paragraph. In taking such action the Board shall take account of the degree of assurance provided by the safeguards measures that have been applied and shall afford the United States every reasonable opportunity to furnish the Board with any necessary reassurance.

Article 19

The United States and the Agency shall, at the request of either, consult about any question arising out of the interpretation or application of this Agreement.

Article 20

The United States shall have the right to request that any question arising out of the interpretation or application of this Agreement be considered by the Board. The Board shall invite the United States to participate in the discussion of any such question by the Board.

Article 21

Any dispute arising out of the interpretation or application of this Agreement, except a dispute with regard to a determination by the Board under Article 18 or an action taken by the Board pursuant to such a determination which is not settled by negotiation or another procedure agreed to by the United States and the Agency shall, at the request of either, be submitted to an arbitral tribunal composed as follows: The United States and the Agency shall each designate one arbitrator, and the two arbitrators so designated shall elect a third, who shall be the Chairman. If, within thirty days of the request for arbitration, either the United States or the Agency has not designated an arbitrator, either the United States or the Agency may request the President of the International Court of Justice to appoint an arbitrator. The same procedure shall apply if, within thirty days of the designation or appointment of the second arbitrator, the third arbitrator has not been elected. A majority of the members of the arbitral tribunal shall constitute a quorum, and all decisions shall require the concurrence of two arbitrators. The arbitral procedure shall be fixed by the tribunal. The decisions of the tribunal shall be binding on the United States and the Agency.

Article 22

The Parties shall institute steps to suspend the application of Agency safeguards in the United States under other safeguards agreements with the Agency while this Agreement is in force. However, the United States and the Agency shall ensure that nuclear material being safeguarded under this Agreement shall be at all times at least equivalent in amount and composition to that which would be subject to safeguards in the United States under the agreements in question. The detailed arrangements for the implementation of this provision shall be specified in the subsidiary arrangements provided for in Article 39, and shall reflect the nature of any undertaking given under such other safeguards agreements.

Article 23

(a) The United States and the Agency shall, at the request of either, consult each other on amendments to this Agreement.

(b) All Amendments shall require the agreement of the United States and the Agency.

Article 24

This Agreement or any amendments thereto shall enter into force on the date on which the Agency receives from the United States written notification that statutory and constitutional requirements of the United States for entry into force have been met.[5]

Article 25

The Director General shall promptly inform all Member States of the Agency of the entry into force of this Agreement, or of any amendments thereto.

Article 26

The Agreement shall remain in force as long as the United States is a party to the Treaty except that the Parties to this Agreement shall, upon the request of either of them, consult and, to the extent mutually agreed, modify this Agreement in order to ensure that it continues to serve the purpose for which it was originally intended. If the Parties are unable after such consultation to agree upon necessary modifications, either Party may, upon six months' notice, terminate this Agreement.

PART II

Article 27

The purpose of this part of the Agreement is to specify the procedures to be applied in the implementation of the safeguards provisions of Part I.

Article 28

The objective of the safeguards procedures set forth in this part of the Agreement is the timely detection of withdrawal, other than in accordance with the terms of this Agreement, of significant quantities of nuclear material from activities in facilities while such material is being safeguarded under this Agreement.

Article 29

For the purpose of achieving the objective set forth in Article 28, material accountancy shall be used as a safeguards measure of fundamental importance, with containment and surveillance as important complementary measures.

Article 30

The technical conclusion of the Agency's

verification activities shall be a statement, in respect of each material balance area, of the amount of material unaccounted for over a specific period, and giving the limits of accuracy of the amounts stated.

Article 31

Pursuant to Article 7, the Agency, in carrying out its verification activities, shall make full use of the United States' system of accounting for and control of all nuclear material subject to safeguards under this Agreement and shall avoid unnecessary duplication of the United States' accounting and control activities.

Article 32

The United States' system of accounting for and control of all nuclear material subject to safeguards under this Agreement shall be based on a structure of material balance areas, and shall make provision, as appropriate and specified in the Subsidiary Arrangements, for the establishment of such measures as:

(a) A measurement system for the determination of the quantities of nuclear material received, produced, shipped, lost or otherwise removed from inventory, and the quantities on inventory.

(b) The evaluation of precision and accuracy of measurements and the estimation of measurement uncertainty;

(c) Procedures for identifying, reviewing and evaluating differences in shipper/receiver measurements;

(d) Procedures for taking a physical inventory;

(e) Procedures for the evaluation of accumulations of unmeasured inventory and unmeasured losses;

(f) A system of records and reports showing, for each material balance area, the inventory of nuclear material and the changes in that inventory including receipts into and transfers out of the material balance area;

---

[5] December 9, 1980

(g)   Provisions to ensure that the accounting procedures and arrangements are being operated correctly; and

(h)   Procedures for the provision of reports to the Agency in accordance with Articles 57 through 63 and 65 through 67.

Article 33

Safeguards under this Agreement shall not apply to material in mining or ore processing activities.

Article 34

The United States may, at any time, notify the Agency of any facility or facilities to be added to or removed from the list provided for in Article 1(b):

(a)   In case of addition to the list, the notification shall specify the facility or facilities to be added to the list and the date upon which the addition is to take effect;

(b)   In the case of removal from the list of a facility or facilities then currently identified pursuant to Articles 2(b) or 39(b):

(i)   The Agency shall be notified in advance and the notification shall specify: the facility or facilities being removed, the date of removal, and the quantity and composition of the nuclear material contained therein at the time of notification. In exceptional circumstances, the United States may remove facilities without giving advance notification;

(ii)   Any facility in respect of which notification has been given in accordance with sub-paragraph (i) shall be removed from the list and the nuclear material contained therein shall cease to be subject to safeguards under this Agreement in accordance with and at the time specified in the notification by the United States.

(c) In the case of removal from the list of a facility or facilities not then currently identified pursuant to Articles 2(b) or 39(b), the notification shall specify the facility or facilities being removed and the date of removal. Such facility or facilities shall be removed from the list at the time specified in the notification by the United States.

Article 35

(a) Safeguards shall terminate on nuclear material subject to safeguards under this Agreement, under the conditions set forth in Article 11. Where the conditions of that Article are not met, but the United States considers that the recovery of safeguarded nuclear material from residues is not for the time being practicable or desirable, the United States and the Agency shall consult on the appropriate safeguards measures to be applied.

(b) Safeguards shall terminate on nuclear material subject to safeguards under this Agreement, under the conditions set forth in Article 13, provided that the United States and the Agency agree that such nuclear material is practicably irrecoverable.

Article 36

At the request of the United States, the Agency shall exempt from safeguards nuclear material, which would otherwise be subject to safeguards under this Agreement, as follows:

(a)   Special fissionable material, when it is used in gram quantities or less as a sensing component in instruments;

(b) Nuclear material, when it is used in non-nuclear activities in accordance with Article 13, if such nuclear material is recoverable; and

(c) Plutonium with an isotopic concentration of plutonium-238 exceeding 80%.

Article 37

At the request of the United States, the Agency shall exempt from safeguards nuclear material that would otherwise be subject to safeguards under this Agreement, provided that the total quantity of nuclear material which has been exempted in the United States in accordance with this Article may not at any time exceed:

(a)   One kilogram in total of special fissionable material, which may consist of one or more of the following:

(i)   Plutonium;

(ii)   Uranium with an enrichment of 0.2 (20%)

and above, taken account of by multiplying its weight by its enrichment; and

(iii) Uranium with an enrichment below 0.2 (20%) and above that of natural uranium, taken account of by multiplying its weight by five times the square of its enrichment.

(b) Ten metric tons in total of natural uranium and depleted uranium with an enrichment above 0.005 (0.5%);

(c) Twenty metric tons of depleted uranium with an enrichment of 0.005 (0.5%) or below; and

(d) Twenty metric tons of thorium;

or such greater amounts as may be specified by the Board for uniform application.

Article 38

If exempted nuclear material is to be processed or stored together with nuclear material subject to safeguards under this Agreement, provision shall be made for the reapplication of safeguards thereto.

Article 39

(a) The United States and the Agency shall make Subsidiary Arrangements which shall:

(i) contain a current listing of those facilities identified by the Agency pursuant to Article 2(b) and thus containing nuclear material subject to safeguards under this Agreement; and

(ii) specify in detail, to the extent necessary to permit the Agency to fulfil its responsibilities under this Agreement in an effective and efficient manner, how the procedures laid down in this Agreement are to be applied.

(b) (i) After entry into force of this Agreement, the Agency shall identify to the United States, from the list provided in accordance with Article 1(b), those facilities to be included in the initial Subsidiary Arrangements listing;

(ii)The Agency may thereafter identify for inclusion in the Subsidiary Arrangements listing additional facilities from the list provided in accordance with Article 1(b) as that list may

have been modified in accordance with Article 34.

(c) The Agency shall also designate to the United States those facilities to be removed from the Subsidiary Arrangements listing which have not otherwise been removed pursuant to notification by the United States in accordance with Article 34. Such facility or facilities shall be removed from the Subsidiary Arrangements listing upon such designation to the United States.

(d) The Subsidiary Arrangements may be extended or changed by agreement between the Agency and the United States without amendment to this Agreement.

Article 40

(a) With respect to those facilities which shall have been identified by the Agency in accordance with Article 39(b)(i), such Subsidiary Arrangements shall enter into force at the same time as, or as soon as possible after, entry into force of this Agreement. The United States and the Agency shall make every effort to achieve their entry into force within 90 days after entry into force of this Agreement; an extension of that period shall require agreement between the United States and the Agency.

(b) With respect to facilities which, after the entry into force of this Agreement, have been identified by the Agency in accordance with Article 39(b)(ii) for inclusion in the Subsidiary Arrangements listing, the United States and the Agency shall make every effort to achieve the entry into force of such Subsidiary Arrangements within ninety days following such identification to the United States; an extension of that period shall require agreement between the Agency and the United States.

(c) Upon identification of a facility by the Agency in accordance with Article 39(b), the United States shall provide the Agency promptly with the information required for completing the Subsidiary Arrangements, and the Agency shall have the right to apply the procedures set forth in this Agreement to the nuclear material listed in the inventory provided for in Article 41, even if the Subsidiary Arrangements have not yet entered into force.

Article 41

The Agency shall establish, on the basis of the initial reports referred to in Article 60(a) below, a unified inventory of all nuclear material in the United States subject to safeguards under this Agreement, irrespective of its origin, and shall maintain this inventory on the basis of subsequent reports concerning those facilities, of the initial reports referred to in Article 60(b), of subsequent reports concerning the facilities listed pursuant to Article 39(b)(ii), and of the results of its verification activities. Copies of the inventory shall be made available to the United States at intervals to be agreed.

Article 42

Pursuant to Article 8, design information in respect of facilities identified by the Agency in accordance with Article 39(b)(i) shall be provided to the Agency during the discussion of the Subsidiary Arrangements. The time limits for the provision of design information in respect of any facility which is identified by the Agency in accordance with Article 39(b)(ii) shall be specified in the Subsidiary Arrangements and such information shall be provided as early as possible after such identification.

Article 43

The design information to be provided to the Agency shall include, in respect of each facility identified by the Agency in accordance with Article 39(b), when applicable:

(a) The identification of the facility, stating its general character, purpose, nominal capacity and geographic location, and the name and address to be used for routine business purposes;

(b) A description of the general arrangement of the facility with reference, to the extent feasible, to the form, location and flow of nuclear material and to the general layout of important items of equipment which use, produce or process nuclear material;

(c) A description of features of the facility relating to material accountancy, containment and surveillance; and

(d) A description of the existing and proposed procedures at the facility for nuclear material accountancy and control, with special reference to material balance areas established by the operator, measurements of flow and procedures for physical inventory taking.

Article 44

Other information relevant to the application of safeguards shall also be provided to the Agency in respect of each facility identified by the Agency in accordance with Article 39(b), in particular on organizational responsibility for material accountancy and control. The United States shall provide the Agency with supplementary information on the health and safety procedures which the Agency shall observe and with which the inspectors shall comply at the facility.

Article 45

The Agency shall be provided with design information in respect of a modification relevant for safeguards purposes, for examination, and shall be informed of any change in the information provided to it under Article 44, sufficiently in advance for the safeguards procedures to be adjusted when necessary.

Article 46

The design information provided to the Agency shall be used for the following purposes:

(a) To identify the features of facilities and nuclear material relevant to the application of safeguards to nuclear material in sufficient detail to facilitate verification;

(b) To determine material balance areas to be used for Agency accounting purposes and to select those strategic points which are key measurement points and which will be used to determine flow and inventory of nuclear material; in determining such material balance areas the Agency shall, inter alia, use the following criteria:

(i) The size of the material balance area shall be related to the accuracy with which the material balance can be established;

(ii) In determining the material balance area, advantage shall be taken of any opportunity to use containment and surveillance to help ensure the completeness of flow measurements and thereby to simplify the application of safeguards and to concentrate measurement efforts at key measurement points;

(iii) A number of material balance areas in use at a facility or at distinct sites may be combined in one material balance area to be used for Agency accounting purposes when the Agency determines that this is consistent with its verification requirements; and

(iv) A special material balance area may be established at the request of the United States around a process step involving commercially sensitive information;

(c) To establish the nominal timing and procedures for taking of physical inventory of nuclear material for Agency accounting purposes;

(d) To establish the records and reports requirements and records evaluation procedures;

(e) To establish requirements and procedures for verification of the quantity and location of nuclear material; and

(f) To select appropriate combinations of containment and surveillance methods and techniques at the strategic points at which they are to be applied.

The results of the examination of the design information shall be included in the Subsidiary Arrangements.

Article 47

Design information shall be re-examined in the light of changes in operating conditions, of developments in safeguards technology or of experience in the application of verification procedures, with a view to modifying the action the Agency has taken pursuant to Article 46.

Article 48

The Agency, in co-operation with the United States, may send inspectors to facilities to verify the design information provided to the Agency pursuant to Article 42 through 45, for the purposes stated in Article 46.

Article 49

In establishing a national system of materials

control as referred to in Article 7, the United States shall arrange that records are kept in respect of each material balance area determined in accordance with Article 46(b). The records to be kept shall be described in the Subsidiary Arrangements.

Article 50

The United States shall make arrangements to facilitate the examination of records referred to in Article 49 by inspectors.

Article 51

Records referred to in Article 49 shall be retained for at least five years.

Article 52

Records referred to in Article 49 shall consist, as appropriate, of:

(a) Accounting records of all nuclear material subject to safeguards under this Agreement; and

(b) Operating records for facilities containing such nuclear material.

Article 53

The system of measurements on which the records used for the preparation of reports are based shall either conform to the latest international standards or be equivalent in quality to such standards.

Article 54

The accounting records referred to in Article 52(a) shall set forth the following in respect of each material balance area determined in accordance with Article 46(b):

(a) All inventory changes, so as to permit a determination of the book inventory at any time;

(b) All measurement results that are used for determination of the physical inventory; and

(c) All adjustments and corrections that have been made in respect of inventory changes, book inventories and physical inventories.

Article 55

For all inventory changes and physical inventories the records referred to in Article 52(a) shall show, in respect of each batch of nuclear material: material identification, batch data and source data. The records shall account for uranium, thorium and plutonium separately in each batch of nuclear material. For each inventory change, the date of the inventory change and, when appropriate, the originating material balance area and the receiving material balance area or the recipient shall be indicated.

Article 56

The operating records referred to in Article 52(b) shall set forth, as appropriate, in respect of each material balance area determined in accordance with Article 46(b):

(a) Those operating data which are used to establish changes in the quantities and composition of nuclear material;

(b) The data obtained from the calibration of tanks and instruments and from sampling and analyses, the procedures to control the quality of measurements and the derived estimates of random and systematic error;

(c) A description of the sequence of the actions taken in preparing for, and in taking, a physical inventory, in order to ensure that it is correct and complete; and

(d) A description of the actions taken in order to ascertain the cause and magnitude of any accidental or unmeasured loss that might occur.

Article 57

The United States shall provide the Agency with reports as detailed in Articles 58 through 67 in respect of nuclear material subject to safeguards under this Agreement.

Article 58

Reports shall be made in English.

Article 59

Reports shall be based on the records kept in accordance with Articles 49 through 56 and shall consist, as appropriate, of accounting reports and special reports.

Article 60

The United States shall provide the Agency with an initial report on all nuclear material contained in each facility which becomes listed in the Subsidiary Arrangements in accordance with Article 39(b):

(a) With respect to those facilities listed pursuant to Article 39(b)(i), such reports shall be dispatched to the Agency within thirty days of the last day of the calendar month in which this Agreement enters into force, and shall reflect the situation as of the last day of that month.

(b) With respect to each facility listed pursuant to Article 39(b)(ii), an initial report shall be dispatched to the Agency within thirty days of the last day of the calendar month in which the Agency identifies the facility to the United States and shall reflect the situation as of the last day of that month.

Article 61

The United States shall provide the Agency with the following accounting reports for each material balance area determined in accordance with Article 46(b):

(a) Inventory change reports showing all changes in the inventory of nuclear material. The reports shall be dispatched as soon as possible and in any event within thirty days after the end of the month in which the inventory changes occurred or were established; and

(b) Material balance reports showing the material balance based on a physical inventory of nuclear material actually present in the material balance area. The reports shall be dispatched as soon as possible and in any event within thirty days after the physical inventory has been taken.

The reports shall be based on data available as of the date of reporting and may be corrected at a later date, as required.

Article 62

Inventory change reports submitted in

accordance with Article 61(a) shall specify identification and batch data for each batch of nuclear material, the date of the inventory change, and, as appropriate, the originating material balance area and the receiving material balance area or the recipient. These reports shall be accompanied by concise notes:

(a) Explaining the inventory changes, on the basis of the operating data contained in the operating records provided for under Article 56(a); and

(b) Describing, as specified in the Subsidiary Arrangements, the anticipated operational programme, particularly the taking of a physical inventory.

Article 63

The United States shall report each inventory change, adjustment and correction, either periodically in a consolidated list or individually. Inventory changes shall be reported in terms of batches. As specified in the Subsidiary Arrangements, small changes in inventory of nuclear materials, such as transfers of analytical samples, may be combined in one batch and reported as one inventory change.

Article 64

The Agency shall provide the United States with semi-annual statements of book inventory of nuclear material subject to safeguards under this Agreement, for each material balance area, as based on the inventory change reports for the period covered by each such statement.

Article 65

Material balance reports submitted in accordance with Article 61(b) shall include the following entries, unless otherwise agreed by the United States and the Agency:

(a) Beginning physical inventory;

(b) Inventory changes (first increases, then decreases);

(c) Ending book inventory;

(d) Shipper/receiver differences;

(e) Adjusted ending book inventory;

(f) Ending physical inventory; and

(g) Material unaccounted for.

A statement of the physical inventory, listing all batches separately and specifying material identification and batch data for each batch, shall be attached to each material balance report.

Article 66

The United States shall make special reports without delay:

(a) If any unusual incident or circumstances lead the United States to believe that there is or may have been loss of nuclear material subject to safeguards under this Agreement that exceeds the limits specified for this purpose in the Subsidiary Arrangements; or

(b) If the containment has unexpectedly changed from that specified in the Subsidiary Arrangements to the extent that unauthorized removal of nuclear material subject to safeguards under this Agreement has become possible.

Article 67

If the Agency so requests, the United States shall provide it with amplifications or clarifications of any report submitted in accordance with Articles 57 through 63, 65 and 66, in so far as relevant for the purpose of safeguards.

Article 68

The Agency shall have the right to make inspections as provided for in Articles 69 through 82.

Article 69

The Agency may make ad hoc inspections in order to:

(a) Verify the information contained in the initial reports submitted in accordance with Article 60;

(b) Identify and verify changes in the situation which have occurred since the date of the relevant initial report; and

(c) Identify and if possible verify the quantity and composition of the nuclear material subject to safeguards under this Agreement in respect of which the information referred to in Article 89(a) has been provided to the Agency.

Article 70

The Agency may make routine inspections in order to:

(a) Verify that reports submitted pursuant to Articles 57 through 63, 65 and 66 are consistent with records kept pursuant to Articles 49 through 56;

(b) Verify the location, identity, quantity and composition of all nuclear material subject to safeguards under this Agreement; and

(c) Verify information on the possible causes of material unaccounted for, shipper/receiver differences and uncertainties in the book inventory.

Article 71

Subject to the procedures laid down in Article 75, the Agency may make special inspections:

(a) In order to verify the information contained in special reports submitted in accordance with Article 66; or

(b) If the Agency considers that information made available by the United States, including explanations from the United States and information obtained from routine inspections, is not adequate for the Agency to fulfill its responsibilities under this Agreement.

An inspection shall be deemed to be special when it is either additional to the routine inspection effort provided for in Articles 76 through 80, or involves access to information or locations in addition to the access specified in Article 74 for *ad hoc* and routine inspections, or both.

Article 72

For the purposes specified in Articles 69 through 71, the Agency may:

(a)   Examine the records kept pursuant to Articles 49 through 56;

(b) Make independent measurements of all nuclear material subject to safeguards under this Agreement;

(c) Verify the functioning and calibration of instruments and other measuring and control equipment;

(d) Apply and make use of surveillance and containment measures; and

(e) Use other objective methods which have been demonstrated to be technically feasible.

Article 73

Within the scope of Article 72, the Agency shall be enabled:

(a) To observe that samples at key measurement points for material balance accountancy are taken in accordance with procedures which produce representative samples, to observe the treatment and analysis of the samples and to obtain duplicates of such samples;

(b) To observe that the measurements of nuclear material at key measurement points for material balance accountancy are representative, and to observe the calibration of the instruments and equipment involved;

(c) To make arrangements with the United States that, if necessary:

(i) Additional measurements are made and additional samples taken for the Agency's use;

(ii) The Agency's standard analytical samples are analyzed;

(iii) Appropriate absolute standards are used in calibrating instruments and other equipment; and

(iv) Other calibrations are carried out;

(d) To arrange to use its own equipment for independent measurement and surveillance, and if so agreed and specified in the Subsidiary Arrangements to arrange to install such equipment;

(e) To apply its seals and other identifying and tamper-indicating devices to containments, if so agreed and specified in the Subsidiary Arrangements; and

(f) To make arrangements with the United States for the shipping of samples taken for the Agency's use.

Article 74

(a) For the purposes specified in Articles 69 (a) and (b) and until such time as the strategic points have been specified in the Subsidiary Arrangements, Agency inspectors shall have access to any location where the initial report or any inspections carried out therewith indicate that nuclear material subject to safeguards under this Agreement is present.

(b) For the purposes specified in Article 69(c), the inspectors shall have access to any facility identified pursuant to Article 2(b) or 39(b) in which nuclear material referred to in Article 69(c) is located.

(c) For the purposes specified in Article 70 the inspectors shall have access only to the strategic points specified in the Subsidiary Arrangements and to the records maintained pursuant to Articles 49 through 56; and

(d) In the event of the United States concluding that any unusual circumstances require extended limitations on access by the Agency, the United States and the Agency shall promptly make arrangements with a view to enabling the Agency to discharge its safeguards responsibilities in the light of these limitations. The Director General shall report each such arrangement to the Board.

Article 75

In circumstances which may lead to special inspections for the purposes specified in Article 71 the United States and the Agency shall consult forthwith. As a result of such consultations the Agency may:

(a) Make inspections in addition to the routine inspection effort provided for in Articles 76 through 80; and

(b) Obtain access, in agreement with the United States, to information or locations in addition to those specified in Article 74. Any disagreement concerning the need for additional access shall be resolved in accordance with Articles 20 and 21; in case action by the United States is essential and urgent, Article 17 shall apply.

Article 76

The Agency shall keep the number, intensity and duration of routine inspections, applying optimum timing, to the minimum consistent with the effective implementation of the safeguards procedures set forth in this Agreement, and shall make the optimum and most economical use of inspection resources available to it.

Article 77

The Agency may carry out one routine inspection per year in respect of facilities listed in the Subsidiary Arrangements pursuant to Article 39 with a content or annual throughput, whichever is greater, of nuclear material not exceeding five effective kilograms.

Article 78

The number, intensity, duration, timing and mode of routine inspections in respect of facilities listed in the Subsidiary Arrangements pursuant to Article 39 with a content or annual throughput of nuclear material exceeding five effective kilograms shall be determined on the basis that in the maximum or limiting case the inspection regime shall be no more intensive than is necessary and sufficient to maintain continuity of knowledge of the flow and inventory of nuclear material, and the maximum routine inspection effort in respect of such facilities shall be determined as follows:

(a) For reactors and sealed storage installations the maximum total of routine inspection per year shall be determined by allowing one sixth of a man-year of inspection for each such facility;

(b) For facilities, other than reactors or sealed storage installations, involving plutonium or uranium enriched to more than 5%, the maximum total of routine inspection per year shall be determined by allowing for each such facility $30 \times \sqrt{E}$ man-days of inspection per year, where E is the inventory or annual throughput of nuclear material, whichever is greater, expressed in effective kilograms. The maximum established for any such facility shall not, however, be less than 1.5 man-years of inspection; and

(c) For facilities not covered by paragraphs (a) or (b), the maximum total of routine inspection per year shall be determined by allowing for each such facility one third of a man-year of inspection plus $0.4 \times E$ man-days of inspection per year, where E is the inventory or annual throughput of nuclear material, whichever is greater, expressed in effective kilograms.

The United States and the Agency may agree to amend the figures for the maximum inspection effort specified in this Article, upon determination by the Board that such amendment is reasonable.

Article 79

Subject to Articles 76 through 78 the criteria to be used for determining the actual number, intensity, duration, timing and mode of routine inspections in respect of any facility listed in the Subsidiary Arrangements pursuant to Article 39 shall include:

(a) The form of the nuclear material, in particular, whether the nuclear material is in bulk form or contained in a number of separate items; its chemical composition and, in the case of uranium, whether it is of low or high enrichment; and its accessibility;

(b) The effectiveness of the United States' accounting and control system, including the extent to which the operators of facilities are functionally independent of the United States' accounting and control system; the extent to which the measures specified in Article 32 have been implemented by the United States; the promptness of reports provided to the Agency; their consistency with the Agency's independent verification; and the amount and accuracy of the material unaccounted for, as verified by the Agency;

(c) Characteristics of that part of the United States fuel cycle in which safeguards are applied under this Agreement, in particular, the number and types of facilities containing nuclear material subject to safeguards under this Agreement, the characteristics of such facilities relevant to safeguards, notably the degree of containment;

the extent to which the design of such facilities facilitates verification of the flow and inventory of nuclear material; and the extent to which information from different material balance areas can be correlated;

(d) International interdependence, in particular the extent to which nuclear material, safeguarded under this Agreement, is received from or sent to other States for use or processing; any verification activities by the Agency in connection therewith; and the extent to which activities in facilities in which safeguards are applied under this Agreement are interrelated with those of other States; and

(e) Technical developments in the field of safeguards, including the use of statistical techniques and random sampling in evaluating the flow of nuclear material.

Article 80

The United States and the Agency shall consult if the United States considers that the inspection effort is being deployed with undue concentration on particular facilities.

Article 81

The Agency shall give advance notice to the United States of the arrival of inspectors at facilities listed in the Subsidiary Arrangements pursuant to Article 39, as follows:

(a) For *ad hoc* inspections pursuant to Article 69(c), at least 24 hours; for those pursuant to Articles 69(a) and (b), as well as the activities provided for in Article 48, at least one week;

(b) For special inspections pursuant to Article 71, as promptly as possible after the United States and the Agency have consulted as provided for in Article 75, it being understood that notification of arrival normally will constitute part of the consultations; and

(c) For routine inspections pursuant to Article 70 at least twenty-four hours in respect of the facilities referred to in Article 78(b) and sealed storage installations containing plutonium or uranium enriched to more than 5% and one week in all other cases.

Such notice of inspections shall include the names of the inspectors and shall indicate the facilities to be visited and the periods during which they will be visited. If the inspectors are to arrive from outside the United States the Agency shall also give advance notice of place and time of their arrival in the United States.

Article 82

Notwithstanding the provisions of Article 81, the Agency may, as a supplementary measure, carry out without advance notification a portion of the routine inspections pursuant to Article 78 in accordance with the principle of random sampling. In performing any unannounced inspections, the Agency shall fully take into account any operational programme provided by the United States pursuant to Article 62(b). Moreover, whenever practicable, and on the basis of the operational programme, it shall advise the United States periodically of its general programme of announced and unannounced inspections, specifying the general periods when inspections are foreseen. In carrying out any unannounced inspections, the Agency shall make every effort to minimize any practical difficulties for the United States and facility operators bearing in mind the relevant provisions of Articles 44 and 87. Similarly the United States shall make every effort to facilitate the task of the inspectors.

Article 83

The following procedures shall apply to the designation of inspectors:

(a) The Director General shall inform the United States in writing of the name, qualifications, nationality, grade and such other particulars as may be relevant, of each Agency official he proposes for designation as an inspector for the United States;

(b) The United States shall inform the Director General within thirty days of the receipt of such a proposal whether it accepts the proposal;

(c) The Director General may designate each official who has been accepted by the United States as one of the inspectors for the United States, and shall inform the United States of such designations; and

(d) The Director General, acting in response to

a request by the United States or on his own initiative, shall immediately inform the United States of the withdrawal of the designation of any official as an inspector for the United States.

However, in respect of inspectors needed for the activities provided for in Article 48 and to carry out ad hoc inspections pursuant to Article 69 (a) and (b) the designation procedures shall be completed if possible within thirty days after the entry into force of this Agreement. If such designation appears impossible within this time limit, inspectors for such purposes shall be designated on a temporary basis.

Article 84

The United States shall grant or renew as quickly as possible appropriate visas, where required, for each inspector designated for United States.

Article 85

Inspectors, in exercising their functions under Article 48 and 69 to 73, shall carry out their activities in a manner designed to avoid hampering or delaying the construction, commissioning or operation of facilities, or affecting their safety. In particular inspectors shall not operate any facility themselves or direct the staff of a facility to carry out any operation. If inspectors consider that in pursuance of paragraphs 72 and 73, particular operations in a facility should be carried out by the operator, they shall make a request therefor.

Article 86

When inspectors require services available in the United States, including the use of the equipment, in connection with the performance of inspections, the United States shall facilitate the procurement of such services and the use of such equipment by inspectors.

Article 87

The United States shall have the right to have inspectors accompanied during their inspections by its representatives, provided that inspectors shall not thereby be delayed or otherwise impeded in the exercise of their functions.

Article 88

The Agency shall inform the United States of:

(a) The results of inspections, at intervals to be specified in the Subsidiary Arrangements; and

(b) The conclusions it has drawn from its verification activities in the United States, in particular by means of statements in respect of each material balance area determined in accordance with Article 46(b) which shall be made as soon as possible after a physical inventory has been taken and verified by the Agency and a material balance has been struck.

Article 89

(a) Information concerning nuclear material exported from and imported into the United States shall be provided to the Agency in accordance with arrangements made with the Agency as, for example, those set forth in INFCIRC/207.

(b) In the case of international transfers to or from facilities identified by the Agency pursuant to Articles 2(b) and 39(b) with respect to which information has been provided to the Agency in accordance with arrangements referred to in paragraph (a), a special report, as envisaged in Article 66, shall be made if any unusual incident or circumstances lead the United States to believe that there is or may have been loss of nuclear material, including the occurrence of significant delay, during the transfer.

DEFINITIONS

Article 90

For the purposes of this Agreement:

A   Adjustment means an entry into an accounting record or a report showing a shipper/receiver difference or material unaccounted for.

B   Annual throughput means, for the purposes of Articles 77 and 78, the amount of nuclear material transferred annually out of a facility working at nominal capacity.

C   Batch means a portion of nuclear material handled as a unit for accounting purposes at a key measurement point and for which the composition and quantity are defined by a single set of specifications or measurements. The nuclear material may be in bulk form or contained in a number of separate items.

D   Batch data means the total weight of each element of nuclear material and, in the case of plutonium and uranium, the isotopic composition when appropriate. The units of account shall be as follows:

(a) Grams of contained plutonium;

(b) Grams of total uranium and grams of contained uranium-235 plus uranium-233 for uranium enriched in these isotopes; and

(c) Kilograms of contained thorium, natural uranium or depleted uranium.

For reporting purposes the weights of individual items in the batch shall be added together before rounding to the nearest unit.

E   Book inventory of a material balance area means the algebraic sum of the most recent physical inventory of that material balance area and of all inventory changes that have occurred since that physical inventory was taken.

F   Correction means an entry into an accounting record or a report to rectify an identified mistake or to reflect an improved measurement of a quantity previously entered into the record or report. Each correction must identify the entry to which it pertains.

G   Effective kilogram means a special unit used in safeguarding nuclear material. The quantity in effective kilograms is obtained by taking:

(a) For plutonium, its weight in kilograms;

(b) For uranium with an enrichment of 0.01 (1%) and above, its weight in kilograms multiplied by the square of its enrichment;

(c) For uranium with an enrichment below 0.01 (1%) and above 0.005 (0.5%), its weight in kilograms multiplied by 0.0001; and

(d) For depleted uranium with an enrichment of

0.005 (0.5%) or below, and for thorium, its weight in kilograms multiplied by 0.00005.

H   Enrichment means the ratio of the combined weight of the isotopes uranium-233 and uranium-235 to that of the total uranium in question.

I Facility means:

   (a) A reactor, a critical facility, a conversion plant, a fabrication plant, a reprocessing plant, an isotope separation plant or a separate storage installation; or

   (b) Any location where nuclear material in amounts greater than one effective kilogram is customarily used.

J   Inventory change means an increase or decrease, in terms of batches, of nuclear material in a material balance area; such a change shall involve one of the following:

   (a) Increases:

        (i) Import;

        (ii) Domestic receipt: receipts from other material balance areas, receipts from a non-safeguarded activity or receipts at the starting point of safeguards;

        (iii) Nuclear production: production of special fissionable material in a reactor; and

        (iv) De-exemption: reapplication of safeguards on nuclear material previously exempted therefrom on account of its use or quantity.

   (b) Decreases:

        (i) Export;

        (ii) Domestic shipment: shipments to other material balance areas or shipments for a non-safeguarded activity;

        (iii) Nuclear loss: loss of nuclear material due to its transformation into other element(s) or isotope(s) as a result of nuclear reactions;

        (iv) Measured discard: nuclear material which has been measured, or estimated on the basis of measurements, and disposed of in such a way that it is not suitable for further nuclear use;

        (v) Retained waste: nuclear material generated from processing or from an operational accident, which is deemed to be unrecoverable for the time being but which is stored;

        (vi) Exemption: exemption of nuclear material from safeguards on account of its use or quantity; and

        (vii) Other loss: for example, accidental loss (that is, irretrievable and inadvertent loss of nuclear material as the result of an operational accident) or theft.

K   Key measurement point means a location where nuclear material appears in such a form that it may be measured to determine material flow or inventory. Key measurement points thus include, but are not limited to, the inputs and outputs (including measured discards) and storages in material balance areas.

L   Man-year of inspection means, for the purposes of Article 78, 300 man-days of inspection, a man-day being a day during which a single inspector has access to a facility at any time for a total of not more than eight hours.

M   Material balance area means an area in or outside of a facility such that:

   (a) The quantity of nuclear material in each transfer into or out of each material balance area can be determined; and

   (b) The physical inventory of nuclear material in each material balance area can be determined when necessary in accordance with specified procedures;

   in order that the material balance for Agency safeguards purposes can be established.

N   Material unaccounted for means the difference between book inventory and physical inventory.

O   Nuclear material means any source or any special fissionable material as defined in Article XX of the statute. The term source material shall not be interpreted as applying to ore or ore residue. Any determination by the Board under Article XX of the statute after the entry into force of this Agreement which adds to the materials considered to be source material or special fissionable material shall have effect under this Agreement only upon acceptance by the United States.

P   Physical inventory means the sum of all the measured or derived estimates of batch quantities of nuclear material on hand at a given time within a material balance area, obtained in accordance with specified procedures.

Q   Shipper/receiver difference means the difference between the quantity of nuclear material in a batch as stated by the shipping material balance area and as measured at the receiving material balance area.

R   Source data means those data, recorded during measurement or calibration or used to derive empirical relationships, which identify nuclear material and provide batch data. Source data may include, for example, weight of compounds, conversion factors to determine weight of element, specific gravity, element concentration, isotopic ratios, relationship between volume and manometer readings and relationship between plutonium produced and power generated.

S   Strategic point means a location selected during examination of design information where, under normal conditions and when combined with the information from all strategic points taken together, the information necessary and sufficient for the implementation of safeguards measures is obtained and verified; a strategic point may include any location where key measurements related to material balance accountancy are made and where containment and surveillance measures are executed.

FOR THE UNITED STATES OF AMERICA:
G.S.

FOR THE INTERNATIONAL OF ATOMIC ENERGY AGENCY:
D.A.V.F.

PROTOCOL TO THE AGREEMENT BETWEEN THE UNITED STATES OF AMERICA AND THE INTERNATIONAL ATOMIC ENERGY AGENCY FOR THE APPLICATION OF SAFEGUARDS IN THE UNITED STATES

Article 1

This Protocol specifies the procedures to be followed with respect to facilities identified by the Agency pursuant to Article 2 of this Protocol.

Article 2

(a) The Agency may from time to time identify to the United States those facilities included in the list, established and maintained pursuant to Articles 1(b) and 34 of the Agreement, of facilities not associated with activities having direct national security significance to the United States, other than those which are then currently identified by the Agency pursuant to Articles 2(b) and 39(b) of the Agreement, to which the provisions of this Protocol shall apply.

(b) The Agency may also include among the facilities identified to the United States pursuant to the foregoing paragraph, any facility which had previously been identified by the Agency pursuant to Articles 2(b) and 39(b) of the Agreement but which had subsequently been designated by the Agency pursuant to Article 39(c) of the Agreement for removal from the Subsidiary Arrangements listing.

(c) In identifying facilities pursuant to the foregoing paragraphs and in the preparation of Transitional Subsidiary Arrangements pursuant to Article 3 of this Protocol, the Agency shall proceed in a manner which the Agency and the United States mutually agree takes into account the requirement of the United States to avoid discriminatory treatment as between United States commercial firms similarly situated.

Article 3

The United States and the Agency shall make Transitional Subsidiary Arrangements which shall:

(a) Contain a current listing of those facilities identified by the Agency pursuant to Article 2 of this Protocol;

(b) Specify in detail how the procedures set forth in this protocol are to be applied.

Article 4

(a) The United States and the Agency shall make every effort to complete the Transitional Subsidiary Arrangements with respect to each facility identified by the Agency pursuant to Article 2 of this Protocol within ninety days following such identification to the United States.

(b) With respect to any facility identified pursuant to Article 2(b) of this Protocol, the information previously submitted to the Agency in accordance with Articles 42 through 45 of the Agreement, the results of the examination of the design information and other provisions of the Subsidiary Arrangements relative to such facility, to the extent that such information, results and provisions satisfy the provisions of this Protocol relating to the submission and examination of information and the preparation of Transitional Subsidiary Arrangements, shall constitute the Transitional Subsidiary Arrangements for such facility, until and unless the United States and the Agency shall otherwise complete Transitional Subsidiary Arrangements for such facility in accordance with the provisions of this Protocol.

Article 5

In the event that a facility currently identified by the Agency pursuant to Article 2(a) of this Protocol is identified by the Agency pursuant to Articles 2(b) and 39(b) of the Agreement, the Transitional Subsidiary Arrangements relevant to such facility shall, to the extent that such Transitional Subsidiary Arrangements satisfy the provisions of the Agreement, be deemed to have been made part of the Subsidiary Arrangements to the Agreement.

Article 6

Design information in respect of each facility identified by the Agency pursuant to Article 2 of this Protocol shall be provided to the Agency during the discussion of the relevant Transitional Subsidiary Arrangements. The information shall include, when applicable:

(a) The identification of the facility, stating its general character, purpose, nominal capacity and geographic location, and the name and address to be used for routine business purpose;

(b) A description of the general arrangement of the facility with reference, to the extent feasible, to the form, location and flow of nuclear material and to the general layout of important items of equipment which use, produce or process nuclear material;

(c) A description of features of the facility relating to material accountancy, containment and surveillance; and

(d) A description of the existing and proposed procedures at the facility for nuclear material accountancy and control, with special reference to material balance areas established by the operator, measurements of flow and procedures for physical inventory taking.

Article 7

Other information relevant to the application of the provisions of this Protocol shall also be provided to the Agency in respect of each facility identified by the Agency in accordance with Article 2 of this Protocol, in particular on organizational responsibility for material accountancy and control. The United States shall provide the Agency with supplementary information on the health and safety procedures which the Agency shall observe and with which inspectors shall comply when visiting the facility in accordance with Article 11 of this Protocol.

Article 8

The Agency shall be provided with design information in respect of a modification relevant to the application of the provisions of this Protocol, for examination, and shall be informed of any change in the information provided to it under Article 7 of this Protocol, sufficiently in advance for the procedures under this Protocol to be adjusted when necessary.

Article 9

The design information provided to the Agency in accordance with the provisions of this Protocol, in anticipation of the application of safeguards under the Agreement, shall be used for the following purposes:

(a) To identify the features of facilities and nuclear material relevant to the application of safeguards to nuclear material in sufficient detail to facilitate verification;

(b) To determine material balance areas to be used for Agency accounting purposes and to select those strategic points which are key measurement points and which will be used to determine flow and inventory of nuclear material; in determining such material balance areas the Agency shall, inter alia, use the following criteria:

(i) The size of the material balance area shall be related to the accuracy with which the material balance can be established;

(ii) In determining the material balance area, advantage shall be taken of any opportunity to use containment and surveillance to help ensure the completeness of flow measurements and thereby to simplify the application of safeguards and to concentrate measurement efforts at key measurement points;

(iii) A number of material balance areas in use at a facility or at distinct sites may be combined in one material balance area to be used for Agency accounting purposes when the Agency determines that this is consistent with its verification requirements; and

(iv) A special material balance area may be established at the request of the United States around a process step involving commercially sensitive information;

(c) To establish the nominal timing and procedures for taking of physical inventory of nuclear material for Agency accounting purposes;

(d) To establish the records and reports requirements and records evaluation procedures;

(e) To establish requirements and procedures for verification of the quantity and location of nuclear material; and

(f) To select appropriate combinations of containment and surveillance methods and techniques and the strategic points at which they are to be applied.

The results of the examination of the design information shall be included in the relevant Transitional Subsidiary Arrangements.

Article 10

Design information provided in accordance with the provisions of this Protocol shall be re-examined in the light of changes in operating conditions, of developments in safeguards technology or of experience in the application of verification procedures, with a view to modifying the action taken pursuant to Article 9 of this Protocol.

Article 11

(a) The Agency, in co-operation with the United States, may send inspectors to facilities identified by the Agency pursuant to Article 2 of this Protocol to verify the design information provided to the Agency in accordance with the provisions of this Protocol, for the purposes stated in Article 9 of this Protocol or for such other purposes as may be agreed between the United States and the Agency.

(b) The Agency shall give notice to the United States with respect to each such visit at least one week prior to the arrival of inspectors at the facility to be visited.

Article 12

In establishing a national system of materials control as referred to in Article 7(a) of the Agreement, the United States shall arrange that records are kept in respect of each material balance area determined in accordance with Article 9(b) of this Protocol. The records to be kept shall be described in the relevant Transitional Subsidiary Arrangements.

Article 13

Records referred to in Article 12 of this Protocol shall be retained for at least five years.

Article 14

Records referred to in Article 12 of this Protocol shall consist, as appropriate, of:

(a) Accounting records of all nuclear material stored, processed, used or produced in each facility; and

(b) Operating records for activities within each facility.

Article 15

The system of measurements on which the records used for the preparation of reports are based shall either conform to the latest international standards or be equivalent in quality to such standards.

Article 16

The accounting records referred to in Article 14(a) of this Protocol shall set forth the following in respect of each material balance area determined in accordance with Article 9(b) of this Protocol:

(a) All inventory changes, so as to permit a determination of the book inventory at any time;

(b) All measurement results that are used for determination of the physical inventory; and

(c) All adjustments and corrections that have been made in respect of inventory changes, book inventories and physical inventories.

Article 17

For all inventory changes and physical inventories the records referred to in Article 14(a) of this Protocol shall show, in respect of each batch of nuclear material: material identification, batch data and source data. The records shall account for uranium, thorium and plutonium separately in each batch of nuclear material. For each inventory change, the date of the inventory change and, when appropriate, the originating material balance area and the receiving material balance area or the recipient, shall be indicated.

Article 18

The operating records referred to in Article 14(b) of this Protocol shall set forth, as appropriate, in respect of each material balance area determined in accordance with Article 9(b) of this Protocol:

(a) Those operating data which are used to establish changes in the quantities and composition of nuclear material;

(b) The data obtained from the calibration of tanks and instruments and from sampling and analyses, the procedures to control the quality of measurements and the derived estimates of random and systematic error;

(c) A description of the sequence of the actions taken in preparing for, and in taking, a physical inventory, in order to ensure that it is correct and complete; and

(d) A description of the actions taken in order to ascertain the cause and magnitude of any accidental or unmeasured loss that might occur.

Article 19

The United States shall provide the Agency with accounting reports as detailed in Articles 20 through 25 of this Protocol in respect of nuclear material in each facility identified by the Agency pursuant to Article 2 of this Protocol.

Article 20

The accounting reports shall be based on the records kept in accordance with Articles 12 to 18 to this Protocol. They shall be made in English.

Article 21

The United States shall provide the Agency with an initial report on nuclear material in each facility identified by the Agency pursuant to Article 2 of this Protocol. Such report shall be dispatched to the Agency within thirty days of the last day of the calendar month in which the facility is identified by the Agency and shall reflect the situation as of the last day of that month.

Article 22

The United States shall provide the Agency with the following accounting reports for each material balance area determined in accordance with Article 9(b) of this Protocol:

(a) Inventory change reports showing all changes in the inventory of nuclear material. The reports shall be dispatched as soon as possible and in any event within thirty days after the end

of the month in which inventory changes occurred or were established; and

(b) Material balance reports showing the material balance based on a physical inventory of nuclear material actually present in the material balance area. The reports shall be dispatched as soon as possible and in any event within thirty days after the physical inventory has been taken.

The reports shall be based on data as of the date of reporting and may be corrected at a later date, as required.

Article 23

Inventory change reports submitted in accordance with Article 22(a) of this Protocol shall specify identification and batch data for each batch of nuclear material, the date of the inventory change, and, as appropriate, the originating material balance area and the receiving material balance area or the recipient. These reports shall be accompanied by concise notes:

(a) Explaining the inventory changes, on the basis of the operating data contained in the operating records provided for in Article 18(a) of this Protocol; and

(b) Describing, as specified in the relevant Transitional Subsidiary Arrangements, the anticipated operational program, particularly the taking of a physical inventory.

Article 24

The United States shall report each inventory change, adjustment and correction, either periodically in a consolidated list or individually. Inventory changes shall be reported in terms of batches. As specified in the relevant Transitional Subsidiary Arrangements, small changes in inventory of nuclear material, such as transfers of analytical samples, may be combined in one batch and reported as one inventory change.

Article 25

Material balance reports submitted in accordance with Article 22(b) of the Protocol shall include the following entries, unless otherwise agreed by the United States and the Agency:

(a)   Beginning physical inventory;

(b)   Inventory changes (first increases, then decreases);

(c)   Ending book inventory;

(d)   Shipper/receiver differences;

(e)   Adjusted ending book inventory;

(f)   Ending physical inventory; and

(g)   Material unaccounted for.

A statement of the physical inventory, listing all batches separately and specifying material identification and batch data for each batch, shall be attached to each material balance report.

Article 26

The Agency shall provide the United States with semi-annual statements of book inventory of nuclear material in facilities identified pursuant to Article 2 of this Protocol, for each material balance area, as based on the inventory change reports for the period covered by each statement.

Article 27

(a) If the Agency so requests, the United States shall provide it with amplifications or clarifications of any report submitted in accordance with Article 19 of this Protocol, in so far as consistent with the purpose of the Protocol.

(b) The Agency shall inform the United States of any significant observations resulting from its examination of reports received pursuant to Article 19 of this Protocol and from visits of inspectors made pursuant to Article 11 of this Protocol.

(c) The United States and the Agency shall, at the request of either, consult about any question arising out of the interpretation or application of this Protocol, including corrective action which, in the opinion of the Agency, should be taken by the United States to ensure compliance with its terms, as indicated by the Agency in its observations pursuant to paragraph (b) of this Article.

Article 28

The definitions set forth in Article 90 of the Agreement shall apply, to the extent relevant, to this Protocol.

DONE in Vienna on the eighteenth day of November 1977, in duplicate, in the English language.

FOR THE UNITED STATES OF AMERICA:
G.S.   **18 November 1977**

FOR THE INTERNATIONAL ATOMIC ENERGY AGENCY:

D.A.V.F.   **18 November 1977**

TREATY BETWEEN THE UNITED STATES OF AMERICA AND THE UNION OF SOVIET SOCIALIST REPUBLICS ON THE LIMITATION OF STRATEGIC OFFENSIVE ARMS

In accordance with Article VII of the Interim Agreement, in which the sides committed themselves to continue active negotiations on strategic offensive arms, the SALT II negotiations began in November 1972. The primary goal of SALT II was to replace the Interim Agreement with a long-term comprehensive Treaty providing broad limits on strategic offensive weapons systems. The principal U.S. objectives as the SALT II negotiations began were to provide for equal numbers of strategic nuclear delivery vehicles for the sides, to begin the process of reduction of these delivery vehicles, and to impose restraints on qualitative developments which could threaten future stability.

Early discussion between the sides focused on the weapon systems to be included, factors involved in providing for equality in numbers of strategic nuclear delivery vehicles, taking into account the important differences between the forces of the two sides, bans on new systems, qualitative limits, and a Soviet proposal to include U.S. forward-based systems. The positions of the sides differed widely on many of these issues.

A major breakthrough occurred at the Vladivostok meeting in November 1974, between President Ford and General Secretary Brezhnev. At this meeting, the sides agreed to a basic framework for the SALT II agreement. Basic elements of the Aide-Memoire, which recorded this agreement, included:

• 2,400 equal aggregate limit on strategic nuclear delivery vehicles (ICBMs, SLBMs, and heavy bombers) of the sides;

• 1,320 equal aggregate limit on MIRV systems;

• ban on construction of new land-based ICBM launchers;

• limits on deployment of new types of strategic offensive arms; and

• important elements of the Interim Agreement (e.g., relating to verification) would be incorporated in the new agreement.

In addition, the Aide-Memoire stated that the duration of the new agreement would be through 1985.

In early 1975, the delegations in Geneva resumed negotiations, working toward an agreement based on this general framework. It was during this time that a Joint Draft Text was first prepared and many limitations were agreed. During the negotiations, however, it became clear that there was fundamental disagreement between the two sides on two major issues: how cruise missiles were to be addressed, and whether the new Soviet bomber known to the United States as Backfire would be considered a heavy bomber and therefore counted in the 2,400 aggregate. While there was disagreement on other issues such as MIRV verification provisions, restrictions on new systems, and missile throw-weight ceilings, progress was made in these areas. However, the issues of cruise missiles and Backfire remained unresolved.

When the new Administration took office in 1977, renewed emphasis was placed on the Strategic Arms Limitation Talks. A comprehensive interagency review of SALT was undertaken. Building on the work of the previous Administration, particularly the Vladivostok accord and the subsequent agreement on many issues in Geneva, the United States made a comprehensive proposal which was presented to the Soviets by Secretary of State Vance in March 1977. This proposal would have added significant reductions and qualitative constraints to the ceilings which were agreed to at Vladivostok. At the same time, the United States also presented an alternative proposal for a SALT II agreement similar to the framework agreed to at Vladivostok, with the Backfire and cruise missile issues deferred until SALT III.

Both proposals were rejected by the Soviets as inconsistent with their understandings of the Vladivostok accord.

In subsequent negotiations, the sides agreed on a general framework for SALT II which accommodated both the Soviet desire to retain the Vladivostok framework for an agreement, and the U.S. desire for more comprehensive limitations in SALT II.

The agreement would consist of three parts:

• A Treaty which would be in force through 1985 based on the Vladivostok accord;

• A Protocol of about three-years' duration which would cover certain issues such as cruise missile constraints, mobile ICBM limits, and qualitative constraints on ICBMs, while deferring further negotiations on these issues to SALT III;

• A Joint Statement of Principles which would be an agreed set of guidelines for future negotiations.

Within this framework, negotiations to resolve the remaining differences continued on several levels. President Carter, Secretary Vance, and Soviet Foreign Minister Gromyko met in Washington in September 1977. Further high-level meetings were held in Washington, Moscow, and Geneva during 1978 and 1979. In addition, the SALT delegations of the United States and Soviet Union in Geneva were in session nearly continuously following the 1974 Vladivostok meeting to work out agreed Treaty language on those issues where agreement in principle had been reached at the ministerial level.

The completed SALT II agreement was signed by President Carter and General Secretary Brezhnev in Vienna on June 18, 1979. President Carter transmitted it to the Senate on June 22 for its advice and consent to ratification.

On January 3, 1980, however, President Carter requested the Senate majority leader to delay consideration of the Treaty on the Senate floor in view of the Soviet invasion of Afghanistan. Although the Treaty remained unratified, each Party was individually bound under the terms of international law to refrain from acts which would defeat the object and purpose of the Treaty, until it had made its intentions clear not to become a party to the Treaty.

In 1980, President Carter announced the United States would comply with the provisions of the Treaty as long as the Soviet Union reciprocated. Brezhnev made a similar statement regarding Soviet intentions.

In May 1982, President Reagan stated he would do nothing to undercut the SALT agreements as long as the Soviet Union showed equal restraint. The Soviet Union again agreed to abide by the unratified Treaty.

Subsequently, in 1984 and 1985, President Reagan declared that the Soviet Union had violated its political commitment to observe the SALT II Treaty. President Reagan decided, however, that an interim framework of mutual restraint remained in the U.S. interest and, in June 1985, declared that the United States would continue to refrain from undercutting existing strategic arms agreements to the extent that the Soviet Union exercised comparable restraint and provided that the Soviet Union actively pursued arms reductions agreements in the Nuclear and Space Talks in Geneva.

On May 26, 1986, President Reagan stated that he had reviewed again the status of U.S. interim restraint policy and that, as he had documented in three detailed reports to the Congress, the Soviet Union had not complied with its political commitment to observe the SALT agreements, including the SALT II Treaty, nor had the Soviet Union indicated its readiness to join in a framework of truly mutual restraint. He declared that, "Given this situation, ... in the future, the United States must base decisions regarding its strategic force structure on the nature and magnitude of the threat posed by Soviet strategic forces and not on standards contained in the SALT structure...." In his statement, President Reagan said that he did not anticipate any appreciable numerical growth in U.S. strategic offensive forces and that, assuming no significant change in the threat, the United States would not deploy more strategic nuclear delivery vehicles or strategic ballistic missile warheads than the Soviets. The United States would, in sum, "...continue to exercise the utmost restraint, while protecting strategic deterrence, in order to help foster the necessary atmosphere for significant reductions in the strategic arsenals of both sides." He again called upon the Soviet Union to join the United States "...in establishing an interim framework of truly *mutual* restraint."

The SALT II Treaty would have provided for:

• an equal aggregate limit on the number of strategic nuclear delivery vehicles -- ICBM and SLBM launchers, heavy bombers, and air-to-surface ballistic missiles (ASBMs). Initially, this ceiling would have been 2,400 as agreed at

Vladivostok. The ceiling would have been lowered to 2,250 at the end of 1981;

• an equal aggregate limit of 1,320 on the total number of launchers of MIRVed ballistic missiles and heavy bombers with long-range cruise missiles;

• an equal aggregate limit of 1,200 on the total number of launchers of MIRVed ballistic missiles; and

• an equal aggregate limit of 820 on launchers of MIRVed ICBMs.

In addition to these numerical limits, the agreement would have included:

• a ban on construction of additional fixed ICBM launchers, and on increases in the number of fixed heavy ICBM launchers;

• a ban on heavy mobile ICBM launchers, and on launchers of heavy submarine-launched ballistic missiles (SLBMs) and air-to-surface ballistic missiles (ASBMs);

• a ban on flight-testing or deployment of new types of ICBMs, with an exception of one new type of light ICBM for each side;

• a ban on increasing the numbers of warheads on existing types of ICBMs, and a limit of 10 warheads on the one new type of ICBM permitted to each Party, a limit of 14 warheads on SLBMs, and 10 warheads on ASBMs. The number of long-range cruise missiles per heavy bomber would have been limited to an average of 28; and the number of long-range cruise missiles per heavy bomber of existing types would have been limited to 20;

• ceilings on the launch-weight and throw-weight of strategic ballistic missiles and a ban on the conversion of light ICBM launchers to launchers of heavy ICBMs;

• a ban on the Soviet SS-16 ICBM;

• a ban on rapid reload ICBM systems;

• a ban on certain new types of strategic offensive systems which were technologically feasible, but which had not yet been deployed. Such systems included long-range ballistic

missiles on surface ships, and ballistic and cruise missile launchers on the seabeds;

• advance notification of certain ICBM test launches; and

• an agreed data base for systems included in various SALT-limited categories.

The Treaty also included detailed definitions of limited systems, provisions to enhance verification, a ban on circumvention of the provisions of the agreement, and a provision outlining the duties of the SCC in connection with the SALT II Treaty. The duration of the Treaty was to have been through 1985.

Verification of the SALT II Treaty would have been by national technical means (NTM) of verification, including photo-reconnaissance satellites. The sides had agreed not to interfere with each others' national technical means of verification, and not to use deliberate concealment measures which would have impeded verification by NTM of compliance with the provisions of the agreement. Because specific characteristics of some SALT-limited systems become apparent during the testing phase, monitoring of testing programs was an important aspect of SALT verification. Such monitoring might have involved collection of electronic signals known as telemetry which are used during tests to transmit information about systems while they are being tested. Therefore, the sides had agreed not to engage in deliberate denial of telemetric information such as through the use of telemetry encryption whenever such denial would have impeded verification of compliance with the provisions of the Treaty.

In addition to these provisions of the Treaty which directly addressed the question of verification, counting and distinguishability rules, as well as some constraints on specific systems, were incorporated into the agreement specifically for verification purposes.

To facilitate verification of the MIRV limits, the sides agreed that once a missile had been tested with MIRVs, then all missiles of that type were to be considered to have been equipped with MIRVs, even if that missile type had also been tested with a non-MIRV payload. Additionally, the sides agreed that once a launcher contained or launched a MIRVed missile, then all launchers of that type would be considered to be launchers of MIRVed missiles and included in the 1,320 limit. Similar counting rules were adopted for cruise missiles and for heavy bombers.

A constraint included for verification purposes was a ban on production, testing, and deployment of the Soviet SS-16 ICBM. The missile appeared to share a number of components with the Soviet SS-20, an intermediate range ballistic missile (IRBM). As the Parties had agreed that land-based launchers of ballistic missiles which are not ICBMs should not be converted into launchers of ICBMs, the United States sought this ban on the SS-16 in order to prevent verification problems which might have arisen if the SS-16 program had gone forward, since in that case distinguishing between SS-16 and SS-20 deployments would have been very difficult.

Pursuant to a Memorandum of Understanding, the sides exchanged data on the numbers of weapons in SALT-limited categories, and agreed to maintain this agreed data base through regular updates at each session of the Standing Consultative Commission. Although the United States did not require (and did not rely upon) this data for verification purposes, maintenance of the agreed data base would have insured that both parties applied the provisions of the Treaty in a consistent manner.

The protocol to the Treaty was to have remained in force until December 31, 1981. In the protocol the sides agreed to ban deployment of mobile ICBM launchers and flight-testing of ICBMs from such launchers. Development of such systems short of flight-testing would have been permitted. (After the protocol period, the Treaty specifically permitted the deployment of mobile ICBM launchers.)

Additionally, the protocol banned deployment, but not testing, of cruise missiles capable of ranges in excess of 600 kilometers on ground- and sea-based launchers. (The protocol would not have limited deployment of such systems after its expiration in 1981.)

Finally, the protocol included a ban on flight testing and deployment of ASBMs.

The Joint Statement of Principles, the third element of the SALT II agreement, would have established a basic framework for the next stage of SALT negotiations, SALT III. The sides agreed on the following general goals to be achieved in the next round of talks:

• significant and substantial reductions in the number of strategic offensive arms;

• further qualitative limitations on strategic offensive arms; and

• resolution of the issues included in the protocol.

The sides would also have considered other steps to enhance strategic stability, and either side could have brought up any other topic relevant to the limitation of strategic arms.

The Joint Statement of Principles also established the principle that cooperative measures might be used to ensure adequate verification of a SALT III agreement, raising the possibility of thus going beyond reliance on national technical means of verification alone.

TREATY BETWEEN THE UNITED STATES OF AMERICA AND THE UNION OF SOVIET SOCIALIST REPUBLICS ON THE LIMITATION OF STRATEGIC OFFENSIVE ARMS, TOGETHER WITH AGREED STATEMENTS AND COMMON UNDERSTANDINGS REGARDING THE TREATY*

Signed at Vienna June 18, 1979

The United States of America and the Union of Soviet Socialist Republics, hereinafter referred to as the Parties,

Conscious that nuclear war would have devastating consequences for all mankind,

Proceeding from the Basic Principles of Relations Between the United States of America and the Union of Soviet Socialist Republics of May 29, 1972,

Attaching particular significance to the limitation of strategic arms and determined to continue their efforts begun with the Treaty on the Limitation of Anti-Ballistic Missile Systems and the Interim Agreement on Certain Measures with Respect to the Limitation of Strategic Offensive Arms, of May 26, 1972,

Convinced that the additional measures limiting strategic offensive arms provided for in this Treaty will contribute to the improvement of relations between the Parties, help to reduce the risk of outbreak of nuclear war and strengthen international peace and security,

Mindful of their obligations under Article VI of the Treaty on the Non-Proliferation of Nuclear Weapons,

Guided by the principle of equality and equal security,

Recognizing that the strengthening of strategic stability meets the interests of the Parties and the interests of international security,

Reaffirming their desire to take measures for the further limitation and for the further reduction of strategic arms, having in mind the goal of achieving general and complete disarmament,

Declaring their intention to undertake in the near future negotiations further to limit and further to reduce strategic offensive arms,

Have agreed as follows:

Article I

Each Party undertakes, in accordance with the provisions of this Treaty, to limit strategic offensive arms quantitatively and qualitatively, to exercise restraint in the development of new types of strategic offensive arms, and to adopt other measures provided for in this Treaty.

Article II

For the purposes of this Treaty:

1. Intercontinental ballistic missile (ICBM) launchers are land-based launchers of ballistic missiles capable of a range in excess of the shortest distance between the northeastern border of the continental part of the territory of the United States of America and the northwestern border of the continental part of the territory of the Union of Soviet Socialist Republics, that is, a range in excess of 5,500 kilometers.

---

* The text of the SALT II Treaty and Protocol, as signed in Vienna, is accompanied by a set of Agreed Statements and Common Understandings, also signed by President Carter and General Secretary Brezhnev, which is prefaced as follows:

In connection with the Treaty Between the United States of America and the Union of Soviet Socialist Republics on the Limitation of Strategic Offensive Arms, the Parties have agreed on the following Agreed Statements and Common Understandings undertaken on behalf of the Government of the United States and the Government of the Union of Soviet Socialist Republics:

As an aid to the reader, the texts of the Agreed Statements and Common Understandings are beneath the articles of the Treaty or Protocol to which they pertain.

First Agreed Statement. The term "intercontinental ballistic missile launchers," as defined in paragraph 1 of Article II of the Treaty, includes all launchers which have been developed and tested for launching ICBMs. If a launcher has been developed and tested for launching an ICBM, all launchers of that type shall be considered to have been developed and tested for launching ICBMs.

First Common Understanding. If a launcher contains or launches an ICBM, that launcher shall be considered to have been developed and tested for launching ICBMs.

Second Common Understanding. If a launcher has been developed and tested for launching an ICBM, all launchers of that type, except for ICBM test and training launchers, shall be included in the aggregate numbers of strategic offensive arms provided for in Article III of the Treaty, pursuant to the provisions of Article VI of the Treaty.

Third Common Understanding. The one hundred and seventy-seven former Atlas and Titan I ICBM launchers of the United States of America, which are no longer operational and are partially dismantled, shall not be considered as subject to the limitations provided for in the Treaty.

Second Agreed Statement. After the date on which the Protocol ceases to be in force, mobile ICBM launchers shall be subject to the relevant limitations provided for in the Treaty which are applicable to ICBM launchers, unless the Parties agree that mobile ICBM launchers shall not be deployed after that date.

2. Submarine-launched ballistic missile (SLBM) launchers are launchers of ballistic missiles installed on any nuclear-powered submarine or launchers of modern ballistic missiles installed on any submarine, regardless of its type.

Agreed Statement. Modern submarine-launched ballistic missiles are: for the United States of America, missiles installed in all nuclear-powered submarines; for the Union of Soviet Socialist Republics, missiles of the type installed in nuclear-powered submarines made operational since 1965; and for both Parties, submarine-launched ballistic missiles first flight-tested since 1965 and installed in any submarine, regardless of its type.

3. Heavy bombers are considered to be:

(a) currently, for the United States of America, bombers of the B-52 and B-1 types, and for the Union of Soviet Socialist Republics, bombers of the Tupolev-95 and Myasishchev types;

(b) in the future, types of bombers which can carry out the mission of a heavy bomber in a manner similar or superior to that of bombers listed in subparagraph (a) above;

(c) types of bombers equipped for cruise missiles capable of a range in excess of 600 kilometers; and

(d) types of bombers equipped for ASBMs.

First Agreed Statement. The term "bombers," as used in paragraph 3 of Article II and other provisions of the Treaty, means airplanes of types initially constructed to be equipped for bombs or missiles.

Second Agreed Statement. The Parties shall notify each other on a case-by-case basis in the Standing Consultative Commission of inclusion of types of bombers as heavy bombers pursuant to the provisions of paragraph 3 of Article II of the Treaty; in this connection the Parties shall hold consultations, as appropriate, consistent with the provisions of paragraph 2 of Article XVII of the Treaty.

Third Agreed Statement. The criteria the Parties shall use to make case-by-case determinations of which types of bombers in the future can carry out the mission of a heavy bomber in a manner similar or superior to that of current heavy bombers, as referred to in subparagraph 3(b) of Article II of the Treaty, shall be agreed upon in the Standing Consultative Commission.

Fourth Agreed Statement. Having agreed that every bomber of a type included in paragraph 3 of Article II of the Treaty is to be considered a heavy bomber, the Parties further agree that:

(a) airplanes which otherwise would be bombers of a heavy bomber type shall not be considered to be bombers of a heavy bomber type if they have functionally related observable differences which indicate that they cannot perform the mission of a heavy bomber;

(b) airplanes which otherwise would be bombers of a type equipped for cruise missiles capable of a range in excess of 600 kilometers shall not be considered to be bombers of a type equipped for cruise missiles capable of a range in excess of 600 kilometers if they have functionally related observable differences which indicate that they cannot perform the mission of a bomber equipped for cruise missiles capable of a range in excess of 600 kilometers, except that heavy bombers of current types, as designated in subparagraph 3(a) of Article II of the Treaty, which otherwise would be of a type equipped for cruise missiles capable of a range in excess of 600 kilometers shall not be considered to be heavy bombers of a type equipped for cruise missiles capable of a range in excess of 600 kilometers if they are distinguishable on the basis of externally observable differences from heavy bombers of a type equipped for cruise missiles capable of a range in excess of 600 kilometers; and

(c) airplanes which otherwise would be bombers of a type equipped for ASBMs shall not be considered to be bombers of a type equipped for ASBMs if they have functionally related observable differences which indicate that they cannot perform the mission of a bomber equipped for ASBMs, except that heavy bombers of current types, as designated in subparagraph 3(a) of Article II of the Treaty, which otherwise would be of a type equipped for ASBMs shall not be considered to be heavy bombers of a type equipped for ASBMs if they are distinguishable on the basis of externally observable differences from heavy bombers of a type equipped for ASBMs.

First Common Understanding. Functionally related observable differences are differences in the observable features of airplanes which indicate whether or not these airplanes can perform the mission of a heavy bomber, or whether or not they can perform the mission of a bomber

equipped for cruise missiles capable of a range in excess of 600 kilometers or whether or not they can perform the mission of a bomber equipped for ASBMs. Functionally related observable differences shall be verifiable by national technical means. To this end, the Parties may take, as appropriate, cooperative measures contributing to the effectiveness of verification by national technical means.

Fifth Agreed Statement. Tupolev-142 airplanes in their current configuration, that is, in the configuration for anti-submarine warfare, are considered to be airplanes of a type different from types of heavy bombers referred to in subparagraph 3(a) of Article II of the Treaty and not subject to the Fourth Agreed Statement to paragraph 3 of Article II of the Treaty. This Agreed Statement does not preclude improvement of Tupolev-142 airplanes as an anti-submarine system, and does not prejudice or set a precedent for designation in the future of types of airplanes as heavy bombers pursuant to subparagraph 3(b) of Article II of the Treaty or for application of the Fourth Agreed Statement to paragraph 3 of Article II of the Treaty to such airplanes.

Second Common Understanding. Not later than six months after entry into force of the Treaty the Union of Soviet Socialist Republics will give its thirty-one Myasishchev airplanes used as tankers in existence as of the date of signature of the Treaty functionally related observable differences which indicate that they cannot perform the mission of a heavy bomber.

Third Common Understanding. The designations by the United States of America and by the Union of Soviet Socialist Republics for heavy bombers referred to in subparagraph 3(a) of Article II of the Treaty correspond in the following manner:

- Heavy bombers of the types designated by the United States of America as the B-52 and the B-1 are known to the Union of Soviet Socialist Republics by the same designations;

- Heavy bombers of the type designated by the Union of Soviet Socialist Republics as the Tupolev-95 are known to the United States of America as heavy bombers of the Bear type; and

- Heavy bombers of the type designated by the Union of Soviet Socialist Republics as the Myasishchev are known to the United States of America as heavy bombers of the Bison type.

---

4. Air-to-surface ballistic missiles (ASBMs) are any such missiles capable of a range in excess of 600 kilometers and installed in an aircraft or on its external mountings.

5. Launchers of ICBMs and SLBMs equipped with multiple independently targetable reentry vehicles (MIRVs) are launchers of the types developed and tested for launching ICBMs or SLBMs equipped with MIRVs.

First Agreed Statement. If a launcher has been developed and tested for launching an ICBM or an SLBM equipped with MIRVs, all launchers of that type shall be considered to have been developed and tested for launching ICBMs or SLBMs equipped with MIRVs.

First Common Understanding. If a launcher contains or launches an ICBM or an SLBM equipped with MIRVs, that launcher shall be considered to have been developed and tested for launching ICBMs or SLBMs equipped with MIRVs.

Second Common Understanding. If a launcher has been developed and tested for launching an ICBM or an SLBM equipped with MIRVs, all launchers of that type, except for ICBM and SLBM test and training launchers, shall be included in the corresponding aggregate numbers provided for in Article V of the Treaty, pursuant to the provisions of Article VI of the Treaty.

Second Agreed Statement. ICBMs and SLBMs equipped with MIRVs are ICBMs and SLBMs of the types which have been flight-tested with two or more independently targetable reentry vehicles, regardless of whether or not they have also been flight-tested with a single reentry vehicle or with multiple reentry vehicles which are not independently targetable. As of the date of signature of the Treaty, such ICBMs and SLBMs are: for the United States of America, Minuteman III ICBMs, Poseidon C-3 SLBMs, and Trident C-4 SLBMs; and for the Union of Soviet Socialist

Republics, RS-16, RS-18, RS-20 ICBMs and RSM-50 SLBMs.

Each Party will notify the other Party in the Standing Consultative Commission on a case-by-case basis of the designation of the one new type of light ICBM, if equipped with MIRVs, permitted pursuant to paragraph 9 of Article IV of the Treaty when first flight-tested; of designations of additional types of SLBMs equipped with MIRVs when first installed on a submarine; and of designations of types of ASBMs equipped with MIRVs when first flight-tested.

Third Common Understanding. The designations by the United States of America and by the Union of Soviet Socialist Republics for ICBMs and SLBMs equipped with MIRVs correspond in the following manner:

- Missiles of the type designated by the United States of America as the Minuteman III and known to the Union of Soviet Socialist Republics by the same designation, a light ICBM that has been flight-tested with multiple independently targetable reentry vehicles;

- Missiles of the types designated by the United States of America as the Poseidon C-3 and known to the Union of Soviet Socialist Republics by the same designation, an SLBM that was first flight-tested in 1968 and that has been flight-tested with multiple independently targetable reentry vehicles;

- Missiles of the type designated by the United States of America as the Trident C-4 and known to the Union of Soviet Socialist Republics by the same designation, an SLBM that was first flight-tested in 1977 and that has been flight-tested with multiple independently targetable reentry vehicles;

- Missiles of the type designated by the Union of Soviet Socialist Republics as the RS-16 and known to the United States of America as the SS-17, a light ICBM that has been flight-tested with a single reentry vehicle and with multiple independently targetable reentry vehicles;

- Missiles of the type designated by the Union of Soviet Socialist Republics as the RS-18 and known to the United States of America as the SS-19, the heaviest in terms of launch-weight and throw-weight of light ICBMs, which has been flight-tested with a single reentry vehicle and with multiple independently targetable reentry vehicles;

- Missiles of the type designated by the Union of Soviet Socialist Republics as the RS-20 and known to the United States of America as the SS-18, the heaviest in terms of launch-weight and throw-weight of heavy ICBMs, which has been flight-tested with a single reentry vehicle and with multiple independently targetable reentry vehicles;

- Missiles of the type designated by the Union of Soviet Socialist Republics as the RSM-50 and known to the United States of America as the SS-N-18, an SLBM that has been flight-tested with a single reentry vehicle and with multiple independently targetable reentry vehicles.

Third Agreed Statement. Reentry vehicles are independently targetable:

(a) if, after separation from the booster, maneuvering and targeting of the reentry vehicles to separate aim points along trajectories which are unrelated to each other are accomplished by means of devices which are installed in a self-contained dispensing mechanism or on the reentry vehicles, and which are based on the use of electronic or other computers in combination with devices using jet engines, including rocket engines, or aerodynamic systems;

(b) if maneuvering and targeting of the reentry vehicles to separate aim points along trajectories which are unrelated to each other are accomplished by means of other devices which may be developed in the future.

Fourth Common Understanding. For the purposes of this Treaty, all ICBM launchers in the Derazhnya and Pervomaysk areas in the Union of Soviet Socialist Republics are included in the aggregate numbers provided for in Article V of the Treaty.

Fifth Common Understanding. If ICBM or SLBM launchers are converted, constructed or undergo significant changes to their principal observable structural design features after entry into force of the Treaty, any such launchers which are launchers of missiles equipped with MIRVs shall be distinguishable from launchers of missiles not equipped with MIRVs, and any such launchers which are launchers of missiles not equipped with MIRVs shall be distinguishable from launchers of missiles equipped with MIRVs, on the basis of externally observable design features of the launchers. Submarines with launchers of SLBMs equipped with MIRVs shall be distinguishable from submarines with launchers of SLBMs not equipped with MIRVs on the basis of externally observable design features of the submarines.

This Common Understanding does not require changes to launcher conversion or construction programs, or to programs including significant changes to the principal observable structural design features of launchers, underway as of the date of signature of the Treaty.

---

6. ASBMs equipped with MIRVs are ASBMs of the types which have been flight-tested with MIRVs.

First Agreed Statement. ASBMs of the types which have been flight-tested with MIRVs are all ASBMs of the types which have been flight-tested with two or more independently targetable reentry vehicles, regardless of whether or not they have also been flight-tested with a single reentry vehicle or with multiple reentry vehicles which are not independently targetable.

Second Agreed Statement. Reentry vehicles are independently targetable:

(a) if, after separation from the booster, maneuvering and targeting of the reentry vehicles to separate aim points along trajectories which are unrelated to each other are accomplished by means of devices which are installed in a self-contained dispensing mechanism or on the reentry vehicles, and which are based on the use of electronic or other computers in combination with devices using jet engines, including rocket engines, or aerodynamic systems;

(b) if maneuvering and targeting of the reentry vehicles to separate aim points along trajectories which are unrelated to each other are accomplished by means of other devices which may be developed in the future.

7. Heavy ICBMs are ICBMs which have a launch-weight greater or a throw-weight greater than that of the heaviest, in terms of either launch-weight or throw-weight, respectively, of the light ICBMs deployed by either Party as of the date of signature of this Treaty.

First Agreed Statement. The launch-weight of an ICBM is the weight of the fully loaded missile itself at the time of launch.

Second Agreed Statement. The throw-weight of an ICBM is the sum of the weight of:

(a) its reentry vehicle or reentry vehicles;

(b) any self-contained dispensing mechanisms or other appropriate devices for targeting one reentry vehicle, or for releasing or for dispensing and targeting two or more reentry vehicles; and

(c) its penetration aids, including devices for their release.

Common Understanding. The term "other appropriate devices," as used in the definition of the throw-weight of an ICBM in the Second Agreed Statement to paragraph 7 of Article II of the Treaty, means any devices for dispensing and targeting two or more reentry vehicles; and any devices for releasing two or more reentry vehicles or for targeting one reentry vehicle, which cannot provide their reentry vehicles or reentry vehicle with additional velocity of more than 1,000 meters per second.

8. Cruise missiles are unmanned, self-propelled, guided, weapon-delivery vehicles which sustain flight through the use of aerodynamic lift over most of their flight path and which are flight-tested from or deployed on aircraft, that is, air-launched cruise missiles, or such vehicles which are referred to as cruise missiles in subparagraph 1(b) of Article IX.

First Agreed Statement. If a cruise missile is capable of a range in excess of 600 kilometers, all cruise missiles of that type shall be considered to be cruise missiles capable of a range in excess of 600 kilometers.

First Common Understanding. If a cruise missile has been flight-tested to a range in excess of 600 kilometers, it shall be considered to be a cruise missile capable of a range in excess of 600 kilometers.

Second Common Understanding. Cruise missiles not capable of a range in excess of 600 kilometers shall not be considered to be of a type capable of a range in excess of 600 kilometers if they are distinguishable on the basis of externally observable design features from cruise missiles of types capable of a range in excess of 600 kilometers.

Second Agreed Statement. The range of which a cruise missile is capable is the maximum distance which can be covered by the missile in its standard design mode flying until fuel exhaustion, determined by projecting its flight path onto the Earth's sphere from the point of launch to the point of impact.

Third Agreed Statement. If an unmanned, self-propelled, guided vehicle which sustains flight through the use of aerodynamic lift over most of its flight path has been flight-tested or deployed for weapon delivery, all vehicles of that type shall be considered to be weapon-delivery vehicles.

Third Common Understanding. Unmanned, self-propelled, guided vehicles which sustain flight through the use of aerodynamic lift over most of their flight path and are not weapon-delivery vehicles, that is, unarmed, pilotless, guided vehicles, shall not be considered to be cruise missiles if such vehicles are distinguishable from cruise missiles on the basis of externally observable design features.

Fourth Common Understanding. Neither Party shall convert unarmed, pilotless, guided vehicles into cruise missiles capable of a range in excess of 600 kilometers, nor shall either Party convert cruise missiles capable of a range in excess of 600 kilometers into unarmed, pilotless, guided vehicles.

Fifth Common Understanding. Neither Party has plans during the term of the Treaty to flight-test from or deploy on aircraft unarmed, pilotless, guided vehicles which are capable of a range in excess of 600 kilometers. In the future, should a Party have such plans, that Party will provide notification thereof to the other Party well in advance of such flight-testing or deployment. This Common Understanding does not apply to target drones.

Article III

1. Upon entry into force of this Treaty, each Party undertakes to limit ICBM launchers, SLBM launchers, heavy bombers, and ASBMs to an aggregate number not to exceed 2,400.

2. Each Party undertakes to limit, from January 1, 1981, strategic offensive arms referred to in paragraph 1 of this Article to an aggregate number not to exceed 2,250, and to initiate reductions of those arms which as of that date would be in excess of this aggregate number.

3. Within the aggregate numbers provided for in paragraphs 1 and 2 of this Article and subject to the provisions of this Treaty, each Party has the right to determine the composition of these aggregates.

4. For each bomber of a type equipped for ASBMs, the aggregate numbers provided for in paragraphs 1 and 2 of this Article shall include the maximum number of such missiles for which a bomber of that type is equipped for one operational mission.

5. A heavy bomber equipped only for ASBMs shall not itself be included in the aggregate numbers provided for in paragraphs 1 and 2 of this Article.

6. Reductions of the numbers of strategic offensive arms required to comply with the provisions of paragraphs 1 and 2 of this Article shall be carried out as provided for in Article XI.

Article IV

1. Each Party undertakes not to start construction of additional fixed ICBM launchers.

2. Each Party undertakes not to relocate fixed ICBM launchers.

3. Each Party undertakes not to convert launchers of light ICBMs, or of ICBMs of older types deployed prior to 1964, into launchers of heavy ICBMs of types deployed after that time.

4. Each Party undertakes in the process of modernization and replacement of ICBM silo launchers not to increase the original internal volume of an ICBM silo launcher by more than thirty-two percent. Within this limit each Party has the right to determine whether such an increase will be made through an increase in the original diameter or in the original depth of an ICBM silo launcher, or in both of these dimensions.

Agreed Statement. The word "original" in paragraph 4 of Article IV of the Treaty refers to the internal dimensions of an ICBM silo launcher, including its internal volume, as of May 26, 1972, or as of the date on which such launcher becomes operational, whichever is later.

Common Understanding. The obligations provided for in paragraph 4 of Article IV of the Treaty and in the Agreed Statement thereto mean that the original diameter or the original depth of an ICBM silo launcher may not be increased by an amount greater than that which would result in an increase in the original internal volume of the ICBM silo launcher by thirty-two percent solely through an increase in one of these dimensions.

---

5. Each Party undertakes:

(a) not to supply ICBM launcher deployment areas with intercontinental ballistic missiles in excess of a number consistent with normal deployment, maintenance, training, and replacement requirements;

(b) not to provide storage facilities for or to store ICBMs in excess of normal deployment requirements at launch sites of ICBM launchers;

(c) not to develop, test, or deploy systems for rapid reload of ICBM launchers.

Agreed Statement. The term "normal deployment requirements," as used in paragraph 5 of Article IV of the Treaty, means the deployment of one missile at each ICBM launcher.

6. Subject to the provisions of this Treaty, each Party undertakes not to have under construction at any time strategic offensive arms referred to in paragraph 1 of Article III in excess

of numbers consistent with a normal construction schedule.

Common Understanding. A normal construction schedule, in paragraph 6 of Article IV of the Treaty, is understood to be one consistent with the past or present construction practices of each Party.

---

7. Each Party undertakes not to develop, test, or deploy ICBMs which have a launch-weight greater or a throw-weight greater than that of the heaviest, in terms of either launch-weight or throw-weight, respectively, of the heavy ICBMs deployed by either Party as of the date of signature of this Treaty.

First Agreed Statement. The launch-weight of an ICBM is the weight of the fully loaded missile itself at the time of launch.

Second Agreed Statement. The throw-weight of an ICBM is the sum of the weight of:

(a) its reentry vehicle or reentry vehicles;

(b) any self-contained dispensing mechanisms or other appropriate devices for targeting one reentry vehicle, or for releasing or for dispensing and targeting two or more reentry vehicles; and

(c) its penetration aids, including devices for their release.

Common Understanding. The term "other appropriate devices," as used in the definition of the throw-weight of an ICBM in the Second Agreed Statement to paragraph 7 of Article IV of the Treaty, means any devices for dispensing and targeting two or more reentry vehicles; and any devices for releasing two or more reentry vehicles or for targeting one reentry vehicle, which cannot provide their reentry vehicles or reentry vehicle with additional velocity or more than 1,000 meters per second.

---

8. Each Party undertakes not to convert land-based launchers of ballistic missiles which are not ICBMs into launchers for launching ICBMs, and not to test them for this purpose.

Common Understanding. During the term of the Treaty, the Union of Soviet Socialist Republics will not produce, test, or deploy ICBMs of the type designated by the Union of Soviet Socialist Republics as the RS-14 and known to the United States of America as the SS-16, a light ICBM first flight-tested after 1970 and flight-tested only with a single reentry vehicle; this Common Understanding also means that the Union of Soviet Socialist Republics will not produce the third stage of that missile, the reentry vehicle of that missile, or the appropriate device for targeting the reentry vehicle of that missile.

---

9. Each Party undertakes not to flight-test or deploy new types of ICBMs, that is, types of ICBMs not flight-tested as of May 1, 1979, except that each Party may flight-test and deploy one new type of light ICBM.

First Agreed Statement. The term "new types of ICBMs," as used in paragraph 9 of Article IV of the Treaty, refers to any ICBM which is different from those ICBMs flight-tested as of May 1, 1979 in any one or more of the following respects:

(a) the number of stages, the length, the largest diameter, the launch-weight, or the throw-weight, of the missile;

(b) the type of propellant (that is, liquid or solid) of any of its stages.

First Common Understanding. As used in the First Agreed Statement to paragraph 9 of Article IV of the Treaty, the term "different," referring to the length, the diameter, the launch-weight, and the throw-weight of the missile, means a difference in excess of five percent.

Second Agreed Statement. Every ICBM of the one new type of light ICBM permitted to each Party pursuant to paragraph 9 of Article IV of the Treaty shall have the same number of stages and the same type of propellant (that is, liquid or solid) of each stage as the first ICBM of the one new type of light ICBM launched by that Party. In addition, after the twenty-fifth launch of an ICBM of that type, or after the last launch before deployment begins of ICBMs of that type, whichever occurs earlier, ICBMs of the one new type of light ICBM permitted to that Party shall not be different in any one or more of the following respects: the length, the largest diameter, the launch-weight, or the throw-weight, of the missile.

A Party which launches ICBMs of the one new type of light ICBM permitted pursuant to paragraph 9 of Article IV of the Treaty shall promptly notify the other Party of the date of the first launch and of the date of either the twenty-fifth or the last launch before deployment begins of ICBMs of that type, whichever occurs earlier.

Second Common Understanding. As used in the Second Agreed Statement to paragraph 9 of Article IV of the Treaty, the term "different," referring to the length, the diameter, the launch-weight, and the throw-weight, of the missile, means a difference in excess of five percent from the value established for each of the above parameters as of the twenty-fifth launch or as of the last launch before deployment begins, whichever occurs earlier. The values demonstrated in each of the above parameters during the last twelve of the twenty-five launches or during the last twelve launches before deployment begins, whichever twelve launches occur earlier, shall not vary by more than ten percent from any other of the corresponding values demonstrated during those twelve launches.

Third Common Understanding. The limitations with respect to launch-weight and throw-weight, provided for in the First Agreed Statement and the First Common Understanding to paragraph 9 of Article IV of the Treaty, do not preclude the flight-testing or the deployment of ICBMs with fewer reentry vehicles, or fewer penetration aids, or both, than the maximum number of reentry vehicles and the maximum number of penetration aids with which ICBMs of that type have been flight-tested as of May 1, 1979, even if this results in a decrease in launch-weight or in throw-weight in excess of five percent.

In addition to the aforementioned cases, those limitations do not preclude a decrease in launch-weight or in throw-weight in excess of five percent, in the case of the flight-testing or the deployment of ICBMs with a lesser quantity of propellant, including the propellant of a

self-contained dispensing mechanism or other appropriate device, than the maximum quantity of propellant, including the propellant of a self-contained dispensing mechanism or other appropriate device, with which ICBMs of that type have been flight-tested as of May 1, 1979, provided that such an ICBM is at the same time flight-tested or deployed with fewer reentry vehicles, or fewer penetration aids, or both, than the maximum number of reentry vehicles and the maximum number of penetration aids with which ICBMs of that type have been flight-tested as of May 1, 1979, and the decrease in launch-weight and throw-weight in such cases results only from the reduction in the number of reentry vehicles, or penetration aids, or both, and the reduction in the quantity of propellant.

Fourth Common Understanding. The limitations with respect to launch-weight and throw-weight, provided for in the Second Agreed Statement and the Second Common Understanding to paragraph 9 of Article IV of the Treaty, do not preclude the flight-testing or the deployment of ICBMs of the one new type of light ICBM permitted to each Party pursuant to paragraph 9 of Article IV of the Treaty with fewer reentry vehicles, or fewer penetration aids, or both, than the maximum number of reentry vehicles and the maximum number of penetration aids with which ICBMs of that type have been flight-tested, even if this results in a decrease in launch-weight or in throw-weight in excess of five percent.

In addition to the aforementioned cases, those limitations do not preclude a decrease in launch-weight or in throw-weight in excess of five percent, in the case of the flight-testing or the deployment of ICBMs of that type with a lesser quantity of propellant, including the propellant of a self-contained dispensing mechanism or other appropriate device, than the maximum quantity of propellant, including the propellant of a self-contained dispensing mechanism or other appropriate device, with which ICBMs of that type have been flight-tested, provided that such an ICBM is at the same time flight-tested or deployed with fewer reentry vehicles, or fewer penetration aids, or both, than the maximum number of reentry vehicles and the maximum number of penetration aids with which ICBMs of that type have been flight-tested, and the decrease in launch-weight and throw-weight in such cases results only from the reduction in the number of reentry vehicles, or penetration aids, or both, and the reduction in the quantity of propellant.

---

10. Each Party undertakes not to flight-test or deploy ICBMs of a type flight-tested as of May 1, 1979 with a number of reentry vehicles greater than the maximum number of reentry vehicles with which an ICBM of that type has been flight-tested as of that date.

First Agreed Statement. The following types of ICBMs and SLBMs equipped with MIRVs have been flight-tested with the maximum number of reentry vehicles set forth below:

For the United States of America

ICBMs of the Minuteman III type -- Seven reentry vehicles;

SLBMs of the Poseidon C-3 type -- Fourteen reentry vehicles;

SLBMs of the Trident C-4 type -- Seven reentry vehicles.

For the Union of Soviet Socialist Republics

ICBMs of the RS-16 type -- Four reentry vehicles;

ICBMs of the RS-18 type -- Six reentry vehicles;

ICBMs of the RS-20 type -- Ten reentry vehicles;

SLBMs of the RSM-50 type -- Seven reentry vehicles.

Common Understanding. Minuteman III ICBMs of the United States of America have been deployed with no more than three reentry vehicles. During the term of the Treaty, the United States of America has no plans to and will not flight-test or deploy missiles of this type with more than three reentry vehicles.

Second Agreed Statement. During the flight-testing of any ICBM, SLBM, or ASBM after May 1, 1979, the number of procedures for releasing or for dispensing may not exceed the

maximum number of reentry vehicles established for missiles of corresponding types as provided for in paragraphs 10, 11, 12, and 13 of Article IV of the Treaty. In this Agreed Statement "procedures for releasing or for dispensing" are understood to mean maneuvers of a missile associated with targeting and releasing or dispensing its reentry vehicles to aim points, whether or not a reentry vehicle is actually released or dispensed. Procedures for releasing anti-missile defense penetration aids will not be considered to be procedures for releasing or for dispensing a reentry vehicle so long as the procedures for releasing anti-missile defense penetration aids differ from those for releasing or for dispensing reentry vehicles.

Third Agreed Statement. Each Party undertakes:

(a) not to flight-test or deploy ICBMs equipped with multiple reentry vehicles, of a type flight-tested as of May 1, 1979, with reentry vehicles the weight of any of which is less than the weight of the lightest of those reentry vehicles with which an ICBM of that type has been flight-tested as of that date;

(b) not to flight-test or deploy ICBMs equipped with a single reentry vehicle and without an appropriate device for targeting a reentry vehicle, of a type flight-tested as of May 1, 1979, with a reentry vehicle the weight of which is less than the weight of the lightest reentry vehicle on an ICBM of a type equipped with MIRVs and flight-tested by that Party as of May 1, 1979; and

(c) not to flight-test or deploy ICBMs equipped with a single reentry vehicle and with an appropriate device for targeting a reentry vehicle, of a type flight-tested as of May 1, 1979, with a reentry vehicle the weight of which is less than fifty percent of the throw-weight of that ICBM.

---

11. Each Party undertakes not to flight-test or deploy ICBMs of the one new type permitted pursuant to paragraph 9 of this Article with a number of reentry vehicles greater than the maximum number of reentry vehicles with which an ICBM of either Party has been flight-tested as of May 1, 1979, that is, ten.

First Agreed Statement. Each Party undertakes not to flight-test or deploy the one new type of light ICBM permitted to each Party pursuant to paragraph 9 of Article IV of the Treaty with a number of reentry vehicles greater than the maximum number of reentry vehicles with which an ICBM of that type has been flight-tested as of the twenty-fifth launch or the last launch before deployment begins of ICBMs of that type, whichever occurs earlier.

Second Agreed Statement. During the flight-testing of any ICBM, SLBM, or ASBM after May 1, 1979 the number of procedures for releasing or for dispensing may not exceed the maximum number of reentry vehicles established for missiles of corresponding types as provided for in paragraphs 10, 11, 12, and 13 of Article IV of the Treaty. In this Agreed Statement "procedures for releasing or for dispensing" are understood to mean maneuvers of a missile associated with targeting and releasing or dispensing its reentry vehicles to aim points, whether or not a reentry vehicle is actually released or dispensed. Procedures for releasing anti-missile defense penetration aids will not be considered to be procedures for releasing or for dispensing a reentry vehicle so long as the procedures for releasing anti-missile defense penetration aids differ from those for releasing or for dispensing reentry vehicles.

---

12. Each Party undertakes not to flight-test or deploy SLBMs with a number of reentry vehicles greater than the maximum number of reentry vehicles with which an SLBM of either Party has been flight-tested as of May 1, 1979, that is, fourteen.

First Agreed Statement. The following types of ICBMs and SLBMs equipped with MIRVs have been flight-tested with the maximum number of reentry vehicles set forth below:

For the United States of America

ICBMs of the Minuteman III type -- Seven reentry vehicles;

SLBMs of the Poseidon C-3 type -- Fourteen reentry vehicles;

SLBMs of the Trident C-4 type -- Seven reentry vehicles.

For the Union of Soviet Socialist Republics

ICBMs of the RS-16 type -- Four reentry vehicles;

ICBMs of the RS-18 type -- Six reentry vehicles;

ICBMs of the RS-20 type -- Ten reentry vehicles;

SLBMs of the RSM-50 type -- Seven reentry vehicles.

Second Agreed Statement. During the flight-testing of any ICBM, SLBM, or ASBM after May 1, 1979 the number of procedures for releasing or for dispensing may not exceed the maximum number of reentry vehicles established for missiles of corresponding types as provided for in paragraphs 10, 11, 12, and 13 of Article IV of the Treaty. In this Agreed Statement "procedures for releasing or dispensing" are understood to mean maneuvers of a missile associated with targeting and releasing or dispensing its reentry vehicles to aim points, whether or not a reentry vehicle is actually released or dispensed. Procedures for releasing anti-missile defense penetration aids will not be considered to be procedures for releasing or for dispensing a reentry vehicle so long as the procedures for releasing anti-missile defense penetration aids differ from those for releasing or for dispensing reentry vehicles.

---

13. Each Party undertakes not to flight-test or deploy ASBMs with a number of reentry vehicles greater than the maximum number of reentry vehicles with which an ICBM of either Party has been flight-tested as of May 1, 1979, that is, ten.

Agreed Statement. During the flight-testing of any ICBM, SLBM, or ASBM after May 1, 1979 the number of procedures for releasing or for dispensing may not exceed the maximum number of reentry vehicles established for missiles of corresponding types as provided for in paragraphs 10, 11, 12, and 13 of Article IV of the Treaty. In this Agreed Statement "procedures for releasing or for dispensing" are understood to mean maneuvers of a missile associated with targeting and releasing or dispensing its reentry vehicles to aim points, whether or not a reentry vehicle is actually released or dispensed. Procedures for releasing anti-missile defense penetration aids will not be considered to be procedures for releasing or for dispensing a reentry vehicle so long as the procedures for releasing anti-missile defense penetration aids differ from those for releasing or for dispensing reentry vehicles.

---

14. Each Party undertakes not to deploy at any one time on heavy bombers equipped for cruise missiles capable of a range in excess of 600 kilometers a number of such cruise missiles which exceeds the product of 28 and the number of such heavy bombers.

First Agreed Statement. For the purposes of the limitation provided for in paragraph 14 of Article IV of the Treaty, there shall be considered to be deployed on each heavy bomber of a type equipped for cruise missiles capable of a range in excess of 600 kilometers the maximum number of such missiles for which any bomber of that type is equipped for one operational mission.

Second Agreed Statement. During the term of the Treaty no bomber of the B-52 or B-1 types of the United States of America and no bomber of the Tupolev-95 or Myasishchev types of the Union of Soviet Socialist Republics will be equipped for more than twenty cruise missiles capable of a range in excess of 600 kilometers.

Article V

1. Within the aggregate numbers provided for in paragraphs 1 and 2 of Article III, each Party undertakes to limit launchers of ICBMs and SLBMs equipped with MIRVs, ASBMs equipped with MIRVs, and heavy bombers equipped for cruise missiles capable of a range in excess of 600 kilometers to an aggregate number not to exceed 1,320.

2. Within the aggregate number provided for in paragraph 1 of this Article, each Party undertakes to limit launchers of ICBMs and SLBMs equipped with MIRVs, and ASBMs equipped with MIRVs to an aggregate number not to exceed 1,200.

3. Within the aggregate number provided for in paragraph 2 of this Article, each Party

undertakes to limit launchers of ICBMs equipped with MIRVs to an aggregate number not to exceed 820.

4. For each bomber of a type equipped for ASBMs equipped with MIRVs, the aggregate numbers provided for in paragraphs 1 and 2 of this Article shall include the maximum number of ASBMs for which a bomber of that type is equipped for one operational mission.

Agreed Statement. If a bomber is equipped for ASBMs equipped with MIRVs, all bombers of that type shall be considered to be equipped for ASBMs equipped with MIRVs.

---

5. Within the aggregate numbers provided for in paragraphs 1, 2, and 3 of this Article and subject to the provisions of this Treaty, each Party has the right to determine the composition of these aggregates.

Article VI

1. The limitations provided for in this Treaty shall apply to those arms which are:

(a) operational;

(b) in the final stage of construction;

(c) in reserve, in storage, or mothballed;

(d) undergoing overhaul, repair, modernization, or conversion.

2. Those arms in the final stage of construction are:

(a) SLBM launchers on submarines which have begun sea trials;

(b) ASBMs after a bomber of a type equipped for such missiles has been brought out of the shop, plant, or other facility where its final assembly or conversion for the purpose of equipping it for such missiles has been performed;

(c) other strategic offensive arms which are finally assembled in a shop, plant, or other facility after they have been brought out of the shop, plant, or other facility where their final assembly has been performed.

3. ICBM and SLBM launchers of a type not subject to the limitation provided for in Article V, which undergo conversion into launchers of a type subject to that limitation, shall become subject to that limitation as follows:

(a) fixed ICBM launchers when work on their conversion reaches the stage which first definitely indicates that they are being so converted;

(b) SLBM launchers on a submarine when that submarine first goes to sea after their conversion has been performed.

Agreed Statement. The procedures referred to in paragraph 7 of Article VI of the Treaty shall include procedures determining the manner in which mobile ICBM launchers of a type not subject to the limitation provided for in Article V of the Treaty, which undergo conversion into launchers of a type subject to that limitation, shall become subject to that limitation, unless the Parties agree that mobile ICBM launchers shall not be deployed after the date on which the Protocol ceases to be in force.

---

4. ASBMs on a bomber which undergoes conversion from a bomber of a type equipped for ASBMs which are not subject to the limitation provided for in Article V into a bomber of a type equipped for ASBMs which are subject to that limitation shall become subject to that limitation when the bomber is brought out of the shop, plant, or other facility where such conversion has been performed.

5. A heavy bomber of a type not subject to the limitation provided for in paragraph 1 of Article V shall become subject to that limitation when it is brought out of the shop, plant, or other facility where it has been converted into a heavy bomber of a type equipped for cruise missiles capable of a range in excess of 600 kilometers. A bomber of a type not subject to the limitation provided for in paragraph 1 or 2 of Article III shall become subject to that limitation and to the limitation provided for in paragraph 1 of Article V when it is brought out of the shop, plant, or other facility where it has been converted into a bomber of a

type equipped for cruise missiles capable of a range in excess of 600 kilometers.

6. The arms subject to the limitations provided for in this Treaty shall continue to be subject to these limitations until they are dismantled, are destroyed, or otherwise cease to be subject to these limitations under procedures to be agreed upon.

Agreed Statement. The procedures for removal of strategic offensive arms from the aggregate numbers provided for in the Treaty, which are referred to in paragraph 6 of Article VI of the Treaty, and which are to be agreed upon in the Standing Consultative Commission, shall include:

(a) procedures for removal from the aggregate numbers, provided for in Article V of the Treaty, of ICBM and SLBM launchers which are being converted from launchers of a type subject to the limitation provided for in Article V of the Treaty, into launchers of a type not subject to that limitation;

(b) procedures for removal from the aggregate numbers, provided for in Articles III and V of the Treaty, of bombers which are being converted from bombers of a type subject to the limitations provided for in Article III of the Treaty or in Articles III and V of the Treaty into airplanes or bombers of a type not so subject.

Common Understanding. The procedures referred to in subparagraph (b) of the Agreed Statement to paragraph 6 of Article VI of the Treaty for removal of bombers from the aggregate numbers provided for in Articles III and V of the Treaty shall be based upon the existence of functionally related observable differences which indicate whether or not they can perform the mission of a heavy bomber, or whether or not they can perform the mission of a bomber equipped for cruise missiles capable of a range in excess of 600 kilometers.

---

7. In accordance with the provisions of Article XVII, the Parties will agree in the Standing Consultative Commission upon procedures to implement the provisions of this Article.

Article VII

1. The limitations provided for in Article III shall not apply to ICBM and SLBM test and training launchers or to space vehicle launchers for exploration and use of outer space. ICBM and SLBM test and training launchers are ICBM and SLBM launchers used only for testing or training.

Common Understanding. The term "testing," as used in Article VII of the Treaty, includes research and development.

2. The Parties agree that:

(a) there shall be no significant increase in the number of ICBM or SLBM test and training launchers or in the number of such launchers of heavy ICBMs;

(b) construction or conversion of ICBM launchers at test ranges shall be undertaken only for purposes of testing and training;

(c) there shall be no conversion of ICBM test and training launchers or of space vehicle launchers into ICBM launchers subject to the limitations provided for in Article III.

First Agreed Statement. The term "significant increase," as used in subparagraph 2(a) of Article VII of the Treaty, means an increase of fifteen percent or more. Any new ICBM test and training launchers which replace ICBM test and training launchers at test ranges will be located only at test ranges.

Second Agreed Statement. Current test ranges where ICBMs are tested are located: for the United States of America, near Santa Maria, California, and at Cape Canaveral, Florida; and for the Union of Soviet Socialist Republics, in the areas of Tyura-Tam and Plesetskaya. In the future, each Party shall provide notification in the Standing Consultative Commission of the location of any other test range used by that Party to test ICBMs.

First Common Understanding. At test ranges where ICBMs are tested, other arms, including those not limited by the Treaty, may also be tested.

Second Common Understanding. Of the eighteen launchers of fractional orbital missiles at the test range where ICBMs are tested in the area of Tyura-Tam, twelve launchers shall be dismantled or destroyed and six launchers may be converted to launchers for testing missiles undergoing modernization.

Dismantling or destruction of the twelve launchers shall begin upon entry into force of the Treaty and shall be completed within eight months, under procedures for dismantling or destruction of these launchers to be agreed upon in the Standing Consultative Commission. These twelve launchers shall not be replaced.

Conversion of the six launchers may be carried out after entry into force of the Treaty. After entry into force of the Treaty, fractional orbital missiles shall be removed and shall be destroyed pursuant to the provisions of subparagraph 1(c) of Article IX and of Article XI of the Treaty and shall not be replaced by other missiles, except in the case of conversion of these six launchers for testing missiles undergoing modernization. After removal of the fractional orbital missiles, and prior to such conversion, any activities associated with these launchers shall be limited to normal maintenance requirements for launchers in which missiles are not deployed. These six launchers shall be subject to the provisions of Article VII of the Treaty and, if converted, to the provisions of the Fifth Common Understanding to paragraph 5 of Article II of the Treaty.

Article VIII

1. Each Party undertakes not to flight-test cruise missiles capable of a range in excess of 600 kilometers or ASBMs from aircraft other than bombers or to convert such aircraft into aircraft equipped for such missiles.

Agreed Statement. For purposes of testing only, each Party has the right, through initial construction or, as an exception to the provisions of paragraph 1 of Article VIII of the Treaty, by conversion, to equip for cruise missiles capable of a range in excess of 600 kilometers or for ASBMs no more than sixteen airplanes, including airplanes which are prototypes of bombers equipped for such missiles. Each Party also has the right, as an exception to the provisions of paragraph 1 of Article VIII of the Treaty, to flight-test from such airplanes cruise missiles capable of a range in excess of 600 kilometers and, after the date on which the Protocol ceases to be in force, to flight-test ASBMs from such airplanes as well, unless the Parties agree that they will not flight-test ASBMs after that date. The limitations provided for in Article III of the Treaty shall not apply to such airplanes.

The aforementioned airplanes may include only:

(a) airplanes other than bombers which, as an exception to the provisions of paragraph 1 of Article VIII of the Treaty, have been converted into airplanes equipped for cruise missiles capable of a range in excess of 600 kilometers or for ASBMs;

(b) airplanes considered to be heavy bombers pursuant to subparagraph 3(c) or 3(d) of Article II of the Treaty; and

(c) airplanes other than heavy bombers which, prior to March 7, 1979, were used for testing cruise missiles capable of a range in excess of 600 kilometers.

The airplanes referred to in subparagraphs (a) and (b) of this Agreed Statement shall be distinguishable on the basis of functionally related observable differences from airplanes which otherwise would be of the same type but cannot perform the mission of a bomber equipped for cruise missiles capable of a range in excess of 600 kilometers or for ASBMs.

The airplanes referred to in subparagraph (c) of this Agreed Statement shall not be used for testing cruise missiles capable of a range in excess of 600 kilometers after the expiration of a six-month period from the date of entry into force of the Treaty, unless by the expiration of that period they are distinguishable on the basis of functionally related observable differences from airplanes which otherwise would be of the same type but cannot perform the mission of a bomber equipped for cruise missiles capable of a range in excess of 600 kilometers.

First Common Understanding. The term "testing," as used in the Agreed Statement to paragraph 1

of Article VIII of the Treaty, includes research and development.

Second Common Understanding. The Parties shall notify each other in the Standing Consultative Commission of the number of airplanes, according to type, used for testing pursuant to the Agreed Statement to paragraph 1 of Article VIII of the Treaty. Such notification shall be provided at the first regular session of the Standing Consultative Commission held after an airplane has been used for such testing.

Third Common Understanding. None of the sixteen airplanes referred to in the Agreed Statement to paragraph 1 of Article VIII of the Treaty may be replaced, except in the event of the involuntary destruction of any such airplane or in the case of the dismantling or destruction of any such airplane. The procedures for such replacement and for removal of any such airplane from that number, in case of its conversion, shall be agreed upon in the Standing Consultative Commission.

---

2. Each Party undertakes not to convert aircraft other than bombers into aircraft which can carry out the mission of a heavy bomber as referred to in subparagraph 3(b) of Article II.

Article IX

1. Each Party undertakes not to develop, test, or deploy:

(a) ballistic missiles capable of a range in excess of 600 kilometers for installation on waterborne vehicles other than submarines, or launchers of such missiles;

Common Understanding to subparagraph (a). The obligations provided for in subparagraph 1(a) of Article IX of the Treaty do not affect current practices for transporting ballistic missiles.

(b) fixed ballistic or cruise missile launchers for emplacement on the ocean floor, on the seabed, or on the beds of internal waters and inland waters, or in the subsoil thereof, or mobile launchers of such missiles, which move only in contact with the ocean floor, the seabed, or the beds of internal waters and inland waters, or missiles for such launchers;

Agreed Statement to subparagraph (b). The obligations provided for in subparagraph 1(b) of Article IX of the Treaty shall apply to all areas of the ocean floor and the seabed, including the seabed zone referred to in Articles I and II of the 1971 Treaty on the Prohibition of the Emplacement of Nuclear Weapons and Other Weapons of Mass Destruction on the Seabed and the Ocean Floor and in the Subsoil Thereof.

(c) systems for placing into Earth orbit nuclear weapons or any other kind of weapons of mass destruction, including fractional orbital missiles;

Common Understanding to subparagraph (c). The provisions of subparagraph 1(c) of Article IX of the Treaty do not require the dismantling or destruction of any existing launchers of either Party.

(d) mobile launchers of heavy ICBMs;

(e) SLBMs which have a launch-weight greater or a throw-weight greater than that of the heaviest, in terms of either launch-weight or throw-weight, respectively, of the light ICBMs deployed by either Party as of the date of signature of this Treaty, or launchers of such SLBMs; or

(f) ASBMs which have a launch-weight greater or a throw-weight greater than that of the heaviest, in terms of either launch-weight or throw-weight, respectively, of the light ICBMs deployed by either Party as of the date of signature of this Treaty.

First Agreed Statement to subparagraphs (e) and (f). The launch-weight of an SLBM or of an ASBM is the weight of the fully loaded missile itself at the time of launch.

Second Agreed Statement to subparagraphs (e) and (f). The throw-weight of an SLBM or of an ASBM is the sum of the weight of:

(a) its reentry vehicle or reentry vehicles;

(b) any self-contained dispensing mechanisms or other appropriate devices for targeting one reentry vehicle, or for releasing or for dispensing and targeting two or more reentry vehicles; and

(c) its penetration aids, including devices for their release.

Common Understanding to subparagraphs (e) and (f). The term "other appropriate devices," as used in the definition of the throw-weight of an SLBM or of an ASBM in the Second Agreed Statement to subparagraphs 1(e) and (f) of Article IX of the Treaty, means any devices for dispensing and targeting two or more reentry vehicles; and any devices for releasing two or more reentry vehicles or for targeting one reentry vehicle, which cannot provide their reentry vehicles or reentry vehicle with additional velocity of more than 1,000 meters per second.

---

2. Each Party undertakes not to flight-test from aircraft cruise missiles capable of a range in excess of 600 kilometers which are equipped with multiple independently targetable warheads and not to deploy such cruise missiles on aircraft.

Agreed Statement. Warheads of a cruise missile are independently targetable if maneuvering or targeting of the warheads to separate aim points along ballistic trajectories or any other flight paths, which are unrelated to each other, is accomplished during a flight of a cruise missile.

Article X

Subject to the provisions of this Treaty, modernization and replacement of strategic offensive arms may be carried out.

Article XI

1. Strategic offensive arms which would be in excess of the aggregate numbers provided for in this Treaty as well as strategic offensive arms prohibited by this Treaty shall be dismantled or destroyed under procedures to be agreed upon in the Standing Consultative Commission.

2. Dismantling or destruction of strategic offensive arms which would be in excess of the aggregate number provided for in paragraph 1 of Article III shall begin on the date of the entry into force of this Treaty and shall be completed within the following periods from that date: four months for ICBM launchers; six months for SLBM launchers; and three months for heavy bombers.

3. Dismantling or destruction of strategic offensive arms which would be in excess of the aggregate number provided for in paragraph 2 of Article III shall be initiated no later than January 1, 1981, shall be carried out throughout the ensuing twelve-month period, and shall be completed no later than December 31, 1981.

4. Dismantling or destruction of strategic offensive arms prohibited by this Treaty shall be completed within the shortest possible agreed period of time, but not later than six months after the entry into force of this Treaty.

Article XII

In order to ensure the viability and effectiveness of this Treaty, each Party undertakes not to circumvent the provisions of this Treaty, through any other state or states, or in any other manner.

Article XIII

Each Party undertakes not to assume any international obligations which would conflict with this Treaty.

Article XIV

The Parties undertake to begin, promptly after the entry into force of this Treaty, active negotiations with the objective of achieving, as soon as possible, agreement on further measures for the limitation and reduction of strategic arms. It is also the objective of the Parties to conclude well in advance of 1985 an agreement limiting strategic offensive arms to replace this Treaty upon its expiration.

Article XV

1. For the purpose of providing assurance of compliance with the provisions of this Treaty, each Party shall use national technical means of verification at its disposal in a manner consistent with generally recognized principles of international law.

2. Each party undertakes not to interfere with the national technical means of verification of the other Party operating in accordance with paragraph 1 of this Article.

3. Each Party undertakes not to use deliberate concealment measures which impede verification by national technical means of compliance with the provisions of this Treaty. This obligation shall not require changes in current construction, assembly, conversion, or overhaul practices.

First Agreed Statement. Deliberate concealment measures, as referred to in paragraph 3 of Article XV of the Treaty, are measures carried out deliberately to hinder or deliberately to impede verification by national technical means of compliance with the provisions of the Treaty.

Second Agreed Statement. The obligation not to use deliberate concealment measures, provided for in paragraph 3 of Article XV of the Treaty, does not preclude the testing of anti-missile defense penetration aids.

First Common Understanding. The provisions of paragraph 3 of Article XV of the Treaty and the First Agreed Statement thereto apply to all provisions of the Treaty, including provisions associated with testing. In this connection, the obligation not to use deliberate concealment measures associated with testing, including those measures aimed at concealing the association between ICBMs and launchers during testing.

Second Common Understanding. Each Party is free to use various methods of transmitting telemetric information during testing, including its encryption, except that, in accordance with the provisions of paragraph 3 of Article XV of the Treaty, neither Party shall engage in deliberate denial of telemetric information, such as through the use of telemetry encryption, whenever such denial impedes verification of compliance with the provisions of the Treaty.

Third Common Understanding. In addition to the obligations provided for in paragraph 3 of Article XV of the Treaty, no shelters which impede verification by national technical means of compliance with the provisions of the Treaty shall be used over ICBM silo launchers.

Article XVI

1. Each Party undertakes, before conducting each planned ICBM launch, to notify the other Party well in advance on a case-by-case basis that such a launch will occur, except for single ICBM launches from test ranges or from ICBM launcher deployment areas, which are not planned to extend beyond its national territory.

First Common Understanding. ICBM launches to which the obligations provided for in Article XVI of the Treaty apply, include, among others, those ICBM launches for which advance notification is required pursuant to the provisions of the Agreement on Measures to Reduce the Risk of Outbreak of Nuclear War Between the United States of America and the Union of Soviet Socialist Republics, signed September 30, 1971, and the Agreement Between the Government of the United States of America and the Government of the Union of Soviet Socialist Republics on the Prevention of Incidents On and Over the High Seas, signed May 25, 1972. Nothing in Article XVI of the Treaty is intended to inhibit advance notification, on a voluntary basis, of any ICBM launches not subject to its provisions, the advance notification of which would enhance confidence between the Parties.

Second Common Understanding. A multiple ICBM launch conducted by a Party, as distinct from single ICBM launches referred to in Article XVI of the Treaty, is a launch which would result in two or more of its ICBMs being in flight at the same time.

Third Common Understanding. The test ranges referred to in Article XVI of the Treaty are those covered by the Second Agreed Statement to paragraph 2 of Article VII of the Treaty.

---

2. The Parties shall agree in the Standing Consultative Commission upon procedures to implement the provisions of this Article.

Article XVII

1. To promote the objectives and implementation of the provisions of this Treaty, the Parties shall use the Standing Consultative Commission established by the Memorandum of Understanding Between the Government of the United States of America and the Government of the Union of Soviet Socialist Republics Regarding the Establishment of a Standing Consultative Commission of December 21, 1972.

2. Within the framework of the Standing Consultative Commission, with respect to this Treaty, the Parties will:

(a) consider questions concerning compliance with the obligations assumed and related situations which may be considered ambiguous;

(b) provide on a voluntary basis such information as either Party considers necessary to assure confidence in compliance with the obligations assumed;

(c) consider questions involving unintended interference with national technical means of verification, and questions involving unintended impeding of verification by national technical means of compliance with the provisions of this Treaty;

(d) consider possible changes in the strategic situation which have a bearing on the provisions of this Treaty;

(e) agree upon procedures for replacement, conversion, and dismantling or destruction, of strategic offensive arms in cases provided for in the provisions of this Treaty and upon procedures for removal of such arms from the aggregate numbers when they otherwise cease to be subject to the limitations provided for in this Treaty, and at regular sessions of the Standing Consultative Commission, notify each other in accordance with the aforementioned procedures, at least twice annually, of actions completed and those in process;

(f) consider, as appropriate, possible proposals for further increasing the viability of this Treaty, including proposals for amendments in accordance with the provisions of this Treaty;

(g) consider, as appropriate, proposals for further measures limiting strategic offensive arms.

3. In the Standing Consultative Commission the Parties shall maintain by category the agreed data base on the numbers of strategic offensive arms established by the Memorandum of Understanding Between the United States of America and the Union of Soviet Socialist Republics Regarding the Establishment of a Data Base on the Numbers of Strategic Offensive Arms of June 18, 1979.

Agreed Statement. In order to maintain the agreed data base on the numbers of strategic offensive arms subject to the limitations provided for in the Treaty in accordance with paragraph 3 of Article XVII of the Treaty, at each regular session of the Standing Consultative Commission the Parties will notify each other of and consider changes in those numbers in the following categories: launchers of ICBMs; fixed launchers of ICBMs; launchers of ICBMs equipped with MIRVs; launchers of SLBMs; launchers of SLBMs equipped with MIRVs; heavy bombers; heavy bombers equipped for cruise missiles capable of a range in excess of 600 kilometers; heavy bombers equipped only for ASBMs; ASBMs; and ASBMs equipped with MIRVs.

Article XVIII

Each Party may propose amendments to this Treaty. Agreed amendments shall enter into force in accordance with the procedures governing the entry into force of this Treaty.

Article XIX

1. This Treaty shall be subject to ratification in accordance with the constitutional procedures of each Party. This Treaty shall enter into force on the day of the exchange of instruments of ratification and shall remain in force through December 31, 1985, unless replaced earlier by an agreement further limiting strategic offensive arms.

2. This Treaty shall be registered pursuant to Article 102 of the Charter of the United Nations.

3. Each Party shall, in exercising its national sovereignty, have the right to withdraw from this Treaty if it decides that extraordinary events related to the subject matter of this Treaty have jeopardized its supreme interests. It shall give notice of its decision to the other Party six months prior to withdrawal from the Treaty. Such notice shall include a statement of the extraordinary events the notifying Party regards as having jeopardized its supreme interests.

DONE at Vienna on June 18, 1979, in two copies, each in the English and Russian languages, both texts being equally authentic.

FOR THE UNITED STATES OF AMERICA:
JIMMY CARTER
President of the United States of America

FOR THE UNION OF SOVIET SOCIALIST REPUBLICS:
L. BREZHNEV
General Secretary of the CPSU, Chairman of the Presidium of the Supreme Soviet of the USSR

PROTOCOL TO THE TREATY BETWEEN THE UNITED STATES OF AMERICA AND THE UNION OF SOVIET SOCIALIST REPUBLICS ON THE LIMITATION OF STRATEGIC OFFENSIVE ARMS, TOGETHER WITH AGREED STATEMENTS AND COMMON UNDERSTANDINGS REGARDING THE PROTOCOL

The United States of America and the Union of Soviet Socialist Republics, hereinafter referred to as the Parties,

Having agreed on limitations on strategic offensive arms in the Treaty,

Having agreed on additional limitations for the period during which this Protocol remains in force, as follows:

Article I

Each Party undertakes not to deploy mobile ICBM launchers or to flight-test ICBMs for such launchers.

Article II

1. Each Party undertakes not to deploy cruise missiles capable of a range in excess of 600 kilometers on sea-based launchers or on land-based launchers.

2. Each Party undertakes not to flight-test cruise missiles capable of a range in excess of 600 kilometers which are equipped with multiple independently targetable warheads from sea-based launchers or from land-based launchers.

Agreed Statement. Warheads of a cruise missile are independently targetable if maneuvering or targeting of the warheads to separate aim points along ballistic trajectories or any other flight paths, which are unrelated to each other, is accomplished during a flight of a cruise missile.

3. For the purposes of this Protocol, cruise missiles are unmanned, self-propelled, guided, weapon-delivery vehicles which sustain flight through the use of aerodynamic lift over most of their flight path and which are flight-tested from or deployed on sea-based or land-based launchers, that is, sea-launched cruise missiles and ground-launched cruise missiles, respectively.

First Agreed Statement. If a cruise missile is capable of a range in excess of 600 kilometers, all cruise missiles of that type shall be considered to be cruise missiles capable of a range in excess of 600 kilometers.

First Common Understanding. If a cruise missile has been flight-tested to a range in excess of 600 kilometers, it shall be considered to be a cruise missile capable of a range in excess of 600 kilometers.

Second Common Understanding. Cruise missiles not capable of a range in excess of 600 kilometers shall not be considered to be of a type capable of a range in excess of 600 kilometers if they are distinguishable on the basis of externally observable design features from cruise missiles of types capable of a range in excess of 600 kilometers.

Second Agreed Statement. The range of which a cruise missile is capable is the maximum distance which can be covered by the missile in its standard design mode flying until fuel exhaustion, determined by projecting its flight path onto the Earth's sphere from the point of launch to the point of impact.

Third Agreed Statement. If an unmanned, self-propelled, guided vehicle which sustains flight through the use of aerodynamic lift over most of its flight path has been flight-tested or deployed for weapon delivery, all vehicles of that type shall be considered to be weapon-delivery vehicles.

Third Common Understanding. Unmanned, self-propelled, guided vehicles which sustain flight through the use of aerodynamic lift over most of their flight path and are not weapon-delivery vehicles, that is, unarmed, pilotless, guided vehicles, shall not be considered to be cruise missiles if such vehicles are distinguishable from cruise missiles on the basis of externally observable design features.

Fourth Common Understanding. Neither Party shall convert unarmed, pilotless, guided vehicles into cruise missiles capable of a range in excess of 600 kilometers, nor shall either Party convert cruise missiles capable of a range in excess of 600 kilometers into unarmed, pilotless, guided vehicles.

Fifth Common Understanding. Neither Party has plans during the term of the Protocol to flight-test from or deploy on sea-based or land-based launchers unarmed, pilotless, guided vehicles which are capable of a range in excess of 600 kilometers. In the future, should a Party have such plans, that Party will provide notification thereof to the other Party well in advance of such flight-testing or deployment. This Common Understanding does not apply to target drones.

Article III

Each Party undertakes not to flight-test or deploy ASBMs.

Article IV

This Protocol shall be considered an integral part of the Treaty. It shall enter into force on the day of the entry into force of the Treaty and shall remain in force through December 31, 1981, unless replaced earlier by an agreement on further measures limiting strategic offensive arms.

DONE at Vienna on June 18, 1979, in two copies, each in the English and Russian languages, both texts being equally authentic.

FOR THE UNITED STATES OF AMERICA:
JIMMY CARTER
President of the United States of America

FOR THE UNION OF SOVIET SOCIALIST REPUBLICS:
L. BREZHNEV
General Secretary of the CPSU, Chairman of the Presidium of the Supreme Soviet of the USSR

MEMORANDUM OF UNDERSTANDING BETWEEN THE UNITED STATES OF AMERICA AND THE UNION OF SOVIET SOCIALIST REPUBLICS REGARDING THE ESTABLISHMENT OF A DATA BASE ON THE NUMBERS OF STRATEGIC OFFENSIVE ARMS

For the purposes of the Treaty Between the United States of America and the Union of Soviet Socialist Republics on the Limitation of Strategic Offensive Arms, the Parties have considered data on numbers of strategic offensive arms and agree that as of November 1, 1978 there existed the following numbers of strategic offensive arms subject to the limitations provided for in the Treaty which is being signed today.

	U.S.A.	USSR
Launchers of ICBMs	1,054	1,398
Fixed launchers of ICBMs	1,054	1,398
Launchers of ICBMs equipped with MIRVs	550	576
Launchers of SLBMs	656	950
Launchers of SLBMs equipped with MIRVs	496	128
Heavy bombers	574	156
Heavy bombers equipped for cruise missiles capable of a range in excess of 600 kilometers	0	0
Heavy bombers equipped only for ASBMs	0	0
ASBMs	0	0
ASBMs equipped with MIRVs	0	0

At the time of entry into force of the Treaty the Parties will update the above agreed data in the categories listed in this Memorandum.

DONE at Vienna on June 18, 1979, in two copies, each in the English and Russian languages, both texts being equally authentic.

FOR THE UNITED STATES OF AMERICA:
RALPH EARLE II
Chief of the United States Delegation to the Strategic Arms Limitation Talks

FOR THE UNION OF SOVIET SOCIALIST REPUBLICS:
V. KARPOV
Chief of the USSR Delegation to the Strategic Arms Limitation Talks

STATEMENT OF DATA ON THE NUMBERS OF STRATEGIC OFFENSIVE ARMS AS OF THE DATE OF SIGNATURE OF THE TREATY

The United States of America declares that as of June 18, 1979 it possesses the following numbers of strategic offensive arms subject to the limitations provided for in the Treaty which is being signed today:

Launchers of ICBMs	1,054
Fixed launchers of ICBMs	1,054
Launchers of ICBMs equipped with MIRVs	550
Launchers of SLBMs	656
Launchers of SLBMs equipped with MIRVs	496
Heavy bombers	573
Heavy bombers equipped for cruise missiles capable of a range in excess of 600 kilometers	3
Heavy bombers equipped only for ASBMs	0
ASBMs	0
ASBMs equipped with MIRVs	0

June 18, 1979
RALPH EARLE II
Chief of the United States Delegation to the Strategic Arms Limitation Talks

I certify that this is a true copy of the document signed by Ambassador Ralph Earle II entitled "Statement of Data on the Numbers of Strategic Offensive Arms as of the Date of Signature of the Treaty" and given to Ambassador V. Karpov on June 18, 1979 in Vienna, Austria.

THOMAS GRAHAM, JR.
General Counsel
United States Arms Control
and Disarmament Agency

**STATEMENT OF DATA ON THE NUMBERS OF
STRATEGIC OFFENSIVE ARMS AS OF THE
DATE OF SIGNATURE OF THE TREATY**

The Union of Soviet Socialist Republics
declares that as of June 18, 1979 it possesses
the following numbers of strategic offensive arms
subject to the limitations provided for in the Treaty
which is being signed today:

Launchers of ICBMs	1,398
Fixed launchers of ICBMs	1,398
Launchers of ICBMs equipped with MIRVs	608
Launchers of SLBMs	950
Launchers of SLBMs equipped with MIRVs	144
Heavy bombers	156
Heavy bombers equipped for cruise missiles capable of a range in excess of 600 kilometers	0
Heavy bombers equipped only for ASBMs	0
ASBMs	0
ASBMs equipped with MIRVs	0

June 18, 1979

V. KARPOV
*Chief of the USSR Delegation to the Strategic
Arms Limitation Talks*

Translation certified by:

W. D. Krimer,
*Senior Language Officer,
Division of Language Services, U.S. Department
of State*

WILLIAM D. KRIMER

**JOINT STATEMENT OF PRINCIPLES AND
BASIC GUIDELINES FOR SUBSEQUENT
NEGOTIATIONS ON THE LIMITATION OF
STRATEGIC ARMS**

The United States of America and the Union
of Soviet Socialist Republics, hereinafter referred
to as the Parties,

Having concluded the Treaty on the Limitation
of Strategic Offensive Arms,

Reaffirming that the strengthening of strategic
stability meets the interests of the Parties and the
interests of international security,

Convinced that early agreement on the further
limitation and further reduction of strategic arms
would serve to strengthen international peace and
security and to reduce the risk of outbreak of
nuclear war,

Have agreed as follows:

First. The Parties will continue to pursue
negotiations, in accordance with the principle of
equality and equal security, on measures for the
further limitation and reduction in the numbers of
strategic arms, as well as for their further
qualitative limitation.

In furtherance of existing agreements
between the Parties on the limitation and
reduction of strategic arms, the Parties will
continue, for the purposes of reducing and
averting the risk of outbreak of nuclear war, to
seek measures to strengthen strategic stability
by, among other things, limitations on strategic
offensive arms most destabilizing to the strategic
balance and by measures to reduce and to avert
the risk of surprise attack.

Second. Further limitations and reductions of
strategic arms must be subject to adequate
verification by national technical means, using
additionally, as appropriate, cooperative
measures contributing to the effectiveness of
verification by national technical means. The
Parties will seek to strengthen verification and to
perfect the operation of the Standing Consultative
Commission in order to promote assurance of
compliance with the obligations assumed by the
Parties.

Third. The Parties shall pursue in the course
of these negotiations, taking into consideration
factors that determine the strategic situation, the
following objectives:

1) significant and substantial reductions in the
numbers of strategic offensive arms;

2) qualitative limitations on strategic offensive
arms, including restrictions on the development,
testing, and deployment of new types of strategic
offensive arms and on the modernization of
existing strategic offensive arms;

3) resolution of the issues included in the
Protocol to the Treaty Between the United States
of America and the Union of Soviet Socialist
Republics on the Limitation of Strategic Offensive
Arms in the context of the negotiations relating to
the implementation of the principles and
objectives set out herein.

Fourth. The Parties will consider other steps
to ensure and enhance strategic stability, to
ensure the equality and equal security of the
Parties, and to implement the above principles
and objectives. Each Party will be free to raise
any issue relative to the further limitation of
strategic arms. The Parties will also consider
further joint measures, as appropriate, to
strengthen international peace and security and to
reduce the risk of outbreak of nuclear war.

Vienna, June 18, 1979

**FOR THE UNITED STATES OF AMERICA:
JIMMY CARTER**
President of the United States of America

**FOR THE UNION OF SOVIET SOCIALIST
REPUBLICS:
L. BREZHNEV**
*General Secretary for the CPSU, Chairman of the
Presidium of the Supreme Soviet of the USSR*

SOVIET BACKFIRE STATEMENT

On June 16, 1979, President Brezhnev handed President Carter the following written statement [original Russian text was attached]:

> The Soviet side informs the U.S. side that the Soviet "Tu-22M" airplane, called "Backfire" in the U.S.A., is a medium-range bomber, and that it does not intend to give this airplane the capability of operating at intercontinental distances. In this connection, the Soviet side states that it will not increase the radius of action of this airplane in such a way as to enable it to strike targets on the territory of the U.S.A. Nor does it intend to give it such a capability in any other manner, including by in-flight refueling. At the same time, the Soviet side states that it will not increase the production rate of this airplane as compared to the present rate.

President Brezhnev confirmed that the Soviet Backfire production rate would not exceed 30 per year.

President Carter stated that the United States enters into the SALT II Agreement on the basis of the commitments contained in the Soviet statement and that it considers the carrying out of these commitments to be essential to the obligations assumed under the Treaty.

CYRUS VANCE

CONVENTION ON THE PHYSICAL PROTECTION OF NUCLEAR MATERIAL

The Convention on the Physical Protection of Nuclear Material provides for certain levels of physical protection during international transport of nuclear material. It also establishes a general framework for cooperation among states in the protection, recovery, and return of stolen nuclear material. Further, the Convention lists certain serious offenses involving nuclear material which state parties are to make punishable and for which offenders shall be subject to a system of extradition or submission for prosecution.

This Convention resulted from a U.S. initiative in 1974, which was subsequently endorsed at the 1975 Non-Proliferation Treaty review conference. Two provisions of the Nuclear Non-Proliferation Act of 1978 call for negotiation of such a convention. Negotiation of the Convention had begun in 1977.

The Convention was adopted at a meeting of government representatives in Vienna on October 26, 1979, and signed by the United States on March 3, 1980. The U.S. Senate provided its advice and consent for the ratification of the Convention on July 30, 1981, by a vote of 98-0. The President ratified it September 4, 1981.

Legislation to implement the Convention was enacted October 18, 1982. The United States deposited its instrument of ratification December 13, 1982. The Convention entered into force February 8, 1987, in accordance with the provision for entry into force 30 days after the deposit of the instrument of ratification by the 21st State, which was Switzerland.

CONVENTION ON THE PHYSICAL PROTECTION OF NUCLEAR MATERIAL

Signed at New York March 3, 1980
Ratification advised by U.S. Senate July 30, 1981
Ratified by U.S. President September 4, 1981
U.S. ratification deposited at Vienna December 13, 1982
Entered into force February 8, 1987

The States Parties to This Convention,

Recognizing the right of all States to develop and apply nuclear energy for peaceful purposes and their legitimate interests in the potential benefits to be derived from the peaceful application of nuclear energy,

Convinced of the need for facilitating international co-operation in the peaceful application of nuclear energy,

Desiring to avert the potential dangers posed by the unlawful taking and use of nuclear material,

Convinced that offenses relating to nuclear material are a matter of grave concern and that there is an urgent need to adopt appropriate and effective measures to ensure the prevention, detection and punishment of such offenses,

Aware of the Need for international co-operation to establish, in conformity with the national law of each State Party and with this Convention, effective measures for the physical protection of nuclear material,

Convinced that this Convention should facilitate the safe transfer of nuclear material,

Stressing also the importance of the physical protection of nuclear material in domestic use, storage and transport,

Recognizing the importance of effective physical protection of nuclear material used for military purposes, and understanding that such material is and will continue to be accorded stringent physical protection,

Have Agreed as follows:

Article 1

For the purposes of this Convention:

(a) "nuclear material" means plutonium except that with isotopic concentration exceeding 80% in plutonium-238; uranium-233; uranium enriched in the isotopes 235 or 233; uranium containing the mixture of isotopes as occurring in nature other than in the form of ore or ore-residue; any material containing one or more of the foregoing;

(b) "uranium enriched in the isotopes 235 or 233" means uranium containing the isotopes 235 or 233 or both in an amount such that the abundance ratio of the sum of these isotopes to the isotope 238 is greater than the ratio of the isotope 235 to the isotope 238 occurring in nature;

(c) "international nuclear transport" means the carriage of a consignment of nuclear material by any means of transportation intended to go beyond the territory of the State where the shipment originates beginning with the departure from a facility of the shipper in that State and ending with the arrival at a facility of the receiver within the State of ultimate destination.

Article 2

1. The Convention shall apply to nuclear material used for peaceful purposes while in international nuclear transport.

2. With the exception of articles 3 and 4 and paragraph 3 of article 5, this Convention shall also apply to nuclear material used for peaceful purposes while in domestic use, storage and transport.

3. Apart from the commitments expressly undertaken by States Parties in the articles covered by paragraph 2 with respect to nuclear material used for peaceful purposes while in domestic use, storage and transport, nothing in this Convention shall be interpreted as affecting the sovereign rights of a State regarding the domestic use, storage and transport of such nuclear material.

Article 3

Each State Party shall take appropriate steps within the framework of its national law and consistent with international law to ensure as far as practicable that, during international nuclear transport, nuclear material within its territory, or on board a ship or aircraft under its jurisdiction insofar as such ship or aircraft is engaged in the transport to or from that State, is protected at the levels described in Annex I.

Article 4

1. Each State Party shall not export or authorize the export of nuclear material unless the State Party has received assurances that such material will be protected during the international nuclear transport at the levels described in Annex I.

2. Each State Party shall not import or authorize the import of nuclear material from a State not party to this Convention unless the State Party has received assurances that such material will during the international nuclear transport be protected at the levels described in Annex I.

3. A State Party shall not allow the transit of its territory by land or internal waterways or through its airports or seaports of nuclear material between States that are not parties to this Convention unless the State Party has received assurances as far as practicable that this nuclear material will be protected during international nuclear transport at the levels described in Annex I.

4. Each State Party shall apply within the framework of its national law the levels of physical protection described in Annex I to nuclear material being transported from a part of that State to another part of the same State through international waters or airspace.

5. The State Party responsible for receiving assurances that the nuclear material will be protected at the levels described in Annex I according to paragraphs 1 to 3 shall identify and inform in advance States which the nuclear material is expected to transit by land or internal waterways, or whose airports or seaports it is expected to enter.

6. The responsibility for obtaining assurances referred to in paragraph 1 may be transferred, by mutual agreement, to the State Party involved in the transport as the importing State.

7. Nothing in this article shall be interpreted as in any way affecting the territorial sovereignty and jurisdiction of a State, including that over its airspace and territorial sea.

Article 5

1. States Parties shall identify and make known to each other directly or through the International Atomic Energy Agency their central authority and point of contact having responsibility for physical protection of nuclear material and for coordinating recovery and response operations in the event of any unauthorized removal, use or alteration of nuclear material or in the event of credible threat thereof.

2. In the case of theft, robbery or any other unlawful taking of nuclear material or of credible threat thereof, States Parties shall, in accordance with their national law, provide co-operation and assistance to the maximum feasible extent in the recovery and protection of such material to any State that so requests. In particular:

(a) a State Party shall take appropriate steps to inform as soon as possible other States, which appear to it to be concerned, of any theft, robbery or other unlawful taking of nuclear material or credible threat thereof and to inform, where appropriate, international organizations;

(b) as appropriate, the States Parties concerned shall exchange information with each other or international organizations with a view to protecting threatened nuclear material, verifying the integrity of the shipping container, or recovering unlawfully taken nuclear material and shall:

(i) co-ordinate their efforts through diplomatic and other agreed channels;

(ii) render assistance, if requested;

(iii) ensure the return of nuclear material stolen or missing as a consequence of the above-mentioned events.

The means of implementation of this co-operation shall be determined by the States Parties concerned.

3. States Parties shall co-operate and consult as appropriate, with each other directly or through international organizations, with a view to obtaining guidance on the design, maintenance and improvement of systems of physical protection of nuclear material in international transport.

Article 6

1. States Parties shall take appropriate measures consistent with their national law to protect the confidentiality of any information which they receive in confidence by virtue of the provisions of this Convention from another State Party or through participation in an activity carried out for the implementation of this Convention. If States Parties provide information to international organizations in confidence, steps shall be taken to ensure that the confidentiality of such information is protected.

2. States Parties shall not be required by this Convention to provide any information which they are not permitted to communicate pursuant to national law or which would jeopardize the security of the State concerned or the physical protection of nuclear material.

Article 7

1. The intentional commission of:

(a) an act without lawful authority which constitutes the receipt, possession, use, transfer, alteration, disposal or dispersal of nuclear material and which causes or is likely to cause death or serious injury to any person or substantial damage to property;

(b) a theft or robbery of nuclear material;

(c) an embezzlement or fraudulent obtaining of nuclear material;

(d) an act constituting a demand for nuclear material by threat or use of force or by any other form of intimidation;

(e) a threat:

(i) to use nuclear material to cause death or serious injury to any person or substantial property damage, or

(ii) to commit an offense described in subparagraph (b) in order to compel a natural or legal person, international organization or State to do or to refrain from doing any act;

(f) an attempt to commit any offense described in paragraphs (a), (b) or (c); and

(g) an act which constitutes participation in any offense described in paragraphs (a) to (f) shall be made a punishable offense by each State Party under its national law.

2. Each State Party shall make the offenses described in this article punishable by appropriate penalties which take into account their grave nature.

Article 8

1. Each State Party shall take such measures as may be necessary to establish its jurisdiction over the offenses set forth in article 7 in the following cases:

(a) when the offense is committed in the territory of that State or on board a ship or aircraft registered in that State;

(b) when the alleged offender is a national of that State.

2. Each State Party shall likewise take such measures as may be necessary to establish its jurisdiction over these offenses in cases where the alleged offender is present in its territory and it does not extradite him pursuant to article 11 to any of the States mentioned in paragraph 1.

3. This Convention does not exclude any criminal jurisdiction exercised in accordance with national law.

4. In addition to the State Parties mentioned in paragraphs 1 and 2, each State Party may, consistent with international law, establish its jurisdiction over the offenses set forth in article 7 when it is involved in international nuclear transport as the exporting or importing State.

Article 9

Upon being satisfied that the circumstances so warrant, the State Party in whose territory the alleged offender is present shall take appropriate measures, including detention, under its national law to ensure his presence for the purpose of prosecution or extradition. Measures taken according to this article shall be notified without delay to the States required to establish jurisdiction pursuant to article 8 and, where appropriate, all other States concerned.

Article 10

The State Party in whose territory the alleged offender is present shall, if it does not extradite him, submit, without exception whatsoever and without undue delay, the case to its competent authorities for the purpose of prosecution, through proceedings in accordance with the laws of that State.

Article 11

1. The offenses in article 7 shall be deemed to be included as extraditable offenses in any extradition Treaty existing between States Parties. States Parties undertake to include those offenses as extraditable offenses in every future extradition Treaty to be concluded between them.

2. If a State Party which makes extradition conditional on the existence of a Treaty receives a request for extradition from another State Party with which it has no extradition Treaty, it may at its option consider this Convention as the legal basis for extradition in respect of those offenses. Extradition shall be subject to the other conditions provided by the law of the requested State.

3. State Parties which do not make extradition conditional on the existence of a Treaty shall recognize those offenses as extraditable offenses between themselves subject to the conditions provided by the law of the requested State.

4. Each of the offenses shall be treated, for the purpose of extradition between States Parties, as if it had been committed not only in the place in which it occurred but also in the territories of the State Parties required to establish their jurisdiction in accordance with paragraph 1 of article 8.

Article 12

Any person regarding whom proceedings are being carried out in connection with any of the offenses set forth in article 7 shall be guaranteed fair treatment at all stages of the proceedings.

Article 13

1. States Parties shall afford one another the greatest measure of assistance in connection with criminal proceedings brought in respect of the offenses set forth in article 7, including the supply of evidence at their disposal necessary for the proceedings. The law of the State requested shall apply in all cases.

2. The provisions of paragraph 1 shall not affect obligations under any other Treaty, bilateral or multilateral, which governs or will govern, in whole or in part, mutual assistance in criminal matters.

Article 14

1. Each State Party shall inform the depositary of its laws and regulations which give effect to this Convention. The depositary shall communicate such information periodically to all States Parties.

2. The State Party where an alleged offender is prosecuted shall, wherever practicable, first communicate the final outcome of the proceedings to the States directly concerned. The State Party shall also communicate the final outcome to the depositary who shall inform all States.

3. Where an offense involves nuclear material used for peaceful purposes in domestic use, storage or transport, and both the alleged offender and the nuclear material remain in the territory of the State Party in which the offense was committed, nothing in this Convention shall be interpreted as requiring that State Party to provide information concerning criminal proceedings arising out of such an offense.

Article 15

The Annexes constitute an integral part of this Convention.

Article 16

1. A conference of States Parties shall be convened by the depositary five years after the entry into force of this Convention to review the implementation of the Convention and its adequacy as concerns the preamble, the whole of the operative part and the annexes in the light of the then prevailing situation.

2. At intervals of not less than five years thereafter, the majority of States Parties may obtain, by submitting a proposal to this effect to the depositary, the convening of further conferences with the same objective.

Article 17

1. In the event of a dispute between two or more States Parties concerning the interpretation or application of this Convention, such States Parties shall consult with a view to the settlement of the dispute by negotiation, or by any other peaceful means of settling disputes acceptable to all parties to the dispute.

2. Any dispute of this character which cannot be settled in the manner prescribed in paragraph 1 shall, at the request of any party to such dispute, be submitted to arbitration or referred to the International Court of Justice for decision. Where a dispute is submitted to arbitration, if, within six months from the date of the request, the parties to the dispute are unable to agree on the organization of the arbitration, a party may request the President of the International Court of Justice or the Secretary-General of the United Nations to appoint one or more arbitrators. In case of conflicting requests by the parties to the dispute, the request to the Secretary-General of the United Nations shall have priority.

3. Each State Party may at the time of signature, ratification, acceptance or approval of this Convention or accession thereto declare that it does not consider itself bound by either or both of the dispute settlement procedures provided for in paragraph 2. The other States Parties shall not be bound by a dispute settlement procedure provided for in paragraph 2, with respect to a State Party which has made a reservation to that procedure.

4. Any State Party which has made a reservation in accordance with paragraph 3 may at any time withdraw that reservation by notification to the depositary.

Article 18

1. This Convention shall be open for signature by all States at the Headquarters of the International Atomic Energy Agency in Vienna and at the Headquarters of the United Nations in New York from 3 March 1980 until its entry into force.

2. This Convention is subject to ratification, acceptance or approval by the signatory States.

3. After its entry into force, this Convention will be open for accession by all States.

4.(a) This Convention shall be open for signature or accession by international organizations and regional organizations of an integration or other nature, provided that any such organization is constituted by sovereign States and has competence in respect of the negotiation, conclusion and application of international agreements in matters covered by this Convention.

(b) In matters within their competence, such organizations shall, on their own behalf, exercise the rights and fulfill the responsibilities which this Convention attributes to States Parties.

(c) When becoming party to this Convention such an organization shall communicate to the depositary a declaration indicating which States are members thereof and which articles of this Convention do not apply to it.

(d) Such an organization shall not hold any vote additional to those of its Member States.

5. Instruments of ratification, acceptance, approval or accession shall be deposited with the depositary.

Article 19

1. This Convention shall enter into force on the thirtieth day following the date of deposit of the twenty-first instrument of ratification, acceptance or approval with the depositary.

2. For each State ratifying, accepting, approving or acceding to the Convention after the date of deposit of the twenty-first instrument of ratification, acceptance or approval, the Convention shall enter into force on the thirtieth day after the deposit by such State of its instrument of ratification, acceptance, approval or accession.

Article 20

1. Without prejudice to article 16 a State Party may propose amendments to this Convention. The proposed amendment shall be submitted to the depositary who shall circulate it immediately to all States Parties. If a majority of States Parties request the depositary to convene a conference to consider the proposed amendments, the depositary shall invite all States Parties to attend such a conference to begin not sooner than thirty days after the invitations are issued. Any amendment adopted at the conference by a two-thirds majority of all States Parties shall be promptly circulated by the depositary to all States Parties.

2. The amendment shall enter into force for each State Party that deposits its instrument of ratification, acceptance or approval of the amendment on the thirtieth day after the date on which two thirds of the States Parties have deposited their instruments of ratification, acceptance or approval with the depositary. Thereafter, the amendment shall enter into force for any other State Party on the day on which that State Party deposits its instrument of ratification, acceptance or approval of the amendment.

Article 21

1. Any State Party may denounce this Convention by written notification to the depositary.

2. Denunciation shall take effect one hundred and eighty days following the date on which notification is received by the depositary.

Article 22

The depositary shall promptly notify all States of:

(a) each signature of this Convention;

(b) each deposit of an instrument of ratification, acceptance, approval or accession;

(c) any reservation or withdrawal in accordance with article 17;

(d) any communication made by an organization in accordance with paragraph 4(c) of article 18;

(e) the entry into force of this Convention;

(f) the entry into force of any amendment to this Convention; and

(g) any denunciation made under article 21.

Article 23

The original of this Convention, of which the Arabic, Chinese, English, French, Russian and Spanish texts are equally authentic, shall be deposited with the Director General of the International Atomic Energy Agency who shall send certified copies thereof to all States.

ANNEX I

LEVELS OF PHYSICAL PROTECTION TO BE APPLIED IN INTERNATIONAL TRANSPORT OF NUCLEAR MATERIAL AS CATEGORIZED IN ANNEX II

1. Levels of physical protection for nuclear material during storage incidental to international nuclear transport include:

(a) For Category III materials, storage within an area to which access is controlled;

(b) For Category II materials, storage within an area under constant surveillance by guards or electronic devices, surrounded by a physical barrier with a limited number of points of entry under appropriate control or any area with an equivalent level of physical protection;

(c) For Category I material, storage within a protected area as defined for Category II above, to which, in addition, access is restricted to persons whose trustworthiness has been determined, and which is under surveillance by guards who are in close communication with appropriate response forces. Specific measures taken in this context should have as their object the detection and prevention of any assault, unauthorized access or unauthorized removal of material.

2. Levels of physical protection for nuclear material during international transport include:

(a) For Category II and III materials, transportation shall take place under special precautions including prior arrangements among sender, receiver, and carrier, and prior agreement between natural or legal persons subject to the jurisdiction and regulation of exporting and importing States, specifying time, place and procedures for transferring transport responsibility;

(b) For Category I materials, transportation shall take place under special precautions identified above for transportation of Category II and III materials, and in addition, under constant surveillance by escorts and under conditions which assure close communication with appropriate response forces;

(c) For natural uranium other than in the form of ore or ore-residue, transportation protection for quantities exceeding 500 kilograms U shall include advance notification of shipment specifying mode of transport, expected time of arrival and confirmation of receipt of shipment.

IN WITNESS WHEREOF, the undersigned, being duly authorized, have signed this Convention, opened for signature at Vienna and at New York on 3 March 1980.

Annex II
Table: Categorization of Nuclear Material

Material	Form	Category		
		I	II	III[3]
1. Plutonium[1] ---	Unirradiated[2] ---	2 kg or more	Less than 2 but more than 500 g	500g or less but more than 15 g
2. Uranium-235 ---	Unirradiated[2] --- —uranium enriched to 20% U 235 or more	5 kg or more	Less than 5 kg but more than 1 kg	1 kg or less but more than 15 g
	—uranium enriched to 10% U 235 but less than 20%	-----------------	10 kg or more	Less than 10 kg but more than 1 kg
	—uranium enriched above natural, but less than 10% U 235	------------------	---------------	10 kg or more
3. Uranium-233 ---	Unirradiated[2] --- but more than 500 g	2 kg or more	Less than 2 kg but more than 500 g	500 g or less but more than 15 g
4. Irradiated fuel -------------------		Depleted or natural uranium, thorium or low-enriched fuel (less than 10% fissile content).[4,5]		

[1] All plutonium except that with isotopic concentration exceeding 80% in plutonium-238.

[2] Material not irradiated in a reactor or material irradiated in a reactor but with a radiation level equal to or less than 100 rads/hour at one metre unshielded.

[3] Quantities not falling in Category III and natural uranium should be protected in accordance with prudent management practice.

[4] Although this level of protection is recommended, it would be open to States, upon evaluation of the specific circumstances, to assign a different category of physical protection.

[5] Other fuel which by virtue of its original fissile material content is classified as Category I and II before irradiation may be reduced one category level while the radiation level from the fuel exceeds 100 rads/hour at one metre unshielded.

Convention on the Physical Protection of Nuclear Material

Country	Date of Signature	Date of Deposit of Ratification	Date of Deposit of Accession
Argentina	02/28/86	05/02/89	
Australia	02/22/84	09/22/87	
Austria	03/03/80	12/22/88	
Belgium	06/13/80		
Brazil	05/15/81	10/17/85	
Bulgaria	06/23/81	04/10/84	
Canada	09/23/80	03/21/86	
China			01/10/89
Czechoslovakia	09/14/81	04/23/82	
Denmark	06/13/80		
Dominican Republic	03/03/80		
Ecuador	06/26/86		
EURATOM	06/13/80		
Finland	06/25/81		
France	06/13/80		
German Democratic Republic	05/21/80	02/05/81	
Germany, Federal Republic of	06/13/80		
Greece	03/03/80		
Guatemala	03/12/80	04/23/85	
Haiti	04/10/80		
Hungary	06/17/80	05/04/84	
Indonesia	07/03/86	11/05/86	
Ireland	06/13/80		
Israel	06/17/83		
Italy	06/13/80		
Japan			10/28/88
Korea, Republic of	12/29/81	04/07/82	
Liechtenstein	01/13/86	11/25/86	
Luxembourg	06/13/80		
Mexico			04/04/88
Mongolia	01/23/86	05/28/86	
Morocco	07/25/80		

Convention on the Physical Protection of Nuclear Material -- Continued

Country	Date of Signature	Date of Deposit of Ratification	Date of Deposit of Accession
Netherlands	06/13/80		
Niger	01/07/85		
Norway	01/26/83	08/15/85	
Panama	03/18/80		
Paraguay	05/21/80	02/06/85	
Philippines	05/19/80	09/21/81	
Poland	08/06/80	10/05/83	
Portugal	09/19/84		
Romania	01/15/81		
South Africa	05/18/81		
Spain	04/07/86		
Sweden	07/02/80	08/01/80	
Switzerland	01/09/87	01/09/87	
Turkey	08/23/83	02/27/85	
Union of Soviet Socialist Republics	05/22/80	05/25/83	
United Kingdom	06/13/80		
United States	03/03/80	12/13/82	
Yugoslavia	07/15/80	05/14/86	
Total	47	24	3

AGREEMENT BETWEEN THE UNITED STATES OF AMERICA AND THE UNION OF SOVIET SOCIALIST REPUBLICS TO EXPAND THE U.S.-USSR DIRECT COMMUNICATIONS LINK

In June 1963 the United States and the Soviet Union agreed in a Memorandum of Understanding to establish a Direct Communications Link, known as the "Hot Line," for use in time of emergency. Each agreed to ensure prompt delivery to its head of government of any communications received over the Direct Communications Link from the other head of government. (See "Hot Line" section.) Eight years later, the "Hot Line" was updated by a September 30, 1971, agreement negotiated by a special working group of the U.S. and Soviet SALT delegations and signed by the U.S. Secretary of State and the Soviet Foreign Minister. This agreement provided for the addition of two satellite circuits to the "Hot Line." Those two circuits became operational in 1978. (See "Hot Line" modernization section.)

In May 1983 President Reagan proposed to upgrade the "Hot Line" by the addition to the existing equipment of a high-speed facsimile transmission capability. This proposal was recommended to the President following a study of possible initiatives for enhancing international stability and reducing the risk of nuclear war. That examination, which involved all concerned U.S. Government agencies, was mandated by the Congress in the Department of Defense Authorization Act of 1983.

As a result of this initiative, negotiations between the United States and USSR on improving bilateral communications links opened in Moscow in August 1983. Subsequent rounds were held in Washington in January 1984, in Moscow in April 1984, and again in Washington in July 1984. Those discussions resulted in an accord, signed on July 17, 1984, to add a facsimile transmission capability to the "Hot Line." This capability became operational in 1986. This agreement was subsequently updated by an exchange of diplomatic notes in Washington, D.C., on June 24, 1988.

The "Hot Line" consists of two satellite circuits and one wire telegraph circuit. Terminals linked to the three circuits in each country are now equipped with teletype and facsimile equipment. Facsimile machines permit the heads of government to exchange messages far more rapidly than they could with the previously existing teletype system. They can also send detailed graphic material such as maps, charts, and drawings by facsimile.

AGREEMENT BETWEEN THE UNITED STATES OF AMERICA AND THE UNION OF SOVIET SOCIALIST REPUBLICS TO EXPAND THE U.S.-USSR DIRECT COMMUNICATIONS LINK

Signed at Washington July 17, 1984
Entered into force July 17, 1984

The Department of State, referring to the Memorandum of Understanding between the United States of America and the Union of Soviet Socialist Republics regarding the Establishment of a Direct Communications Link, signed June 20, 1963; to the Agreement on Measures to Improve the Direct Communications Link, signed September 30, 1971; and to the exchange of views between the two parties in Moscow and Washington during which it was deemed desirable to arrange for facsimile communication in addition to the current teletype Direct Communications Link, proposes that for this purpose the parties shall:

1. Establish and maintain three transmission links employing INTELSAT and STATSIONAR satellites and cable technology with secure orderwire circuit for operational monitoring. In this regard:

(a) Each party shall provide communications circuits capable of simultaneously transmitting and receiving 4800 bits per second.

(b) Operation of facsimile communication shall begin with the test operation over the INTELSAT satellite channel as soon as development, procurement and delivery of the necessary equipment by the sides are completed.

(c) Facsimile communication via STATSIONAR shall be established after transition of the Direct Communications Link teletype circuit from MOLNIYA to STATSIONAR using mutually agreeable transition procedures and after successful tests of facsimile communication via INTELSAT and cable.

2. Employ agreed-upon information security devices to assure secure transmission of facsimile materials. In this regard:

(a) The information security devices shall consist of microprocessors that will combine the digital facsimile output with buffered random data read from standard 5¼ inch floppy disks. The

American side shall provide a specification describing the key data format and necessary keying material resident on a floppy disk for both parties until such time as the Soviet side develops this capability. Beyond that time, each party shall provide necessary keying material to the other.

(b) The American side shall provide to the Soviet side the floppy disk drives integral to the operation of the microprocessor.

(c) The necessary security devices as well as spare parts for the said equipment shall be provided by the American side to the Soviet side in return for payment of costs thereof by the Soviet side.

3. Establish and maintain at each operating end of the Direct Communications Link facsimile terminals of the same make and model. In this regard:

(a) Each party shall be responsible for the acquisition, installation, operation and maintenance of its own facsimile machines, the related information security devices, and local transmission circuits appropriate to the implementation of this understanding, except as otherwise specified.

(b) A Group III facsimile unit which meets CCITT Recommendations T.4 and T.30 and operates at 4800 bits per second shall be used for this purpose.

(c) The necessary facsimile equipment as well as spare parts for the said equipment shall be provided to the Soviet side by the American side in return for payment of costs thereof by the Soviet side.

4. Establish and maintain secure orderwire communications necessary for coordination of facsimile operation. In this regard:

(a) The orderwire terminals used with the information security devices described in Paragraph 2(a) shall incorporate standard USSR Cyrillic and United States Latin keyboards and cathode ray tube displays to permit telegraphic exchange of information between operators. The specific layout of the Cyrillic keyboard shall be as specified by the Soviet side.

(b) To coordinate the work of the facsimile equipment operators, an orderwire shall be configured so as to permit, prior to the transmission and reception of facsimile messages, the exchange of all information pertinent to the coordination of such messages.

(c) Orderwire messages concerning facsimile transmissions shall be encoded using the same information security devices specified in Paragraph 2(a).

(d) The orderwire shall use the same modem and communications link as used for facsimile transmission.

(e) A printer shall be included to provide a record copy of all information exchanged on the orderwire.

(f) The necessary orderwire equipment as well as spare parts for the said equipment shall be provided by the American side to the Soviet side, in return for payment of costs thereof by the Soviet side.

5. Ensure the exchange of information necessary for the operation and maintenance of the facsimile system.

6. Take all possible measures to assure the continuous, secure and reliable operation of the facsimile equipment, information security devices and communications links including orderwire, for which each party is responsible in accordance with this agreement.

The Department of State also proposes that the parties, in consideration of the continuing advances in information and communications technology, conduct reviews as necessary regarding questions concerning improvement of the Direct Communications Link and its technical maintenance.

It is also proposed to note that the Memorandum of Understanding between the United States of America and the Union of Soviet Socialist Republics regarding the Establishment of a Direct Communications Link, signed on June 20, 1963, with the Annex thereto; the Agreement between the United States of America and the Union of the Soviet Socialist Republics on Measures to Improve the Direct Communications Link, with the Annex thereto, signed on September 30, 1971; those Understandings, with Attached Annexes, reached between the United States and Union of Soviet Socialist Republics delegations of technical specialists and experts signed on September 11, 1972, December 10, 1973, March 22, 1976, and the exchange of notes at Moscow on March 20 and April 29, 1975, constituting an Agreement Amending the Agreement of September 30, 1971, remain in force, except to the extent that their provisions are modified by this agreement.

If the foregoing is acceptable to the Soviet side, it is proposed that this note, together with the reply of the Embassy of the Union of Soviet Socialist Republics, shall constitute an agreement, effective on the date of the Embassy's reply.

Kenneth W. Dean
Department of State,

Washington, July 17, 1984[1]

---

[1] Note: Soviet Charge d' affaires Isakov initialed the Soviet diplomatic note and the notes were exchanged on July 17, 1984.

DOCUMENT OF THE STOCKHOLM CONFERENCE ON CONFIDENCE- AND SECURITY-BUILDING MEASURES AND DISARMAMENT IN EUROPE CONVENED IN ACCORDANCE WITH THE RELEVANT PROVISIONS OF THE CONCLUDING DOCUMENT OF THE MADRID MEETING OF THE CONFERENCE ON SECURITY AND COOPERATION IN EUROPE

On September 19*, 1986, the Conference on Confidence- and Security-Building Measures and Disarmament in Europe (CDE) reached agreement on a set of confidence- and security-building measures (CSBMs) designed to increase openness and predictability about military activities in Europe, with the aim of reducing the risk of armed conflict in Europe.

Security Aspects of CSCE

The CDE is a substantial and integral part of the Conference on Security and Cooperation in Europe (CSCE), which was established in the early 1970s, but whose origins date back to the 1950s.

In 1954 Soviet Foreign Minister Molotov proposed an all-European Treaty on collective security with the goal of ensuring the status quo in Europe and establishing a collective European security agreement, with the United States having "observer" status. Between 1954 and 1969, the Soviet Union and its allies presented several variations of this initial proposal. In response, NATO members of the North Atlantic Alliance established several preconditions for an agreement to an all-European security forum, including: the participation of the United States and Canada as full partners; the inclusion, as integral elements of such a security framework, of issues such as human rights, human contacts, and cultural and educational exchanges; the peaceful resolution of the status of Berlin; and the initiation of talks on force reductions in Central Europe, the Mutual and Balanced Force Reductions (MBFR) talks. Agreement was eventually reached on these preconditions.

Preparatory talks began in November 1972, and the Conference on Security and Cooperation in Europe (CSCE) opened in Helsinki in July 1973. From September 18, 1973 to July 21, 1975, the Conference was held in Geneva.

The Concluding Document of the Conference, the Helsinki Final Act, was signed on August 1, 1975 in Helsinki by the 35 participating countries (the United States, Canada, and all European states except Albania). This launched what has come to be known as the "Helsinki process" or "CSCE process," which calls for balanced progress in three subject areas, called "Baskets." Basket One concerns questions of security in Europe, including principles guiding relations among participating states and confidence-building measures; Basket Two concerns cooperation in the field of economics, science and technology, and the environment; Basket Three concerns cooperation in humanitarian and other fields. The Final Act represents a political commitment that is not legally binding upon the parties.

CSCE Confidence-Building Measures (CBMs)

Included in Basket One of the Helsinki Final Act is a document on Confidence-Building Measures and Certain Aspects of Security and Disarmament. The document contains a series of modest confidence-building measures designed to reduce the "dangers of armed conflict and of misunderstanding or miscalculation of military activities which could give rise to apprehension...." The centerpiece is the commitment to provide notification, twenty-one days in advance, of major military maneuvers involving more than 25,000 troops (to include amphibious and airborne troops) taking place "on the territory, in Europe, of any participating state as well as, if applicable, in the adjoining sea area and air space." In addition, the document encourages voluntary notification of smaller scale military maneuvers, major military movements, and the invitation of observers to maneuvers.

---

* The actual date of adoption was September 22. The clock at the Conference was stopped by common consent in the early evening of September 19 when it was judged that extra time would be required to finalize the agreement. This was necessary to satisfy the stipulation of the Madrid Mandate that the Conference end on September 19.

Madrid CSCE Followup Meeting

The Helsinki Final Act calls for periodic CSCE followup meetings, designed to review implementation of the provisions and principles of the Final Act, and to consider new proposals. The second follow-up meeting, held in Madrid from November 1980 to September 1983, considered a variety of proposals for a new conference to develop further the Helsinki CBMs. The concluding document of the Madrid meeting called for a special meeting, titled the Conference on Confidence- and Security-Building Measures and Disarmament in Europe, whose aim was to "undertake in stages, new, effective and concrete actions designed to make progress in strengthening confidence and security and in achieving disarmament, so as to give effect and expression to the duty of states to refrain from the threat or use of force in their mutual relations." It stipulated that the first conference would be held in Stockholm, Sweden, and would be devoted to the negotiation and adoption of a set of mutually complementary confidence- and security-building measures designed to reduce the risk of military confrontation in Europe. The mandate specified that these CSBMs would be militarily significant, politically binding, verifiable, and applicable to the whole of Europe. The extension of the area of applicability to the entire European part of Soviet territory (i.e., to the Ural Mountains) was a significant step, since the CBMs in the 1975 Helsinki Final Act were applicable in Soviet territory only to a depth of 250 kilometers from its European borders.

Conference on Confidence- and Security-Building Measures and Disarmament in Europe (CDE)

The CDE opened in Stockholm on January 17, 1984. Seven days later, the 16 members of NATO tabled a package of six concrete and mutually complementary confidence- and security-building measures, providing for: exchange of information about the organization and location of military forces in the area of applicability; exchange of annual forecasts of notifiable military activities; 45-day advance notification of military exercises at significantly lower thresholds than the Helsinki CBMs; invitation of observers to all notified activities; on-site inspection to help verify compliance; and improved means of communication.

The first eighteen months of the conference were dominated by debate on the purpose of the conference, that is, whether it would adopt a largely declaratory approach to confidence-building as advocated by the Soviet Union and its allies, or the concrete approach of the NATO allies. The conference formed itself into working groups at the end of 1985, which facilitated serious work, and received political impetus from the Geneva Summit meeting between President Reagan and General Secretary Gorbachev. But it was not until late summer of 1986, when the Soviet Union indicated willingness to accept on-site inspection, that it became evident that a substantive outcome that met the criteria of the Madrid mandate might be possible.

At the closing plenary, the conference adopted by consensus the Stockholm Document. Principal measures call for the following:

- *Notification*: 42-day prior notification of military activities taking place within the whole of Europe whenever they involve a divisional structure or two or more brigades/regiments and at least 13,000 troops or 300 tanks.

- *Observation*: mandatory invitation of observers from all participating states to attend notified military activities above a threshold of 17,000 troops.

- *Forecasting*: exchange of annual forecasts of all notifiable military activities. Activities involving more than 40,000 troops are prohibited unless announced a year in advance and activities involving more than 75,000 troops are prohibited unless forecast two years in advance.

- *Inspection*: on-site inspection from the air or ground or both to verify compliance with agreed measures, with no right of refusal.

The conference's reaffirmation of the non-use of force principle includes language on human rights, anti-terrorism, and compliance with international commitments and denying the validity of the so-called Brezhnev doctrine.

In January 1989, the third follow-up meeting of the CSCE, held in Vienna, Austria, issued the Vienna Concluding Document. Among its provisions as a mandate to resume the negotiations in CSBMs. These negotiations among the 35 CSCE states opened in Vienna on March 9, 1989. The concluding document also noted that new negotiations among the 23 members of NATO and the Warsaw Treaty Organization would be conducted "within the framework of the CSCE process." These negotiations also opened in Vienna on March 1, 1989.

DOCUMENT OF THE STOCKHOLM
CONFERENCE ON CONFIDENCE- AND
SECURITY-BUILDING MEASURES AND
DISARMAMENT IN EUROPE CONVENED IN
ACCORDANCE WITH THE RELEVANT
PROVISIONS OF THE CONCLUDING
DOCUMENT OF THE MADRID MEETING OF
THE CONFERENCE ON SECURITY AND
COOPERATION IN EUROPE

Signed at Stockholm September 19, 1986

(1) The representatives of the participating
States of the Conference on Security and
Co-operation in Europe (CSCE), Austria, Belgium,
Bulgaria, Canada, Cyprus, Czechoslovakia,
Denmark, Finland, France, the German
Democratic Republic, the Federal Republic of
Germany, Greece, the Holy See, Hungary,
Iceland, Ireland, Italy, Liechtenstein, Luxembourg,
Malta, Monaco, the Netherlands, Norway, Poland,
Portugal, Romania, San Marino, Spain, Sweden,
Switzerland, Turkey, the Union of Soviet Socialist
Republics, the United Kingdom, the United States
of America and Yugoslavia, met in Stockholm
from 17 January 1984 to 19 September 1986, in
accordance with the provisions relating to the
Conference on Confidence- and Security-Building
Measures and Disarmament in Europe contained
in the Concluding Document of the Madrid
Followup Meeting of the CSCE.

(2) The participants were addressed by the
Prime Minister of Sweden, the late Olof Palme,
on 17 January 1984.

(3) Opening statements were made by the
Ministers of Foreign Affairs and other Heads of
Delegation. The Prime Minister of Spain as well
as Ministers and senior officials of several other
participating States addressed the Conference
later. The Minister for Foreign Affairs of Sweden
addressed the Conference on 19 September
1986.

(4) The Secretary-General of the United Nations
addressed the Conference on 6 July 1984.

(5) Contributions were made by the following
non-participating Mediterranean States: Algeria,
Egypt, Israel, Lebanon, Libya, Morocco, Syria and
Tunisia.

(6) The participating States recalled that the
aim of the Conference on Confidence- and
Security-Building Measures and Disarmament in
Europe is, as a substantial and integral part of the
multilateral process initiated by the Conference on
Security and Co-operation in Europe, to
undertake, in stages, new, effective and concrete
actions designed to make progress in
strengthening confidence and security and in
achieving disarmament, so as to give effect and
expression to the duty of States to refrain from
the threat or use of force in their mutual relations
as well as in their international relations in
general.

(7) The participating States recognized that the
set of mutually complementary confidence- and
security-building measures which are adopted in
the present document and which are in
accordance with the Madrid mandate serve by
their scope and nature and by their
implementation to strengthen confidence and
security in Europe and thus to give effect and
expression to the duty of States to refrain from
the threat or use of force.

(8) Consequently the participating States have
declared the following:

REFRAINING FROM THE THREAT OR USE OF FORCE

(9) The participating States, recalling their
obligation to refrain, in their mutual relations as
well as in their international relations in general,
from the threat or use of force against the
territorial integrity or political independence of any
State, or in any other manner inconsistent with
the purposes of the United Nations, accordingly
reaffirm their commitment to respect and put into
practice the principle of refraining from the threat
or use of force, as laid down in the Final Act.

(10) No consideration may be invoked to serve
to warrant resort to the threat or use of force in
contravention of this principle.

(11) They recall the inherent right of individual
or collective self-defence if an armed attack
occurs, as set forth in the Charter of the United
Nations.

(12) They will refrain from any manifestation of force for the purpose of inducing any other State to renounce the full exercise of its sovereign rights.

(13) As set forth in the Final Act, no occupation or acquisition of territory resulting from the threat or use of force in contravention of international law, will be recognized as legal.

(14) They recognize their commitment to peace and security. Accordingly they reaffirm that they will refrain from any use of armed forces inconsistent with the purposes and principles of the Charter of the United Nations and the provisions of the Declaration on Principles Guiding Relations between Participating States, against another participating State, in particular from invasion of or attack on its territory.

(15) They will abide by their commitment to refrain from the threat or use of force in their relations with any State, regardless of that State's political, social, economic, or cultural system and irrespective of whether or not they maintain with that State relations of alliance.

(16) They stress that non-compliance with the obligation of refraining from the threat or use of force, as recalled above, constitutes a violation of international law.

(17) They stress their commitment to the principle of peaceful settlement of disputes as contained in the Final Act, convinced that it is an essential complement to the duty of States to refrain from the threat or use of force, both being essential factors for the maintenance and consolidation of peace and security. They recall their determination and the necessity to reinforce and to improve the methods at their disposal for the peaceful settlement of disputes. They reaffirm their resolve to make every effort to settle exclusively by peaceful means any dispute between them.

(18) The participating States stress their commitment to the Final Act and the need for full implementation of all its provisions, which will further the process of improving security and developing co-operation in Europe, thereby contributing to international peace and security in the world as a whole.

(19) They emphasize their commitment to all the principles of the Declaration on Principles Guiding Relations between Participating States and declare their determination to respect and put them into practice irrespective of their political, economic or social systems as well as of their size, geographical location or level of economic development.

(20) All these ten principles are of primary significance and, accordingly, they will be equally and unreservedly applied, each of them being interpreted taking into account the others.

(21) Respect for and the application of these principles will enhance the development of friendly relations and co-operation among the participating States in all fields covered by the provisions of the Final Act.

(22) They reconfirm their commitment to the basic principle of the sovereign equality of States and stress that all States have equal rights and duties within the framework of international law.

(23) They reaffirm the universal significance of human rights and fundamental freedoms. Respect for and the effective exercise of these rights and freedoms are essential factors for international peace, justice and security, as well as for the development of friendly relations and co-operation among themselves as among all States, as set forth in the Declaration on Principles Guiding Relations between Participating States.

(24) They reaffirm that, in the broader context of world security, security in Europe is closely linked with security in the Mediterranean area as a whole; in this context, they confirm their intention to develop good neighborly relations with all States in the region, with due regard to reciprocity, and in the spirit of the principles contained in the Declaration on Principles Guiding Relations between Participating States, so as to promote confidence and security and make peace prevail in the region in accordance with the provisions contained in the Mediterranean chapter of the Final Act.

(25) They emphasize the necessity to take resolute measures to prevent and to combat terrorism, including terrorism in international relations. They express their determination to take effective measures, both at the national level and through international co-operation, for the prevention and suppression of all acts of

terrorism. They will take all appropriate measures in preventing their respective territories from being used for the preparation, organization or commission of terrorist activities. This also includes measures to prohibit on their territories illegal activities, including subversive activities, of persons, groups and organizations that instigate, organize or engage in the perpetration of acts of terrorism, including those directed against other States and their citizens.

(26) They will fulfill in good faith their obligations under international law; they also stress that strict compliance with their commitments within the framework of the CSCE is essential for building confidence and security.

(27) The participating States confirm that in the event of a conflict between the obligations of the members of the United Nations under the Charter of the United Nations and their obligations under any Treaty or other international agreement, their obligations under the Charter will prevail, in accordance with Article 103 of the Charter of the United Nations.

(28) The participating States have adopted the following measures:

PRIOR NOTIFICATION OF CERTAIN MILITARY ACTIVITIES

(29) The participating States will give notification in writing through diplomatic channels in an agreed form of content, to all other participating States 42 days or more in advance of the start of notifiable[1] military activities in the zone of application for confidence- and security-building measures (CSBMs).[2]

(30) Notification will be given by the participating State on whose territory the activity in question is planned to take place even if the forces of that State are not engaged in the activity or their strength is below the notifiable level. This will not relieve other participating States of their obligation to give notification, if their involvement in the planned military activity reaches the notifiable level.

(31) Each of the following military activities in the field conducted as a single activity in the zone of application for CSBMs at or above the levels defined below, will be notified.

(31.1) The engagement of formations of land forces* of the participating States in the same exercise activity conducted under a single operational command independently or in combination with any possible air or naval components.

(31.1.1) This military activity will be subject to notification whenever it involves at any time during the activity:

• at least 13,000 troops, including support troops, or

• at least 300 battle tanks

if organized into a divisional structure or at least two brigades/regiments, not necessarily subordinate to the same division.

(31.1.2) The participation of air forces of the participating States will be included in the notification if it is foreseen that in the course of the activity 200 or more sorties by aircraft, excluding helicopters, will be flown.

(31.2) The engagement of military forces either in an amphibious landing or in a parachute assault by airborne forces in the zone of application for CSBMs.

(31.2.1) These military activities will be subject to notification whenever the amphibious landing involves at least 3,000 troops or whenever the parachute drop involves at least 3,000 troops.

(31.3) The engagement of formations of land forces of the participating States in a transfer from outside the zone of application for CSBMs to arrival points in the zone, or from inside the zone of application for CSBMs to points of concentration in the zone, to participate in a notifiable exercise activity or to be concentrated.

(31.3.1) The arrival or concentration of these forces will be subject to notification whenever it involves, at any time during the activity:

---

* In this context, the term land forces includes amphibious, air-mobile and airborne forces.

• at least 13,000 troops, including support troops, or

• at least 300 battle tanks

if organized into a divisional structure or at least two brigades/regiments, not necessarily subordinate to the same division.

(31.3.2) Forces which have been transferred into the zone will be subject to all provisions of agreed CSBMs when they depart their arrival points to participate in a notifiable exercise activity or to be concentrated within the zone of application for CSBMs.

(32) Notifiable military activities carried out without advance notice to the troops involved, are exceptions to the requirement for prior notification to be made 42 days in advance.

(32.1) Notification of such activities, above the agreed thresholds, will be given at the time the troops involved commence such activities.

(33) Notification will be given in writing of each notifiable military activity in the following agreed form:

(34) **A - General Information**

(34.1) The designation of the military activity;

(34.2) The general purpose of the military activity;

(34.3) The names of the States involved in the military activity;

(34.4) The level of command, organizing and commanding the military activity;

(34.5) The start and end dates of the military activity.

(35) **B - Information on different types of notifiable military activities**

(35.1) The engagement of land forces of the participating States in the same exercise activity conducted under a single operational command independently or in combination with any possible air or naval components:

(35.1.1) The total number of troops taking part in the military activity (i.e., ground troops, amphibious troops, airmobile and airborne troops) and the number of troops participating for each State involved, if applicable;

(35.1.2) Number and type of divisions participating for each State;

(35.1.3) The total number of battle tanks for each State and the total number of anti-tank guided missile launchers mounted on armored vehicles;

(35.1.4) The total number of artillery pieces and multiple rocket launchers (100 mm calibre or above);

(35.1.5) The total number of helicopters, by category;

(35.1.6) Envisaged number of sorties by aircraft, excluding helicopters;

(35.1.7) Purpose of air missions;

(35.1.8) Categories of aircraft involved;

(35.1.9) The level of command, organizing and commanding the air force participation;

(35.1.10) Naval ship-to-shore gunfire;

(35.1.11) Indication of other naval ship-to-shore support;

(35.1.12) The level of command, organizing and commanding the naval force participation.

(35.2) The engagement of military forces either in an amphibious landing or in a parachute assault by airborne forces in the zone of application for CSBMs;

(35.2.1) The total number of amphibious troops involved in notifiable amphibious landings, and/or the total number of airborne troops involved in notifiable parachute assaults;

(35.2.2) In the case of a notifiable amphibious landing, the point or points of embarkation, if in the zone of application for CSBMs.

(35.3) The engagement of formations of

land forces of the participating States in a transfer from outside the zone of application for CSBMs to arrival points in the zone, or from inside the zone of application for CSBMs to points of concentration in the zone, to participate in a notifiable exercise activity or to be concentrated:

(35.3.1) The total number of troops transferred;

(35.3.2) Number and type of divisions participating in the transfer;

(35.3.3) The total number of battle tanks participating in a notifiable arrival of concentration;

(35.3.4) Geographical co-ordinates for the points of arrival and for the points of concentration.

(36) C - The envisaged area and timeframe of the activity

(36.1) The area of the military activity delimited by geographic features together with geographic coordinates, as appropriate;

(36.2) The start and end dates of each phase (transfers, deployment, concentration of forces, active exercise phase, recovery phase) of activities in the zone of application for CSBMs of participating formations, the tactical purpose and corresponding geographical areas (delimited by geographical co-ordinates) for each phase;

(36.3) Brief description of each phase.

(37)   D - Other information

(37.1) Changes, if any, in relation to information provided in the annual calendar regarding the activity;

(37.2) Relationship of the activity to other notifiable activities.

OBSERVATION OF CERTAIN MILITARY ACTIVITIES

(38) The participating States will invite observers from all other participating States to the following notifiable military activities:

(38.1) The engagement of formations of land forces* of the participating States in the same exercise activity conducted under a single operational command independently or in combination with any possible air or naval components;

(38.2) The engagement of military forces either in an amphibious landing or in a parachute assault by airborne forces in the zone of application for CSBMs;

(38.3) In the case of the engagement of formations of land forces of the participating States in a transfer from outside the zone of application for CSBMs to arrival points in the zone, or from inside the zone of application for CSBMs to points of concentration in the zone, to participate in a notifiable exercise activity or to be concentrated, the concentration of these forces. Forces which have been transferred into the zone will be subject to all provisions of agreed confidence- and security-building measures when they depart their arrival points to participate in a notifiable exercise activity or to be concentrated within the zone of application for CSBMs;

(38.4)   The above-mentioned activities will be subject to observation whenever the number of troops engaged meets or exceeds 17,000 troops, except in the case of either an amphibious landing or a parachute assault by airborne forces, which will be subject to observation whenever the number of troops engaged meets or exceeds 5,000 troops.

(39) The host State will extend the invitations in writing through diplomatic channels to all other participating States at the time of notification. The host State will be the participating State on whose territory the notified activity will take place.

(40) The host State may delegate some of its responsibilities as host to another participating State engaged in the military activity on the territory of the host State. In such cases, the host State will specify the allocation of responsibilities in its invitation to observe the activity.

(41) Each participating State may send up to two observers to the military activity to be observed.

---

* In this context, the term land forces includes amphibious, air-mobile and airborne forces.

(42) The invited State may decide whether to send military and/or civilian observers, including members of its personnel accredited to the host State. Military observers will, normally, wear their uniforms and insignia while performing their tasks.

(43) Replies to the invitation will be given in writing not later than 21 days after the issue of the invitation.

(44) The participating State accepting an invitation will provide the names and ranks of their observers in their reply to the invitation. If the invitation is not accepted in time, it will be assumed that no observers will be sent.

(45) Together with the invitation the host State will provide a general observation programme, including the following information:

(45.1) the date, time and place of assembly of observers;

(45.2) planned duration of the observation programme;

(45.3) languages to be used in interpretation and/or translation;

(45.4) arrangements for board, lodging and transportation of the observers;

(45.5) arrangements for observation equipment which will be issued to the observers by the host State;

(45.6) possible authorization by the host State of the use of special equipment that the observers may bring with them;

(45.7) arrangements for special clothing to be issued to the observers because of weather or environmental factors.

(46) The observers may make requests with regard to the observation programme. The host State will, if possible, accede to them.

(47) The host State will determine a duration of observation which permits the observers to observe a notifiable military activity from the time that agreed thresholds for observation are met or exceeded until, for the last time during the

activity, the thresholds for observation are no longer met.

(48) The host State will provide the observers with transportation to the area of the notified activity and back. This transportation will be provided from either the capital or another suitable location to be announced in the invitation, so that the observers are in position before the start of the observation programme.

(49) The invited State will cover the travel expenses for its observers to the capital, or another suitable location specified in the invitation, of the host State, and back.

(50) The observers will be provided equal treatment and offered equal opportunities to carry out their functions.

(51) The observers will be granted, during their mission, the privileges and immunities accorded to diplomatic agents in the Vienna Convention on Diplomatic Relations.

(52) The host State will not be required to permit observation of restricted locations, installations or defence sites.

(53) In order to allow the observers to confirm that the notified activity is non-threatening in character and that it is carried out in conformity with the appropriate provisions of the notification, the host State will:

(53.1) at the commencement of the observation programme give a briefing on the purpose, the basic situation, the phases of the activity and possible changes as compared with the notification and provide the observers with a map of the area of the military activity with a scale of 1 to not more than 500,000 and an observation programme with a daily schedule as well as a sketch indicating the basic situation;

(53.2) provide the observers with appropriate observation equipment; however, the observers will be allowed to use their personal binoculars, which will be subject to examination and approval by the host State;

(53.3) in the course of the observation programme give the observers daily briefings with the help of maps on the various phases of the military activity and their development and inform the observers about their positions geographically; in the case of a land force activity conducted in combination with air or naval components, briefings will be given by representatives of these forces;

(53.4) provide opportunities to observe directly forces of the State/States engaged in the military activity so that the observers get an impression of the flow of the activity; to this end, the observers will be given the opportunity to observe major combat units of the participating formations of a divisional or equivalent level and, whenever possible, to visit some units and communicate with commanders and troops; commanders or other senior personnel of participating formations as well as of the visited units will inform the observers of the mission of their respective units;

(53.5) guide the observers in the area of the military activity; the observers will follow the instructions issued by the host State in accordance with the provisions set out in this document;

(53.6) provide the observers with appropriate means of transportation in the area of the military activity;

(53.7) provide the observers with opportunities for timely communication with their embassies or other official missions and consular posts; the host State is not obligated to cover the communication expenses of the observers;

(53.8) provide the observers with appropriate board and lodging in a location suitable for carrying out the observation programme and, when necessary, medical care.

(54) The participating States need not invite observers to notifiable military activities which are carried out without advance notice to the troops involved unless these notifiable activities have a duration of more than 72 hours. The continuation of these activities beyond this time will be subject to observation while the agreed thresholds for observation are met or exceeded. The observation programme will follow as closely as practically possible all the provisions for observation set out in this document.

ANNUAL CALENDARS

(55) Each participating State will exchange, with all other participating States, an annual calendar of its military activities subject to prior notification,* within the zone of application for CSBMs, forecast for the subsequent calendar year. It will be transmitted every year, in writing, through diplomatic channels, not later than 15 November for the following year.

(56) Each participating State will list the above-mentioned activities chronologically and will provide information on each activity in accordance with the following model:

(56.1) type of military activity and its designation;

(56.2) general characteristics and purpose of the military activity;

(56.3) States involved in the military activity;

(56.4) area of the military activity, indicated by appropriate geographic features and/or defined by geographic co-ordinates;

(56.5) planned duration of the military activity and the 14-day period, indicated by dates, within which it is envisaged to start;

**(56.6) the envisaged total number of troops engaged in the military activity;

(56.7) the types of armed forces involved in the military activity;

(56.8) the envisaged level of command, under which the military activity will take place;

(56.9) the number and type of divisions whose participation in the military activity is envisaged;

---

* As defined in the provisions on Prior Notification of Certain Military Activities.
** As defined in the provisions on Prior Notification of Certain Military Activities.

(56.10) any additional information concerning, *inter alia*, components of armed forces, which the participating State planning the military activity considers relevant.

(57) Should changes regarding the military activities in the annual calendar prove necessary, they will be communicated to all other participating States no later than in the appropriate notification.

(58) Information on military activities subject to prior notification not included in an annual calendar will be communicated to all participating States as soon as possible, in accordance with the model provided in the annual calendar.

CONSTRAINING PROVISIONS

(59) Each participating State will communicate, in writing, to all other participating States, by 15 November each year, information concerning military activities subject to prior notification* involving more than 40,000 troops,* which it plans to carry out in the second subsequent calendar year. Such communication will include preliminary information on each activity, as to its general purpose, timeframe and duration, area, size and States involved.

(60) Participating States will not carry out military activities subject to prior notification involving more than 75,000 troops, unless they have been the object of communication as defined above.

(61) Participating States will not carry out military activities subject to prior notification involving more than 40,000 troops unless they have been included in the annual calendar, not later than 15 November each year.

(62) If military activities subject to prior notification are carried out in addition to those contained in the annual calendar, they should be as few as possible.

COMPLIANCE AND VERIFICATION

(63) According to the Madrid Mandate, the confidence- and security-building measures to be agreed upon "will be provided with adequate forms of verification which correspond to their content."

(64) The participating States recognize that national technical means can play a role in monitoring compliance with agreed confidence- and security-building measures.

(65) In accordance with the provisions contained in this document each participating State has the right to conduct inspections on the territory of any other participating State within the zone of application for CSBMs.

(66) Any participating State will be allowed to address a request for inspection to another participating State on whose territory, within the zone of application for CSBMs, compliance with the agreed confidence- and security-building measures is in doubt.

(67) No participating State will be obliged to accept on its territory, within the zone of application for CSBMs, more than three inspections per calendar year.

(68) No participating State will be obliged to accept more than one inspection per calendar year from the same participating State.

(69) An inspection will not be counted if, due to *force majeure*, it cannot be carried out.

(70) The participating State which requests an inspection will state the reasons for such a request.

(71) The participating State which has received such a request will reply in the affirmative to the request within the agreed period of time, subject to the provisions contained in paragraphs (67) and (68).

(72) Any possible dispute as to the validity of the reasons for a request will not prevent or delay the conduct of an inspection.

(73) The participating State which requests an inspection will be permitted to designate for inspection on the territory of another State within the zone of application for CSBMs, a specific area. Such an area will be referred to as the

---

* As defined in the provisions on Prior Notification of Certain Military Activities.

"specified area." The specified area will comprise terrain where notifiable military activities are conducted or where another participating State believes a notifiable military activity is taking place. The specified area will be defined and limited by the scope and scale of notifiable military activities but will not exceed that required for an army level military activity.

(74) In the specified area the representatives of the inspecting State accompanied by the representatives of the receiving State will be permitted access, entry and unobstructed survey, except for areas or sensitive points to which access is normally denied or restricted, military and other defence installations, as well as naval vessels, military vehicles and aircraft. The number and extent of the restricted areas should be as limited as possible. Areas where notifiable military activities can take place will not be declared restricted areas, except for certain permanent or temporary military installations which, in territorial terms, should be as small as possible, and consequently those areas will not be used to prevent inspection of notifiable military activities. Restricted areas will not be employed in a way inconsistent with the agreed provisions on inspection.

(75) Within the specified area, the forces of participating States other than the receiving State will also be subject to the inspection conducted by the inspecting State.

(76) Inspection will be permitted on the ground, from the air, or both.

(77) The representatives of the receiving State will accompany the inspection team, including when it is in land vehicles and an aircraft from the time of their first employment until the time they are no longer in use for the purposes of inspection.

(78) In its request, the inspecting State will notify the receiving State of:

(78.1) the reasons for the request;

(78.2) the location of the specified area defined by geographical co-ordinates;

(78.3) the preferred point(s) of entry for the inspection team;

(78.4) mode of transport to and from the point(s) of entry and, if applicable, to and from the specified area;

(78.5) where in the specified area the inspection will begin;

(78.6) whether the inspection will be conducted from the ground, from the air, or both simultaneously;

(78.7) whether aerial inspection will be conducted using an airplane, a helicopter, or both;

(78.8) whether the inspection team will use land vehicles provided by the receiving State or, if mutually agreed, its own vehicles;

(78.9) information for the issuance of diplomatic visas to inspectors entering the receiving State.

(79) The reply to the request will be given in the shortest possible period or time, but within not more than 24 hours. Within 36 hours after the issuance of the request, the inspection team will be permitted to enter the territory of the receiving State.

(80) Any request for inspection as well as the reply thereto will be communicated to all participating States without delay.

(81) The receiving State should designate the point(s) of entry as close as possible to the specified area. The receiving State will ensure that the inspection team will be able to reach the specified area without delay from the point(s) of entry.

(82) All participating States will facilitate the passage of the inspection teams through their territory.

(83) Within 48 hours after the arrival of the inspection team at the specified area, the inspection will be terminated.

(84) There will be no more than four inspectors in an inspection team. While conducting the inspection the inspection team may divide into two parts.

(85) The inspectors and, if applicable, auxiliary personnel, will be granted during their mission the privileges and immunities in accordance with the Vienna Convention on Diplomatic Relations.

(86) The receiving State will provide the inspection team with appropriate board and lodging in a location suitable for carrying out the inspection, and, when necessary, medical care; however this does not exclude the use by the inspection team of its own tents and rations.

(87) The inspection team will have use of its own maps, own photo cameras, own binoculars and own dictaphones, as well as own aeronautical charts.

(88) The inspection team will have access to appropriate telecommunications equipment of the receiving State, including the opportunity for continuous communication between the members of an inspection team in an aircraft and those in a land vehicle employed in the inspection.

(89) The inspecting State will specify whether aerial inspection will be conducted using an airplane, a helicopter or both. Aircraft for inspection will be chosen by mutual agreement between the inspecting and receiving States. Aircraft will be chosen which provide the inspection team a continuous view of the ground during the inspection.

(90) After the flight plan, specifying, *inter alia*, the inspection team's choice of flight path, speed and altitude in the specified area, has been filed with the competent air traffic control authority the inspection aircraft will be permitted to enter the specified area without delay. Within the specified area, the inspection team will, at its request, be permitted to deviate from the approved flight plan to make specific observations provided such deviation is consistent with paragraph (74) as well as flight safety and air traffic requirements. Directions to the crew will be given through a representative of the receiving State on board the aircraft involved in the inspection.

(91) One member of the inspection team will be permitted, if such a request is made, at any time to observe data on navigational equipment of the aircraft and to have access to maps and charts used by the flight crew for the purpose of determining the exact location of the aircraft during the inspection flight.

(92) Aerial and ground inspectors may return to the specified area as often as desired within the 48-hour inspection period.

(93) The receiving State will provide for inspection purposes land vehicles with cross country capability. Whenever mutually agreed taking into account the specific geography relating to the area to be inspected, the inspecting State will be permitted to use its own vehicles.

(94) If land vehicles or aircraft are provided by the inspecting State, there will be one accompanying driver for each land vehicle, or accompanying aircraft crew.

(95) The inspecting State will prepare a report of its inspection and will provide a copy of that report to all participating States without delay.

(96) The inspection expenses will be incurred by the receiving State except when the inspecting State uses its own aircraft and/or land vehicles. The travel expenses to and from the point(s) of entry will be borne by the inspecting State.

(97) Diplomatic channels will be used for communications concerning compliance and verification.

(98) Each participating State will be entitled to obtain timely clarification from any other participating State concerning the application of agreed confidence- and security-building measures. Communications in this context will, if appropriate, be transmitted to all other participating States.

(99) The participating States stress that these confidence- and security-building measures are designed to reduce the dangers of armed conflict and misunderstanding or miscalculation of military activities and emphasize that their implementation will contribute to these objectives.

(100) Reaffirming the relevant objectives of the Final Act, the participating States are determined to continue building confidence, to lessen military confrontation and to enhance security for all. They are also determined to achieve progress in disarmament.

(101) The measures adopted in this document are politically binding and will come into force on 1 January 1987.

(102) The Government of Sweden is requested to transmit the present document to the follow-up meeting of the CSCE in Vienna and to the Secretary-General of the United Nations. The Government of Sweden is also requested to transmit the present document to the Governments of the non-participating Mediterranean States.

(103) The text of this document will be published in each participating State, which will disseminate it and make it known as widely as possible.

(104) The representatives of the participating States express their profound gratitude to the Government and people of Sweden for the excellent arrangements made for the Stockholm Conference and the warm hospitality extended to the delegations which participated in the Conference.

Stockholm, 19 September 1986

ANNEX I

Under the terms of the Madrid mandate, the zone of application for CSBMs is defined as follows:

"On the basis of equality of rights, balance and reciprocity, equal respect for the security interests of all CSCE participating States, and of their respective obligations concerning confidence- and security-building measures and disarmament in Europe, these confidence- and security-building measures will cover the whole of Europe as well as the adjoining sea area[5] and air space. They will be of military significance and politically binding and will be provided with adequate forms of verification which correspond to their content.

"As far as the adjoining sea area* and air space is concerned, the measures will be applicable to the military activities of all the participating States taking place there whenever these activities affect security in Europe as well as constitute a part of activities taking place within the whole of Europe as referred to above, which they will agree to notify. Necessary specifications will be made through the negotiations on the confidence- and security-building measures at the Conference.

"Nothing in the definition of the zone given above will diminish obligations already undertaken under the Final Act. The confidence- and security-building measures to be agreed upon at the Conference will also be applicable in all areas covered by any of the provisions in the Final Act relating to confidence-building measures and certain aspects of security and disarmament."

ANNEX II

Chairman's Statement

It is understood that, taking into account the agreed date of entry into force of the agreed confidence- and security-building measures and the provisions contained in them concerning the timeframes of certain advance notifications, and expressing their interest in an early transition to the full implementation of the provisions of this document, the participating States agree to the following:

The annual calendars concerning military activities subject to prior notification and forecast for 1987 will be exchanged not later than 15 December 1986.

Communications, in accordance with agreed provisions, concerning military activities involving more than 40,000 troops planned for the calendar year 1988 will be exchanged by 15 December 1986. Participating States may undertake activities involving more than 75,000 troops during the calendar year 1987 provided that they are included in the annual calendar exchanged by 15 December 1986.

Activities to begin during the first 42 days after 1 January 1987 will be subject to the relevant provisions of the Final Act of the CSCE. However, the participating States will make every effort to apply to them the provisions of this document to the maximum extent possible.

* In this context, the notion of adjoining sea area is understood to refer also to ocean areas adjoining Europe.

This statement will be an annex to the Document of the Stockholm Conference and will be published with it.

Stockholm, 19 September 1986

ANNEX III

Chairman's Statement

It is understood that each participating State can raise any question consistent with the mandate of the Conference on Confidence- and Security-Building Measures and Disarmament in Europe at any stage subsequent to the Vienna CSCE Follow-up Meeting.

This statement will be an annex to the Document of the Stockholm Conference and will be published with it.

Stockholm, 19 September 1986

ANNEX IV

Chairman's Statement

It is understood that the participating States recall that they have the right to belong or not to belong to international organizations, to be or not to be a party to bilateral or multilateral treaties including the right to be or not to be a party to treaties of alliance; they also have the right of neutrality. In this context, they will not take advantage of these rights to circumvent the purposes of the system of inspection, and in particular the provision that a participating State will be obliged to accept on its territory within the zone of application for CSBMs, more than three inspections per calendar year.

Appropriate understandings between participating States on this subject will be expressed in interpretative statements to be included in the journal of the day.

The statement will be an annex to the Document of the Stockholm Conference and will be published with it.

Stockholm, 19 September 1986

---

[1] In this document, the term notifiable means subject to notification [text in original].

[2] See Annex I [text in original].

[3] In this context, the term land forces includes amphibious, airmobile, and airborne forces [text in original].

[4] As defined in the provisions on Prior Notification of Certain Military Activities [text in original].

[5] "In this context, the notion of adjoining sea area is understood to refer also to ocean areas adjoining Europe" [quoted text in original].

(Whenever the term "the zone of application for CSBMs" is used in this document, the above definition will apply [text in original].)

AGREEMENT BETWEEN THE UNITED STATES OF AMERICA AND THE UNION OF SOVIET SOCIALIST REPUBLICS ON THE ESTABLISHMENT OF NUCLEAR RISK REDUCTION CENTERS (AND PROTOCOLS THERETO)

As the result of a U.S. initiative, President Reagan and General Secretary Gorbachev agreed at the November 1985 Geneva Summit to have experts explore the possibility of establishing centers to reduce the risk of nuclear war. The impetus for this initiative grew out of consultations between the Executive Branch and Congress, particularly Senators Sam Nunn and John Warner. U.S. and Soviet experts held informal meetings in Geneva on May 5-6 and August 25, 1986. In October 1986, at their meeting in Reykjavik, President Reagan and General Secretary Gorbachev indicated satisfaction with the progress made at the experts meetings and agreed to begin formal negotiations to establish Nuclear Risk Reduction Centers. Those negotiations were held in Geneva on January 13 and May 3-4, 1987.

The negotiations resulted in the Agreement that was signed in Washington September 15, 1987, by Secretary of State Shultz and Foreign Minister Shevardnadze.

Under the Agreement, which is of unlimited duration, each party agreed to establish a Nuclear Risk Reduction Center in its capital and to establish a special facsimile communications link between these Centers. These Nuclear Risk Reduction Centers became operational on April 1, 1988. The American National Center (known as the NRRC) is located in Washington, D.C. in the Department of State. The Soviet National Center became the Russian National Center with the dissolution of the Soviet Union and is located in Moscow in the Russian Federation Ministry of Defense.

The Centers are intended to supplement existing means of communication and provide direct, reliable, high-speed systems for the transmission of notifications and communications at the Government-to-Government level. The Centers communicate by direct satellite links that can transmit rapidly full texts and graphics. In this respect, the Centers have a communications capability very similar to -- but separate from -- the modernized "Hot Line," which is reserved for Heads of Government.

The Nuclear Risk Reduction Centers do not replace normal diplomatic channels of communication or the "Hot Line," nor are they intended to have a crisis management role. The principal function of the Centers is to exchange information and notifications as required under various arms control treaties and other confidence-building agreements.

There are two protocols to the NRRC Agreement. Protocol I identifies the notifications the parties agreed to exchange. These include ballistic missile launches required under Article 4 of the 1971 Agreement on Measures to Reduce the Risk of Outbreak of Nuclear War and under paragraph 1 of Article VI of the 1972 Agreement on the Prevention of Incidents on and over the High Seas.

The Agreement provides that the list of notifications transmitted through the Centers may be altered by agreement between the Parties as relevant new agreements are reached. Since the Agreement was signed, the Parties have additionally agreed to exchange through the Centers inspection and compliance notifications, as well as other information, required under the INF Treaty, and notifications called for under the Ballistic Missile Launch Notification Agreement.[1]

The Centers may be used for the transmission by either side of additional communications as a display of "good-will" and with a view to building confidence.

---

[1] Additionally, the Parties have agreed to use the Nuclear Risk Reduction Centers to transmit notifications under the following: the Agreement on Advance Notification of Major Strategic Exercises; the START I and START II Treaties, the Wyoming MOU; the Threshold Test Ban Treaty; and the Underground Nuclear Explosions for Peaceful Purposes Treaty. Both the American and Russian Centers have also assumed responsibility for their governments in transmitting messages related to the CFE Treaty, the CSBM notifications under Vienna Document 94 and the Open Skies Treaty via the Organization for Security and Cooperation in Europe (OSCE) Communications Network.

Protocol II establishes the technical specifications of the communications and facsimile links, the operating procedures to be employed, and the terms for transfer of, and payment for, equipment required by the system.[2]

To help ensure the smooth operation of the Centers, the Agreement calls for regular meetings at least once a year between representatives of the two national centers to discuss operation of the system.

---

[2] Both Parties have agreed to a modernization of communications equipment that updates the terminal equipment (replacing the facsimile capability with scanned files transfer) and should become fully operational in late 1995. Under separate agreements with Belarus, Kazakstan, and Ukraine, the U.S. NRRC operates similar communications links with those countries in support of the START I and INF Treaties.

AGREEMENT BETWEEN THE UNITED STATES OF AMERICA AND THE UNION OF SOVIET SOCIALIST REPUBLICS ON THE ESTABLISHMENT OF NUCLEAR RISK REDUCTION CENTERS

Signed at Washington September 15, 1987
Entered into force September 15, 1987

The United States of America and the Union of Soviet Socialist Republics, hereinafter referred to as the Parties,

Affirming their desire to reduce and ultimately eliminate the risk of outbreak of nuclear war, in particular, as a result of misinterpretation, miscalculation, or accident,

Believing that a nuclear war cannot be won and must never be fought,

Believing that agreement on measures for reducing the risk of outbreak of nuclear war serves the interests of strengthening international peace and security,

Reaffirming their obligations under the Agreement on Measures to Reduce the Risk of Outbreak of Nuclear War between the United States of America and the Union of Soviet Socialist Republics of September 30, 1971, and the Agreement between the Government of the United States of America and the Government of the Union of Soviet Socialist Republics on the Prevention of Incidents on and over the High Seas of May 25, 1972,

Have agreed as follows:

Article 1

Each Party shall establish, in its capital, a national Nuclear Risk Reduction Center that shall operate on behalf of and under the control of its respective Government.

Article 2

The Parties shall use the Nuclear Risk Reduction Centers to transmit notifications identified in Protocol I which constitutes an integral part of this Agreement.

In the future, the list of notifications transmitted through the Centers may be altered by agreement between the Parties, as relevant new agreements are reached.

Article 3

The Parties shall establish a special facsimile communications link between their national Nuclear Risk Reduction Centers in accordance with Protocol II which constitutes an integral part of this Agreement.

Article 4

The Parties shall staff their national Nuclear Risk Reduction Centers as they deem appropriate, so as to ensure their normal functioning.

Article 5

The Parties shall hold regular meetings between representatives of the Nuclear Risk Reduction Centers at least once each year to consider matters related to the functioning of such Centers.

Article 6

This Agreement shall not affect the obligations of either Party under other agreements.

Article 7

This Agreement shall enter into force on the date of its signature.

The duration of this Agreement shall not be limited.

This Agreement may be terminated by either Party upon 12 months written notice to the other Party.

DONE at Washington on September 15, 1987, in two copies, each in the English and Russian languages, both texts being equally authentic.

FOR THE UNITED STATES OF AMERICA:
George P. Shultz

FOR THE UNION OF SOVIET SOCIALIST REPUBLICS:
Eduard A. Shevardnadze

PROTOCOL I TO THE AGREEMENT BETWEEN THE UNITED STATES OF AMERICA AND THE UNION OF SOVIET SOCIALIST REPUBLICS ON THE ESTABLISHMENT OF NUCLEAR RISK REDUCTION CENTERS

Pursuant to the provisions and in implementation of the Agreement between the United States of America and the Union of Soviet Socialist Republics on the Establishment of Nuclear Risk Reduction Centers, the Parties have agreed as follows:

Article 1

The Parties shall transmit the following types of notifications through the Nuclear Risk Reduction Centers:

(a) notifications of ballistic missile launches under Article 4 of the Agreement on Measures to Reduce the Risk of Outbreak of Nuclear War between the United States of America and the Union of Soviet Socialist Republics of September 30, 1971;

(b) notifications of ballistic missile launches under paragraph 1 of Article VI of the Agreement between the Government of the United States of America and the Government of the Union of Soviet Socialist Republics on the Prevention of Incidents on and over the High Seas of May 25, 1972.

Article 2

The scope and format of the information to be transmitted through the Nuclear Risk Reduction Centers shall be agreed upon.

Article 3

Each Party also may, at its own discretion as a display of good will and with a view to building confidence, transmit through the Nuclear Risk Reduction Centers communications other than those provided for under Article 1 of this Protocol.

Article 4

Unless the Parties agree otherwise, all communications transmitted through and communications procedures of the Nuclear Risk Reduction Centers' communication link will be confidential.

Article 5

This Protocol shall enter into force on the date of its signature and shall remain in force as long as the Agreement between the United States of America and the Union of Soviet Socialist Republics on the Establishment of Nuclear Risk Reduction Centers of September 15, 1987, remains in force.

DONE at Washington on September 15, 1987, in two copies, each in the English and Russian languages, both texts being equally authentic.

FOR THE UNITED STATES OF AMERICA:
George P. Shultz

FOR THE UNION OF SOVIET AMERICA SOCIALIST REPUBLICS:
Eduard A. Shevardnadze

**PROTOCOL II TO THE AGREEMENT
BETWEEN THE UNITED STATES OF AMERICA
AND THE UNION OF SOVIET SOCIALIST
REPUBLICS ON THE ESTABLISHMENT OF
NUCLEAR RISK REDUCTION CENTERS**

Pursuant to the provisions and in
implementation of the Agreement between the
United States of America and the Union of Soviet
Socialist Republics on the Establishment of
Nuclear Risk Reduction Centers, the Parties have
agreed as follows:

Article 1

To establish and maintain for the purpose of
providing direct facsimile communications
between their national Nuclear Risk Reduction
Centers, established in accordance with Article 1
of this Agreement, hereinafter referred to as the
national Centers, an INTELSAT satellite circuit
and a STATSIONAR satellite circuit, each with a
secure orderwire communications capability for
operational monitoring. In this regard:

(a) There shall be terminals equipped for
communication between the national Centers;

(b) Each Party shall provide communications
circuits capable of simultaneously transmitting
and receiving 4800 bits per second;

(c) Communication shall begin with test
operation of the INTELSAT satellite circuit, as
soon as purchase, delivery and installation of the
necessary equipment by the Parties are
completed. Thereafter, taking into account the
results of test operations, the Parties shall agree
on the transition to a fully operational status;

(d) To the extent practicable, test operation of
the STATSIONAR satellite circuit shall begin
simultaneously with test operation of the
INTELSAT satellite circuit. Taking into account
the results of test operations, the Parties shall
agree on the transition to a fully operational
status.

Article 2

To employ agreed-upon information security
devices to assure secure transmission of
facsimile messages. In this regard:

(a) The information security devices shall
consist of microprocessors that will combine the
digital message output with buffered random data
read from standard 5 1/4 inch floppy disks;

(b) Each Party shall provide, through its
Embassy, necessary keying material to the other.

Article 3

To establish and maintain at each operating
end of the two circuits, facsimile terminals of the
same make and model. In this regard:

(a) Each Party shall be responsible for the
purchase, installation, operation and maintenance
of its own terminals, the related information
security devices, and local transmission circuits
appropriate to the implementation of this Protocol;

(b) A Group III facsimile unit which meets
CCITT Recommendations T.4 and T.30 and
operates at 4800 bits per second shall be used;

(c) Direct facsimile messages from the USSR
national Center to the U.S. national Center shall
be transmitted and received in the Russian
language, and from the U.S. national Center to
the USSR national Center in the English
language;

(d) Transmission and operating procedures
shall be in conformity with procedures employed
on the Direct Communications Link and adapted
as necessary for the purpose of communications
between the national Centers.

Article 4

To establish and maintain a secure orderwire
communications capability necessary to
coordinate facsimile operation. In this regard:

(a) The orderwire terminals used with the
information security devices described in
paragraph (a) of Article 2 shall incorporate
standard USSR Cyrillic and United States Latin
keyboards and cathode ray tube displays to
permit the exchange of messages between
operators. The specific layout of the Cyrillic
keyboard shall be as specified by the Soviet side;

(b) To coordinate the work of operators, the
orderwire shall be configured so as to permit,

prior to the transmission and reception of messages, the exchange of all information pertinent to the coordination of such messages;

(c) Orderwire messages concerning transmissions shall be encoded using the same information security devices specified in paragraph (a) of Article 2;

(d) The orderwire shall use the same modem and communications link as used for facsimile message transmission;

(e) A printer shall be included to provide a record copy of all information exchanged on the orderwire.

Article 5

To use the same type of equipment and the same maintenance procedures as currently in use for the Direct Communications Link for the establishment of direct facsimile communications between the national Centers. The equipment, security devices, and spare parts necessary for telecommunications links and the orderwire shall be provided by the United States side to the Soviet side in return for payment of costs thereof by the Soviet side.

Article 6

To ensure the exchange of information necessary for the operation and maintenance of the telecommunication system and equipment configuration.

Article 7

To take all possible measures to assure the continuous, secure and reliable operation of the equipment and communications link, including the orderwire, for which each Party is responsible in accordance with this Protocol.

Article 8

To determine, by mutual agreement between technical experts of the Parties, the distribution and calculation of expenses for putting into operation the communication link, its maintenance and further development.

Article 9

To convene meetings of technical experts of the Parties in order to consider initially questions pertaining to the practical implementation of the activities provided for in this Protocol and, thereafter, by mutual agreement and as necessary for the purpose of improving telecommunications and information technology in order to achieve the mutually agreed functions of the national Centers.

Article 10

This Protocol shall enter into force on the date of its signature and shall remain in force as long as the Agreement Between the United States of America and the Union of Soviet Socialist Republics on the Establishment of Nuclear Risk Reduction Centers of September 15, 1987, remains in force.

DONE at Washington on September 15, 1987, in two copies, each in the English and Russian languages, both texts being equally authentic.

FOR THE UNITED STATES OF AMERICA:
George P. Shultz

FOR THE UNION OF SOVIET SOCIALIST REPUBLICS:
Eduard A. Shevardnadze

TREATY BETWEEN THE UNITED STATES OF AMERICA AND THE UNION OF SOVIET SOCIALIST REPUBLICS ON THE ELIMINATION OF THEIR INTERMEDIATE-RANGE AND SHORTER-RANGE MISSILES

The Treaty Between the United States of America and the Union of Soviet Socialist Republics on the Elimination of Their Intermediate-Range and Shorter-Range Missiles, commonly referred to as the INF (Intermediate-Range Nuclear Forces) Treaty, requires destruction of the Parties' ground-launched ballistic and cruise missiles with ranges of between 500 and 5,500 kilometers, their launchers and associated support structures and support equipment within three years after the Treaty enters into force.

In the mid-1970s the Soviet Union achieved rough strategic parity with the United States. Shortly thereafter, the Soviet Union began replacing older intermediate-range SS-4 and SS-5 missiles with a new intermediate-range missile, the SS-20, bringing about what was perceived as a qualitative and quantitative change in the European security situation. The SS-20 was mobile, accurate, and capable of being concealed and rapidly redeployed. It carried three independently targetable warheads, as distinguished from the single warheads carried by its predecessors. The SS-20's 5,000 kilometer range permitted it to cover targets in Western Europe, North Africa, the Middle East, and, from bases in the eastern Soviet Union, most of Asia, Southeast Asia, and Alaska.

In late 1977, NATO's Nuclear Planning Group ordered a study of the Alliance's long-term INF modernization needs, consistent with the doctrine of flexible response. In the spring of 1979, NATO established the Special Consultative Group to formulate guiding principles for future arms control efforts involving INF. That summer, NATO produced the Integrated Decision Document, which set forth the basic aims of the Alliance's INF policy. It called for complementary programs of force modernization and arms control.

On November 12, 1979, the NATO ministers unanimously adopted a "dual track" strategy to counter Soviet SS-20 deployments. One track called for arms control negotiations between the United States and the Soviet Union to reduce INF

forces to the lowest possible level; the second track called for deployment in Western Europe, beginning in December 1983, of 464 single-warhead U.S. ground-launched cruise (GLCM) missiles and 108 Pershing II ballistic missiles.

Initially the Soviet Union refused to engage in preliminary talks, unless NATO revoked its deployment decision; however, by July 1980, the Soviet position changed, and preliminary discussions began in Geneva in the fall of 1980.

The U.S. approach to the negotiations, developed through extensive consultations within NATO, required that any INF agreement must: (1) provide for equality both in limits and rights between the United States and the Soviet Union; (2) be strictly bilateral and thus exclude British and French systems; (3) limit systems on a global basis; (4) not adversely affect NATO's conventional defense capability; and (5) be effectively verifiable.

Agreement to begin formal talks was reached on September 23, 1981. On November 18, President Reagan announced a negotiating proposal in which the United States would agree to eliminate its Pershing IIs and GLCMs if the Soviet Union would dismantle all of its SS-20s, SS-4s, and SS-5s. This proposal became known as the "zero-zero offer."

At the beginning of the talks, the Soviet Union opposed the deployment of any U.S. INF missiles in Europe and proposed a ceiling of 300 "medium-range" missiles and nuclear-capable aircraft for both sides, with British and French nuclear forces counting toward the ceiling for the West.

During the first two years of the talks, which ended with a Soviet walkout on November 23, 1983, the United States continued to emphasize its preference for the "zero option" even while introducing the concept of an interim agreement based on equally low numbers of INF systems.

During 1984 there were no INF negotiations. U.S. deployments were carried out as planned in the Federal Republic of Germany, Italy, and the United Kingdom, while preparations for deployment continued in Belgium.

In January 1985, Secretary of State George Shultz and Soviet Foreign Minister Andrey Gromyko agreed to separate but parallel negotiations on INF, strategic arms (START), and defense and space issues as part of a new bilateral forum called the Nuclear and Space Talks (NST). The United States and the Soviet Union agreed that all questions regarding these three areas would be considered in their interrelationship. Negotiations would be conducted by a single delegation from each side, divided into three groups -- one for defense and space, one for START, and one for INF. Formal talks resumed in March 1985 in all three areas.

In the fall of 1985, the Soviet Union hinted at the possibility of an INF agreement independent of START or defense and space issues. As U.S. GLCM deployments continued, the Soviet Union outlined an interim INF agreement that would permit some U.S. GLCMs in Europe, but which would permit SS-20 warheads equal to the sum of all warheads on U.S., British, and French systems combined. The Soviets also offered to freeze INF systems in Asia -- contingent on U.S. acceptance of their proposals and provided the Asian strategic situation did not change.

In November of 1985, President Reagan and General Secretary Gorbachev met in Geneva, where they issued a joint statement calling for an "interim accord on intermediate-range nuclear forces." At the end of 1985, the United States proposed a limit of 140 launchers in Europe for both sides and proportionate reductions in Asia while emphasizing collateral constraints on shorter-range missiles, since these systems can cover the same targets as longer-range systems.

On January 15, 1986, General Secretary Gorbachev announced a Soviet proposal for a three-stage program to ban nuclear weapons by the year 2000, which included elimination of all U.S. and Soviet INF missiles in Europe.

In late February 1986, the United States proposed a limit of 140 INF launchers in Europe and concurrent proportionate reductions in Asia. This proposal also called for both sides to reduce their INF missile launchers remaining in Europe and Asia by an additional 50 percent in 1988 and, finally, to eliminate all INF weapons by the end of 1989. There would be no constraints on British and French nuclear forces. Moreover, as of the end of 1987, shorter-range missiles would be limited equally either to current Soviet levels existing on January 1, 1982, or to a lower level. The United States also presented an outline for comprehensive verification.

A series of high-level discussions took place in August and September 1986 followed by a meeting between President Reagan and General Secretary Gorbachev in Reykjavik, Iceland, in October 1986, where the sides agreed to equal global ceilings of systems capable of carrying 100 INF missile warheads, none of which would be deployed in Europe. The Soviet Union also proposed a freeze on shorter-range missile deployments and agreed in principle to intrusive on-site verification.

Several months later, on February 28, 1987, the Soviet Union announced that it was prepared to reach a separate INF agreement. On March 4, 1987, the United States tabled a draft INF Treaty text, which reflected the agreement reached at Reykjavik, and submitted a comprehensive verification regime. In April the Soviet Union presented its own draft Treaty, and by July, it had agreed in principle to some of the provisions in the U.S. comprehensive verification regime, including data exchange, on-site observation of elimination, and on-site inspection of INF missile inventories and facilities. In a major shift, however, the Soviet side proposed the inclusion of U.S.-owned warheads on the West German Pershing IA missile systems. The United States responded by restating that the INF negotiations were bilateral, covering only U.S. and Soviet missiles, and could not involve third-country systems or affect existing patterns of cooperation.

During April meetings with Secretary Shultz in Moscow, General Secretary Gorbachev proposed the possible elimination of U.S. and Soviet shorter-range missiles. At the June 1987 meeting of the North Atlantic Council, NATO foreign ministers announced support for the global elimination of all U.S. and Soviet intermediate-range and shorter-range missile systems. On June 15, President Reagan proposed the elimination of all U.S. and Soviet shorter-range missile systems.

On July 22, 1987, General Secretary Gorbachev agreed to a "double global zero" Treaty to eliminate intermediate-range and shorter-range missiles.

On August 26, 1987, Chancellor Kohl announced the Federal Republic of Germany would dismantle its 72 Pershing IA missiles and not replace them with more modern weapons if the United States and the Soviet Union scrapped all of their INF missiles as foreseen in the emerging Treaty. This was a unilateral declaration by the FRG and is not part of the INF Treaty, which is a bilateral U.S.-Soviet agreement.

In September, the two sides reached agreement in principle to complete the Treaty before the end of the year. On December 8, 1987, the Treaty was signed by President Reagan and General Secretary Gorbachev at a summit meeting in Washington. At the time of its signature, the Treaty's verification regime was the most detailed and stringent in the history of nuclear arms control, designed both to eliminate all declared INF systems entirely within three years of the Treaty's entry into force and to ensure compliance with the total ban on possession and use of these missiles.

The Treaty the United States and the Soviet Union signed at Washington on December 8 includes the Memorandum of Understanding (MOU) on Data,[1] the Protocol on Inspections, and the Protocol on Elimination. Because of concerns raised by the Senate during the ratification hearings, and because of issues that arose during technical consultations between the United States and the Soviet Union during the spring of 1988, this package was augmented by three exchanges of diplomatic notes (one on May 12, 1988 and two on May 21, 1988) and an agreed minute signed May 12, 1988. The Senate resolution of ratification required the President, prior to exchanging instruments of ratification, to obtain Soviet agreement that the four documents "are of the same force and effect as the provisions of the Treaty." This was done through an exchange of notes on May 28, 1988. The Treaty entered into force upon the exchange of instruments of ratification in Moscow on June 1, 1988.

The May 12 and May 28 exchanges of notes, as well as the May 12 agreed minute, are included herein following the texts of the Treaty, the MOU and the Protocols. The May 21 exchange of notes, which corrected errors in the site diagrams and Treaty text, are not included,

but the textual corrections are listed following the text of the Treaty, MOU and protocols.

Article XIII established the Special Verification Commission (SVC). The SVC serves as a forum for discussing and resolving implementation and compliance issues, for considering additional procedures to improve the viability and effectiveness of the Treaty, and for determining the characteristics and methods of use of inspection equipment as anticipated by Section VI of the Protocol on Inspection. The sides resolved many of those issues during the first SVC session and agreed to utilize the agreements reached until such time as a document embodying them was signed by the two sides.

During the third session of the SVC (December 1988), the sides signed an Agreed Statement on inspection procedures at the continuous monitoring inspection site at Votkinsk and a Memorandum of Understanding on operating procedures for the SVC.

To confirm the declared inventory of INF systems throughout the three-year elimination period and for ten years thereafter, the INF Treaty established various types of on-site inspections, among these are, baseline inspections, to confirm the initial data update; closeout inspections of facilities and missile operation bases at which INF activity ceased; short-notice (quota) inspections of declared and formerly declared facilities, and elimination inspections to confirm elimination of INF systems in accordance with agreed procedures. In addition the United States also received the right to monitor, on a continuous basis for up to 13 years, the access (or portals) to any Soviet facility manufacturing a ground-launched ballistic missile (GLBM), not covered under the INF Treaty, which has a stage outwardly similar to a stage of a GLBM limited by the Treaty. The Soviets received a similar right to monitor the U.S. facility that previously produced the Pershing rocket motor.

---

[1] A comprehensive data exchange took place at the time the Treaty was signed. This MOU included the numbers and locations of all Treaty-limited items, as well as their technical characteristics. All categories of data in the MOU are updated at six-month intervals for the duration of the Treaty.

The U.S. On-Site Inspection (OSIA) was established January 15, 1988, *inter alia*, to coordinate and implement the inspection provisions of the Treaty. Baseline inspections were conducted in 1988 by U.S. and Soviet inspectors to verify the data provided by the United States and Soviet Union on the number and locations of their respective INF systems and facilities.

In late April and early May 1991, the United States eliminated its last ground-launched cruise missile and ground-launched ballistic missile covered under the INF Treaty. The last declared Soviet SS-20 was eliminated on May 11, 1991. A total of 2,692 missiles was eliminated after the Treaty's entry-into-force.

Following the December 25, 1991, dissolution of the Soviet Union, the United States sought to secure continuation of full implementation of the INF Treaty regime and to multilateralize the INF Treaty with twelve former Soviet republics which the United States considers INF Treaty successors.[2] Of the twelve successor states, six -- Belarus, Kazakstan, Russia, Turkmenistan, Ukraine, and Uzbekistan -- have inspectable INF facilities on their territory. Of these six, four -- Belarus, Kazakstan, Russia, and Ukraine -- are active participants in the process of implementing the Treaty. With the agreement of the other Parties, Turkmenistan and Uzbekistan, each with only one inspectable site on its territory, while participants, have assumed a less active role, foregoing attendance at sessions of the SVC and participation in inspections.

The multilateralizing of what was previously a bilateral U.S.-Soviet INF Treaty required establishing agreements between the United States and the governments of the relevant Soviet successor states on numerous issues. In the SVC and through diplomatic contacts with the actively participating successor states, the United States worked to secure agreements to ensure continuation of the viability of the Treaty regime and to assure the exercise by the United States of its rights under the Treaty. Among the tasks undertaken were: arrangements for the settlement of costs connected with implementation activities in the new, multilateral Treaty context; the establishment of new points of entry (POE's) in Belarus, Kazakstan, and Ukraine through which to conduct inspections of the former INF facilities in those countries; and the establishment of communications links between the United States and those countries for transmission of various Treaty-related notifications. Other issues that have been discussed in the SVC include multilateral operating procedures for the SVC's concurrent continuous monitoring under the START I and INF Treaties, and inspection procedures for new missiles exiting from the Votkinsk Machine Building Plant in Russia.

---

[2] The United States did not consider the Baltic states to be successors, since it had never recognized the legality of their incorporation into the Soviet Union.

TREATY BETWEEN THE UNITED STATES OF AMERICA AND THE UNION OF SOVIET SOCIALIST REPUBLICS ON THE ELIMINATION OF THEIR INTERMEDIATE-RANGE AND SHORTER-RANGE MISSILES

Signed at Washington December 8, 1987
Ratification advised by U.S. Senate May 27, 1988
Instruments of ratification exchanged June 1, 1988
Entered into force June 1, 1988
Proclaimed by U.S. President December 27, 1988

The United States of America and the Union of Soviet Socialist Republics, hereinafter referred to as the Parties,

Conscious that nuclear war would have devastating consequences for all mankind,

Guided by the objective of strengthening strategic stability,

Convinced that the measures set forth in this Treaty will help to reduce the risk of outbreak of war and strengthen international peace and security, and

Mindful of their obligations under Article VI of the Treaty on the Non-Proliferation of Nuclear Weapons,

Have agreed as follows:

Article I

In accordance with the provisions of this Treaty which includes the Memorandum of Understanding and Protocols which form an integral part thereof, each Party shall eliminate its intermediate-range and shorter-range missiles, not have such systems thereafter, and carry out the other obligations set forth in this Treaty.

Article II

For the purposes of this Treaty:

1. The term "ballistic missile" means a missile that has a ballistic trajectory over most of its flight path. The term "ground-launched ballistic missile (GLBM)" means a ground-launched ballistic missile that is a weapon-delivery vehicle.

2. The term "cruise missile" means an unmanned, self-propelled vehicle that sustains flight through the use of aerodynamic lift over most of its flight path. The term "ground-launched cruise missile (GLCM)" means a ground-launched cruise missile that is a weapon-delivery vehicle.

3. The term "GLBM launcher" means a fixed launcher or a mobile land-based transporter-erector-launcher mechanism for launching a GLBM.

4. The term "GLCM launcher" means a fixed launcher or a mobile land-based transporter-erector-launcher mechanism for launching a GLCM.

5. The term "intermediate-range missile" means a GLBM or a GLCM having a range capability in excess of 1000 kilometers but not in excess of 5500 kilometers.

6. The term "shorter-range missile" means a GLBM or a GLCM having a range capability equal to or in excess of 500 kilometers but not in excess of 1000 kilometers.

7. The term "deployment area" means a designated area within which intermediate-range missiles and launchers of such missiles may operate and within which one or more missile operating bases are located.

8. The term "missile operating base" means:

(a) in the case of intermediate-range missiles, a complex of facilities, located within a deployment area, at which intermediate-range missiles and launchers of such missiles normally operate, in which support structures associated with such missiles and launchers are also located and in which support equipment associated with such missiles and launchers is normally located; and

(b) in the case of shorter-range missiles, a complex of facilities, located any place, at which shorter-range missiles and launchers of such missiles normally operate and in which support equipment associated with such missiles and launchers is normally located.

9. The term "missile support facility," as regards intermediate-range or shorter-range missiles and launchers of such missiles, means a missile production facility or a launcher production facility, a missile repair facility or a launcher repair facility, a training facility, a missile storage facility or a launcher storage facility, a test range, or an elimination facility as those terms are defined in the Memorandum of Understanding.

10. The term "transit" means movement, notified in accordance with paragraph 5(f) of Article IX of this Treaty, of an intermediate-range missile or a launcher of such a missile between missile support facilities, between such a facility and a deployment area or between deployment areas, or of a shorter-range missile or a launcher of such a missile from a missile support facility or a missile operating base to an elimination facility.

11. The term "deployed missile" means an intermediate-range missile located within a deployment area or a shorter-range missile located at a missile operating base.

12. The term "non-deployed missile" means an intermediate-range missile located outside a deployment area or a shorter-range missile located outside a missile operating base.

13. The term "deployed launcher" means a launcher of an intermediate-range missile located within a deployment area or a launcher of a shorter-range missile located at a missile operating base.

14. The term "non-deployed launcher" means a launcher of an intermediate-range missile located outside a deployment area or a launcher of a shorter-range missile located outside a missile operating base.

15. The term "basing country" means a country other than the United States of America or the Union of Soviet Socialist Republics on whose territory intermediate-range or shorter-range missiles of the Parties, launchers of such missiles or support structures associated with such missiles and launchers were located at any time after November 1, 1987. Missiles or launchers in transit are not considered to be "located."

Article III

1. For the purposes of this Treaty, existing types of intermediate-range missiles are:

(a) for the United States of America, missiles of the types designated by the United States of America as the Pershing II and the BGM-109G, which are known to the Union of Soviet Socialist Republics by the same designations; and

(b) for the Union of Soviet Socialist Republics, missiles of the types designated by the Union of Soviet Socialist Republics as the RSD-10, the R-12 and the R-14, which are known to the United States of America as the SS-20, the SS-4 and the SS-5, respectively.

2. For the purposes of this Treaty, existing types of shorter-range missiles are:

(a) for the United States of America, missiles of the type designated by the United States of America as the Pershing IA, which is known to the Union of Soviet Socialist Republics by the same designation; and

(b) for the Union of Soviet Socialist Republics, missiles of the types designated by the Union of Soviet Socialist Republics as the OTR-22 and the OTR-23, which are known to the United States of America as the SS-12 and the SS-23, respectively.

Article IV

1. Each Party shall eliminate all its intermediate-range missiles and launchers of such missiles, and all support structures and support equipment of the categories listed in the Memorandum of Understanding associated with such missiles and launchers, so that no later than three years after entry into force of this Treaty and thereafter no such missiles, launchers, support structures or support equipment shall be possessed by either Party.

2. To implement paragraph 1 of this Article, upon entry into force of this Treaty, both Parties shall begin and continue throughout the duration of each phase, the reduction of all types of their deployed and non-deployed intermediate-range missiles and deployed and non-deployed launchers of such missiles and support structures and support equipment associated with such missiles and launchers in accordance with the

provisions of this Treaty. These reductions shall be implemented in two phases so that:

(a) by the end of the first phase, that is, no later than 29 months after entry into force of this Treaty:

(i) the number of deployed launchers of intermediate-range missiles for each Party shall not exceed the number of launchers that are capable of carrying or containing at one time missiles considered by the Parties to carry 171 warheads;

(ii) the number of deployed intermediate-range missiles for each Party shall not exceed the number of such missiles considered by the Parties to carry 180 warheads;

(iii) the aggregate number of deployed and non-deployed launchers of intermediate-range missiles for each Party shall not exceed the number of launchers that are capable of carrying or containing at one time missiles considered by the Parties to carry 200 warheads;

(iv) the aggregate number of deployed and non-deployed intermediate-range missiles for each Party shall not exceed the number of such missiles considered by the Parties to carry 200 warheads; and

(v) the ratio of the aggregate number of deployed and non-deployed intermediate-range GLBMs of existing types for each Party to the aggregate number of deployed and non-deployed intermediate-range missiles of existing types possessed by that Party shall not exceed the ratio of such intermediate-range GLBMs to such intermediate-range missiles for that Party as of November 1, 1987, as set forth in the Memorandum of Understanding; and

(b) by the end of the second phase, that is, no later than three years after entry into force of this Treaty, all intermediate-range missiles of each Party, launchers of such missiles and all support structures and support equipment of the categories listed in the Memorandum of Understanding associated with such missiles and launchers, shall be eliminated.

Article V

1. Each Party shall eliminate all its shorter-range missiles and launchers of such missiles, and all support equipment of the categories listed in the Memorandum of Understanding associated with such missiles and launchers, so that no later than 18 months after entry into force of this Treaty and thereafter no such missiles, launchers or support equipment shall be possessed by either Party.

2. No later than 90 days after entry into force of this Treaty, each Party shall complete the removal of all its deployed shorter-range missiles and deployed and non-deployed launchers of such missiles to elimination facilities and shall retain them at those locations until they are eliminated in accordance with the procedures set forth in the Protocol on Elimination. No later than 12 months after entry into force of this Treaty, each Party shall complete the removal of all its non-deployed shorter-range missiles to elimination facilities and shall retain them at those locations until they are eliminated in accordance with the procedures set forth in the Protocol on Elimination.

3. Shorter-range missiles and launchers of such missiles shall not be located at the same elimination facility. Such facilities shall be separated by no less than 1000 kilometers.

Article VI

1. Upon entry into force of this Treaty and thereafter, neither Party shall:

(a) produce or flight-test any intermediate-range missiles or produce any stages of such missiles or any launchers of such missiles; or

(b) produce, flight-test or launch any shorter-range missiles or produce any stages of such missiles or any launchers of such missiles.

2. Notwithstanding paragraph 1 of this Article, each Party shall have the right to produce a type of GLBM not limited by this Treaty which uses a stage which is outwardly similar to, but not interchangeable with, a stage of an existing type of intermediate-range GLBM having more than one stage, providing that that Party does not produce any other stage which is outwardly

similar to, but not interchangeable with, any other stage of an existing type of intermediate-range GLBM.

Article VII

For the purposes of this Treaty:

1. If a ballistic missile or a cruise missile has been flight-tested or deployed for weapon delivery, all missiles of that type shall be considered to be weapon-delivery vehicles.

2. If a GLBM or GLCM is an intermediate-range missile, all GLBMs or GLCMs of that type shall be considered to be intermediate-range missiles. If a GLBM or GLCM is a shorter-range missile, all GLBMs or GLCMs of that type shall be considered to be shorter-range missiles.

3. If a GLBM is of a type developed and tested solely to intercept and counter objects not located on the surface of the earth, it shall not be considered to be a missile to which the limitations of this Treaty apply.

4. The range capability of a GLBM not listed in Article III of this Treaty shall be considered to be the maximum range to which it has been tested. The range capability of a GLCM not listed in Article III of this Treaty shall be considered to be the maximum distance which can be covered by the missile in its standard design mode flying until fuel exhaustion, determined by projecting its flight path onto the earth's sphere from the point of launch to the point of impact. GLBMs or GLCMs that have a range capability equal to or in excess of 500 kilometers but not in excess of 1000 kilometers shall be considered to be shorter-range missiles. GLBMs or GLCMs that have a range capability in excess of 1000 kilometers but not in excess of 5500 kilometers shall be considered to be intermediate-range missiles.

5. The maximum number of warheads an existing type of intermediate-range missile or shorter-range missile carries shall be considered to be the number listed for missiles of that type in the Memorandum of Understanding.

6. Each GLBM or GLCM shall be considered to carry the maximum number of warheads listed for a GLBM or GLCM of the type in the Memorandum of Understanding.

7. If a launcher has been tested for launching a GLBM or a GLCM, all launchers of that type shall be considered to have been tested for launching GLBMs or GLCMs.

8. If a launcher has contained or launched a particular type of GLBM or GLCM, all launchers of that type shall be considered to be launchers of that type of GLBM or GLCM.

9. The number of missiles each launcher of an existing type of intermediate-range missile or shorter-range missile shall be considered to be capable of carrying or containing at one time is the number listed for launchers of missiles of that type in the Memorandum of Understanding.

10. Except in the case of elimination in accordance with the procedures set forth in the Protocol on Elimination, the following shall apply:

(a) for GLBMs which are stored or moved in separate stages, the longest stage of an intermediate-range or shorter-range GLBM shall be counted as a complete missile;

(b) for GLBMs which are not stored or moved in separate stages, a canister of the type used in the launch of an intermediate-range GLBM, unless a Party proves to the satisfaction of the other Party that it does not contain such a missile, or an assembled intermediate-range or shorter-range GLBM, shall be counted as a complete missile; and

(c) for GLCMs, the airframe of an intermediate-range or shorter-range GLCM shall be counted as a complete missile.

11. A ballistic missile which is not a missile to be used in a ground-based mode shall not be considered to be a GLBM if it is test-launched at a test site from a fixed land-based launcher which is used solely for test purposes and which is distinguishable from GLBM launchers. A cruise missile which is not a missile to be used in a ground-based mode shall not be considered to be a GLCM if it is test-launched at a test site from a fixed land-based launcher which is used solely for test purposes and which is distinguishable from GLCM launchers.

12. Each Party shall have the right to produce and use for booster systems, which might otherwise be considered to be intermediate-range or shorter-range missiles, only existing types of booster stages for such booster systems. Launches of such booster systems shall not be considered to be flight-testing of intermediate-range or shorter-range missiles provided that:

(a) stages used in such booster systems are different from stages used in those missiles listed as existing types of intermediate-range or shorter-range missiles in Article III of this Treaty;

(b) such booster systems are used only for research and development purposes to test objects other than the booster systems themselves;

(c) the aggregate number of launchers for such booster systems shall not exceed 35 for each Party at any one time; and

(d) the launchers for such booster systems are fixed, emplaced above ground and located only at research and development launch sites which are specified in the Memorandum of Understanding.

Research and development launch sites shall not be subject to inspection pursuant to Article XI of this Treaty.

Article VIII

1. All intermediate-range missiles and launchers of such missiles shall be located in deployment areas, at missile support facilities or shall be in transit. Intermediate-range missiles or launchers of such missiles shall not be located elsewhere.

2. Stages of intermediate-range missiles shall be located in deployment areas, at missile support facilities or moving between deployment areas, between missile support facilities or between missile support facilities and deployment areas.

3. Until their removal to elimination facilities as required by paragraph 2 of Article V of this Treaty, all shorter-range missiles and launchers of such missiles shall be located at missile operating bases, at missile support facilities or shall be in transit. Shorter-range missiles or launchers of

such missiles shall not be located elsewhere.

4. Transit of a missile or launcher subject to the provisions of this Treaty shall be completed within 25 days.

5. All deployment areas, missile operating bases and missile support facilities are specified in the Memorandum of Understanding or in subsequent updates of data pursuant to paragraphs 3, 5(a) or 5(b) of Article IX of this Treaty. Neither Party shall increase the number of, or change the location or boundaries of, deployment areas, missile operating bases or missile support facilities, except for elimination facilities, from those set forth in the Memorandum of Understanding. A missile support facility shall not be considered to be part of a deployment area even though it may be located within the geographic boundaries of a deployment area.

6. Beginning 30 days after entry into force of this Treaty, neither Party shall locate intermediate-range or shorter-range missiles, including stages of such missiles, or launchers of such missiles at missile production facilities, launcher production facilities or test ranges listed in the Memorandum of Understanding.

7. Neither Party shall locate any intermediate-range or shorter-range missiles at training facilities.

8. A non-deployed intermediate-range or shorter-range missile shall not be carried on or contained within a launcher of such a type of missile, except as required for maintenance conducted at repair facilities or for elimination by means of launching conducted at elimination facilities.

9. Training missiles and training launchers for intermediate-range or shorter-range missiles shall be subject to the same locational restrictions as are set forth for intermediate-range and shorter-range missiles and launchers of such missiles in paragraphs 1 and 3 of this Article.

Article IX

1. The Memorandum of Understanding contains categories of data relevant to obligations undertaken with regard to this Treaty and lists all intermediate-range and shorter-range missiles,

launchers of such missiles, and support structures and support equipment associated with such missiles and launchers, possessed by the Parties as of November 1, 1987. Updates of that data and notifications required by this Article shall be provided according to the categories of data contained in the Memorandum of Understanding.

2. The Parties shall update that data and provide the notifications required by this Treaty through the Nuclear Risk Reduction Centers, established pursuant to the Agreement Between the United States of America and the Union of Soviet Socialist Republics on the Establishment of Nuclear Risk Reduction Centers of September 15, 1987.

3. No later than 30 days after entry into force of this Treaty, each Party shall provide the other Party with updated data, as of the date of entry into force of this Treaty, for all categories of data contained in the Memorandum of Understanding.

4. No later than 30 days after the end of each six-month interval following the entry into force of this Treaty, each Party shall provide updated data for all categories of data contained in the Memorandum of Understanding by informing the other Party of all changes, completed and in process, in that data, which have occurred during the six-month interval since the preceding data exchange, and the net effect of those changes.

5. Upon entry into force of this Treaty and thereafter, each Party shall provide the following notifications to the other Party:

(a) notification, no less than 30 days in advance, of the scheduled date of the elimination of a specific deployment area, missile operating base or missile support facility;

(b) notification, no less than 30 days in advance, of changes in the number or location of elimination facilities, including the location and scheduled date of each change;

(c) notification, except with respect to launches of intermediate-range missiles for the purpose of their elimination, no less than 30 days in advance, of the scheduled date of the initiation of

the elimination of intermediate-range and shorter-range missiles, and stages of such missiles, and launchers of such missiles and

support structures and support equipment associated with such missiles and launchers, including:

(i) the number and type of items of missile systems to be eliminated;

(ii) the elimination site;

(iii) for intermediate-range missiles, the location from which such missiles, launchers of such missiles and support equipment associated with such missiles and launchers are moved to the elimination facility; and

(iv) except in the case of support structures, the point of entry to be used by an inspection team conducting an inspection pursuant to paragraph 7 of Article XI of this Treaty and the estimated time of departure of an inspection team from the point of entry to the elimination facility;

(d) notification, no less than ten days in advance, of the scheduled date of the launch, or the scheduled date of the initiation of a series of launches, of intermediate-range missiles for the purpose of their elimination, including:

(i) the type of missiles to be eliminated;

(ii) the location of the launch, or, if elimination is by a series of launches, the location of such launches and the number of launches in the series;

(iii) the point of entry to be used by an inspection team conducting an inspection pursuant to paragraph 7 of Article XI of this Treaty; and

(iv) the estimated time of departure of an inspection team from the point of entry to the elimination facility;

(e) notification, no later than 48 hours after they occur, of changes in the number of intermediate-range and shorter-range missiles, launchers of such missiles and support structures and support equipment associated with such missiles and launchers resulting from elimination as described in the Protocol on Elimination, including:

(i) the number and type of items of a missile system which were eliminated; and

(ii) the date and location of such elimination; and

(f) notification of transit of intermediate-range or shorter-range missiles or launchers of such missiles, or the movement of training missiles or training launchers for such intermediate-range and shorter-range missiles, no later than 48 hours after it has been completed, including:

(i) the number of missiles or launchers;

(ii) the points, dates, and times of departure and arrival;

(iii) the mode of transport; and

(iv) the location and time at that location at least once every four days during the period of transit.

6. Upon entry into force of this Treaty and thereafter, each Party shall notify the other Party, no less than ten days in advance, of the scheduled date and location of the launch of a research and development booster system as described in paragraph 12 of Article VII of this Treaty.

Article X

1. Each Party shall eliminate its intermediate-range and shorter-range missiles and launchers of such missiles and support structures and support equipment associated with such missiles and launchers in accordance with the procedures set forth in the Protocol on Elimination.

2. Verification by on-site inspection of the elimination of items of missile systems specified in the Protocol on Elimination shall be carried out in accordance with Article XI of this Treaty, the Protocol on Elimination and the Protocol on Inspection.

3. When a Party removes its intermediate-range missiles, launchers of such missiles and support equipment associated with such missiles and launchers from deployment areas to elimination facilities for the purpose of their elimination, it shall do so in complete deployed

organizational units. For the United States of America, these units shall be Pershing II batteries and BGM-109G flights. For the Union of Soviet Socialist Republics, these units shall be SS-20 regiments composed of two or three battalions.

4. Elimination of intermediate-range and shorter-range missiles and launchers of such missiles and support equipment associated with such missiles and launchers shall be carried out at the facilities that are specified in the Memorandum of Understanding or notified in accordance with paragraph 5(b) of Article IX of this Treaty, unless eliminated in accordance with Sections IV or V of the Protocol on Elimination. Support structures, associated with the missiles and launchers subject to this Treaty, that are subject to elimination shall be eliminated *in situ*.

5. Each Party shall have the right, during the first six months after entry into force of this Treaty, to eliminate by means of launching no more than 100 of its intermediate-range missiles.

6. Intermediate-range and shorter-range missiles which have been tested prior to entry into force of this Treaty, but never deployed, and which are not existing types of intermediate-range or shorter-range missiles listed in Article III of this Treaty, and launchers of such missiles, shall be eliminated within six months after entry into force of this Treaty in accordance with the procedures set forth in the Protocol on Elimination. Such missiles are:

(a) for the United States of America, missiles of the type designated by the United States of America as the Pershing IB, which is known to the Union of Soviet Socialist Republics by the same designation; and

(b) for the Union of Soviet Socialist Republics, missiles of the type designated by the Union of Soviet Socialist Republics as the RK-55, which is known to the United States of America as the SSC-X-4.

7. Intermediate-range and shorter-range missiles and launchers of such missiles and support structures and support equipment associated with such missiles and launchers shall be considered to be eliminated after completion of the procedures set forth in the Protocol on Elimination and upon the notification provided for

in paragraph 5(e) of Article IX of this Treaty.

8. Each Party shall eliminate its deployment areas, missile operating bases and missile support facilities. A Party shall notify the other Party pursuant to paragraph 5(a) of Article IX of this Treaty once the conditions set forth below are fulfilled:

(a) all intermediate-range and shorter-range missiles, launchers of such missiles and support equipment associated with such missiles and launchers located there have been removed;

(b) all support structures associated with such missiles and launchers located there have been eliminated; and

(c) all activity related to production, flight-testing, training, repair, storage or deployment of such missiles and launchers has ceased there.

Such deployment areas, missile operating bases and missile support facilities shall be considered to be eliminated either when they have been inspected pursuant to paragraph 4 of Article XI of this Treaty or when 60 days have elapsed since the date of the scheduled elimination which was notified pursuant to paragraph 5(a) of Article IX of this Treaty. A deployment area, missile operating base or missile support facility listed in the Memorandum of Understanding that met the above conditions prior to entry into force of this Treaty, and is not included in the initial data exchange pursuant to paragraph 3 of Article IX of this Treaty, shall be considered to be eliminated.

9. If a Party intends to convert a missile operating base listed in the Memorandum of Understanding for use as a base associated with GLBM or GLCM systems not subject to this Treaty, then that Party shall notify the other Party, no less than 30 days in advance of the scheduled date of the initiation of the conversion, of the scheduled date and the purpose for which the base will be converted.

Article XI

1. For the purpose of ensuring verification of compliance with the provisions of this Treaty, each Party shall have the right to conduct on-site inspections. The Parties shall implement on-site inspections in accordance with this Article, the

Protocol on Inspection and the Protocol on Elimination.

2. Each Party shall have the right to conduct inspections provided for by this Article both within the territory of the other Party and within the territories of basing countries.

3. Beginning 30 days after entry into force of this Treaty, each Party shall have the right to conduct inspections at all missile operating bases and missile support facilities specified in the Memorandum of Understanding other than missile production facilities, and at all elimination facilities included in the initial data update required by paragraph 3 of Article IX of this Treaty. These inspections shall be completed no later than 90 days after entry into force of this Treaty. The purpose of these inspections shall be to verify the number of missiles, launchers, support structures and support equipment and other data, as of the date of entry into force of this Treaty, provided pursuant to paragraph 3 of Article IX of this Treaty.

4. Each Party shall have the right to conduct inspections to verify the elimination, notified pursuant to paragraph 5(a) of Article IX of this Treaty, of missile operating bases and missile support facilities other than missile production facilities, which are thus no longer subject to inspections pursuant to paragraph 5(a) of this Article. Such an inspection shall be carried out within 60 days after the scheduled date of the elimination of that facility. If a Party conducts an inspection at a particular facility pursuant to paragraph 3 of this Article after the scheduled date of the elimination of that facility, then no additional inspection of that facility pursuant to this paragraph shall be permitted.

5. Each Party shall have the right to conduct inspections pursuant to this paragraph for 13 years after entry into force of this Treaty. Each Party shall have the right to conduct 20 such inspections per calendar year during the first three years after entry into force of this Treaty, 15 such inspections per calendar year during the subsequent five years, and ten such inspections per calendar year during the last five years. Neither Party shall use more than half of its total number of these inspections per calendar year within the territory of any one basing country. Each Party shall have the right to conduct:

(a) inspections, beginning 90 days after entry into force of this Treaty, of missile operating bases and missile support facilities other than elimination facilities and missile production facilities, to ascertain, according to the categories of data specified in the Memorandum of Understanding, the numbers of missiles, launchers, support structures and support equipment located at each missile operating base or missile support facility at the time of the inspection; and

(b) inspections of former missile operating bases and former missile support facilities eliminated pursuant to paragraph 8 of Article X of this Treaty other than former missile production facilities.

6. Beginning 30 days after entry into force of this Treaty, each Party shall have the right, for 13 years after entry into force of this Treaty, to inspect by means of continuous monitoring:

(a) the portals of any facility of the other Party at which the final assembly of a GLBM using stages, any of which is outwardly similar to a stage of a solid-propellant GLBM listed in Article III of this Treaty, is accomplished; or

(b) if a Party has no such facility, the portals of an agreed former missile production facility at which existing types of intermediate-range or shorter-range GLBMs were produced.

The Party whose facility is to be inspected pursuant to this paragraph shall ensure that the other Party is able to establish a permanent continuous monitoring system at that facility within six months after entry into force of this Treaty or within six months of initiation of the process of final assembly described in subparagraph (a). If, after the end of the second year after entry into force of this Treaty, neither Party conducts the process of final assembly described in subparagraph (a) for a period of 12 consecutive months, then neither Party shall have the right to inspect by means of continuous monitoring any missile production facility of the other Party unless the process of final assembly as described in subparagraph (a) is initiated again. Upon entry into force of this Treaty, the facilities to be inspected by continuous monitoring shall be: in accordance with subparagraph (b), for the United States of America, Hercules Plant

Number 1, at Magna, Utah; in accordance with subparagraph (a), for the Union of Soviet Socialist Republics, the Votkinsk Machine Building Plant, Udmurt Autonomous Soviet Socialist Republic, Russian Soviet Federative Socialist Republic.

7.   Each Party shall conduct inspections of the process of elimination, including elimination of intermediate-range missiles by means of launching, of intermediate-range and shorter-range missiles and launchers of such missiles and support equipment associated with such missiles and launchers carried out at elimination facilities in accordance with Article X of this Treaty and the Protocol on Elimination. Inspectors conducting inspections provided for in this paragraph shall determine that the processes specified for the elimination of the missiles, launchers and support equipment have been completed.

8.   Each Party shall have the right to conduct inspections to confirm the completion of the process of elimination of intermediate-range and shorter-range missiles and launchers of such missiles and support equipment associated with such missiles and launchers eliminated pursuant to Section V of the Protocol on Elimination, and of training missiles, training missile stages, training launch canisters and training launchers eliminated pursuant to Sections II, IV and V of the Protocol on Elimination.

Article XII

1. For the purpose of ensuring verification of compliance with the provisions of this Treaty, each Party shall use national technical means of verification at its disposal in a manner consistent with generally recognized principles of international law.

2. Neither Party shall:

(a) interfere with national technical means of verification of the other Party operating in accordance with paragraph 1 of this Article; or

(b) use concealment measures which impede verification of compliance with the provisions of this Treaty by national technical means of verification carried out in accordance with paragraph 1 of this Article. This obligation does not apply to cover or concealment practices, within a deployment area, associated with normal training, maintenance and operations, including the use of environmental shelters to protect missiles and launchers.

3. To enhance observation by national technical means of verification, each Party shall have the right until a Treaty between the Parties reducing and limiting strategic offensive arms enters into force, but in any event for no more than three years after entry into force of this Treaty, to request the implementation of cooperative measures at deployment bases for road-mobile GLBMs with a range capability in excess of 5500 kilometers, which are not former missile operating bases eliminated pursuant to paragraph 8 of Article X of this Treaty. The Party making such a request shall inform the other Party of the deployment base at which cooperative measures shall be implemented. The Party whose base is to be observed shall carry out the following cooperative measures:

(a) no later than six hours after such a request, the Party shall have opened the roofs of all fixed structures for launchers located at the base, removed completely all missiles on launchers from such fixed structures for launchers and displayed such missiles on launchers in the open without using concealment measures; and

(b) the Party shall leave the roofs open and the missiles on launchers in place until twelve hours have elapsed from the time of the receipt of a request for such an observation.

Each Party shall have the right to make six such requests per calendar year. Only one deployment base shall be subject to these cooperative measures at any one time.

Article XIII

1. To promote the objectives and implementation of the provisions of this Treaty, the Parties hereby establish the Special Verification Commission. The Parties agree that, if either Party so requests, they shall meet within the framework of the Special Verification Commission to:

(a) resolve questions relating to compliance with the obligations assumed; and

(b) agree upon such measures as may be

necessary to improve the viability and effectiveness of this Treaty.

2. The Parties shall use the Nuclear Risk Reduction Centers, which provide for continuous communication between the Parties, to:

(a) exchange data and provide notifications as required by paragraphs 3, 4, 5 and 6 of Article IX of this Treaty and the Protocol on Elimination;

(b) provide and receive the information required by paragraph 9 of Article X of this Treaty;

(c) provide and receive notifications of inspections as required by Article XI of this Treaty and the Protocol on Inspection; and

(d) provide and receive requests for cooperative measures as provided for in paragraph 3 of Article XII of this Treaty.

Article XIV

The Parties shall comply with this Treaty and shall not assume any international obligations or undertakings which would conflict with its provisions.

Article XV

1. This Treaty shall be of unlimited duration.

2. Each Party shall, in exercising its national sovereignty, have the right to withdraw from this Treaty if it decides that extraordinary events related to the subject matter of this Treaty have jeopardized its supreme interests. It shall give notice of its decision to withdraw to the other Party six months prior to withdrawal from this Treaty. Such notice shall include a statement of the extraordinary events the notifying Party regards as having jeopardized its supreme interests.

Article XVI

Each Party may propose amendments to this Treaty. Agreed amendments shall enter into force in accordance with the procedures set forth in Article XVII governing the entry into force of this Treaty.

Article XVII

1. This Treaty, including the Memorandum of Understanding and Protocols, which form an integral part thereof, shall be subject to ratification in accordance with the constitutional procedures of each Party. This Treaty shall enter into force on the date of the exchange of instruments of ratification.

2. This Treaty shall be registered pursuant to Article 102 of the Charter of the United Nations.

DONE at Washington on December 8, 1987, in two copies, each in the English and Russian languages, both texts being equally authentic.

FOR THE UNITED STATES OF AMERICA:

Ronald Reagan

President of the United States of America

FOR THE UNION OF SOVIET SOCIALIST REPUBLICS:

Mikhail Gorbachev

General Secretary of the Central Committee of the CPSU

MEMORANDUM OF UNDERSTANDING REGARDING THE ESTABLISHMENT OF THE DATA BASE FOR THE TREATY BETWEEN THE UNION OF SOVIET SOCIALIST REPUBLICS AND THE UNITED STATES OF AMERICA ON THE ELIMINATION OF THEIR INTERMEDIATE-RANGE AND SHORTER-RANGE MISSILES

Pursuant to and in implementation of the Treaty Between the Union of Soviet Socialist Republics and the United States of America on the Elimination of Their Intermediate-Range and Shorter-Range Missiles of December 8, 1987, hereinafter referred to as the Treaty, the Parties have exchanged data current as of November 1, 1987, on intermediate-range and shorter-range missiles and launchers of such missiles and support structures and support equipment associated with such missiles and launchers.

I. Definitions

For the purposes of this Memorandum of Understanding, the Treaty, the Protocol on Elimination, and the Protocol on Inspection:

1. The term "missile production facility" means a facility for the assembly or production of solid-propellant intermediate-range or shorter-range GLBMs, or existing types of GLCMs.

2. The term "missile repair facility" means a facility at which repair or maintenance of intermediate-range or shorter-range missiles takes place other than inspection and maintenance conducted at a missile operating base.

3. The term "launcher production facility" means a facility for final assembly of launchers of intermediate-range or shorter-range missiles.

4. The term "launcher repair facility" means a facility at which repair or maintenance of launchers of intermediate-range or shorter-range missiles takes place other than inspection and maintenance conducted at a missile operating base.

5. The term "test range" means an area at which flight-testing of intermediate-range or shorter-range missiles takes place.

6. The term "training facility" means a facility, not at a missile operating base, at which personnel are trained in the use of intermediate-range or shorter-range missiles or launchers of such missiles and at which launchers of such missiles are located.

7. The term "missile storage facility" means a facility, not at a missile operating base, at which intermediate-range or shorter-range missiles or stages of such missiles are stored.

8. The term "launcher storage facility" means a facility, not at a missile operating base, at which launchers of intermediate-range or shorter-range missiles are stored.

9. The term "elimination facility" means a facility at which intermediate-range or shorter-range missiles, missile stages and launchers of such missiles or support equipment associated with such missiles or launchers are eliminated.

10. The term "support equipment" means unique vehicles and mobile or transportable equipment that support a deployed intermediate-range or shorter-range missile or a launcher of such a missile. Support equipment shall include full-scale inert training missiles, full-scale inert training missile stages, full-scale inert training launch canisters, and training launchers not capable of launching a missile. A listing of such support equipment associated with each existing type of missile, and launchers of such missiles, except for training equipment, is contained in Section VI of this Memorandum of Understanding.

11. The term "support structure" means a unique fixed structure used to support deployed intermediate-range missiles or launchers of such missiles. A listing of such support structures associated with each existing type of missile, and launchers of such missiles, except for training equipment, is contained in Section VI of this Memorandum of Understanding.

12. The term "research and development launch site" means a facility at which research and development booster systems are launched.

II. Total Numbers of Intermediate-Range and Shorter-Range Missiles and Launchers of Such Missiles Subject to the Treaty

1. The numbers of intermediate-range missiles and launchers of such missiles for each Party are as follows:

	USA	USSR
Deployed missiles	429	470
Non-deployed missiles	260	356
Aggregate number of deployed and non-deployed missiles	689	826
Aggregate number of second stages	236	650
Deployed launchers	214	484
Non-deployed launchers	68	124
Aggregate number of deployed and non-deployed launchers	282	608

2. The numbers of shorter-range missiles and launchers of such missiles for each Party are as follow:

	USA	USSR
Deployed missiles	0	387
Non-deployed missiles	170 [*]	539
Aggregate number of deployed and non-deployed missiles	170 [*]	926
Aggregate number of second stages	175 [*]	726
Deployed launchers	0	197
Non-deployed launchers	1	40
Aggregate number of deployed and non-deployed launchers	1	237

[Whereas the printed numbers match the previous edition, the changes marked match the Treaty as it will be printed in T.I.A.S. by State/Legal.]

III. Intermediate-Range Missiles, Launchers of Such Missiles and Support Structures and Support Equipment Associated With Such Missiles and Launchers

1. Deployed

The following are the deployment areas, missile operating bases, their locations and the numbers, for each Party of all deployed intermediate-range missiles listed as existing types in Article III of the Treaty, launchers of such missiles and the support structures and support equipment associated with such missiles and launchers. Site diagrams, to include boundaries and center coordinates, of each listed missile operating base are appended to this Memorandum of Understanding. The boundaries of deployment areas are indicated by specifying geographic coordinates, connected by straight lines or linear landmarks, to include national boundaries, rivers, railroads or highways.

	Missiles	Launchers	Support Structures and Equipment

(a) UNITED STATES OF AMERICA

(i) Pershing II

Deployment Area One

The Federal Republic of Germany

Boundaries: The territory of The Federal Republic of Germany bounded on the north by 51 degrees 00 minutes 00 seconds north latitude; on the east by 012 degrees 00 minutes 00 seconds east longitude; on the south by 48 degrees 00 minutes 00 seconds north latitude; and within the national boundaries of The Federal Republic of Germany.

Missile Operating Bases

	Missiles	Launchers	Support Structures and Equipment
Schwaebisch-Gmuend 48 48 54 N 009 48 29 E	40 (includes 4 spares)	36	Launch Pad Shelter-0 Training Missile Stage-24
Neu Ulm 48 22 40 N 010 00 45 E	40 (includes 4 spares)	43 (includes 7 spares)	Launch Pad Shelter-0 Training Missile Stage-24
Waldheide-Neckarsulm 49 07 45 N 009 16 31 E	40 (includes 4 spares)	36	Launch Pad Shelter-0 Training Missile Stage-24

	Missiles	Launchers	Support Structures and Equipment

(ii) BGM-109G

Deployment Area One

The United Kingdom of Great Britain and Northern Ireland

Boundaries: The territory of The United Kingdom bounded on the north by 52 degrees 40 minutes 00 seconds north latitude; on the west by 003 degrees 30 minutes 00 seconds west longitude; on the south by the English Channel; and on the east by the English Channel and the North Sea.

Missile Operating Base

	Missiles	Launchers	Support Structures and Equipment
Greenham Common 51 22 35 N 001 18 12 W	101 with launch canister (includes 5 spares)	29 (includes 5 spares)	Training Missile-0 Training Launch Canister-7

Deployment Area Two

The United Kingdom of Great Britain and Northern Ireland

Boundaries: The territory of The United Kingdom bounded on the north by 53 degrees 45 minutes 00 seconds north latitude; on the west by 002 degrees 45 minutes 00 seconds west longitude; on the south by 51 degrees 05 minutes 00 seconds north latitude; and on the east by the English Channel and the North Sea.

Missile Operating Base

	Missiles	Launchers	Support Structures and Equipment
Molesworth	18* with launch canister	6*	Training Missile-0 Training Launch Canister-7

*In preparation for operational status.

Deployment Area

The Republic of Italy

Boundaries: The territory of The Republic of Italy within the boundaries of the Island of Sicily.

Missile Operating Base

	Missiles	Launchers	Support Structures and Equipment
Comiso 36 59 44 N 014 36 34 E	108 with launch canister (includes 12 spares)	31 (includes 7 spares)	Training Missile-0 Training Launch Canister-7

	Missiles	Launchers	Support Structures and Equipment

Deployment Area

The Kingdom of Belgium

Boundaries: The territory of The Kingdom of Belgium.

Missile Operating Base

Florennes 50 13 35 N 004 39 00 E	20 with launch canister (includes 4 spares)	12 (includes 8 spares)	Training Missile-0 Training Launch Canister-7

Deployment Area Two

The Federal Republic of Germany

Boundaries: The territory of The Federal Republic of Germany bounded on the north by 51 degrees 25 minutes 00 seconds north latitude; on the east by 009 degrees 30 minutes 00 seconds east longitude; on the south by 48 degrees 43 minutes 00 seconds north latitude; and on the west by the national boundaries of The Federal Republic of Germany.

Missile Operating Base

Wueschheim 50 02 33 N 007 25 40 E	62 with launch canister (includes 14 spares)	21 (includes 9 spares)	Training Missile-1 Training Launch Canister-10

Deployment Area

The Kingdom of the Netherlands

Boundaries: The territory of The Kingdom of the Netherlands bounded on the north by 52 degrees 30 minutes 00 seconds north latitude and within the national boundaries of The Kingdom of the Netherlands.

	Missiles	Launchers	Support Structures and Equipment

Missile Operating Base

Woensdrecht
51 26 12 N   004 21 15 E

	Missiles	Launchers	Support Structures and Equipment
Woensdrecht 51 26 12 N 004 21 15 E	0 with launch canister	0	Training Missile-0 Training Launch Canister-0

(b) UNION OF SOVIET SOCIALIST REPUBLICS

(i) SS-20

Deployment Area

Postavy
55 12 13 N 027 00 00 E
54 52 47   026 41 18
54 43 58   026 04 07
55 01 13   026 03 43

Missile Operating Base

	Missiles	Launchers	Support Structures and Equipment
Postavy 55 09 47 N 026 54 21 E	9	9	Launch Canister-9 Missile Transporter Vehicle-0 Fixed Structure for Launcher-9 Training Missile-0

Deployment Area

Vetrino
55 28 44 N 028 42 29 E
55 01 03   028 15 03
55 01 16   027 48 46
55 16 22   027 49 05

Missile Operating Base

	Missiles	Launchers	Support Structures and Equipment
Vetrino 55 24 19 N 028 33 29 E	9	9	Launch Canister-9 Missile Transporter Vehicle-0 Fixed Structure for Launcher-9 Training Missile-0

Deployment Area

Polotsk
55 37 36 N 028 23 49 E
55 28 07   029 20 25
54 32 15   029 09 47
54 39 32   028 10 40

	Missiles	Launchers	Support Structures and Equipment
Missile Operating Base			
Polotsk 55 22 34 N 028 44 17 E	9	9	Launch Canister-9 Missile Transporter Vehicle-0 Fixed Structure for Launcher-9 Training Missile-0
Deployment Area			
Smorgon' 54 37 43 N 026 52 34 E 54 22 37 026 52 37 54 37 18 025 41 58 54 45 21 026 15 13			
Missile Operating Base			
Smorgon' 54 36 16 N 026 23 05 E	9	9	Launch Canister-9 Missile Transporter Vehicle-0 Fixed Structure for Launcher-9 Training Missile-0
Deployment Area			
Smorgon' 54 29 01 N 026 26 40 E 54 05 04 025 53 59 54 24 14 025 31 18 54 35 27 026 19 10			
Missile Operating Base			
Smorgon' 54 31 36 N 026 17 20 E	9	9	Launch Canister-9 Missile Transporter Vehicle-0 Fixed Structure for Launcher-9 Training Missile-0
Deployment Area			
Lida 53 45 24 N 025 29 02 E 53 34 00 024 49 35 53 42 25 024 38 15 53 58 05 025 10 17			
Missile Operating Base			
Lida 53 47 39 N 025 20 27 E	9	9	Launch Canister-9 Missile Transporter Vehicle-0 Fixed Structure for Launcher-9 Training Missile-0

	Missiles	Launchers	Support Structures and Equipment

Deployment Area

Gezgaly
53 38 53 N   025 25 38 E
53 23 48   025 26 12
53 12 46   025 08 38
53 22 57   024 35 43

Missile Operating Base

Gezgaly 53 32 50 N 025 16 48 E	6	6	Launch Canister-6 Missile Transporter Vehicle-0 Fixed Structure for Launcher-6 Training Missile-0

Deployment Area

Slonim
52 58 15 N   025 55 42 E
52 45 02   025 31 08
53 04 08   025 09 00
53 08 45   025 30 20

Missile Operating Base

Slonim 52 55 54 N 025 21 59 E	9	9	Launch Canister-9 Missile Transporter Vehicle-0 Fixed Structure for Launcher-9 Training Missile-0

Deployment Area

Ruzhany
52 55 21 N 024 58 40 E
52 46 32   024 48 25
52 45 52   024 16 26
53 07 34   024 22 14

Missile Operating Base

Ruzhany 52 49 29 N 024 45 45 E	6	6	Launch Canister-6 Missile Transporter Vehicle-0 Fixed Structure for Launcher-6 Training Missile-0

	Missiles	Launchers	Support Structures and Equipment

Deployment Area

Zasimovichi
52 37 55 N 024 48 50 E
52 22 00   024 10 52
52 32 36   023 56 54
52 45 52   024 16 26

Missile Operating Base

| Zasimovichi 52 30 38 N 024 08 43 E | 6 | 6 | Launch Canister-6 **Missile Transporter Vehicle-0** **Fixed Structure for Launcher-6** **Training Missile-0** |

Deployment Area

Mozyr'
52 05 31 N 029 13 04 E
51 39 05   029 39 31
51 42 00   029 01 30
51 52 57   028 51 32

Missile Operating Base

| Mozyr' 52 02 27 N 029 11 15 E | 9 | 9 | Launch Canister-9 **Missile Transporter Vehicle-0** **Fixed Structure for Launcher-9** **Training Missile-0** |

Deployment Area

Petrikov
52 16 29 N 029 03 04 E
52 08 06   028 48 40
52 08 33   028 13 37
52 27 47   028 28 17

Missile Operating Base

| Petrikov 52 10 29 N 028 34 52 E | 6 | 6 | Launch Canister-6 **Missile Transporter Vehicle-0** **Fixed Structure Launcher-6** **Training Missile-0** |

	Missiles	Launchers	Support Structures and Equipment

Deployment Area

Zhitkovichi
52 23 40 N 028 10 31 E
52 08 35   028 10 07
52 08 55   027 14 01
52 24 01   027 14 06

Missile Operating Base

| Zhitkovichi
52 11 36 N 027 48 07 E | 6 | 6 | Launch Canister-6
Missile Transporter Vehicle-0
Fixed Structure for Launcher-6
Training Missile-0 |

Deployment Area

Rechitsa
52 26 34 N 030 21 10 E
52 05 27   030 43 26
51 47 47   030 23 27
52 13 08   030 00 53

Missile Operating Base

| Rechitsa
52 11 58 N 030 07 11 E | 6 | 6 | Launch Canister-6
Missile Transporter Vehicle-0
Fixed Structure for Launcher-6
Training Missile-0 |

Deployment Area

Slutsk
53 28 29 N 027 57 50 E
53 02 31   028 07 59
53 13 35   027 25 09
53 28 40   027 28 55

Missile Operating Base

| Slutsk
53 14 20 N 027 42 15 E | 9 | 9 | Launch Canister-9
Missile Transporter Vehicle-0
Fixed Structure for Launcher-9
Training Missile-0 |

	Missiles	Launchers	Support Structures and Equipment

Deployment Area

Lutsk
51 08 14 N 025 54 51 E
50 50 45   025 34 49
51 16 24   025 16 49
51 20 51   025 26 59

Missile Operating Base

| Lutsk
50 56 07 N 025 36 26 E | 9 | 9 | Launch Canister-9
Missile Transporter Vehicle-0
Fixed Structure for Launcher-9
Training Missile-0 |

Deployment Area

Lutsk
51 10 05 N 025 27 21 E
50 43 54   025 07 49
50 47 35   024 33 38
51 11 22   024 35 49

Missile Operating Base

| Lutsk
50 50 06 N 025 04 02 E | 9 | 9 | Launch Canister-9
Missile Transporter Vehicle-0
Fixed Structure for Launcher-9
Training Missile-0 |

Deployment Area

Brody
50 14 00 N 025 29 11 E
50 00 46   025 09 30
50 17 32   024 41 55
50 22 10   024 58 33

Missile Operating Base

| Brody
50 06 09 N 025 12 14 E | 9 | 9 | Launch Canister-9
Missile Transporter Vehicle-0
Fixed Structure for Launcher-9
Training Missile-0 |

	Missiles	Launchers	Support Structures and Equipment

Deployment Area

Chervonograd
50 41 07 N   024 33 58 E
50 13 10   024 38 45
50 19 02   024 11 30
50 36 26   024 17 15

Missile Operating Base

Chervonograd 50 22 45 N 024 18 16 E	9	9	Launch Canister-9 Missile Transporter Vehicle-0 Fixed Structure for Launcher-9 Training Missile-0

Deployment Area

Slavuta
50 18 55 N   027 03 22 E
50 08 07   027 03 21
50 07 59   026 16 22
50 29 38   026 29 34

Missile Operating Base

Slavuta 50 17 05 N 026 41 31 E	9	9	Launch Canister-9 Missile Transporter Vehicle-0 Fixed Structure for Launcher-9 Training Missile-0

Deployment Area

Belokorovichi
51 10 19 N   028 12 04 E
50 51 05   027 51 07
51 21 28   027 01 43
51 21 22   027 37 54

Missile Operating Base

Belokorovichi 51 10 45 N 028 03 20 E	9	9	Launch Canister-9 Missile Transporter Vehicle-0 Fixed Structure for Launcher-9 Training Missile-0

	Missiles	Launchers	Support Structures and Equipment

Deployment Area

Lipniki
51 11 38 N 029 10 28 E
50 52 28   028 55 56
51 05 53   028 22 14
51 20 57   028 26 07

Missile Operating Base

| Lipniki
51 12 22 N 028 26 37 E | 9 | 9 | Launch Canister-9
Missile Transporter Vehicle-0
Fixed Structure for Launcher-9
Training Missile-0 |

Deployment Area

Vysokaya Pech'
50 29 13 N 028 21 10 E
50 09 49   028 20 37
50 10 10   027 40 19
50 29 33   027 43 58

Missile Operating Base

| Vysokaya Pech'
50 10 11 N 028 16 22 E | 6 | 6 | Launch Canister-6
Missile Transporter Vehicle-0
Fixed Structure for Launcher-6
Training Missile-0 |

Deployment Area

Vysokaya Pech'
50 13 33 N   029 01 05 E
49 56 07   029 10 23
49 52 42   028 06 47
50 07 39   028 20 33

Missile Operating Base

| Vysokaya Pech'
50 05 43 N   028 22 09 E | 6 | 6 | Launch Canister-6
Missile Transporter Vehicle-0
Fixed Structure for Launcher-6
Training Missile-0 |

	Missiles	Launchers	Support Structures and Equipment

Deployment Area

Korosten'
50 54 31 N   029 02 51 E
50 41 34   029 02 16
50 42 05   028 28 20
50 55 01   028 28 44

Missile Operating Base

Korosten' 50 52 22 N 028 31 17 E	6	6	Launch Canister-6 Missile Transporter Vehicle-0 Fixed Structure for Launcher-6 Training Missile-0

Deployment Area

Lebedin
50 35 26 N   034 41 41 E
50 12 10   034 00 31
50 14 25   033 50 28
50 35 42   034 21 21

Missile Operating Base

Lebedin 50 33 06 N 034 26 02 E	9	9	Launch Canister-9 Missile Transporter Vehicle-0 Fixed Structure for Launcher-9 Training Missile-0

Deployment Area

Glukhov
52 02 16 N   033 52 28 E
51 36 21   033 55 26
51 34 22   033 27 42
52 02 21   033 38 28

Missile Operating Base

Glukhov 51 41 00 N 033 30 56 E	9	9	Launch Canister-9 Missile Transporter Vehicle-0 Fixed Structure for Launcher-9 Training Missile-0

	Missiles	Launchers	Support Structures and Equipment

Deployment Area

Glukhov
51 42 59 N 033 27 47 E
51 23 31   033 37 56
51 23 37   032 56 33
51 43 02   033 10 25

Missile Operating Base

Glukhov 51 36 44 N 033 29 17 E	9	9	Launch Canister-9 Missile Transporter Vehicle-0 Fixed Structure for Launcher-9 Training Missile-0

Deployment Area

Akhtyrka
50 17 58 N 034 54 32 E
49 49 59   034 50 05
50 10 03   033 57 06
50 18 24   034 24 13

Missile Operating Base

Akhtyrka 50 16 01 N 034 49 53 E	9	9	Launch Canister-9 Missile Transporter Vehicle-0 Fixed Structure for Launcher-9 Training Missile-0

Deployment Area

Akhtyrka
50 10 43 N 035 34 34 E
49 54 08   035 00 16
50 18 14   034 24 13
50 26 42   034 48 07

Missile Operating Base

Akhtyrka 50 21 59 N 034 57 03 E	9	9	Launch Canister-9 Missile Transporter Vehicle-0 Fixed Structure for Launcher-9 Training Missile-0

	Missiles	Launchers	Support Structures and Equipment

Deployment Area

Novosibirsk
55 51 09 N   083 52 28 E
55 14 33   083 49 49
55 21 52   083 08 41
55 30 29   083 09 09

Missile Operating Base

| Novosibirsk
55 22 05 N   083 13 52 E | 9 | 9 | Launch Canister-9
Missile Transporter Vehicle-0
Fixed Structure for Launcher-9
Training Missile-0 |

Deployment Area

Novosibirsk
55 06 17 N   083 34 11 E
54 57 40   083 33 38
55 04 53   082 52 45
55 24 16   082 53 40

Missile Operating Base

| Novosibirsk
55 22 57 N   082 55 16 E | 9 | 9 | Launch Canister-9
Missile Transporter Vehicle-0
Fixed Structure for Launcher-9
Training Missile-0 |

Deployment Area

Novosibirsk
55 31 47 N   084 08 57 E
55 13 26   082 56 55
55 20 01   082 49 41
55 40 13   084 00 42

Missile Operating Base

| Novosibirsk
55 19 32 N   082 56 18 E | 9 | 9 | Launch Canister-9
Missile Transporter Vehicle-0
Fixed Structure for Launcher-9
Training Missile-0 |

	Missiles	Launchers	Support Structures and Equipment

Deployment Area

Novosibirsk
55 08 01 N 083 53 07 E
54 52 56   083 52 02
55 11 17   082 56 49
55 22 00   083 01 07

Missile Operating Base

| Novosibirsk
55 18 44 N   083 01 38 E | 9 | 9 | Launch Canister-9
Missile Transporter Vehicle-0
Fixed Structure for Launcher-9
Training Missile-0 |

Deployment Area

Novosibirsk
55 03 58 N 084 18 27 E
54 53 12   084 19 10
55 04 49   082 56 30
55 22 00   083 01 07

Missile Operating Base

| Novosibirsk
55 19 07 N 083 09 59 E | 9 | 9 | Launch Canister-9
Missile Transporter Vehicle-0
Fixed Structure for Launcher-9
Training Missile-0 |

Deployment Area

Drovyanaya
51 44 02 N 113 08 33 E
51 22 28   113 07 32
51 22 49   112 46 52
51 44 16   112 54 39

Missile Operating Base

| Drovyanaya
51 27 20 N 113 03 42 E | 9 | 9 | Launch Canister-9
Missile Transporter Vehicle-0
Fixed Structure for Launcher-9
Training Missile-0 |

	Missiles	Launchers	Support Structures and Equipment
Deployment Area			
Drovyanaya			
51 37 34 N 113 08 14 E			
51 22 28 113 07 32			
51 18 39 112 36 23			
51 27 14 112 40 08			
Missile Operating Base			
Drovyanaya	9	9	Launch Canister-9
51 26 10 N 113 02 43 E			Missile Transporter Vehicle-0
			Fixed Structure for Launcher-9
			Training Missile-0
Deployment Area			
Drovyanaya			
51 24 52 N 112 53 51 E			
51 20 36 112 50 13			
51 18 54 112 15 44			
51 23 13 112 15 51			
Missile Operating Base			
Drovyanaya	9	9	Launch Canister-9
51 22 59 N 112 49 55 E			Missile Transporter Vehicle-0
			Fixed Structure for Launcher-9
			Training Missile-0
Deployment Area			
Drovyanaya			
51 26 54 N 113 00 50 E			
51 18 13 113 03 54			
51 18 47 112 26 03			
51 29 39 112 19 29			
Missile Operating Base			
Drovyanaya	9	9	Launch Canister-9
51 20 18 N 113 00 54 E			Missile Transporter Vehicle-0
			Fixed Structure for Launcher-9
			Training Missile-0

	Missiles	Launchers	Support Structures and Equipment

Deployment Area

Drovyanaya
51 33 19 N 113 04 35 E
51 22 32   113 04 05
51 22 49   112 46 52
51 33 36   112 47 17

Missile Operating Base

| Drovyanaya
51 23 49 N 112 52 13 E | 9 | 9 | Launch Canister-9
Missile Transporter Vehicle-0
Fixed Structure for Launcher-9
Training Missile-0 |

Deployment Area

Barnaul
53 54 32 N 084 01 02 E
53 43 46   084 01 48
53 35 30   083 43 07
53 44 16   083 36 24

Missile Operating Base

| Barnaul
53 46 08 N 083 57 11 E | 9 | 9 | Launch Canister-9
Missile Transporter Vehicle-0
Fixed Structure for Launcher-9
Training Missile-0 |

Deployment Area

Barnaul
53 29 21 N 084 31 45 E
52 58 43   083 47 57
53 13 47   083 48 56
53 29 02   084 17 18

Missile Operating Base

| Barnaul
53 18 21 N   084 08 47 E | 9 | 9 | Launch Canister-9
Missile Transporter Vehicle-0
Fixed Structure for Launcher-9
Training Missile-0 |

	Missiles	Launchers	Support Structures and Equipment

Deployment Area

Barnaul
53 16 38 N 084 43 16 E
52 59 32   084 51 20
52 55 09   084 47 58
53 16 02   084 14 31

Missile Operating Base

Barnaul   9   9   Launch Canister-9
53 13 29 N 084 40 10 E   Missile Transporter Vehicle-0
                                                 Fixed Structure for Launcher-9
                                                 Training Missile-0

Deployment Area

Barnaul
53 27 33 N 084 49 55 E
53 16 42   084 46 52
53 16 02   084 14 31
53 26 58   084 21 02

Missile Operating Base

Barnaul   9   9   Launch Canister-9
53 18 47 N 084 30 27 E   Missile Transporter Vehicle-0
                                                 Fixed Structure for Launcher-9
                                                 Training Missile-0

Deployment Area

Kansk
56 32 14 N 096 12 14 E
56 15 16   095 34 54
56 28 30   095 20 13
56 34 39   095 36 13

Missile Operating Base

Kansk   9   9   Launch Canister-9
56 22 31 N 095 28 35 E   Missile Transporter Vehicle-0
                                                 Fixed Structure for Launcher-9
                                                 Training Missile-0

	Missiles	Launchers	Support Structures and Equipment

Deployment Area

Kansk
56 30 47 N   095 12 33 E
56 19 53   095 19 41
56 13 45   094 59 58
56 31 03   094 56 58

Missile Operating Base

Kansk 56 20 09 N 095 16 34 E	9	9	Launch Canister-9 Missile Transporter Vehicle-0 Fixed Structure for Launcher-9 Training Missile-0

Deployment Area

Kansk
56 19 29 N   096 20 56 E
56 08 43   096 21 41
56 08 17   096 02 24
56 19 14   095 50 42

Missile Operating Base

Kansk 56 11 19 N 096 03 13 E	9	9	Launch Canister-9 Missile Transporter Vehicle-0 Fixed Structure for Launcher-9 Training Missile-0

Deployment Area

Kansk
56 14 50 N   096 05 46 E
55 59 57   096 14 35
55 59 41   096 03 03
56 15 00   095 46 30

Missile Operating Base

Kansk 56 02 19 N 096 04 58 E	9	9	Launch Canister-9 Missile Transporter Vehicle-0 Fixed Structure for Launcher-9 Training Missile-0

	Missiles	Launchers	Support Structures and Equipment

(ii) SS-4

Deployment Area

Sovetsk
55 05 33 N   021 52 38 E
55 03 22   021 56 20
54 57 04   021 29 58
55 01 23   021 26 16

Missile Operating Base

Sovetsk 54 59 07 N 021 36 36 E	5	6 (Launch Stand)	Missile Transporter Vehicle-11 Missile Erector-7 Propellant Tank-52 Training Missile-6

Deployment Area

Gusev
54 46 02N   022 07 07 E
54 24 14   022 28 42
54 20 01   022 21 10
54 43 58   021 55 53

Missile Operating Base

Gusev 54 43 59 N 022 03 27 E	5	7 (Launch Stand)	Missile Transporter Vehicle-12 Missile Erector-7 Propellant Tank-52 Training Missile-7

Deployment Area

Malorita
51 53 50 N 024 05 39 E
51 43 09   024 09 49
51 42 59   023 57 07
51 53 45   023 57 50

Missile Operating Base

Malorita 51 51 47 N 024 01 55 E	5	6 (Launch Stand)	Missile Transporter Vehicle-14 Missile Erector-7 Propellant Tank-48 Training Missile-5

	Missiles	Launchers	Support Structures and Equipment
Deployment Area			
Pinsk			
52 15 03 N 025 49 43 E			
52 04 09 025 39 30			
52 03 56 025 22 00			
52 14 54 025 35 40			
Missile Operating Base			
Pinsk	5	5	Missile Transporter Vehicle-13
52 10 56 N 025 41 27 E		(Launch	Missile Erector-6
		Stand)	Propellant Tank-47
			Training Missile-6
Deployment Area			
Vyru			
57 49 33 N 027 00 00 E			
57 43 05 027 00 00			
57 43 04 026 43 54			
57 49 32 026 43 51			
Missile Operating Base			
Vyru	5	6	Missile Transporter Vehicle-11
57 45 47 N 026 47 13 E		(Launch	Missile Erector-5
		Stand)	Propellant Tank-51
			Training Missile-6
Deployment Area			
Aluksne			
57 25 51 N 026 56 00 E			
57 21 32 026 56 01			
57 17 12 026 40 06			
57 25 49 026 40 01			
Missile Operating Base			
Aluksne	5	6	Missile Transporter Vehicle-12
57 25 04 N 026 49 46 E		(Launch	Missile Erector-6
		Stand)	Propellant Tank-45
			Training Missile-6

	Missiles	Launchers	Support Structures and Equipment

Deployment Area

Ostrov
57 38 21 N 028 20 22 E
57 21 04   028 23 43
57 21 14   028 07 47
57 38 28   028 08 19

Missile Operating Base

Ostrov 57 31 53 N 028 12 19 E	5	8 (Launch Stand)	Missile Transporter Vehicle-12 Missile Erector-7 Propellant Tank-48 Training Missile-6

Deployment Area

Karmelava
55 06 12 N 024 22 04 E
54 57 49   024 33 51
54 55 00   024 04 05
55 01 28   024 03 36

Missile Operating Base

Karmelava 55 00 51 N 024 14 16 E	5	5 (Launch Stand)	Missile Transporter Vehicle-13 Missile Erector-6 Propellant Tank-47 Training Missile-6

Deployment Area

Ukmerge
55 17 41 N 024 59 06 E
55 04 25   024 40 58
55 08 35   024 33 12
55 19 43   024 51 26

Missile Operating Base

Ukmerge 55 07 51 N 024 38 36 E	5	6 (Launch Stand)	Missile Transporter Vehicle-14 Missile Erector-7 Propellant Tank-50 Training Missile-6

	Missiles	Launchers	Support Structures and Equipment
Deployment Area			
Taurage			
55 18 07 N 022 30 42 E			
55 09 30 022 30 22			
55 03 10 022 18 52			
55 13 35 022 21 01			
Missile Operating Base			
Taurage	5	5 (Launch Stand)	Missile Transporter Vehicle-12 Missile Erector-6 Propellant Tank-47 Training Missile-6
55 04 58 N 022 19 38 E			
Deployment Area			
Kolomyya			
48 45 01 N 024 55 59 E			
48 36 23 024 56 20			
48 36 04 024 40 04			
48 44 42 024 39 40			
Missile Operating Base			
Kolomyya	5	6 (Launch Stand)	Missile Transporter Vehicle-12 Missile Erector-6 Propellant Tank-46 Training Missile-7
48 39 32 N 024 48 04 E			
Deployment Area			
Stryy			
49 19 59 N 023 58 46 E			
49 11 22 023 58 29			
49 21 09 023 31 57			
49 29 46 023 32 24			
Missile Operating Base			
Stryy	5	7 (Launch Stand)	Missile Transporter Vehicle-12 Missile Erector-7 Propellant Tank-49 Training Missile-7
49 25 23 N 023 34 56 E			

	Missiles	Launchers	Support Structures and Equipment
Deployment Area			
Skala-Podol'skaya			
48 54 37 N 026 17 26 E			
48 48 09 026 17 32			
48 48 02 026 01 12			
48 54 30 026 01 04			
Missile Operating Base			
Skala-Podol'skaya	5	6	Missile Transporter Vehicle-12
48 51 02 N 026 08 36 E		(Launch Stand)	Missile Erector-6
			Propellant Tank-46
			Training Missile-5

2. Non-Deployed

The following are missile support facilities, their locations and the numbers, for each Party of all non-deployed intermediate-range missiles listed as existing types in Article III of the Treaty, launchers of such missiles and support structures and support equipment associated with such missiles and launchers. Site diagrams for agreed missile support facilities, to include boundaries and center coordinates, are appended to this Memorandum of Understanding.

(a) UNITED STATES OF AMERICA

(i) Pershing II

Missile Production Facilities:			
Hercules Plant #1	0	0	Launch Pad Shelter-0
Magna, Utah			Training Missile Stage-0
40 39 40 N 112 03 14 W			

Launcher Production Facilities:			
Martin Marietta	0	0	Launch Pad Shelter-0
Middle River, Maryland			Training Missile Stage-0
39 35 N 76 24 W			

Missile Storage Facilities:			
Pueblo Depot Activity	11	0	Launch Pad Shelter-0
Pueblo, Colorado			Training Missile Stage-4
38 19 N 104 20 W			

	Missiles	Launchers	Support Structures and Equipment
Redstone Arsenal Huntsville, Alabama 34 36 N 086 38 W	1	0	Launch Pad Shelter-0 Training Missile Stage-20
Weilerbach Federal Republic of Germany 49 27 N 007 38 E	12	0	Launch Pad Shelter-0 Training Missile Stage-0

Launcher Storage Facilities:

	Missiles	Launchers	Support Structures and Equipment
Redstone Arsenal Huntsville, Alabama 34 35 N 086 37 W	0	1	Launch Pad Shelter-0 Training Missile Stage-0

Missile/Launcher Storage Facilities:

NONE

Missile Repair Facilities:

	Missiles	Launchers	Support Structures and Equipment
Pueblo Depot Activity Pueblo, Colorado 38 18 N 104 19 W	0	0	Launch Pad Shelter-0 Training Missile Stage-0

Launcher Repair Facilities:

	Missiles	Launchers	Support Structures and Equipment
EMC Hausen Frankfurt, Federal Republic of Germany 50 08 N 008 38 E	0	0	Launch Pad Shelter-0 Training Missile Stage-0
Redstone Arsenal Huntsville, Alabama 34 37 N 086 38 W	0	10	Launch Pad Shelter-0 Training Missile Stage-0
Ft. Sill Ft. Sill, Oklahoma 34 40 N 098 24 W	0	2	Launch Pad Shelter-0 Training Missile Stage-0

	Missiles	Launchers	Support Structures and Equipment
Pueblo Depot Activity Pueblo, Colorado 38 19 N 104 20 W	0	0	Launch Pad Shelter-0 Training Missile Stage-0

Missile/Launcher Repair Facilities:

NONE

Test Ranges:

	Missiles	Launchers	Support Structures and Equipment
Complex 16 Cape Canaveral, Florida 28 29 N 080 34 W	3	0	Launch Pad Shelter-0 Training Missile Stage-0

Training Facilities:

	Missiles	Launchers	Support Structures and Equipment
Ft. Sill Ft. Sill, Oklahoma 34 41 N 098 34 W	0	38	Launch Pad Shelter-0 Training Missile Stage-78

Elimination Facilities:
(Not determined)

	Missiles	Launchers	Support Structures and Equipment
Missiles, Launchers, and Support Equipment in Transit:	0	0	Training Missile Stage-4

(ii) BGM-109G

Missile Production Facilities:

	Missiles	Launchers	Support Structures and Equipment
McDonnell-Douglas Titusville, Florida 28 32 N 080 40 W	52 with launch canister	0	Training Missile-0 Training Launch Canister-0

	Missiles	Launchers	Support Structures and Equipment
General Dynamics Kearney Mesa, California 32 50 N 117 08 W	48 with launch canister	0	Training Missile-0 Training Launch Canister-0

Launcher Production Facilities:

Air Force Plant 19 San Diego, California 32 45 N 117 12 W	2 with launch canister	4	Training Missile-0 Training Launch Canister-0

Missile Storage Facilities:

NONE

Launcher Storage Facilities:

NONE

Missile/Launcher Storage Facilities:

NONE

Missile Repair Facilities:

SABCA Gosselies, Belgium 50 27 N 004 27 E	16 with launch canister	0	Training Missile-0 Training Launch Canister-0

Launcher Repair Facilities:

NONE

Missile/Launcher Repair Facilities:

NONE

	Missiles	Launchers	Support Structures and Equipment

Test Ranges:

| Dugway Proving Grounds, Utah 40 22 N 113 04 W | 0 with launch canister | 0 | Training Missile-0 Launch Training Canister-0 |

Training Facilities:

| Davis-Monthan AFB Tucson, Arizona 32 11 N 110 53 W | 0 with launch canister | 7 | Training Missile-2 Training Launch Canister-27 |
| Ft. Huachuca Ft. Huachuca, Arizona 31 29 N 110 19 W | 0 with launch canister | 6 | Training Missile-0 Training Launch Canister-8 |

Elimination Facilities:
(Not determined)

| Missiles, Launchers, and Support Equipment in Transit: | 15 with launch canister | 0 | Training Missile-0 Training Launch Canister-2 |

(b) UNION OF SOVIET SOCIALIST REPUBLICS

(i) SS-20

Missile Production Facilities:

| Votkinsk Machine Building Plant Udmurt ASSR, RSFSR 57 01 30 N 054 08 00 E | 36* | 0 | Launch Canister-36 Missile Transporter Vehicle-0 Fixed Structure for Launcher-0 Training Missile-0 |

* In various stages of manufacture.

	Missiles	Launchers	Support Structures and Equipment
Launcher Production Facilities:			
Barrikady Plant Volgograd 48 44 N 044 32 E	0	1	Launch Canister-0 Missile Transporter Vehicle-0 Fixed Structure for Launcher-0 Training Missile-0
Missile Storage Facilities:			
NONE			
Launcher Storage Facilities:			
NONE			
Missile/Launcher Storage Facilities:			
Postavy 55 10 N 026 55 E	2	3	Launch Canister-3 Missile Transporter Vehicle-10 Fixed Structure for Launcher-0 Training Missile-1
Gezgaly 53 36 N 025 28 E	2	2	Launch Canister-6 Missile Transporter Vehicle-10 Fixed Structure for Launcher-0 Training Missile-4
Mozyr' 52 03 N 029 11 E	2	2	Launch Canister-4 Missile Transporter Vehicle-10 Fixed Structure for Launcher-0 Training Missile-2
Lutsk 50 53 N 025 30 E	1	1	Launch Canister-3 Missile Transporter Vehicle-10 Fixed Structure for Launcher-0 Training Missile-2
Belokorovichi 51 09 N 028 00 E	2	2	Launch Canister-3 Missile Transporter Vehicle-10 Fixed Structure for Launcher-0 Training Missile-1

	Missiles	Launchers	Support Structures and Equipment
Lebedin 50 36 N 034 25 E	2	1	Launch Canister-5 Missile Transporter Vehicle-10 Fixed Structure for Launcher-0 Training Missile-3
Novosibirsk 55 16 N 083 02 E	1	1	Launch Canister-3 Missile Transporter Vehicle-10 Fixed Structure for Launcher-0 Training Missile-2
Drovyanaya 51 30 N 113 03 E	2	2	Launch Canister-4 Missile Transporter Vehicle-10 Fixed Structure for Launcher-0 Training Missile-2
Kansk 56 16 N 095 39 E	1	1	Launch Canister-2 Missile Transporter Vehicle-1 Fixed Structure for Launcher-0 Training Missile-1
Barnaul 53 34 N 083 48 E	1	1	Launch Canister-1 Missile Transporter Vehicle-3 Fixed Structure for Launcher-0 Training Missile-0
Kolosovo 53 31 N 026 55 E	144	0	Launch Canister-144 Missile Transporter Vehicle-0 Fixed Structure for Launcher-0 Training Missile-0
Zherebkovo 47 51 N 029 54 E	20	0	Launch Canister-21 Missile Transporter Vehicle-2 Fixed Structure for Launcher-0 Training Missile-1

Missile Repair Facilities:

NONE

	Missiles	Launchers	Support Structures and Equipment

Launcher Repair Facilities:

NONE

Missile/Launcher Repair Facilities:

| Bataysk
47 08 N 039 47 E | 0 | 11 | Launch Canister-2
Missile Transporter Vehicle-4
Fixed Structure for Launcher-0
Training Missile-2 |

Test Ranges:

| Kapustin Yar
48 37 N 046 18 E | 0 | 8 | Launch Canister-0
Missile Transporter Vehicle-3
Fixed Structure for Launcher-1
Training Missile-0 |

Training Facilities:

| Serpukhov
54 54 N 037 28 E | 0 | 6 | Launch Canister-4
Missile Transporter Vehicle-1
Fixed Structure for Launcher-0
Training Missile-4 |

| Krasnodar
40 03 N 038 58 E | 0 | 1 | Launch Canister-2
Missile Transporter Vehicle-1
Fixed Structure for Launcher-0
Training Missile-2 |

| Training Center at
Test Range
  Kapustin Yar
48 38 N 046 10 E | 0 | 7 | Launch Canister-12
Missile Transporter Vehicle-1
Fixed Structure for Launcher-3
Training Missile-12 |

Elimination Facilities:

| Sarny
52 21 N 026 35 E | 29 | 68 | Launch Canister-32
Missile Transporter Vehicle-35
Fixed Structure for Launcher-0
Training Missile-3 |

	Missiles	Launchers	Support Structures and Equipment
Aral'sk 46 50 N 61 18 E	0	0	Launch Canister-0 Missile Transporter Vehicle-0 Fixed Structure for Launcher-0 Training Missile-0
Chita 52 22 N 113 17 E	0	0	Launch Canister-0 Missile Transporter Vehicle-0 Fixed Structure for Launcher-0 Training Missile-0
Kansk 56 20 N 095 06 E	0	0	Launch Canister-0 Missile Transporter Vehicle-0 Fixed Structure for Launcher-0 Training Missile-0

Missiles, Launchers, and Support
Equipment in Transit:

NONE

(ii) SS-4

Missile Production Facilities:

NONE

Launch Production Facilities:

NONE

Missile Storage Facilities:

NONE

Launcher Storage Facilities:

NONE

	Missiles	Launchers	Support Structures and Equipment
Missile/Launcher Storage Facilities:			
Kolosovo 53 31 N 026 55 E	35	1 (Launch Stand)	Missile Transporter Vehicle-9 Missile Erector-10 Propellant Tank-59 Training Missile-31
Zherebkovo 47 51 N 029 54 E	56	3 (Launch Stand)	Missile Transporter Vehicle-5 Missile Erector-4 Propellant Tank-11 Training Missile-30
Missile Repair Facilities:			
Bataysk 47 08 N 039 47 E	0	0 (Launch (Stand)	Missile Transporter Vehicle-0 Missile Erector-0 Propellant Tank-0 Training Missile-6
Launcher Repair Facilities:			
NONE			
Missile/Launcher Repair Facilities:			
NONE			
Test Ranges:			
Kapustin Yar 48 35 N 046 18 E	14	2 (Launch Stand)	Missile Transporter Vehicle-4 Missile Erector-2 Propellant Tank-4 Training Missile-1
Training Facilities:			
NONE			
Elimination Facilities:			
Lesnaya 52 59 N 025 46 E	0	0 (Launch Stand)	Missile Transporter Vehicle-0 Missile Erector-0 Propellant Tank-0 Training Missile-0
Missiles, Launchers, and Support Equipment in Transit:			
NONE			

	Missiles	Launchers	Support Structures and Equipment

(iii) SS-5

Missile Production Facilities:

NONE

Launcher Production Facilities:

NONE

Missile Storage Facilities:

Kolosovo	6	0

53 31 N 026 55 E

Launcher Storage Facilities:

NONE

Missile/Launcher Storage Facilities:

NONE

Missile Repair Facilities:

NONE

Launcher Repair Facilities:

NONE

Missile/Launcher Repair Facilities:

NONE

Test Ranges:

NONE

	Missiles	Launchers	Support Structures and Equipment

Training Facilities:

NONE

Elimination Facilities:

| Lesnaya | 0 | 0 |
| 52 59 N 025 46 E | | |

Missiles, Launchers, and Support
Equipment in Transit:

NONE

3. Training Launchers

In addition to the support equipment listed in paragraphs 1 and 2 of this Section, the Parties possess vehicles, used to train drivers of launchers of intermediate-range missiles, which shall be considered for purposes of this Treaty to be training launchers. The number of such vehicles for each Party is:

(a) for the United States of America--29; and
(b) for the Union of Soviet Socialist Republics--65.

Elimination of such vehicles shall be carried out in accordance with procedures set forth in the Protocol on Elimination.

IV. **Shorter-Range Missiles, Launchers of Such Missiles and Support Equipment Associated With Such Missiles and Launchers**

1. Deployed

The following are the missile operating bases, their locations and the numbers, for each Party, of all deployed shorter-range missiles listed as existing types in Article III of the Treaty, and launchers of such missiles, and the support equipment associated with such missiles and launchers. Site diagrams, to include boundaries and center coordinates, of each listed missile operating base are appended to this Memorandum of Understanding.

	Missiles	Launchers	Support Structures and Equipment

(a) UNITED STATES OF AMERICA

(i) Pershing IA

Missile Operating Base:

NONE

	Missiles	Launchers	Support Structures and Equipment

(b) UNION OF SOVIET SOCIALIST REPUBLICS

(i) SS-12

Missile Operating Bases:

	Missiles	Launchers	Support Structures and Equipment
Koenigsbrueck, German Democratic Republic 51 16 40 N 013 53 20 E	19	11	Missile Transporter Vehicle-9 Training Missile-10
Bischofswerda, German Democratic Republic 51 08 33 N 014 12 18 E	8	5	Missile Transporter Vehicle-0 Training Missile-4
Waren, German Democratic Republic 53 32 40 N 012 37 30 E	22	12	Missile Transporter Vehicle-9 Training Missile-7
Wokuhl, German Democratic Republic 53 16 20 N 013 15 50 E	5	6	Missile Transporter Vehicle-0 Training Missile-7
Hranice, Czechoslovak Socialist Republic 49 33 00 N 017 45 00 E	39	24	Missile Transporter Vehicle-15 Training Missile-13
Pashino 55 16 37 N 082 59 42 E	0	4	Missile Transporter Vehicle-1 Training Missile-5
Gornyy 51 33 10 N 113 01 30 E	36	14	Missile Transporter Vehicle-4 Training Missile-10
Lapichi 53 25 30 N 028 30 00 E	9	5	Missile Transporter Vehicle-1 Training Missile-10
Kattakurgan 39 38 18 N 065 58 40 E	9	5	Missile Transporter Vehicle-1 Training Missile-6

	Missiles	Launchers	Support Structures and Equipment
Saryozek 44 31 58 N 077 46 20 E	36	15	Missile Transporter Vehicle-3 Training Missile-16
Novosysoyevka 44 11 58 N 133 26 05 E	37	14	Missile Transporter Vehicle-5 Training Missile-17

(ii) SS-23

Missile Operating Bases:

	Missiles	Launchers	Support Structures and Equipment
Weissenfels, German Democratic Republic 51 11 50 N 011 59 50 E	6	4	Missile Transporter Vehicle-3 Training Missile-18
Jena-Forst, German Democratic Republic 50 54 55 N 011 32 40 E	47	12	Missile Transporter Vehicle-8 Training Missile-3
Stan'kovo 53 38 30 N 027 13 20 E	40	18	Missile Transporter Vehicle-18 Training Missile-10
Tsel' 53 23 38 N 028 28 06 E	26	12	Missile Transporter Vehicle-11 Training Missile-9
Slobudka 52 30 30 N 024 31 30 E	26	12	Missile Transporter Vehicle-12 Training Missile-10
Bayram-Ali 37 36 18 N 062 10 40 E	0	12	Missile Transporter Vehicle-12 Training Missile-0
Semipalatinsk 50 23 00 N 080 09 30 E	22	12	Missile Transporter Vehicle-12 Training Missile-4

2. Non-Deployed

The following are missile support facilities, their locations and the numbers, for each Party of all non-deployed shorter-range missiles listed as existing types in Article III of the Treaty, and launchers of such missiles and support equipment associated with such missiles and launchers. Site diagrams for agreed missile support facilities, to include boundaries and center coordinates, are appended to this Memorandum of Understanding.

	Missiles	Launchers	Support Structures and Equipment

(a) UNITED STATES OF AMERICA

(i) Pershing IA

Missile Production Facilities:

| Longhorn Army
  Ammunition Plant
Marshall, Texas
32 39 N 094 08 W | 0 | 0 | Training Missile Stage-0 |

Launcher Production Facilities:

| Martin Marietta
  Middle River, Maryland
39 35 N 076 24 W | 0 | 0 | Training Missile Stage-0 |

Missile Storage Facilities:

| Pueblo Depot Activity
  Pueblo, Colorado
38 19 N 104 20 W | 169 | 0 | Training Missile Stage-53 |

Launcher Storage Facilities:

NONE

Missile/Launcher Storage Facilities:

NONE

Missile Repair Facilities:

NONE

Launcher Repair Facilities:

| Pueblo Depot Activity
  Pueblo, Colorado
38 19 N 104 20 W | 0 | 1 | Training Missile Stage-0 |

	Missiles	Launchers	Support Structures and Equipment

Missile/Launcher Repair Facilities:

NONE

Test Ranges:

NONE

Training Facilities:

NONE

Elimination Facilities:
(Not determined)

| Missiles, Launchers, and Support Equipment in Transit: | 1 | 0 | Training Missile Stage-0 |

(b) UNION OF SOVIET SOCIALIST REPUBLICS

(i) SS-12

Missile Production Facilities:

| Votkinsk Machine Building Plant   Udmurt ASSR, RSFSR 57 01 30 N 054 08 00 E | 0 | 0 | Missile Transporter Vehicle-0 Training Missile-0 |

Launcher Production Facilities:

| Barrikady Plant   Volgograd 48 46 50 N 044 35 44 E | 0 | 0 | Missile Transporter Vehicle-0 Training Missile-0 |

Missile Storage Facilities:

| Lozovaya 48 55 N 036 22 E | 126 | 0 | Missile Transporter Vehicle-0 Training Missile-12 |

	Missiles	Launchers	Support Structures and Equipment
Ladushkin 54 35 N 020 12 E	72	0	Missile Transporter Vehicle-0 Training Missile-18
Bronnaya Gora 52 37 N 025 04 E	170	0	Missile Transporter Vehicle-0 Training Missile-3
Balkhash 46 50 N 075 36 E	138	0	Missile Transporter Vehicle-0 Training Missile-47

Launcher Storage Facilities:

Berezovka 50 20 N 028 26 E	0	15	Missile Transporter Vehicle-10 Training Missile-0

Missile/Launcher Storage Facilities:

NONE

Missile Repair Facilities:

NONE

Launcher Repair Facilities:

NONE

Missile/Launcher Repair Facilities:

NONE

Test Ranges:

NONE

Training Facilities:

Saratov 51 34 N 046 01 E	0	3	Missile Transporter Vehicle-2 Training Missile-0

	Missiles	Launchers	Support Structures and Equipment
Kazan' 55 58 N 049 11 E	0	2	Missile Transporter Vehicle-2 Training Missile-0
Kamenka 53 11 N 044 04 E	0	0	Missile Transporter Vehicle-0 Training Missile-0

Elimination Facilities:

Saryozek (Missiles) 44 32 N 077 46 E	0	0	Missile Transporter Vehicle-0 Training Missile-0
Stan'kovo (Launchers and Missile Transporter Vehicles) 53 38 N 027 13 E	0	0	Missile Transporter Vehicle-0 Training Missile-0

Missiles, Launchers, and Support Equipment in Transit:

NONE

(ii) SS-23

Missile Production Facilities:

Votkinsk Machine Building Plant Udmurt ASSR, RSFSR 57 01 30 N 054 06 00 E	0	0	Missile Transporter Vehicle-0 Training Missile-0

Launcher Production Facilities:

V.I. Lenin Petropavlovsk Heavy Machine Building Plant Petropavlovsk 54 51 N 069 09 E	0	0	Missile Transporter Vehicle-0 Training Missile-0

Missile Storage Facilities:

Ladushkin 54 35 N 020 12 E	33	0	Missile Transporter Vehicle-0 Training Missile-42

	Missiles	Launchers	Support Structures and Equipment
Launcher Storage Facilities:			
Berezovka 50 20 N 028 26 E	0	13	Missile Transporter Vehicle-5 Training Missile-0
Missile/Launcher Storage Facilities:			
NONE			
Missile Repair Facilities:			
NONE			
Launcher Repair Facilities:			
NONE			
Missile/Launcher Repair Facilities:			
NONE			
Test Ranges:			
NONE			
Training Facilities:			
Saratov 51 34 N 046 01 E	0	3	Missile Transporter Vehicle-2 Training Missile-0
Kazan' 55 58 N 049 11 E	0	3	Missile Transporter Vehicle-2 Training Missile-0
Kamenka 53 11 N 044 04 E	0	1	Missile Transporter Vehicle-1 Training Missile-0

	Missiles	Launchers	Support Structures and Equipment
Elimination Facilities:			
Saryozek (Missiles) 44 32 N 077 46 E	0	0	Missile Transporter Vehicle-0 Training Missile-0
Stan'kovo (Launchers and Missile Transporter Vehicles) 53 38 N 027 13 E	0	0	Missile Transporter Vehicle-0 Training Missile-0

Missiles, Launchers, and Support Equipment in Transit:

NONE

V. Missile Systems Tested, But Not Deployed, Prior to Entry into Force of the Treaty

The following are the missile support facilities, their locations and the numbers, for each Party of all intermediate-range and shorter-range missiles, and launchers of such missiles, which were tested prior to entry into force of the Treaty, but were never deployed, and which are not existing types of intermediate-range or shorter-range missiles listed in Article III of the Treaty. Site diagrams for agreed missile support facilities, to include boundaries and center coordinates, are appended to this Memorandum of Understanding.

	Missiles	Launchers	Support Structures and Equipment

(a) UNITED STATES OF AMERICA

(i) Pershing IB

Missile Production Facilities:

NONE

Launcher Production Facilities:

NONE

Missile Storage Facilities:

NONE

	Missiles	Launchers	Support Structures and Equipment

Launcher Storage Facilities:

NONE

Missile/Launcher Storage Facilities:

NONE

Missile Repair Facilities:

NONE

Launcher Repair Facilities:

NONE

Missile/Launcher Repair Facilities:

NONE

Test Ranges:

NONE

Training Facilities:

NONE

Elimination Facilities:

NONE

Missiles, Launchers, and Support Equipment in Transit:

NONE

	Missiles	Launchers	Support Structures and Equipment

(b) UNION OF SOVIET SOCIALIST REPUBLICS

(i) SSC-X-4

Missile Production Facilities:

NONE

Launcher Production Facilities:

	Missiles	Launchers
Experimental Plant of the Amalgamated Production Works "M.I. Kalinin Machine Building Plant," Sverdlovsk 56 47 24 N 060 47 03 E	0 with launch canister	0

Missile Storage Facilities:

NONE

Launcher Storage Facilities:

NONE

Missile/Launcher Storage Facilities:

	Missiles	Launchers
Jelgava 56 40 N 024 06 E	84 with launch canister	6

	Missiles	Launchers	Support Structures and Equipment

Missile Repair Facilities:

NONE

Launcher Repair Facilities:

NONE

Missile/Launcher Repair Facilities:

NONE

Test Ranges:

NONE

Training Facilities:

NONE

Elimination Facilities:

| Jelgava 56 40 N 024 06 E | 0 with launch canister | 0 | |

Missiles, Launchers, and Support Equipment in Transit:

NONE

VI. Technical Data

Following are agreed categories of technical data for missiles and launchers subject to the Treaty, support structures and support equipment associated with such missiles and launchers and the relevant data for each of these categories. Photographs of missiles, launchers, support structures and support equipment listed below are appended to this Memorandum of Understanding.

	P-II	BGM-109G	SS-20	SS-4	SS-5	SSC-X-4

1. Intermediate-Range Missiles

(a) Missile Characteristics:

	P-II	BGM-109G	SS-20	SS-4	SS-5	SSC-X-4
(i) Maximum number of warheads per missile	1	1	3	1	1	1
(ii) Length of missile, with front section (meters)	10.61	6.40	16.49	22.77	24.30	8.09
(iii) Length of 1st stage 2nd stage (meters)	3.68 2.47	---- ----	8.58 4.60	18.60 ----	21.62 ----	---- ----
(iv) Maximum diameter of	----	0.53	----	1.65	2.40	0.51
1st stage	1.02	----	1.79	----	----	-----
2nd stage (meters)	1.02	----	1.47	----	----	-----
(v) Weight of GLBM, in metric tons (without front section; for liquid-fueled missiles, empty weight)	6.78	----	----	3.35	4.99	-----
1st stage	4.15	----	26.63	----	----	-----
2nd stage	2.63	----	8.63	----	----	-----
Missile in canister	----	----	42.70	----	----	-----
(vi) Weight of assembled GLCM, in metric tons (with fuel)						
In canister	----	1.71	----	----	----	2.44
Without canister	----	1.47	----	----	----	1.70

		P-II	BGM-109G	SS-20	SS-4	SS-5	SSC-X-4
(b)	**Launcher Characteristics:**						
(i)	Dimensions (maximum length, width, height in meters)	9.60 2.49 2.86	10.64 2.44 2.64	16.81 3.20 2.94	3.02 3.20 3.27	---- ---- ----	12.80 3.05 3.80
(ii)	Maximum number of missiles each launcher is capable of carrying or containing at one time	1	4	1	1	----	6
(iii)	Weight (in metric tons)	12.04	14.30	40.25	6.90	----	29.10

(c) Characteristics of Support Structures Associated With Such Missiles and Launchers:

Dimensions of support structures are as follows (maximum length, width, height in meters):

		P-II	BGM-109G	SS-20	SS-4	SS-5	SSC-X-4
(i)	Fixed structure for a launcher	----	----	27.70 9.07 6.82	----	----	----
(ii)	Launch pad shelter	74.00 14.60 10.00	----	----	----	----	----

(d) Characteristics of Support Equipment Associated With Such Missiles and Launchers:

Dimensions of support equipment are as follows (maximum length, width, height in meters):

		P-II	BGM-109G	SS-20	SS-4	SS-5	SSC-X-4
(i)	Launch canister (Diameter)	----	6.94 0.53	19.32 2.14	----	----	8.39 0.65
(ii)	Missile transporter vehicle (number of missiles per vehicle)	----	----	17.33 3.20 2.90 (1)	22.85 2.72 2.50 (1)	----	----

	P-II	BGM-109G	SS-20	SS-4	SS-5	SSC-X-4
(iii) Missile erector	----	----	----	15.62 3.15 3.76	----	----
(iv) Propellant tank (Transportable)						
Fuel	----	----	----	11.38 2.63 2.96	----	----
Oxidizer	----	----	----	10.70 2.63 3.35	----	----

	Pershing IA	Pershing IB	SS-12	SS-23
2. Shorter-Range Missiles				
(a) Missile Characteristics:				
(i) Maximum number of warheads per missile	1	1	1	1
(ii) Length of missile, with front section (meters)	10.55	8.13	12.38	7.52
(iii) Length of 1st stage 2nd stage (meters)	2.83 2.67	3.68 ----	4.38 5.37	5.17 ----
(iv) Maximum diameter of 1st stage 2nd stage (meters)	1.02 1.02	1.02 ----	1.01 1.01	0.97 ----
(v) Weight of GLBM, in metric tons (without front section) 1st stage 2nd stage	4.09 2.45 1.64	4.15 ---- ----	8.80 4.16 4.64	3.99 ---- ----

	Pershing IA	Pershing IB	SS-12	SS-23
(b) Launcher Characteristics:				
(i) Dimensions	9.98	9.60	13.26	11.76
(maximum length,	2.44	2.49	3.10	3.13
width, height in meters)	3.35	2.86	3.45	3.00
(ii) Maximum number of missiles each launcher is capable of carrying or containing at one time	1	1	1	1
(iii) Weight (in metric tons)	8.53	12.04	30.80	24.07

(c) Characteristics of Support Equipment Associated With Such Missile and Launchers:

Dimensions of support equipment are as follows (maximum length, width, height in meters):

	Pershing IA	Pershing IB	SS-12	SS-23
Missile transporter	----	----	13.15	11.80
vehicle (number of			3.10	3.13
missiles per vehicle)			3.50	3.00
			(1)	(1)

VII. Research and Development Booster Systems

Following are the numbers and locations for each Party of launchers of research and development booster systems.

1. Research and Development Launch Sites   Number of Launchers

(a) UNITED STATES OF AMERICA

Eastern Test Range, Florida   1
   28 27 N 080 42 W

Eglin AFB, Florida   5
   30 36 N 086 48 W

White Sands Missile Range, New Mexico   4
   32 30 N 106 30 W

Green River, Utah   2
   38 00 N 109 30 W

Poker Flats Research Range, Alaska   6
  65 07 N 147 29 W

Roi Namur, Kwajalein   3
  09 25 N 167 28 E

Barking Sands, Kauai, Hawaii   4
  22 06 N 159 47 W

Western Test Range, California   1
  34 37 N 120 37 W

Cape Cod, Massachusetts   1
  42 01 N 070 07 W

Wake Island   2
  19 18 N 166 37 E

Wallops Island, Virginia   1
  37 51 N 075 28 W

(b) UNION OF SOVIET SOCIALIST REPUBLICS

Plesetskaya   3
  62 53 N 040 52 E

Kapustin Yar   2
  48 32 N 046 18 E

Each Party, in signing this Memorandum of Understanding, acknowledges it is responsible for the accuracy of only its own data. Signature of this Memorandum of Understanding constitutes acceptance of the categories of data and inclusion of the data contained herein.

This Memorandum of Understanding is an integral part of the Treaty. It shall enter into force on the date of entry into force of the Treaty and shall remain in force so long as the Treaty remains in force.

DONE at Washington on December 8, 1987, in two copies, each in the English and Russian languages, both texts being equally authentic.

FOR THE UNITED STATES OF AMERICA:	FOR THE UNION OF SOVIET SOCIALIST REPUBLICS:
Ronald Reagan	**Mikhail Gorbachev**
President of the United States of America	**General Secretary of the Central Committee of the CPSU**

PROTOCOL ON PROCEDURES GOVERNING THE ELIMINATION OF THE MISSILE SYSTEMS SUBJECT TO THE TREATY BETWEEN THE UNITED STATES OF AMERICA AND THE UNION OF SOVIET SOCIALIST REPUBLICS ON THE ELIMINATION OF THEIR INTERMEDIATE-RANGE AND SHORTER-RANGE MISSILES

Pursuant to and in implementation of the Treaty Between the United States of America and the Union of Soviet Socialist Republics on the Elimination of Their Intermediate-Range and Shorter-Range Missiles of December 8, 1987, hereinafter referred to as the Treaty, the Parties hereby agree upon procedures governing the elimination of the missile systems subject to the Treaty.

I.   Items of Missile Systems Subject to Elimination

The specific items for each type of missile system to be eliminated are:

1. For the United States of America:

Pershing II: missile, launcher and launch pad shelter;

BGM-109G: missile, launch canister and launcher;

Pershing IA: missile and launcher; and

Pershing IB: missile.

2. For the Union of Soviet Socialist Republics:

SS-20:   missile, launch canister, launcher, missile transporter vehicle and fixed structure for a launcher;

SS-4:   missile, missile transporter vehicle, missile erector, launch stand and propellant tanks;

SS-5:   missile;

SSC-X-4:   missile, launch canister and launcher;

SS-12:   missile, launcher and missile transporter vehicle; and

SS-23:   missile, launcher and missile transporter vehicle.

3. For both Parties, all training missiles, training missile stages, training launch canisters and training launchers shall be subject to elimination.

4. For both Parties, all stages of intermediate-range and shorter-range GLBMs shall be subject to elimination.

5. For both Parties, all front sections of deployed intermediate-range and shorter-range missiles shall be subject to elimination.

II.   Procedures for Elimination at Elimination Facilities

1. In order to ensure the reliable determination of the type and number of missiles, missile stages, front sections, launch canisters, launchers, missile transporter vehicles, missile erectors and launch stands, as well as training missiles, training missile stages, training launch canisters and training launchers, indicated in Section I of this Protocol, being eliminated at elimination facilities, and to preclude the possibility of restoration of such items for purposes inconsistent with the provisions of the Treaty, the Parties shall fulfill the requirements below.

2. The conduct of the elimination procedures for the items of missile systems listed in paragraph 1 of this Section, except for training missiles, training missile stages, training launch canisters and training launchers, shall be subject to on-site inspection in accordance with Article XI of the Treaty and the Protocol on Inspection. The Parties shall have the right to conduct on-site inspections to confirm the completion of the elimination procedures set forth in paragraph 11 of this Section for training missiles, training missile stages, training launch canisters and training launchers. The Party possessing such a training missile, training missile stage, training launch canister or training launcher shall inform the other Party of the name and coordinates of the elimination facility at which the on-site inspection may be conducted as well as the date on which it may be conducted. Such information shall be provided no less than 30 days in advance of that date.

3. Prior to a missile's arrival at the elimination facility, its nuclear warhead device and guidance elements may be removed.

4. Each Party shall select the particular technological means necessary to implement the procedures required in paragraphs 10 and 11 of this Section and to allow for on-site inspection of the conduct of the elimination procedures required in paragraph 10 of this Section in accordance with Article XI of the Treaty, this Protocol and the Protocol on Inspection.

5. The initiation of the elimination of the items of missile systems subject to this Section shall be considered to be the commencement of the procedures set forth in paragraph 10 or 11 of this Section.

6. Immediately prior to the initiation of the elimination procedures set forth in paragraph 10 of this Section, an inspector from the Party receiving the pertinent notification required by paragraph 5(c) of Article IX of the Treaty shall confirm and record the type and number of items of missile systems, listed in paragraph 1 of this Section, which are to be eliminated. If the inspecting Party deems it necessary, this shall include a visual inspection of the contents of launch canisters.

7. A missile stage being eliminated by burning in accordance with the procedures set forth in paragraph 10 of this Section shall not be instrumented for data collection. Prior to the initiation of the elimination procedures set forth in paragraph 10 of this Section, an inspector from the inspecting Party shall confirm that such missile stages are not instrumented for data collection. Those missile stages shall be subject to continuous observation by such an inspector from the time of that inspection until the burning is completed.

8. The completion of the elimination procedures set forth in this Section, except those for training missiles, training missile stages, training launch canisters and training launchers, along with the type and number of items of missile systems for which those procedures have been completed, shall be confirmed in writing by the representative of the Party carrying out the elimination and by the inspection team leader of the other Party. The elimination of a training missile, training missile stage, training launch canister or training launcher shall be considered to have been completed upon completion of the procedures set forth in paragraph 11 of this Section and notification as required by paragraph 5(e) of Article IX of the Treaty following the date specified pursuant to paragraph 2 of this Section.

9. The Parties agree that all United States and Soviet intermediate-range and shorter-range missiles and their associated reentry vehicles shall be eliminated within an agreed overall period of elimination. It is further agreed that all such missiles shall, in fact, be eliminated fifteen days prior to the end of the overall period of elimination. During the last fifteen days, a Party shall withdraw to its national territory reentry vehicles which, by unilateral decision, have been released from existing programs of cooperation and eliminate them during the same timeframe in accordance with the procedures set forth in this Section.

10. The specific procedures for the elimination of the items of missile systems listed in paragraph 1 of this Section shall be as follows, unless the Parties agree upon different procedures to achieve the same result as the procedures identified in this paragraph:

For the Pershing II:

Missile:

(a) missile stages shall be eliminated by explosive demolition or burning;

(b) solid fuel, rocket nozzles and motor cases not destroyed in this process shall be burned, crushed, flattened or destroyed by explosion; and

(c) front section, minus nuclear warhead device and guidance elements, shall be crushed or flattened.

Launcher:

(a) erector-launcher mechanism shall be removed from launcher chassis;

(b) all components of erector-launcher mechanism shall be cut at locations that are not assembly joints into two pieces of approximately equal size;

(c) missile launch support equipment, including external instrumentation compartments, shall be removed from launcher chassis; and

(d) launcher chassis shall be cut at a location that is not an assembly joint into two pieces of approximately equal size.

For the BGM-109G:

Missile:

(a) missile airframe shall be cut longitudinally into two pieces;

(b) wings and tail section shall be severed from missile airframe at locations that are not assembly joints; and

(c) front section, minus nuclear warhead device and guidance elements, shall be crushed or flattened.

Launch Canister:

launch canister shall be crushed, flattened, cut into two pieces of approximately equal size or destroyed by explosion.

Launcher:

(a) erector-launcher mechanism shall be removed from launcher chassis;

(b) all components of erector-launcher mechanism shall be cut at locations that are not assembly joints into two pieces of approximately equal size;

(c) missile launch support equipment, including external instrumentation compartments, shall be removed from launcher chassis; and

(d) launcher chassis shall be cut at a location that is not an assembly joint into two pieces of approximately equal size.

For the Pershing IA:

Missile:

(a) missile stages shall be eliminated by explosive demolition or burning;

(b) solid fuel, rocket nozzles and motor cases not destroyed in this process shall be burned, crushed, flattened or destroyed by explosion; and

(c) front section, minus nuclear warhead device and guidance elements, shall be crushed or flattened.

Launcher:

(a) erector-launcher mechanism shall be removed from launcher chassis;

(b) all components of erector-launcher mechanism shall be cut at locations that are not assembly joints into two pieces of approximately equal size;

(c) missile launch support equipment, including external instrumentation compartments, shall be removed from launcher chassis; and

(d) launcher chassis shall be cut at a location that is not an assembly joint into two pieces of approximately equal size.

For the Pershing IB:

Missile:

(a) missile stage shall be eliminated by explosive demolition or burning;

(b) solid fuel, rocket nozzle and motor case not destroyed in this process shall be burned, crushed, flattened or destroyed by explosion; and

(c) front section, minus nuclear warhead device and guidance elements, shall be crushed or flattened.

For the SS-20:

Missile:

(a) missile shall be eliminated by explosive demolition of the missile in its launch canister or by burning missile stages;

(b) solid fuel, rocket nozzles and motor cases not destroyed in this process shall be burned, crushed, flattened or destroyed by explosion; and

(c) front section, including reentry vehicles, minus nuclear warhead devices, and instrumentation compartment, minus guidance elements, shall be crushed or flattened.

Launch Canister:

launch canister shall be destroyed by explosive demolition together with a missile, or shall be destroyed separately by explosion, cut into two pieces of approximately equal size, crushed or flattened.

Launcher:

(a) erector-launcher mechanism shall be removed from launcher chassis;

(b) all components of erector-launcher mechanism shall be cut at locations that are not assembly joints into two pieces of approximately equal size;

(c) missile launch support equipment, including external instrumentation compartments, shall be removed from launcher chassis;

(d) mountings of erector-launcher mechanism and launcher leveling supports shall be cut off launcher chassis;

(e) launcher leveling supports shall be cut at locations that are not assembly joints into two pieces of approximately equal size; and

(f) a portion of the launcher chassis, at least 0.78 meters in length, shall be cut off aft of the rear axle.

Missile Transporter Vehicle:

(a) all mechanisms associated with missile loading and mounting shall be removed from transporter vehicle chassis;

(b) all mountings of such mechanisms shall be cut off transporter vehicle chassis;

(c) all components of the mechanisms associated with missile loading and mounting shall be cut at locations that are not assembly joints into two pieces of approximately equal size;

(d) external instrumentation compartments

shall be removed from transporter vehicle chassis;

(e) transporter vehicle leveling supports shall be cut off transporter vehicle chassis and cut at locations that are not assembly joints into two pieces of approximately equal size; and

(f) a portion of the transporter vehicle chassis, at least 0.78 meters in length, shall be cut off aft of the rear axle.

For the SS-4:

Missile:

(a) nozzles of propulsion system shall be cut off at locations that are not assembly joints;

(b) all propellant tanks shall be cut into two pieces of approximately equal size;

(c) instrumentation compartment, minus guidance elements, shall be cut into two pieces of approximately equal size; and

(d) front section, minus nuclear warhead device, shall be crushed or flattened.

Launch Stand:

launch stand components shall be cut at locations that are not assembly joints into two pieces of approximately equal size.

Missile Erector:

(a) jib, missile erector leveling supports and missile erector mechanism shall be cut off missile erector at locations that are not assembly joints; and

(b) jib and missile erector leveling supports shall be cut into two pieces of approximately equal size.

Missile Transporter Vehicle:

mounting components for a missile and for a missile erector mechanism as well as supports for erecting a missile onto a launcher shall be cut off transporter vehicle at locations that are not assembly joints.

For the SS-5:

Missile:

(a) nozzles of propulsion system shall be cut off at locations that are not assembly joints;

(b) all propellant tanks shall be cut into two pieces of approximately equal size; and

(c) instrumentation compartment, minus guidance elements, shall be cut into two pieces of approximately equal size.

For the SSC-X-4:

Missile:

(a) missile airframe shall be cut longitudinally into two pieces;

(b) wings and tail section shall be severed from missile airframe at locations that are not assembly joints; and

(c) front section, minus nuclear warhead device and guidance elements, shall be crushed or flattened.

Launch Canister:

launch canister shall be crushed, flattened, cut into two pieces of approximately equal size or destroyed by explosion.

Launcher:

(a) erector-launcher mechanism shall be removed from launcher chassis;

(b) all components of erector-launcher mechanism shall be cut at locations that are not assembly joints into two pieces of approximately equal size;

(c) missile launch support equipment, including external instrumentation compartments, shall be removed from launcher chassis;

(d) mountings of erector-launcher mechanism and launcher leveling supports shall be cut off launcher chassis;

(e) launcher leveling supports shall be cut at locations that are not assembly joints into two pieces of approximately equal size; and

(f) the launcher chassis shall be severed at a location determined by measuring no more than 0.70 meters rearward from the rear axle.

For the SS-12:

Missile:

(a) missile shall be eliminated by explosive demolition or by burning missile stages;

(b) solid fuel, rocket nozzles and motor cases not destroyed in this process shall be burned, crushed, flattened or destroyed by explosion; and

(c) front section, minus nuclear warhead device, and instrumentation compartment, minus guidance elements, shall be crushed, flattened or destroyed by explosive demolition together with a missile.

Launcher:

(a) erector-launcher mechanism shall be removed from launcher chassis;

(b) all components of erector-launcher mechanism shall be cut at locations that are not assembly joints into two pieces of approximately equal size;

(c) missile launch support equipment, including external instrumentation compartments, shall be removed from launcher chassis;

(d) mountings of erector-launcher mechanism and launcher leveling supports shall be cut off launcher chassis;

(e) launcher leveling supports shall be cut at locations that are not assembly joints into two pieces of approximately equal size; and

(f) a portion of the launcher chassis, at least 1.10 meters in length, shall be cut off aft of the rear axle.

Missile Transporter Vehicle:

(a) all mechanisms associated with missile loading and mounting shall be removed from transporter vehicle chassis;

(b) all mountings of such mechanisms shall be cut off transporter vehicle chassis;

(c) all components of the mechanisms associated with missile loading and mounting shall be cut at locations that are not assembly joints into two pieces of approximately equal size;

(d) external instrumentation compartments shall be removed from transporter vehicle chassis;

(e) transporter vehicle leveling supports shall be cut off transporter vehicle chassis and cut at locations that are not assembly joints into two pieces of approximately equal size; and

(f) a portion of the transporter vehicle chassis, at least 1.10 meters in length, shall be cut off aft of the rear axle.

For the SS-23:

Missile:

(a) missile shall be eliminated by explosive demolition or by burning the missile stage;

(b) solid fuel, rocket nozzle and motor case not destroyed in this process shall be burned, crushed, flattened or destroyed by explosion; and

(c) front section, minus nuclear warhead device, and instrumentation compartment, minus guidance elements, shall be crushed, flattened, or destroyed by explosive demolition together with a missile.

Launcher:

(a) erector-launcher mechanism shall be removed from launcher body;

(b) all components of erector-launcher mechanism shall be cut at locations that are not assembly joints into two pieces of approximately equal size;

(c) missile launch support equipment shall be removed from launcher body;

(d) mountings of erector-launcher mechanism and launcher leveling supports shall be cut off launcher body;

(e) launcher leveling supports shall be cut at locations that are not assembly joints into two pieces of approximately equal size;

(f) each environmental cover of the launcher body shall be removed and cut into two pieces of approximately equal size; and

(g) a portion of the launcher body, at least 0.85 meters in length, shall be cut off aft of the rear axle.

Missile Transporter Vehicle:

(a) all mechanisms associated with missile loading and mounting shall be removed from transporter vehicle body;

(b) all mountings of such mechanisms shall be cut off transporter vehicle body;

(c) all components of mechanisms associated with missile loading and mounting shall be cut at locations that are not assembly joints into two pieces of approximately equal size;

(d) control equipment of the mechanism associated with missile loading shall be removed from transporter vehicle body;

(e) transporter vehicle leveling supports shall be cut off transporter vehicle body and cut at locations that are not assembly joints into two pieces of approximately equal size; and

(f) a portion of the transporter vehicle body, at least 0.85 meters in length, shall be cut off aft of the rear axle.

11. The specific procedures for the elimination of the training missiles, training missile stages, training launch canisters and training launchers indicated in paragraph 1 of this Section shall be as follows:

Training Missile and Training Missile Stage:

training missile and training missile stage shall be crushed, flattened, cut into two pieces of approximately equal size or destroyed by explosion.

Training Launch Canister:

training launch canister shall be crushed, flattened, cut into two pieces of approximately equal size or destroyed by explosion.

Training Launcher:

training launcher chassis shall be cut at the same location designated in paragraph 10 of this Section for launcher of the same type of missile.

III. Elimination of Missiles by Means of Launching

1. Elimination of missiles by means of launching pursuant to paragraph 5 of Article X of the Treaty shall be subject to on-site inspection in accordance with paragraph 7 of Article XI of the Treaty and the Protocol on Inspection. Immediately prior to each launch conducted for the purpose of elimination, an inspector from the inspecting Party shall confirm by visual observation the type of missile to be launched.

2. All missiles being eliminated by means of launching shall be launched from designated elimination facilities to existing impact areas for such missiles. No such missile shall be used as a target vehicle for a ballistic missile interceptor.

3. Missiles being eliminated by means of launching shall be launched one at a time, and no less than six hours shall elapse between such launches.

4. Such launches shall involve ignition of all missile stages. Neither Party shall transmit or recover data from missiles being eliminated by means of launching except for unencrypted data used for range safety purposes.

5. The completion of the elimination procedures set forth in this Section, and the type and number of missiles for which those procedures have been completed, shall be confirmed in writing by the representative of the Party carrying out the elimination and by the inspection team leader of the other Party.

6. A missile shall be considered to be eliminated by means of launching after completion of the procedures set forth in this Section and upon notification required by paragraph 5(e) of Article IX of the Treaty.

IV. Procedures for Elimination *In Situ*

1. Support Structures

(a) Support structures listed in Section I of this Protocol shall be eliminated *in situ*.

(b) The initiation of the elimination of support structures shall be considered to be the commencement of the elimination procedures required in paragraph 1(d) of this Section.

(c) The elimination of support structures shall be subject to verification by on-site inspection in accordance with paragraph 4 of Article XI of the Treaty.

(d) The specific elimination procedures for support structures shall be as follows:

(i) the superstructure of the fixed structure or shelter shall be dismantled or demolished, and removed from its base or foundation;

(ii) the base or foundation of the fixed structure or shelter shall be destroyed by excavation or explosion;

(iii) the destroyed base or foundation of a fixed structure or shelter shall remain visible to national technical means of verification for six months or until completion of an on-site inspection conducted in accordance with Article XI of the Treaty; and

(iv) upon completion of the above requirements, the elimination procedures shall be considered to have been completed.

2. Propellant Tanks for SS-4 Missiles

Fixed and transportable propellant tanks for SS-4 missiles shall be removed from launch sites.

3. Training Missiles, Training Missile Stages, Training Launch Canisters and Training Launchers

(a) Training missiles, training missile stages, training launch canisters and training launchers not eliminated at elimination facilities shall be eliminated *in situ*.

(b) Training missiles, training missile stages,

training launch canisters and training launchers being eliminated *in situ* shall be eliminated in accordance with the specific procedures set forth in paragraph 11 of Section II of this Protocol.

(c) Each Party shall have the right to conduct on-site inspection to confirm the completion of the elimination procedures for training missiles, training missile stages, training launch canisters and training launchers.

(d) The Party possessing such a training missile, training missile stage, training launch canister or training launcher shall inform the other Party of the place-name and coordinates of the location at which the on-site inspection provided for in paragraph 3(c) of this Section may be conducted as well as the date on which it may be conducted. Such information shall be provided no less than 30 days in advance of that date.

(e) Elimination of a training missile, training missile stage, training launch canister or training launcher shall be considered to have been completed upon the completion of the procedures required by this paragraph and upon notification as required by paragraph 5(e) of Article IX of the Treaty following the date specified pursuant to paragraph 3(d) of this Section.

V. Other Types of Elimination

1. Loss or Accidental Destruction

(a) If an item listed in Section I of this Protocol is lost or destroyed as a result of an accident, the possessing Party shall notify the other Party within 48 hours, as required in paragraph 5(e) of Article IX of the Treaty, that the item has been eliminated.

(b) Such notification shall include the type of the eliminated item, its approximate or assumed location and the circumstances related to the loss or accidental destruction.

(c) In such case, the other Party shall have the right to conduct an inspection of the specific point at which the accident occurred to provide confidence that the item has been eliminated.

2. Static Display

(a) The Parties shall have the right to eliminate missiles, launch canisters and

launchers, as well as training missiles, training launch canisters and training launchers, listed in Section I of this Protocol by placing them on static display. Each Party shall be limited to a total of 15 missiles, 15 launch canisters and 15 launchers on such static display.

(b) Prior to being placed on static display, a missile, launch canister or launcher shall be rendered unusable for purposes inconsistent with the Treaty. Missile propellant shall be removed and erector-launcher mechanisms shall be rendered inoperative.

(c) The Party possessing a missile, launch canister or launcher, as well as a training missile, training launch canister or training launcher that is to be eliminated by placing it on static display shall provide the other Party with the place-name and coordinates of the location at which such a missile, launch canister or launcher is to be on static display, as well as the location at which the on-site inspection provided for in paragraph 2(d) of this Section, may take place.

(d) Each Party shall have the right to conduct an on-site inspection of such a missile, launch canister or launcher within 60 days of receipt of the notification required in paragraph 2(c) of this Section.

(e) Elimination of a missile, launch canister or launcher, as well as a training missile, training launch canister or training launcher, by placing it on static display shall be considered to have been completed upon completion of the procedures required by this paragraph and notification as required by paragraph 5(e) of Article IX of the Treaty.

This Protocol is an integral part of the Treaty. It shall enter into force on the date of the entry into force of the Treaty and shall remain in force so long as the Treaty remains in force. As provided for in paragraph 1(b) of Article XIII of the Treaty, the Parties may agree upon such measures as may be necessary to improve the viability and effectiveness of this Protocol. Such measures shall not be deemed amendments to the Treaty.

DONE at Washington on December 8, 1987, in two copies, each in the English and Russian languages, both texts being equally authentic.

FOR THE UNITED STATES OF AMERICA:
RONALD REAGAN
President of the United States of America

FOR THE UNION OF SOVIET SOCIALIST REPUBLICS:
M.S. GORBACHEV
General Secretary of the Central Committee of the CPSU

PROTOCOL REGARDING INSPECTIONS RELATING TO THE TREATY BETWEEN THE UNITED STATES OF AMERICA AND THE UNION OF SOVIET SOCIALIST REPUBLICS ON THE ELIMINATION OF THEIR INTERMEDIATE-RANGE AND SHORTER-RANGE MISSILES

Pursuant to and in implementation of the Treaty Between the United States of America and the Union of Soviet Socialist Republics on the Elimination of Their Intermediate-Range and Shorter-Range Missiles of December 8, 1987, hereinafter referred to as the Treaty, the Parties hereby agree upon procedures governing the conduct of inspections provided for in Article XI of the Treaty.

I. Definitions

For the purposes of this Protocol, the Treaty, the Memorandum of Understanding and the Protocol on Elimination:

1.   The term "inspected Party" means the Party to the Treaty whose sites are subject to inspection as provided for by Article XI of the Treaty.

2.   The term "inspecting Party" means the Party to the Treaty carrying out an inspection.

3.   The term "inspector" means an individual designated by one of the Parties to carry out inspections and included on that Party's list of inspectors in accordance with the provisions of Section III of this Protocol.

4.   The term "inspection team" means the group of inspectors assigned by the inspecting Party to conduct a particular inspection.

5.   The term "inspection site" means an area, location or facility at which an inspection is carried out.

6.   The term "period of inspection" means the period of time from arrival of the inspection team at the inspection site until its departure from the inspection site, exclusive of time spent on any pre- and post-inspection procedures.

7.   The term "point of entry" means: Washington, D.C., or San Francisco, California, the United States of America; Brussels (National Airport), The Kingdom of Belgium; Frankfurt (Rhein Main Airbase), The Federal Republic of Germany; Rome (Ciampino), The Republic of Italy; Schiphol, The Kingdom of the Netherlands; RAF Greenham Common, The United Kingdom of Great Britain and Northern Ireland; Moscow, or Irkutsk, the Union of Soviet Socialist Republics; Schkeuditz Airport, the German Democratic Republic; and International Airport Ruzyne, the Czechoslovak Socialist Republic.

8.   The term "in-country period" means the period from the arrival of the inspection team at the point of entry until its departure from the country through the point of entry.

9.   The term "in-country escort" means individuals specified by the inspected Party to accompany and assist inspectors and aircrew members as necessary throughout the in-country period.

10. The term "aircrew member" means an individual who performs duties related to the operation of an airplane and who is included on a Party's list of aircrew members in accordance with the provisions of Section III of this Protocol.

II. General Obligations

1.   For the purpose of ensuring verification of compliance with the provisions of the Treaty, each Party shall facilitate inspection by the other Party pursuant to this Protocol.

2.   Each Party takes note of the assurances received from the other Party regarding understandings reached between the other Party and the basing countries to the effect that the basing countries have agreed to the conduct of inspections, in accordance with the provisions of this Protocol, on their territories.

III. Pre-Inspection Requirements

1.   Inspections to ensure verification of compliance by the Parties with the obligations assumed under the Treaty shall be carried out by inspectors designated in accordance with paragraphs 3 and 4 of this Section.

2.   No later than one day after entry into force of the Treaty, each Party shall provide to the other Party: a list of its proposed aircrew members; a list of its proposed inspectors who will carry out inspections pursuant to paragraphs

3, 4, 5, 7 and 8 of Article XI of the Treaty; and a list of its proposed inspectors who will carry out inspection activities pursuant to paragraph 6 of Article XI of the Treaty. None of these lists shall contain at any time more than 200 individuals.

3.   Each Party shall review the lists of inspectors and aircrew members proposed by the other Party. With respect to an individual included on the list of proposed inspectors who will carry out inspection activities pursuant to paragraph 6 of Article XI of the Treaty, if such an individual is unacceptable to the Party reviewing the list, that Party shall, within 20 days, so inform the Party providing the list, and the individual shall be deemed not accepted and shall be deleted from the list. With respect to an individual on the list of proposed aircrew members or the list of proposed inspectors who will carry out inspections pursuant to paragraphs 3, 4, 5, 7 and 8 of Article XI of the Treaty, each Party, within 20 days after the receipt of such lists, shall inform the other Party of its agreement to the designation of each inspector and aircrew member proposed. Inspectors shall be citizens of the inspecting Party.

4.   Each Party shall have the right to amend its lists of inspectors and aircrew members. New inspectors and aircrew members shall be designated in the same manner as set forth in paragraph 3 of this Section with respect to the initial lists.

5.   Within 30 days of receipt of the initial lists of inspectors and aircrew members, or of subsequent changes thereto, the Party receiving such information shall provide, or shall ensure the provision of, such visas and other documents to each individual to whom it has agreed as may be required to ensure that each inspector or aircrew member may enter and remain in the territory of the Party or basing country in which an inspection site is located throughout the in-country period for the purpose of carrying out inspection activities in accordance with the provisions of this Protocol. Such visas and documents shall be valid for a period of at least 24 months.

6.   To exercise their functions effectively, inspectors and aircrew members shall be accorded, throughout the in-country period, privileges and immunities in the country of the inspection site as set forth in the Annex to this Protocol.

7.   Without prejudice to their privileges and immunities, inspectors and aircrew members shall be obliged to respect the laws and regulations of the State on whose territory an inspection is carried out and shall be obliged not to interfere in the internal affairs of that State. In the event the inspected Party determines that an inspector or aircrew member of the other Party has violated the conditions governing inspection activities set forth in this Protocol, or has ever committed a criminal offense on the territory of the inspected Party or a basing country, or has ever been sentenced for committing a criminal offense or expelled by the inspected Party or a basing country, the inspected Party making such a determination shall so notify the inspecting Party, which shall immediately strike the individual from the lists of inspectors or the list of aircrew members. If, at that time, the individual is on the territory of the inspected Party or a basing country, the inspecting Party shall immediately remove that individual from the country.

8.   Within 30 days after entry into force of the Treaty, each Party shall inform the other Party of the standing diplomatic clearance number for airplanes of the Party transporting inspectors and equipment necessary for inspection into and out of the territory of the Party or basing country in which an inspection site is located. Aircraft routings to and from the designated point of entry shall be along established international airways that are agreed upon by the Parties as the basis for such diplomatic clearance.

IV. Notifications

1.   Notification of an intention to conduct an inspection shall be made through the Nuclear Risk Reduction Centers. The receipt of this notification shall be acknowledged through the Nuclear Risk Reduction Centers by the inspected Party within one hour of its receipt.

(a)   For inspections conducted pursuant to paragraphs 3, 4 or 5 of Article XI of the Treaty, such notifications shall be made no less than 16 hours in advance of the estimated time of arrival of the inspection team at the point of entry and shall include:

(i)   the point of entry;

(ii)   the date and estimated time of arrival at the point of entry;

(iii) the date and time when the specification of the inspection site will be provided; and

(iv) the names of inspectors and aircrew members.

(b) For inspections conducted pursuant to paragraphs 7 or 8 of Article XI of the Treaty, such notifications shall be made no less than 72 hours in advance of the estimated time of arrival of the inspection team at the point of entry and shall include:

(i) the point of entry;

(ii) the date and estimated time of arrival at the point of entry;

(iii) the site to be inspected and the type of inspection; and

(iv) the names of inspectors and aircrew members.

2. The date and time of the specification of the inspection site as notified pursuant to paragraph 1(a) of this Section shall fall within the following time intervals:

(a) for inspections conducted pursuant to paragraphs 4 or 5 of Article XI of the Treaty, neither less than four hours nor more than 24 hours after the estimated date and time of arrival at the point of entry; and

(b) for inspections conducted pursuant to paragraph 3 of Article XI of the Treaty, neither less than four hours nor more than 48 hours after the estimated date and time of arrival at the point of entry.

3. The inspecting Party shall provide the inspected Party with a flight plan, through the Nuclear Risk Reduction Centers, for its flight from the last airfield prior to entering the airspace of the country in which the inspection site is located to the point of entry, no less than six hours before the scheduled departure time from that airfield. Such a plan shall be filed in accordance with the procedures of the International Civil Aviation Organization applicable to civil aircraft. The inspecting Party shall include in the remarks section of each flight plan the standing diplomatic clearance number and the notation: "Inspection aircraft. Priority clearance processing required."

4. No less than three hours prior to the scheduled departure of the inspection team from the last airfield prior to entering the airspace of the country in which the inspection is to take place, the inspected Party shall ensure that the flight plan filed in accordance with paragraph 3 of this Section is approved so that the inspection team may arrive at the point of entry by the estimated arrival time.

5. Either Party may change the point or points of entry to the territories of the countries within which its deployment areas, missile operating bases or missile support facilities are located, by giving notice of such change to the other Party. A change in a point of entry shall become effective five months after receipt of such notification by the other Party.

V. Activities Beginning Upon Arrival at the Point of Entry

1. The in-country escort and a diplomatic aircrew escort accredited to the Government of either the inspected Party or the basing country in which the inspection site is located shall meet the inspection team and aircrew members at the point of entry as soon as the airplane of the inspecting Party lands. The number of aircrew members for each airplane shall not exceed ten. The in-country escort shall expedite the entry of the inspection team and aircrew, their baggage, and equipment and supplies necessary for inspection, into the country in which the inspection site is located. A diplomatic aircrew escort shall have the right to accompany and assist aircrew members throughout the in-country period. In the case of an inspection taking place on the territory of a basing country, the in-country escort may include representatives of that basing country.

2. An inspector shall be considered to have assumed his duties upon arrival at the point of entry on the territory of the inspected Party or a basing country, and shall be considered to have ceased performing those duties when he has left the territory of the inspected Party or basing country.

3. Each Party shall ensure that equipment and supplies are exempt from all customs duties.

4. Equipment and supplies which the inspecting Party brings into the country in which an inspection site is located shall be subject to

examination at the point of entry each time they are brought into that country. This examination shall be completed prior to the departure of the inspection team from the point of entry to conduct an inspection. Such equipment and supplies shall be examined by the in-country escort in the presence of the inspection team members to ascertain to the satisfaction of each Party that the equipment and supplies cannot perform functions unconnected with the inspection requirements of the Treaty. If it is established upon examination that the equipment or supplies are unconnected with these inspection requirements, then they shall not be cleared for use and shall be impounded at the point of entry until the departure of the inspection team from the country where the inspection is conducted. Storage of the inspecting Party's equipment and supplies at each point of entry shall be within tamper-proof containers within a secure facility. Access to each secure facility shall be controlled by a "dual key" system requiring the presence of both Parties to gain access to the equipment and supplies.

5. Throughout the in-country period, the inspected Party shall provide, or arrange for the provision of, meals, lodging, work space, transportation and, as necessary, medical care for the inspection team and aircrew of the inspecting Party. All the costs in connection with the stay of inspectors carrying out inspection activities pursuant to paragraph 6 of Article XI of the Treaty, on the territory of the inspected Party, including meals, services, lodging, work space, transportation and medical care shall be borne by the inspecting Party.

6. The inspected Party shall provide parking, security protection, servicing and fuel for the airplane of the inspecting Party at the point of entry. The inspecting Party shall bear the cost of such fuel and servicing.

7. For inspections conducted on the territory of the Parties, the inspection team shall enter at the point of entry on the territory of the inspected Party that is closest to the inspection site. In the case of inspections carried out in accordance with paragraphs 3, 4 or 5 of Article XI of the Treaty, the inspection team leader shall, at or before the time notified, pursuant to paragraph 1(a)(iii) of Section IV of this Protocol, inform the inspected Party at the point of entry through the in-country escort of the type of inspection and the inspection site, by place-name and geographic coordinates.

VI. General Rules for Conducting Inspections

1. Inspectors shall discharge their functions in accordance with this Protocol.

2. Inspectors shall not disclose information received during inspections except with the express permission of the inspecting Party. They shall remain bound by this obligation after their assignment as inspectors has ended.

3. In discharging their functions, inspectors shall not interfere directly with on-going activities at the inspection site and shall avoid unnecessarily hampering or delaying the operation of a facility or taking actions affecting its safe operation.

4. Inspections shall be conducted in accordance with the objectives set forth in Article XI of the Treaty as applicable for the type of inspection specified by the inspecting Party under paragraph 1(b) of Section IV or paragraph 7 of Section V of this Protocol.

5. The in-country escort shall have the right to accompany and assist inspectors and aircrew members as considered necessary by the inspected Party throughout the in-country period. Except as otherwise provided in this Protocol, the movement and travel of inspectors and aircrew members shall be at the discretion of the in-country escort.

6. Inspectors carrying out inspection activities pursuant to paragraph 6 of Article XI of the Treaty shall be allowed to travel within 50 kilometers from the inspection site with the permission of the in-country escort, and as considered necessary by the inspected Party, shall be accompanied by the in-country escort. Such travel shall be taken solely as a leisure activity.

7. Inspectors shall have the right throughout the period of inspection to be in communication with the embassy of the inspecting Party located within the territory of the country where the inspection is taking place using the telephone communications provided by the inspected Party.

8. At the inspection site, representatives of the inspected facility shall be included among the in-country escort.

9. The inspection team may bring onto the inspection site such documents as needed to conduct the inspection, as well as linear measurement devices; cameras; portable weighing devices; radiation detection devices; and other equipment, as agreed by the Parties. The characteristics and method of use of the equipment listed above, shall also be agreed upon within 30 days after entry into force of the Treaty. During inspections conducted pursuant to paragraphs 3, 4, 5(a), 7 or 8 of Article XI of the Treaty, the inspection team may use any of the equipment listed above, except for cameras, which shall be for use only by the inspected Party at the request of the inspecting Party. During inspections conducted pursuant to paragraph 5(b) of Article XI of the Treaty, all measurements shall be made by the inspected Party at the request of the inspecting Party. At the request of inspectors, the in-country escort shall take photographs of the inspected facilities using the inspecting Party's camera systems which are capable of producing duplicate, instant development photographic prints. Each Party shall receive one copy of every photograph.

10. For inspections conducted pursuant to paragraphs 3, 4, 5, 7 or 8 of Article XI of the Treaty, inspectors shall permit the in-country escort to observe the equipment used during the inspection by the inspection team.

11. Measurements recorded during inspections shall be certified by the signature of a member of the inspection team and a member of the in-country escort when they are taken. Such certified data shall be included in the inspection report.

12. Inspectors shall have the right to request clarifications in connection with ambiguities that arise during an inspection. Such requests shall be made promptly through the in-country escort. The in-country escort shall provide the inspection team, during the inspection, with such clarifications as may be necessary to remove the ambiguity. In the event questions relating to an object or building located within the inspection site are not resolved, the inspected Party shall photograph the object or building as requested by the inspecting Party for the purpose of clarifying its nature and function. If the ambiguity cannot be removed during the inspection, then the question, relevant clarifications and a copy of any

photographs taken shall be included in the inspection report.

13. In carrying out their activities, inspectors shall observe safety regulations established at the inspection site, including those for the protection of controlled environments within a facility and for personal safety. Individual protective clothing and equipment shall be provided by the inspected Party, as necessary.

14. For inspections pursuant to paragraphs 3, 4, 5, 7 or 8 of Article XI of the Treaty, pre-inspection procedures, including briefings and safety-related activities, shall begin upon arrival of the inspection team at the inspection site and shall be completed within one hour. The inspection team shall begin the inspection immediately upon completion of the pre-inspection procedures. The period of inspection shall not exceed 24 hours, except for inspections pursuant to paragraphs 6, 7 or 8 of Article XI of the Treaty. The period of inspection may be extended, by agreement with the in-country escort, by no more than eight hours. Post-inspection procedures, which include completing the inspection report in accordance with the provisions of Section XI of this Protocol, shall begin immediately upon completion of the inspection and shall be completed at the inspection site within four hours.

15. An inspection team conducting an inspection pursuant to Article XI of the Treaty shall include no more than ten inspectors, except for an inspection team conducting an inspection pursuant to paragraphs 7 or 8 of that Article, which shall include no more than 20 inspectors and an inspection team conducting inspection activities pursuant to paragraph 6 of that Article, which shall include no more than 30 inspectors. At least two inspectors on each team must speak the language of the inspected Party. An inspection team shall operate under the direction of the team leader and deputy team leader. Upon arrival at the inspection site, the inspection team may divide itself into subgroups consisting of no fewer than two inspectors each. There shall be no more than one inspection team at an inspection site at any one time.

16. Except in the case of inspections conducted pursuant to paragraphs 3, 4, 7 or 8 of Article XI of the Treaty, upon completion of the post-inspection procedures, the inspection team

shall return promptly to the point of entry from which it commenced inspection activities and shall then leave, within 24 hours, the territory of the country in which the inspection site is located, using its own airplane. In the case of inspections conducted pursuant to paragraphs 3, 4, 7 or 8 of Article XI of the Treaty, if the inspection team intends to conduct another inspection it shall either:

(a) notify the inspected Party of its intent upon return to the point of entry; or

(b) notify the inspected Party of the type of inspection and the inspection site upon completion of the post-inspection procedures. In this case it shall be the responsibility of the inspected Party to ensure that the inspection team reaches the next inspection site without unjustified delay. The inspected Party shall determine the means of transportation and route involved in such travel.

With respect to subparagraph (a), the procedures set forth in paragraph 7 of Section V of this Protocol and paragraphs 1 and 2 of Section VII of this Protocol shall apply.

VII.   Inspections Conducted Pursuant to Paragraphs 3, 4 or 5 of Article XI of the Treaty

1. Within one hour after the time for the specification of the inspection site notified pursuant to paragraph 1(a) of Section IV of this Protocol, the inspected Party shall implement pre-inspection movement restrictions at the inspection site, which shall remain in effect until the inspection team arrives at the inspection site. During the period that pre-inspection movement restrictions are in effect, missiles, stages of such missiles, launchers or support equipment subject to the Treaty shall not be removed from the inspection site.

2. The inspected Party shall transport the inspection team from the point of entry to the inspection site so that the inspection team arrives at the inspection site no later than nine hours after the time for the specification of the inspection site notified pursuant to paragraph 1(a) of Section IV of this Protocol.

3. In the event that an inspection is conducted in a basing country, the aircrew of the inspected Party may include representatives of the basing country.

4. Neither Party shall conduct more than one inspection pursuant to paragraph 5(a) of Article XI of the Treaty at any one time, more than one inspection pursuant to paragraph 5(b) of Article XI of the Treaty at any one time, or more than 10 inspections pursuant to paragraph 3 of Article XI of the Treaty at any one time.

5. The boundaries of the inspection site at the facility to be inspected shall be the boundaries of that facility set forth in the Memorandum of Understanding.

6. Except in the case of an inspection conducted pursuant to paragraphs 4 or 5(b) of Article XI of the Treaty, upon arrival of the inspection team at the inspection site, the in-country escort shall inform the inspection team leader of the number of missiles, stages of missiles, launchers, support structures and support equipment at the site that are subject to the Treaty and provide the inspection team leader with a diagram of the inspection site indicating the location of these missiles, stages of missiles, launchers, support structures and support equipment at the inspection site.

7. Subject to the procedures of paragraphs 8 through 14 of this Section, inspectors shall have the right to inspect the entire inspection site, including the interior of structures, containers or vehicles, or including covered objects, whose dimensions are equal to or greater than the dimensions specified in Section VI of the Memorandum of Understanding for the missiles, stages of such missiles, launchers or support equipment of the inspected Party.

8. A missile, a stage of such a missile or a launcher subject to the Treaty shall be subject to inspection only by external visual observation, including measuring, as necessary, the dimensions of such a missile, stage of such a missile or launcher. A container that the inspected Party declares to contain a missile or stage of a missile subject to the Treaty, and which is not sufficiently large to be capable of containing more than one missile or stage of such a missile of the inspected Party subject to the Treaty, shall be subject to inspection only by external visual observation, including measuring, as necessary, the dimensions of such a container to confirm that

it cannot contain more than one missile or stage of such a missile of the inspected Party subject to the Treaty. Except as provided for in paragraph 14 of this Section, a container that is sufficiently large to contain a missile or stage of such a missile of the inspected Party subject to the Treaty that the inspected Party declares not to contain a missile or stage of such a missile subject to the Treaty shall be subject to inspection only by means of weighing or visual observation of the interior of the container, as necessary, to confirm that it does not, in fact, contain a missile or stage of such a missile of the inspected Party subject to the Treaty. If such a container is a launch canister associated with a type of missile not subject to the Treaty, and declared by the inspected Party to contain such a missile, it shall be subject to external inspection only, including use of radiation detection devices, visual observation and linear measurement, as necessary, of the dimensions of such a canister.

9. A structure or container that is not sufficiently large to contain a missile, stage of such a missile or launcher of the inspected Party subject to the Treaty shall be subject to inspection only by external visual observation including measuring, as necessary, the dimensions of such a structure or container to confirm that it is not sufficiently large to be capable of containing a missile, stage of such a missile or launcher of the inspected Party subject to the Treaty.

10. Within a structure, a space which is sufficiently large to contain a missile, stage of such a missile or launcher of the inspected Party subject to the Treaty, but which is demonstrated to the satisfaction of the inspection team not to be accessible by the smallest missile, stage of a missile or launcher of the inspected Party subject to the Treaty shall not be subject to further inspection. If the inspected Party demonstrates to the satisfaction of the inspection team by means of a visual inspection of the interior of an enclosed space from its entrance that the enclosed space does not contain any missile, stage of such a missile or launcher of the inspected Party subject to the Treaty, such an enclosed space shall not be subject to further inspection.

11. The inspection team shall be permitted to patrol the perimeter of the inspection site and station inspectors at the exits of the site for the duration of the inspection.

12. The inspection team shall be permitted to inspect any vehicle capable of carrying missiles, stages of such missiles, launchers or support equipment of the inspected Party subject to the Treaty at any time during the course of an inspection and no such vehicle shall leave the inspection site during the course of the inspection until inspected at site exits by the inspection team.

13. Prior to inspection of a building within the inspection site, the inspection team may station subgroups at the exits of the building that are large enough to permit passage of any missile, stage of such a missile, launcher or support equipment of the inspected Party subject to the Treaty. During the time that the building is being inspected, no vehicle or object capable of containing any missile, stage of such a missile, launcher or support equipment of the inspected Party subject to the Treaty shall be permitted to leave the building until inspected.

14. During an inspection conducted pursuant to paragraph 5(b) of Article XI of the Treaty, it shall be the responsibility of the inspected Party to demonstrate that a shrouded or environmentally protected object which is equal to or larger than the smallest missile, stage of a missile or launcher of the inspected Party subject to the Treaty is not, in fact, a missile, stage of such a missile or launcher of the inspected Party subject to the Treaty. This may be accomplished by partial removal of the shroud or environmental protection cover, measuring, or weighing the covered object or by other methods. If the inspected Party satisfies the inspection team by its demonstration that the object is not a missile, stage of such a missile or launcher of the inspected Party subject to the Treaty, then there shall be no further inspection of that object. If the container is a launch canister associated with a type of missile not subject to the Treaty, and declared by the inspected Party to contain such a missile, then it shall be subject to external inspection only, including use of radiation detection devices, visual observation and linear measurement, as necessary, of the dimensions of such a canister.

VIII.   Inspections Conducted Pursuant to Paragraphs 7 or 8 of Article XI of the Treaty

1. Inspections of the process of elimination of items of missile systems specified in the Protocol on Elimination carried out pursuant to paragraph 7 of Article XI of the Treaty shall be conducted in accordance with the procedures set forth in this paragraph and the Protocol on Elimination.

(a) Upon arrival at the elimination facility, inspectors shall be provided with a schedule of elimination activities.

(b) Inspectors shall check the data which are specified in the notification provided by the inspected Party regarding the number and type of items of missile systems to be eliminated against the number and type of such items which are at the elimination facility prior to the initiation of the elimination procedures.

(c) Subject to paragraphs 3 and 11 of Section VI of this Protocol, inspectors shall observe the execution of the specific procedures for the elimination of the items of missile systems as provided for in the Protocol on Elimination. If any deviations from the agreed elimination procedures are found, the inspectors shall have the right to call the attention of the in-country escort to the need for strict compliance with the above-mentioned procedures. The completion of such procedures shall be confirmed in accordance with the procedures specified in the Protocol on Elimination.

(d) During the elimination of missiles by means of launching, the inspectors shall have the right to ascertain by visual observation that a missile prepared for launch is a missile of the type subject to elimination. The inspectors shall also be allowed to observe such a missile from a safe location specified by the inspected Party until the completion of its launch. During the inspection of a series of launches for the elimination of missiles by means of launching, the inspected Party shall determine the means of transport and route for the transportation of inspectors between inspection sites.

2. Inspections of the elimination of items of missile systems specified in the Protocol on Elimination carried out pursuant to paragraph 8 of Article XI of the Treaty shall be conducted in accordance with the procedures set forth in Sections II, IV, and V of the Protocol on Elimination or as otherwise agreed by the Parties.

IX. Inspection Activities Conducted Pursuant to Paragraph 6 of Article XI of the Treaty

1. The inspected Party shall maintain an agreed perimeter around the periphery of the inspection site and shall designate a portal with not more than one rail line and one road which shall be within 50 meters of each other. All vehicles which can contain an intermediate-range GLBM or longest stage of such a GLBM of the inspected Party shall exit only through this portal.

2. For the purposes of this Section, the provisions of paragraph 10 of Article VII of the Treaty shall be applied to intermediate-range GLBMs of the inspected Party and the longest stage of such GLBMs.

3. There shall not be more than two other exits from the inspection site. Such exits shall be monitored by appropriate sensors. The perimeter of and exits from the inspection site may be monitored as provided for by paragraph 11 of Section VII of this Protocol.

4. The inspecting Party shall have the right to establish continuous monitoring systems at the portal specified in paragraph 1 of this Section and appropriate sensors at the exits specified in paragraph 3 of this Section and carry out necessary engineering surveys, construction, repair and replacement of monitoring systems.

5. The inspected Party shall, at the request of and at the expense of the inspecting Party, provide the following:

(a) all necessary utilities for the construction and operation of the monitoring systems, including electrical power, water, fuel, heating and sewage;

(b) basic construction materials including concrete and lumber;

(c) the site preparation necessary to accommodate the installation of continuously operating systems for monitoring the portal specified in paragraph 1 of this Section, appropriate sensors for other exits specified in paragraph 3 of this Section and the center for collecting data obtained during inspections. Such preparation may include ground excavation, laying of concrete foundations, trenching between equipment locations and utility connections;

(d) transportation for necessary installation tools, materials and equipment from the point of entry to the inspection site; and

(e) a minimum of two telephone lines and, as necessary, high frequency radio equipment capable of allowing direct communication with the embassy of the inspecting Party in the country in which the site is located.

6. Outside the perimeter of the inspection site, the inspecting Party shall have the right to:

(a) build no more than three buildings with a total floor space of not more than 150 square meters for a data center and inspection team headquarters, and one additional building with floor space not to exceed 500 square meters for the storage of supplies and equipment;

(b) install systems to monitor the exits to include weight sensors, vehicle sensors, surveillance systems and vehicle dimensional measuring equipment;

(c) install at the portal specified in paragraph 1 of this Section equipment for measuring the length and diameter of missile stages contained inside of launch canisters or shipping containers;

(d) install at the portal specified in paragraph 1 of this Section non-damaging image producing equipment for imaging the contents of launch canisters or shipping containers declared to contain missiles or missile stages as provided for in paragraph 11 of this Section;

(e) install a primary and back-up power source; and

(f) use, as necessary, data authentication devices.

7. During the installation or operation of the monitoring systems, the inspecting Party shall not deny the inspected Party access to any existing structures or security systems. The inspecting Party shall not take any actions with respect to such structures without consent of the inspected Party. If the Parties agree that such structures are to be rebuilt or demolished, either partially or completely, the inspecting Party shall provide the necessary compensation.

8. The inspected Party shall not interfere with the installed equipment or restrict the access of the inspection team to such equipment.

9. The inspecting Party shall have the right to use its own two-way systems of radio communication between inspectors patrolling the perimeter and the data collection center. Such systems shall conform to power and frequency restrictions established on the territory of the inspected Party.

10. Aircraft shall not be permitted to land within the perimeter of the monitored site except for emergencies at the site and with prior notification to the inspection team.

11. Any shipment exiting through the portal specified in paragraph 1 of this Section which is large enough and heavy enough to contain an intermediate-range GLBM or longest stage of such a GLBM of the inspected Party shall be declared by the inspected Party to the inspection team before the shipment arrives at the portal. The declaration shall state whether such a shipment contains a missile or missile stage as large or larger than and as heavy or heavier than an intermediate-range GLBM or longest stage of such a GLBM of the inspected Party.

12. The inspection team shall have the right to weigh and measure the dimensions of any vehicle, including railcars, exiting the site to ascertain whether it is large enough and heavy enough to contain an intermediate-range GLBM or longest stage of such a GLBM of the inspected Party. These measurements shall be performed so as to minimize the delay of vehicles exiting the site. Vehicles that are either not large enough or not heavy enough to contain an intermediate-range GLBM or longest stage of such a GLBM of the inspected Party shall not be subject to further inspection.

13. Vehicles exiting through the portal specified in paragraph 1 of this Section that are large enough and heavy enough to contain an intermediate-range GLBM or longest stage of such a GLBM of the inspected Party but that are declared not to contain a missile or missile stage as large or larger than and as heavy or heavier than an intermediate-range GLBM or longest

stage of such a GLBM of the inspected Party shall be subject to the following procedures.

(a) The inspecting Party shall have the right to inspect the interior of all such vehicles.

(b) If the inspecting Party can determine by visual observation or dimensional measurement that, inside a particular vehicle, there are no containers or shrouded objects large enough to be or to contain an intermediate-range GLBM or longest stage of such a GLBM of the inspected Party, then that vehicle shall not be subject to further inspection.

(c) If inside a vehicle there are one or more containers or shrouded objects large enough to be or to contain an intermediate-range GLBM or longest stage of such a GLBM of the inspected Party, it shall be the responsibility of the inspected Party to demonstrate that such containers or shrouded objects are not and do not contain intermediate-range GLBMs or the longest stages of such GLBMs of the inspected Party.

14. Vehicles exiting through the portal specified in paragraph 1 of this Section that are declared to contain a missile or missile stage as large or larger than and as heavy or heavier than an intermediate-range GLBM or longest stage of such a GLBM of the inspected Party shall be subject to the following procedures.

(a) The inspecting Party shall preserve the integrity of the inspected missile or stage of a missile.

(b) Measuring equipment shall be placed only outside of the launch canister or shipping container; all measurements shall be made by the inspecting Party using the equipment provided for in paragraph 6 of this Section. Such measurements shall be observed and certified by the in-country escort.

(c) The inspecting Party shall have the right to weigh and measure the dimensions of any launch canister or of any shipping container declared to contain such a missile or missile stage and to image the contents of any launch canister or of any shipping container declared to contain such a missile or missile stage; it shall have the right to view such missiles or missile stages contained in launch canisters or shipping containers eight times per calendar year. The

in-country escort shall be present during all phases of such viewing. During such interior viewing:

(i) the front end of the launch canister or the cover of the shipping container shall be opened;

(ii) the missile or missile stage shall not be removed from its launch canister or shipping container; and

(iii) the length and diameter of the stages of the missile shall be measured in accordance with the methods agreed by the Parties so as to ascertain that the missile or missile stage is not an intermediate-range GLBM of the inspected Party, or the longest stage of such a GLBM, and that the missile has no more than one stage which is outwardly similar to a stage of an existing type of intermediate-range GLBM.

(d) The inspecting Party shall also have the right to inspect any other containers or shrouded objects inside the vehicle containing such a missile or missile stage in accordance with the procedures in paragraph 13 of this Section.

X. Cancellation of Inspection

An inspection shall be cancelled if, due to circumstances brought about by *force majeure*, it cannot be carried out. In the case of a delay that prevents an inspection team performing an inspection pursuant to paragraphs 3, 4, or 5 of Article XI of the Treaty, from arriving at the inspection site during the time specified in paragraph 2 of Section VII of this Protocol, the inspecting Party may either cancel or carry out the inspection. If an inspection is cancelled due to circumstances brought about by *force majeure* or delay, then the number of inspections to which the inspecting Party is entitled shall not be reduced.

XI. Inspection Report

1. For inspections conducted pursuant to paragraphs 3, 4, 5, 7, or 8 of Article XI of the Treaty, during post-inspection procedures, and no later than two hours after the inspection has been completed, the inspection team leader shall provide the in-country escort with a written inspection report in both the English and Russian

languages. The report shall be factual. It shall include the type of inspection carried out, the inspection site, the number of missiles, stages of missiles, launchers and items of support equipment subject to the Treaty observed during the period of inspection and any measurements recorded pursuant to paragraph 11 of Section VI of this Protocol. Photographs taken during the inspection in accordance with agreed procedures, as well as the inspection site diagram provided for by paragraph 6 of Section VII of this Protocol, shall be attached to this report.

2. For inspection activities conducted pursuant to paragraph 6 of Article XI of the Treaty, within 3 days after the end of each month, the inspection team leader shall provide the in-country escort with a written inspection report both in the English and Russian languages. The report shall be factual. It shall include the number of vehicles declared to contain a missile or stage of a missile as large or larger than and as heavy or heavier than an intermediate-range GLBM or longest stage of such a GLBM of the inspected Party that left the inspection site through the portal specified in paragraph 1 of Section IX of this Protocol during that month. The report shall also include any measurements of launch canisters or shipping containers contained in these vehicles recorded pursuant to paragraph 11 of Section VI of this Protocol. In the event the inspecting Party, under the provisions of paragraph 14(c) of Section IX of this Protocol, has viewed the interior of a launch canister or shipping container declared to contain a missile or stage of a missile as large or larger than and as heavy or heavier than an intermediate-range GLBM or longest stage of such a GLBM of the inspected Party, the report shall also include the measurements of the length and diameter of missile stages obtained during the inspection and recorded pursuant to paragraph 11 of Section VI of this Protocol. Photographs taken during the inspection in accordance with agreed procedures shall be attached to this report.

3. The inspected Party shall have the right to include written comments in the report.

4. The Parties shall, when possible, resolve ambiguities regarding factual information contained in the inspection report. Relevant clarifications shall be recorded in the report. The report shall be signed by the inspection team leader and by one of the members of the in-country escort. Each Party shall retain one copy of the report.

This Protocol is an integral part of the Treaty. It shall enter into force on the date of entry into force of the Treaty and shall remain in force as long as the Treaty remains in force. As provided for in paragraph 1(b) of Article XIII of the Treaty, the Parties may agree upon such measures as may be necessary to improve the viability and effectiveness of this Protocol. Such measures shall not be deemed amendments to the Treaty.

DONE at Washington on December 8, 1987, in two copies, each in the English and Russian languages, both texts being equally authentic.

FOR THE UNITED STATES OF AMERICA:
RONALD REAGAN
President of the United States of America

FOR THE UNION OF SOVIET SOCIALIST REPUBLICS:
M.S. GORBACHEV
General Secretary of the Central Committee of the CPSU

ANNEX PROVISIONS ON PRIVILEGES AND IMMUNITIES OF INSPECTORS AND AIRCREW MEMBERS

In order to exercise their function effectively, for the purpose of implementing the Treaty and not for their personal benefit, the inspectors and aircrew members referred to in Section III of this Protocol shall be accorded the privileges and immunities contained in this Annex. Privileges and immunities shall be accorded for the entire in-country period in the country in which an inspection site is located, and thereafter with respect to acts previously performed in the exercise of official functions as an inspector or aircrew member.

1. Inspectors and aircrew members shall be accorded the inviolability enjoyed by diplomatic agents pursuant to Article 29 of the Vienna Convention on Diplomatic Relations of April 18, 1961.

2. The living quarters and office premises occupied by an inspector carrying out inspection activities pursuant to paragraph 6 of Article XI of the Treaty shall be accorded the inviolability and protection accorded the premises of diplomatic agents pursuant to Article 30 of the Vienna Convention on Diplomatic Relations.

3. The papers and correspondence of inspectors and aircrew members shall enjoy the inviolability accorded to the papers and correspondence of diplomatic agents pursuant to Article 30 of the Vienna Convention on Diplomatic Relations. In addition, the aircraft of the inspection team shall be inviolable.

4. Inspectors and aircrew members shall be accorded the immunities accorded diplomatic agents pursuant to paragraphs 1, 2 and 3 of Article 31 of the Vienna Convention on Diplomatic Relations. The immunity from jurisdiction of an inspector or an aircrew member may be waived by the inspecting Party in those cases when it is of the opinion that immunity would impede the course of justice and that it can be waived without prejudice to the implementation of the provisions of the Treaty. Waiver must always be express.

5. Inspectors carrying out inspection activities pursuant to paragraph 6 of Article XI of the Treaty shall be accorded the exemption from dues and taxes accorded to diplomatic agents pursuant to Article 34 of the Vienna Convention on Diplomatic Relations.

6. Inspectors and aircrew members of a Party shall be permitted to bring into the territory of the other Party or a basing country in which an inspection site is located, without payment of any customs duties or related charges, articles for their personal use, with the exception of articles the import or export of which is prohibited by law or controlled by quarantine regulations.

7. An inspector or aircrew member shall not engage in any professional or commercial activity for personal profit on the territory of the inspected Party or that of the basing countries.

8. If the inspected Party considers that there has been an abuse of privileges and immunities specified in this Annex, consultations shall be held between the Parties to determine whether such an abuse has occurred and, if so determined, to prevent a repetition of such an abuse.

CORRIGENDA

The following are corrections to the text of the Treaty that were agreed between the Parties in an exchange of diplomatic notes on May 21, 1988.

1. In the Memorandum of Understanding (MOU) regarding the establishment of a data base for the Treaty, Section II, paragraph 1, concerning intermediate-range missiles and launchers, for the United States: the number of non-deployed missiles should read "266," the aggregate number of deployed and non-deployed missiles should read "695," and the aggregate number of second stages should read "238."

2. In the MOU, Section III, paragraph 1(A)(II), for missile operating base Wueschheim -- the geographic coordinates should read, in the pertinent part, 007 25 40 E., and the number of launchers should read "21."

3. In the MOU, Section III, paragraph 2(A)(I), for launcher production facilities: Martin Marietta -- the geographic coordinates should read, in the pertinent part, 39 19 N. For missile storage facilities: Pueblo Depot activity -- the number of missiles should read "120"; Redstone Arsenal -- the number of training missile stages should read "0"; Weilerbach -- the number of missiles should read "9." For launcher storage facilities: Redstone Arsenal -- the number of training stages should read "4." For launcher repair facilities: Redstone Arsenal --the number of training missile stages should read "20"; Ft. Sill -- the number of launchers should read "1"; Pueblo Depot activity -- the geographic coordinates should read, in the pertinent part, 38 17 N. For training facilities: Ft. Sill -- the number of training missile stages should read "76."

4. In paragraph 2(b)(i) of Section III and in paragraph 2(b)(i) of Section IV of the Memorandum of Understanding, the geographic coordinates for the Barrikady Plant, Volgograd, should be 48° 46' 50" N and 44° 35' 44" E.

5. In paragraph 2(b)(i) of Section III of the Memorandum of Understanding, the Elimination Facility at Aral'sk with the coordinates 46° 50' N and 61° 18' E should be changed to the Elimination Facility at Kapustin Yar with the coordinates 48° 46'N and 45° 59' E.

6. In the MOU, Section VI, paragraph 2(A)(I), for missile production facilities: Longhorn Army Ammunition Plant -- the number of missiles should read "8" and the number of training missile stages should read "1." For launcher production facilities: Martin Marietta -- the geographic coordinates should read, in the pertinent part, 39 19 N. For missile storage facilities: Pueblo Depot activity -- the number of missiles should read "162" and the number of training missile stages should read "63." For missiles, launchers, and support equipment in transit the number of missiles should read "0" and the number of training missile stages should read "6."

7. In paragraph 2(b)(ii) of Section IV of the Memorandum of Understanding, the geographic coordinates for the V.I. Lenin Petropavlovsk Heavy Machine Building Plant, Petropavlovsk, should be 54° 54' 20" N and 69° 09' 58" E.

8. In the MOU, Section VI, paragraph 1(A)(IV) for the BGM 109G, the maximum diameter of the missile should read "0.52."

9. In the MOU, Section VI, paragraph 1(B)(I), for the BGM 109G launcher the maximum length should read "10.80" and the maximum height should read "3.5."

10. In the MOU, Section VI, paragraph 1(D)(I) for the BGM 109G launch canister the maximum length should read "6.97" and the maximum diameter should read "0.54."

11. In the Protocol Regarding Inspections, paragraph 7 of Section I regarding points of entry for the Union of Soviet Socialist Republics should read "Moscow or Ulan Ude."

12. In the Protocol Regarding Inspections, Section XI, paragraph 1, the reference to "paragraph 10 of Section VI of this protocol" should read "paragraph 11 of Section VI of this protocol."

AGREED MINUTE

Geneva

May 12, 1988

Representatives of the United States of America and the Union of Soviet Socialist Republics discussed the following issues related to the Treaty Between the United States of America and the Union of Soviet Socialist Republics on the Elimination of Their Intermediate-Range and Shorter-Range Missiles, signed in Washington on 8 December, 1987, during the meeting between Secretary Shultz and Foreign Minister Shevardnadze in Geneva on 11-12 May 1988. As a result of these discussions, the Parties agreed on the points that follow.

1. In accordance with paragraph 7 of Section VII of the Inspection Protocol, during baseline, close-out and short-notice inspections, the Parties will be inspecting the entire inspection site, including the interior of structures, containers or vehicles, or including covered objects, capable of containing: for the United States -- the second stage of the Pershing II, and the BGM-109G cruise missile; for the USSR -- the first stage of the SS-12 missile, the stage of the SS-23 missile, the SSC-X-4 cruise missile and the SS-4 launch stand.

2. Regarding the second stages of United States GLBMs, the aggregate numbers of these stages are listed in the Memorandum of Understanding and will be updated in accordance with Article IX of the Treaty no later than 30 days after entry into force of the Treaty and at six-month intervals thereafter. Except in the case of close-out inspections and inspections of formerly declared facilities, the United States in-country escort is obliged to provide the Soviet inspection team leader with the number of such second stages at the inspection site as well as a diagram of the inspection site indicating the location of those stages. Finally, as set forth in the Elimination Protocol, Soviet inspectors will observe the elimination of all the stages of United States GLBMs.

3. The entire area of an inspection site, including all buildings, within the outer boundaries depicted on the site diagrams are subject to

inspection. In addition, anything depicted outside these outer boundaries on the site diagrams is subject to inspection. Any technical corrections to the site diagrams appended to the Memorandum of Understanding will be made via the corrigendum exchange of notes prior to entry into force of the Treaty. Such corrections will not involve the exclusion of buildings, structures or roads within or depicted outside the outer boundaries depicted on the site diagrams currently appended to the Memorandum of Understanding.

4. The Soviet side assured the United States side that, during the period of continuous monitoring of facilities under the Treaty, no shipment shall exit a continuous monitoring facility on the territory of the USSR whose dimensions are equal to or greater than the dimensions of the SS-20 missile without its front section but less than the dimensions of an SS-20 launch canister, as those dimensions are listed in the Memorandum of Understanding. For the purposes of this assurance, the length of the SS-20 missile without its front section will be considered to be 14.00 meters. In the context of this assurance, the United States side will not be inspecting any shipment whose dimensions are less than those of an SS-20 launch canister, as listed in the Memorandum of Understanding.

5. Inspection teams may bring to the inspection site the equipment provided for in the Inspection Protocol. Use of such equipment will be implemented in accordance with the procedures set forth in that Protocol. For example, if the inspecting Party believes that an ambiguity has not been removed, upon request the inspected Party shall take a photograph of the object or building about which a question remains.

6. During baseline inspections, the Parties will have the opportunity, on a one-time basis, to verify the technical characteristics listed in Section VI of the Memorandum of Understanding, including the weights and dimensions of SS-20 stages, at an elimination facility. Inspectors will select at random one of each type of item to weigh and measure from a sample presented by the inspected Party at a site designated by the inspected Party. To ensure that the items selected are indeed representative, the sample presented by the inspected Party must contain an adequate number of each item (i.e., at least 8-12,

except in the case of the United States Pershing IA launcher, only one of which exists).

7. Immediately prior to the initiation of elimination procedures, an inspector shall confirm and record the type and number of items of missile systems which are to be eliminated. If the inspecting Party deems it necessary, this shall include a visual inspection of the contents of launch canisters. This visual inspection can include looking into the launch canister once it is opened at both ends. It can also include use of the equipment and procedures that will be used eight times per year at Votkinsk and Magna to measure missile stages inside launch canisters (i.e., an optical or mechanical measuring device). If it should turn out, in particular situations, that the inspector is unable to confirm the missile type using the above techniques, the inspected Party is obligated to remove the inspector's doubts so that the inspector is satisfied as to the contents of the launch canister.

8. The length of the SS-23 missile stage will be changed, in a corrigendum to the Memorandum of Understanding, to 4.56 meters. The length of the SS-12 first stage will continue to be listed as 4.38 meters, which includes an interstage structure.

9. The sides will exchange additional photographs no later than May 15, 1988. For the United States side, these photographs will be of the Pershing IA missile and the Pershing II missile with their front sections attached and including a scale. For the Soviet side, these photographs will be of the SS-23, SS-12, and SS-4 with their front sections attached, and of the front section of the SS-20.

10. In providing notifications of transit points in accordance with paragraph 5(f)(iv) of Article IX of the Treaty, the Parties will specify such intermediate locations by providing the place-name and its center coordinates in minutes.

11. The United States side has informed the Soviet side that Davis Monthan Air Force Base, Arizona will serve as the elimination facility for the United States BGM-109G cruise missile. In order to address Soviet concerns on a related matter, the United States will formally inform the Soviet side before entry into force of the Treaty, of an elimination facility for each of its Treaty-limited items.

These points reflect the understandings of the two Parties regarding their obligations under the Treaty.

Ambassador Maynard W. Glitman
United States Chief Negotiator
on Intermediate-Range Nuclear Forces

Colonel General N. Chervov
Chief of Directorate General Staff
of the Soviet Armed Forces

NOTE OF THE GOVERNMENT OF THE UNITED STATES OF AMERICA TO THE GOVERNMENT OF THE UNION OF SOVIET SOCIALIST REPUBLICS

In light of the discussions between the Secretary of State of the United States of America and the Foreign Minister of the Union of Soviet Socialist Republics in Geneva and Moscow on April 14 and April 21-22, 1988, and the Foreign Minister's letter to the Secretary of State, dated April 15, 1988, the Government of the United States of America wished to record in an agreement concluded by exchange of notes the common understanding reached between the two Governments as to the application of the Treaty Between the United States of America and the Union of Soviet Socialist Republics on the Elimination of Their Intermediate-range and Shorter-range Missiles (hereinafter referred to as "the Treaty"), signed at Washington on December 8, 1987, to intermediate-range and shorter-range missiles flight-tested or deployed to carry weapons based on either current or future technologies and as to the related question of the definition of the term "weapon-delivery vehicle" as used in the Treaty.

It is the position of the Government of the United States of America that the Parties share a common understanding that all their intermediate-range and shorter-range missiles as defined by the Treaty, both at present and in the future, are subject to the provisions of the Treaty.

In this connection, it is also the position of the Government of the United States of America that the Parties share a common understanding that the term "weapon-delivery vehicle" in the Treaty means any ground-launched ballistic or cruise missile in the 500 kilometer to 5500 kilometer range that has been flight-tested or deployed to carry or be used as a weapon -- that is, any warhead, mechanism or device, which, when directed against any target, is designed to damage or destroy it. Therefore, the Treaty requires elimination and bans production and flight-testing of all such missiles tested or deployed to carry or be used as weapons based on either current or future technologies, with the exception of missiles mentioned in paragraph 3 of Article VII of the Treaty. It is also the position of the Government of the United States of America

that the Parties share a common understanding that the Treaty does not cover non-weapon-delivery vehicles.

It is the understanding of the Government of the United States of America that the above reflects the common view of the two Governments on these matters. If so, the Government of the United States of America proposes that this note and the Soviet reply note confirming that the Government of the Union of Soviet Socialist Republics shares the understanding of the Government of the United States of America, as set forth above, shall constitute an agreement between the Government of the United States of America and the Government of the Union of Soviet Socialist Republics.

Max M. Kampelman

Geneva, May 12, 1988

NOTE OF THE GOVERNMENT OF THE UNION OF SOVIET SOCIALIST REPUBLICS TO THE GOVERNMENT OF THE UNITED STATES OF AMERICA

The Government of the Union of Soviet Socialist Republics acknowledges receipt of the note of the Government of the United States of America of May 12, 1988, as follows:

"In light of the discussion between the Secretary of State of the United States of America and the Foreign Minister of the Union of Soviet Socialist Republics in Geneva and Moscow on April 14 and April 21-22, 1988, and the Foreign Minister's letter to the Secretary of State, dated April 15, 1988, the Government of the United States of America wished to record in an agreement concluded by exchange of notes the common understanding reached between the two Governments as to the application of the Treaty Between the United States of America and the Union of Soviet Socialist Republics on the Elimination of Their Intermediate-range and Shorter-range Missiles (hereinafter referred to as "the Treaty"), signed at Washington on December 8, 1987, to intermediate-range and shorter-range missiles flight-tested or deployed to carry weapons based on either current or future technologies and as to the related question of the definition of the term "weapon-delivery vehicle" as used in the Treaty.

It is the position of the Government of the United States of America that the Parties share a common understanding that all their intermediate-range and shorter-range missiles as defined by the Treaty, both at present and in the future, are subject to the provisions of the Treaty.

In this connection, it is also the position of the Government of the United States of America that the Parties share a common understanding that the term "weapon-delivery vehicle" in the Treaty means any ground-launched ballistic or cruise missile in the 500 kilometer to 5500 kilometer range that has been flight-tested or deployed to carry or be used as a weapon -- that is, any warhead, mechanism or device, which, when directed against any target, is designed to damage or destroy it. Therefore, the Treaty requires elimination and bans production and flight-testing of all such missiles tested or deployed to carry or be used as weapons based on either current or future technologies, with the exception of missiles mentioned in paragraph 3 of Article VII of the Treaty. It is also the position of the Government of the United States of America that the Parties share a common understanding that the Treaty does not cover non-weapon-delivery vehicles.

It is the understanding of the Government of the United States of America that the above reflects the common view of the two Governments on these matters. If so, the Government of the United States of America proposes that this note and the Soviet reply note confirming that the Government of the Union of Soviet Socialist Republics shares the understanding of the Government of the United States of America, as set forth above, shall constitute an agreement between the Government of the United States of America and the Government of the Union of Soviet Socialist Republics."

The Government of the Union of Soviet Socialist Republics states that it is in full accord with the text and contents of the note of the Government of the United States of America as quoted above and fully shares the understanding of the Government of the United States of America set forth in the above note.

The Government of the Union of Soviet Socialist Republics agrees that the note of the Government of the United States of America of May 12, 1988, and this note in reply thereto, constitute an agreement between the Government of the Union of Soviet Socialist Republics and the Government of the United States of America that the Treaty Between the United States of America and the Union of Soviet Socialist Republics on the Elimination of Their Intermediate-range and Shorter-range Missiles is applicable to intermediate-range and shorter-range missiles flight-tested or deployed to carry weapons based on either current or future technologies, and also regarding the related question of the definition of the term "weapon-delivery vehicle" as used in the Treaty.

Geneva, May 12, 1988

EXCHANGE OF NOTES AT MOSCOW MAY 28,
1988 IDENTIFYING AND CONFIRMING WHICH
DOCUMENTS, IN ADDITION TO THE TREATY,
HAVE THE SAME FORCE AND EFFECT AS
THE TREATY

EMBASSY OF THE UNITED STATES OF AMERICA

MOSCOW, MAY 28, 1988

No. MFA/148/88

The Government of the United States of America has the honor to refer:

1) to the notes exchanged in Geneva on May 12, 1988, between the United States and the Union of Soviet Socialist Republics concerning the application of the Treaty Between the United States of America and the Union of Soviet Socialist Republics on the Elimination of Their Intermediate-range and Shorter-range Missiles (the INF Treaty);

2) to the agreed minute concluded in Geneva on May 12, 1988, concerning certain issues related to the Treaty; and

3) to the agreements concluded by exchanges of notes, signed on May 21, 1988, in Vienna and Moscow, respectively, correcting the site diagrams and certain technical errors in the Treaty.

The Government of the United States proposes, in connection with the exchange of the instruments of ratification of the INF Treaty, that the two Governments signify their agreement that these documents are of the same force and effect as the provisions of the Treaty, and that this note together with the reply of the Union of Soviet Socialist Republics, shall constitute an agreement between the two Governments to that effect.

John M. Joyce

Charge d'Affaires a.i.

UNION OF SOVIET SOCIALIST REPUBLICS,

MAY 29, 1988

The Government of the Union of Soviet Socialist Republics confirms receipt of U.S. Government Note no. MFA/148/88, which reads as follows:

[The Russian text of Note no. MFA/148/88 of May 28, 1988, agrees in all substantive respects with the original English text]

The Government of the Union of Soviet Socialist Republics agrees that documents mentioned in U.S. Government Note no. MFA/148/88 of May 28, 1988, are of the same force and effect as the provisions of the Treaty Between the Union of Soviet Republics and the United States of America on the Elimination of Their Intermediate-Range and Shorter-Range Missiles, and that this note and the reply thereto shall constitute an agreement between the Governments of the Union of Soviet Socialist Republics and the United States of America to that effect.

Moscow
May 29, 1988

[S.] V. Karpov

/Seal of the Ministry of Foreign Affairs of the USSR/

Translation by Division of Language Services, U.S. Department of State.

AGREEMENT BETWEEN THE UNITED STATES OF AMERICA AND THE UNION OF SOVIET SOCIALIST REPUBLICS ON NOTIFICATIONS OF LAUNCHES OF INTERCONTINENTAL BALLISTIC MISSILES AND SUBMARINE-LAUNCHED BALLISTIC MISSILES

The Agreement on Notifications of ICBM and SLBM Launches, signed during the 1988 Moscow Summit, reflects the continuing interest of the United States and the Soviet Union in reducing the risk of nuclear war as a result of misinterpretation, miscalculation, or accident.

A number of earlier U.S.-Soviet agreements address advance notification of some, but not all, strategic ballistic missile launches.

■ The 1971 "Accidents Measures" Agreement requires each Party to notify the other in advance of any planned missile launches if such launches will extend beyond its national territory in the direction of the other Party.

■ The 1972 "Incidents at Sea" Agreement provides for advance notice, through Notices to Airmen and Mariners of actions on the high seas which represent a hazard to navigation or aircraft in flight. Planned ballistic missile launches which will take place in international waters represent such a hazard, and, under the "Incidents at Sea" Agreement, notification must be provided. The Notices to Airmen and Mariners, however, consist of warnings which announce "closure areas" due to a hazard to navigation or aircraft in flight; they need not identify the nature of the hazard.

■ Article XVI of the SALT II Treaty, which was never ratified, would have obligated each Party to notify the other well in advance before conducting multiple ICBM launches, or single ICBM launches planned to extend beyond its national territory. There was no obligation, however, to notify single launches not intended to extend beyond national territory. There were also no provisions in the SALT II Treaty for the notification of SLBM launches.

None of these earlier agreements, therefore, provided total coverage of all strategic ballistic missile (ICBM and SLBM) launches. In 1982, President Reagan proposed a number of new confidence-building measures for discussion at the U.S.-Soviet Strategic Arms Reductions Talks (START). Among these was a proposal for prior notification of all launches of ICBMs and SLBMs. During the course of the START negotiations, both sides drafted similar launch notification procedures which were incorporated into the joint draft of the START agreement text.

In May 1988, the United States proposed to the Soviets that, as a confidence-building measure, the sides conclude a separate agreement calling for advance notification of ICBM and SLBM launches. The Soviets agreed, and on May 31, 1988, in Moscow, U.S. Secretary of State Shultz and Soviet Foreign Minister Shevardnadze signed the Agreement on Notifications of ICBM and SLBM Launches. The Agreement provides for notification, no less than 24 hours in advance, of the planned date, launch area, and area of impact for any launch of an ICBM or SLBM. The Agreement also provides that these notifications be provided through the Nuclear Risk Reduction Centers. The Agreement entered into force on the date it was signed.

The U.S.-Soviet Joint Statement issued following the Moscow Summit included the following statement:

> The agreement between the United States and the USSR on notifications of launches of Inter-continental Ballistic Missiles and Submarine-Launched Ballistic Missiles, signed during the Moscow summit, is a practical new step, reflecting the desire of the sides to reduce the risk of outbreak of nuclear war, in particular as a result of misinterpretation, miscalculation, or accident.

Afterwards, the START I Treaty was signed in 1991. This Treaty contains an obligation to notify any flight test of an ICBM or SLBM, including those used to launch objects into the upper atmosphere or space. In addition to the requirements under the Ballistic Missile Launch Notification Agreement (i.e., that the notifying Party provide planned launch date, launch area, and reentry impact area), the START I Treaty requires that the notifying Party must also specify the telemetry broadcast frequencies to be used, modulation types and information as to whether the flight test is to employ encapsulation or encryption.

AGREEMENT BETWEEN THE UNITED STATES
OF AMERICA AND THE UNION OF SOVIET
SOCIALIST REPUBLICS ON NOTIFICATIONS
OF LAUNCHES OF INTERCONTINENTAL
BALLISTIC MISSILES AND SUBMARINE-
LAUNCHED BALLISTIC MISSILES

Signed at Moscow May 31, 1988
Entered into Force May 31, 1988

The United States of America and the Union
of Soviet Socialist Republics, hereinafter referred
to as the Parties,

Affirming their desire to reduce and ultimately
eliminate the risk of outbreak of nuclear war, in
particular, as a result of misinterpretation,
miscalculation, or accident,

Believing that a nuclear war cannot be won
and must never be fought,

Believing that agreement on measures for
reducing the risk of outbreak of nuclear war
serves the interests of strengthening international
peace and security,

Reaffirming their obligations under the
Agreement on Measures to Reduce the Risk of
Outbreak of Nuclear War between the United
States of America and the Union of Soviet
Socialist Republics of September 30, 1971, the
Agreement between the Government of the
United States of America and the Government of
the Union of Soviet Socialist Republics on the
Prevention of Incidents on and over the High
Seas of May 25, 1972, and the Agreement
between the United States of America and the
Union of Soviet Socialist Republics on the
Establishment of Nuclear Risk Reduction Centers
of September 15, 1987,

Have agreed as follows:

Article I

Each Party shall provide the other Party
notification, through the Nuclear Risk Reduction
Centers of the United States of America and the
Union of Soviet Socialist Republics, no less than
twenty-four hours in advance, of the planned
date, launch area, and area of impact for any
launch of a strategic ballistic missile: an
intercontinental ballistic missile (hereinafter
"ICBM") or a submarine-launched ballistic missile
(hereinafter "SLBM").

Article II

A notification of a planned launch of an ICBM
or an SLBM shall be valid for four days counting
from the launch date indicated in such a
notification. In case of postponement of the
launch date within the indicated four days, or
cancellation of the launch, no notification thereof
shall be required.

Article III

1. For launches of ICBMs or SLBMs from
land, the notification shall indicate the area from
which the launch is planned to take place.

2. For launches of SLBMs from submarines,
the notification shall indicate the general area
from which the missile will be launched. Such
notification shall indicate either the quadrant
within the ocean (that is, the ninety-degree sector
encompassing approximately one-fourth of the
area of the ocean) or the body of water (for
example, sea or bay) from which the launch is
planned to take place.

3. For all launches of ICBMs or SLBMs, the
notification shall indicate the geographic
coordinates of the planned impact area or areas
of the reentry vehicles. Such an area shall be
specified either by indicating the geographic
coordinates of the boundary points of the area, or
by indicating the geographic coordinates of the
center of a circle with a radius specified in
kilometers or nautical miles. The size of the
impact area shall be determined by the notifying
Party at its discretion.

Article IV

The Parties undertake to hold consultations,
as mutually agreed, to consider questions relating
to implementation of the provisions of this
Agreement, as well as to discuss possible
amendments thereto aimed at furthering the
implementation of the objectives of this
Agreement. Amendments shall enter into force in
accordance with procedures to be agreed upon.

Article V

This Agreement shall not affect the obligations of either Party under other agreements.

Article VI

This Agreement shall enter into force on the date of its signature.

The duration of this Agreement shall not be limited.

This Agreement may be terminated by either Party upon 12 months written notice to the other Party.

DONE at Moscow on May 31, 1988, in two copies, each in the English and Russian languages, both texts being equally authentic.

FOR THE UNITED STATES OF AMERICA:
George P. Shultz

FOR THE UNION OF SOVIET SOCIALIST REPUBLICS:
Eduard A. Shevardnadze

Footnotes

1 Dates given are the earliest dates on which countries signed the agreements or deposited their ratifications or accessions -- whether in Washington, London, Moscow, or New York. In the case of a country that was a dependent territory which became a party through succession, the date given is the date on which the country gave notice that it would continue to be bound by the terms of the agreement.

2 The United States regards the signature and ratification by the Byelorussian S.S.R. and the Ukrainian S.S.R. as already included under the signature and ratification of the Union of Soviet Socialist Republics.

3 This total does not include actions by the Byelorussian S.S.R. and the Ukrainian S.S.R. (See footnote 2.)

4 Effective January 1, 1979, the United States recognized the Government of the People's Republic of China as the sole government of China.